GYNAECOLOGY

To my wife Mae whose tolerance now extends through three editions of the book, and whose support has been essential

R.W.S.

To my wife Winnie, and children Liz and Eleanor

W.P.S.

To my wife Julia, and children Claire, Talia, Jo, Tamara and Noah

S.L.S.

GYNAECOLOGY

Third edition

Edited by

Robert W. Shaw CBE MD FRCOG FRCS(Ed) FRANZCOG(Hon) FACOG (Hon) FRCPI(Hon)

Professor of Obstetrics and Gynaecology, Nottingham University, Derby City General Hospital, Derby, UK

W. Patrick Soutter MD MSc FRCOG

Reader in Gynaecological Oncology, Imperial College School of Medicine, Hammersmith Hospital, London, UK

Stuart L. Stanton FRCS FRCOG FRANZCOG(Hon)

Consultant Urogynaecologist, Pelvic Reconstruction & Urogynaecology Unit, St George's Hospital Medical School, London, UK

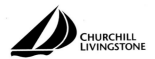
CHURCHILL LIVINGSTONE

CHURCHILL LIVINGSTONE
An imprint of Elsevier Science Limited

First edition 1992
Second edition 1997
Third edition 2003

ISBN 0 4430 7029 6

British Library Cataloguing in Publication Data
A catalogue record for this book is available from the British Library

Library of Congress Cataloging in Publication Data
A catalog record for this book is available from the Library of Congress

Note
Medical knowledge is constantly changing. As new information becomes available, changes in treatment, procedures, equipment and the use of drugs become necessary. The contributors and the publishers have taken care to ensure that the information given in this text is accurate and up to date. However, readers are strongly advised to confirm that the information, especially with regard to drug usage, complies with the latest legislation and standards of practice.

your source for books,
journals and multimedia
in the health sciences
www.elsevierhealth.com

The
publisher's
policy is to use
**paper manufactured
from sustainable forests**

Printed in China by the RDC Group Ltd

Commissioning Editor: Judith Fletcher
Project Development Manager: Hilary Hewitt
Project Manager: Cheryl Brant
Illustration Manager: Mick Ruddy
Design Manager: Jayne Jones
Illustrator: Marion Tasker

Contents

Contributors

D. Robert E. Abayasekara BSc(Hons) PhD
Lecturer in Physiology, Reproduction and Development
Group, Department of Veterinary Basic Sciences, Royal
Veterinary College, London, UK

Nazar N. Amso PhD FRCOG
Senior Lecturer in Obstetrics & Gynaecology, Department of
Obstetrics & Gynaecology, University of Wales College of
Medicine, Cardiff, UK

Richard A. Anderson PhD MD MRCOG
Clinical Consultant, MRC Human Reproductive Sciences
Unit, Centre for Reproductive Biology, Edinburgh, UK

Adam Balen MB BS MD MRCOG
Consultant Reproductive Medicine and Surgery, Assisted
Conception Unit, Department of Obstetrics & Gynaecology,
Leeds General Infirmary, Leeds, UK

Susan Bewley MD MA FRCOG
Clinical Director, Womens Health Services, Guy's and St
Thomas' Hospitals NHS Trust, St Thomas' Hospital, London,
UK

Siladitya Bhattacharya MD MRCOG
Senior Lecturer (Honorary Consultant), Department of
Obstetrics & Gynaecology, Aberdeen Maternity Hospital and
Aberdeen University, Aberdeen, UK

Tom Bourne MB BS MRCOG PhD
Consultant Gynaecologist, Early Pregnancy, Gynaecological
Ultrasound and MAS Unit, St George's Hospital, London, UK

William Buckett MB BS MRCOG
Consultant Gynaecologist, St Mary's Hospital, London;
Honorary Senior Lecturer, Imperial College, London, UK

Helen Cameron MB BS FRCOG
Consultant Obstetrician & Gynaecologist, Department of
Obstetrics & Gynaecology, Sunderland Royal Hospital,
Sunderland, UK

Linda Cardozo MD FRCOG
Professor of Urogynaecology; Consultant, Department of
Obstetrics & Gynaecology, King's College Hospital, London,
UK

Susan V. Carr MFFP DRCOG MPhil
Consultant in Family Planning & Reproductive Healthcare,
The Sandyford Initiative, Glasgow, UK

Charlotte Chaliha MA MBBChiv MRCOG MD
Specialist Registrar in Obstetrics & Gynaecology, Royal
Surrey County Hospital, Guildford, UK

Stephen Charnock-Jones BSc PhD
University Lecturer, Department of Obstetrics &
Gynaecology, University of Cambridge, Cambridge, UK

Tara Cooper MRCOG
Consultant Obstetrician & Gynaecologist, West Lothian
Healthcare NHS Trust, St Johns Hospital at Howden,
Livingstone, UK

David O. Cosgrove BA BM BCh MRCP MSc
Professor of Clinical Ultrasound, Imaging Services
Department, Clinical Sciences Division, Imperial College
Hammersmith Hospital Campus, London, UK

Hilary O.D. Critchley BSc MBChB MD FRCOG FRANZCOG
Professor of Reproductive Medicine, University of
Edinburgh; Honorary Consultant Gynaecologist, Royal
Infirmary, Edinburgh, UK

Jack Cuzick PhD
Principal Scientist, Department of Mathematics, Statistics
and Eidemiology, Cancer Research UK, London, UK

Camille de San Lazaro MB BS DCH FRCP FRCPCH
Senior Lecturer in Paediatric Forensic Medicine, Department
of Child Health, University of Newcastle upon Tyne Medical
School, Newcastle upon Tyne, UK

Nandita de Souza MB BS MD FRCP
Consultant Radiologist, Department of Imaging Services,
Hammersmith Hospital, London, UK

Paul W. Dimmock BSc(Hons) PhD
Research Fellow, Academic Obstetrics & Gynaecology, Keele
University, Keele, UK

Roberto Dina MD
Consultant Cytopathologist/Histopathologist, Department of
Histopathology, Hammersmith Hospital, London, UK

Ovrang Djahanbakhch FRCOG MD
Professor of Obstetrics & Gynaecology, Academic
Department of Obstetrics & Gynaecology, Newham Campus,
Queen Mary and Westfield College, University of London,
London, UK

Sheila L.B. Duncan MD FRCOG DHMSA
Former Reader in Obstetrics & Gynaecology, University of Sheffield, Sheffield, UK

Peter Dwyer MB BS FRANZCOG FRCOG
Head, Urogynaecology Department, Mercy Hospital for Women and Royal Women's Hospital, Melbourne, Victoria, Australia

Keith Edmonds FRCOG FRANZCOG
Clinical Director and Consultant Obstetrician & Gynaecologist, Department of Obstetrics & Gynaecology, Queen Charlottes and Chelsea Hospital, London, UK

Abigail A. Evans BSc MD FRCS
Consultant Surgeon, Poole Hospital NHS Trust, Poole, UK

Alan J. Farthing MD MRCOG
Consultant Obstetrician & Gynaecologist, Department of Gynaecology, St Mary's Hospital, London, UK

Stephen Franks MD FRCP HonMD(Uppsala)
Professor of Reproductive Endocrinology; Head, Department of Reproductive Science & Medicine, Imperial College School of Medicine, London, UK

Michelle Fynes MD MRCOG DU
Urogynaecology Fellow, Pelvic Reconstruction and Urogynaecology Unit
St George's Hospital, London, UK

Carole Gilling-Smith PhD MRCOG
Consultant Gynaecologist; Director of the Assisted Conception Unit, Chelsea and Westminster Hospital, London, UK

Joanna C. Girling MA MRCP MRCOG
Senior Registrar, Department of Obstetrics & Gynaecology, Hammersmith Hospital, London, UK

Anna F. Glasier MB ChB BSc MD FRCOG MFFP
Director or Family Planning & Well Women Services, Lothian Primary Care NHS Trust; Senior Lecturer, Department of Obstetrics & Gynaecology, University of Edinburgh, Edinburgh, UK

Rob J. Gornall MD MRCOG
Gynaelogical Oncology, Cheltenham & Gloucester Hospital, Cheltenham & Gloucester, UK

Jurgis Geddes Grudzinskas MD FRCOG FRACOG
Professor of Obstetrics & Gynaecology, Department of Obstetrics & Gynaecology
(Reproductive Physiology Laboratory), St Bartholomew's Hospital and Royal London Hospital School of Medicine and Dentistry, University of London, London, UK

Dimitrios Haidopoulos MB ChB
Visiting Fellow, Gynaecological Oncology Centre, Hammersmith Hospital, London, UK

Aidan Halligan MB BCh BAO BA MRCOG MA MD MRCPI
Director of Clinical Governance for the NHS; Head of the NHS Clinical Governance Support Team; Professor of Fetal Maternal Medicine, University of Leicester, Leicester, UK

Phillip Hay MB BS FRCP
Consultant and Senior Lecturer in Genito-urinary Medicine, Department of Genito-urinary Medicine, St George's Hospital, London, UK

David L. Healy BMed Sci MB BS(Hons) PhD FRANZCOG CREI
Professor and Departmental Chairman, Department of Obstetrics & Gynaecology, Monash University, Victoria, Australia

Mary Hepburn BSc MD MRCGP FRCOG
Senior Lecturer in Women's Reproductive Health, Princess Royal Maternity Hospital, Glasgow, UK

Alexander G. Heriot MD FRCS FRCSEd
Colorectal Fellow, St Vincent's Hospital, Melbourne, Australia

Paul Hilton MD FRCOG
Consultant Gynaecologist and Subspecialist in Urogynaecology, Directorate of Women's Services, Royal Victoria Infirmary, Newcastle-upon-Tyne, UK

Pak Chung Ho MD FRCOG FHKAM(O&G) FHKCOG
Professor and Chair of Obstetrics & Gynaecology, Department of Obstetrics & Gynaecology, The University of Hong Kong, Queen Mary Hospital, Hong Kong

Stewart Irvine BSc MD FRCOG
Clinical Consultant, MRC Human Reproductive Sciences Unit, Centre for Reproductive Biology, Edinburgh, UK

Khaled M.K. Ismail MBBCh, MD MRCOG
Clinical Lecturer in Obstetrics & Gynaecology, Academic Department of Obstetrics & Gynaecology, Maternity Unit, City General Hospital, Stoke-on-Trent, UK

Ian Jacobs MD MRCOG
Professor of Gynaecological Oncology, Gynaecological Oncology Unit and Cancer Research UK Translational Oncology Laboratory, St Bartholomew's & Royal London School of Medicine, London, UK

Karen Jermy MB BS MRCOG
Clinical Research Fellow, Early Pregnancy, Gynaecological Ultrasound and MAS Unit, St George's Hospital Medical School, London, UK

Margaret Johnson MD FRCP
Clinical Director of HIV/AIDS Services, Royal Free Hampstead NHS Trust, London, UK

Bleddyn Jones MA MSc MD FRCR FRCP
Reader in Oncology, Imperial College School of Medicine, London, UK

Mickey M Karram MD
Associate Professor of Obstetrics & Gynecology, Department of Obstetrics & Gynecology, Good Samaritan Hospital and the University of Cincinnati, Cincinnati, Ohio, USA

Con J. Kelleher MD MRCOG
Consultant Obstetrician & Gynaecologist, Guys and St Thomas' Hospitals NHS Trust, London, UK

Vikram Khullar BSc MB BS
Senior Lecturer, Department of Obstetrics & Gynaecology,
St Mary's Hospital,
London

Henry Kitchener MD FRCS FRCOG
Professor of Gynaecological Oncology, Academic Unit of
Obstetrics & Gynaecology, St Mary's Hospital, Manchester,
UK

Lukas D. Klentzeris MD FRCOG
Consultant Gynaecologist and Director, Cardiff Assisted
Reproduction Unit, University Hospital of Wales, Cardiff,
UK

Devinder Kumar PhD FRCS
Colorectal and General Surgeon, St George's Hospital,
London

Gary E. Lemack MD
Assistant Professor of Urology; Director of Neurourology,
Department of Urology, University of Texas, Southwestern
Medical Center, Dallas, Texas, USA

Adrian M. Lower BMedSc BM BS MRCOG
Consultant Gynaecologist, St Bartholomew's & The Royal
London Hospitals, London, UK

Mary Ann Lumsden MB BS MD FRCOG
Reader in Obstetrics & Gynaecology, University Department
of Obstetrics & Gynaecology, The Queen Mother's Hospital,
Glasgow, UK

John Lynn MS FRCS
Consultant Endocrine & Breast Surgeon, Department of
Surgery, Hammersmith Hospital, London, UK

Allan MacLean BMedSc MD FRCOG
Professor of Obstetrics & Gynaecology, Royal Free and
University College Medical Schook, Royal Free Campus,
London, UK

Sandeep Mane MB BS DGO DICOG FCPS MD MRCOG
Consultant Gynaecologist, Department of Minimal Access
Surgery, P.D. Hinduja National Hospital, Mumbai, India;
Visiting Lecturer, Welsh Institute for Minimal Access
Therapy, Cardiff Medicentre, Cardiff, UK

Neil McClure MD FRCOG
Professor of Obstetrics & Gynaecology, Institute of Clinical
Science, School of Medicine, The Queen's University of
Belfast, Belfast, UK

Jay McGavigan MB BS
Specialist Registrar, University Department of Obstetrics
& Gynaecology, The Queen Mother's Hospital, Glasgow,
UK

G. Angus McIndoe PhD FRCS MRCOG
Consultant in Gynaecological Oncology, Hammersmith
Hospital; Honorary Senior Lecturer, Imperial College School
of Medicine, London, UK

Christine McManus BA(Hons)
Solicitor, Hempsons, London, UK

Anthony E. Michael BSc(Hons) PhD
Senior Lecturer in Biochemistry and Molecular Biology,
Department of Biochemistry and Molecular Biology, Royal
Free and University College Medical School, University
College London, London, UK

Pontus Molander MD
Clinical Scientist, Department of Obstetrics & Gynecology,
University of Helsinki, Helsinki, Finland

Ash K. Monga BM MS MRCOG
Consultant Gynaecologist, Urogynaecology Unit, The
Princess Anne Hospital, Southampton, UK

Antonia Moore MSc MRCOG MB ChB
Clinical Research Fellow, Centre for HIV Studies and
Department of Primary Care and Population Sciences, Royal
Free and University College Medical School, London, UK

Nick J. Naftalin OBE MB ChB FRCOG
Consultant Gynaecologist, The University of Leicester NHS
Trust, Leicester Royal Infirmary, Leicester, UK

Edward S. Newlands PhD FRCP
Professor of Cancer Medicine; Co-Director of the
Gestational Trophoblastic Disease Unit, Department of
Medical Oncology; Charing Cross Hospital, London, UK

Ernest Hung Yu Ng MB BS MRCOG
Associate Professor, Department of Obstetrics &
Gynaecology, The University of Hong Kong, Queen Mary
Hospital, Hong Kong

Susanna Nicholls BA(Hons) MB ChB
Medical Support Physician, Procter & Gamble
Pharmaceuticals Ltd, Staines, UK

P.M Shaugh O'Brien MB BCh MD FRCOG
Professor and Head, Academic Obstetrics & Gynaecology,
Keele University, Keele, UK

Jorma Paavonen MD
Professor of Obstetrics & Gynecology, Department of
Obstetrics & Gynecology, University of Helsinki, Helsinki,
Finland

R. John Parsons BScTech PhD FIPEMB
Head of Department of Medical Physics and Biomedical
Engineering, Derriford Hospital, Plymouth, UK

Richard J.A. Penketh BSc MB BS MD MRCOG
Consultant Obstetrician & Gynaecologist, Department of
Gynaecology, University Hospital of Wales, Cardiff, UK

Paramoporn Prasarttong-Osoth MD MSc FRCS(Glas)
Laboratory Research Fellow, Department of Surgery,
Hammersmith Hospital, London, UK

Michael A. Quinn MB ChB MGO MRCP(UK) FRCOG FRANZCOG
Director of Oncology, Oncology and Dysplasia Unit, The
Royal Women's Hospital, Melbourne, Victoria, Australia

Margaret Rees MB BS
Honorary Senior Clinical Lecturer, Nuffield Department of
Obstetrics & Gynaecology, John Radcliffe Hospital, Oxford,
UK

Lesley Regan MD MB BS FRCOG
Professor of Obstetrics & Gynaecology, Department of
Reproductive Science and Medicine, Imperial College
School of Medicine, London, UK

Dudley Robinson MRCOG
Sub-specialty Trainee in Urogynaecology, Department of
Urogynaecology, Kings College Hospital, London, UK

Gordon Rustin MD MSc FRCP
Consultant Medical Oncologist, Mount Vernon Hospital,
Northwood, UK

Ertan Saridogan PhD MRCOG
Consultant in Reproductive Medicine and Minimal Access
Surgery, Department of Obstetrics & Gynaecology,
University College London Hospitals, London, UK

Peter Sasieni PhD
Senior Scientist, Department of Mathematics, Statistics and
Epidemiology, Cancer Research UK, London, UK

Michael J. Seckl PhD FRCP
Reader in Cancer Medicine; Co-Director of the Gestational
Trophoblastic Disease Unit, Department of Medical
Oncology; Charing Cross Hospital, London, UK

D. Gwyn Seymour MB ChB BSc MD FRCP
Professor of Medicine (Care of the Elderly), Department of
Medicine for the Elderly, Foresterhill Health Centre,
Aberdeen, UK

Robert W. Shaw MD FRCOG FRCS(Ed) MFFP
Professor of Obstetrics and Gynaecology, Nottingham
University, Derby City General Hospital, Derby, UK

Anthony I. Skene BM FRCS MS
Consultant Surgeon, Royal Bournemouth Hospital,
Bournemouth, UK

Anthony R.B. Smith MD FRCOG
Consultant Gynaecologist, Department of Urological
Gynaecology, Saint Mary's Hospital for Women & Children,
Manchester, UK

Stephen K. Smith MB BS MD DSc FIBiol FMedSci
Professor of Obstetrics & Gynaecology, Department of
Obstetrics & Gynaecology, University of Cambridge,
Cambridge, UK

W. Patrick Soutter MD MSc FRCOG
Reader in Gynaecological Oncology, Imperial College
School of Medicine, Hammersmith Hospital, London, UK

Stuart L. Stanton FRCS FRCOG FRANZCOG(Hon)
Consultant Urogynaecologist, Pelvic Reconstruction &
Urogynaecology Unit, St George's Hospital Medical School,
London, UK

R. William Stones MD FRCOG
Senior Lecturer in Obstetrics & Gynaecology, Princess Anne
Hospital, Southampton, UK

Abdul Sultan MB ChB MRCOG MD
Consultant Obstetrician &Gynaecologist, Mayday University
Hospital, Croydon, UK

Karen Summerville
Gynaecological Oncology Specialist Nurse, Hammersmith
Hospital, London, UK

William E. Svensson LRCPSI FRCSI FRCR
Consultant Radiologist and Honorary Senior Consultant,
Hammersmith Hospital and Ealing Hospitals, London, UK

Allan Templeton MD FRCOG
Professor of Obstetrics & Gynaecology, Department of
Obstetrics & Gynaecology, University of Aberdeen,
Aberdeen, UK

Hilary Thomas MA(Camb), MBBS, PhD, FRCP, FRCR
Professor of Clinical Oncology, Royal Surrey County
Hospital, Guildford, Surrey

Philippe Van Trappen MD
Fellow in Gynaecological Oncology, Gynaecological
Oncology Unit and Cancer Research UK Translational
Oncology Laboratory, John Vane Science Centre, London,
UK

Brett Vassallo MD
Assistant Professor of Obstetrics & Gynecology, Department
of Obstetrics & Gynecology, University of Chicago
Hospitals, Chicago, Illinois, USA

Beverly Vollenhoven MB BS PhD CREI FRANZCOG
Senior Lecturer, Department of Obstetrics & Gynaecology,
Monash Medical Centre, Clayton, Victoria, Australia

Gareth Weston MB BS Grad Dip(Epid)
Doctoral Resident, Department of Obstetrics & Gynaecology,
Monash University, Clayton, Victoria, Australia

Tamsin E. Wilton DPhil MSc PGCE BA(hons)
Reader in Sociology, Faculty of Economics and Social
Science, University of West England, Frenchay Campus,
Bristol, UK

Philippe E. Zimmern MD FACS
Professor of Urology; Director, Bladder & Incontinence
Center, Department of Urology, University of Texas,
Southwestern Medical Center, Dallas, Texas, USA

Preface

Gynaecology in the 21st Century continues to reflect the major advances in the practice and science of gynaecology, the social community in which we live and work, and the globalization of medicine.

All the chapters in the new edition of *Gynaecology* have been substantially revised with key points to focus on and summarize chapter contents and up-to-date references. Many chapters are inter-disciplinary, acknowledging the increasing collaboration and reliance we place on other disciplines.

Our successful philosophy in the first and second editions of a combination of general and subspecialty-based gynaecology continues. The book has been enhanced by a 30% increase in new contributors, 13% of whom practise outside the United Kingdom and have given the text greater internationalization. General gynaecological advances are prominent in the chapters on laparoscopy and imaging. Gynaecology in old age is a multi-disciplinary approach to that most important and growing section of our patients who need more specialized and relevant care. The increased focus by many agencies including our own internal audit systems and clinical governance, the Department of Health, patient organizations and our professional colleagues, the lawyers, emphasize the important role of chapters on evidence based care and risk management.

Four new chapters include *molecular biology*, the core of much of medical science and fundamental to our own understanding of gynaecology. Improvements in ultrasonography and a medicine-wide change from in patient to out patient care has given the impetus to *one-stop gynaecology*, where emergency and many routine gynaecological patients are managed on a one-stop rapid basis. Changing social patterns and mores have been the driving force behind *violence against women* - a sad and increasingly publicized unacceptable aspect of our society where there is a role for us in its recognition and management. The appreciation of health concepts, a different lifestyle and, most importantly, the need to effectively communicate are dealt with in *lesbian health issues*.

Unravelling the molecular basis of some of the major benign gynaecological disorders is beginning to have an impact on the way we approach and treat many reproductive diseases. The understanding of the mechanisms of cell dysfunction in the polycystic ovary syndrome, endometriosis and menorrhagia have opened up the prospect for new novel pharmacological approaches to conditions which previously have predominantly been treated by surgical approaches. These will offer patients the potential for less invasive treatment approaches and more importantly the option to retain reproductive capacity.

Utilizing the techniques and expertise of our interventional radiology colleagues has resulted in the introduction of uterine artery embolization for the treatment of symptomatic uterine leiomyomas. Long-term follow-up and appropriate case selection will be the key to successful use of this form of therapy that further exemplifies the move to non-surgical approaches within reproductive medicine.

Within the field of infertility refinements of current techniques have further improved success rates. However, some might say that the widespread introduction of intracytoplasmic sperm injection (ICSI) across the spectrum of male infertility may have had the deleterious effect of inhibiting research into the various causes. That being so, ICSI has without doubt further expanded the indication for assisted reproduction technologies. The success rates following embryo transfer have universally improved such that there is now little or no justification to transfer more than two embryos, thus allowing the opportunity to reduce the risk of high order multiple pregnancy with its associated increased perinatal loss and morbidity potentials. To further advance results of infertility treatment requires concentrating on the mechanisms of implantation failure to open up new avenues of investigation and management in infertile couples.

The new technology brings new problems with increasing numbers of women being referred with asymptomatic pelvic cysts. The role of laparoscopy in the management of women with gynaecological cancer remains controversial. Is it a gimmick or does it offer genuine advantages that do not compromise the effectiveness of treatment? Taxanes now seem to offer less to women with ovarian cancer than had been hoped and new technologies are just beginning to reach the clinic for trial. What role might HPV vaccines play in the eradication of cervical cancer? While these exciting developments are being investigated, it is worth remembering that we could improve the survival of our patients with gynaecological cancer by making full use of the treatments already at our disposal.

Urogynaecological advances include the importance of quality of life issues as relevant outcome measures, and the recognition that the pelvic floor and urinary and anal sphincters are no longer historically or anatomically divided into separate disciplines, but should be one pathophysiological unit managed by clinicians who have training in urology, gynaecology and colorectal surgery. New approaches to the overactive (unstable) bladder, with a greater emphasis on conservative treatments, and the innovative tension-free vaginal tape (TVT), which has altered our concept of the mechanism of continence, now provide reliable day case treatments for continence. The role of synthetic mesh and biological tissues and a re-evaluation of abdominal and vaginal approaches are exciting topics in prolapse surgery.

This edition sees a fundamental change in the training of our junior staff. Coming into line with Europe, we have a shorter working week and fewer years in training. This has meant a radical re-think of the way in which we teach and how we learn, with a greater emphasis now on structured training as they have had in the USA for many years. Our book is directed towards trainees and consultants, for whom we hope it will provide stimulating, clear guidelines and teaching on the core subject of gynaecology, and on issues that affect the way we practise medicine today.

We acknowledge our past reviewers and readers whose criticisms have helped shape this new edition and for whose views

we are grateful. We also thank our many trainees, research fellows and colleagues who have stimulated our writing with their comments and suggestions. We would like to express our sincere gratitude to our secretaries Eileen Gomez, Penny Quayle and Wendy Nash, and finally, the staff of Elsevier Science, particularly Miranda Bromage, Kim Benson, Cheryl Brant and more recently Judith Fletcher, whose professional skills and tactful reminders we have all appreciated.

R.W.S.
W.P.S.
S.L.S.
London 2002

Section 1
BASIC PRINCIPLES AND INVESTIGATIONS

1

Embryology of the female genital tract: its genetic defects and congenital anomalies

Sheila L. B. Duncan

INTRODUCTION

The mechanisms by which the gender-differential urogenital system is established long before birth are complex and remarkable. They are also easily pertubed. Advances in knowledge in genetics and in steroidogenesis, together with painstaking experimental work on mammalian embryos, have combined to improve our understanding of some of the derangements of the female genital tract seen in clinical practice. Errors of sexual development are distressing but their careful study has provided knowledge out of proportion to their frequency.

In this chapter key events in the development of the female genital tract are discussed, especially related to clinical abnormalities. Genetic conditions and congenital abnormalities of the genital tract affecting gynaecological practice are outlined. Some knowledge of the development of the gut and urogenital system is assumed, as is an understanding of the formation of gametes, cell division and the topography of female and male chromosomes. This chapter does not include disorganized development incompatible with life, nor does it deal with conditions diagnosed in infancy and primarily dealt with by the paediatric surgeon. Reference is made to male development only in relation to understanding developmental problems in the female or female phenotype. Thus, most disturbances of virilization or of spermatogenesis in phenotypic males are not included.

EMBRYOLOGY

Development of the mesonephros, paramesonephric ducts and kidneys

The urinary and genital systems develop from a common mesodermal ridge running along the posterior abdominal wall. During the 5th week of embryonic life (timed from fertilization) the nephrogenic cord develops from the mesoderm and forms the urogenital ridge and mesonephric duct (later to form the wolffian duct). The mesonephros consists of a comparatively large ovoid organ on each side of the midline with the developing gonad on the medial side of its lower portion. The paramesonephric duct, later to form the müllerian system, develops as an ingrowth of coelomic epithelium anterolateral to the mesonephric duct. Primordial germ cells migrate from the yolk sac along the dorsal mesentery of the hindgut and reach the primitive gonad by the end of the 6th

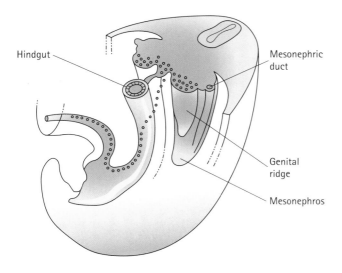

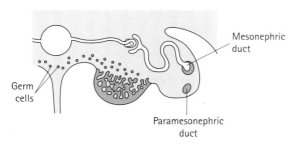

Fig. 1.1   Cross-sectional diagram of posterior abdominal wall in embryo. **Top** Migration of germ cells into genital ridge, overlying the mesonephros, with mesonephric duct on lateral aspect. **Bottom** Paramesonephric (müllerian) duct lying anterolaterally to the mesonephric duct.

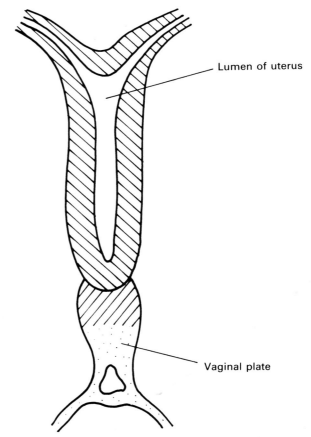

Fig. 1.2   The fused lower paramesonephric ducts form the uterus, cervix and upper vagina. The characteristic shape of the uterus is created by the junction of the fused and unfused portions.

week (42 days; Fig. 1.1). The fate of the mesonephric and paramesonephric ducts is critically dependent on gonadal secretion. In female development, the two paramesonephric ducts extend caudally to project but not open into the posterior wall of the urogenital sinus as the müllerian tubercle. There is degeneration of the wolffian system. The lower ends of the müllerian system fuse, later to form the uterus, cervix and upper vagina, while the cephalic ends remain separate, forming the fallopian tubes (Fig. 1.2).

The ureter develops as an outgrowth of the mesonephric duct close to its lower end, and grows outward and upward to penetrate the metanephric mesoderm which ultimately forms the definitive kidney. Unilateral renal aplasia is usually due to degeneration of the ureteric bud and this failure is frequently associated with failure of müllerian development on the same side, since both are dependent on adequate development of the mesonephric system. Splitting of the ureteric bud results in partial or complete duplication of the ureter. If a developing ureter fails to connect with the bladder it may retain its connection with the wolffian duct and thus open into the vagina or vestibule. This is more likely to occur if there has been splitting of the bud and abnormal ureteric development. The kidney starts off much more caudally than the gonads and failure to ascend accounts for its occasional pelvic location and for supernumerary renal vessels which result from the persistence of embryonic vessels.

The cloaca

Meanwhile, and usually before the 7th week, the urorectal septum divides the cloaca into the urogenital sinus and the anorectal canal. When the urogenital septum reaches the cloacal membrane, the perineum is formed (Figs 1.3 and 1.4). An ectodermal anal pit forms to meet the anorectal canal and an opening forms here during the 9th embryonic week. Thus, the lower third of the anal canal forms from ectoderm, consists of stratified squamous epithelium and is supplied by the internal pudendal artery. Where the anal pit fails to form or there is atresia of the lower end of the rectum, the thickness of the intervening layer is very variable. Sometimes the rectal opening is in the perineum or even in the vagina (Fig. 1.5).

The urogenital sinus may be divided into:

- an upper part which forms the urinary bladder. The early connection superiorly with the allantois obliterates and forms the urachus which connects the apex of the bladder to the umbilicus. If mesoderm fails to invade the cloacal membrane anteriorly, extrophy of the bladder results
- a pelvic part which forms the urethra and lower vagina. This is intimately connected with the development of the lower part of the müllerian system.

Duplication or failure of fusion at uterine level

Fusion of the ducts occurs at an early stage of müllerian development before organ differentiation into cervix or uterine body. Thus, there is no point at which a formed uterus and cervix fuse. True duplication of the uterus, cervix and tubes

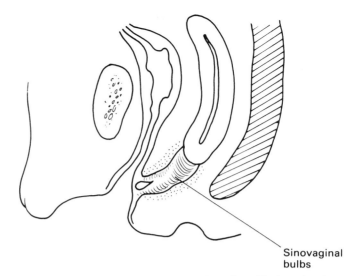

Sinovaginal bulbs

Fig. 1.4 A later stage in development where the müllerian tubercle and the sinovaginal bulbs (not yet canalized), forming the 'vaginal plate', are elongating within the urorectal septum. In this diagram, the anorectal canal has failed to connect with the anal pit; this would later present as an imperforate anus.

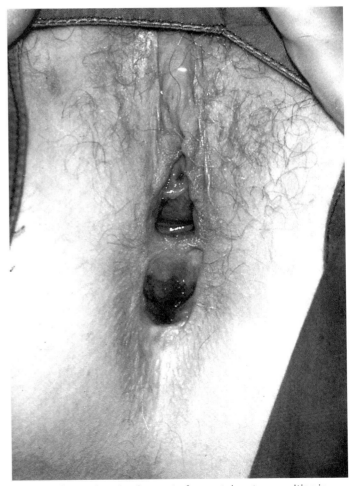

Fig. 1.5 Incomplete development of urorectal septum resulting in perineal anus with deficient perineum.

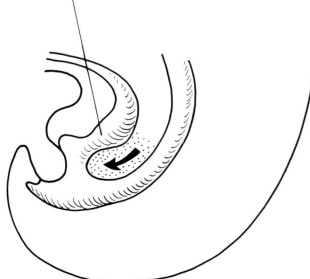

Primary urogenital sinus

Fig. 1.3 Development of the urorectal septum (arrowed), eventually separating the bladder and vagina from the rectum.

involves splitting of the müllerian duct at an early stage. This can occur on one or both sides but is rare. More common is incomplete development of the fused ducts, i.e. incomplete fusion of two halves. These variations form a series of well-recognized uterine anomalies (American Fertility Society 1988).

Development of the vagina

The müllerian ducts, usually now fused in their lower part, reach and invaginate the urogenital sinus in the 9th week (30 mm stage). The solid, single end forms the müllerian tubercle which does not open into the sinus but makes contact with solid outgrowths of the sinus, the sinovaginal bulbs. This solid vaginal plate is thus formed by intermingling of the lower ends of the müllerian ducts and sinus cells. As the hind part of the fetus unfolds, the pelvic structures, including the vaginal plate, elongate, providing length for the future vagina (see Fig. 1.4). Thereafter lacunae appear which join up to canalize the future vagina. Complete canalization of the vagina is a comparatively late event (occurring at about 22 menstrual weeks or later).

There has long been dispute among embryologists about the exact contribution of the urogenital sinus to the vaginal plate and hence to the length of the vagina and whether the stratified squamous epithelium of the vagina is formed by upward migration of sinus epithelium or by metaplasia of epithelium originally from the paramesonephric ducts (see O'Rahilly 1977). When there is vaginal atresia with normal development of a uterus and cervix, there is usually a patent upper vagina though the epithelium is fragile and often shows adenosis. Where there is müllerian agenesis, the urogenital sinus still forms but does not lengthen and the vagina is short, though of variable length and entirely lined with stratified squamous epithelium. Similarly, in girls with complete androgen insensitivity, where the müllerian element has regressed, the vagina is also of variable length and similarly lined. These clinical observations support the view that, normally, the urogenital sinus contributes to the epithelium and the length of the vagina is mainly from müllerian tissue though contributed to by both (Ulfelder & Robboy 1976). There is acceptance of the view that there is some urogenital sinus contribution above the level of the anatomical hymen. One or both müllerian ducts may fail to make contact with the urogenital sinus. Failure of complete canalization of the vagina can leave a variety of septae: transverse, sagittal, coronal or oblique of varying thicknesses (Fig. 1.6). The mildest abnormality of this sort to cause complete obstruction is a lower vaginal transverse membrane (imperforate hymen) which is generally just above the anatomical hymen. Partial obstruction may result in apareunia or inability to insert a tampon but no obstruction to menstrual flow (Fig. 1.7).

Mechanism and timescale of gonadal development

To understand the development of the external genitalia and derangements of internal structures, it is necessary to consider the factors which control gonadal development. This complex area has been much clarified by the studies of many workers in recent decades, notably Jost & Wachtel (for references see

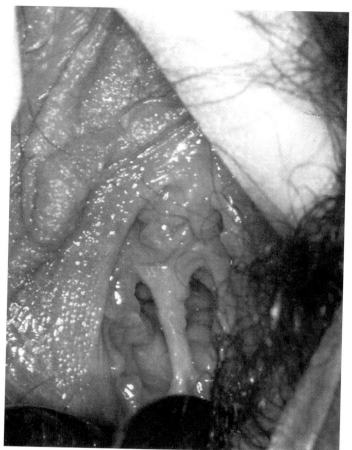

Fig. 1.6   Anteroposterior septum at introitus.

Wilson et al 1981a). Sexual differentiation is dealt with in Chapter 14 but reference here is necessary to understand the importance of timing in deviations of embryological development. The basic sequence is chromosomal sex, gonadal differentiation and phenotype. In essence, whatever chromosome complement is present, it is the effects of gonadal production which determine phenotype.

If germ cells fail to reach the genital ridge by the end of the 6th week of embryonic development, the gonad forms only a fibrous streak. Provided they do by then, the gonad contains primordial germ cells, connective tissue of the genital ridge and covering epithelium and has cortical and medullary potential. What happens then depends on whether there is a testicular component to induce somatic cells to form all or part of a male system. The testis-determining factor was localized to the short arm of the Y chromosome (Yp) and by progressive molecular genetic analysis of smaller fragments, the major gene for testicular development, SRY (sex-determining region of Y) was located (Sinclair et al 1990) to a very specific region near the tip (Yp 11.3) (for discussion and references, see McElreavy & Fellous 1999, Yding Anderson & Byskov 1996). Even in exceptions, such as 46 XX males, the SRY gene is present, usually on the short arm of the X by accidental interchange of X and Y material during paternal meiosis. When SRY is present, cortical regression and medullary growth start,

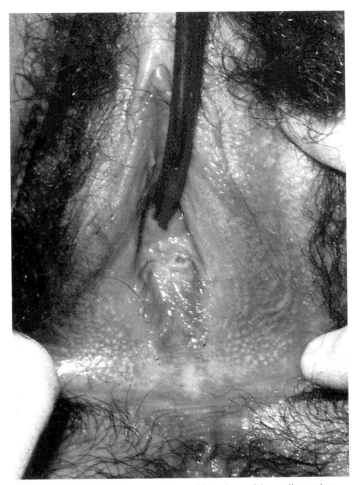

Fig. 1.7 Almost complete occlusion of introitus with small opening about 2 cm posterior to the urethra (catheter) and slightly to the left. There had been no obstruction to menstrual flow but there was apareunia and inability to insert a tampon.

leading to the development of spermatic cords, seminiferous tubules and Leydig and Sertoli cells. This process does not occur without the protein product of the SRY gene. However, even if present, male development can fail at some other stage downstream. Individuals with Y chromosome components can have female or ambiguous phenotypes. Females with gonadal dysgenesis who have 46 XY chromosomes usually have the SRY gene, so their gonadal failure is not because SRY is missing (Behzadian et al 1991).

Normally, in female development, the SRY gene is absent and the indifferent embryonic gonad develops into an ovary by development of the cortical zone with the germ cells, while the medullary zone regresses to form a compressed aggregation of tubules and Leydig cells in the hilus of the ovary. This is not a simple passive matter. Full ovarian function is an active process involving loci on the X chromosome and on autosomes (Simpson 1995). Only one X is required for ovarian differentiation but more X material is needed for maintenance of ovarian follicles beyond birth. Also, other factors can lead to ovarian failure (for discussion and references, see Simpson & Rajkovic 1999). Morphological development of the ovary

starts about 2 weeks later than the testis and proceeds more slowly. Development of the female internal duct system is not dependent on ovarian formation and proceeds ahead of development of the germ cells. Nevertheless, oestrogen is produced from the ovary prior to germ cell growth and it is presumed that the primitive Leydig cells produce oestrogen by conversion from testosterone – a process that has been shown to occur before differentiation. The germ cells divide and by 20 weeks of gestation there are primordial follicles with oocytes. The peak formation of primordial follicles occurs at about this time, reaching about 5–7 million by 20 weeks. Atresia starts around that time and by birth there are about 1–2 million germ cells surrounded by a layer of follicular cells. The germ cells enter the first meiotic division and are arrested in prophase.

Development of the duct systems

It is the differentiation of the gonad which determines the hormonal environment and, hence, the differentiation of the internal duct system, the external genitalia and perhaps the embryonic brain (Wilson et al 1981b). Because testicular development is very early, differences in timing between the genders occur. The Sertoli cells produce anti-müllerian hormone and HCG stimulates the Leydig cells so that testosterone synthesis is under way by 9 weeks from fertilization. The timing of the various steps is shown in Figure 1.8.

Provided that the genital ridge develops, all embryos have wolffian and müllerian systems. What actually happens to duct development is controlled by the fetal gonad. Continued development of the wolffian system requires sufficient androgens. Development of the müllerian system will usually occur unless positively inhibited. The first interactive event between gonad and duct system is the production of müllerian inhibition. The hormone involved, formerly called müllerian-inhibiting factor (MIF), is now characterized as a glycoprotein, anti-müllerian hormone (AMH) formed by the Sertoli cells of the spermatogenic tubules very early in the development of the fetal testis (Josso et al 1993). The fetal müllerian duct is sensitive to AMH for only a short, critical phase soon after the start of sexual differentiation. If this function fails, a female genital tract will form internally regardless of chromosomal sex. Equally, exposure to AMH in a female fetus at the critical phase results in regression of the system. The production of AMH precedes, and is separate from, androgen production. It acts locally and deficiency can be unilateral. A hereditary disorder, usually autosomal recessive, of persistent müllerian duct syndrome exists, where a fallopian tube and hemiuterus may occur on one or both sides and coexist with normal wolffian development in an otherwise normal genetic and phenotypic male.

Mutations in the gene for AMH have been shown in some but not all cases studied (Belville et all 1999) and some may be due to unresponsive target cells. Suboptimal testicular function is probable since there is often failure of testicular descent, though this could also be secondary to the anatomical presence of müllerian structures. Another feature indicative of the independence of these processes is that there is usually regression of the müllerian ducts even when defective testosterone synthesis

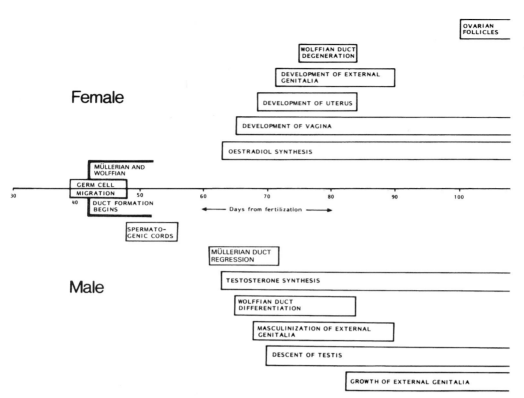

Fig. 1.8 Timing of anatomical, gonadal and endocrine events. Data from Coulam (1979) and Wilson et al (1981b). A closed box indicates that the event has a critical period for development.

results in an undermasculinized male. However, if there is no functional testis, no AMH is produced, the müllerian system develops and there is no stimulation of the wolffian system. This is the normal event in the female and proceeds whether there is a normal ovary or not. The distal portion of the regressing wolffian duct may leave remnants in the mesovarium (epoopheron) or in the cervical or vaginal walls (Gartner's duct) which may form cysts. The incidence of some remnant is estimated to be about 20%, but clinical significance is less.

Development of the external genitalia

The two genital duct systems and the urinary tract have a common opening between the genital folds. Their fate depends on the formation of the external genitalia. There is overlap in the timing of the formation of the external genitalia and the internal duct system (Fig. 1.9). There is a common indifferent stage, consisting of two genital folds, two genital swellings and a midline, anterior genital tubercle. The female development is a simple progression from these structures:

genital tubercle → clitoris
genital folds → labia minora
genital swellings → labia majora.

In the male, the genital folds elongate and fuse:

genital tubercle → glans
genital folds → penis and urethra
genital swelling → scrotum.

This process is normally dependent on fetal testosterone production. Agents or inborn errors that prevent the synthesis

or action of androgens inhibit formation of the external genitalia. By the end of the first trimester of pregnancy, fusion of the genital folds has occurred in the male but with little differential growth. Hence at this stage of gestation inspection of the genitalia may be misleading. It is during the second trimester that most of the differential male growth occurs.

The external genitalia are very sensitive to androgen effects during development, the end-result depending on both androgen availability and local tissue sensitivity. If sufficient local androgen activity is not achieved by the 10th week from fertilization, incompletely masculinized genitalia will result in the male. This can account for a variable degree of ambiguity of the female phenotype. Equally, exposure to sufficient androgens can result in a very similar appearance in the female. In congenital adrenal hyperplasia in the female, the degree of masculinization is variable (Fig. 1.10) but full scrotal and penile development may take place. However, the timing of adrenal development means that the androgenic stimulus arrives too late to affect the internal duct system. Once the external genitalia are fully developed, future androgen stimulus in the female will cause clitoral hypertrophy but not fusion of the labia.

Defective virilization resulting in female phenotype

There are several mechanisms by which defective virilization in a genetic male may occur. They are of importance to the gynaecologist where the end-result is one of female or ambiguous external genitalia. There are several subgroups.

1. Chromosomal variations, e.g. some cases of 45X/46XY and XY gonadal dysgenesis.

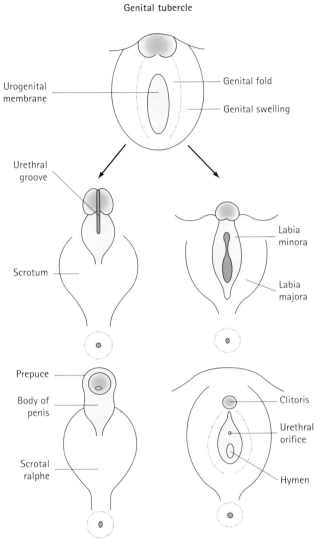

Fig. 1.9   Development of male and female external genitalia.

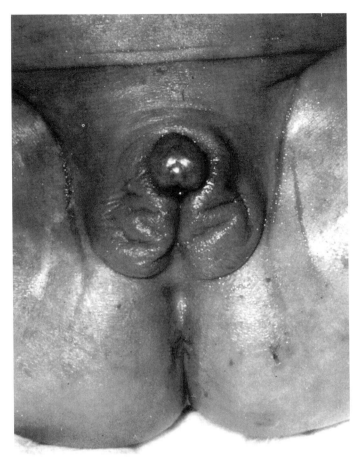

Fig. 1.10   Masculinized female genitalia in congenital adrenal hyperplasia.

2. Gonadal failure: testicular regression due to, for example, viral infection or vascular accident.
3. Defect of testosterone biosynthesis; enzyme defects.
4. End-organ resistance: complete androgen insensitivity, incomplete androgen insensitivity, 5α-reductase deficiency, androgen receptor failure.

The deviations from the normal in these conditions depend on the exact timing of stimuli as well as on the basic cause and this can contribute to the wide variation in clinical effects. For example, in the spectrum of conditions of gonadal failure, the outcome depends on the embryonic stage at the time of testicular failure (Coulam 1979). Many of these conditions are discussed in Chapter 14 and the following section illustrates the critical effect of timing only in the subgroup of individuals with a Y chromosome who are agonadal by the time of birth.

The clinical effect depends on whether, if there is a fetal testis, it produced enough AMH to suppress the müllerian system and whether there was enough androgen production to develop both the wolffian system and male external genitalia. There are different clinical entities (Table 1.1). To have a female phenotype there has to be failure of testicular development before androgen is secreted, but AMH may already have been produced. Such a girl would not be expected to have wolffian duct development. Whether or not there is a female genital tract depends on whether there was AMH (or enough AMH) before gonadal failure occurred. To have ambiguous or male genitalia, there must have been some secretion of androgen before gonadal failure occurred. The amount and duration of androgen production determine the anatomical result. Müllerian and wolffian ducts can coexist if gonadal failure occurred before müllerian regression was complete yet after androgen secretion had started. The clinical effects can be seen as a consequence of loss of testicular function at different stages of intrauterine development. The possible range extends from complete failure of development of the genital ridge, and therefore no internal duct system of either kind, to a male phenotype with anorchia.

The cause of these testicular insults is not usually known. They can be experimentally induced by drugs such as cyproterone acetate. In the human some may be viral or a consequence of torsion or vascualr occlusion. This group of

Table 1.1 Classification of XY agonadal individuals

Timing	Embryonic testicular regression		Fetal testicular regression				
	Early	Late	Early			Mid	Late
Days from fertilization	43	60	69	75	84	120	
Embryological consequence of testicular failure	No genital ridge development	Müllerian regression not yet started; no testosterone production	Müllerian regression not complete; testosterone synthesis *just* started	Müllerian regression still not complete; testosterone enough for duct development	Müllerian regression complete; testosterone production too little to develop duct system but some for external genitalia	Müllerian regression complete; wolffian development complete; incomplete external genitalia; rudimentary testes	Complete wolffian duct system; complete external genitalia; no testes or epididymis
Müllerian system	–	+	+	+	–	–	–
Wolffian system	–	–	–	+	–	+	+
External genitalia	Female	Female	Ambiguous	Ambiguous	Ambiguous	Ambiguous Male	Male

Adpated form Coulam (1979).

conditions is best described as the testicular regression syndrome, classified further according to the timing of the failure in development (see Table 1.1). Disordered development with a Y chromosome, gonadal formation but some abnormality of testosterone production or effect are not discussed further here. Yet, some of these latter abnormalities, e.g. androgen insensitivity syndrome, result in an entirely female phenotype and are relevant to disorders of puberty.

GENETICS – SEX CHROMOSOME ANOMALIES

Sexual development is essentially gonadal but is, of course, highly dependent on the exact genetic complement. There are many derangements of the X and Y chromosomes and some have important anatomical and functional effects. Variations may occur in the number or in the structure of the chromosomes in mosaic or non-mosaic form. The main non-mosaic forms are summarized in Table 1.2 in order of the number of X chromosomes and of extra Y chromosomes.

Aneuploidy

Aneuploidy may result from non-disjunction of either meiotic division in either parent or in an early cleavage of the zygote. Some are more common in older women (e.g. 47XXX and 47XXY) and the non-disjunction is presumed to arise mainly in maternal meiosis. The occurrence of 45X does not seem to be related to maternal age.

Although there is a wide range of clinical effects, some generalizations can be made.

Table 1.2 Identified non-mosaic patterns of sex chromosomes; normal male and female karyotypes highlighted

Female phenotype	Male phenotype	Barr bodies
45X	**46XY** 47XYY 48XYYY	0
46XX	46XX 47XXY 48XXYY 49XXYYY	1
47XXX	48XXXY 49XXXYY	2
48XXXX	49XXXXY	3
49XXXXX		4

- If there is a Y chromosome, the phenotype is usually male.
- If the number of sex chromosomes increases beyond three (i.e. more than one extra), there is a strong tendency to some degree of mental retardation.
- Additional Y chromosome material tends to increase height.
- Provided there is at least one Y chromosome, one or more extra chromosomes result in hypogonadism.
- In each somatic cell, only one X chromosome is active. Others are inactivated (lyonized).

Both Klinefelter's syndrome (XXY) and XYY occur in about 1 in 700 newborn males. The clinical features are well recognized but are outside the scope of this chapter. Higher-order anomalies with a male phenotype are very rare.

X chromosome aneuploidy with a female phenotype

Many of the abnormal X chromosomal complements are associated with gonadal dysgenesis and abnormalities of stature.

One X less

The 45X chromosome constitution accounts for more than half of the number of girls with Turner's syndrome. The overall incidence of this condition is about 1 in 2500 live female births but nearly half have a mosaic pattern or some other X chromosome aberration. Short stature is invariable in 45X; gonadal failure is usual and other somatic features such as webbed neck, low hairline, cubitus valgus, pigmented naevi and cardiovascular anomalies are variably expressed but useful in alerting clinicians to the diagnosis. There is no systematic impairment of IQ, at least by verbal testing, but scoring on spatial ability tends to be lower. Classically, by the time of birth (or puberty) the gonads are non-functioning streaks but ovarian function has been described in about 3% and even fertility (especially in those with mosaicism). Pregnancy loss and karyotype anomalies of the fetus are common when pregnancy does occur.

One extra X

Triple X arises in about 1 in 1200 live female births and often passes unnoticed. There is no consistent clinical syndrome, thus accounting for the lack of ascertainment, but an increased incidence of psychosis has been noted. Phenotype, puberty and initial fertility are normal though there is a higher incidence of secondary amenorrhoea and early menopause. There is a tendency to increased height. Conception could result in XXX or XXY (or mosaic) progeny, but this occurs much less often than the predicted 50% and it is clear that in the meiotic division of the oocyte, the extra X chromosome ends up in the polar body more often than would be predicted by chance.

Two or more extra X

This is rare. Dysmorphism and mental retardation are usual but psychosis and aggression are not features. Phenotype, external genitalia and puberty are usually normal. Menstrual disorders are common. Fertility is possible and the incidence of chromosomal abnormalities in the progeny, though not well assessed, is likely to be high.

Mosaicism

This is more common for sex chromosomes than for autosomes. Two cell lines can arise from a single zygote due to non-disjunction in an early mitosis. The commonest are 46XX or 46XY accompanied by a 45X cell line, but an enormous variety is possible and there can be more than two cell lines. The clinical effects are wide ranging and especially complex when there is both an XX and an XY cell line. The relative proportion of the different cell lines tends to determine the phenotype, but this can vary in different organs and some result in hermaphrodite or intersex states.

Structural abnormalities of X chromosomes

Apart from the number of X chromosomes and mosaic cell lines, there are many possible variations within the X chromosome in the female. The basic conventions of banding and nomenclature of chromosomes (Mueller & Young 1998) with respect to deletion and isochromy should be understood (Figs 1.11 and 1.12). Note that the X chromosome carries many genes for metabolic and developmental disorders and that the gene map is being constantly updated. If there is one normal X and the other is abnormal, then usually inactivation of the abnormal X occurs in the somatic cells and this tends to diminish the effect of the abnormality, except in the ovary. Although only one X chromosome is sufficient for early fetal ovarian development, germ cell maintenance requires several loci on the second X and on autosomes (for discussion and references, see Simpson 1997). Developments in molecular

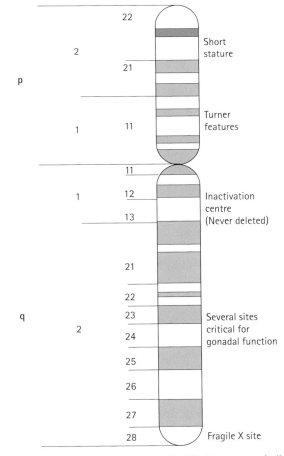

Fig. 1.11 Diagram of banded chromatid of X chromosome indicating the main numerical locations, on the left. On the right, phenotypic effects of some sites affected by deletions or variations are noted (based on data in Therman & Susman 1993 and Simpson 1999).

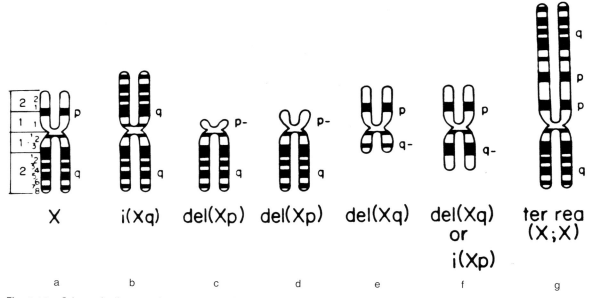

Fig. 1.12 Schematic diagram of some structural abnormalities of the X chromosome. **a** nomal; **b** isochrome for long arm; **c** deletion of most of the short arm; **d** probable interstitial deletion of the middle portion of the short arm; **e** interstitial deletion of the long arm; **f** deletion of a portion of the long arm; **g** short-arm end-to-end terminal rearrangement. Note that i(Xp) is thought not to occur since the inactivation centre, close to the centromere on Xq, is essential. (From de la Chapelle 1983, with permission.)

Table 1.3 General effects of structural abnormalities of X chromosomes

	Aspects of phenotype affected	Effect of loss of material	Effect of extra material
Short arm	Ovarian function	Gonadal dysgenesis	
	Somatic features of Turner's	Turner's phenotype	
	Growth	Short stature	
Long arm	Ovarian function	Gonadal dysgenesis	
	Growth	Reduced growth	Increased growth

genetic techniques of studying DNA sequences have enabled the identification of loci on the X chromosome, determining gonadal and somatic features (Fig. 1.11), but there is not a direct karyotype-phenotype effect in variations and rearrangements. Table 1.3 summarizes generalizations in relation to clinical effects. It does not appear that localization is highly specific since multiple loci are necessary. Location of responsible genes has largely been deduced from study of individuals with deletions of some or all of the short or long arm of one X (Simpson 1995). If the loci at 11.2–11.4 on the short arm are missing, ovarian maintenance is unlikely. More distal deletions are associated with infertility and secondary amenorrhoea. Deletions in the proximal to mid region of the long arm (Xq11.3–2.1) are also associated with ovarian failure and more terminal deletions with secondary amenorrhoea (Simpson & Rajkjovic 1999). If most or all of the short arm is deleted, then short stature and Turner's features are usual.

Deletion of most or all of the long arm is nearly always associated with gonadal dysgenesis. It seems likely that a proportion of women with premature ovarian failure have quite small and subtle deletions of the distal part of Xq (Marozzi et al 2000).

A ring chromosome can form if part of both ends is missing. The clinical effect will depend on the amount of genetic material lost but the effect tends to be less than if a whole arm is absent. Isochromy, due to misdivision at the centromere, can result in two long arms i(Xq) instead of a short (p) and a long (q) arm. In the whole cell, this results in three long arms and one short one and the effect on gonadal function and stature is the same as 45X. Thus, gonadal determinants appear to be located on both arms and it is not a question of total amount, since duplication of one fails to compensate for loss of the other, so each arm must carry different functions. There appear to be genes determining stature on both arms but loss of short arm material seems to result more consistently in short stature. This area remains complex and only partially understood, but some prediction of stature and potential for gonadal function can be made from consideration of the karyotype (Table 1.4).

XX gonadal dysgenesis

Gonadal dysgenesis can occur without demonstrable abnormality of either X chromosome. The gonads and genitalia look the same in this condition as in 45X, though most such girls are of normal stature without other Turner features. This condition is usually inherited in an autosomal recessive way and may have a range of causes, including defects in germ cell migration or in ovarian receptors. It may be part of syndromes

Table 1.4   Correlation of X karyotype, phenotype and gonadal development

Problem	Example of karyotype	Stature	Primary amenorrhoea	Breast development
Monosomy for X	45X	Short	Almost certain	Absent or minimal
Short arm material missing				
Isochromy of long arm	46X, i(Xq) or 45X/46X, i(Xq)	Short	Almost certain	Absent or minimal
Most of short arm	46X, del (X)(p11)	Short	Variable	May be some
Terminal part of short arm	46X, del (X)(p22)	Short	Not likely	Usually some
Long arm material missing				
Most of long arm	46X, del (X)(q13)	Reduced	Likely	Slight
Terminal part of long arm	46X, del (X)(q22)	Reduced	Likely	Slight
Mosaic*	45X/46XX	Variable	Variable	Variable
	46XX/range of deletions/isochromy	Variable	Variable	Variable

* The clinical effects of a mosaic karyotype depend on the proportion and distribution of the normal cell line. (Compiled from data in Therman & Susman 1993 and Simpson 1995).

with other somatic anomalies. It may also be of non-genetic origin, e.g. autoimmune or infection (Simpson 1995).

Translocations

Translocation can occur between an X chromosome and an autosome. If the normal X is inactivated in all autosomal cells and the parts of the other X attached to the autosome remain active, the affected woman may be overtly normal but there are implications for any progeny. However, the X inactivation is liable to be more patchy and mental retardation is likely. If the translocation is unbalanced there is mental retardation and ovarian failure (Gardner & Sutherland 1996).

X–X translocations

One X chromosome may be replaced by a long X consisting of two X chromosomes attached by either their long or short arms (Zakharov & Baranovskaya 1983). This results in a variable amount of X material being deleted or being present in a double dose. Where long arm material is lost there is usually gonadal dysgenesis, despite the extra X material. The abnormal X is late replicating and it is the structurally normal X which is genetically active. In an example of such an X chromosome (Fig. 1.13) the girl had tall stature, gonadal dysgenesis and dysmorphism (Barnes et al 1988).

True hermaphrodites

This condition is characterized by the demonstration of both ovarian and testicular tissue. Genetically, it is heterogeneous. The most common single chromosome pattern is 46XX but there is often more than one cell line and this may be due to chimaerism (two cell lines at fertilization) or mitotic non-disjunction. Recognized cell lines include 46XX/46XY and 46XX/47XXY. Essentially, the more testicular tissue there is, the more likely is gonadal descent. Usually there is at least a hemiuterus and if ovarian tissue is present, it is more likely to be on the left side. The management depends on the phenotype. Ovulation and, where the anatomy is appropriate, conception and delivery can occur.

CONGENITAL ABNORMALITIES OF FEMALE DEVELOPMENT

This section deals with anatomical disorders of the genital tract in the phenotypic female. Fetal diagnosis, although possible for some conditions, is not considered further here. Conditions with a genetic but no anatomical genital abnormality, e.g. 45X, and other conditions presenting with primary amenorrhoea, e.g. complete androgen insensitivity, are discussed elsewhere. Many anomalies of the female genital tract relate to failure of development of all or some of the müllerian ducts, failure of lateral fusion or incomplete canalization. The urinary system is often involved. Some of the resulting conditions involve the paediatric surgeon (e.g. cloacal anomalies), the urologist (e.g. bladder extrophy, abnormal ureters) or the paediatrician (e.g. disorders of growth). There is necessarily overlap between specialties in conditions such as ambiguous genitalia and disorders of puberty. Most disorders of the female genital tract are not associated with apparent chromosome variations. Some appear to have familial aggregates, though this may be due to reporting bias and developmental genes may well be involved. Some are part of syndromes associated with multiple skeletal and sensory disorders (Simpson 1999).

Some of the anatomical abnormalities are an arrest of a stage of normal development, e.g. vaginal atresia, while others, e.g. bladder extrophy, do not represent a stage through which the normal fetus passes. Common times of presentation are:

- newborn, if there are external abnormalities or obstruction of bladder or bowel
- childhood, if there is disturbance of function
- puberty, particularly if menstrual function is affected
- at attempted coitus, if there is relative obstruction
- adulthood, because of infertility or pregnancy

It is not possible to estimate a true incidence of most genital tract anomalies, since the age of ascertainment, the thoroughness of surveillance and the inclusion of minor anomalies will influence this. In pregnancy, an incidence of müllerian anomalies of 1 in 600 women has been estimated but this

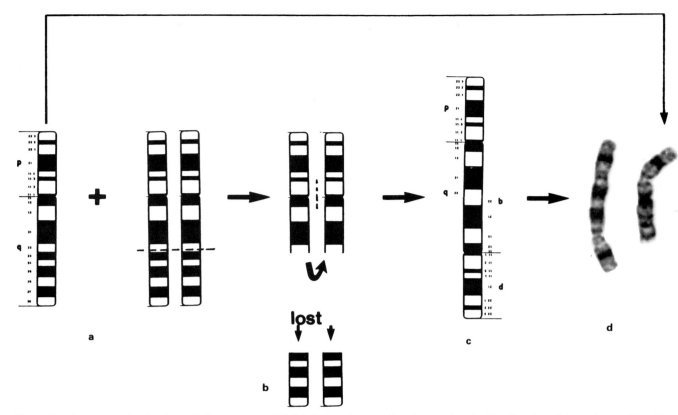

Fig. 1.13 Formation of an isodicentric X chromosome idic(x)q(22). **a** chromatid breakage at band q22. **b** Reunion of sister chromatids with loss of acentric segment. **c** Division of centromere to form end-to-end fusion chromosome. One centromere becomes inactive. **d** Chromosomes form a 46X idic(X)(q22) cell. The other X chromosome, extreme right and left, is normal.

excludes the very important groups who present earlier or who cannot conceive. Perhaps a reasonable estimate would be some abnormality of the genital tract in 1% of phenotypic females.

The neonate or child

Neonates and children with congenital abnormalities of female development may present by:

- ambiguous genitalia
- imperforate vagina, with an abdominal mass due to muco-colpos
- duplication of the vulva
- cloaca (often involving spinal defects)
- ectopia vesicae
- imperforate anus
- disorders of renal system affecting micturition or drainage.

Need for gynaecological assessment

Abnormalities of the urinary or bowel systems in the female child are often associated with anomalies of the genital tract. There are several reasons why a gynaecologist should be involved as well as a paediatrician and paediatric surgeon.

- Study of the original anatomy aids comprehension of the problem.
- Familiarity with the surgery in the infant helps with reconstructive surgery at puberty or later.

- Where there are anomalies of the urinary or bowel systems, good liaison improves investigation of the genital tract.
- Diagnosis of the abnormal vulva is not easy and improves with practice

Multiple abnormalities

These include persistent cloaca (Fig. 1.14), bladder exstrophy and ectopic ureter. Investigation by endoscopy, ultrasound, contrast vaginogram (sinogram), magnetic resonance imaging (MRI) and, where necessary, laparotomy should clarify the structure of the genital tract. Free drainage of the genital tract is important and careful recording of its anatomy is valuable for prognosis and later reference.

Imperforate vagina

Mucocolpos due to an imperforate vagina is important in the differential diagnosis of an abdominal mass in a newborn girl.

Duplication of vulva

Full paediatric surgical investigation is required to establish other abnormalities and effective drainage. A didelphic uterus is likely. If there is no functional problem, an acceptable cosmetic effect would be the aim.

Ambiguous genitalia

Ambiguity of gender at birth is an emergency matter requiring integrated management. It occurs in:

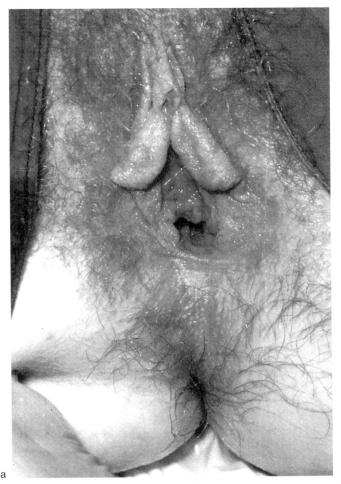
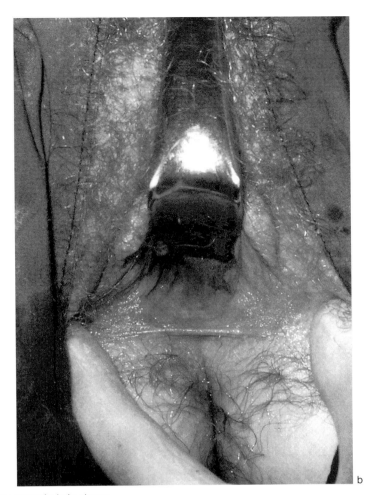

a

b

Fig. 1.14 Cloaca: **a** single opening with absence of anus; **b** rectal columns posteriorly in cloaca.

- virilized females, e.g. congenital adrenal hyperplasia, high maternal androgen levels, maternal drug ingestion
- undermasculinized males
- true hermaphrodites.

When a female gender role is agreed, sufficient surgical correction should be effected in infancy for social acceptability. Newer techniques (e.g. Passerini-Glazel 1994) may give better results in future than infancy surgery in the past.

Puberty or later

Müllerian agenesis

There is no corpus, cervix or upper vagina (Fig. 1.15). There may be fallopian tubes representing the upper separate ends of the müllerian duct system. There may also be remnants of müllerian tissue. The condition has been reported in siblings but not with enough consistency to suggest that it is due to a single gene defect. Müllerian agenesis accounts for over 80% of occurrences of absent vagina.

Vaginal atresia

There is development of the müllerian system with consequent menstrual obstruction. There is no reporting of family aggregates except where the atresia is part of multiple anomalies. The failure of the urogenital sinus to form the lower vagina may be complete or there may be a short lower vagina with an obstruction of variable thickness in the mid-portion.

True duplication

This is rare and is due to splitting of the müllerian duct or even of the genital ridge early in embryogenesis. It does not have any family aggregates.

Incomplete fusion

This may occur at various levels and may be symmetrical or asymmetrical. It may be one component of a congenitally determined multiple malformation. Even if it occurs as the only abnormality, incomplete fusion seems to have a polygenic or multifactorial basis resulting in some family aggregation.

Presentation

Abnormalities not diagnosed in infancy may become of clinical relevance around the time of puberty or later and are more likely to affect the vagina or upper genital tract. Vulvar abnormalities, however, may become evident because of hormonal stimulation. Where there is primary amenorrhoea

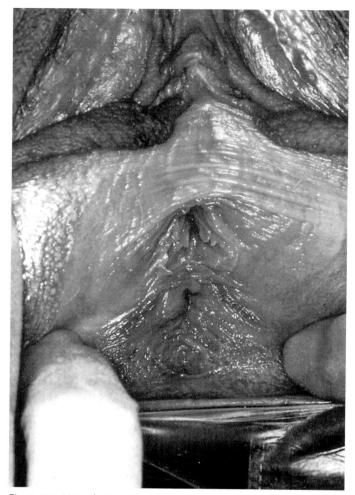

Fig. 1.15   Vulva (labia widely retracted) of a girl with müllerian agenesis. The urethra is abnormally patulous and there is very little formation of the urogenital sinus portion of the vagina.

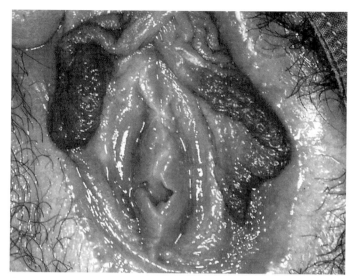

Fig. 1.16   Normal-looking vulva of a girl with vaginal atresia and haematocolpos and haematometra. There was a short lower vagina.

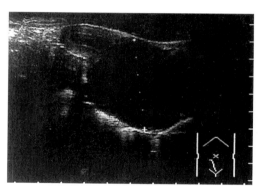

Fig. 1.17   Ultrasound scan of the same girl, showing distended upper vagina and distended uterus.

with secondary sexual development, absence of the uterus or obstruction to menstrual flow should be considered. Other presenting complaints include apareunia or inability to insert a tampon.

Vaginal atresia or obstruction

Where this condition has not been diagnosed in infancy, failure to menstruate is the likeliest presenting symptom. The crucial clinical question is whether or not there is haematocolpos. Higher levels of obstruction, at the cervix or upper vagina, will tend to cause symptoms early and also cause more serious backflow and endometriosis. Any recurrent abdominal pain (not necessarily regular or monthly) in a pubertal girl with secondary sexual development should be investigated adequately. Ultrasound of the pelvis and kidneys is very useful. Inspection of the introitus, although important, may be misleading where there is a high obstruction (Figs 1.16–1.19).

Where the obstruction is low and thin, usually just above the hymen, a simple but adequate cruciate incision to allow free drainage of retained menses is all that is required initially. After two or three further periods, which allows time for any

distortion or swelling to subside, laparoscopy is indicated to diagnose and treat any endometriosis. The anatomy of the renal tract should be established.

Where there is vaginal atresia, management can be difficult. If it is not possible to reach the upper vagina from the perineum, an abdominoperineal approach may be required. Achieving drainage is not usually difficult and should be effected from the vagina if possible. The difficulty is to maintain subsequent patency. Much patience and ingenuity may be required. Continuous oestrogen/progestogen treatment may provide a respite.

Atresia of the cervix

This condition is due to failure of development of the cervical portion of the fused müllerian ducts. It is rare and serious. The uterus may be normal or bicornuate. Creation of a cervical opening and successful pregnancy have proved possible (Edmond 1994) but if initial attempts are not effective it may be better to resort to hysterectomy before serious intraperitoneal infection occurs. The tubes are susceptible to infective damage even before presentation and diagnosis.

The presentation is generally with amenorrhoea and well-developed secondary sex characteristics. Care is required to establish for certain whether or not there is a functioning uterus or remnant. If not, the question of a neovagina is best deferred until there is an interest in sexual activity. A range of techniques is available (Edmonds 1994) but the extent to which a small vagina can be enlarged by non-surgical means should not be underestimated where motivation is high.

Where there is a short blind vagina and müllerian agenesis, androgen insensitivity must be included in the differential diagnosis. Small breasts and poorly developed axillary and pubic hair are important accompanying features. There may be a family history. Virilization at puberty is a feature of partial androgen insensitivity. Chromosome analysis is helpful in these circumstances and should be done when there is müllerian agenesis without well-developed secondary sexual characteristics.

Persistent urogenital sinus

A common genitourinary channel is the normal arrangement in a male infant and occurs to some degree during development in all female infants. Failure of development and caudal

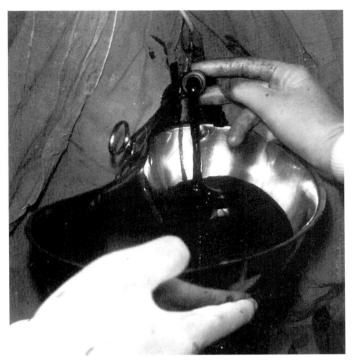

Fig. 1.18 Drainage of haematocolpos required dissection and insertion of a trocar.

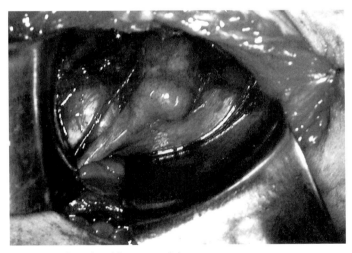

Fig. 1.19 Associated haematosalpinx.

Vaginal agenesis as part of müllerian agenesis

Where vaginal agenesis is part of müllerian duct failure, the clinical picture is different. The introitus may look normal or there may be hypoplasia of the urogenital sinus component. Usually there is a short (1–2 cm) vagina. The incidence is about 1 in 10 000 female births. Ureterorenal anomalies occur in about 50%. A rudimentary uterus is quite common but it may be just a remnant on one or both sides and is not usually canalized. The appearances on ultrasound have sometimes been deceptive but with better resolution a false impression of canalization is less likely. However, it should be noted that ultrasound of the uterus is more difficult where there is no vagina.

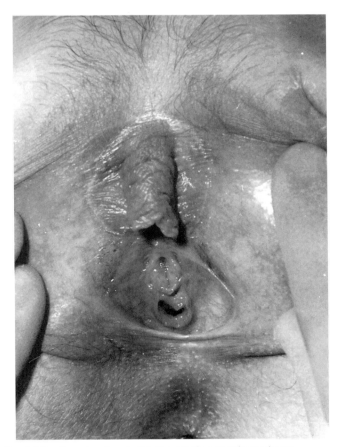

Fig. 1.20 Hypertrophy of clitoris occurring at puberty due to oestrogen administration, in an otherwise phenotypic female (XY). There had been minimal hypertrophy in infancy associated with intersex (mainly scrotal development with testes) and the gonads had been removed in the neonatal period. Note that the androgenic stimulus in utero had not been sufficient to fuse the genital folds.

movement of the lower vagina results in a higher common channel than usual. The confluence of the vagina and urethra may be at a very variable level. The condition is present in most girls with infantile congenital adrenal hyperplasia, all those with an intersex condition brought up as girls and can sometimes occur without obvious cause or associated features.

The presentation depends on whether there is, or has been, virilization (not necessarily a feature) and on prior surgery, possibly in infancy. The typical feature is a small, single opening with no visible separate urethra and fusion of the labia majora. Even a minor degree of the condition may interfere with coitus or use of tampons. When severe, surgery is necessary to enable coitus.

Virilization occurring at puberty
There are a number of causes.

- An intersex problem rectified in infancy but leaving a slightly enlarged clitoris. This tends to enlarge at puberty during spontaneous or replacement hormone stimulation, even only by oestrogens (Fig. 1.20).
- Incomplete androgen insensitivity; there may have been only slight clitoral enlargement which responds further to the greater androgen boost at puberty.
- 5α-reductase deficiency; which is always relative and the puberty levels of testosterone cause enlargement of the external genitalia.
- Gonadoblastoma in a dysgenetic gonad.

The hormonal, gonadal and anatomical status must be completely evaluated. Inappropriate androgen secretion must be removed, except in some cases of 5α-reductase deficiency, where reinforcement of the male gender has been successful. If clitoral hypertrophy remains a problem, it is unlikely to regress if oestrogen replacement is effected even if the androgenic stimulus is no longer present. Some form of clitoral reduction should be offered (Duncan 2000).

Uterine anomalies
Fusion anomalies are more common than absence of the uterus and result in a variety of uterine shapes (Fig. 1.21). Where there is atresia of one of the paramesonephric ducts there is a unicornuate uterus with a single tube. The kidney on the side of the defective duct is often absent. If the unilateral atresia is partial, the rudimentary part may be an appendage to the well-developed side and, if it fails to communicate, the rudimentary horn causes complications. Where there is a didelphic uterus, the uterine cavities are completely separate (Fig. 1.22) but the two cervices are often united externally. The vagina may or may not be septate. In this condition, asymmetry of the vagina may result in complete closure of one half, with subsequent crytopmenorrhoea and haematometra but with apparently normal menstrual function (Figs 1.23–1.25). Curiously, when this condition occurs, the occluded side is nearly always on the right. There is ipsilateral absence of the kidney (Rock & Jones 1980). Failure of complete müllerian formation and failure to form a ureter are both a consequence of a defective mesonephric duct.

Provided there is no obstruction to menstrual flow, these uterine anomalies present few problems in the absence of

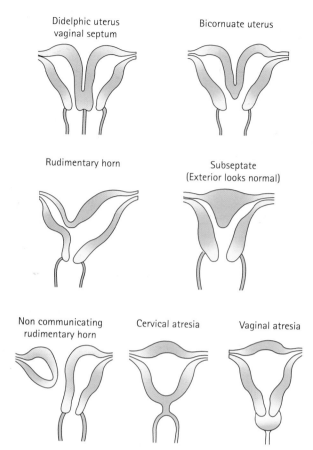

Fig. 1.21   Varieties of uterine anomaly.

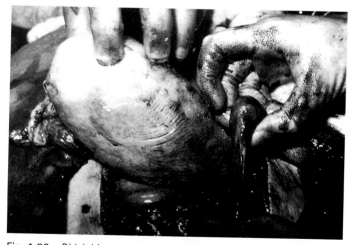

Fig. 1.22   Didelphic uterus at the time of caesarean section. The non-pregnant right uterus is attached externally at the cervix.

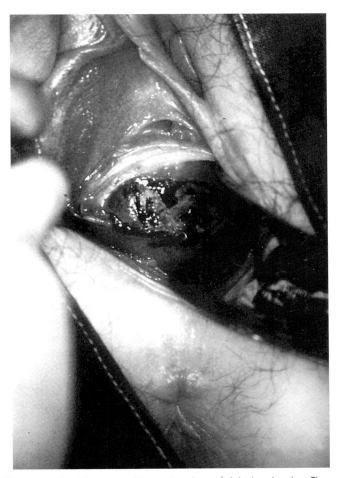

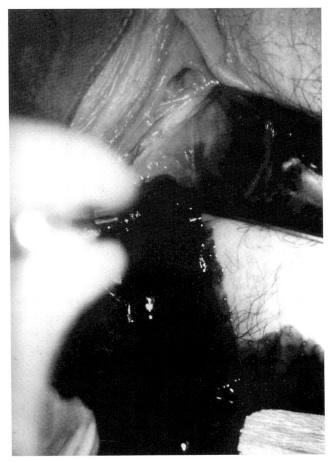

Fig. 1.24   Incision and drainage.

Fig. 1.23   Partially exposed haematocolpos of right hemivagina. The speculum is in the normal left hemivagina.

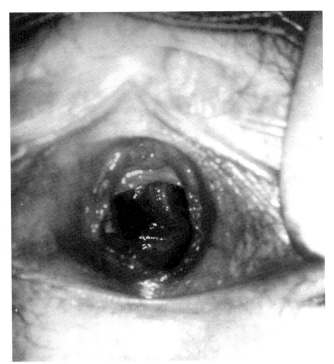

Fig. 1.25   Septum in the same girl after drainage.

pregnancy. An increased incidence of miscarriage, poor fetal growth, malpresentation and placental adherence is recognized. The incidence of abnormalities and the complication rate are ill defined since ascertainment is higher where there are complications and operative delivery (Rock & Schlaff 1985). Pregnancy may occur in a non-communicating rudimentary horn by transperitoneal sperm passage and can result in a difficult diagnostic and management problem.

For many of the anatomical congenital anomalies, the event which caused developmental failure is not clear even if the stage of arrest can be recognized. Much is continuing to be discovered about inducer substances and cellular mechanisms and gradually further elucidation of the picture will occur.

KEY POINTS

1. The nephrogenic cord develops from the mesoderm and forms the urogenital ridge and mesonephric duct (later to form the wolffian duct).
2. The paramesonephric duct, later to form the müllerian system, develops as an ingrowth of coelomic epithelium anterolateral to the mesonephric duct.
3. In the normal female, the wolffian system degenerates and the lower ends of the müllerian system fuse to form the uterus, cervix and upper vagina while the cephalic ends remain separate, forming the fallopian tubes.
4. Unilateral renal aplasia is frequently associated with failure of müllerian development on the same side, since both are dependent on adequate development of the mesonephric system.
5. If the tubular portions of the müllerian ducts develop to form a uterus and cervix, there is usually a patent upper vagina.
6. Where there is müllerian agenesis, the urogenital sinus still forms but does not lengthen and the vagina is short, though variable.
7. Chromosomal sex determines the development of the gonad and this, in turn, ordains the sexual phenotype.
8. The wolffian system is dependent on androgens for its development.
9. The müllerian system will develop in the absence of anti-müllerian hormone (AMH) and does not require a normal ovary.
10. The development of male external genitalia depends upon both the presence of androgens and local tissue sensitivity to androgens, regardless of chromosomal sex.
11. Although the second X chromosome is usually inactivated, both X chromosomes are required for fertility.
12. Gonadal dysgenesis can occur in an XX individual.
13. In the management of pelvic abnormalities recognized in childhood involving bladder and bowel, free drainage of the genital tract is important, as obstruction is often a feature and permanent damage may result if this is not corrected before puberty.
14. Müllerian agenesis is the most common cause for an absent vagina in girls.
15. Recurrent abdominal pain in a pubertal girl with definite secondary sexual development should be investigated to exclude haematocolpos. Ultrasound of the pelvis and kidneys is very useful.
16. If correction of cervical atresia is unsuccessful, hysterectomy should be employed to avoid the serious peritonitis that may result.
17. Virilizing features at puberty require thorough investigation and sensitive management.
18. Haematocolpos and haematometra can occur despite normal menstruation.

REFERENCES

American Fertility Society 1988 The American Fertility Society classifications of adnexal adhesions, distal tubal occlusion, tubal occlusion secondary to tubal ligations, tubal pregnancies, Müllerian anomalies and intrauterine adhesions. Fertility and Sterility 49:944–954

Barnes ICS, Curtis D, Duncan SLB 1988 A duplication/deficient X chromosome in a girl with mental retardation and dysmorphic features. Journal of Medical Genetics 25:267–267

Belville C, Josso N, Picard J-Y 1999 Persistance of mullerian derivatives in males. American Journal of Medical Genetics. (Seminars in Medical Genetics) 89:218–223

Behzadian MA, Tho SPT, McDonough PG 1991 The presence of the testicular determining sequence SRY in 46.XY females with gonadal dysgenesis (Swyer syndrome). American Journal of Obstetrics and Gynecology 165:1887–1890

Coulam CB 1979 Testicular regression syndrome. Obstetrics and Gynecology 53:44–49

de la Chapelle A 1983 Sex chromosome anomalies. In: Emery AEH, Rimoin DL (eds) Principles and practice of medical genetics. Churchill Livingstone, Edinburgh, p 197

Duncan SLB 2000 Congenital abnormalities: gynaecological aspect. In: Stanton SL, Monga AK (eds) Clinical urogynaecology, 2nd edn. Churchill Livingstone, London, pp 294–308

Edmonds DK 1994 Sexual developmental anomalies and their reconstruction: upper and lower tracts. In: Sanfilippo JS, Muram D, Lee PA, Dewhurst J (Eds) Pediatric and adolescent gynecology. W B Saunders, Philadelphia, pp 535–566

Gardner RJM, Sutherland G R 1996 Sex chromosome translocations. In: Chromosome abnormalities and genetic counselling, 2nd edn. Oxford monographs on medical genetics no 29. Oxford University Press, Oxford, pp 95–114

Josso N, Lamarre I, Picard J-Y et al 1993 Anti-mullerian hormone in early human development: Early Human Development 33:91–99

Marozzi A, Manfredi E, Tibiletti MG et al 2000 Molecular definition of Xq common–deleted region in patients affected by premature ovarian failure. Human Genetics 107:304–311

McElreavy K, Fellous M 1999 Sex differentiation and the Y chromosome. American Journal of Medical Genetics. (Seminars in Medical Genetics) 89:176–185

Mueller RF, Young ID 1998 Chromosomes. In: Mueller RF, Young ID (eds) Emery's elements of medical genetics, 10th edn. Churchill Livingstone, Edinburgh, pp 52–53

O'Rahilly R 1977 The development of the vagina in the human. In: Blandau RJ, Bergsma D (eds) Morphogenesis and malformation of the genital system. Birth Defects. The National Foundation. Alan R Liss, New York, pp 123–136

Passerini-Glazel G 1994 Combined cliteroplasty and vaginoplasty. In: Hinman Jr F (ed) Atlas of pediatric urologic surgery. W B Saunders, Philadelphia, pp 644–648

Rock JA, Jones HW 1980 The double uterus associated with an obstructed hemivagina and ipsilateral renal agenesis. American Journal of Obstetrics and Gynecology 138:339–342

Rock JA, Schlaff WD 1985 The obstetric consequences of uterovaginal anomalies. Fertility and Sterility 43:681–692

Simpson JL 1995 Genetic control of ovarian development In: Grudzinkas JG, Yovich JL (Eds) Gametes – the oocyte. Cambridge reviews in human reproduction. Cambridge University Press, Cambridge, pp 108–118

Simpson JL 1997 Ovarian maintenance determinants on the X-chromosome and on its autosomes In: Coutifaris, Mastroianni L (Eds) New horizons in reproductive medicine. Parthenon Publishing Group, New York, pp 439–443

Simpson JL 1999 Genetics of the female reproductive ducts. American Journal of Medical Genetics. (Seminars in Medical Genetics) 89:224–239

Simpson JL, Rajkovic A 1999 Ovarian differentiation and gonadal failure. American Journal of Medical Genetics. (Seminars in Medical Genetics) 89:186–200

Sinclair AH, Berta P, Palmer MS et al 1990 A gene from the human sex-determining region encodes a protein with homology to conserved DNA-binding motif. Nature 346:240–244

Therman E, Susman M 1993 Abnormal human sex chromosome constitutions. In: Human chromosomes; structure, behavior and effects, 3rd edn. Springer Verlag, New York, pp 220–227

Ulfelder H, Robboy SJ 1976 The embryologic development of the human vagina. American Journal of Obstetrics and Gynecology 126:769–775

Wilson JD, Griffin JE, George FW, Leshin M 1981a The role of gonadal steroids in sexual differentiation. Recent Progress in Hormone Research 37:1–39

Wilson JD, George FW, Griffin JE 1981b The hormonal control of sexual development. Science 211:1278–1284

Yding Andersen C, Byskov A G 1966 Gonadal differentiation. In: Hillier SG, Kitchener HC, Neilson JP (Eds) Scientific essentials of reproductive medicine. W B Saunders, London, pp 105–119

Zakharov AF, Baranovskaya LI 1983 X-X chromosome translocations and their karyotype-phenotype correlations. In: Sandbert AA (ed) Cytogenetics of the mammalian X chromosome. Part B. Alan R Liss, New York, pp 261–279

FURTHER READING

Gilbert S F 1997 Developmental biology, 5th edn. Sinauer Associates, Sunderland, Massachusetts

Moore K L, Persaud T V N 1998 The developing human. Clinically orientated embryology, 6th edn. W B Saunders, Philadelphia

Mueller R F, Young I D (Eds) 1998 Emery's clements of medical genetics, 10th edn. Churchill Livingstone, Edinburgh

Sadler T W 2000 Langman's medical embryology, 8th edn. Lippincott Williams and Wilkins, Baltimore

Sanfilipo J S, Muran D, Lee P A, Dewhurst I (eds) 1994 Pediatric and adolescent gynaecology. W B Saunders, Philadelphia

Stanton S L, Monga A K 2000 Clinical urogynaecology, 2nd edn Churchill Livingstone, London

2

Surgical anatomy

Adrian M. Lower

INTRODUCTION

A clear understanding of the anatomy of the female pelvis is essential to successful gynaecological surgery and the avoidance or surgical morbidity. The close relationships between the reproductive, urinary and gastrointestinal tracts must be appreciated together with the pelvic musculofascial support, vascular and lymphatic circulations and neurological innervation. It is important to understand the effect of pneumoperitoneum on the anatomy and relationships of the pelvis and the opportunities afforded by a retroperitoneal approach in minimal access techniques.

THE OVARY

The size and appearance of the ovaries depend on both age and the stage of the menstrual cycle. In the young adult, they are almond shaped, solid and white in colour, 3 cm long, 1.5 cm wide and about 1 cm thick. The long axis is normally vertical before childbirth; after this there is a wide range of variation, presumably due to considerable displacement in the first pregnancy.

The ovary is the only intra-abdominal structure not to be covered by peritoneum. Each ovary is attached to the cornu of the uterus by the ovarian ligament, and at the hilum to the broad ligament by the mesovarium, which contains its supply of vessels and nerves. Laterally, each is attached to the suspensory ligament of the ovary with folds of peritoneum which become continuous with that over the psoas major.

Structure

The ovary has a central vascular medulla, consisting of loose connective tissue containing many elastin fibres and non-striated muscle cells, and an outer thicker cortex, denser than the medulla and consisting of networks of reticular fibres and fusiform cells, although there is no clear-cut demarcation between the two. The surface of the ovary is covered by a single layer of cuboidal cells, the germinal epithelium. Beneath this is an ill-defined layer of condensed connective tissue, the tunica albuginea, which increases in density with age. At birth, numerous primordial follicles are found, mostly in the cortex but some in the medulla. With puberty, some form each month into graafian follicles which at later stages of their development form corpora lutea and ultimately atretic follicles, the corpora albicantes (Fig. 2.1).

Relations

Anteriorly lie the fallopian tubes, the superior portion of bladder and uterovesical pouch; posteriorly is the pouch of Douglas. The broad ligament and its content are related inferiorly whilst superior to the ovaries are bowel and omentum. The lateral surface of the ovary is in contact with the parietal peritoneum and the pelvic side walls.

Vestigial structures

The vestigial remains of the mesonephric duct and tubules are always present in young children, but are variable structures in adults. The epoophoron, a series of parallel blind tubules, lies in the part of the broad ligament between the mesovarium and the fallopian tube, the mesosalpinx. The tubules run to the rudimentary duct of the epoophoron, which runs parallel to the lateral fallopian tube. Situated in the broad ligament, between the epoophoron and the uterus, are occasionally seen a few rudimentary tubules, the paroophoron.

In a few individuals, the caudal part of the mesonephric duct is well developed, running alongside the uterus to the internal os. This is the duct of Gartner.

Age-related changes

During early fetal life, the ovaries are situated in the lumbar region near the kidneys. They gradually descend into the lesser pelvis and during childhood they are small and situated near the pelvic brim. They are packed with primordial follicles. The ovary grows in size until puberty by an increase in the stroma. Ova are first shed around the time of onset of menstruation and ovulation is usually established within a couple of years.

After the menopause, the ovary atrophies and assumes a smaller, shrivelled appearance. The fully involuted ovary of old age contains practically no germinal elements.

Blood supply

The main vascular supply to the ovaries is the ovarian artery, which arises from the anterolateral aspect of the aorta just below the origin of the renal arteries. The right artery crosses the anterior surface of the vena cava, the lower part of the abdominal ureter and then, lateral to the ureter, enters the pelvis via the infundibulopelvic ligament. The left artery crosses the ureter almost immediately after its origin and then travels lateral to it, crossing the bifurcation of the common iliac artery at the pelvic brim to enter the infundibulopelvic ligament. Both arteries then divide to send branches to the ovaries through the mesovarium. Small branches pass to the ureter and fallopian

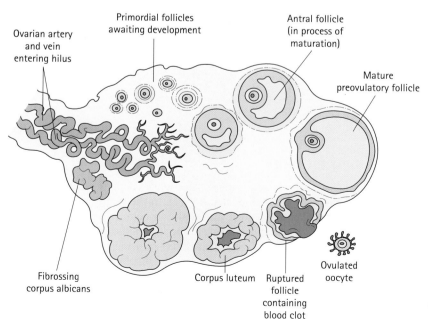

Ovarian artery and vein entering hilus

Primordial follicles awaiting development

Antral follicle (in process of maturation)

Mature preovulatory follicle

Fibrossing corpus albicans

Corpus luteum

Ruptured follicle containing blood clot

Ovulated oocyte

Fig. 2.1 Diagrammatic section of an ovary and schematic representation of the cycle of follicular maturations.

tube and one branch passes to the cornu of the uterus where it freely anastomoses with branches of the uterine artery to produce a continuous arterial arch (see Fig. 2.12).

The ovarian and uterine trunks drain into a pampiniform plexus of veins in the broad ligament near the mesovarium, which can occasionally become varicose. The right ovarian vein drains into the inferior vena cava, the left usually into the left renal vein.

THE FALLOPIAN TUBE

The uterine or fallopian tubes are two oviducts originating at the cornu of the uterus which travel a rather tortuous course along the upper margins of the broad ligament. They are around 10 cm in length and end in the peritoneal cavity close to the ovary. This abdominal opening is situated at the end of a trumpet-shaped lateral portion of tube, the infundibulum. This opening is fringed by a number petal-like processes, the fimbriae, which closely embrace the tubal end of the ovary. This fimbriated end has an important role in fertility.

Medial to the infundibulum is the ampulla which is thin-walled and tortuous and comprises at least half the length of the tube. The medial third of the tube, the isthmus, is relatively straight. The tube has narrowed at this point, from around 3 mm at the abdominal opening to 1–2 mm. The final centimetre, the interstitial portion, is within the uterine wall.

Structure

The tubes are typical of many hollow viscera in that they contain three layers. The outer serosal layer consists of peritoneum and underlying areolar tissue. This covers the whole tube apart from the fimbriae at one end and the interstitial portion at the other. The middle muscular layer consists of outer longitudinal fibres and inner circular ones. This is fairly thick at the isthmus and thins at the ampulla.

The mucous membrane is thrown into a series of plicae or folds, especially at the infundibular end. It is lined with columnar epithelium, much of which contains cilia which, together with the peristaltic action of the tube, help in sperm and ovum transport. Secretory cells are also present as well as a third group of intercalary cells of uncertain function.

Relations (Fig. 2.2)

These are similar to those of the ovary (see above). Medially, the fallopian tube, after arching over the ovary, curves around its tubal extremity and passes down its free border.

Blood supply

The fallopian tube is supplied by branches from the vascular arcade formed by the ovarian artery laterally and a branch of the uterine artery medially.

THE UTERUS

The uterus is shaped like an inverted pear, tapering inferiorly to the cervix and, in the non-pregnant state, is situated entirely within the lesser pelvis. It is hollow and has thick muscular walls. Its maximal external dimensions are about 9 cm long, 6 cm wide and 4 cm thick. The upper expanded part of the uterus is termed the body or corpus. The area of insertion of each fallopian tube is termed the cornu and that part of the body above the cornu, the fundus. The uterus tapers to a small central constricted area, the isthmus, and below this is the cervix, which projects obliquely into the vagina and can be divided into vaginal and supravaginal portions (Fig. 2.3).

The cavity of the uterus has the shape of an inverted triangle when sectioned coronally; the fallopian tubes open at the upper lateral angles (Fig. 2.4). The lumen is apposed anteroposteriorly. The constriction at the isthmus where the corpus joins the cervix is the anatomical internal os.

Structure

The uterus consists of three layers – the outer serous layer (peritoneum), the middle muscular layer (myometrium) and the inner mucous layer (endometrium).

The peritoneum covers the body of the uterus and posteriorly, the supravaginal portion of the cervix. This serous coat is intimately attached to a subserous fibrous layer, except

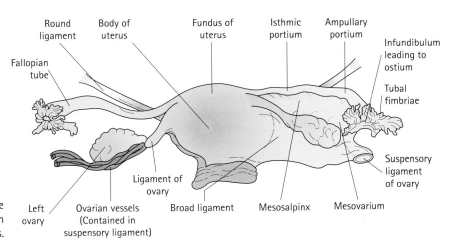

Fig. 2.2 Posterosuperior aspect of the uterus and the broad ligament. This is the view as seen laparoscopically from the umbilicus.

Round ligament
Body of uterus
Fundus of uterus
Isthmic portium
Ampullary portium
Fallopian tube
Infundibulum leading to ostium
Tubal fimbriae
Suspensory ligament of ovary
Ligament of ovary
Left ovary
Ovarian vessels (Contained in suspensory ligament)
Broad ligament
Mesosalpinx
Mesovarium

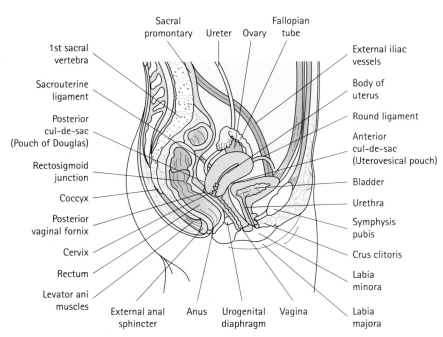

Fig. 2.3 Median sagittal section through a female pelvis.

Labels (clockwise from top): Sacral promontary, Ureter, Ovary, Fallopian tube, External iliac vessels, Body of uterus, Round ligament, Anterior cul-de-sac (Uterovesical pouch), Bladder, Urethra, Symphysis pubis, Crus clitoris, Labia minora, Labia majora, Vagina, Urogenital diaphragm, Anus, External anal sphincter, Levator ani muscles, Rectum, Cervix, Posterior vaginal fornix, Coccyx, Rectosigmoid junction, Posterior cul-de-sac (Pouch of Douglas), Sacrouterine ligament, 1st sacral vertebra

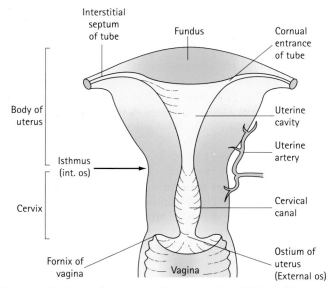

Fig. 2.4 Sectional diagram showing the interior divisions of the uterus and its continuity with the vagina.

Labels: Interstitial septum of tube, Fundus, Cornual entrance of tube, Body of uterus, Uterine cavity, Uterine artery, Isthmus (int. os), Cervix, Cervical canal, Fornix of vagina, Vagina, Ostium of uterus (External os)

laterally where it spreads out to form the leaves of the broad ligament.

The muscular myometrium forms the main bulk of the uterus and comprises interlacing smooth muscle fibres intermingling with areolar tissue, blood vessels, nerves and lymphatics. Externally these are mostly longitudinal but the larger intermediate layer has interlacing longitudinal, oblique and transverse fibres. Internally, they are mainly longitudinal and circular.

The endometrium forms the inner layer and is not sharply separated from the myometrium: the tubular glands dip into the innermost muscle fibres. A single layer of columnar epithelium covers the endometrium. Ciliated prior to puberty, this columnar epithelium is mostly lost due to the effects of pregnancy and menstruation. The endometrium undergoes cyclical histological changes during menstruation and varies in thickness between 1 and 5 mm.

The cervix

The cervix is cylindrical in shape, narrower than the body of the uterus and around 2.5 cm in length. It can be divided into the upper, supravaginal and lower vaginal portions. Due to anteflexion or retroflexion, the long axis of the cervix is rarely the same as the long axis of the body. Anterior and lateral to the supravaginal portion is cellular connective tissue, the parametrium. The posterior aspect is covered by peritoneum of the pouch of Douglas. The ureter runs about 1 cm laterally to the supravaginal cervix. The vaginal portion projects into the vagina to form the fornices.

The upper part of the cervix mostly consists of involuntary muscle, whereas the lower part is mainly fibrous connective tissue.

The mucous membrane of the endocervix has anterior and posterior columns from which folds radiate out, the arbor vitae. It has numerous deep glandular follicles which secrete a clear alkaline mucus, the main component of physiological vaginal discharge. The epithelium of the endocervix is cylindrical and also ciliated in its upper two-thirds, and changes to stratified squamous epithelium around the region of the external os. This change may be abrupt or there may be a transitional zone up to 1 cm in width.

Position

The longitudinal axis of the uterus is approximately at right angles to the vagina and normally tilts forwards: this is termed anteversion. The uterus is usually also flexed forwards on itself at the isthmus – anteflexion. In around 20% of women, this tilt is not forwards but backward – retroversion and retroflexion, respectively. In most cases, this does not have a pathological significance and the uterus is mobile.

Relations

Anteriorly, the uterus is related to the bladder and is separated from it by the uterovesical pouch of peritoneum. Posteriorly is the pouch of Douglas plus coils of small intestine, pelvic colon and upper rectum. Laterally, the relations are the broad ligament and that contained within it. Of special importance are the uterine artery and also the ureter, running close to the supravaginal cervix.

Age-related changes

The disappearance of maternal oestrogenic stimulation after birth causes the uterus to decrease in length by around one-third and in weight by about half. The cervix is then around twice the length of the body of the uterus. At puberty, however, the corpus grows much faster and the size ratio reverses; the body becomes twice the length of the cervix. After the menopause, the uterus undergoes atrophy, the mucosa becomes very thin, the glands almost disappear and the walls become relatively less muscular. These changes affect the cervix more than the corpus so that the cervical lips disappear and the external os becomes more or less flush with the vault.

THE VAGINA

The vagina is a fibromuscular tube which extends postero-superiorly from the vestibule to the uterine cervix. It is longer in its posterior wall (around 9 cm) than anteriorly (around 7.5 cm). The vaginal walls are normally in contact except superiorly, at the vault, where they are separated by the cervix. The vault of the vagina is divided into four fornices – posterior, anterior and two lateral. These increase in depth posteriorly. The mid-vagina is a transverse slit and the lower portion has an H-shape in transverse section.

Structure

The skin of the vagina is firmly attached to the underlying muscle and consists of stratified squamous epithelium. There are no epithelial glands present and the vagina is lubricated by mucus secretion from the cervix and Bartholin's glands. The epithelium is thick and rich in glycogen, which increases in the postovulatory phase of the cycle. Doderlein's bacillus is a normal commensal of the vagina, breaking down the glycogen to form lactic acid and producing a pH of around 4.5. This pH has a protective role for the vagina in decreasing the incidence of pyogenic infection.

The muscle layers consist of an outer longitudinal and inner circular layer, but these are not distinctly separate and are mostly spirally arranged and interspersed with elastic fibres.

The hymen

The hymen is a thin fold of mucous membrane across the entrance to the vagina. It has no known function. There are usually one or more openings in it to allow menses to escape. If these are not present a haematocolpos will form with the commencement of menstruation. The hymen is usually, but not always, torn with first intercourse but can also be torn digitally or with tampons. It is certainly destroyed in childbirth and only small tags remain – carunculae myrtiformes.

Relations

The upper posterior vaginal wall forms the anterior peritoneal reflection of the pouch of Douglas. The middle third is separated from the rectum by pelvic fascia and the lower third abuts the perineal body.

Anteriorly, the upper vagina is in direct contact with the base of the bladder whilst the urethra runs down the lower half in the midline to open into the vestibule; its muscles fuse with the anterior vaginal wall.

Laterally, at the fornices, the vagina is related to the attachment of the cardinal ligaments. Below this are levator ani muscles and the ischiorectal fossa. Near the vaginal orifice, the lateral relations include the vestibular bulb, bulbospongiosus muscles and Bartholin's gland.

Age-related changes

Immediately after birth, the vagina is under the influence of maternal oestrogen so the epithelium is well developed. Acidity is similar to that of an adult and Doderlein's bacilli are present. After a couple of weeks, the effects of maternal oestrogen disappear, the pH rises to 7 and the epithelium atrophies.

At puberty, the reverse occurs. The pH becomes acid again, the epithelium undergoes oestrogenization and the numbers of Doderlain's bacilli markedly increase. The vagina undergoes stretching during coitus, and especially childbirth, and the rugae tend to disappear.

At the menopause, the vagina tends to shrink and the epithelium atrophies.

THE VULVA

The female external genitalia, commonly referred to as the vulva, include the mons pubis, the labia majora and minora, the vestibule, the clitoris and the greater vestibular glands (Fig. 2.5).

Labia majora

The labia majora are two prominent folds of skin with under-lying adipose tissue bounding either side of the vaginal opening. They contain numerous sweat and sebaceous glands and correspond to the scrotum of the male. Anteriorly, they fuse together over the symphysis pubis to form a deposition of fat known as the mons pubis. Posteriorly, they merge with the perineum. From puberty onwards, the lateral aspects of the labia majora and the mons pubis are covered with coarse hair.

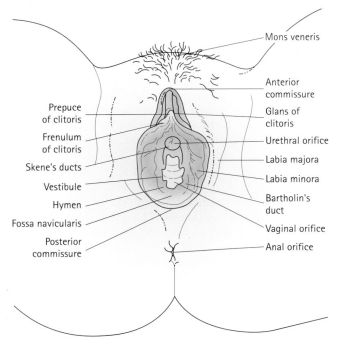

Fig. 2.5 Female external genitalia, with the labia majora and minora separated.

The inner aspects are smooth but have numerous sebaceous follicles.

Labia minora

The labia minora are two small vascular folds of skin, containing sebaceous glands but devoid of adipose tissue, which lie within the labia majora. Anteriorly they divide into two to form the prepuce and frenulum of the clitoris. Posteriorly they fuse to form a fold of skin called the fourchette. They are not well developed before puberty and atrophy after the menopause. Their vascularity allows them to become turgid during sexual excitement.

Clitoris

This is a small erectile structure, about 2.5 cm long, homologous with the penis but not containing the urethra. The body of the clitoris contains two crura, the corpora cavernosa, which are attached to the inferior border of the pubic rami. The clitoris is covered by ischiocavernosus muscle, whilst bulbospongiosus muscle inserts into its root. The clitoris has a highly developed cutaneous nerve supply and is the most sensitive organ during sexual arousal.

Vestibule (Fig. 2.6)

The vestibule is the cleft between the labia minora. Into it open the vagina, urethra, the paraurethral (Skene's) duct and the ducts of the greater vestibular (Bartholin's) glands. The vestibular bulbs are two masses of erectile tissue on either side of the vaginal opening and contain a rich plexus of veins within bulbospongiosus muscle. Bartholin's glands, each about the size of a small pea, lie at the base of each bulb and open via a 2 cm duct into the vestibule between the hymen and the labia minora. These are mucus secreting, producing copious amounts during intercourse to act as a lubricant. They are compressed by contraction of the bulbospongiosus muscle.

Perineal body

This is a fibromuscular mass occupying the area between the vagina and the anal canal. It supports the lower part of the vagina and is of variable length. It is frequently torn during childbirth.

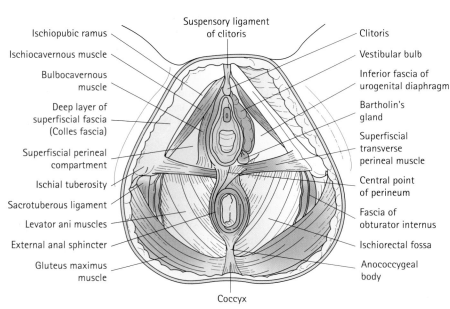

Fig. 2.6 Dissection of the female perineum to show the bulb of the vestibule and greater vestibular gland on the right; on the left side of the body the muscles superficial to these structures have been left in situ.

Age-related changes

In infancy, the vulva is devoid of hair and there is considerable adipose tissue in the labia majora and mons pubis which is lost during childhood but reappears during puberty, at which time hair grows. The vaginal opening tends to widen and sometimes shorten after childbirth. After the menopause, the skin atrophies and becomes thinner and drier. The labia minora shrink, subcutaneous fat is lost and the vaginal orifice becomes smaller.

THE URETER

The ureters are a pair of muscular tubes which convey urine to the bladder by peristaltic action. They are between 25 and 30 cm in length, about half abdominally and half within the pelvis. Each has a diameter of around 3 mm but there are slight constrictions as they cross the brim of the lesser pelvis and when they enter the bladder.

Structure

The ureter has three layers. The outer fibrous coat merges inferiorly with the bladder wall. The middle muscular one has outer circular and inner longitudinal non-striated fibres plus a further outer longitudinal layer along the lower third of the ureter. The inner mucous coat is lined with transitional epithelium and is continuous with the mucous membrane of the bladder below.

Relations and course

Throughout its abdominal course, the ureter travels retroperitoneally along the anteromedial aspect of psoas major and is crossed by the ovarian vessels. The right ureter passes down just laterally to the inferior vena cava and must be carefully retracted away if dissection of the nodes of the inferior vena cava is necessary.

The ureter enters the pelvis anterior to the sacroiliac joints and crosses the bifurcation of the common iliac artery. It then passes along the posterolateral aspect of the pelvis, running in front of and below the internal iliac artery and its anterior division, medial to the obturator vessels and nerves.

On reaching the true pelvis, the ureter turns forwards and medially, passing lateral to the uterosacral ligaments. It then travels through the base of the broad ligament and, lateral to the cervix, is crossed superiorly from the lateral to the medial side by the uterine artery. It continues, running about 1.5 cm lateral to the cervix, anterolateral to the upper part of the vagina and, passing slightly medially, enters the bladder at the trigone.

Surgical injury

The ureter can be damaged during gynaecological surgery at a number of points in its course. It can be injured near the pelvic brim where it is adjacent to the ovarian vessels or lower, near the cervix, where it crosses beneath the uterine vessels. The dangers are greater when the pelvis is distorted by fibroids or ovarian cysts or the ureter's course is displaced by a broad ligament cyst. Damage can occur through the ureter being cut, crushed or ligated and occasionally it may be devitalized by extensive dissection, especially at Wertheim's hysterectomy. Occasionally, it is injured by high sutures near the cervix in a pelvic floor repair.

THE BLADDER

The bladder is a muscular reservoir capable of altering its size and shape depending on the amount of fluid within it. It is a retroperitoneal viscus and lies behind the symphysis pubis. When empty it is the shape of a tetrahedron, with a triangular base or fundus and a superior and two inferolateral surfaces. The two inferolateral surfaces meet to form the rounded border which joins the superior surface at the apex. The base and the inferolateral surface meet at the urethral orifice to form the bladder neck. As the bladder fills, it expands upwards and outwards and becomes more rounded. Normal bladder capacity is between 300 and 600 ml but it can, in cases of urinary retention, contain several litres and extend as far as the umbilicus.

Vesical interior

The mucous membrane of the bladder is only loosely attached to the underlying muscular coat, so that it becomes irregularly folded when the bladder is empty. A triangular area, the trigone, is immediately above and behind the urethral openings; the posterolateral angles are formed by the ureteric orifices (Fig. 2.7). The mucous membrane here is redder in colour, smooth and attached firmly to the underlying muscle. The superior boundary is slightly curved – the interureteric ridge.

The ureteric orifices are slit-like and about 2.5 cm apart in the contracted bladder. They enter the bladder at an oblique angle which helps to prevent reflux of urine during filling.

Structure

The wall of the bladder is in three layers. The outer serous coat, the peritoneal covering, is only present over the fundus. The muscular layer, the detrusor muscle, consists of three layers of non-striated muscle, inner and outer longitudinal layers and a middle circular layer.

The mucous membrane is entirely covered by transitional epithelium which is responsive to ovarian hormonal stimulation. There are no true glands in this layer.

Relations

Superiorly, the bladder is covered by peritoneum. This extends forwards on to the anterior abdominal wall and sideways on to the pelvic side walls where there is a peritoneal depression, the paravesical fossa. As the bladder fills the peritoneum is displaced upwards anteriorly, so that suprapubic catheterization of the full bladder can take place without the peritoneal cavity being entered. Anteriorly, below the peritoneal reflection is the loose cellular tissue of the cave of Retzius.

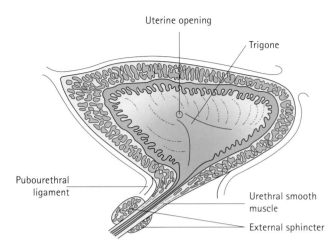

Fig. 2.7 Except where it is fixed at its base, the bladder is a highly distensible structure and urinary continence probably depends on the physical relations of the fixed/mobile junction.

Posteriorly the base of the bladder is separated from the upper vagina by pubocervical fascia. Above this is the supravaginal portion of the cervix. The peritoneal reflection is at the isthmus of the uterus to form a slight recess, the uterovesical pouch, which often contains coils of intestine.

Surgical injury

The bladder may occasionally be opened during abdominal hysterectomy. The trigone, being in close relation with the upper vagina and anterior fornix, is fortunately rarely damaged and perforation is usually 3–4 cm above it and can be easily repaired without damage to the ureter. If the injury is not noted, however, a vesicovaginal fistula may result. Damage may also occur during anterior colporrhaphy or vaginal hysterectomy, especially if a previous repair has been performed.

THE URETHRA

The urethra begins at the internal meatus of the bladder and runs anteroinferiorly behind the symphysis pubis, immediately related to the anterior vaginal wall. It is around 4 cm long and about 6 mm in diameter. It crosses the perineal membrane and ends at the external urethral orifice in the vestibule, about 2.5 cm behind the clitoris. Skene's tubules, draining the paraurethral glands, open into the lower urethra. These glands are homologous to the male prostate.

There are no true anatomical sphincters to the urethra. The decussation of vesical muscle fibres at the urethrovesical junction acts as a form of internal sphincter and continence is normally maintained at this level. Urethral resistence is mostly due to the tone and elasticity of the involuntary muscles of the urethral wall and this keeps it closed except during micturition. About 1 cm from its lower end, before it crosses the perineal membrane, the urethra is encircled by voluntary muscle fibres, arising from the inferior pubic ramus, to form the so-called external sphincter. This sphincter allows the voluntary arrest of urine flow.

Structure

The urethra has mucous and muscular coats. Near the bladder the mucous membrane is lined by transitional epithelium which gradually converts into non-keratinizing stratified squamous epithelium as it approaches the external urethral meatus. The muscular layer, consisting of inner longitudinal and outer circular fibres, is continuous with those of the bladder.

Relations

Anteriorly, the urethra is separated from the symphysis pubis by loose cellular tissue. Posteriorly is the anterior vaginal wall plus Skene's tubules. Laterally is the urogenital diaphragm, bulbospongiosus muscle and the vestibular bulb.

THE SIGMOID COLON

The pelvic or sigmoid colon is continuous with the descending colon and commences at the brim of the pelvis. It forms a loop around 40 cm in length and lies in the lesser pelvis behind the broad ligament. It is entirely covered by peritoneum, which forms a mesentery, the sigmoid mesocolon, which diminishes in length at either end and is largest at mid-segment. The lower end of the colon is continuous with the rectum at the level of the 3rd sacral vertebra.

Structure

The mucous membrane of the colon is thrown into irregular folds and is covered by non-ciliated columnar epithelium. Separated from this layer by areolar tissue is the muscle layer. This is arranged as an inner circular layer and outer longitudinal layer which has three narrow bands, the taeniae coli. These bands are shorter than the general surface of the colon and therefore give it its typical sacculated appearance. The serous coat has attached to is a series of small pieces of fat, the appendices epiploicae.

Relations

The position and shape of the pelvic colon vary considerably and hence so do its relations. Inferiorly it rests on the uterus and bladder. Above and on the right are the coils of ileum; below and on the left is the rectum. Posterior relations also include the ureter, the internal iliac vessels, piriformis muscle and the sacral plexus, all on the left side. Lateral relations include the ovary, external iliac vessels and the obturator nerve.

THE RECTUM

The rectum, which begins at the level of the 3rd sacral vertebra, moulds to the concavity of the sacrum and coccyx: its antero-posterior curve forms the sacral flexure of the rectum. It is around 12 cm in length. The lower end dilates to form the ampulla which bulges into the posterior vaginal wall and then continues as the anal canal. When distended, the rectum has three lateral curves: the upper and lower are usually convex to the right and the middle convex to the left. Peritoneum covers the front and sides of the upper third of the rectum and the front of the middle third. The lower third is devoid of peritoneum.

Structure

Unlike the sigmoid colon, there are no sacculations, appendices epiploicae or mesentery. The taeniae coli blend about 5 cm above the junction of the rectum and colon and form two bands, anterior and posterior, which descend the rectal wall. When the rectum is empty the mucous membrane is thrown into longitudinal folds which disappear with distension. Permanent horizontal folds are also present and are more pronounced during distension. The lining is of mucus-secreting columnar epithelium.

Anal canal

The anal canal is around 3 cm long and passes downwards and backwards from the rectum. It is slit-like when empty but distends greatly during defaecation. This is aided by the presence of fat laterally in the ischiorectal fossa. Anteriorly the anal canal is related to the perineal body and lower vagina; posteriorly to the anococcygeal body.

For most of its length it is surrounded by sphincteric muscles which are involved in the control of defaecation. The action of the levator ani muscles which surround it are also important in the control mechanism. The internal sphincter is involuntary and is a thickening of the circular muscle of the gut wall enclosing the anal canal just above the anorectal junction. The external sphincter is voluntary and composed of three layers of striated muscle.

Relations

The relations of the rectum are particularly important because they can be felt on digital examination. Posteriorly are the lower three sacral vertebrae, the coccyx, median sacral and superior rectal vessels. Posterolateral relations are piriformis, coccygeus and levator ani muscles, plus 3rd, 4th and 5th sacral and coccygeal nerves. Below and lateral to the levator ani muscle is the ischiorectal fossa (Fig. 2.8).

Anteriorly, above the peritoneal reflection lie the uterus and adnexa, upper vagina and pouch of Douglas with it contents. Below the reflection it is related to the lower vagina.

PELVIC MUSCULOFASCIAL SUPPORT

Pelvic peritoneum

Posteriorly, the peritoneum is reflected from the rectum on to the posterior wall of the vagina, at which point it is in close contact with the outside world, a fact that can be used both diagnostically and therapeutically. It then passes upwards over the cervix and uterus to form the rectouterine pouch, the pouch of Douglas.

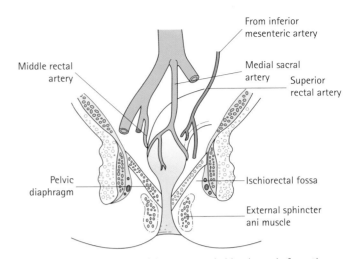

Fig. 2.8 The rectum has a rich anastomotic blood supply from the median sacral, the internal iliac and the inferior mesenteric arteries and this arrangement is reflected in its venous drainage.

The peritoneum then passes over the fundus of the uterus and down its anterior wall to reach the junction of the body and cervix, where it reflects over the anterior wall of the bladder, forming a shallow recess, the uterovesical pouch. The peritoneum in front of the bladder is loosely applied to the anterior abdominal wall so that it strips away as the bladder fills. Suprapubic catheterization of the distended bladder can therefore be perfomed without entering the peritoneal cavity.

On either side of the uterus a double fold of peritoneum passes to the lateral pelvic side walls, the broad ligament. These two layers, anteroinferior and posterosuperior, enclose loose connective tissue, the parametrium. At the upper border, between the two layers, is the fallopian tube. The mesentery between the broad ligament and the fallopian tube is the mesosaplpinx and to the ovary, the mesovarium (see Fig. 2.2). Beyond the fallopian tube, the upper edge of the broad ligament, as it passes to the pelvic side wall, forms the infundibulopelvic ligament, or suspensory ligament of ovary, and contains the ovarian blood vessels and nerves. Between the fallopian tube and the ovary, the mesosalpinx contains the vestigial epoophoron and paroophoron. After crossing the ureter, the uterine vessels pass between the layers of the broad ligament at its inferior border. They then ascend the ligament medially and anastomose with the ovarian vessels.

Pelvic ligaments

The round ligaments, a mixture of smooth muscle and fibrous tissue, are two narrow flat bands which arise from the lateral angles of the uterus and then pass laterally, deep to the anterior layer of the broad ligament, towards the lateral pelvic side wall. They then turn forwards towards the deep inguinal ring, crossing medial to the vesical vessels, obturator vessels and nerve, obliterated umbilical artery and the external iliac vessels. They finally pass through the inguinal canal to end in the subcutaneous tissue of the labia majora. Together with the uterosacral ligaments, the round ligaments help to keep the uterus in a position of anteversion and anteflexion.

The ovarian ligaments, which are fibromuscular cords of similar structure to the round ligament, lie within the broad ligament and each runs from the cornu of the uterus to the medial border of the ovary. The round and ovarian ligaments together form the homologue of the gubernaculum testis of the male.

In addition, there are also condensations of pelvic fascia on the upper surface of the levator ani muscles, the so-called 'fascial ligaments', composed of elastic tissue and smooth muscle. They are attached to the uterus at the level of the supravaginal cervix and, being extensive and strong, have an important supporting role. The transverse cervical or cardinal ligaments pass laterally to the pelvic side wall and their posterior reflection continues around the lateral margins of the rectum as the uterosacral ligaments. They insert into the periostium of the 4th sacral vertebra. These ligaments provide the major support to the uterus above the pelvic diaphragm, helping to prevent uterine descent. The uterosacrals also help to pull the supravaginal cervix backwards in the pelvis, to assist in anteflexion. Anteriorly, the pubocervical fascia is more of a fascial plane than a distinct ligament. It extends beneath the base of the blader, passing around the urethra and inserting into the body of the pubic. It supports the bladder base and the anterior vaginal wall.

Pelvic musculature (Figs 2.9 and 2.10)

The levator ani and coccygeus muscles on either side, together with their fascial coverings, form the pelvic diaphragm which separates the structures in the pelvis from the perineum and ischiorectal fossa. This diaphragm, together with all the tissue between the pelvic cavity and the perineum, makes up the pelvic floor. In lower mammals, the diaphragm represents the abductor and flexor muscles of the tail; in humans, who have an erect attitude, these muscle help provide support to the pelvic viscera.

Levator ani is a wide, thin curved sheet of muscle which arises anteriorly from the pelvic surface of the body of the pubic bone, the ischial spine and the tendinous arch of the obturator fascia between the two. The muscle fibres converge across the midline. Levator ani can be divided into three parts: *puborectalis*, which is most medial, encircling the rectum and vagina and acting as support and additional sphincter for both; *pubococcygeus*, the strongest part of the muscular component, which is slung from the pubis to the coccyx; and *iliococcygeus*, the most posterior, also attached to the coccyx.

The posterior part of the pelvic floor is made up of coccygeus muscle, a thin flat triangular muscle, lying on the same plane as the iliococcygeal portion of levator ani. It arises from the ischial spine and inserts into the lower sacrum and upper coccyx. Like levator ani, it acts by supporting the pelvic viscera.

Most of the side wall of the lesser pelvis is covered by the fan-shaped obturator internus muscle which is attached to the obturator membrane and the neighbouring bone. The fibres run backwards and turn laterally at a right angle to emerge through the lesser sciatic foramen. The side wall is covered medially by obturator fascia (Fig. 2.11).

The ischiorectal fossa, the wedge-shaped space lateral to the anus, is bounded laterally by obturator internus and superomedially by the external surface of levator ani. The base is the perineal skin. The fossa extends forwards, almost to the pubis, and backwards almost to the sacrum, where it is widest and deepest. The posterior boundary is made up by sacrotuberous ligament and gluteus maximus muscle and the anterior boundary by the upper surface of the deep fascia of the sphincter urethrae muscle. It crosses the midline in front of the anal canal.

The musculature of the urogenital region can be divided into two groups, the superficial and deep muscles. Superficially, there are three: *bulbospongiosus*, the sphincter vaginae, which surrounds the vaginal orifice, posteriorly being continuous with the perineal body and anteriorly attaching to the corpora cavernosa of the clitoris; *ischiocavernosus*, covering the un-attached surface of the crus of the clitoris; and *superficial transverse* perineal muscle. More deeply are the deep transverse perineal muscle, starting from the inner surface of the

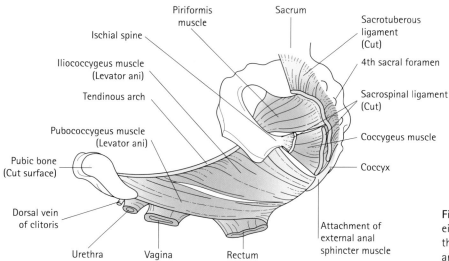

Fig. 2.9 Pelvic musculature. Muscles leave the pelvis either above the superior ramus of the pubis or through the greater or lesser sciatic foramina. Nerves and vessels also leave via the obturator foramen.

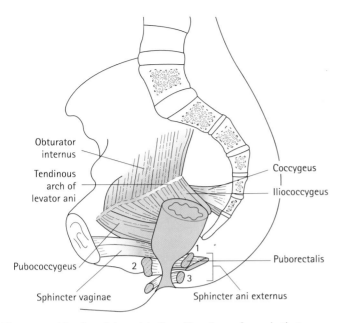

Fig. 2.10   Muscles of the pelvic floor. The slings of muscle that surround and separate the major body effluents have an important role as sphincters.

ischial ramus and passing to the perineal body, and sphincter urethrae, surrounding the membranous urethra. These layers, and their fascial component, constitute the urogenital diaphragm.

The perineal body or central perineal tendon is a fibromuscular mass lying between the anal canal and the vagina. Superficially it contains insertions of transverse perineal muscles and fibres of the external anal sphincter and on a deeper plane,

levator ani muscle. It supports the lower part of the vagina and is frequently torn during childbirth.

BLOOD SUPPLY TO THE PELVIS

Abdominal aorta

The abdominal portion of the aorta commences as it passes between the crura of the diaphragm at the level of the body of the 12th thoracic vertebra. It runs downwards to the left of the midline along the front of the vertebral column and bifurcates at the level of the body of the 4th lumbar vertebra to form the right and left common iliac arteries. The inferior vena cava runs immediately on its right. In the lower part of its course, ovarian and inferior mesenteric branches arise from the front of the aorta and median sacral and lumbar branches arise from the back.

Inferior mesenteric artery

The inferior mesenteric artery arises 3–4 cm above the bifurcation of the aorta. It descends at first in front of the aorta, then to the left of it, to cross the left common iliac artery medial to the left ureter and continues in the mesentery of the sigmoid colon into the lesser pelvis. During its course, it gives off a left colic branch which supplies the left half of the transverse colon and descending colon and a sigmoid branch supplying the sigmoid colon. In the lesser pelvis, it continues as the superior rectal artery, supplying upper rectum and anastomosing with the middle and inferior rectal branches. The inferior mesenteric artery can occasionally be traumatized during para-aortic lymph node dissection and will bleed freely. Transection, however, is not

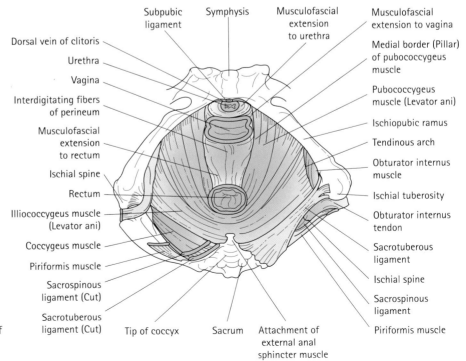

Fig. 2.11   The urogenital diaphragm. The floor of the pelvis slopes steeply forwards and plays an important role in continence and childbirth.

of serious consequence to the blood supply to the lower bowel due to considerable anastomotic connections.

Common iliac artery

After the aortic bifurcation, the two common iliac arteries run a distance of 4–5 cm before again bifurcating to form internal and external iliac branches on either side. The left artery runs partly lateral and partly in front of the corresponding iliac vein. On the right side, the slightly longer artery runs in front of the lowermost portion of inferior vena cava and the terminations of the two common iliac veins and then anterior to the right common iliac vein. The bifurcation of the common iliac artery is in front of the sacroiliac joint. The ureter lies in front of the bifurcation at this point.

External iliac artery and its branches

These are larger than the internal iliac vessels and run obliquely and laterally down the medial border of psoas major. At a point midway between the anterior superior iliac spine and the symphysis pubis the artery enters the thigh behind the inguinal ligament and becomes the femoral artery. At this point it is lateral to the femoral vein but medial to the nerve. The ovarian vessels cross in front of the artery just below the bifurcation, as does the round ligament. The external iliac vein is partly behind the upper part of the artery, but medial in its lower part.

The external iliac artery gives off two main branches. The inferior epigastric artery ascends obliquely along the medial margin of the deep inguinal ring, pierces transversalis fascia and runs up between rectus abdominis muscle and its posterior sheath, supplying the muscle and sending branches to the skin. It anastomoses with the superior epigastric artery above the level of the umbilicus. The deep circumflex artery runs posteroinferior to the inguinal ligament to the anterior superior iliac spine and then pierces and supplies transversus abdominis and internal oblique muscles.

Once the external iliac artery has pierced the thigh and become the femoral artery it almost immediately gives off an external pudendal branch which supplies much of the skin of the vulva, anastomosing with the labial branches of the internal pudendal artery.

Internal iliac artery and its branches

The internal iliac arteries are both 4 cm long and descend to the upper margin of the greater sciatic foramen where they divide into anterior and posterior divisions (Fig. 2.12). In the fetus they are twice as large as the external iliac vessels and ascend the anterior wall to the umbilicus to form the umbilical artery. After birth, with the cessation of the placental circulation, only the pelvic portion remains patent; the remainder becomes a fibrous cord, the lateral umbilical ligament. The ureter runs anteriorly down the artery and the internal iliac vein runs behind.

The posterior division has three branches which mainly supply the musculature of the buttocks. The iliolumbar artery ascends deep to psoas muscle and divides to supply iliacus and quadratus lumborum. The lateral sacral arteries descend in front of the sacral rami and supply the structures of the sacral canal. The superior gluteal artery is the direct continuation and leaves the lesser pelvis through the greater sciatic foramen to supply much of the gluteal musculature.

The anterior division has seven main branches. The superior vesical artery runs anteroinferiorly between the side of the bladder and the pelvic side wall to supply the upper part of the bladder. The obturator artery passes to the obturator canal and thence to the adductor compartment of the thigh. Inside the pelvis it sends off iliac, vesical and pubic branches (Table 2.1).

The vaginal artery corresponds to the inferior vesical artery of the male. It descends inwards, low in the broad ligament to supply the upper vagina, base of the bladder and adjacent rectum. It anastomoses with branches of the uterine artery to form two median longitudinal vessels, the azygos arteries of the vagina, one descending in front and the other behind.

The uterine artery passes along the root of the broad ligament and about 2 cm from the cervix crosses above and in front of the ureter. It then runs tortuously along the lateral margin of the uterus between the layers of the broad ligament. It supplies the cervix and body of the uterus, part of the bladder and one branch anastomoses with the vaginal artery to produce the azygos arteries. It ends by anastomosing with the ovarian artery (Fig. 2.13). The branches of the uterine artery pass circumferentially around the myometrium, giving off coiled radial branches which end as basal arteries supplying the endometrium.

The middle rectal artery is a small branch passing medially to the rectum to vascularize the muscular tissue of the lower rectum and anastomose with the superior and inferior rectal arteries.

The internal pudendal artery, the smaller of the two terminal trunks of the internal iliac artery, descends anterior to piriformis and, piercing the pelvic fascia, leaves the pelvis through the inferior part of the greater sciatic foramen, crosses the gluteal aspect of the ischial spine and enters the perineum through the lesser sciatic foramen (Fig. 2.14). It then traverses

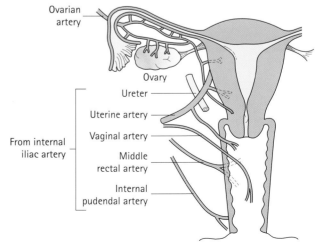

Fig. 2.12 The blood supply to the pelvic viscera is derived in the main from the internal iliac artery.

Table 2.1 Arterial supply of the pelvic organs

Organ	Artery	Origin
Ovary	Ovarian	Aorta
	Uterine	Internal iliac
Fallopian tube	Ovarian	Aorta
	Uterine	Internal iliac
Uterus	Uterine	Internal iliac
	Ovarian	Aorta
Vagina	Vaginal	Internal iliac
	Uterine	Internal iliac
	Internal pudendal	Internal iliac
	Middle rectal	Internal iliac
Vulva	Internal pudendal	Internal iliac
	External pudendal	Internal iliac
Ureter	Renal	Aorta
	Ovarian	Aorta
	Uterine	Internal iliac
	Superior vesical	Internal iliac
	Inferior vesical	Internal iliac
Bladder	Superior vesical	Internal iliac
	Inferior vesical	Internal iliac
Urethra	Inferior vesical	Internal iliac
	Internal pudendal	Internal iliac
Sigmoid colon	Left colic	Inferior mesenteric
Rectum	Superior rectal	Inferior mesenteric
	Middle rectal	Internal iliac
	Inferior rectal	Internal pudendal (internal iliac)

the pudendal canal, with the pudendal nerve, about 4 cm above the ischial tuberosity. It then proceeds forwards above the inferior fascia of the urogenital diaphragm and divides into a number of branches. The inferior rectal branch supplies skin and musculature of the anus and anastomoses with the superior and middle rectal arteries: the perineal artery supplies much of the perineum and small branches supply the labia, vestibular bulbs and vagina. The artery terminates as the dorsal artery of the clitoris.

The inferior gluteal artery, the larger terminal trunk, descends behind the internal pudendal artery, traverses the lower part of the greater sciatic foramen and, with the superior gluteal artery, supplies much of the buttock and back of the thigh.

NERVE SUPPLY TO THE PELVIS

Autonomic nerves (see Fig. 2.14)

The internal pelvic organs are supplied by both the sympathetic and the parasympathetic autonomic nervous system and this is their sole innervation. As they descend into the pelvis, branches from the lower part of the lumbar sympathetic trunk join the aortic plexus of sympathetic nerves and ganglia as it continues downwards over the bifurcation of the aorta to form the superior hypogastric plexus. This then divides to form the right and left inferior hypogastric or pelvic plexuses, which lie lateral to the rectum and further subdivide into two – anteriorly innervating the base of the bladder and urethra and posteriorly innervating the uterus, cervix, vagina, sigmoid colon and rectum.

The parasympathetic nerves enter the pelvis through the 2nd, 3rd and 4th sacral nerves. The preganglionic fibres are distributed through the pelvic plexus and the parasympathetic ganglia are situated close to, or in the walls of, the viscera concerned. With the exception of the ovaries and fallopian tube, which are supplied directly by nerves from the preaortic

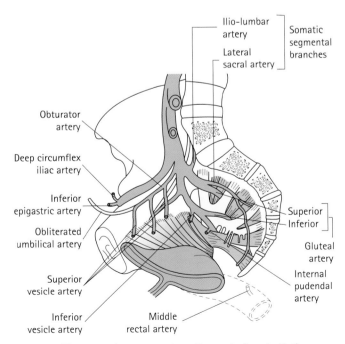

Fig. 2.13 The uterus has an anastomotic supply from both the ovarian and uterine arteries, both vessels running in the broad ligament.

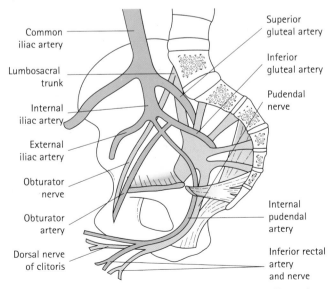

Fig. 2.14 Pelvic nerves and blood supply of the pudenda. The major nerve is the pudendal, but it is supplemented by the posterior cutaneous nerve of the thigh and the ilioinguinal and genitofemoral nerves.

plexus travelling along the ovarian vessels, all internal pelvic organs are supplied via the pelvic plexuses.

Somatic nerves

The lumbar plexus is formed by the anterior primary rami of the first three lumbar nerves, part of the fourth and a contribution from the 12th thoracic (subcostal) nerve. It lies on the surface of psoas major and gives off a number of major branches.

The iliohypogastric and ilioinguinal nerves both arise from the 1st lumbar nerve. The former gives branches to the buttock, while the latter supplies the skin of the mons pubis and surrounding vulva. The genitofemoral nerve arises from the 1st and 2nd lumbar nerves, its femoral branch supplying the upper thigh, whilst its genital branch supplies the skin of the labium majus. The lateral femoral cutaneous nerve arises from the 2nd and 3rd lumbar nerves and also supplies the thigh.

The femoral nerve is the largest branch, coming from 2nd, 3rd and 4th lumbar nerves. It descends in the groove between psoas and iliacus muscles and enters the thigh deep to the inguinal ligament, lateral to the femoral sheath, to supply the flexors of the hip, the extensors of the knee and numerous cutaneous branches including the saphenous nerve. The obturator nerve also comes from the 2nd, 3rd and 4th lumbar nerves and passes downwards medial to psoas into the pelvis, to supply the adductor muscles of the hip.

The lumbosacral trunk comes from the 4th and 5th lumbar nerves passes medial to psoas into the pelvis to join the anterior primary rami of the first three sacral nerves to form the sacral plexus in front of piriformis muscle. From this

plexus, a number of branches emerge. The most important of these are the sciatic nerves – a large nerve formed from the 4th and 5th lumbar and the 1st, 2nd and 3rd sacral nerves – which leaves the pelvis through the lower part of the greater sciatic foramen to supply the muscles of the back of the thigh and the lower limb, and the pudendal nerve, which forms from the 2nd, 3rd and 4th sacral nerves.

The pudendal nerve leaves the pelvis between piriformis and coccygeus muscles and curls around the ischial spine to re-enter the pelvis through the lesser sciatic foramen where, medial to the internal pudendal artery, it lies in the pudendal canal on the lateral wall of the ischiorectal fossa. The point where the nerve circles the ischial spine is the region in which a pudendal block of local anaesthetic is injected.

The pudendal nerve gives a number of terminal branches. The inferior rectal nerve gives motor and sensory fibres to the external anal sphincter, anal canal and skin around the anus. The perineal nerve passes forwards below the internal pudendal artery to give labial branches, supplying the skin of the labia majora, the deep perineal nerve supplying the perineal muscles and the bulb of the vestibule. The dorsal vein of the clitoris passes through the pudendal canal, giving a branch to the crus and piercing the perineal membrane 1–2 cm from the symphysis pubis. It supplies the clitoris and surrounding skin.

LYMPHATIC DRAINAGE TO THE PELVIS

In the pelvis, as elsewhere in the body, the lymph nodes are arranged along the blood vessels. The lateral aortic lymph nodes lie on either side of the aorta; their efferents form a lumbar

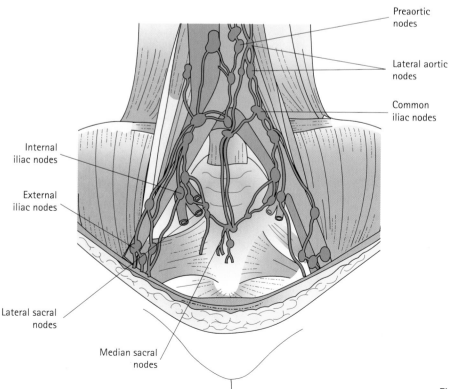

Fig. 2.15   The lymph vessels and nodes of the pelvis.

Table 2.2 Lymphatic drainage of the pelvis

Organ	Lymph nodes	Organ	Lymph nodes
Ovary	Lateral aortic nodes	Lower vagina	Superficial inguinal nodes
Fallopian tube	Lateral aortic nodes Superficial inguinal nodes External and internal iliac nodes	Vulva	Superficial inguinal nodes Internal iliac nodes (deep tissues)
		Ureter	Lateral aortic nodes Internal iliac nodes
Corpus uteri	External and internal iliac nodes Superficial inguinal nodes Lateral aortic nodes	Bladder	External and internal iliac nodes
Cervix	External and internal iliac nodes Obturator node Sacral nodes	Urethra	Internal iliac nodes
		Sigmoid colon	Preaortic nodes
		Upper rectum	Preaortic nodes
Upper vagina	External and internal iliac nodes Obturator node Sacral nodes	Lower rectum and canal	Internal iliac nodes
		Anal orifice	Superficial inguinal nodes

trunk on either side which terminates at the cisterna chylia. Those structures which receive their blood supply directly from branches of the aorta, i.e. ovary, fallopian tube, upper ureter and, in view of arterial anastomoses, uterine fundus, drain directly into the lateral aortic group of nodes.

The lymph drainage of most other structures within the pelvis is via more outlying groups of lymph nodes associated with the iliac vessels. The common iliac lymph nodes are grouped around the common iliac artery and usually arranged in medial, lateral and intermediate chains. They receive efferents from the external and internal iliac nodes and send efferents to the lateral aortics (Fig. 2.15).

The external iliac nodes lie on the external iliac vessels and are in three groups: lateral, medial and anterior. They collect from the cervix, upper vagina, bladder, deeper lower abdominal wall and from the inguinal lymph nodes. Inferior epigastric and circumflex iliac nodes are associated with these vessels and can be considered to be outlying members of the external iliac group (Table 2.2).

The internal iliac nodes, which surround the internal iliac artery, receive afferents from all the pelvic viscera, deeper perineum and muscles of the thigh and buttock. The obturator lymph node, sometimes present in the obturator canal, and the sacral lymph nodes on the median and lateral sacral vessels can be considered to be outlying members of this group (Fig. 2.16).

The upper group of superficial inguinal lymph nodes forms a chain immediately below the inguinal ligament. The lateral members receive afferents from the gluteal region and adjoining lower anterior abdominal wall. The medial members drain the

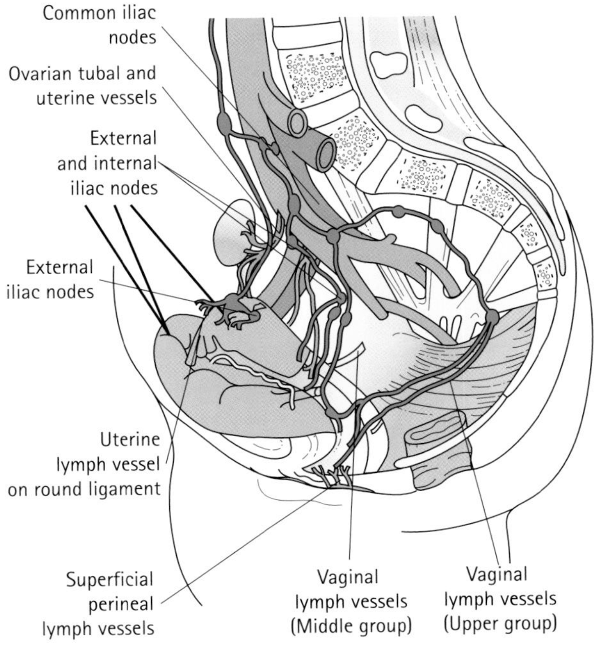

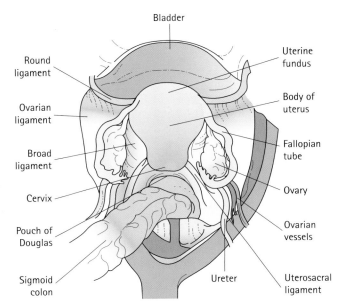

Fig. 2.16 The lymphatic drainage of the female reproductive organs (semi-diagrammatic after Cunéo & Marcille).

Fig. 2.17 Overview of pelvis as seen from the umbilicus at laparoscopy.

35

vulva and perineum, lower vagina, lower anal canal, adjoining anterior abdominal wall and also from the uterus owing to lymph vessels that accompany the round ligament to the anterior abdominal wall. The lymphatics on either side of the vulva communicate freely, emphasizing the importance of removing the whole vulva in cases of malignant disease. The superficial lymph nodes send their efferents to the external iliac lymph nodes, passing around the femoral vessels or traversing the femoral canal.

The deep inguinal (femoral) lymph nodes, varying from one to three, are on the medial side of the femoral vein. They receive efferents from the deep femoral vessels, some from the superficial inguinal nodes; one, the node of Cloquet, is thought to drain the clitoris. Efferents from the deep nodes pass through the femoral canal to the external iliac group.

KEY POINTS

1. Knowing the course of pelvic migration of the ovaries is important in understanding the consequences of maldescent.
2. The sizes of the uterus and cervix, and their ratio, change with age and parity.
3. The uterine artery is a branch of the internal iliac artery that crosses above the ureter and passes medially in the base of the broad ligament to reach the supravaginal portion of the cervix. It divides to pass superiorly alongside the body of the uterus and inferiorly to supply the vagina and cervix.
4. The ovarian artery arises from the aorta at the level of the 2nd lumbar vertebra. The right ovarian vein drains into the inferior vena cava while the left ovarian vein drains into the left renal vein.
5. The inferior epigastric artery is a branch of the external iliac artery and ascends between the rectus muscle and the posterior rectus sheath, where it should be avoided during insertion of laparoscopic cannulae.
6. The ureter crosses the pelvic brim at the bifurcation of the common iliac artery and descends on the lateral pelvic side wall, where it is at risk during oophorectomy.
7. The ureter runs beneath the uterine vessels in the base of the broad ligament and emerges close to the supravaginal portion of the cervix (1.0–1.5 cm), where it is at risk during the ligation of pedicles at hysterectomy.
8. The internal urethral sphincter comprises two loops of smooth muscle fibres that pass around the vesical neck.
9. The term external urethral sphincter refers to paraurethral striated muscle that is under voluntary control and includes the external, circular layer of urethral muscle together with the compressor urethrae and urethrovaginal sphincter.
10. The pudendal nerve leaves the pelvis between the piriformis and coccygeus muscles, passes around the ischial spine and re-enters the pelvis via the lesser sciatic foramen, where it lies medial to the internal pudendal artery in the lateral wall of the ischiorectal fossa.

3
Hysteroscopy
Sandeep Mane   Richard Penketh

INTRODUCTION

Abnormal uterine bleeding, which affects 64% of women at some stage of their lives, coupled with the burden of infertility necessitates diagnostic assessment of the genital tract in the majority of women (Grainger & de Cherney 1989). The ability to view the uterine cavity has enabled the accurate diagnosis and treatment of numerous conditions. The quest to improve diagnostic and therapeutic capabilities has led to the widespread acceptance of modern gynaecological endoscopy.

Bozzini was the first to look into the cavity of a hollow organ, the bladder, in 1805. This was achieved with long tubes assisted by external illumination. In 1853, Desormeaux made the first satisfactory endoscope, but it was Panteleoni who performed the first satisfactory hysteroscopy in 1869 (Panteleoni 1869). Inability to distend the uterus and lack of proper illumination caused poor visualization and lack of widespread acceptance until Lindemann renewed Rubin's attempts to use carbon dioxide in the 1970s (Lindemann 1972).

Over the last two decades, improved optics and video-monitoring systems have encouraged gynaecologists to learn this skill. Increased use of lasers and better understanding of electrosurgery have enabled significant developments in operative hysteroscopy. Smaller diameter hysteroscopes have enabled hysteroscopy without anaesthesia and outpatient hysteroscopy is now established. 'See and treat' on outpatient basis is a reality in modern gynaecological practice.

DIAGNOSTIC INDICATIONS

Abnormal uterine bleeding

Menstrual abnormality is one of the most common referrals to the gynaecological outpatients department. Menometrorrhagia, dysmenorrhoea and intermenstrual bleeding are the most common presentations. After the menarche, such problem are usually dysfunctional and hysteroscopy is rarely indicated. In the postmenopause, bleeding is an alarming symptom and warrants urgent attention as the patient is anxious to exclude endometrial cancer. Outpatient hysteroscopy offers rapid diagnosis and reassurance. In the reproductive age group, abnormal uterine bleeding can be associated with hormonal disturbances or pathology such as fibroids and polyps. Cervical polyps may be associated with endometrial polyps in 26.7% of the patients (Coeman 1993).

Infertility

The numerous causes for inabillity to conceive include unfavourable endometrium, fibroid, polyp or intrauterine adhesions. Congenital anomalies are infrequent but are associated with infertility (Donnez et al 2001). Hysteroscopy complements laparoscopy in the early assessment of the infertile woman. Abnormalities of the endometrium and organic intrauterine pathologies are important causes of failed IVF-ET cycles (Dicker 1992).

Intrauterine synaechiae – Asherman's syndrome
Intrauterine adhesions can lead to infertility, recurrent miscarriage, hypomenorrhoea or amenorrhoea. Adhesions are caused by trauma to the endometrial basal layer during evacuation of retained products of conception (Schenker & Margalioth 1982) or may be secondary to infections, e.g. tuberculosis. Hysterosalpingography allows assessment of the severity of adhesions.

Fibroids and polyps
Fibroids and polyps, which occlude the cervix or the tubal openings, may hamper sperm progression and interfere with implantation.

Tubal cannulation
Under hysteroscopic guidance tubal cannulation can provide valuable information about the tubal patency and the mucosal lining. Up to 40% of proximal tubal obstructions seen on hysterosalpingography are false positives due to mucus plugs or tubal spasm. Of these, 92% can be successfully cannulated under hysteroscopic guidance combined with laparoscopy, with 39% becoming pregnant in 3–7 months (Flood & Grow 1993).

Müllerian anomalies
Patients may have normal fertility or present with infertility. Hysteroscopy may reveal arcuate, subseptate, septate, bicornuate or uterus didelphis. Hysterosalphingography and laparoscopy are additional valuable tools to investigate these patients.

Recurrent miscarriage
The aetiology of recurrent miscarriage is poorly understood. Intrauterine pathology such as fibroids, polyps, Asherman's syndrome or congenital abnormalities is detected in up to 33% of infertile couples (Romano 1994). Implantation of an embryo over the septum or fibroid can also fail due to the poor blood supply.

Foreign body

Missing threads of an IUCD or a deeply embedded coil may need to be removed under hysteroscopic guidance (Siegler &

Kemmann 1976, Valle et al 1977). Apart from anxiety, these patients may present with menstrual irregularities and pain.

Chronic pelvic pain

Patients with chronic pain can pose a difficult challenge to the gynaecologist. In adolescents, laparoscopy reveals endometriosis in up to 52% of these patients (Goldstein et al 1980). Obstructive uterine anomaly may be associated in 40% (Schifrin et al 1973). Concomitant hysteroscopy may reveal polyps, fibroids, adhesions and septate uterus.

CONTRAINDICATIONS

Infection

Hysteroscopy in the presence of acute pelvic infection can lead to spread of infection. The distension medium flowing through the tubes can spread the infection to the peritoneal cavity. Infection is even more likely when an operative procedure is anticipated and prophylactic antibiotics are advised.

Hysteroscopy in the presence of vaginitis and cervicitis can also lead to spread of infection to the endometrial or peritoneal cavity. The only exception is when infection is secondary to a lost IUCD which should be removed hysteroscopically under antibiotic cover.

Pregnancy

This is a relative contraindication, although embryoscopy prior to 10 weeks gestation was performed as an aid to prenatal diagnosis. Pregnancy leads to increased uterine softening and vascularity. If the CO_2 insufflation does not exceed a flow rate of 30 cc/min and a maximum intrauterine pressure of 40–50 mmHg, then the risk of gas embolism and bleeding is minimized (Gallinat 1964).

Hysteroscopy during pregnancy may be performed to remove a coil. If miscarriage occurs in patients with congenital uterine anomalies, retained products of conception may pose a difficult clinical dilemma. Transvaginal ultrasound scan is able to reliably detect retained products of conception but in difficult cases, hysteroscopic assessment of the uterine cavity can facilitate guided evacuation.

Cervical cancer

Hysteroscopy in such patients may cause trauma to lymphatics and blood vessels. Systemic dissemination of malignant cells can follow (Taylor & Gordon 1993). Malignant cells will also be carried to the endometrial cavity. A friable cervical lesion can lead to excessive bleeding during cervical grasping and introduction of the hysteroscope. The spread of endometrial cancer is also a concern, but evidence does not confirm this fear (Sugimoto 1975).

Bleeding

Diagnostic hysteroscopy may be performed in the presence of bleeding, but the view is likely to be poor. Minimal uterine bleeding may allow adequate visualization of the endometrial cavity. Hysteroscopy is best performed in the proliferative phase when the endometrium is thinnest. If this is difficult to arrange, then preoperative hormonal treatment with progesterone can help to postpone or control bleeding.

It is even more difficult to perform operative procedures in the presence of bleeding. Preoperative endometrial thinning agents help by decreasing the thickness and vascularity of the endometrium. This allows good visualization of the endometrial cavity, improves success rates and reduces fluid absorption, particularly when the procedure is prolonged. If hysteroscopy is performed during bleeding, continuous-flow uterine distension enables better visualization by removing the blood (Steffensen & Schuster 1995). The pressure of the distension medium decreases the flow of bleeding as the distension pressure reaches arterial pressure.

Cardiopulmonary disorders

Patients with these medical conditions are at a higher anaesthetic risk when recognized hysteroscopic complications such as gas embolism and fluid overload occur. Carbon dioxide embolism is a known risk and can be fatal. Fluid overload can cause high-output cardiac failure, pulmonary oedema and death.

Cervical stenosis

Patients who have a history of cervical surgery or difficult uterine entry in the past are at an increased risk of cervical trauma, perforation and false passage. Prostaglandins inserted 2 hours before the hysteroscopy help to soften the cervix, allowing easy dilatation and entry into the uterine cavity (Preutthipaan & Herabutya 1999).

Inexperienced surgeon and inadequate equipment

The majority of the complications during hysteroscopy are avoidable. Every aspiring hysteroscopist must undergo formal training, before undertaking complex hysteroscopic operations.

Inadequate instrumentation resulting in poor visualization and reduced safety is not only dangerous but amounts to negligence. Good-quality hysteroscopes, camera and drive unit are a basic requirement for good visualization of the uterine cavity. Appropriate fluid monitoring systems and energy sources such as laser or diathermy are essential for operative hysteroscopy.

INSTRUMENTATION

Before commencing any hysteroscopic procedure, one must ensure that the stack system (Fig. 3.1) is fully functional. This includes the telescope, surgical instruments, camera drive unit, camera head, light source, light lead, monitor, electrosurgical generator and the image-recording equipment. If a simultaneous laparoscopy is required, then two stack systems should be made available. Apart from checking the availability of the instruments needed, the hysteroscopist is also responsible for checking the insulation. It is essential to assemble the equipment to ensure that it works. The distension medium,

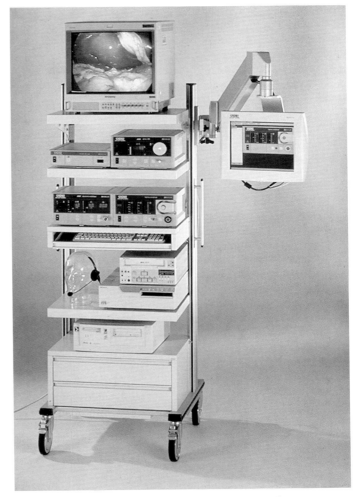

Fig. 3.1 Stack system (courtesy of Karl Storz, Germany).

suction machine, fluid measurement apparatus and the connecting tubing must be checked. Fluid should be allowed to flow through the giving set to remove all air bubbles.

Optical systems

Rigid telescopes
Panoramic hysteroscopy is performed with the help of a distension medium and is common practice. The majority of hysteroscopists use rigid telescopes. Improved technology has allowed significant reduction in the outer diameter (as low as 2.5 mm, including the inflow sheath). The outer diameter of operative hysteroscopes using monopolar electrosurgery may be up to 10 mm. This includes the telescope with the working element, the inflow sheath (inner) and the outflow sheath (outer). Smaller diameter operative scopes (Fig. 3.2) measure 5 mm and consist of an operative channel of 5 French communicating with the outflow sheath. This allows instruments of 5 F diameter, e.g. the bipolar electrode, laser fibre or the mechanical scissors and grasper, to be introduced down the operative channel. The telescopes may be forward view (0°) or oblique view (angled scopes – 12°, 30°, 70° or 90°).

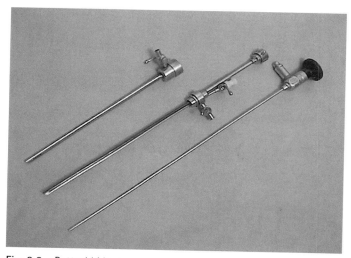

Fig. 3.2 Bettochhi hysteroscope.

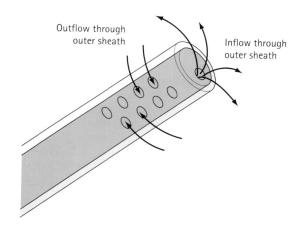

Fig. 3.3 Continuous flow concept.

Flexible telescopes

Flexible hysteroscopes offer the advantage of negotiating the scope along the uterine cavity with a 'no touch' technique. The tip can bend up to 110°, allowing easy uterine entry with minimal discomfort. Improved optics mean that the image quality is comparable to small rigid scopes. The risk of uterine perforation is reduced as the scope is able to negotiate the angle between cervix and uterus. The disadvantage is that currently, continuous-flow irrigation is not available for flexible hysteroscopy.

Contact hysteroscopy

Colpohysteroscopy and colpomicrohysteroscopy offer magnified examination off the endometrial and cervical epithelium for diagnostic purposes only. The uterine cavity is not distended and the endometrium is assessed without any intrauterine pressure. The cellular and vascular patterns are assessed by contact with the hysteroscope, giving high magnification. This form of hysteroscopy is not widely practised.

Hysteroscopic sheaths

For diagnostic panoramic hysteroscopy, a single sheath for inflow is sufficient. This enables a smaller outer diameter and outpatient hysteroscopy without anaesthesia. Operative hysteroscopy needs separate sheaths for inflow and outflow. The inflow sheath carries the distension medium to the tip of the telescope from where it is withdrawn via the outer sheath (Fig. 3.3). Fluid circulates over the tip of the telescope to maintain a clear view.

Camera and the stack system

The hysteroscopic image is visualized on a monitor with the help of a camera connected to a camera drive unit. The image clarity of a single chip camera is perfectly adequate. Special weighted cameras are available and facilitate orientation, but the same camera as is used for laparoscopy is equally appropriate. It is important to white balance the camera system to ensure the colours are displayed correctly.

Light source

A minimum power of 150 W is essential to obtain a clear image. It is essential to have a spare bulb and know how to change it, as it can fail in the middle of a procedure. Between cases, if the light source is not going to be used for a short while, then the bulb intensity should be turned down. Switching the light source on and off frequently reduces the bulb life.

Light lead

The optic fibres running along the light lead need careful handling and should never be rolled or kinked as the fibres break. Damaged fibres do not transmit light from the source and give rise to poor illumination. The light lead should be checked before starting any procedure.

Monitor

The wiring and controls of the camera drive unit are often complex. The hysteroscopist should be familiar with the setting up of the system and be able to rectify simple faults. Always check that the monitor is displaying the appropriate image before commencing the procedure.

Image-recording equipment

Images taken before and after the procedure can help patients to understand their clinical condition and allow comparison with images obtained at a later date. Recorded images can serve as evidence in defence if there is a claim of medical negligence against the surgeon. Recordings of various hysteroscopic procedures can become useful teaching aids for trainees.

DISTENSION MEDIUM

The anterior and posterior uterine walls are in apposition. In order to obtain a view, the uterine cavity has to be distended with gas or fluid. Carbon dioxide can be effective for diagnosis and is delivered via a pressure reduction system or Hysteroflator which is designed to give a flow rate of a maximum of 100 ml per minute and a maximum pressure of 200 mmHg (NB: the Laproflator must not be used). An alternative is to use a liquid distension medium, e.g. normal saline or Hartmann's solution which are appropriate for diagnosis and some operative procedures. Monopolar electrosurgery requires a non-conductive distension medium such as 1.5% glycine. It should be remembered, however, that once the solution becomes contaminated with blood its function as an insulator is reduced. Fluid can be pressurized via a roller pump with a maximum flow rate of 500 ml/min and maximum pressure of 200 mmHg, by gravity or a pressure infusion bag cuff system. For diagnosis, gravity or a 50 ml syringe connected to a giving set via a three-way tap provides very good control of the distension pressure. Dextran 70 (Hyskon) is no longer used owing to anaphylactoid reactions.

IMAGING OF THE UTERUS BEFORE DIAGNOSTIC HYSTEROSCOPY

Hysterosalpingography (the instillation of radio-opaque dye into the uterine cavity and imaging via X-rays) is associated with increased incidence of infection and discomfort compared with outpatient hysteroscopy (Finikiotos 1994). Transvaginal ultrasound (Fig. 3.4a) has been used for many years to investigate women with abnormal uterine bleeding. In many units, it is being supplemented by sonohysterography where saline or contrast media are instilled into the cavity and imaged using ultrasound (Fig. 3.4b). These techniques are being used to assess tubal patency in the infertile and also give a good view of the relationship of a uterine lesion to the endometrial cavity. Polyps and fibroids suspected on ultrasound can be clearly defined when saline is instilled into the uterine cavity, resulting in improved diagnositc abilities (Schwarzler et al 1998). Such techniques are suggested by some to be a replacement for diagnostic hysteroscopy. Indeed, ultrasound examination extends beyond the uterus and allows assessment of the ovaries which adds information to the clinical picture. Patients presenting with an episode of postmenopausal bleeding who have an endometrial thickness of 4 mm or less may be spared a diagnostic hysteroscopy or endometrial biopsy

provided their symptoms do not recur (Karlsson et al 1995). The authors firmly believe that hysteroscopic examination remains the gold standard for assessment of the endometrial cavity and is complemented by ultrasound examination.

CLINICAL ANATOMY OF THE UTERUS

The uterine cavity is flat in its anterior/posterior dimension as, when not distended, the anterior and posterior endometrial surfaces are apposed to each other. The cervical canal is essentially round but once the cavity is entered the lateral dimension widens until it is at its broadest at the fundus. The cavity extends laterally towards the tubal ostia (see Fig. 3.5). The fundal dome may be flat, concave or convex on its interior surface. Indeed, a proportion of uteri have a pronounced fundal convexity – a so-called arcuate deformity. It must be remembered that the hysteroscope is only able to look at one side of the uterine wall. Complementary laparoscopy is required to examine the fundal dome where uterine malformation is suspected.

TECHNIQUE OF DIAGNOSTIC HYSTEROSCOPY

Endometrial preparation

A diagnostic hysteroscopic examination is best performed without medical preparation of the endometrium. The endometrium will be at its thinnest in the immediate postmenstrual phase and at its most vascular premenstrually. Abnormal bleeding is a common indication for diagnosis and whilst it is often possbile to time the examination such that bleeding is not occurring, light bleeding need not preclude successful examination of the endometrial cavity. When prolonged heavy bleeding occurs, norethisterone 5 mg three times a day for 7–10 days may be given prior to the examination. It is rarely necessary to use a GnRH analogue prior to a diagnostic procedure but one to three doses are employed prior

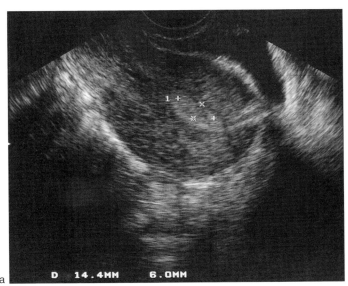

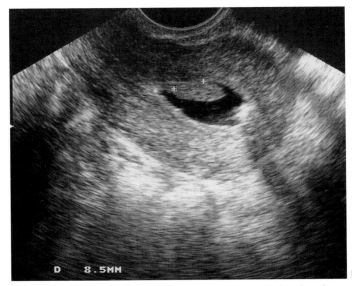

a   b

Fig. 3.4 **a** Transvaginal sonography showing polyp. **b** Sonohysterography with polyp clearly outlined (courtesy of Mr Nazar Amso, University of Wales, Cardiff).

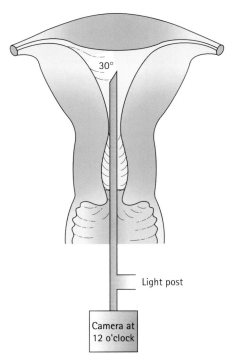

30°

Light post

Camera at
12 o'clock

Fig. 3.5 Clinical anatomy of the uterus, showing the relation between the angle of the telescope, the light lead and the camera orientation.

to endometrial ablation or to shrink a vascular fibroid prior to operative hysteroscopy.

Anaesthesia

The smallest modern diagnostic hysteroscopes in the majority of cases require no anaesthetic whatsoever. A crucial factor is good communication between the gynaecologist and the patient with thorough preoperative counselling and the support of a skilled nurse who is able to complement the operator in explaining things to the patient. The role of local anaesthetic gels is open to question. They are inexpensive and certainly lubricate and cause the external os to open. They probably have little anaesthetic effect other than as a psychological adjunct to the gynaecologist's reassurance.

Where facilities do not exist for outpatient hysteroscopy, the procedure is carried out in the operating theatre. Whilst a 5 mm rigid diagnostic hysteroscope can be passed through the cervix in the majority of women in the reproductive age range, this can prove extremely difficult in the postmenopausal woman and cervical dilatation is often needed. This requires a paracervical block, a regional anaesthetic or a general anaesthetic. The choice of anaesthetic method will of course be decided in conjunction with the anaesthetist and the patient and will in part be determined by the patient's state of health and whether any additional procedures are planned. It must be remembered, however, that those patients who are at risk of endometrial cancer in the post menopausal period are often considerably obese and suffer from cardiovascular and airways disease which put them at high risk from the anaesthetic point of view. Such patients provided a major

stimulus to the establishment of outpatient diagnostic and in some cases therapeutic hysteroscopy services.

Positioning

Hysteroscopy can be performed on a general operating table equipped with lithotomy poles or Lloyd Davies supports. Care must be taken to avoid excessive pressure from the leg supports on neurovascular structures and if there is limitation of joint movement owing to pathology, the final position of the patient will have to be modified. In the outpatient setting a colposcopy chair is desirable. This allows a comfortable modified lithotomy position with minimum loss of dignity. Of course, the patient should be kept covered until the examination is due to start.

Procedure

A pelvic examination is performed in order to determine the size and direction of the uterus. The vulva and vagina are cleansed with antiseptic solution and the anterior lip of the cervix is grasped with a vulsellum forceps. The majority of rigid hysterosocopes offer a fore/oblique view ranging from 12° to 90°. By convention, the direction of the view is away from the light post. The camera system is attached to the scope with the camera orientated correctly and the light post either up or down such that the angled view is in the vertical plane. It is easier to follow the cervical canal if the scope is orientated to view along the direction of the canal, i.e. forwards and downwards in a retroverted retroflexed uterus. Crucial to obtaining a thorough hysteroscopic examination is an understanding of how rotation of the hysteroscope allows the area of uterine wall under inspection to be changed. We suggest holding the camera in one hand and maintaining the position of the camera fixed in relation to the vertical plane. Rotation of the scope by manipulating the light post with the other hand then allows the view to be manipulated appropriately.

Insertion of the hysteroscope through the cervical canal should be performed under direct vision and in the first instance without cervical dilatation or the passage of a sound. This allows examination of the cervical canal and inspection of undamaged endometrium. Once instruments have been passed into the uterine cavity, they cause damage to and stripping of the endometrium which can then give appearances suggestive of polyp formation. The image of the cervical canal during passage of the scope is, of course, dependent on the viewing angle of the scope. A 0° scope requires the cervical canal to be kept in the middle of the field of view during insertion to maintain the direction of travel of the scope parallel to the direction of the cervical canal. When an angled viewing scope is used, the position of the cervical canal in the field of view has to be offset in order to maintain the direction of travel of the hysteroscope parallel with the direction of the cervical canal. This is why orientation of the light post relative to the orientation of the camera is a crucial step in the assembly of the equipment, which is often overlooked (Fig. 3.5).

Once the cervical canal is passed, a panoramic view of the uterine cavity is obtained. Uterine distension at a flow rate of 40–60 cc/min with pressure between 40–80 mmHg achieves good visualization. The scope is then advanced towards the fundus and rotated to allow inspection of the tubal ostia. It can then be withdrawn and readvanced whilst rotating the scope to enable a systematic inspection of each uterine wall in turn.

Potential problems include blood accumulating in the cavity and obscuring the view. This can occur during diagnosis when the seal between the hysteroscope and the cervix is very tight, preventing outflow of distension medium. The passage of a dilator to 1 mm greater than the outer diameter of the hystero-scope allows flow and clearance of the contaminating blood. If a large polyp is present in the endometrial cavity, it is possible to inspect the cavity without realizing that the polyp is there because the polyp fills the cavity and the scope has been passed beyond the tip of the polyp before inspection begins. Suspicion should be aroused if the endometrial surfaces are different in colour and careful inspection of the panoramic view of the cavity during insertion and removal of the scope will prevent missing a large polyp as the tip of it will be seen. A thorough examination of the uterine cavity should allow inspection of both tubal ostia. A record of this in the operation note demonstrates that the operator has obtained a good view.

Postoperative

The majority of the recovery process after a diagnostic hystersocopy relates to the anaesthetic used. A small amount of vaginal bleeding is not unusual following hysteroscopy and the patient should be warned about this. Occasionally cramping period-like pains are experienced which should settle within 48 hours and respond to paracetamol or an NSAID such as mefenamic acid. Persistent pain and bleeding may suggest a complication such as endometritis and the patient should seek medical help. The provision of a post-procedure information leaflet is good practice.

OUTPATIENT HYSTEROSCOPY CLINIC

A hysteroscopy service in outpatients provides a very efficient method of performing diagnostic hysteroscopy. As mentioned earlier, many patients who require a hysteroscopy pose significant risk for general anaesthesia and are best managed under local or no anaesthetic (Valli et al 1998). In addition, there are many advantages to the patient, including shorter time at the hospital and more rapid return to normal activity. There are also cost advantages to the hospital as an outpatient clinic is clearly a less expensive environment than an operating theatre. The trade-off, if the outpatient service is purely diagnostic, is the proportion of cases in which pathology is found, necessitating a second procedure.

Choice of equipment will vary with the prior experience of the operator and the facilities available for disinfection and sterilization of the instruments. Rod lens hysteroscopes may be autoclaved, necessitating the provision of an adequate number of scopes for a session of activity. Fibreoptic hysteroscopes, whether rigid or flexible, cannot be autoclaved and must be sterilized with ethylene oxide or liquid disinfection system such as Cidex or NuCidex. Sterilization solutions require adequate ventilation to avoid staff exposure to the fumes and a closed system may be required.

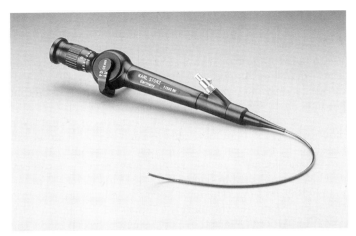

Fig. 3.6   Flexible hysteroscope.

Proponents of outpatient hysteroscopy declare significant advantages for their chosen scopes. In reality, there are dis-advantages and advantages with every system. Rigid auto-clavable scopes tend to be of larger diameter, necessitating cervical dilatation in a proportion of cases. The advantage is clarity of view and a fore/oblique view allowing easier examination of the cornua. Flexible scopes are delicate and more expensive, but permit steering through the cervical canal and angulation to allow full inspection of the uterine cavity without any anaesthesia (Kremer et al 1998) (Fig. 3.6). Fibreoptic rigid scopes can be of very small diameter (1.2 mm in a 2.5 mm diagnostic sheath). They are 0°, so viewing of the cornua is more difficult, but are relatively easy to pass through stenosed postmenopausal cervices, leading to a very low failure rate. The Versascope system provides a disposable sheath, which can be distended by the passage of a 5 F instrument. This means that a change of sheath is not required to convert a diagnostic procedure into an operative one.

In the outpatient setting the authors favour a Cusco's speculum to bring the cervix into veiw prior to introduction of the hysteroscope. This allows manipulation of the position of the cervix with the speculum as the scope is inserted to straighten the cervical canal. Rarely it is necessary to grasp the cervix with a single-toothed tenaculum. Others use no speculum at all, performing vaginoscopy and then locating the cervix before inserting the hysteroscope into it.

With the patient awake and the gynaecologist concentrating on passing the scope through a difficult cervix, the role of the attending nurse is paramount (Prather & Wolfe 1995). She should have a good knowledge of the procedure, excellent communication skills and be able to maintain a rapport with the patient during the procedure. Pre-procedure explanation leaflets and a brief discussion help to reassure the patient who often finds that the procedure causes less discomfort than is anticipated. Patients vary as to their wish to see the television screen during the procedure but the majority find it reassuring and helpful to be able to view the image of the uterine cavity. This also allows easier explanation of any pathology found.

Endometrial sampling, which yields only a small percentage of the endometrium, causes discomfort often greater than that of the hysteroscopy. It is not indicated in all cases and in-particular should be avoided in patients with postmenopausal bleeding in whom the endometrium is found to be atrophic on hysteroscopy. An 'inadequate diagnosis – malignancy cannot be excluded' report on histology confounds the picture and leads to further unnecessary procedures. Hysteroscopically-directed biopsy often results in a sample which is so small that it is difficult for the pathologist to orientate.

The availability of outpatient hysteroscopy enables a diagnostic assessment for problems such as postmenopausal bleeding to be accomplished in one clinical visit. History, examination scan if necessary and diagnostic hysteroscopy can be accomplished in one visit to the clinic lasting approximately half an hour. The most advanced clinics are allowing GPs to refer patients who meet the clinic's criteria via the NHS computer network. Once the appointment has been made, the patient information leaflet is then printed in the referring doctor's surgery and handed to the patient (Gupta 2000).

PATHOLOGY SEEN AT DIAGNOSTIC HYSTEROSCOPY

Diagnostic hysteroscopists should familiarize themselves with the normal appearances of the endometrium both during the phases of the endometrial cycle and during the menopause (Fig. 3.7). The endometrium should be assessed for colour, texture, vascularity and thickness. An impression of thickness can be gained by pressing the surface of the endometrium with the end of the hysteroscope. Postmenopausal atrophy is characterized by very thin, pale endometrium, often accompanied by a ridged appearance.

Endometrial polyps (Fig. 3.8a) can vary considerably in appearance and the observer should define the position and size of the base of the polyp to aid subsequent operative hysteroscopy. Fibroids (Fig. 3.8b) have a characteristic whitish appearance and often have clearly visible surface vessels. Submucous fibroids, which are significantly bulging into the uterine cavity, may remain covered with endometrium but often have a similar appearance to a fibroid polyp. An assessment should be made of the relative proportion of the fibroid which is bulging into the endometrial cavity, as this determines whether it is likely to be resectable during a single operative procedure or may require multiple attempts. Uterine septum (Fig. 3.8c) may be seen dividing the cavity into two halves, while intrauterine adhesions (Fig. 3.8d) can lead to complete disruption of the cavity. Intrauterine contraceptive devices (IUCD) (Fig. 3.8e) are the most common foreign body seen at diagnostic hysteroscopy.

Hyperplastic endometrium is thickened and often polypoid and has increased vascularity. Endometrial cancer is often friable, sometimes has a lobed appearance and may appear necrotic. It should be suspected in postmenopausal patients where only a poor view is obtained owing to excessive bleeding. Tamoxifen causes a specific pattern of hyperplasia associated with a vesicular appearance (Fig. 3.9).

HYSTEROSCOPIC SKILLS

The RCOG Report on Minimal Access Surgery (RCOG 1994) categorized skill levels in training in both laparoscopy and hysteroscopy. Hysteroscopic procedures were divided into

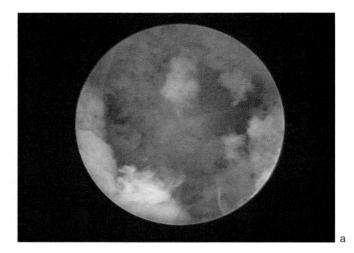

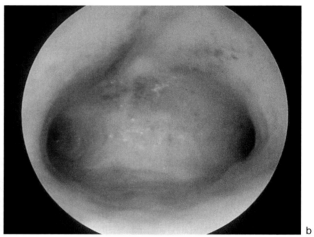

Fig. 3.7   a Premenstrual endometrium. b Postmenstrual endometrium.

three levels with the first level covering diagnostic and simple procedures such as the removal of a foreign body (Table 3.1). The second category contained operative procedures such as resection or ablation of the endometrium and removal of polyps and fibroids. Advanced procedures include repeated resection or ablation and treatment of extensive uterine synechiae. The RCOG established a subcommittee of the Training Committee to supervise training in MAS. Accreditation in hysteroscopic surgery is gained by submitting a log of procedures performed, a number of which must be under the supervision of an RCOG-recognized preceptor. To date, there are 70 recognized preceptors for hysteroscopic training in the UK and several individuals have achieved recognition of their training.

TRAINING AND LEARNING CURVE

Hysteroscopy is a relatively simple surgical skill to learn provided the surgeon undergoes a structured training process. It is clear that familiarity with equipment and knowledge of the basic underlying principles should be imparted early in the training process. To this end the Basic Skills course in O & G has been developed and an RCOG-franchised course is soon to be launched. Manipulating hysteroscopes and camera systems on models allows an early grasp of the basic principles of

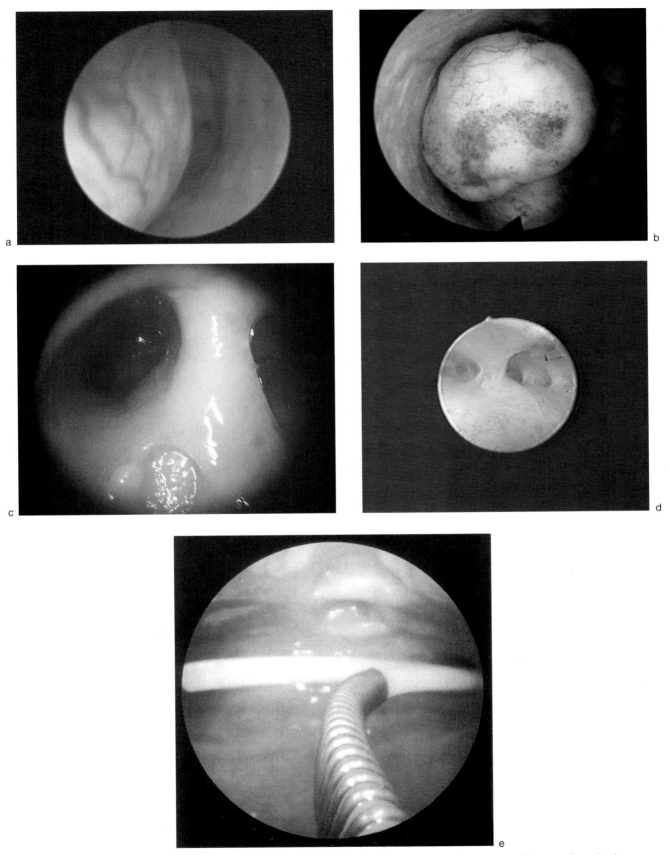

Fig. 3.8 a Versapoint spring electrode at the base of a polyp. b Submucous fibroid polyp. c Intrauterine septum. d Intrauterine adhesion. e Intrauterine foreign body.

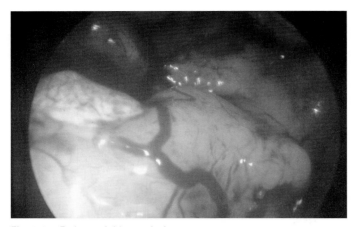

Fig. 3.9   Endometrial hyperplasia.

Table 3.1   Stratification of hysteroscopic procedures by level of training

Level 1   Diagnostic procedures
Diagnostic hysteroscopy, plus target biopsy
Removal of simple polyps
Removal of intrauterine contraceptive devices (IUCDs)

Level 2   Minor operative procedures
Proximal fallopian tube cannulation
Minor Asherman's syndrome
Removal of pedunculated fibroid or large polyp

*Level 3   More complex operative procedures requiring additional
            training*
Division/resection of uterine septum
Endoscopic surgery for major Asherman's syndrome
Endometrial resection or ablation
Resection of submucous leiomyoma
Repeat endometrial resection or ablation

Reproduced with permission from RCOG (1994)

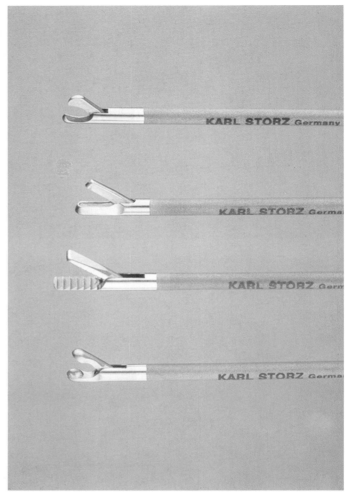

Fig. 3.10   Mechanical instruments for operative hysteroscopy
(courtesy of Karl Storz, Germany).

orientation and permits the trainee to progress rapidly to successful diagnostic hysteroscopy on anesthetized patients. Outpatient diagnostic hysteroscopy requires considerable skill, confidence and familiarity with the equipment. It should be reserved for consultants and senior trainees with a specific interest.

Operative hysteroscopy experience should begin with Level 1 procedures and progressively aim towards competence at Level 3 (see Table 3.1). Attendance at an endoscopic surgery training course may help to acquire knowledge, as would training in a laboratory setting on inanimate models. There is no substitute for 'hands-on' clinical experience, which should begin with direct supervision.

A national survey of outpatient hysteroscopy revealed that in 1994–95, over 100 000 diagnostic procedures were undertaken for menorrhagia in England alone, with only 30 000 of these performed in outpatient settings. A questionnaire was sent to 1148 consultant gynaecologists in the UK, of which 629 (55%) responded. Of the respondents, 48% had an interest in MAS. Of these, 54% had outpatient hysteroscopy available to them and of the ones with no facility, 76% would like it instituted (Rogerson & Duffy 2000).

OPERATIVE HYSTEROSCOPY

Operative hysteroscopy generally requires a larger instrument and a continuous flow sheath. In addition, a source of energy is used to perform the required manipulations. Operators should familiarize themselves with the use of a variety of energy systems so that they can use an alternative if their chosen system fails.

Mechanical

Scissors and grasping forceps are passed down the operating channel of the hysteroscope and can be used to cut the stalk of simple polyps, which are then grasped with forceps for removal (Fig. 3.10). Lost foreign bodies such as IUCDs can be removed in a similar fashion.

Monopolar electrical

Monopolar electrosurgery requires the flow of radiofrequency electric current from the active tip of the instrument through the patient to the large surface area return plate. The electrical effect depends on both current density and the waveform

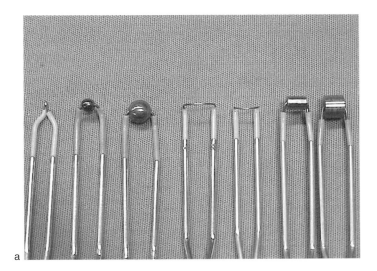

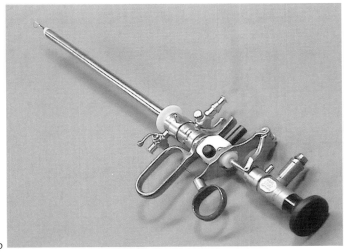

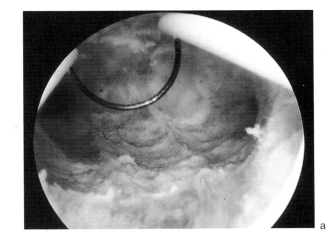

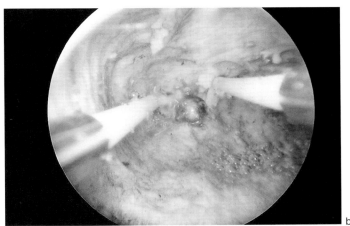

Fig. 3.11 a Working elements for operative hysteroscopy. b Assembled resectoscope (courtesy of Karl Storz, Germany).

provided by the generator. Simple instruments for use with monopolar diathermy include a polyp snare and simple electrodes, which can be passed down a 5 F operating channel. A dedicated continuous-flow hysteroscope is required for more sophisticated operative instruments including a resection loop, knife and rollerball and cylinder (Fig. 3.11).

Transcervical resection of the endometrium is a popular technique for endometrial destruction in which the loop is used to cut away the prepared endometrium down to the myometrium. Figure 3.12 demonstrates the loop in use and the transverse myometrial fibres can be clearly seen. Movement of the loop within the hysteroscope sheath and withdrawal of the scope itself allow long strips of endometrium to be resected. Removal of the tissue strips maintains a clear view. Most operators start with the posterior wall so that the resected tissue strips do not obscure the working area. Considerable training is needed to ensure safe use of this technique. Difficult areas to treat include the cornua, where the myometrium is thin, and the fundus, where the resection loop has to be bent forwards in order to achieve a cutting effect in front of the hysteroscope tip. Cornual endometrium may be ablated with rollerball and

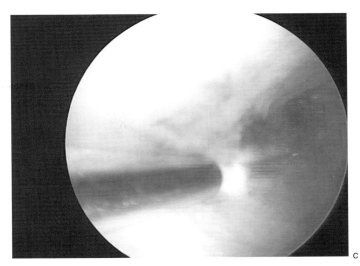

Fig. 3.12 a Endometrial resection. b Rollerball ablation. c Laser ablation.

combined with resection of the remaining endometrium (Fig. 3.12b). Broadbent & Magos (1994) reported that more than 80% of patients in their series were satisfied with endometrial resection, at 2.5 years after the procedure. Daniell et al (1992) reviewed 64 women 6 months after rollerball ablation. Of these women, 80% were satisfied with the outcome and 30% had amenorrhoea.

The same instrument is used for resection of submucous fibroids and fibroid polyps. The knife is employed for the treatment of Asherman's Syndrome and uterine septae. The resectoscope system is inexpensive as it uses reuseable electrodes, which are autoclavable. A careful watch must be kept on the fluid balance during the procedure as overload of 1.5% glycine solution may lead to significant complications. More than 1 litre of solution lost into the patient poses significant risk and the procedure should be abandoned if such levels of fluid loss are significantly exceeded.

Laser

The neodymium yttrium argon garnet laser (Nd:YAG for short) delivers high-energy laser light into the uterus via a flexible fibre. The energy is invisible to the eye and a helium neon beam is also directed down the fibre so that the operator knows that the fibre is active and can see where the energy will be delivered. The uterus is distended with saline when the laser is used. This still requires observation of the fluid loss but is less likely to cause complications as fluid overload is amenable to treatment with diuretics.

The laser can be used in non-contact mode, for example to coagulate the endometrium around the tubal ostia, or in contact mode where the laser fibre is dragged along the surface of the endometrium, cutting a groove down to the level of the myometrium (Fig. 3.13c). There is lateral spread of the laser energy such that if adjacent grooves are cut as far apart as the size of the laser fibre, the basal layer of endometrium between the grooves will be destroyed.

A multicentre collaborative study involving 859 women undergoing laser ablation was reported by Garry et al in 1991. Of these, 479 women were followed up for over 6 months. A satisfactory result was reported for 97%, although 8% needed a second treatment. Amenorrhoea occurred in 60% of the patients. Erian (1994) studied 2342 women undergoing laser ablation of whom 1866 were followed up for over a year. Successful outcome was reported in 93% and amenorrhoea in 56% of the women.

The Nd:YAG laser can also be used to destroy fibroids and cut through the stalk of polyps. It provides a very controllable energy source, which can be used to divide synechiae or uterine septae.

Bipolar electrosurgery

A recent development and introduction to the hysteroscopic surgeon's armamentarium is a bipolar electrosurgery system known as Versapoint (Fig. 3.13a). Three 5 F electrode forms require a dedicated electrosurgery generator which pulses the electrical energy through the saline irrigation medium from the active electrode tip to the larger return sleeve (Fig. 3.13b). This creates a vapour pocket around the active eletrode and when tissue enters the vapour pocket, the high current density causes vaporization of the tissue. This device has been used for vaporizing fibroids and polyps. It is suitable for use under local anaesthetic, particularly in conjunction with the Versascope. The Versapoint resection system, a larger version using similar technology, is suitable for the removal of larger fibroids under general anaesthetic (Fig. 3.13c).

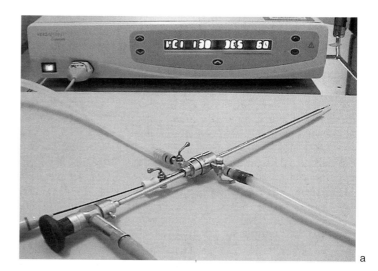

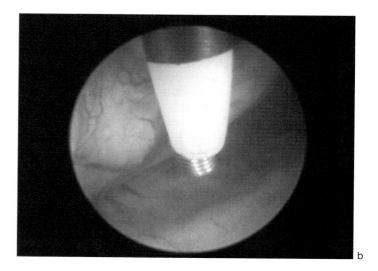

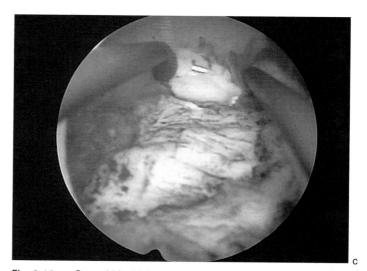

Fig. 3.13   a Bettochhi with Versapoint. b Versapoint spring electrode at polyp base. c Versapoint resection system.

Endometrial preparation

The in vivo studies of Duffy and colleagues (1992) demonstrate that rollerball coagulation results in thermal necrosis to a depth of 3.3–3.7 mm. The depth of cut with a resection loop is 3–4 mm and tissue is destroyed to a depth of 4–5 mm using the Nd:YAG laser. Endometrial thickness, however, varies from 3 to 12 mm during the menstrual cycle. Therefore satisfactory ablation can only be achieved if surgery is performed in the immediate postmenstrual phase. This would cause difficulty in scheduling operations, hence endometrial thinning is necessary. This leads to shorter duration and greater ease of surgery and a high rate of postoperative amenorrhoea (Sowter et al 2001).

A national survey of the complications of endometrial destruction for menstrual disorders, the MISTLETOE study (Overton et al 1997), compared the different surgical techniques for endometrial destruction. Combined diathermy resection appeared safer than resection alone, but laser and rollerball ablation were the safest. Fibroids were associated with increased operative haemorrhage. Increasing operative experience was associated with fewer uterine perforations in the loop resection alone group but had no effect on operative haemorrhage in any group. Cumulative failure rate at 1 year for combined resection and rollerball was lowest at 15%, compared with 20% for resection or rollerball alone and 32% for laser ablation.

Comparison of endometrial destruction methods with hysterectomy revealed that they have less postoperative morbidity, shorter hospital stay, quicker return to work, quicker return to normal acitivity and sexual intercourse compared to hysterectomy, but patient satisfaction may be slightly higher following hysterectomy (Pinion et al 1994).

As with all ablation techniques success is dependent on the proximity of the menopause, with postoperative amenorrhoea rates being highest in the older age group. Adenomyosis is a major cause of failure. Non-operative methods of endometrial ablation and the use of the levonorgestrel-releasing intrauterine device (LNG IUS) for the treatment of menorrhagia have decreased the use of endometrial resection to treat dysfunctional uterine bleeding. The LNG IUS results in a smaller mean reduction in menstrual blood loss than transcervical resection of endometrium and women are not as likely to become amenorrhoeic, but there is no difference in the rate of satisfaction with treatment (Lethaby et al 2001).

Hysteroscopic polypectomy and myomectomy are dependent on the experience of the operator and the size and position of the fibroid. Removal of the polyp can be as difficult as detaching it. If the polyp is small enough, grasping it with forceps and pulling it against the end of the scope and then withdrawing the whole scope can be effective. An alternative is to remove the detached polyp blindly using polyp forceps. This is often difficult and serves to illustrate the futility of blind techniques. Fibroids under 2 cm in size can be resected in one sitting. For larger fibroids or those where more than half is intramural, a two-stage procedure may be necessary (Donnez et al 1990). At stage 1 the protruding portion of the fibroid is removed followed by transhysteroscopic myolysis of the intramural portion (Donnex & Nisdle 1992). Subsequently, GnRH agonist therapy given for 8 weeks which shrinks the uterine cavity, thus

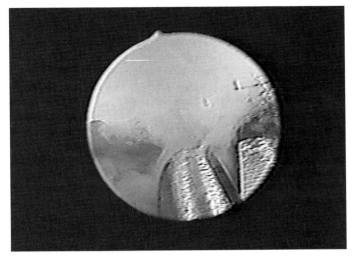

Fig. 3.14 Division of intrauterine synechiae with scissors.

extruding the intraumural portion of the fibroid, which is then easily removed at the second stage to complete the myomectomy. Complete removal of the fibroid is associated with improved long-term results (Wamstaker et al 1993).

The division of dense uterine synechiae (Fig. 3.14) and uterine septae requires considerable skill and is often performed under laparoscopic guidance which ensures that thermal or electrical energy is not allowed to penetrate through the myometrium and to damage the adjacent bowel. Careful assessment prior to division of uterine septae is essential to prevent perforation at the fundus. The hysteroscopic appearances of a septae uterus and a uterus didelphis can be similar and clearly any attempt to resect the septum will lead to disaster in the latter case. Careful ultrasound evaluation helps to differentiate the two but has not yet replaced laparoscopic assessment. After adhesiolysis, an IUD may be inserted for 3 months to prevent re-formation of the adhesions. Similarly, postoperative hormone therapy may be initiated to help endometrial development and prevent further adhesion formation (Gordon et al 1995).

Hysteroscopic sterilization

The different methods tried to occlude the fallopian tubes include use of sclerosing agents, destruction of the interstitial portion of the tubes and occlusion using plugs. Silicone plugs have a high rate of expulsion and return of fertility after removing the plugs is not guaranteed due to the tubal scarring. These methods are not widely accepted as they have an unacceptably high failure rate and are less efficient than other options currently available (Cooper 1992).

COMPLICATIONS

Surgeon related

Inadequate training and lack of equipment can lead to avoidable but potentially major complications, such as uterine perforation, haemorrhage and other visceral injuries. One must start learning the skill in a laboratory setting under supervision. The first patient experience is best obtained as a diagnostic procedure under general anaesthetic in the presence of an experienced surgeon. Gradual progression to the outpatient setting will help reduce the number of such complications. The surgeon should make a special effort to understand the basic working principles of the instruments in use.

Distension medium

There are different types of distension media used for hysteroscopy. Carbon dioxide may lead to gas embolism, which can lead to hypotension, tachycardia and arrhythmias which can be fatal. Fortunately this is a rare complication and should not occur provided the correct pressure insufflator is used.

Numerous gadgets are available to measure fluid deficit as rough estimation of fluid loss during hysteroscopic surgery is grossly inaccurate. Careful assessment of fluid input and output is critical, particularly if glycine is used, to avoid complications of uterine distension. Fluid absorption through patent fallopian tubes has been found to be of relatively little importance (Bent & Ostergard 1990).

Excessive deficit of non-electrolytic liquid distension medium such as 1.5% glycine can lead to hypervolaemia and hyponatraemia (Baumann et al 1990); deficit of 1 litre requires caution and the surgery should be discontinued at 1.5 litres. If the patient is asymptomatic with normal serum electrolytes and haematocrit, then observation is sufficient. Patients may, however, develop bradycardia, hypertension, nausea, vomiting, headache, confusion, agitation and visual disturbances. This is due to water moving across the blood–brain barrier, leading to cerebral oedema. If hyponatraemia is present with haemodilution, a loop diuretic, e.g. furosemide, and restricted fluid intake may be helpful. This symptom complex has been described in the past as 'post TURP syndrome'.

Haemorrhage

Bleeding during hysteroscopy is caused either by inadvertent trauma or by the operative steps disturbing the endometrium. Thick and vascular endometrium is likely to cause heavy bleeding. Preoperative endometrial thinning to decrease the vascularity is recommended practice. Bleeding can be controlled intraoperatively by coagulating the vessels under direct vision or postoperatively by inflating a Foley balloon in the uterine cavity with 5 ml of normal saline. The balloon is then deflated 6 hours after surgery. If bleeding has settled, leave the catheter in place for 1–2 hours, before discharging the patient. If not, the balloon can be left for a maximum of 24 hours. If bleeding continues despite tamponade by the Foley balloon, then hysterectomy may become necessary. In the MISTLETOE study (Overton et al 1997), 1% of women undergoing endometrial resection required an emergency hysterectomy.

Bleeding is likely to occur during endometrial ablation, myomectomy, adhesiolysis and septum resection. Polyps are unlikely to bleed significantly. Arterial bleeding is pulsatile and should be stopped immediately using laser or electrosurgery. Distension medium can suppress venous ooze (Fig. 3.15). The

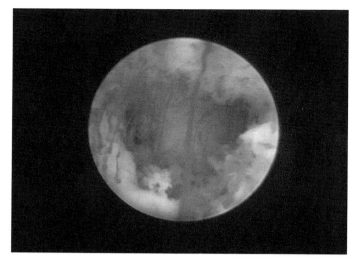

Fig. 3.15   Suppression of venous ooze with intrauterine pressure.

cavity should be viewed after the pressure is reduced, to check for haemostasis after operative hysteroscopy, and the hysteroscopist should always be prepared to control bleeding, which can happen unexpectedly.

Trauma

At the beginning of any hysteroscopy, due care must be taken while grasping the cervical lip as a good grip ensures that the tenaculum does not cut through. Dilatation of the cervix, if needed, is a blind procedure. If one is not careful, a false passage may be created and occasionally perforation of the cervical canal. This is more likely to occur when the cervix is scarred and stenosed following previous surgery and some surgeons prefer to soften the cervix with vaginal prostaglandin 2 hours preoperatively. Rarely, the dilator can give way suddenly to perforate the fundus.

Introducing the hysteroscope under direct vision, as described above, minimizes the chance of cervical trauma or uterine perforation, during the introduction of the scope.

Uterine perforation

This occurs in about 1% of women undergoing endometrial ablation (Lewis 1994). It can happen due to entry of the scope into a false passage or when the scope is against the fundus or while using the energy sources without visualizing the electrode. It is suspected if excessive bleeding is noted before the procedure is commenced, if the scope goes freely into the uterine cavity, if the fluid distension pressure stays low or decreases suddenly. Rarely a loop of bowel or omentum may be seen.

The energy source should only be activated while withdrawing the active tip, keeping the working element constantly under vision, which decreases the risk of perforation.

The distension medium tends to stretch the uterine wall, which is normally 2–2.5 cm thick. This has to be understood while performing operative hysteroscopy to avoid myometrial damage and decrease the risk of perforation. Extra care should be taken while operating near the uterine cornu as this is the thinnest portion of the uterine wall. Cornual injuries are likely to be full thickness with an additional risk to bladder, bowel and pelvic vessels.

As soon as perforation is suspected, the procedure should be stopped. Diagnostic hysteroscopy may be attempted, but the visualization will be poor due to inadequate distension and bleeding. Laparoscopy will help in assessment of the perforation site. The majority of injuries can be managed conservatively. In the event of heavy bleeding, haemostasis should be achieved by coagulating or by suturing the perforation. Diagnostic hysteroscopy may be completed under laparoscopic control. If perforation occurs during an operative hysteroscopy, then it is wise to defer the procedure.

Infections

Diagnostic hysteroscopy is less likely to cause infection. During operative hysteroscopy, blood and tissue debris becomes a focus of infection. Energy applied to tissue leads to necrotic tissue in the uterine cavity. Infection leads to bloodstained offensive discharge, which is accompanied by fever, generally feeling unwell and raised white cell count. A high degree of suspicion in postoperative patients with deteriorating symptoms is crucial for early diagnosis. Prophylactic antibiotics should be considered for operative hysteroscopy.

Anaesthetic and energy source–related complications

These are rare, but still need to be discussed with the patients. Patients at high anaesthetic risk will need a thorough explanation of the risks involved and performing the procedure under local anaesthetic offered as an alternative.

Late complications

Infertility
Neosynechiae formation after hysteroscopic surgery may lead to Asherman's syndrome and adhesions can re-form after adhesiolysis. Infertility may persist despite treatment of the suspected cause.

Abnormal menstrual bleeding
Hysteroscopic surgery performed in the younger age group (40–45 years) is more likely to fail than in later age groups. This is due to the possibility of concomitant hormonal imbalance in these patients. In the peri- and postmenopausal patients, the success of hysteroscopic surgery is well above 90%. Counselling to ensure realistic postoperative expectations is crucial to improve patient satisfaction.

Pregnancy
Patients undergoing endometrial ablation should be made aware of the need to practise contraception. Intrauterine and extrauterine pregnancies can occur following endometrial ablation, even after months of amenorrhoea (Lam et al 1992). Unexpected and unplanned pregnancy can have significant implications. Miscarriage is commonly seen in these patients,

due to uterine scarring and fibrosis. Cervical scarring can lead to abnormalities of labour. Detailed documentation of the procedure and any complications is absolutely vital. Uterine rupture in labour has been reported in patients with past history of uterine perforation during hysteroscopic surgery (Gurgan et al 1996). Placental localization at the site of damaged endometrium can lead to placenta accreta and its consequences.

Sterilization at the time of endometrial ablation prevents loss of distension fluid through the tube and offers permanent contraception.

Cancer
As explained earlier, cervical cancer is a contraindication for hysteroscopy but endometrial cancer is not. Failure of endometrial ablation and lack of endometrial thinning, despite agents such as GnRH analogues and danazol, should raise suspicion. Inability to shrink a fibroid by preoperative GnRH analogue treatment is another cause for concern.

There is no evidence of retrograde spread with the fluid or gaseous distension media or of any adverse effects on the activity of the malignant cells.

Endometrial cancer seen at hysteroscopy may be either suspected, as in patients presenting with postmenopausal bleeding, or a total surprise, as in younger women with abnormal uterine bleeding. For this reason, histological assessment of the endometrium is very important prior to endometrial ablation. It is crucial to obtain tissue for histology during hysteroscopic surgery to ensure that the diagnosis is not accidentally missed.

Similarly, histology of all specimens obtained at hysteroscopic surgery must be reviewed. Sarcomatous change in a fibroid occurs in <1% of patients, but must be ruled out. Endometrial chips obtained at resection may occasionally reveal malignancy.

Haematometra and pyometra
Collection of blood in the uterine cavity followed by infection can occur after hysteroscopic surgery, due to cervical stenosis. This can be prevented by avoiding ablation near the internal os. Occasionally, haematometra may occur after commencement of hormone replacement therapy (Dwyer et al 1991).

Postablation sterilization syndrome
Endometrial ablation in women with a history of sterilization can occasionally lead to postoperative pain. Active endometrium between the scarred uterine cavity and the tubal block leads to haemorrhagic tubal distension, during menses. This causes stretching of the intramural and isthmic portion of the tube with resultant pain. The presentation of this condition can be similar to an ectopic pregnancy.

PREOPERATIVE CONSENT ISSUES

Complications can occur during any treatment procedure, in spite of all due precautions, and can lead to patient dissatisfaction. It is annoying for patients when they are not warned about such possibilities, however rare they may be. Thorough preoperative explanation and counselling, including detailed explanation of the pathophysiology of the underlying gynaecological condition, treatment options available and their risks and benefits, are essential to ensure a successful operative experience for the patient as well as the surgeon. This is best started during the outpatient consultation when the decision for hysteroscopy is taken and followed by giving an information leaflet with a helpline where any further doubts can be clarified.

NEW DEVELOPMENTS AND THE FUTURE

The latest development in hysteroscopy is the successful use of this skill in gynaecological outpatient clinics, under local or no anaesthesia.

Bipolar equipment of 5 F diameter, used through a hysteroscope of 5 mm outer diameter, has made 'see and treat' possible in the outpatient clinic. The challenge for the majority of hysteroscopists is to improve their confidence and competence at obtaining a clear view at diagnostic procedures and to extend their operative repertoire. No doubt new technology will improve our ability to manage with smaller instruments, but the challenge for hysteroscopy for the next decade is to extend its effective use more widely.

KEY POINTS

1. Hysteroscopy is a well-established tool in modern gynaecology due to its unique advantage of direct visualization of the uterine cavity.
2. Advantages include decreased morbidity and quicker recovery for the patient, ability for diagnosis and treatment in the outpatient department for the surgeon and resultant cost benefits for the healthcare system.
3. Contraindications include cervical cancer, pelvic infection, heavy uterine bleeding, pregnancy and inexperienced or untrained surgeon.
4. Uterine distension, essential for panoramic hysteroscopy, is achieved using media such as carbon dioxide, normal saline, Ringer's lactate, 5% dextrose, sorbitol or 1.5% glycine.
5. Pathology such as fibroids, polyps, adhesions or uterine septum can be seen and then treated using mechanical scissors, laser or electrosurgery–monopolar or bipolar.
6. Hysteroscopic myomectomy is successful in controlling menorrhagia in about 93% of women. Adhesiolysis causes improved fertility in 60.5% and menstruation in over 80%.
7. Abnormal uterine bleeding is the most common indication for hysteroscopy. Partial or complete endometrial ablation can be performed using a resection loop, rollerball, bipolar technology or laser.
8. Endometrial ablation offers a conservative alternative to hysterectomy, although one would like to improve the current amenorrhoea rates of 15–40% and success rates of 70–75%.
9. Preoperative endometrial thinning with danazol or GnRH analogues helps by shrinking the tissue and decreasing vascularity, thereby leading to reduced blood loss, reduced operating time and decreased fluid absorption.

KEY POINTS (CONTINUED)

10. Histological assessment of the tissue obtained at endometrial ablation, myomectomy or polypectomy is important to detect the occasional underlying malignancy.
11. Endometrial histology is also essential before any form of endometrial ablation and desirable for patients with postmenopausal bleeding.
12. Technological development has enabled hysteroscopy in the outpatients setting, which has led to the widespread introduction of one-stop hysteroscopy clinics, where patients with abnormal uterine bleeding are clerked, assessed and investigated fully at the same visit.
13. Other indications for hysteroscopy include infertility, foreign body and chronic pelvic pain.
14. Transvaginal sonography, hysterosonography and hysterosalpingography are useful diagnostic adjuncts to hysteroscopy.
15. Complication during hysteroscopy include cervical or uterine trauma, haemorrhage, infection, fluid overload, gas embolism and uterine perforation with injury to other pelvic viscera. Important late complications include failure to relieve presenting symptoms, infertility, pregnancy with associated complications and cancer.
16. The above complications are rare and avoidable but potentially serious and hence the surgeon must understand the working principles of the hysteroscopic equipment, including the energy source used, and undergo a structured training programme.
17. Adequate explanation and consent improve patient satisfaction and decrease litigation when complications occur.
18. The training process includes acquiring knowledge, working on laboratory models, attending a recognized structured course and assisting experts. Initial procedures are undertaken under general anaesthesia, followed by day case procedures under local anaesthesia and finally performing diagnostic and then operative hysteroscopy in the outpatient set-up.

REFERENCES

Baumann R, Magos AL, Kay JDS et al 1990 Absorption of glycine irrigating solution during transcervical resection of endometrium. British Medical Journal 300:304–305
Bent AE, Ostergard DR 1990 Endometrial ablation with the neodymium: YAG laser. Obsterics and Gynecology 75:923–925
Broadbent JAM, Magos AL 1994 Transcervical resection of the endometrium. In: Sutton C, Diamond M (eds) Endoscopic surgery of gynaecologists. W B Saunders, London
Coeman D 1993 Hysteroscopic findings in patients with a cervical polyp. American Journal of Obstetrics and Gynecology 169:1563
Cooper JM 1992 Hysteroscopic sterilization. Clinical Obstetrics and Gynecology 35:282–298
Daniell JF, Kurtz BR, Raymond W 1992 Hysteroscopic endometrial ablation using rollerball electrode. Obstetrics and Gynecology 49:48–54
Dicker D 1992 The value of repeat hysteroscopic evaluation in patients with failed in vitro fertilization transfer cycles. Fertility and Sterility 58(4):833
Donnez J, Nisolle M 1992 Hysteroscopic surgery. Current Opinion in Obstetrics and Gynecology 4:439

Donnez J, Nisolle M, Smets M et al 2001 Hysteroscopy in the diagnosis of specific disorders. In: Donnez J, Nisolle M (eds) An atlas of operative laparoscopy and hysteroscopy. Parthenon, Lancs

Donnez J, Gillerot S, Bourgonjon D et al 1990 Neodymium:YAG laser hysteroscopy in large submuous fibroids. Fertility and Sterility 54:999

Duffy S, Reid PC, Sharp F 1992 In vivo studies of uterine electrosurgery. British Journal of Obstetrics and Gynaecology 99:579–582

Dwyer N, Fox R, Mills M et al 1991 Haematometra caused by hormone replacement therapy after endometrial resection. Lancet 338:1205

Erian J 1994 Endometrial ablation in the treatment of menorrhagia. British Journal of Obstetrics and Gynaecology 101(suppl 11):19–22

Finikiotos G 1994 Hysteroscopy: a review. Obstetrics and Gynecology Survey 49(4):273

Flood JT, Grow DR 1993 Transcervical tubal cannulation: a review. Obstetrics and Gynecology Survey 48(11):768

Gallinat A 1964 Hysteroscopy in early pregnancy. In: Siegler AM (eds) Hysteroscopy principles and management. Lippincott, Philadelphia

Garry R, Erian J, Grochmal SA 1991 A multi-centre collaborative study into the treatment of menorrhagia by Nd-YAG laser ablation of the endometrium. British Journal of Obstetrics and Gynaecology 98:357–362

Goldstein DP, Decholnoky C, Emans SJ et al 1980 Laparoscopy in the diagnosis and management of pelvic pain in adolescents. Journal of Reproductive Medicine 24:251

Gordon AG, Lewis BV, De Cherney AH 1995 Gynecologic endoscopy, 2nd edn. Mosby Wolfe, London

Grainger DA, de Cherney AH 1989 Hysteroscopic management of uterine bleeding. Baillière's Clinical Obstetrics and Gynaecology 3:403–414

Gupta JK 2000 Rapid access ambulatory diagnostic (RAAD) clinic internet link between primary and secondary care. Millennium Annual Meeting of British Society for Gynaecological Endoscopy

Gurgan T, Yarali H, Urman B et al 1996 Uterine rupture following hysteroscopic lysis of synechiae due to tuberculosis and uterine perforation. Human Reproduction 11(2):291–293

Karlsson B, Granberg S, Wikland M et al 1995 Transvaginal ultrasonography of the endometrium in women with postmenopausal bleeding: a Nordic multicenter study. American Journal of Obstetrics and Gynecology 172:1488–1494

Kremer C, Barik S, Duffy S 1998 Flexible outpatient hysteroscopy without anaesthesia: a safe, successful and well tolerated procedure. British Journal of Obstetric and Gynaecology 105(6):672–676

Lam AM, Al-Jumaily RY, Holt EM 1992 Ruptured ectopic pregnancy in an amenorrhoeic woman after transcervical resection of the endometrium. Australia and New Zealand Journal of Obstetrics and Gynaecology 32:81–82

Lethaby AE, Cooke I, Rees M 2001 Progesterone releasing intrauterine systems versus either placebo or any other medication for heavy menstrual bleeding. Cochrane Database of Systematic Reviews Issue 1. Update Software, Oxford

Lewis BV 1994 Guidelines for endometrial ablation. British Journal of Obstetrics and Gynaecology 101:470–473

Lindemann HJ 1972 The use of CO2 in the uterine cavity for hysteroscopy. International Journal of Fertility 17:221

Overton C, Hargreaves J, Maresh M 1997 A national survey of the complications of endometrial destruction for menstrual disorders: the MISTLETOE study. Minimally invasive surgical techniques – laser, endothermal or endoresection. British Journal of Obstetrics and Gynaecology 104(12):1351–1359

Panteleoni D 1869 On endoscopic examination of the cavity of the womb. Med Press Circ 8:26–27

Pinion SB, Parkin DE, Amramovich DR et al 1994 Randomised trial of hysterectomy, endometrial laser ablation and transcervical endometrial resection for dysfunctional uterine bleeding. British Medical Journal 309:979–983

Prather C, Wolfe A 1995 The nurse's role in office hysteroscopy. Journal of Obstetrical, Gynecological and Neonatal Nursing 24(9):813–816

Preutthipaan S, Herabutya Y 1999 A randomized controlled trial of vaginal misoprostol for cervical priming before hysteroscopy. Obstetrics and Gynecology 94:427

Rogerson L, Duffy S 2000 National survey of outpatient hysteroscopy. Millennium Annual Meeting of British Society for Gynaecological Endoscopy

Romano F 1994 Sonohysteroscopy versus hysteroscopy for diagnosing endouterine abnormalities in fertile women. International Journal of Gynecology and Obstetrics 45:253

Royal College of Obstetricians and Gynaecologists (RCOG) 1994 Report of the RCOG working party on training in gynaecological endoscopic surgery. RCOG Press, London

Schenker JG, Margalioth EJ 1982 Intrauterine adhesions: an updated appraisal. Fertility and Sterility 37:593

Schifrin BS, Erez S, Moore JG 1973 Teenage endometriosis. American Journal of Obstetrics and Gynaecology 116:973

Schwarzler P, Concin H, Bosch H et al 1998 An evaluation of sono-hysterography and diagnostic hysteroscopy for the assessment of intrauterine pathology. Ultrasound in Obstetrics and Gynecology 11:337–342

Siegler AM, Kemmann E 1976 Location and removal of misplaced or embedded intrauterine devices by hysteroscopy. Journal of Reproductive Medicine 16:139

Sowter MC, Singla AA, Lethaby A 2001 Pre-operative endometrial thinning agents before hysteroscopic surgery for heavy menstrual bleeding. Cochrance Database of Systematic Reviews. Issue 1

Steffensen AJ, Schuster M 1995 Continuous flow hysteroscopy. An improved endoscopic method for examination of the uterine cavity. Tidsskrift for den Norske Laegeforening 115(10):1228–1229

Sugimoto O 1975 Hysteroscopic diagnosis of endometrial carcinoma: a report of fifty-three cases examined at Women's clinic of Kyoto University Hospital. American Journal of Obstetrics and Gynecology 121:105

Taylor PJ, Gordon AG 1993 Diagnostic hysteroscopy. In: Taylor PJ, Gordon AG (eds) Practical hysteroscopy. Blackwell, Oxford

Valle RF, Sciarra JJ, Freeman DW 1977 Hysteroscopic removal of intrauterine devices with missing filaments. Obstetrics and Gynecology 49:55

Valli E, Zupi E, Marconi D et al 1998 Outpatient diagnostic hysteroscopy. Journal of the American Association of Gynecological Laparoscopy 5(4):397–402

Wamstaker K, Emanuel MH, de Kruif JH 1993 Transcervical hysteroscopic resection of submucous fibroids for abnormal uterine bleeding: results regarding the degree of intramural extension. Obstetrics and Gynecology 82:736–740

4

Laparoscopy

Alan Farthing

INTRODUCTION

Laparoscopy (Greek *lapar* meaning flank) is a technique utilized by surgical gynaecologists around the world to great effect. Advances in the technique over the past two decades have revolutionized gynaecological surgery and provided a vastly improved service for patients. At the same time some of these advances have been associated with considerable controversy and many opinions are forcefully expressed without much factual basis. This chapter aims to discuss the basics of laparoscopy and its application, providing some of the evidence from the literature where possible.

HISTORY

Examination of the body cavities using instrumentation has been practised by clinicians over many centuries. Most of the early techniques involved inspection of the bladder and urethra (Bozzini 1805). Light sources were introduced initially with alcohol flames (Desmoreaux 1865) and subsequently the incandescent light bulb and the first inspection of the peritoneal cavity was through the posterior fornix in the early 20th centrury (von Ott 1901). Examination of other cavities was described soon afterwards (Jacobaeus 1910) with CO_2 used for insufflation more than a decade later (Zollikoffer 1924). The first diagnosis of an ectopic pregnancy followed (Hope 1937) as did female sterilizations. Veress first reported the spring-loaded insufflation needle as a technique for introducing a pneumothorax in patients with tuberculosis (Veress 1938).

Further advances were relatively slow with few clinicians inspired by the new techniques. The first description of sterilization in English was not until 25 years later (Steptoe 1967). Few therapeutic procedures were performed laparoscopically although the technique gained widespread support for diagnosis.

The revolution in therapeutic techniques probably started with the report of the first laparoscopic hysterectomy (Reich et al 1989) and, with advances in instrumentation, light sources and camera systems, continued apace throughout the 1990s. However, a few practitioners attempted procedures that were beyond either their surgical training or ability and responsible bodies rapidly concluded that regulation was required. The RCOG established its training guidelines in 1994 with certification for those trained to perform at different levels. This was modified in 1999 to bring the UK training into line with the practice in other European countries.

As technology improves and evidence-based medicine, together with audit, becomes a greater part of the clinician's practice there are likely to be further changes over the next few years. The so-called 'star wars' defence programmes have spawned robotics techniques that have yet to be assessed for their use in surgery but may provide further advances in the future. One certainty is that this area of medical practice will continue to change well into this next century.

Box 4.1   Therapeutic procedures that should routinely be performed laparoscopically

Laser ablation of endometriosis (Sutton et al 1994)

Salpingectomy (Yao & Tulandi 1997)

Removal of ovarian cysts (Audebert M 1998)

Minor adhesiolysis

Sterilization

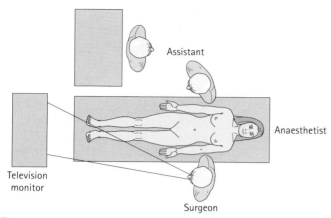

Fig. 4.1 Theatre set-up is important. The monitor should be in the same plane as the surgical field, i.e. a straight line from the surgeon through the surgical field also passes through the monitor.

THEATRE SET-UP

When setting up a theatre for laparoscopic surgery, a number of factors need to be taken into consideration. First, both the surgeon and the assistant need to have an excellent view of the operating area. Second, the surgeon needs to be in a comfortable position and third, the instrumentation needs to be systematically and consistently arranged.

The author believes that the television screen should be placed between the patient's legs if the camera is inserted at the umbilicus. Figure 4.1 demonstrates that the view obtained by the surgeon on a television screen is in an exact straight line with the direction in which the surgeon is operating. Many experienced surgeons place the television screen directly in front of themselves and behind the assistant. Under these circumstances, the surgeon is operating in a different direction to which he or she is looking; not only is this uncomfortable and ergonomically disadvantageous, but all images have to be transposed through 90°, adding to the difficulties of hand–eye co-ordination. The additional advantage of placing the television monitor between the patient's legs is that only one screen is required.

The scrub nurse should stand in a consistent position and instrumentation such as bipolar diathermy, scissors, graspers and suction irrigation should be placed consistently and within easy reach of the surgeon. The scrub nurse should be within sight of the television screen, enabling an experienced assistant to anticipate the next instrument required. A protective bar placed across the table prevents the assistant's arm from resting on the upper part of the patient and potentially dislodging the endotracheal tube (Fig. 4.2).

EQUIPMENT

Laparoscopic surgeons are totally dependent on their equipment. Any laparoscopic procedure can only be performed safely if clear images are presented to the surgeon. The quality of the image is dependent on the weakest link in a long series of technologically advanced items. It is essential that laparoscopic surgeons are familiar with the function and adjustments of the imaging systems that they use and it is this complicated equipment that provides the majority of the cost of laparoscopic surgery.

It is primarily the vast improvement in technology that has led to the increase in the number of procedures performed using laparoscopic techniques; however, there is scope for further improvement in laparoscopic equipment and robotics. Three-dimensional viewing systems and automated assistants may enhance the current instrumentation.

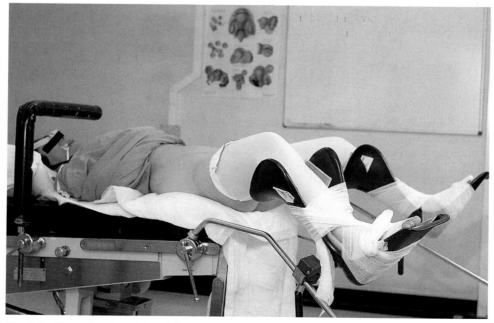

Fig. 4.2 The patient is positioned flat on the table with legs supported. A bar is placed over the endotracheal tube to protect this from being dislodged and to give the assistant's arm support.

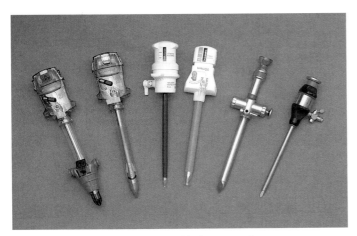

Fig. 4.3 A selection of trocars used in laparoscopic surgery.

The following items are essential.

Trocars

There are many different types of trocar available which vary in size, length and design of the tip (Fig. 4.3). The most commonly utilized trocars in gynaecological surgery are the 12 mm, 10 mm and 5 mm. When performing complicated surgery, there can be many changes of instrument down any individual port. For this reason, the trocars have to be able to grip the abdominal wall and there are various designs to facilitate this. Some of the more modern trocars have a type of 'fish scale' whilst other utilize a screw thread which can grip more effectively but increases the diameter of the incision. The trocar tip can be conical, pyramidal or a single flat blade in design. They create different sized and shaped incisions in the fascia, with the single flat blade and conical dilating tip producing the smallest defect. Trocars may be disposable or reusable. Many laparoscopic surgeons have been persuaded to use disposable trocars because of their constantly sharp tips, the so-called safety devices to retract the tip when through the full thickness of the abdominal wall and to avoid contamination between patients. However, most surgical units find the costs of disposable trocars prohibitive for use with every case.

Laparoscopes

The laparoscopes most commonly used in gynaecological surgery are of 10 mm, 5 mm or occasionally 3 mm diameter. The 10 mm laparoscopes provide the largest images with the optimal illumination, although the new generation of 5 mm laparoscopes can provide an image equal to their 10 mm relatives from only a few years ago. The laparoscope is a high-precsion engineered instrument which requires careful handling, both during operations and in the sterilization process between cases. It contains both a fibreoptic bundle for light transmission and a series of lenses to transfer the image back to the eyepiece. Modern laparoscopes consist of a hybrid rod lens system although the 3 mm laparoscope utilizes a high-quality fibreoptic bundle. The hybrid rod lens system at 3 mm diameter would be too easily damaged. Most surgeons utilize a laparoscope which projects an image that appears at 0° to the shaft of the scope; however, laparoscopes that project an image from 30° or 70°

are also available. Although these laparoscopes rarely cause problems for the surgeon, they can cause difficulty in co-ordination of the image by the assistant who is holding the laparoscope and camera device.

Light source and lead

The weakest link in the endoscopic equipment chain is often the light lead. This fibreoptic cable is often used for months or years after many of its cables are damaged. It also requires careful maintenance and will inevitably require replacement in time. A number of light sources exist and many surgeons still utilize the halogen system even though this has been superseded by the more powerful xenon light source.

Camera system

Modern camera systems are an essential part of the laparoscopic surgeon's equipment. There are few surgeons around the world who continue to operate by looking directly down the eyepiece of the laparoscope even for minor diagnostic procedures. There is a clear advantage in being able to project the image onto a television screen that is visible to all members of the surgical team. Together with the ergonomic advantages of not having to stoop over the patient, this means that camera systems are now commonplace. The image seen through the eyepiece of the laparoscope is converted into electrical signals by a charge-coupled device (CCD) housed in the camera head. These electrical signals are then processed by the camera control facility which is in turn connected to the television monitor. Cameras may contain a single CCD or three CCDs, each of which is colour specific, recording only one of the three primary colours. Some camera heads incorporate remote buttons to allow the operator to control various features of the imaging system, such as taking prints, operating the video recorder or white balancing. Some cameras are autoclavable but the majority of surgeons will place the camera system inside a sterile plastic sheath before connecting to the endoscope (Fig. 4.4).

Recording equipment

The modern laparoscopic surgery theatre should contain a video recorder and still photo facility for the purpose of producing images of any procedure. Many educational and training videos have been produced and are extremely valuable. Patients may appreciate a copy of their operation and some surgeons believe it is important to create a medico-legal record of the procedure for possible future reference. There is no reason why laparoscopic surgery should be treated any differently to open surgery and surgeons not recording their procedures on a video can hardly be regarded as neglecting the medical records. Within gynaecology, the majority of medico-legal claims are connected with laparoscopic sterilization and most surgeons would regard photographs of the clips occluding each fallopian tube to be a sensible precaution.

TV monitor

Many different TV monitors are available, but the majority are 20" in size. The monitor should be the last piece of equipment that is adjusted if the image is of poor quality and is possibly

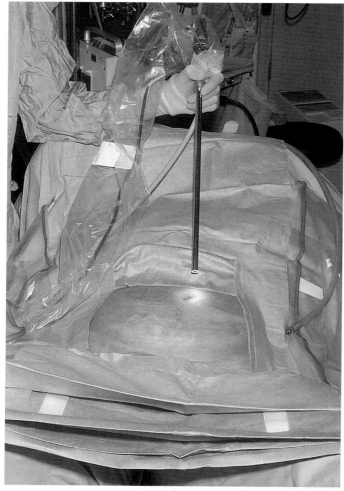

Fig. 4.4   A sterile bag can be used for placement of the camera head and cable.

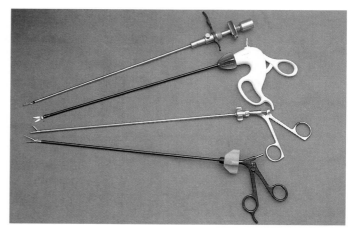

Fig. 4.5   A selection of laparoscopic scissors, graspers and bipolar diathermy of 5 mm diameter.

the least important in determining a good view of the surgical field.

Insufflator

As laparoscopic surgical techniques have advanced, there has been a significant improvement in the technology of insufflators. They should provide a maximum flow rate of around 35 litres/min with a continuous monitoring of the volume, flow rate and intra-abdominal pressure. Safety devices should ensure that the maximum pressure setting is not exceeded and most modern insufflators have an alarm to notify the surgeon. Some insufflators additionally provide smoke evacuation, either controlled by the surgeon with a foot pedal or with a direct link through to the diathermy or laser device. The insufflator needs to have simple and easily interpreted display panels. The laparoscopic surgeon will refer to the insufflator when creating the pneumoperitoneum and at this vital part of the procedure, needs to know where to look for the information he or she is seeking.

Operating instruments

There are innumerable varieties of operating instruments and individual surgeons will have their own preferences.

Essentially, the instruments can be divided into the jaws, the shaft and the handles. Jaws have been designed which mimic all the instrumentation available at open surgery, plus many others. Examples are shown in Figure 4.5. The shafts may be of 10, 5 or 3 mm diameter and may or may not contain a diathermy attachment. For non-disposable instrumentation, it is often the shaft that is the most difficult part of the instrument to keep clean and maintain. Handles come in a variety of ergonomic designs, according to surgeon preference. Handles may be ratcheted or non-racheted in a variety of ways. Most non-disposable instruments have a detachable handle in order to convert an instrument into one with or without a ratchet. Surgeons have their favourite graspers and as with most situations, it is more important to be familiar with an instrument and know its limitations than it is to have a wide varity of instrumentation that is less familiar.

Laparoscopic operating equipment is expensive and has a relatively short shelf-life in comparison to open instrumentation. It is essential that any theatre budget takes this into consideration and that laparoscopic surgeons are not asked to continue working with blunt and non-functioning instruments. The more complex problems of decontamination and sterilization of these precision instruments mean that they require careful maintenance by a specialist team.

PORT ENTRY

There are a variety of techniques described for insufflation in order to allow the surgeon to view the pelvic and abdominal contents through the laparoscope. A great deal of discussion has occurred, particularly in medico-legal circles, about which is the safest technique. Complication rates for laparoscopy are so relatively low that individual surgeons are unlikely to be able to evaluate the various entry techniques in their own practice. However, the number of laparoscopies performed is so high that the overall effect of an inferior technique could be significant for a number of patients around the country each year. Traditionally, gynaecologists are familiar with the closed technique, having performed many diagnostic laparoscopies in their training. General surgeons perform many fewer laparo-

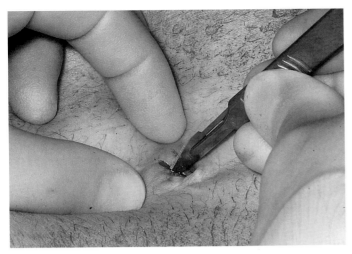

Fig. 4.6   An incision is made intraumbilically.

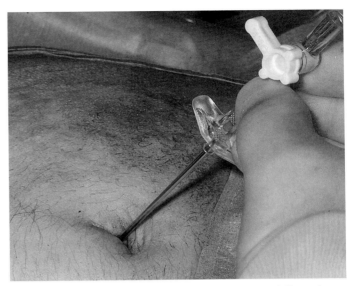

Fig. 4.7   The Veress needle is placed intraumbilically and directed towards the pouch of Douglas during insertion.

scopies each and these are usually for major procedures. They are usually more familiar with the open technique. Each technique has it persuasive advocates basing their arguments on a combination of scientific evidence and personal bias. Recent reviews comprehensively cover this subject and are recommended reading (Bonjer et al 1997, Garry 2000).

Site of entry

There are three main sites of entry into the peritoneal cavity. The most common site is at the umbilicus with some clinicians using a suprapubic approach and others utilizing Palmer's point (in the mid-clavicular line in the 9th intercostal space).

At the umbilicus the abdominal wall is at its thinnest. A subumbilical incision is preferred by some clinicians, but there appears to be no logic to this. If the umbilicus is to be used, then there is little point in inserting either the Veress needle or primary trocar at a point where the abdominal wall has expanded. In addition, an intraumbilical incision is cosmetically superior (Fig. 4.6). The left upper quadrant of the peritoneal cavity is where the fewest intraperitoneal adhesions occur. For this reason, Palmer suggested the 9th intercostal space as an insertion point for insufflation and brief inspection of the peritoneal cavity. A number of clinicians utilize this entry point when they suspect periumbilical adhesions may be present.

Closed laparoscopy

A vertical incision is made intraumbilically and a Veress needle inserted with the tip aiming towards the pouch of Douglas (Fig. 4.7). Most clinicians stabilize the anterior abdominal wall by grasping it with the left hand, while the right hand inserts the Veress needle. Experienced laparoscopists can feel the Veress neddle pass through the layers of the anterior abdominal wall and will usually be able to tell whether the Veress is correctly positioned. At this point, a number of techniques have been described to assist in demonstrating that the Veress needle is correctly positioned. A syringe can be used to aspirate from the Veress needle to identify visceral contents. Alternatively, a droplet of water or saline can

be placed on the end of the Veress needle and the negative intra-abdominal pressure causes this to be sucked in. A syringe placed on the end of the Veress needle and containing water or saline, but without its plunger, will usually allow the solution to drip into the peritoneal cavity if correctly positioned. Once insufflation is commenced, the filling pressure can be observed and uniform distension of the abdominal cavity determined by percussion. In particular, the area over the liver becomes resonant to percussion when a pneumoperitoneum is created.

It is important to create a pneumoperitoneum of a set pressure, not volume. The size of the intraperitoneal cavity varies greatly between individuals. The purpose of the insufflation is to provide a cushion between the anterior abdominal wall and the important underlying structures when the primary trocar is inserted. Phillips et al (1999) demonstrated that intraperitoneal pressure of 25 mmHg was necessary in order to maintain the gas bubble during insertion of the primary trocar. It is extremely important that this pressure is then reduced to 15 mmHg or less for the rest of the operation. Ventilation difficulties are not encountered at this initial filling pressure, as the patient is flat and the pressure of this level is maintained for only a short period of time.

Direct trocar insertion without pneumoperitoneum has been suggested, but there is limited knowledge about its level of safety (Dingfelder 1978). Few laparoscopists practise this particular technique as any inadvertent visceral perforation is guaranteed to be of significant size, unlike damage caused by the Veress needle.

Open laparoscopy

The Hasson entry technique was first described in 1971 (Hasson 1971). A vertical incision is placed intraumbilically and the various layers of the abdominal wall incised using two Langenbeck retractors on either side to assist with visualization. Once the rectus sheath is incised, a suture is inserted either side of the incision into the sheath. The peritoneum is opened and a blunt Hasson cannula inserted direct into the peritoneal cavity and insufflation commenced. A seal is usually created utilizing the sutures in the rectus sheath and tightening around a cone attached to the Hasson cannula.

Comparison of complications

A vast number of laparoscopies using the closed technique have been performed over many years. A recent collection of over 350 000 procedures has calculated the risk of bowel damage to be 0.4/1000 and the risk of major vessel injury to be 0.2/1000. The most common bowel injury is to the transvese colon, while the most common vascular injury is to the right common iliac artery (Clements 1995).

There are no comparable data on such a large number of patients utilizing open laparoscopy. One rationale of the Hasson technique is to identify intraperitoneal and bowel adhesions at entry into the peritoneal cavity, so avoiding blind insertion of a trocar into this visceral structure. More logically, the Hasson technique avoids major vessel damage. Population-based studies are an inappropriate way of comparing the two techniques, as many clinicians will only use the open laparoscopy approach if they think there is a danger of intraperitoneal adhesions. They are therefore selecting a high-risk group of patients on which to perform this technique while those studies that have been published with large numbers suggest the bowel damage in the open laparoscopy group is equivalent to that in the closed laparoscopy group (Chapron et al 1998).

Advocates of the open laparoscopy approach maintain that the time taken to achieve pneumoperitoneum is the equivalent to that of the closed laparoscopy approach (Pickersgill et al 1999).

Ten per cent of patients will have intra-abdominal adhesions with 5% having severe adhesions containing bowel around the umbilicus. Ninety-two percent of these patients with severe adhesions will have had a previous laparotomy with the vast majority following midline incisions (Garry 2000). Although not all visceral perforations caused by laparoscopy are the result of negligence, it would seem prudent that clinicians take into consideration the previous midline laparotomies when performing a laparoscopy. It is important that those advocates of closed laparoscopy are able to perform open laparoscopy when their own technique fails. There is currently no conclusive proof that one technique is safer than the other and a huge randomized controlled trial would be necessary to detect small safety differences between the two.

TEACHING AND LEARNING

The Royal College of Obstetricians and Gynaecologists recognized at an early stage that teaching and learning laparoscopic surgery was important for safe practice. A system of recognized preceptors who are qualified to teach laparoscopic techniques has been established and is maintained by the RCOG. Laparoscopic procedures are divided into procedures of three levels.

- Level 1 or basic skills include procedures that every

Box 4.2 RCOG classification of laparoscopic procedures

Level 1   Diagnostic and minor laparoscopic procedures
Diagnostic laparoscopy
Laparoscopic sterilization
Laparoscopic needle aspiration of simple cysts
Laparoscopic ovarian biopsy

Level 2   More extensive procedures requiring additional training
Minor adhesiolysis for filmy adhesions
Linear salpingotomy or salpingectomy for ectopic pregnancy
Laser/diathermy to polycystic ovaries
Laser/diathermy or excision of mild endometriosis (revised AFS Stage I and II)
Laparoscopic pedunculated myomectomy
Laparoscopic uterosacral nerve ablation
Laparoscopic salpingostomy for infertility
Laparoscopic salpingo-oophorectomy
Laparoscopic ovarian cystectomy
Laparoscopic/laser management of endometrioma
Laparoscopically assisted vaginal/subtotal hysterectomy without significant associated pathology

Level 3   Extensive endoscopic procedures requiring subspecialist or advanced/tertiary level endoscopic skills
Laparoscopic adhesiolysis for thick adhesions
Laparoscopic hysterectomy with associated pathology
Total laparoscopic hysterectomy
Laparoscopic intramural myomectomy
Laparoscopic surgery for endometriosis (revised AFS Stage III and IV (invasive disease)) and dissection of pouch of Douglas
Pelvic and aortic lymphadenectomy
Pelvic side wall/ureteric dissection
Presacral neurectomy
Laparoscopic incontinence procedures
Laparoscopic suspension procedures

Box 4.3 Skills required for each level of laparoscopic expertise

Level 1
Basic hand-eye co-ordination
Various port entry techniques
Understanding of potential complications
Ability to care for postoperative surgical patients

Level 2
All of the above
Understanding of diathermy and lasers
Experience of haemostasis techniques
Use of staples, scissors, specimen retrieval systems

Level 3
Expertise and experience of retroperitoneal dissections
Experience of suturing techniques
Subspecialty training or experience in oncology or urogynaecology

---

trainee gynaecologist will be able to perform proficiently. These include laparoscopic sterilization and diagnostic laparoscopy.
- Level 2 procedures are those that would otherwise be referred to as intermediate. They may be performed on a routine basis by those with specific training, but not specialized gynaecologists. Examples include laparoscopic

tubal surgery, simple adhesiolysis and laparoscopic oophorectomy or ovarian cystectomy.

- Advanced laparoscopic surgery is classified as level 3. Qualification to perform this level of surgery will be gained after prolonged training to obtain surgical competence. Examples of level 3 procedures include pelvic and para-aortic lymphadenectomy, colposuspension and vaginal vault suspension procedures.

There are recognized level 1 and 2 laparoscopy training courses around the country, the details of which can be obtained from the RCOG. Many trainers have recognized the value of simulating exercises in the training of laparoscopic surgeons so laboratories have been established to teach and assess practical skills in a variety of centres around the country. Hand–eye co-ordination exercises are now widespread and many are quite imaginative.

Computer simulations will play an increasing part in the training of laparoscopic surgeons. Already simple exercises based on surgical procedures are available through the MistVR® system. More complicated simulators are being developed so that surgeons can learn techniques in virtual reality systems in an attempt to avoid some of the learning curve encountered with patients. It is perfectly logical to assume that surgeons will in the future have to demonstrate their competence on these virtual reality systems before being allowed to operate on patients. Reproducible tests of dextrous ability can be used as part of the assessment process when determining which candidate should be appointed to a particular specialty post.

SPECIALIST TECHNIQUES

Laparoscopic suturing

Laparoscopic suturing can be avoided in many procedures, but is an important skill for the advanced laparoscopic surgeon. Many experienced open surgeons are reluctant to pass through the sometimes humiliating learning curve required in order to master suturing techniques. However, it is simply a matter of 'practice making perfect' and laparoscopic suturing is an ideal exercise for the simulator.

Sutures are usually introduced through the accessory ports and care needs to be taken to ensure the needle is observed the entire time it is in the peritoneal cavity. Laparoscopic suturing is less forgiving than suturing at open surgery and this is classically demonstrated with the curved needle. The correct surgical technique is to insert the tip of the needle into the tissue and then rotate the needle through the tissue in an arc that follows the exact curve of the needle. The needle-holder needs to be at right angles to the needle in order to fulfil this task. Poor surgical technique at open surgery often involves surgeons pushing a curved needle in a straight line through the tissues rather than rotating it through.

Some surgeons prefer to use a straight needle when suturing laparoscopically as this passes through the ports more easily. The principle of suture insertion remains the same by passing the needle through the tissues in a direction that mimics the shape of the needle.

Once the suture is appropriately placed, a knot can be tied either intracorporeally or extracorporeally, according to the

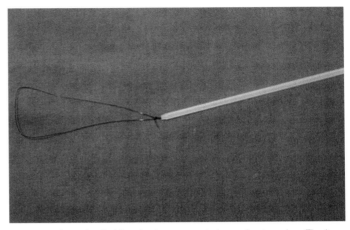

Fig. 4.8 A ready-tied Roeder knot mounted on a knot pusher. The loop is placed over the pedicle and the knot pushed tight by advancing the plastic pusher.

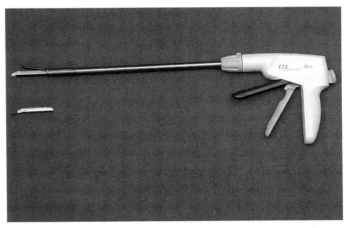

Fig. 4.9 The stapling device. The white handle is fixed, the grey lever closes the instrument and the black lever fires the staples and knife.

individual surgeon's preference and familiarity. Adequate strength knots can be tied by either method. An excellent review of both intracorporeal and extracorporeal knot tying is available at www.ethicon.com through links to their endo-surgery division.

Pretied sutures

The endo-loop is a simple technique for applying a suture to a pedicle, pushing down a pretied knot (Fig. 4.8). These pretied sutures employ a Roeder knot and are extremely useful either as a time-saving device or for less experienced laparoscopic surgeons.

Stapling

Mechanical stapling devices have helped revolutionize laparoscopic surgery and encouraged a generation of surgeons to utilize these precision instruments (Figs 4.9 and 4.10). The device usually inserts three lines of carefully arranged titanium

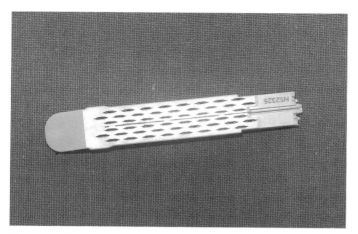

Fig. 4.10 The cartridge of the stapling device shows six rows of titanium staples separated in the centre by the knife tract.

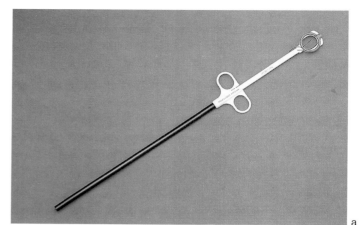

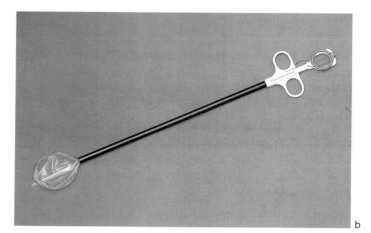

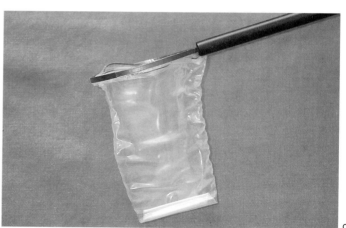

Fig. 4.11 The bag specimen retrieval system. Advancing the white plunger pushes the bag out of the introducer. The wire around the neck of the bag springs open.

staples, either side of a knife tract which allows the tissue to be divided when the staples are fired. It is an extremely efficient and rapid instrument which is particularly useful on the ovarian blood supply. Their major disadvantage is their expense and the diameter of the instrument which ensures a 12 mm port is required. They do need to be applied with great care and the surgeon needs to ensure that only the desired tissue is secure within the jaws of the device. In the use of this instrument the surgeon has to be particularly aware that the view on the monitor is only provided in two dimensions. The tips of the stapling device must be visualized before firing.

Specimen removal

Many laparoscopic operations are initially straightforward, such as an oophorectomy for a large ovarian cyst. The pedicle is well defined and a stapling device placed over this removes the organ from its attachments with ease. Very often, the most difficult part of the procedure is actually removing the specimen without increasing the size of the incisions on the abdominal wall. A number of devices have been employed in order to make this extraction easier. The most commonly used specimen retrieval system utilizes a bag such as the Endo-catch bag in Figure 4.11. The bag comes prefolded and once inserted into the abdominal cavity, springs open, allowing the specimen to be inserted. The edges of the bag are brought to the surface and the specimen removed without spilling its contents into the peritoneal cavity. A large cyst can be deflated extracorporeally for easy removal.

For larger cysts and for more solid structures, such as fibroids, alternative methods of specimen removal may be necessary. A posterior colpotomy can be extended with ease to 4 or 5 cm diameter without increasing discomfort or recovery time for the patient. Large-volume specimen bags can be inserted through the posterior fornix and wrapped around large ovarian cysts or fibroids. The neck of the bag can be brought through the incision in the posterior fornix and the specimen either morcellated or deflated through a much larger incision than is required for the abdominal ports. Figures 4.12–4.20 demonstrate the removal of a 7 cm pedunculated fibroid using a pos-

terior colpotomy. Initially, the fibroid is fixed with a suture to avoid it being displaced into the upper abdomen under the influence of gravity once it is disconnected from the uterus (Fig. 4.13). A straightforward Endo-GIA staple disconnects the fibroid from the uterus and the fibroid is brought down to the posterior colpotomy by pulling on the suture (Figs 4.15, 4.16, 4.17). Transvaginally, the posterior colpotomy is extended and

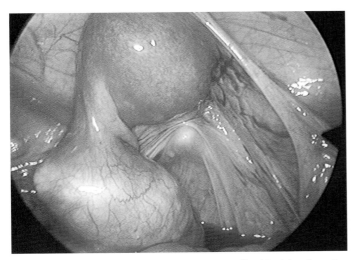

Fig. 4.12   This uterus has a pedunculated 7 cm fibroid arising from the left side of the fundus. An instrument can be seen causing an indentation in the posterior fornix.

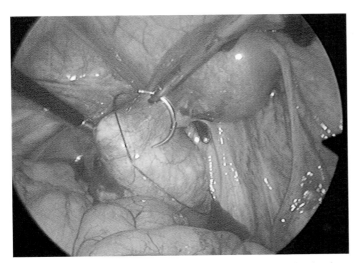

Fig. 4.13   A suture has been introduced through the posterior fornix and is passed through the fibroid to fix the specimen.

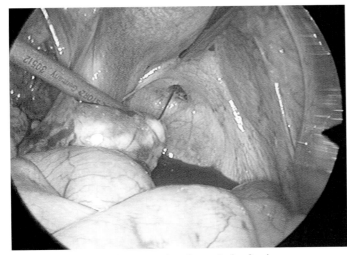

Fig. 4.14   The suture is returned to the posterior fornix.

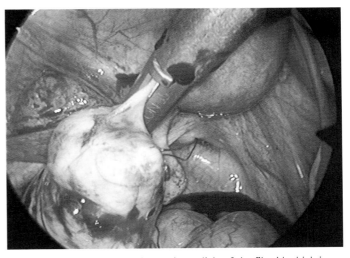

Fig. 4.15   A staple is placed over the pedicle of the fibroid which is divided.

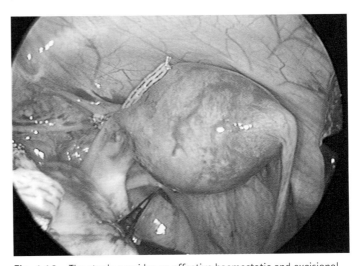

Fig. 4.16   The staple provides an effective haemostatic and excisional device. Despite the patient being in steep Trendelenburg tilt, the separated fibroid remains fixed by the suture through the posterior fornix.

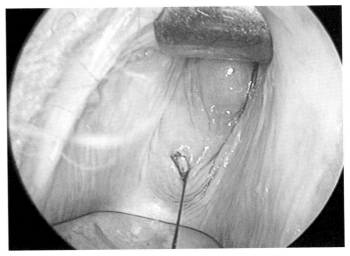

Fig. 4.17   The view vaginally shows the suture passing through into the peritoneal cavity.

the fibroid morcellated to remove the specimen (Figs 4.18, 4.19). The posterior colpotomy is repaired either vaginally or laparoscopically with precision.

Mechanical morcellators are an alternative way of removing the fibroids or the fundus and body of the uterus if a subtotal hysterectomy is performed. Extreme care needs to be taken with mechanical morcellators as they are dangerous if the wrong tissue is grasped inadvertently. They require considerable patience and are another piece of expensive theatre equipment.

Lasers and electrodiathermy

The use of lasers and electrodiathermy is covered elsewhere in this text (see Chapter 5). Progress in this area of technology has allowed many diagnostic laparoscopies to be converted into effective therapeutic treatment.

Gasless laparoscopy

It is possible to operate within the peritoneal cavity without distending it using carbon dioxide (Chin et al 1993, Wood et al 1994). A rigid mechanical support is required in order to elevate the anterior abdominal wall so that the viscera can be identified. The advantage of gasless laparoscopy is the avoidance of insufflators and their possible complications and the use of simpler trocars. The possibility of gas emboli is abolished and there is some evidence that carbon dioxide insufflation encourages the dissemination of metastatic intraperitoneal tumour. For this reason, some oncology procedures are performed without carbon dioxide distension.

However, most gasless laparoscopy techniques require extra portals in order to insert the mechanical device for visualization. It is not a technique that has become widespread.

COMPLICATIONS OF LAPAROSCOPY

The complications associated with port entry have already been mentioned earlier in this chapter and generally this is the most dangerous time for the patient. However, laparoscopic surgery can have many of the same complications as open surgery, depending on the complexity of any procedure. A list of possible complications is seen in Box 4.4.

Once access has been obtained and the laparoscope inserted then accessory ports have to be placed. These need to avoid the inferior epigastric vessels which supply the anterior abdominal wall. They can invariably be visualized even in the most obese of patients by remembering they originate from the external iliac vessels as they enter the femoral canal and then run laterally to the obliterated umbilical vessels. The author usually places a left accessory port lateral to the inferior epigastric vessels and a further right-sided port medial to the inferior epigastrics. This allows the right-handed surgeon to operate in a straight line whilst opposing the instruments sufficiently for them to work together. Placing the right port lateral to the inferior epigastric vessels means the surgeon will have to reach over the patient to an instrument that is then aimed back towards the pelvis. This position is uncomfortable for long procedures.

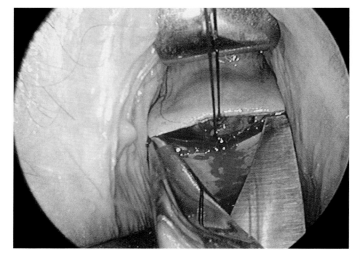

Fig. 4.18   The incision in the posterior fornix is enlarged to 3–4 cm.

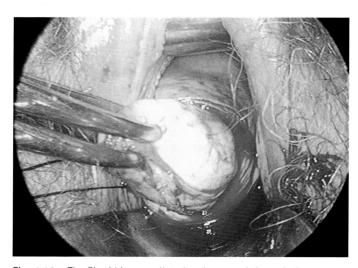

Fig. 4.19   The fibroid is morcellated and removed through the posterior fornix incision.

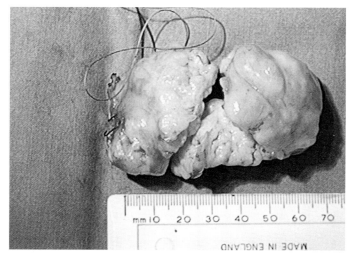

Fig. 4.20   Although morcellated, the fibroid is completely removed without the need to extend the abdominal incisions.

Box 4.4   Complications of laparoscopy

Primary trocar insertion
Bowel injury: transverse colon, small bowel
Vessel injury: common iliac arteries or veins, aorta, inferior vena cava
Bladder perforation
Damage to omentum
Surgical emphysema from extraperitoneal gas
Vasovagal reflex during gas insertion

Secondary trocar insertion
Inferior epigastric vessels
Bowel injury

During the procedure
Anaesthetic complications: ventilatory problems, CO_2 absorption
Visceral injury: recognized, unrecognized, direct, secondary to diathermy, etc., contamination of operative field
Haemorrhage: circulatory compromise, visual loss
Equipment failure: cameras, lighting, diathermy, staples, sutures, etc.

Postoperative
Fluid balance
Pain relief
Thromboembolic
Unrecognized visceral injury
Port site hernia

Once the accessory trocars are inserted complications will depend on the procedure and will be similar to open surgery. During steep Trendelenburg tilt the pressure required to ventilate the patient will increase and carbon dioxide absorption can be a problem in those with borderline pulmonary function. As with any type of surgery, trust and understanding between anaesthetist and surgeon are essential.

Damage to visceral structures can occur during any procedure but with laparoscopic surgery they can be more difficult to recognize. Dense adhesions may involve bowel and therefore the use of diathermy should be limited. Inadvertent diathermy damage by direct current transfer, direct or capacitive coupling may occur.

Postoperatively patients should be more mobile and make a quicker recovery as a result of smaller abdominal wounds. Serious complications such as unrecognized visceral injury may occur in the first few days and it is essential that these are immediately rectified. All surgeons get complications and any surgeon who does not believe it possible that their patient could sustain a complication from a laparoscopic procedure is a potentially dangerous surgeon. As a general rule, all patients should continue to improve from 24 hours after any laparoscopic procedure. If this does not occur then consideration should be given to intraoperative visceral injury and the patient investigated further with possible return to theatre before they collapse.

Medium- and long-term laparoscopic complications are rare. Incisional hernias have been reported particularly in slim patients where larger (10–12 mm) ports are used lateral to the rectus muscle. These can usually be avoided by closure of the rectus sheath and ensuring that when removing the primary trocars at the same time as the pneumoperitoneum no omentum has become drawn into the wound.

USES OF LAPAROSCOPY

Diagnostic

All gynaecologists perform diagnostic laparoscopies for multiple indications. It is a common investigation for pelvic pain, infertility, assessment of pelvic masses and in trials to assess clinical efficacy of treatment. There is virtually no indication for a diagnostic laparotomy in current medical practice. All clinicians would agree that the diagnostic laparoscopy is a quick, easy and safe way of assessing the peritoneal cavity, while causing minimal discomfort and allowing the patient rapid recovery.

Therapeutic

If a therapeutic laparoscopic procedure can be performed with ease and without putting the patient in increased danger then there is no question about its efficacy. Clinicians would agree that a diagnostic laparotomy is unnecessary, has a long recovery period and significant minor morbidity. It is therefore logical to extend this principle into the area of therapeutics. There are many procedures that are clearly better performed laparoscopically and these should be made available to all patients. It is the responsibility of health authorities, hospital administration and local clinicians to ensure that this logical and sensible approach is available for their patients. Examples of procedures that should normally be performed laparoscopically are given in Box 4.1.

The debate about laparoscopic surgery becomes more involved when examining more complex gynaecological procedures. There is no doubt that the vast majority of procedures *can* be performed laparoscopically but that not all procedures *should* be performed laparoscopically. The dilemma is in determining which patient fits into which category and that will sometimes depend on who their surgeon is. This is not the place to discuss at length the use of laparoscopy in various operations. Laparoscopy is merely the route by which a procedure is performed. It is the appropriate operation rather than the route that is perhaps more important.

The debate concerning the route most suitable for a hysterectomy is an excellent example of the difficulties in determining where laparoscopic surgery is best used. For many years, the surgeon has had a choice of the vaginal or the abdominal route for removing the patient's uterus. The rates of vaginal hysterectomy vary enormously depending on which country the patient is treated in. However, we are still unclear about many of the circumstances in which a vaginal or abdominal hysterectomy is most suitable.

The frequently quoted paper from Dicker et al (1982), where a third of hysterectomies were performed vaginally, demonstrates a faster recovery time and lower minor morbidity rate by this route. The major morbidity was infrequent in both groups, but considerably higher in the vaginal hysterectomy group. It seems logical that an easy vaginal hysterectomy would have minimal major complications and provide the patient with the shortest recovery period. However, as the procedure becomes more difficult, then the possibility of major complications increases. Judging when to dismiss the advantages of shorter recovery and look for the lower major morbidity rate is a problem not standardized.

It is most desirable to perform a vaginal hysterectomy under the easiest circumstances, but when the procedure is extremely difficult, an abdominal hysterectomy would be preferred. At some point between these two extremes, the lines cross. Laparoscopic hysterectomy was introduced as an attempt to make some of the more difficult vaginal hysterectomies easier. As a consequence, many patients who would have otherwise had an abdominal hysterectomy were offered a laparoscopic hysterectomy or a laparoscopic-assisted vaginal hysterectomy. Minor morbidity and recovery times for these patients are significantly reduced. Nevertheless, the question is raised as to whether the major morbidity is increased for a small minority. Certainly, at the early stages of some surgeons' learning curves, this was shown to be the case.

With a decreased number of hysterectomies being performed and significantly reduced surgical experience as a trainee, the opportunity to learn these techniques is limited. The vast majority of gynaecologists performing this surgery are inevitably self-taught. There are no scientifically reproducible data to show which factors should determine whether a patient has a vaginal, laparoscopic-assisted vaginal or abdominal hysterectomy. Indeed, the indications would be different for individual surgeons with varied surgical expertise – hence the debate continues.

There will obviously be some instances where one procedure is clearly preferred. Where prolapse exists, a vaginal hysterectomy is preferable. Where multiple intraperitoneal adhesions are expected or ovarian malignancy diagnosed, then clearly an abdominal approach is superior. For most stage I endometrial cancers where the peritoneal cavity needs to be inspected, washings taken, ovaries removed and possibly lymph node sampling performed, than a laparoscopic hysterectomy is superior.

As with the majority of situations, the real truth lies somewhere between the two extremes. Clinicians who have avoided learning laparoscopic surgical techniques need to accept that they have significantly improved the care of many patients and should be readily available. Conversely, some of the proponents of laparoscopic surgery need to accept that there is nothing clever about a procedure that results in increased serious morbidity.

KEY POINTS

1. As a result of smaller incisions, uncomplicated operations performed laparoscopically result in faster recovery and less postoperative pain.
2. The equipment required for laparoscopic surgery should be of good quality and well maintained.
3. Systematic training of surgeons is required using courses and simulators and a log of the case load.
4. The single most dangerous time in any laparoscopic procedure should be the insertion of the primary trocar. An understanding of anatomy and surgical principles is necessary in order to minimize the risk.

KEY POINTS (CONTINUED)

5. Various techniques are available to make laparoscopic surgery easier. These include staples, pretied knots, specimen retrieval bags and in the future may utilize robotics.
6. Virtually all operations can be performed laparoscopically but not all should be performed laparoscopically.

REFERENCES

Audebert AJM 1998 Laparoscopic ovarian surgery and ovarian torsion. In: Sutton C, Diamond MP (Eds) Endoscopic surgery for Gynecologists. W B Saunders, Philadelphia

Bonjer HJ, Hazebrook EJ, Kazemier G, Giuffrida MC, Meijer WS, Lange JF 1997 Open versus closed establishment of pneumoperitoneum in laparoscopic surgery. British Journal of Surgery 84:599–602

Bozzini P 1805 Der lichtleiter odere beschreibung einer eingachen vorrichtung und ihrer anwendung zur erleuchung innerer hohlen und zwischeraume deslebenden animaleschen corpses. Landes-Industrie-Comptoi, Weimer

Chapron C, Querleu D, Bruhat M A et al 1998 Surgical complications of diagnostic and operative gynaecological laparoscopy: a series of 29,966 cases. Human Reproduction 13:867–872

Chin A K, Moll F H, McColl M B, Reiv H 1993 Mechanical peritoneal retraction as a replacement for carbon dioxide pneumoperitoneum. Journal of the American Association of Gynecologic Laparoscopists 1:62–66

Clements R V 1995 Major vessel injury. Clinical Risk 1:112–115

Dicker R C, Scally MJ, Greenspan JR et al 1982 Hysterectomy amoung women of reproductive age – trends in USA 1970–78 JAMA 248:323–327

Desmoreaux AJ 1865 De l'endoscopie et de sas applications au diagnostic et au traitement des affections de l'uretre et de la vessie. Baillière, Paris

Dingfelder JR 1978 Direct laparoscopic trocar insertion without prior pneumoperitoneum. Journal of Reproductive Medicine 21:45–47

Garry R 2000 Towards evidence based laparoscopic entry techniques: clinical problems and dilemmas. Gynaecological Endoscopy 8(6):315–326

Hasson HM 1971 A modified instrument and method for laparoscopy. American Journal of Obstetrics and Gynecology 110:886–887

Hope R 1937 The differential diagnosis of ectopic pregnancy in peritoneoscopy. Surgery, Gynecology and Obstetrics 64:229–234

Jacobaeus HC 1910 Uber due Moglichkeil die Zystoskopie bei Untersuchlung seroser Hohlungen anzerwerden. Munchener Medizinische Wochenschrift 57:2090–2092

Phillips G, Garry R, Kumar C, Reich H 1999 How much gas is required for initial insufflation at laparoscopy? Gynaecological Endoscopy 8:369–374

Pickersgill A, Slade RJ, Falconer GF, Attwood S 1999 Open laparoscopy: the way forward. British Journal of Gynaecology and Obstetrics 106:1116–1119

Reich H, DeCaprio J, McGlynn F 1989 Laparoscopic hysterectomy. Journal of Gynecologic Surgery 5:213–216

Steptoe PC 1967 Laparoscopy in gynaecology. E&S Livingstone, Edinburgh

Sutton CJG, Ewen SP, Whitelaw N, Haines P 1994 Prospective, randomised, double-blind controlled trial of laser laparoscopy in the treatment of pelvic pain associated with minimal, mild, and moderate endometriosis. Fertility and Sterility 62:696–700

Veress J 1938 Neues instrument fur ausfuhrung von brust–oder brachpunktionen und pneumothoraxbehandlung. Deutsche Medizinische Wochenschrift 104:1480–1481

von Ott D 1901 Ventroscopic illumination of the abdominal cavity in pregnancy. Zhurnal Akrestierstova I Zhenskikh Boloznei 15:7–8

Wood G, Maher P, Hill D 1994 Current states of laparoscopic associated hysterectomy. Gynaecological Endoscopy 3:75–84

Yao M, Tulandi T 1997 Current status of surgical and nonsurgical management of ectopic pregnancy. Fertility and Sterility 67:421–433

Zollikofer R 1924 Zur Laparoskopie. Schweizerische Medizinische Wochenschrift 15:264–265

5
Diathermy and lasers
Anthony R.B. Smith   John Parsons

INTRODUCTION

For many years diathermy was the technique of choice for tissue resection and destruction in both gynaecology and general surgery. The advent of the laser in the 1960s threatened this supremacy but during the last decade advances in diathermy have led to a more balanced position between the two modalities. The aim of this chapter is to explain briefly the operation of these instruments, tissue effects, common system types, some of the safety aspects involved and practical clinical use of both techniques in gynaecology.

DIATHERMY

Diathermy has been used in surgical procedures for over 100 years (d'Arsonval 1893) for cutting and coagulation of tissues. Harvey Cushing pioneered the use of electrosurgery in neurosurgery, using a generator designed by Bovie in the 1920s, and this name is still synonymous with diathermy to some surgeons.

Although diathermy is still a much-used tool in surgical practice few surgeons have received formal training in its use. Operating theatres will often have a variety of diathermy units for which 'standard' settings are used without reference to the operating conditions. In conventional open surgery this has presented only a few hazards. The development of laparoscopic and hysteroscopic surgery has greatly increased the number of applications for electrosurgery and has presented new dangers. Only by having an understanding of the principles of this energy source will surgeons avoid the risk of injury to the patient, theatre staff and themselves.

Electrosurgery refers to both types of diathermy, monopolar or bipolar, in which current passes through the patient's tissue. In monopolar diathermy the active electrode and return electrode are some distance apart. In bipolar diathermy two electrodes are only millimetres apart. Electrocautery refers to the use of a heating element in which no current passes through the patient.

Monopolar diathermy

In monopolar diathermy, one electrode is applied to the patient who becomes part of the circuit. The surface area of the electrode plate is much greater than the contact area of the diathermy instrument to ensure that heating effects are confined to the end of the active electrode (Fig. 5.1). The advantage of monopolar diathermy is that it can be used to cut as well as to coagulate tissues.

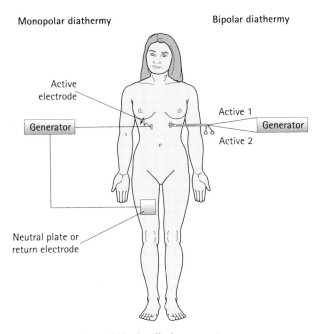

Fig. 5.1   Monopolar and bipolar diathermy systems.

Tissue effects of diathermy

When household electrical current of 50 Hz frequency passes through the body it causes an irreversible depolarization of cell membranes. If the current is sufficiently large, depolarization of cardiac muscles will occur and death may result. If household current is modified to a higher frequency, above 200 Hz, depolarization does not occur; instead, ions are excited to produce a thermal effect. This is the basis of diathermy. Figure 5.2 illustrates how the frequency of a current influences the effects on the body.

Factors which influence the effect of diathermy

1. The diathermy current
   - Current density
   - Size of the current
2. The current waveform
   - Cutting and coagulation current
3. The type of tissue
   - Tissue moisture
4. Duration of application
5. Size and shape of diathermy electrode

The diathermy current

The amount of damage or thermal injury diathermy produces is determined by the current density and the size of the current.

The current density at the tip of a needle electrode will be very high because the current is concentrated into a small point. The plate used for the return electrode in monopolar diathermy has a large surface area of contact, resulting in a much lower current density. Any thermal effect will therefore be widely dissipated. This highlights the need for the whole surface of the plate to be attached securely to the body. If the plate becomes partially detached the current density will be greater in the remaining attached part and a burn may result.

The size of the current is influenced by the voltage potential and the resistance to current flow according to the following equation:

Current (amps) = potential (volts)/impedance or tissue resistance (ohms)

Turning up the power output of an electrosurgical unit will increase the size of the diathermy current if the resistance remains constant. Some electrosurgical units can automatically alter the voltage potential to keep the current constant if the resistance changes.

The resistance of tissue varies particularly with its water content. Dry tissue produces a high resistance and moist tissue a lower resistance. Thus, during diathermy of an area of tissue, it is dessicated by the thermal effect and its resistance will increase. To prevent the current flow falling some modern electrosurgical units will increase the voltage output. The surgeon should be aware of this because there are additional hazards to working with higher voltages. Insulation failure, capacitance coupling and direct coupling are all more likely with a higher voltage.

Cutting and coagulation

Coagulation or cutting can be achieved by changing the area of contact or the waveform of the current. The cutting waveform is a low-voltage, higher frequency current but area of contact is the main factor and a cutting effect is achieved when the cutting electrode is not quite in contact with the tissue so that an electrical arc is formed. This causes the water in the cells to vaporize and the cells to explode as they come into contact with the arc. The power and current levels will rise when cutting takes place inside a liquid-filled cavity such as the bladder or uterus. The surgeon must be aware that if the resistance increases when using cutting current (for example, when cutting through the cervix with a wire loop) some generators will produce a higher voltage to maintain current flow against the increased resistance.

When the electrode is brought into direct contact with tissue and the waveform is modulated, coagulation rather than vaporization occurs. An intermittent waveform is used and thus bursts of thermal energy are insterspersed with periods of no energy (Fig. 5.3). For the power delivered to the tissue to remain constant, the electrosurgical unit must deliver a higher voltage to compensate for the episodes when no energy is delivered (up to 90% of the time with pure coagulation current). Thus whilst cutting current at 50 W power will produce a high-frequency current of 500–1000 V, a coagulation current will produce over 3000 volts to deliver the same wattage to the tissue. The coagulating effects is produced by slower desiccation and shrinkage of adjacent tissue, producing haemostasis. The higher voltage produced by coagulation current carries a higher risk of inadvertent discharge of energy.

If a mixture of the two types of waveform is employed then the advantages of both techniques are exploited. This is normally termed 'blended' output and many combinations are possible.

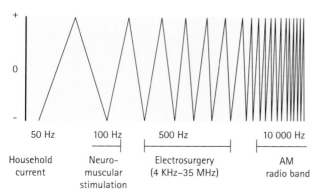

Fig. 5.2 Current frequency spectrum.

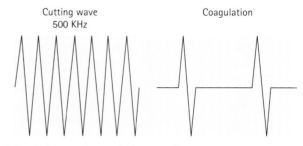

Fig. 5.3 Cutting and coagulation waveforms.

The type of tissue

Tissue moisture is the major factor affecting tissue resistance; the higher the moisture content, the lower the resistance and the higher the current flow. The cervix in a postmenopausal woman will have a lower water content than that of a young nulliparous woman. A lower wattage will be required to perform a loop biopsy in the latter case.

Duration of application

The longer the duration of application of electrosurgical current, the greater the extent of thermal injury. Research on uterine tissue shows that the duration of exposure of the tissue to current, rather than the wattage used, was the most important factor in producing tissue damage (Duffy et al 1991).

Size and shape of the diathermy electrode

The smaller the point of contact, the greater will be the current density. Thus, if the points of diathermy scissors are brought close to tissue, a cutting effect will result whilst if the convex part of the scissor blades is used, a lower current density will result with a coagulating effect. Similarly, when using a wire loop to biopsy the cervix, the thickness of the wire will influence the current; a thicker wire will need a higher current than a finer wire to produce a cutting effect because of the lower current density.

Heat and tissue injury

Diathermy current produces thermal injury to tissues. The temperature generated will dictate the degree of injury (Table 5.1). If carbon is seen on the tip of the diathermy electrode the surgeon can assume that at some stage a temperature of 200°C has been reached.

Bipolar diathermy

In bipolar diathermy, the current flows between two electrodes a short distance apart because both contacts are on the surgical instrument. Lower power is employed since high power would damage the tips of the instrument. This is safer because the current flow is limited to a small area and lower power is used but a cutting effect cannot be achieved. These features encourage some surgeons to employ bipolar diathermy exclusively in the laparoscopic environment. However, there is still a risk of aberrant current flow because the patient, table and diathermy machine are all earthed. In addition, the tissue temperatures are much higher (340°C) and this itself can cause unexpected effects.

Bipolar current produces tissue desiccation and has been used commonly in tubal sterilization. More recently, in laparosopic surgery its value in coagulating major vascular pedicles has led to its use in laparoscopic hysterectomy and laparoscopic salpingectomy for ectopic pregnancy. The lower power employed also leads to less heat spread to adjacent tissues, which reduces the risk of injury to nearby delicate structures. Engineers are endeavouring to produce reliable bipolar dissectors and scissors to compete with the range of monopolar diathermy instruments available.

Bipolar instrumentation has also been introduced into hysteroscopic surgery. A bipolar electrode may be employed in the outpatient setting for removal of endometrial polyps although such instrumentation is somewhat expensive.

Short-wave diathermy

Electrode redesign has led to an interest in the use of short-wave diathermy for tissue destructive effect (Phipps et al 1990). In this the two electrodes form a capacitor in the output circuit with the patient providing the dielectric medium between the two plates. Frequencies of around 27 MHz are employed with power levels of about 500 W. By altering the shape and size of the electrodes, heating effects may be localized or diffused as required. However, care must be exercised as the effects are not always predictable.

Diathermy safety

Three major safety issues with the use of monopolar diathermy have become apparent with the evolution of electro-surgery in laparoscopic surgery. They each involve inadvertent discharge of diathermy current.

- Insulation failure
- Direct coupling
- Capacitative coupling.

Insulation failure

Defects in insulation are most likely to cause a discharge of current when higher power is employed. The use of 'coagulation current' carries a greater risk than 'cutting current'. Insulation failure can occur at any point from the electrosurgical unit to the active electrode. The most common site of failure is in the instrument that contains the active electrode. With conventional surgical instruments the most common site is the joint on diathermy graspers where repeated use wears away the insulation material. Any insulation breakdown, seen as sparks from the joint area, is usually clearly visible because the whole instrument is within the surgeon's field of view. This contrasts with laparoscopic surgery where the field of view is much smaller and only a small part of the instrument containing the active electrode may be visible. Repeated discharges from a break in the insulation may occur without the surgeon being aware of it. Damage to insulation most commonly occurs when moving an instrument through the laparoscopic port. Although the port valve may cause damage the most likely cause is scraping against the sharp edge of the inner end of the port, particularly one constructed of metal.

Concern about insulation failure has fuelled the debate about disposable and reusable instruments. Disposable instruments clearly have an advantage in that the insulation

Table 5.1 The degree of injury caused at different temperatures

Temperature °C	Tissue effect
44	Necrosis
70	Coagulation
90	Dessication
200	Carbonization

sheath does not have to withstand both repeated use and repeated cleaning cycles. However, the disposable instruments are built to much less robust specifications and the insulating material may not withstand harsh treatment in a long case. It is important that surgeons and theatre nurses are constantly vigilant for evidence of trauma to insulation and reusable instruments must be checked on a regular basis both during and between cases.

Whilst a metal port may cause more trauma to the instruments passing through it, it will allow discharge of diathermy current in the event of an insulation failure. The large area of port contact with the skin should enable the current to be dissipated without serious thermal injury. A plastic port would not facilitate such a discharge and the current might therefore flow to adjacent bowel, causing damage that may not be recognized at the time. Sigmoid colon is the most vulnerable piece of bowel because of its proximity to a left lateral port. If a metal port cannula is used a plastic retaining sleeve must not be used because this prevents any discharged diathermy current passing through the skin back to the ground plate.

Direct coupling

Direct coupling involves the transmission of diathermy current from one instrument to another. Many surgeons use direct coupling to coagulate small vessels which have been grasped with a small forceps, when opening a wound for example. The diathermy instrument is then placed against the small forceps and the pedal pressed. Such a practice carries a real risk of a diathermy burn to the surgeon or assistant. If the surgeon's glove has a perforation the diathermy current may flow through the surgeon to ground either through the feet or through contact with the operating table. The surgeon should also be aware that theatre gowns do not provide insulations against high-frequency diathermy current.

The risk of direct coupling will be reduced in laparoscopic surgery if only insulated instruments are used when diathermy is employed. Since many instruments, such as needle-holders, are not commonly produced with insulation this may restrict instrument choice. The risk of direct coupling to a metal port is increased when the working part of the laparoscopic instrument is large. The surgeon must always try to keep the whole of the metal part visible when using diathermy so that any inadvertent discharge will be seen.

Capacitative coupling

The concept of capacitative coupling is new to most gynaecologists. A capacitor consists of two conductors separated by an insulator. A metal instrument surrounded by an insulated sheath passing through a metal port is a capacitor. When a current passes through the instrument a capacitative current may develop in the metal port, particularly if it is insulated from the skin. The higher the current passing through the instrument, the greater will be the capacitative current. If the port is insulated from the skin (by a plastic sleeve) capacitative current may be discharged to adjacent bowel, causing thermal injury. In common with insulation failure, the sigmoid colon is most vulnerable to capacitative current injury due to its proximity to a left lateral port.

A capacitative current can also develop in a gloved hand holding a non-insulated instrument through which diathermy current is passed. This risk is greater if the hand is moist and there is contact between the surgeon and the operating table or the floor.

Other safety issues

Current flow to adjacent organs The current will follow the path of least resistance and if a non-target tissue like bowel lies in contact with target tissue, the current will flow through the tissue with least impedence. In addition, the impedence will rise as the target vessels dessicate and current may then flow to an alternative earth, usually but not necessarily in contact with the pedicle. If the current flows through bowel, damage will result which may not be recognized at the time.

Surgical clothing Operating theatre gowns do not provide insulation against high-frequency electrosurgical currents. This means that there is always a risk of discharge of electrosurgical current through to the operating table.

Operating theatre footwear used to provide 'antistatic' protection. Antistatic theatre shoes were used to prevent build-up of static electricity, which could spark and ignite volatile anaesthetic gases. Since such agents are no longer employed in anaesthesia there is no need for antistatic footwear. Non-antistatic footwear will generally provide a higher resistance between the surgeon and ground and will therefore reduce the risk of discharge through the surgeon to ground.

Electrosurgical unit The surgeon should be familiar with the electrosurgical unit in the theatre. Many departments have different units available with different settings and features. The power delivered by a numerical setting may vary greatly in different machines. Many units divide the power output in settings from 1 to 10. Position 5 in one unit may represent a different power output to position 5 in another unit. In addition, there will not always be equal differences between the unit settings so that there may be a different change in output between 1 and 2 than between 8 and 9. Modern units have overcome this hazard by indicating the power setting on a digital display.

Changes in electrosurgical unit Prior to 1970 all electrosurgical units had a 'grounded design' which provided numerous potential alternative pathways for the discharge of diathermy current to ground, e.g. ECG leads. In 1970 isolated electrosurgery units were introduced. This meant that the ground electrode discharge returned to the electrosurgical unit. Thus the whole circuit of electrosurgical current passed through the unit. Whilst this arrangement reduced the risk of inappropriate grounding routes it did not solve the risk of burns from poor contact of the ground electrode with the patient. Poor contact leads to the development of high current density areas and a subsequent heating effect.

After 1980 electrosurgical units employed a return electrode monitoring system, which detects failure of contact of the ground electrode. Ground plate burns will be avoided with this system.

Since 1990 the growth of minimal access surgery has increased the risks of inadvertent discharge from the active electrode through insulation failure or capacitative coupling.

The Active Electrode Monitoring system now marketed by Encision provides an additional protective shield on the active electrode instrument, which picks up discharge of current from any point other than the active part of the electrode and inactivates the unit if such current is detected.

Electrosurgical equipment set-up　It is critically important to be certain that the diathermy ground plate is securely attached in the correct postion. Whilst modern machines will give a warning signal when the plate is incorrectly attached, many machines will function if there is partial attachment. Partial attachment may lead to severe burns.

The positioning of the diathermy leads to and from the operating table needs care and attention. Capacitance current can develop alongside the diathermy lead delivering current to the active electrode anywhere along its length. Diathermy leads should not be secured with metal clips to the theatre gowns covering the patients.

Theatre staff must be trained in the use of electrosurgical equipment. Protocols for who attaches the equipment and who switches the machine on should be in place. If a patient's position is changed during the course of an operation the electrosurgical unit should be switched off prior to the move and the attachment of the ground electrode should be checked after repositioning.

Risk of fire/explosion　Flammable materials should not be used for skin preparation in gynaecological surgery. Theatre gowns can soak up such solutions which may also pool in the vagina or under the buttocks. Fires have been reported caused by sparks from diathermy current igniting flammable cleansing material.

Pacemakers　Monopolar diathermy should be avoided in patients with internal or external catheter pacemakers. There is a risk of inducing a rhythm disturbance, damage to the device or even electrical burns around the device. If monopolar diathermy is used, short bursts in the cutting mode are advisable. The pacemaker should not lie in the pathway of the diathermy current but this will not guarantee safety as it is known that radiofrequency current can radiate away from a straight pathway. The electrosurgical unit should be placed as far away from the pacemaker as possible because of the risk of 'noise' from the generator. When diathermy is required a bipolar instrument should be used whenever possible.

Keloid scarring　Keloid scarring has a high tissue resistance so the diathermy ground electrode should not be placed over an area of keloid.

Joint prostheses　The joint prosthesis most commonly encountered by a gynaecologist is in the hip joint. If the prosthesis is unilateral the diathermy ground plate should be sited on the opposite side. If bilateral prostheses are present the ground plate should be placed on the flank. If a ground plate is sited over a prosthesis, current may be concentrated through the prosthesis in a preferential pathway and also in the tissue between the plate and the prosthesis and a thermal injury may occur.

LASERS

A laser is a device capable of producing near-parallel beams of monochromatic light, either visible or invisible, at controlled intensities. This light can be focused, thus concentrating its energy, so that it can then be utilized to treat various conditions. The term 'laser' is an acronym for "Light Amplification by the Stimulated Emission of Radiation". The process of stimulated emission was foreshadowed by Einstein at the turn of the century but it was not until 1960 that the first optical device was constructed (Maiman 1960). Since that time many lasers have been made but comparatively few have found their way into gynaecological practice.

Basic laser physics

A laser consists of three main elements: a power supply, an excitable medium and an optical resonator (Fig. 5.4). Atoms or molecules within the medium are raised to high-energy states (Fig. 5.5a) by the power supply and under normal circumstances these would decay to the ground state by the emission of the energy as photons (Fig. 5.5b). By confining the process to an optical cavity and restricting the decay paths, stimulated emission (Fig. 5.5c) can take place. This process produces a build-up of photons (light) at a particular wavelength inside

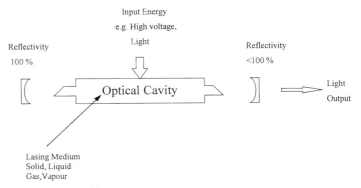

Fig. 5.4　Typical laser systems.

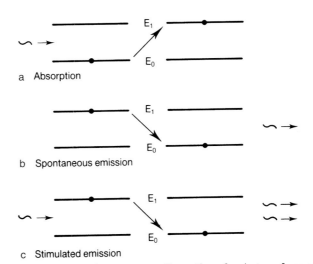

Fig. 5.5　Basic atomic processes. **a** Absorption of a photon of energy; **b** spontaneous emission of a photon; **c** stimulated emission of an additional photon of energy, $\sim$, photon; E_0, lower energy state; E_1, higher energy state; ●, particle.

the cavity. The laser output is a small fraction of this which is allowed to escape from one end of the cavity.

Many substances have been found to be suitable laser media–solids, liquids, gases or metallic vapours–but the basic principles remain the same. A more detailed explanation of laser physics is provided elsewhere (Carruth & McKenzie 1986).

The radiation emitted is monochromatic (if only one decay path is involved), coherent and collimated. Collimation, or the near-parallel nature of laser light, can be exploited in many ways and it is the main feature which makes such devices useful in the medical world. A single convex lens placed in the beam will bring it to a sharp focus, the size of which is dependent upon the width of the collimated beam. The use of different lenses or varying the lens-to-tissue distance alters the diameter of the beam at the point of contact with the tissue (Fig. 5.6). This is referred to as changing the spot size.

The most important determinant of the effects of a laser upon tissue is the power density (PD). This can be calculated roughly as:

$$PD = 100 \times W/D^2 \text{ watts/cm}^2$$

where PD is power density, W is power output in watts and D is the effective diameter of the spot in millimetres. D can be measured by firing a short low-power pulse at a suitable target. The power density can be altered by changing either the power or the spot size but the latter has the greater effect.

Light–tissue interaction

Light impinging on tissue is subject to the normal laws of physics. Some of the light is reflected and some is transmitted through the air–tissue barrier and passes into the tissue where it is scattered or absorbed. Obviously the extent to which each process dominates is dependent upon the physical properties of the light and the tissue. The theory of light–tissue interaction is not as well developed as that of ionizing radiation (Wall et al 1988) but enough is known to explain the macroeffects upon which most laser treatments depend.

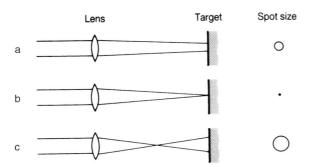

Fig. 5.6 Changing the focal length of the focusing lens while keeping the lens-to-tissue distance constant alters the spot size, the diameter of the beam at the point of contact with the tissue. **a** The focal length of the lens is greater than the lens-to-tissue distance; **b** the focal length of the lens is the same as the lens-to-tissue distance, i.e. the laser is focused on the tissue; **c** the focal length of the lens is less than the lens-to-tissue distance.

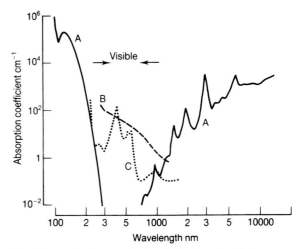

Fig. 5.7 Absorption characteristics of **A** water; **B** melanin; **C** haemoglobin at different wavelengths. After Boulnois (1986).

At very low-energy density levels (power density × time), say below 4 J/cm², a stimulating effect on cells has been observed but above this level the effect is reversed and suppression occurs (Mester et al 1968). As the energy density rises to 40 J/cm², indirect cell damage can take place if any sensitizing agents present become activated (e.g. haemato-porphyrin derivative). Direct tissue damage does not take place until about 400 J/cm² when the first thermal effects appear and photocoagulation occurs. Another 10-fold increase in energy density results in complete tissue destruction as it is sufficient to raise the cell temperature rapidly to 100°C, causing tissue vaporization. Obviously these are general observations and other properties of the incident beam will have an influence but the general 10-fold relationship alluded to above holds even though other parameters may be varied. Amongst the most important of these are the wavelength and the pulsatile nature of the radiation involved.

The wavelength absorption characteristics of various body tissues are reasonably well understood, qualitatively if not quantitatively. Figure 5.7 shows the absorption curves for water, melanin and haemoglobin which, to a large extent, will determine the curves for tissue as a whole. In the ultraviolet and the middle-to-far infrared spectrum, absorption by water predominates whereas melanin and haemoglobin effects take over in the visible range. From this graph it is easy to see that a particular laser, operating at a fixed wavelength, will be preferentially absorbed by one tissue constituent and its effects will be different from those to another laser with a different wavelength.

So far it is implied that the laser is operated continuously for long enough for thermal effects to appear (continuous wave or CW mode). However, it is relatively simple, by means of a shutter or a controllable power supply, to switch the energy on and off rapidly – the pulse mode. In general the medical definition of a pulse is a burst of energy lasting 0.25 s or less. This does not correspond to the physics definition of a pulse and care must be taken to avoid confusion. Methods of generating these pulses differ between lasers and the tissue effects can also vary. The reason for this phenomenon is shown in Figure 5.8.

Minton JP, Carlton DM, Dearman JR et al 1965 An evaluation of the physical response of malignant tumour implants to pulsed laser radiation. Surgery, Gynecology and Obstetrics 121:538–544

Phipps JH, Lewis BV, Roberts T et al 1990 Treatment of functional menorrhagia by radiofrequency-induced thermal endometrial ablation. Lancet 335:374–376

Spikes JD, Jori G 1987 Photodynamic therapy of tumours and other diseases using porphyrins. Lasers in Medical Science 2:3–15

Stamp JM 1983 An introduction to medical lasers. Clinical Physics and Physiological Measurement 4:267–290

Wall BF, Harrison RM, Spiers FN 1988 Patient dosimetry techniques in diagnostic radiology. Institute of Physical Sciences in Medicine, York

6

Imaging techniques in gynaecology

Nandita deSouza   *David Cosgrove*

INTRODUCTION

Since the discovery of X-rays by Roentgen in 1895, there has been an explosion in technology for imaging the human body; not only ionizing radiation but also high-frequency sound (Wade 1999), radiolabelled pharmaceuticals and non-ionizing radiation in strong magnetic fields are used. The parallel expansion in computer technology has enabled the development of cross-sectional imaging using computed tomographic (CT) techniques and three-dimensional imaging using magnetic resonance (MR) imaging data.

METHODOLOGY

X-ray techniques

Standard radiographs are obtained by placing the patient between an X-ray source and a photographic film. Images are produced by the attenuation of X-ray photons by the patient. As a result, structures of interest are often obscured by the attenuation of photons by other overlying structures. A basic limitation of the standard X-ray technique is the effect of scattered photons adding to the image noise and degrading the quality of the final image. Various manoeuvres have been adopted to reduce this effect, for example scatter grids. The linear tomograph is obtained by the synchronous movement of the X-ray tube and the film, causing a blurring of the overlying and underlying structures while leaving the plane of interest in focus. This procedure increases the detection of lesions such as chest metastases.

Contrast studies

To increase contrast in the soft tissues, an iodine-containing agent may be injected into the lumen of a cavity such as the uterus and fallopian tubes (hysterosalpingogram) or blood vessels (angiogram). Such contrast agents are widely available in both ionic and more expensive non-ionic forms. The less toxic non-ionic preparations are preferred.

Ultrasound

In 1950 Ian Donald used an industrial flaw detector, designed for testing the integrity of steel boilers, to demonstrate that the massive abdominal swelling of one of his patients was fluid and not solid (Kurjak 2000). A large ovarian cyst that proved to be benign was subsequently removed. Since then, the rapid and continuing evolution of ultrasound technology has lead to a proliferation of applications in almost all aspects of medicine and surgery.

Ultrasound waves are generated by a piezoelectric crystal mounted in a transducer housing, the whole construction being referred to as a probe. Piezo materials respond to an applied voltage by changing thickness and correspondingly, they produce electrical signals of a few millivolts when compressed. While in the final image, the resolution along the beam is determined by the wavelength, resolution across it depends on the width of the beam, which is improved by focusing, using combinations of lenses and electronic mechanisms.

The time from the transmission of the ultrasound pulse to the receipt of an echo is translated into depth using the speed of sound in tissue. Echoes arise wherever the pulse of ultrasound encounters an interface between tissues of different acoustic impedance which may simplistically be regarded as changes in density. Thus, homogeneous materials such as clear fluids are echo free, while low-level echoes are given by the interfaces between the various components of soft tissue structures. Stronger echoes result from the interface between fibrous tissue (high impedance) and fatty tissues (low impedance) and maximal echoes are given by interfaces between soft tissues and bone or gas, both of which are effectively opaque to ultrasound. To form a real-time image, the beam is electronically swept through a region of tissue and the images are pie shaped (sector probes) or rectangular (linear probes).

The choice of frequency is a compromise between the spatial resolution and the depth of penetration required. The higher the frequency, the better the resolution but the greater the attenuation of the beam within the tissues. Hence, for abdominal scanning, frequencies of between 3.5 and 5 MHz are commonly employed. Probes designed for intracavitary and intraoperative use employ higher frequencies (8–15 MHz) because the organs of interest are closer to the transducer. This enables higher resolution images to be obtained and also allows study of the movement of structures when pressure is applied to the probe; this gives important diagnostic clues on their relative mobility. The drawbacks of transvaginal scanning are practical (intolerance of the probe by the very young and old and in the presence of scarring) and diagnostic (the depth of view is limited to about 70 mm) (Bennett & Richards 2000).

The interactivity of ultrasound is an important feature: it is almost an extension of clinical examination. Ultrasound also provides numerous views during real-time examination and facilitates guided needle biopsies. However, it has many limitations that frustrate its application, notably the variable image quality. An important problem is the complete barrier posed by bowel gas. That is why a full bladder is required for transabdominal scanning of the pelvis.

Doppler operates by detecting the change in frequency of ultrasound echoes caused by movement of the target. In the simplest system, this is done continuously with only minimal control of the beam direction. Continuous-wave Doppler is well suited to fetal heart monitoring, especially because movements of the fetus do not interrupt the signal. In gynaecology, the vessels of interest are small so that precise placement of the Doppler sample is a prerequisite. This can be achieved with pulsed Doppler. The Doppler gate is superimposed on a real-time image that allows the target to be pinpointed (Fig. 6.1). The Doppler signal depicts a range of blood velocities occurring in the selected vessel over time. Output can be audio or as a strip chart on which intensity indicates the strength of the signal at each velocity in the spectrum. A variety of measurements can be made from these tracings, the most useful of which are systolic/diastolic velocity ratios. These are measures of the arteriolar resistance to flow, with a low value indicating low vasomotor tone, typical of the placenta and the corpus luteum. This pattern also occurs in inflammation and malignancy. High indices are typical of inactive tissue, such as the resting uterus. Doppler can be used to measure fetal and uteroplacental blood flow, thereby producing physiological information from what was previously an anatomical imaging technique (Brinkman & Wladimiroff 2000).

In colour Doppler scanning the same process is applied across an area of interest. The velocity signals are presented as a colour-coded overlay, superimposed on the real-time scan (Fig. 6.2). Though the Doppler information is less rich than with spectral Doppler (only the mean velocity or the amount of flow is depicted), the angiogram-like map provides information

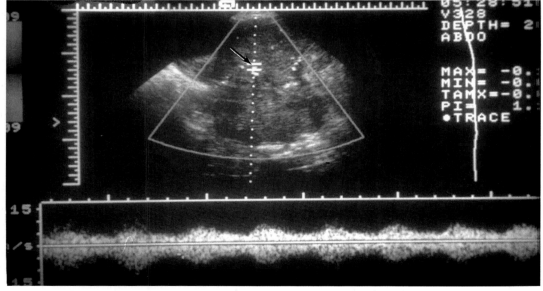

Fig. 6.1 Spectral Doppler. In this scan of an ovarian cancer, the Doppler gate (arrow) has been positioned on the tumour. The spectral tracing is in the lower portion of the figure and shows the typical low-resistance pattern of malignant neovascularization with marked diastolic flow.

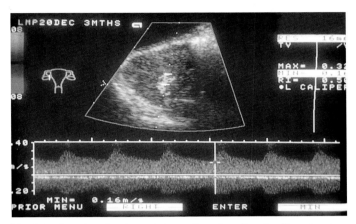

Fig. 6.2 Doppler of a corpus luteum. On colour Doppler, flow signals are colour coded for direction and velocity. The neovascularization in this corpus luteum is shown as a knot of colour. Apart from providing a graphic display of vascularity, a useful feature of colour Doppler is to guide placement of the gate for spectral Doppler tracings. Shown in the lower portion of the figure is a low impedance trace with flow throughout diastole. This is typical of growing tissue.

on the morphological arrangement of the vascular tree and its sensitivity allows vessels as small as a millimetre or so in diameter to be detected. Often colour Doppler is used to locate a vessel to guide placement of the spectral Doppler gate for haemodynamic analysis.

A recent advance has been the introduction of contrast agents for ultrasound in the form of microbubbles for injection. Not only does the signal improvement they produce allow smaller vessels to be detected but they can be visualized on grey scale to reveal regions of flow in real time. In addition, they can be used as tracers by tracking a bolus as it crosses a tissue of interest and this may yield valuable functional information.

Computed tomography

The sensitivity of conventional radiography may be improved by using a radiation detector such as a scintillation crystal and a photomultiplier tube. By measuring the attenuation of a finely collimated beam of radiation, passing through the patient at multiple angles, it has been possible to produce images of very high quality. A computer uses the attenuation of each beam passing through the patient to calculate the attenuation coefficient for each area of tissue in the cross-section of interest. The final images are reconstructed using a filtered back-projection technique and displayed in a grey scale as a series of attenuation units (with values between +500 and −500) in a matrix of 512×512 or 1024×1024 elements. The reconstruction of data is limited to the transverse (transaxial) plane. This technique of imaging revolutionized modern medicine in the 1970s but its impact on gynaecology has been less marked.

Magnetic resonance (MR) imaging

MR imaging depends upon the magnetic properties of certain atomic nuclei which, when placed within a magnetic field and stimulated by radio waves of a specific frequency, will absorb

and then re-emit some of this energy as a radio signal. This phenomenon of nuclear magnetic resonance (NMR) was first described by Felix Bloch and Edward Purcell in 1946. NMR as a basis for an imaging technique was proposed some 30 years later by Lauterbur.

Nuclei possessing magnetic properties have an odd number of protons or neutrons. The charged particles are spinning, which causes them to behave as tiny bar magnets. If placed within a magnetic field, a majority of protons will line up in the direction of the magnetic field. In addition, their axes are tilted and caused to rotate like small gyroscopes. the frequency of this precessional movement is directly proportional to the strength of the applied field and is called the Larmor frequency. The hydrogen proton gives a relatively high signal due to its abundance in biological tissues. Other potential NMR isotopes include ^{13}C, ^{23}Na, ^{19}F and ^{31}p.

If a pulse of radio waves is imposed on the nuclei, a strong interaction of 'resonance' will occur when the frequency coincides with the precessional frequency of the nuclei. The energy absorbed by the nuclei is then re-emitted as a signal that can be detected in a receiver coil situated around the sample. The initial strength of this signal is proportional to the proton density of the sample. It will then decay in an exponential fashion as the disturbed protons relax back to their original state. The T_1 relaxation time is described as the time taken for the stimulated protons to return to their initial state. The T_2 relaxation time is that taken for the precessing nuclei to get out of step with one another. A variety of sequences of radio-wave pulses have been devised so that the resulting signal is weighted to different degrees by the proton density and the T_1 and T_2 relaxation times.

The contrast between different tissues in MR imaging can be manipulated by altering the pattern of radio waves applied. This is done by changing the time constants associated with the different sequences of radio waves: the repetition time (TR), echo time (TE) or inversion time (TI). A further advantage of MR imaging is the ability to obtain images in multiple planes, such as sagittal, coronal or oblique planes, without moving the patient.

The female pelvis is suitable for MR imaging examination because of the minimal effect of respiratory motion on the pelvic organs. By placing the receiver coil adjacent to the tissue of interest (e.g. endovaginally to maximize signal from the cervix), very high resolution images of an area of interest may be obtained. However, as the data to produce a set of images are accumulated over 5–10 minutes patients are required to remain still during this time. If multiple sequences and multiple planes are employed the total imaging time may exceed 30 minutes which reduces patient tolerance. However, newer, faster pulse sequences with breath-hold techniques and improved computer software are greatly reducing scan times.

Recently, open-design MR scanners and production of MR-compatible equipment have produced an explosion in the field of 'interventional MR imaging'. This has expanded the applications of MR imaging from being purely diagnostic to its use during treatment, e.g. for placing brachytherapy implants (Popowski et al 2000) or for monitoring thermal ablative therapy.

Radionuclide imaging

Unlike the other imaging modalities, radionuclide imaging provides physiological rather than anatomical detail. Modern gamma cameras are capable of accurately imaging the distribution of administered radiopharmaceuticals and the use of tomographic systems for single photon emission tomography (SPECT) has improved image resolution. In gynaecological oncology, radiolabelled monoclonal antibodies may be employed in the localization of malignancies (radioimmunoscintigraphy) and in their treatment (radioimmunotherapy).

The purity and specificity of monoclonal antibodies give them an important role in tumour detection and possibly in the targeting of antitumour agents. A murine monoclonal antibody (791T/36), initially developed for colorectal cancer, has subsequently been shown to localize in gynaecological cancers (Powell et al 1986a). Another monoclonal antibody produced against a cell surface antigen, CA125, is also proving invaluable for imaging ovarian cancer. Different anticytokeratin antibodies may help in distinguishing a primary ovarian adenocarcinoma from a metastatic adenocarcinoma, especially of colorectal origin (McCluggage 2000). These antibodies have also helped to clarify the origin of the peritoneal disease in most cases of pseudomyxoma peritonei. In recent years, several studies have also investigated the value of a variety of monoclonal antibodies in the diagnosis of ovarian sex cord stromal tumours and in the distinction between these neoplasms and their histological mimics. Of these, anti-α inhibin and CD99 appear to be of most diagnostic value (Choi et al 2000). Antibodies should always be used as part of a larger panel and not in isolation.

The antibodies or antibody fragments are radiolabelled with a γ-emitting radionuclide such as ^{99m}Tc, ^{131}I, ^{123}I or ^{111}In. A subcutaneous test dose is no longer given because of the immune response it may generate in the patient. If ^{131}I or ^{123}I is employed, oral potassium iodide is given to block thyroid uptake of free radioactive iodide. In addition, blood pool subtraction techniques are required for ^{131}I studies to simulate the non-tumour distribution of labelled antibody. This is not necessary for ^{123}I- or ^{111}In-labelled preparations.

Following injection of the antibody, a gamma camera provides serial images of the distribution and uptake of radiolabelled antibody between 18 and 72 hours after the antibody has been administered. The radionuclide ^{111}In is ideally suited for tomographic studies using images produced by a gamma camera mounted on a gantry which rotates through 360°. The images are reconstructed by computer in the same manner as X-ray CT. ^{111}In tomography localizes the antibody uptake site more accurately and may reduce the false-positive results. Figure 6.3 is an example of a ^{131}I-labelled antibody study of a patient with a palpable mass in the left iliac fossa, suspected to be recurrent ovarian tumour. This was subsequently confirmed by laparoscopy.

False-positive ^{131}I-imaging can arise as a result of incomplete subtraction of radio-iodide in the urinary bladder. ^{111}In-labelled antibody has a different biodistribution with uptake of radiolabel into the liver, spleen, bone marrow and occasionally the adrenal glands. Excretion of ^{111}In into the bladder has not been a problem. An example of an ^{111}In study is shown in Figure 6.4. A central area of increased uptake is apparent at the site of a primary ovarian cancer. ^{111}In is a more suitable radiolabel than ^{131}I and, together with ^{123}I and ^{99m}Tc, has largely replaced ^{131}I. However, ^{111}In is taken up by the reticuloendothelial system into the liver and spleen, preventing its use for the detection of liver metastases. Non-specific bowel uptake sometimes seen with ^{111}In may account for some false-positive results.

Angiography

Diagnostic and therapeutic angiography has made great strides in recent years, with the development of catheters whose tips can be manipulated. This allows considerable control over the guidance of these catheters into selected vessels. In parallel with this, ingenious devices have been devised which can be introduced via these catheters for purposes as diverse as angioplasty and embolization.

In gynaecological practice, the main use of angiography is for the control of pelvic bleeding but both the diagnosis of pelvic venous thrombosis and the prevention of subsequent pulmonary embolism are important roles for this valuable technique. Embolization of the uterine arteries in the treatment of fibroids is an emerging application with promising short-term results (see below). Pelvic arteriovenous malformations are most readily diagnosed and treated with angiography and pelvic varices causing chronic pain may be managed in the same way. Selective sampling of gonadal venous blood and steroid hormone assay can be most valuable in the preoperative assessment of phenotypic women with chromosomal abnormalities and intra-abdominal gonads of uncertain nature.

CLINICAL APPLICATIONS

Normal anatomy and variations

Uterus
The normal uterine cavity is delineated as a triangular structure on hysterosalpingography, with the cornua and the internal cervical os as the corners. Intracavitary abnormalities, both congenital and acquired, such as internal septations and divisions, may be defined using this technique (Fig. 6.5). Similar information can be acquired with ultrasound following instillation of saline into the uterine cavity (hysterosonography) (van den Brule et al 1998).

On ultrasound, the uterine cavity is normally represented by a bright line of apposition of the endometrial layers, though occasionally a trace of fluid can be seen at menstruation. Persistent fluid or fluid in a non-menstruating woman is abnormal. In adolescence, it may be caused by vaginal atresia, where the upper vagina dilates more than the uterus so that haematocolpos dominates the picture, while in postmenopausal women cervical stenosis, either fibrotic or malignant, must be considered. Ultrasound is also useful in detecting the position of an IUCD; provided the coil lies in the uterus it is easily located (Fig. 6.6) but a coil that has penetrated through the myometrium is obscured by echoes from bowel gas.

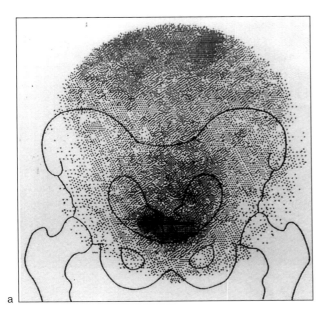
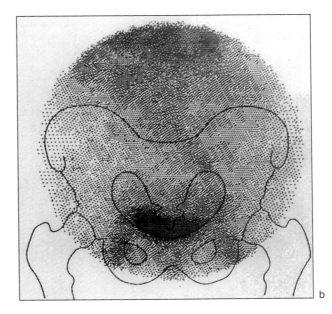
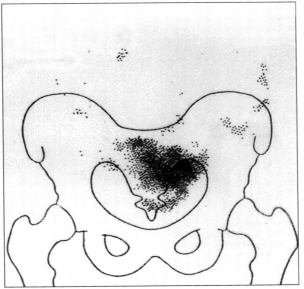

Fig. 6.3 Radionuclide scan of recurrent ovarian cancer. Anterior views of the pelvis with 80 Mbq ^{131}I-labelled antibody 791T/36. **a** The image before **b** subtraction of the ^{99m}Tc-labelled blood pool image; **c** after subtraction with an area of increased antibody uptake on the patient's left.

The entire uterus can be imaged using ultrasound (Fig. 6.7) and its size measured accurately. This is useful in precocious or delayed puberty and in planning brachytherapy. The endometrium is seen as an echogenic layer of uniform texture, often with a fine echo-poor margin. Its thickness varies through the menstrual cycle from 12 mm premenstrually (double-layer thickness) to a thin line after menstruation. The endometrium gradually thins after menopause unless supported by hormones.

The morphology of the normal uterus, however, is best defined on MR imaging where its zonal architecture may be recognized (Hricak et al 1983). On T_2-weighted images the endometrium is seen as a central high-signal stripe which increases in thickness in the secretory phase of the menstrual cycle. The inner myometrium (junctional zone) is of lower signal intensity than the outer myometrium on T_2 weighting and histologically correlates with a layer of more densely packed smooth muscle.

Fallopian tubes
The patency of the fallopian tubes may be demonstrated on hysterosalpingography where filling and free spill into the peritoneal cavity may be seen (see Fig. 6.5). To reduce the radiation dose to the ovaries in patients trying to conceive, ultrasound contrast salpingography is currently being evaluated. Normal uterine tubes cannot be demonstrated on ultrasound, but instillation of microbubble contrast agents into the uterus and tubes permits their visualization and can be used as an initial screening test for tubal patency. Though the anatomical

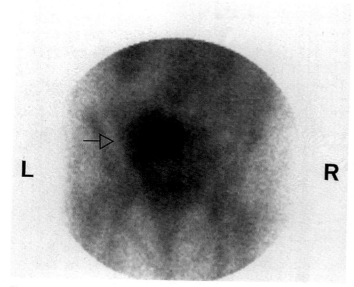

Fig. 6.4 Radionuclide scan: primary ovarian carcinoma. Anterior view of the pelvis with 80 Mbq ^{111}In-labelled OC-125.

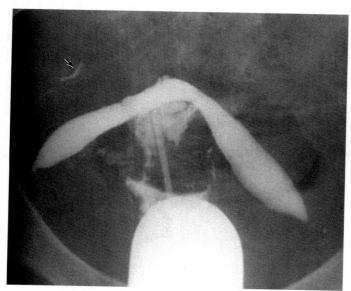

Fig. 6.5 Hysterosalpingogram: contrast outlining the cavities of a bicornuate uterus. Free spill into the peritoneal cavity can be seen on the right (arrow).

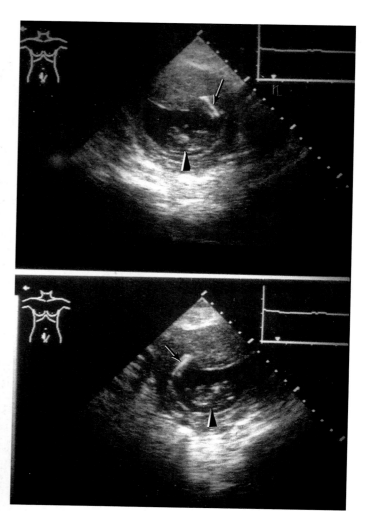

Fig. 6.6 Two views of an IUCD in the uterine cavity (arrows) with a coexisting pregnancy (arrowheads).

detail is less than that offered by conventional X-ray salpingography, and false-positive results occur, this technique of ultrasound salpingography seems likely to find an important role as an initial screen. If the tubes are demonstrated to be patent, no further investigation is necessary and this should result in a reduction of radiation exposure.

The normal fallopian tubes are too small in calibre and of too variable a course to be reliably imaged using a cross-sectional technique such as CT or MRI.

Ovaries

The ovaries are best imaged with ultrasound (either trans-abdominal or preferably transvaginal). Changes in their

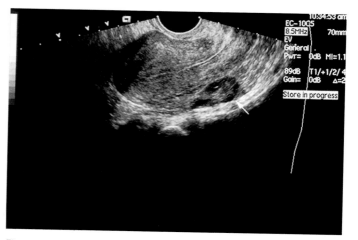

Fig. 6.7 Transvaginal scan of the uterus. In this scan, taken in the luteal phase of the cycle, the secretory endometrium is seen as an echogenic band by comparison with the relatively echo-poor myometrium. The arrow indicates a normal ovary.

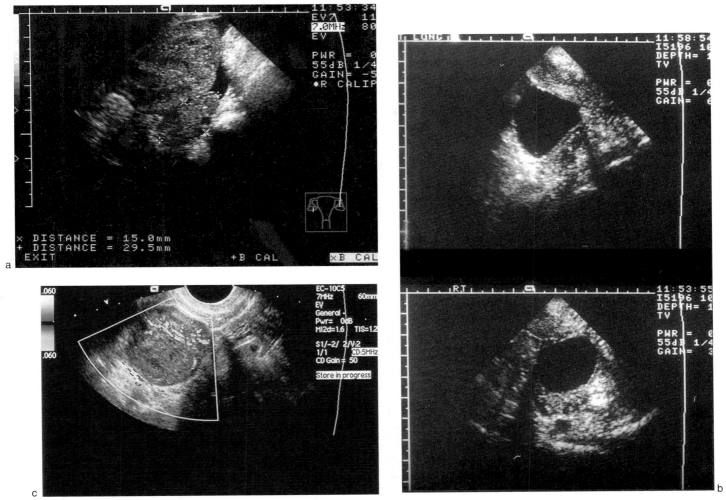

Fig. 6.8 Transvaginal scans of the ovary. **a** An inactive ovary is indicated by the calliper marks. It is surrounded by a small amount of free fluid and contains minute developing follicles. **b** Two views of an ovary containing a 3 cm simple cystic structure which presumably represents an unruptured follicle. **c** An ovary in the luteal phase containing a solid corpus luteum.

appearances can be correlated with their functional status. Infantile ovaries are small (except in the neonate when hypertrophy and follicles stimulated by maternal hormones may be a surprising finding) and they enlarge before puberty. Follicular development begins before menstruation but these cycles and those at the menopause are often imperfect, so that follicles may persist and continue enlarging for several months. Normally ovulation occurs at a follicle size of 20–25 mm diameter and the echo-free follicle is replaced by a corpus luteum which can be cystic or solid. Corpora lutea produce a confusing variety of appearances, whose only consistent feature is their transience (Fig. 6.8). In doubtful cases, a re-scan at 6 weeks to image them at a different phase of the cycle may be needed to resolve their identity. The postmenopausal ovary may be too small to identify with ultrasound.

On CT and MRI, the normal ovaries are sometimes difficult to define but may be recognized on short inversion recovery (STIR) MRI sequences as very high signal foci in the adnexae.

Ovarian varices

The pelvic congestion syndrome is one of many causes of chronic pelvic pain and is associated with the presence of large varices within the broad ligaments (Hobbs 1990). When pelvic symptoms are severe there may be gross dilatation of the ovarian veins, with reflux down into the pelvis and often into the legs. These vessels are best demonstrated by selective ovarian venography although they may also be imaged with Doppler ultrasound (Haag & Manhes 1999). Venography is performed via a femoral or internal jugular venous approach and the ovarian veins are selectively catheterized with an appropriately shaped angiographic catheter. Satisfactory retrograde opacification of pelvic varices is achieved by injecting contrast medium through the selectively placed catheter with the patient almost upright on a tilting table, while Valsalva manoeuvre is performed.

Treatment of this condition is primarily surgical and consists of venous ligation. Symptomatic relief has been reported following transcatheter ovarian vein embolization (Sichlau et al 1994).

Investigation of female infertility

The success of in vitro fertilization (IVF) has been due in part to the correct timing of ovulation and subsequent oocyte recovery which ultrasound can provide. Using transabdominal scanning, ovarian follicles of 3–5 mm diameter can be visualized. They appear as echo-free structures amidst the more echogenic ovarian tissue. Their rate of growth is linear and the mean diameter prior to ovulation is 20 mm (range 18–24 mm; Bryce et al 1982). Structures within the follicle such as the cumulus oophorus can also be visualized. Following ovulation, internal echoes appear because of bleeding. Free fluid may also be observed in the pouch of Douglas.

Transvaginal sonography has largely replaced the trans-abdominal approach in infertility practice because of the superior anatomical display and because it allows precisely guided aspiration of follicles and of fluid in the pouch of Douglas. More precise measurement of follicles is possible and the corpus luteum is easily recognized. In the mid-luteal phase it appears as an oval structure of 30–35 mm in length and 20–25 mm wide with a wide variety of sonographic appearances (Timor–Tritsch et al 1988). Endometrial reflectivity patterns have been proposed as another way to assess ovulation (Randall et al 1989). Ultrasound can only provide presumptive evidence of ovulation/pregnancy. The collection of secondary oocytes constitutes definitive evidence of ovulation. The appearance of internal echoes before the follicle reaches 18 mm or continuous enlargement to 30–40 mm indicate follicular failure.

Ultrasound is also useful for accurate timing of artificial insemination, while a postcoital test can help differentiate between inadequate sperm penetration and poor mucus production in the presence of immature follicles. Ultrasound scanning is also employed to monitor patients on clomiphene therapy and there is good correlation between follicular diameter and plasma oestradiol concentration. The hyperstimulation syndrome is uncommon if gonadotrophin therapy is monitored by ultrasound in conjunction with measurements of plasma oestradiol levels.

The waveforms of blood flow in vessels supplying the ovaries of women undergoing IVF have been studied using transvaginal pulsed Doppler ultrasound (Barber et al 1988). The observation of blood flow patterns may help in the prediction of implantation failure.

MR imaging is valuable in the investigation of infertility where uterine pathology is suspected and it provides a particularly high diagnostic yield in patients with dysmenorrhoea and menorrhagia (deSouza et al 1995). It should be part of the investigation of patients with persistent unexplained infertility awaiting costly procedures such as gamete intrafallopian transfer (GIFT) and IVF. MR imaging should also be used before myomectomy in order to differentiate between leiomyoma and adenomyoma as attempts to perform a myomectomy on a localized adenomyoma often result in extensive uterine damage.

Adenomyosis and endometriosis

The diagnosis of adenomyosis is often suggested by symptoms of hypermenorrhoea and dysmenorrhoea but similar symptoms are also produced by leiomyomas. Hysterosalpingography may show multiple small tracks of contrast extending into the myometrium but the results are often equivocal (Marshall & Eliasoph 1955) and the dose of pelvic radiation must be taken into consideration in patients trying to conceive. Laparoscopy may reveal a nodular, sometimes injected-looking uterine serosa. Myometrial biopsies taken at laparoscopy may be negative in focal disease and the diagnosis of adenomyosis may be missed. Ultrasound in skilled hands may be useful (Fedele et al 1992).

Adenomyosis is best demonstrated on T_2-weighted MR images, with which two patterns, a focal and a diffuse one, can be recognized (Byun et al 1999, Hricak et al 1992, Togashi et al 1988). In focal adenomyosis there is a localized ill-defined mixed signal intensity mass (adenomyoma) within the myometrium (Fig. 6.9). Diffuse adenomyosis presents with diffuse or irregular thickening of the junctional zone, often with underlying high-signal foci (Fig. 6.10). Pathologically this represents smooth muscle hypertrophy and hyperplasia surrounding a focus of basal endometrium (Noval & deLima 1948). It is the smooth muscle changes that are easily recognized by MR rather than the foci of heterotopic glandular epithelium. Values for junctional zone thickness from >5 to >12 mm have been suggested for the diagnosis of adenomyosis: use of 12 mm as a cut-off (Reinhold et al 1996) results in low sensitivity but good specificity. In our experience, however, the thickening of the junctional zone that is described in adenomyosis (Reinhold et al 1999, Togashi et al 1988) is not diagnostic of adenomyosis on its own; it may be seen in hypermenorrhoea where no pathological evidence for adenomyosis has subsequently been shown. In these instances, absolute values for junctional zone widths are unhelpful (Kang et al 1996) and

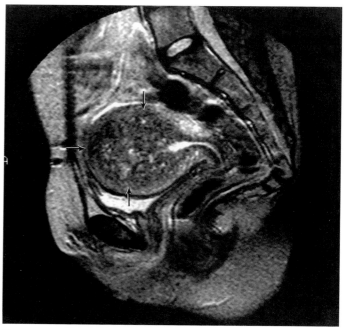

Fig. 6.9 Focal adenomyoma. T_2-weighted spin echo (SE2500/80) midline sagittal section through the uterus, demonstrating a large ill-defined mixed-signal intensity mass characteristic of an adenomyoma (arrows).

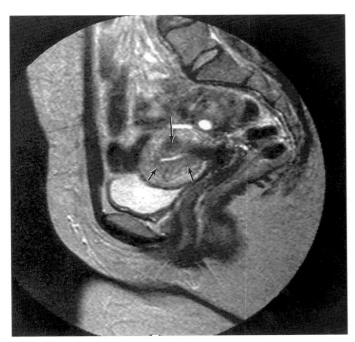

Fig. 6.10 Diffuse adenomyosis. T_2-weighted spin echo (SE2500/80) midline sagittal section through the uterus, showing thickening and irregularity of the low signal band of junctional zone (short arrows). Diffuse infiltration of a mixed-signal lesion (long arrow) is seen in the posterior wall.

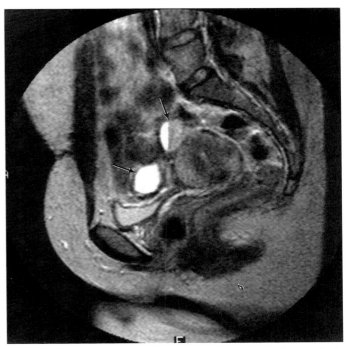

Fig. 6.11 Endometriotic deposits. T_2-weighted spin echo (SE2500/80) midline sagittal image; fluid levels are seen in cystic lesions with mixed signal intensity suggestive of haemorrhage (arrows).

ratios to the width of the outer myometrium or the cervical stroma may be more meaningful (Hricak et al 1983).

The lesions of endometriosis are difficult to detect with imaging techniques, mainly because of their small size. Only larger endometriomas can be detected on ultrasound and are seen as well-defined spaces, most commonly in the adnexal region. The role of MR imaging in the diagnosis of endometriosis also depends on the site of the endometriotic implants (Fig. 6.11): deposits on the ovarian cortex are much more readily identified than small peritoneal deposits. The latter are recognized at laparoscopy but may be missed on MR imaging (Brosens 1993). Endoscopic ultrasound has been advocated to improve the diagnosis of endometriotic infiltrates of the digestive tract (Dumontier et al 2000). MR imaging is particularly valuable in detecting deep enclosed endometriosis typically found in the uterosacral ligaments and rectovaginal septum (Fig. 6.12) commonly associated with pelvic pain. Deep pelvic endometriosis consists mainly of fibromuscular rather than endometrial tissue (Hamlin et al 1985) and, because of its position, often goes undetected on visual inspection of the pelvic cavity. However, MR imaging lacks sensitivity in detecting rectal endometriosis if the rectum is not distended (Kinkel et al 1999). More recently, there have been isolated reports correlating an increased junctional zone thickness with endometriosis in patients with infertility (Kunz et al 2000).

Leiomyomas

Diagnosis

The commonest cause of disturbance of the normal uniform

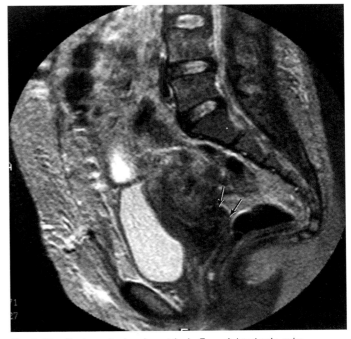

Fig. 6.12 Rectovaginal endometriosis. T_2-weighted spin echo (SE2500/80) sagittal section demonstrating a rectovaginal mass (arrows) in a patient with laparoscopically proven endometriosis. This was not detected at laparoscopy because it is retroperitoneal.

echo texture of the myometrium is fibroids. Generally, a focal thickening occurs and their position in the uterus can be determined. Submucosal fibroids, or the polyps they may produce, can be mistaken for endometrial thickening, though occasionally the way they move with normal uterine contractions is diagnostic. Instillation of saline into the uterine cavity, a form of ultrasound contrast, provides much more information about intracavitary lesions. Pedunculated or broad ligament fibroids frequently masquerade as extrauterine masses. The echo texture of fibroids is very variable in accordance with their histological spectrum. A characteristic is calcification which is easily recognized on ultrasound as intensely reflective foci with accompanying acoustic shadowing.

MR imaging has been reported to be superior to ultrasound for the diagnosis of leiomyomas (Ascher et al 1994, Hamlin et al 1985, Hricak et al 1992). Characteristic well-defined, low-intensity masses are seen within the myometrium on T_2-weighted scans, often with high-signal foci within them. There are no completely reliable features that distinguish fibroids from leiomyosarcomas on ultrasound or MR imaging and even Doppler has proved disappointing. In those patients presenting with more advanced disease, alterations in the uterine configuration may suggest malignant change.

Embolization of fibroids

Uterine arterial embolization is gaining popularity as a safe and cost-effective way of treating leiomyomas that produce symptoms of menorrhagia or sensation of pressure or a mass (Bradley et al 1998, Goodwin et al 1999, Hutchins et al 1999, McLucas et al 2001, Ravina et al 1995). Selective catheterization of both uterine arteries in turn is done usually via a femoral approach. Embolization is achieved by injecting polyvinyl alcohol with a particle size of 355–500 microns into each uterine artery until flow ceases.

Severe pain may result, requiring intravenous opiates, by either regular bolus or patient-controlled pump. Most patients are admitted for at least 24–48 hours for pain relief and stays of up to 4 days are not uncommon. Infection in the necrotic fibroid is a real risk. Many now prescribe prophylactic antibiotics. Deaths have been reported following embolization (Vashist et al 2000).

Although the procedure obliterates flow in both uterine arteries, clinical follow-up suggests that the perfusion of the myometrium recovers, with reports of successful full-term pregnancies (Pelage et al 2000). MR imaging clearly demonstrates differential changes in perfusion between myometrium and leiomyomas after bilateral uterine artery embolization (deSouza & Williams 2002). At 1 month there is recovery of myometrial perfusion but perfusion of the leiomyoma remains depressed. The reasons for this are poorly understood but it is likely that the normal myometrial vascular beds recover following the embolization process while the abnormal vessels of the leiomyoma do not.

It may be possible to predict clinical response from MR perfusion data immediately following embolization (deSouza & Williams 2002). An initial large reduction in leiomyoma enhancement correlates with a good clinical response at 1 year. Cellular leiomyomas, identified by a relatively higher signal intensity on T_2-weighted images, undergo a significantly greater volume reduction following embolization. Dynamic MR imaging may thus be used to predict clinical response, while T_2-weighted signal intensity predicts volume reduction.

Ectopic pregnancy

Traditionally, ultrasound has been used to exclude an ectopic pregnancy by demonstrating an intrauterine pregnancy but this sign is unreliable in assisted pregnancy because the likelihood of coexistent intra- and extrauterine pregnancies is not negligible. The positive diagnosis of ectopic pregnancy requires the demonstration of an extrauterine fetal heart. Secondary features that may be recognized are an adnexal mass with peritrophoblastic Doppler signals, free fluid in the pelvis and increased endometrial thickness. With a combination of these features the negative predictive value of an ultrasound examination may be 96%. This figure is improved further with the addition of the measurement of β-HCG (Emerson et al 1992). However, significant problems can arise in distinguishing an ectopic pregnancy with a pseudogestational sac from an early normal or failed intrauterine pregnancy.

The role of ultrasound in the diagnosis of ectopic gestations has been strengthened by the use of transvaginal probes and the introduction of Doppler. A weakness of transabdominal scanning was the difficulty in demonstrating the sac itself, because of gas in overlying or adherent bowel. With transvaginal scanning, the adnexal sac can be demonstrated and women at high risk can be monitored through the first few weeks of pregnancy (Fig. 6.13). Early ectopic sacs can be treated by injection of potassium chloride or methotrexate under ultrasound guidance. This approach is especially useful in IVF programmes where sparing the uterine tubes is so important.

Infections

Ultrasound is useful in the diagnosis and management of ovarian abscesses, where shaggy-walled cavities can be demonstrated in the adnexal region (Fig. 6.14). They usually have a vascular pseudocapsule that can be demonstrated on colour Doppler (Fig. 6.15). However, in pelvic inflammatory disease without abscess formation, the ultrasonic changes are too subtle to make this a useful technique. Monitoring the effects of antibiotic treatment on tubo-ovarian abscesses may

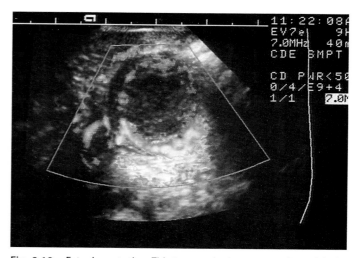

Fig. 6.13 Ectopic gestation. This transvaginal scan was taken with the energy mode of colour Doppler, a more sensitive type of signal processing which shows colour signals around the ectopic sac.

Fig. 6.14 Tubo-ovarian abscess. The irregular walls of this cavity are vascularized as part of the inflammatory response.

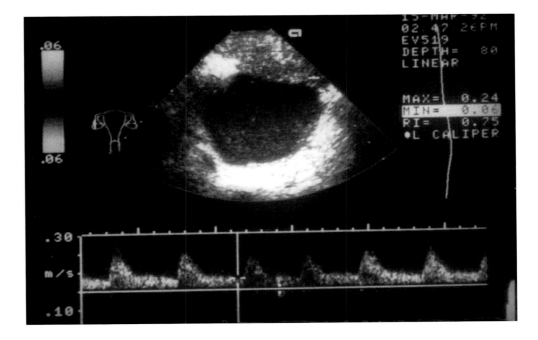

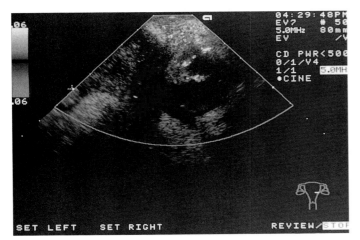

Fig. 6.15 Tubo-ovarian abscess. The marked signals within and around this abscess cavity are indicators of its inflammatory nature.

be useful, although in some cases sterile cavities persist for many weeks after signs of infection have been controlled. The hydrosalpinx that complicates pelvic inflammatory disease (PID) is seen as a funnel-shaped cavity in the adnexal region with thin walls and no internal echoes.

Venous thrombosis

Diagnosis

A relatively common complication of pregnancy and gynaecological malignancies, deep venous thrombosis is most easily diagnosed using colour Doppler ultrasound and this should be the investigation of first choice. Visualization of the iliac veins may be difficult and some patients will have to proceed to contrast venography. If colour Doppler ultrasound has shown the femoral veins to be clear of thrombus, this is most easily performed by puncturing these vessels directly which allows

Box 6.1 Indications for inferior vena cava filter placement

Recurrent pulmonary emboli despite anticoagulation
Pulmonary embolic disease in a patient in whom anticoagulation is contraindicated
Free-floating pelvic or inferior vena caval thrombus
Prophylaxis during surgery (see text)
Previous life-threatening pulmonary embolism

excellent opacification of the iliac veins and thus a confident diagnosis or exclusion of thrombosis, which can be difficult when contrast is injected into foot veins.

Inferior vena cava filter insertion

The indications for insertion of an inferior vena cava filter are listed in Box 6.1. The procedure is easily performed via femoral or jugular venous punctures and some devices may even be inserted through a sheath introduced into an antecubital fossa vein. The majority of these filters are inserted permanently; short-term placement is possible, however, and is most commonly indicated in the late stages of pregnancy (when free-floating thrombus is demonstrated or when a recent pulmonary embolus has occurred) or prior to surgical removal of a large pelvic tumour which has caused compression and thrombosis of one or both iliac veins. Two types of short-term filter may be used.

1. *Temporary filters* are mounted on a long catheter and are placed via an internal jugular or antecubital fossa venous approach into the infrarenal inferior vena cava above the thrombus (Fig. 6.16). The device is then sutured in place. They can only be left in situ for approximately 10 days and should then be removed because of the risk of infection.
2. *Retrievable filters* are designed for permanent placement and are inserted via an internal jugular venous approach. One such device is the Günther Tulip filter (William Cook Europe, Bjaeverskov, Denmark) which has a hook on its

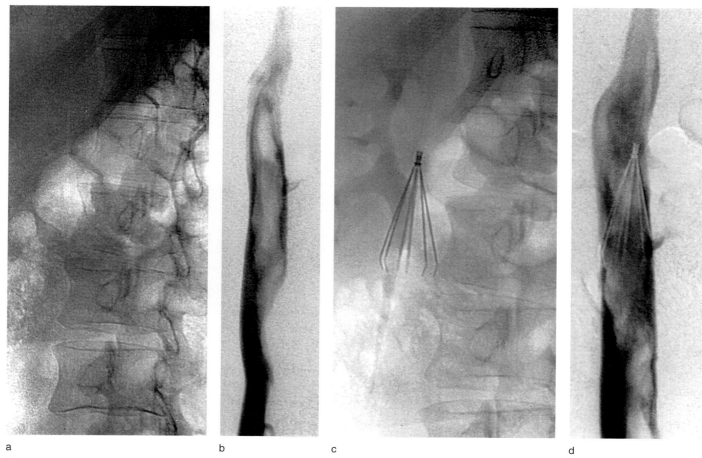

a   b   c   d

Fig. 6.16 Temporary vena caval filter insertion above free-floating thrombus. **a** Control film. **b** Inferior vena cavogram using digital subtraction demonstrates a large free-floating thrombus. **c, d** A temporary filter has been placed on top of the thrombus using a right internal jugular approach. The plastic catheter on which the filter is mounted is barely visible.

superior aspect. This may be grasped with a loop snare and withdrawn into a sheath prior to its removal. These devices can be removed after 10 days, but this is associated with more potential complications, as some endothelialization of the filters is likely to have occurred at this time and the filter limbs may be partially fixed to the caval wall.

Haemorrhage

Haemorrhage from the genital tract may complicate parturition or may be associated with benign (e.g. uterine arteriovenous malformation) or malignant (e.g. cevical carcinoma) disease. Traditional surgical therapy of severe pelvic haemorrhage consists most commonly of unilateral or bilateral internal iliac artery ligation, although in the case of primary postpartum haemorrhage (PPH) hysterectomy is more often performed (Shingawa 1964). In the largest series devoted to internal iliac artery ligation, however, the technique was successful in only eight out of 19 cases (Clark et al 1985).

There is a strong argument in favour of angiography and embolization prior to arterial ligation or hysterectomy in hospitals having the necessary expertise. Bleeding sites are often impossible to localize at surgery (hence the necessity for non-specific ligation of the internal iliac artery) but are usually easily identified at angiography; selective occlusion of the haemorrhaging vessel can then be performed with a much higher likelihood of controlling bleeding (Fig. 6.17). Previous internal iliac artery ligation does not necessarily prevent successful arterial embolization but may make the procedure technically more difficult (Collins & Jackson 1995, Duggan et al 1991).

Embolization is very successful in a variety of gynaecological disorders complicated by bleeding (Collins & Jackson 1995). For certain conditions (e.g. uterine arteriovenous malformations, bleeding from recurrent cervical carcinoma) this should be considered as the procedure of first choice (Fig. 6.18). In others it may be life-saving when more conventional treatment has failed.

Cervical carcinoma

The cervix

In cervical carcinoma, precise staging of the primary disease provides a prognosis, allows the institution of correct treatment and permits comparison of different treatment protocols. Clinical staging, applied according to the system of the

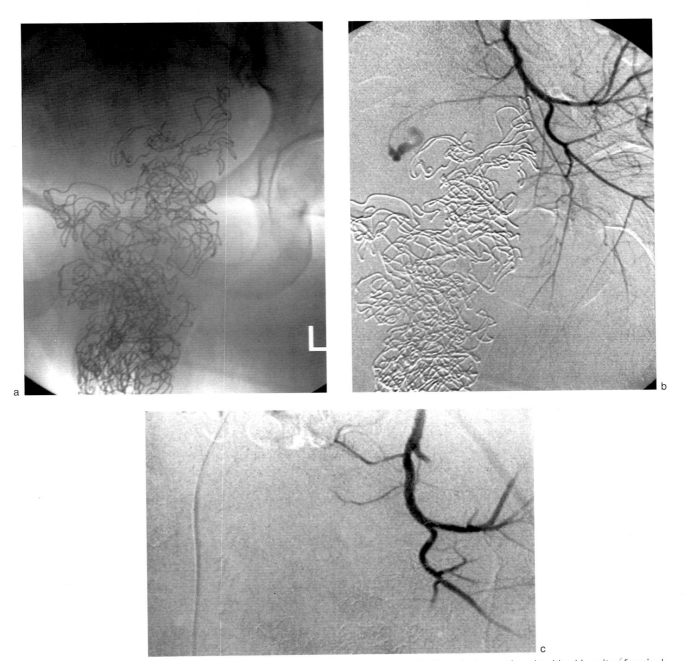

Fig. 6.17 Severe postpartum haemorrhage in a patient who had been explored twice vaginally and who continued to bleed in spite of vaginal packing. **a** Control film showing a large pack in pelvis. **b** Selective internal iliac arteriogram demonstrates brisk extravasation of contrast from a branch of the anterior division. This was selectively catheterized and occluded with polyvinyl alcohol particles. **c** Postembolization arteriogram demonstrates occlusion of the bleeding vessel with no further extravasation of contrast.

Federation International de Gynaecologie et Obstetrique (FIGO), is subjective and is notoriously poor, so that some centres use pretreatment laparotomy as the staging method of choice (Levenback et al 1992). Imaging with ultrasound does not improve the accuracy of clinical staging (Levenback et al 1992) so transabdominal ultrasound is of little value in the assessment of patients with cervical cancer. Poor image quality and difficulty in interpretation are the major problems. Transrectal ultrasound produces clearer views of the cervix but definition of tumour from normal cervix is still poor. The same difficulty limits the value of CT because the normal cervix and cervical carcinomas have similar attenuation values, so that the tumour can only be recognized if it alters the contour or size of the cervix (Subak et al 1995).

Several studies have confirmed the accuracy of MRI in the staging of early cervical cancer in comparison to surgical staging (Powell et al 1986b, Togashi et al 1987). The primary tumour is best assessed using T_2-weighted MR imaging which

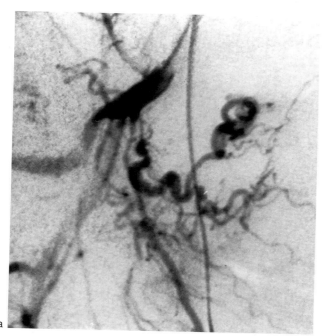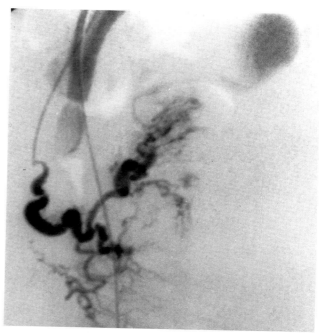

a

b

Fig. 6.18 Embolization of an area of neovascularity in the right side of the pelvis due to recurrent carcinoma of the cervix in a patient with persistent bleeding. **a** Selective right internal iliac arteriogram using digital subtraction shows encasement of the origin of the right uterine artery which supplies an extensive area of neovascularity. **b** The right uterine artery has been selectively catheterized prior to embolization. Note the marked irregularity of this vessel due to involvement by tumour. Embolization performed with polyvinyl alcohol particles gave excellent control of bleeding.

is superior to CT in detection (sensitivity 75 vs 51%, $p < 0.005$) and in staging (accuracy 75–77% vs 32–69%, $p < 0.025$) (Ho et al 1992, Kim et al 1993).

The resolution of the primary tumour on MR imaging may be further improved by using intracavitary receiver coils. Endorectal coils give high-resolution images of the posterior cervix, but the anterior margin of the tumour and its relation to the bladder base are often difficult to define because of drop-off of signal. Endovaginal coils give very high-resolution images of the cervix and adjacent parametrium (deSouza et al 1996). The distortion of the low-signal ring of inner stroma may be apparent and any breaks in the ring representing tumour extension may be identified (Fig. 6.19).

With MR imaging, the invasion of cervical cancer may be assessed in three planes: the coronal and axial planes are used for determining parametrial invasion, the axial plane for determining extension into the bladder and rectum and the sagittal plane for extension into the uterine body, bladder and rectum (Fig. 6.20) (Goto et al 1990). Fast spin-echo sequences further improve the quality of the images. MR imaging is also accurate in the prediction of myometrial tumour involvement and in showing the relationship of the tumour to the internal os and hence the patient's suitability for trachelectomy (Peppercorn et al 1999). Volume (3-D) imaging also provides the information necessary to calculate tumour volumes, which is of prognostic significance (deSouza et al 1998). Volumes obtained with MR imaging correlate well with those obtained by histomorphometric methods but only weakly with clinical stage (Burghardt et al 1989). The volumetry of the tumour also gives a more accurate prediction of parametrial invasion

and lymph node involvement (Burghardt et al 1992). Latterly, dynamic contrast-enhanced studies have been used for assessment of tumour angiogenesis (Hawighorst et al 1999) and the rate of contrast uptake shown to correlate with microvessel density in the tumour. However, no correlation with tumour aggressiveness has been demonstrated (Postema et al 1999).

Parametrium

Transrectal ultrasound, CT (Fig. 6.21) and MRI have all been used to assess parametrial spread. In a series of 180 patients, good correlation was found between the ultrasound and surgical findings, but significant problems arose in distinguishing between inflammatory or fibrotic change and tumour invasion (Yuhara et al 1987). Similarly, false-positive diagnoses may arise from misinterpreting inflammatory parametrial soft tissue strands associated with a tumour as actual tumour invasion, on both CT and MR imaging. A comparison of the assessment by these modalities with histological findings after radical hysterectomy showed an accuracy rate for parametrial involvement of 87–90% for MR imaging, 55–80% for CT and 82.5% for examination under anaesthesia (Ho et al 1992, Kim et al 1993). Extracervical extension on MR imaging is best defined using T_2-weighted fast spin-echo sequences transverse to the cervix. Fat suppression techniques do not provide additional benefits (Lam et al 2000). MR therefore yields valuble information for treatment planning (deSouza et al 1998, Sironi et al 1991) and should be used routinely in conjunction with clinical staging to determine the appropriate therapy in patients with cervical carcinoma.

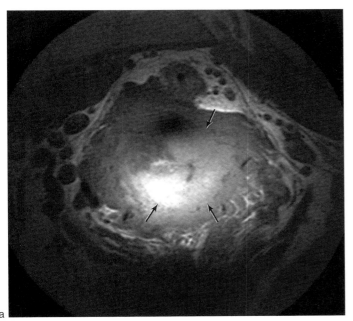 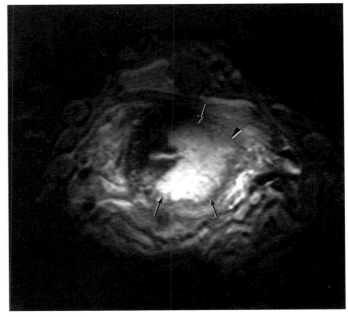

a   b

Fig. 6.19 Carcinoma of the cervix. **a** T$_1$-weighted (SE780/20) and **b** T$_2$-weighted (SE2500/80) transverse spin–echo through the cervix showing a large intermediate signal intensity mass mainly on the left. There is distortion and displacement of the normal low signal band of inner stroma (arrows). A break in this stromal ring indicating parametrial extension is seen on the T$_2$-weighted images (arrowhead in **b**).

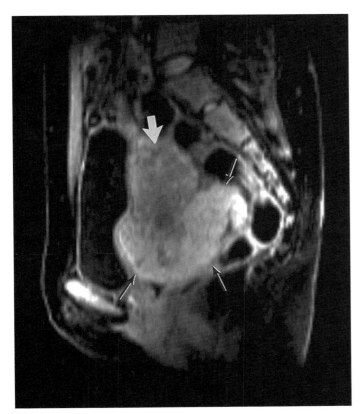

Fig. 6.20 Carcinoma of the cervix: a sagittal MRI image using a newly developed double inversion recovery sequence through the pelvis. A large carcinoma is seen (arrows) abutting but not invading the bladder base anteriorly and the rectal wall posteriorly. The uterus lies immediately cranial (large arrow).

An intravenous urogram (IVU) is still used as part of the staging process although it is increasing superseded by MR imaging. It may sometimes demonstrate partial or complete ureteric obstruction or displacement and distortion of the bladder outline. The IVU is abnormal in 2.1% of apparent stage I cases, 5.1% in stage II, 26.8% in stage III and 48.9% in stage IV (Griffin et al 1976). The finding of hydronephrosis or a non-functioning kidney resulting from tumour invasion of the ureter puts the patient into stage III, even if, according to the other findings, the case should be allotted to an earlier stage.

Barium enema abnormalities are rare in cervical cancer and proctoscopy is also positive if an abnormality is observed on the enema.

Nodal involvement

The role of lymphangiography in the staging of cervical cancer is obsolete, with up to 71% false positives and 16% false negatives. Percutaneous fine needle aspiration biopsy of nodes had been used to improve the results obtained with pelvic lymphangiography but has been replaced by CT. The major drawback for epithelial tumours is that nodes must be enlarged to be detectable. Thus metastases less than 2 cm in diameter will not be identified.

Some studies have shown an improvement in pelvic lymph node evaluation with MR imaging compared to CT (accuracy 88% vs 83%, $p <0.01$) (Kim et al 1993). However, like CT, it relies on changes in the size of the lymph nodes since the tumour deposits themselves are not highlighted. Although an in vitro study has shown that lymph nodes containing metastases have a significantly longer T$_2$ than do normal or hyperplastic nodes (Weiner et al 1986), in vivo tissue characterization based on relaxation times or signal intensities does not support these data.

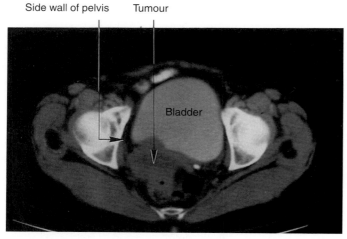

Side wall of pelvis   Tumour

Bladder

Fig. 6.21   CT scan of stage IIIb cervical carcinoma.

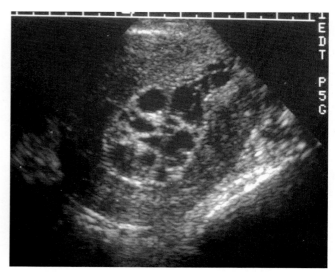

Fig. 6.22   Transvaginal ultrasound image of cystic hyperplasia of the endometrium: the grossly thickened endometrium is clearly seen, together with the cystic spaces, in this patient on tamoxifen.

A small clinical study suggested that ^{123}I-labelled epidermal growth factor may be used to recognize cervical cancer lymph node metastases because these tumours express high levels of the receptor (Schatten et al 1992).

The role of positron emission tomography (PET) in detecting metastatic pelvic lymph nodes remains unproven. A recent study of 35 patients claimed a 91% sensitivity and 100% specificity for detecting nodes involved with tumour (Reinhardt et al 2001), while results from other studies are much less optimistic (Williams et al 2001). Urinary residues of [18]FDG in the ureters remain a source of false-positive results.

Distant spread

Even with advanced pelvic spread, involvement of distant sites is the exception rather than the rule. In only one of 160 patients was a bone scan positive and this patient had stage IV disease with liver metastases (Hirnle et al 1990). Patients with stage I and II cervical cancer do not need to have bone scans.

A chest X-ray is a routine pretreatment investigation but the yield of lung metastases at first presentation is likely to be no more than 2%.

Assessing response and recurrence

In conjunction with clinical examination, MR imaging can provide an objective assessment of the effects of surgery or radiotherapy. Serial MR imaging may be used before and after primary radiation therapy to assess tumour response (Flueckiger et al 1992). Primary tumours with a volume of >50 cm^3 are likely to have a poor or delayed response (Flueckiger et al 1992). An early (2–3 months) and significant decrease in the signal intensity and volume of tumour indicates a favourable response.

With the increased use of cytotoxic regimes for primary and recurrent tumour, accurate imaging techniques become more important. CT and ultrasound have limited ability to differentiate between fibrosis and tumour. While some say that infiltration of the parametrium may be easily recognizable, it is difficult to differentiate fibrosis after treatment from tumour recurrence. Although isolated reports promote MR imaging in distinguishing post-treatment fibrosis and recurrent pelvic neoplasm by measuring signal intensities from the different tissues on T$_2$-weighted pulse sequences (Ebner et al 1988), in individual cases fibrosis is often impossible to differentiate from recurrence.

Endometrial carcinoma

Primary tumour

Thickening of the endometrium is characteristic of endometrial carcinoma and is well demonstrated on transvaginal ultrasound (Fig. 6.22). Because of its high negative predictive value, ultrasound plays a major role in the management of women with postmenopausal bleeding (Smith-Bindman et al 1998). However, specificity is low, making it quite unsuitable for screening the general population. Doppler may help distinguish hormonal causes of thickening (weak signals) and malignancy, which gives marked colour and spectral Doppler signals (Weber et al 1998).

In patients already proven to have an endometrial cancer, myometrial extension has important prognostic and therapeutic implications. Myometrial invasion may be classified as absent, superficial or deep and this can be assessed with high-resolution ultrasound probes. In a study of 20 patients, 70% of the ultrasound estimations of invasion depth were within 10% of the actual pathological measurement (Fleischer et al 1987). Errors occurred when the tumour was exophytic and had significant extension into the uterine cavity. False positives also occur if the uterine cavity is distended with pus or blood when a subendometrial hypoechoic halo may be seen. Ultrasound assessment of the integrity of the echo-poor layer can be improved by the use transvaginal or transrectal sonography.

Changes in uterine blood flow have been used to detect endometrial cancer using endometrial thickness (including tumour) and the pulsatility index (PI) derived from flow velocity waveforms recorded from both uterine arteries and from within the tumour. Bourne et al (1991) found an overlap in endometrial thickness between women with endometrial cancer

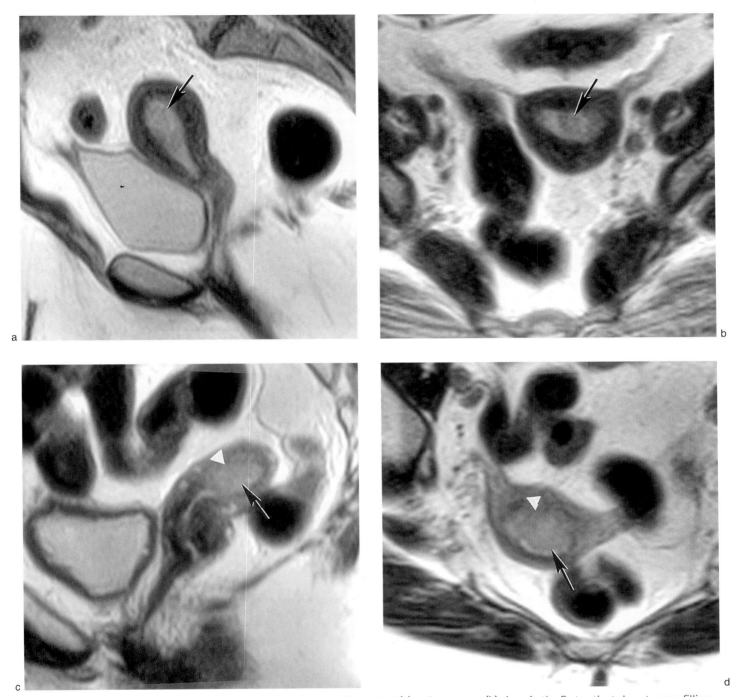

Fig. 6.23 MRI scans (T$_2$) of two patients with endometrial cancer. The sagittal (a) and transverse (b) views in the first patient show tumour filling the endometrial cavity (arrows) but the surrounding low signal-intensity junctional zone is intact. In the second patient, the sagittal (c) and transverse (d) views show tumour filling the endometrial cavity (arrows) with breach of the low-intensity junctional zone (arrowheads) and extension of tumour into the myometrium.

and those without, but the PI was invariably lower in women with postmenopausal bleeding caused by endometrial cancer than in those with other reasons for bleeding. Blood flow impedance is inversely related to the stage of the cancer. However, although PI values in healthy women increase slightly with age, they decrease with oestrogen replacement therapy, so although Doppler studies may be helpful in the

detection of endometrial cancer, allowance must be made for oestrogen replacement therapy.

CT may also be used to stage endometrial cancer which is seen as a hypodense lesion in the uterine parenchyma (Suzuki 1989) or as a fluid-filled uterus due to tumour obstruction of the endocervical canal or vagina. These findings, however, are non-specific and are easily confused with leiomyomata, intrauterine fluid collections and extension of a cervical carcinoma into the uterine body. In addition, a central lucency may occur in normal postmenopausal women. Newer helical CT approaches do not provide any improvement in the sensitivity and specificity for preoperative staging of endometrial cancer (Hardesty et al 2001).

MR imaging represents the best method of assessing a patient with an endometrial cancer, with advantages over other radiological techniques in stage I and II disease, but is probably equal to CT in usefulness in the patient with a more advanced tumour (Powell et al 1986a). Figure 6.23 is a series of MR imaging scans of patients with endometrial cancer. On the T_2-weighted pulse sequence, the tumour has a signal intensity similar to that of normal endometrium, but showing some degree of variability. The high signal makes the tumour quite distinct from the surrounding myometrium, which possesses an intermediate signal intensity. In a premenopausal uterus, however, it may be difficult to differentiate tumour from adenomatous hyperplasia or indeed from the high signal of normal endometrium. Contrast-enhanced T_1-weighted MR imaging improves the ability to assess the depth of myometrial invasion by endometrial tumour (Frei et al 2000, Sironi et al 1992a). MR imaging has been found to have a sensitivity of 57% and a specificity of 96% for tumour confined to the endometrium, a sensitivity and specificity of 74% for superficial invasion and a sensitivity and specificity of 88% and 85% respectively for deep penetration (Sironi et al 1992b). However, the degree of invasiveness may be overestimated for exophytic polypoid tumours with significant extraluminal extension (Gordon et al 1989, Lien et al 1991). Powell et al (1986a) found the low-signal band of inner myometrium to be thinned or absent in those patients with deeply invasive tumours and this correlated well with the pathological measurement of myometrial invasion.

The sagittal plane is the most appropriate for examination of a patient with primary endometrial cancer, as this provides a longitudinal view of the uterus which include both corpus and cervix. Using the sagittal plane also provides the opportunity to assess anterior invasion of the tumour into the bladder and posteriorly to the rectum.

Recurrent disease

Transrectal sonography has been investigated in cases where recurrent endometrial cancer is suspected (Squillaci et al 1988). Physical examination may be difficult because of post-surgical fibrosis. Infiltration into the surrounding connective tissues and organs such as the rectum and bladder can be identified and transrectal ultrasound can be used to guide transvaginal or transperineal fine needle biopsy. CT (Balfe et al 1986) or MR imaging may also be used to detect recurrent disease and metastatic carcinoma to omentum or lymph nodes.

Ovarian carcinoma

In patients with ovarian cancer, the dramatic difference in cure between those with local disease (80–90%) and those with distant disease (15–25%) means that imaging to detect ovarian cancer early is desirable.

The ovary

Ultrasound is being explored as a screening method for carcinoma of the ovary, in the attempt to detect early disease (Menon & Jacobs 2000, Sato et al 2000). Out of 5479 women screened in one study (Campbell et al 1989), five women with primary stage I cancer and four with metastatic disease to the ovary were diagnosed. The overall rate of false positives was 2.3% and the likelihood of a positive scan being a primary ovarian cancer was 1 in 67. The improved resolution of transvaginal scanning permits a more detailed morphological examination (Fig. 6.24). A scoring system has been evolved which reduces the number of false positives which otherwise result from confusion with unusual-appearing corpora lutea and with benign tumours (Bourne et al 1993, Timmerman et al 1999). Benign lesions are unilocular or multilocular with

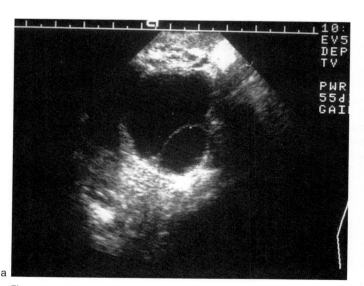
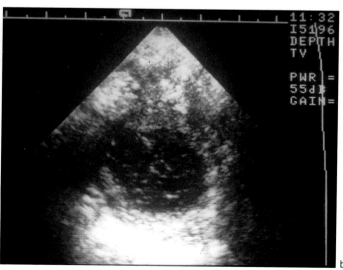

Fig. 6.24 Ultrasound scan of ovarian tumours. The smooth walls and echo-free contents of the benign cystic mass in **a** are very different from the complex appearance of the carcinoma in **b**.

thin septae and no nodules, whereas malignant lesions are often multilocular with thick septae and nodules. Uniformly echogenic lesions are less likely to be malignant than those of mixed echogenicity. In postmenopausal women, anechoic lesions less than 5 cm in diameter are unlikely to be malignant but those greater than 5 cm in diameter carry a 1 in 10 chance of malignancy (Andolf & Jorgenson 1989). Campbell et al (1989) were unable to identify any morphological characteristics to differentiate reliably between ovarian tumour-like conditions, benign ovarian tumours and early malignant tumours.

Bourne et al (1989) proposed that the false-positive rate may be reduced by the use of transvaginal colour flow imaging, but these studies have been variously reported as disappointing (Hata et al 1992) or useful (Kawai et al 1992). Initially a low resistance index (less than 0.4) was advocated as the best discriminator but this has proved unreliable and a high peak velocity may be a better feature.

At present the role of ultrasound in screening, though attractive, remains unproven (Taylor & Schwartz 1994). A pilot study of CA125 estimation combined with ultrasound as the second test has shown encouraging results in a population of 21 935 women of average risk (Bourne et al 1994). The results of larger trials are awaited. Despite these reservations, a transvaginal scan is accepted as a reasonable way to monitor the ovaries in patients with a high risk of ovarian carcinoma, such as those with a family history of the disease. Because of the risk of interval cancers, the screening interval should be less than 2 years (Bourne et al 1993).

As a tumour arising from a non-essential organ that is initially confined to the peritoneal cavity, ovarian cancer makes an attractive target for monoclonal antibodies. In the last decade, tumour imaging has improved progressively when one compares the best examples of early studies, performed with ^{131}I heterosera, to the best of modern images obtained with ^{123}I-, ^{99m}Tc- or ^{111}In-labelled monosera. Several monoclonal antibodies have been developed that have actual or potential clinical use for monitoring the course of disease. An antibody to CA125 has been widely assessed in monitoring the course of the disease (Fayers et al 1993). However, these antibodies are limited by problems that include antibody specificity, stability and immunoreactivity as well as patient reaction to the antibodies used.

Methods have therefore been developed to label with ^{198}Au a human monoclonal antibody (TC5) developed against an ovarian cell surface antigen (Chaudhuri et al 1994) which has a high sensitivity and specificity for detecting ovarian cancer. Antibodies coupled to drugs or biological toxins are also under investigation. Some antibodies may have direct antitumour effects through binding to biologically active receptors or through immune receptor functions. The use of antibody fragments, chimeric antibodies and genetically engineered antibodies is also under active investigation (Rubin 1993). Monoclonal antibodies therefore have enormous potential for improving the diagnosis and monitoring the response to therapy in the treatment of ovarian cancer.

The potential of PET to distinguish benign from malignant tumours is being evaluated by comparing the results of F^{18}-fluro-2-deoxyglucose (F^{18}-FDG) PET scans with surgical findings.

The positive predictive value from one such study was 86% and, more importantly, the negative predictive value was 76% (Hubner et al 1993). It may be possible, using such techniques, to identify metabolically active tumours that do not appear on morphological studies.

Pelvic and abdominal spread

Computed tomography is the most useful imaging modality for demonstrating macroscopic recurrence and can spare patients a second-look laparotomy. A variety of manifestations can be seen with CT, each of which can have a spectrum of appearances including ascites, peritoneal seeding and visceral and nodal metastases (Lee et al 1994). Ultrasound may also be used to detect ascites and liver metastases. MR imaging should be performed in women with questionable macroscopic recurrent tumour and negative CT examination. In a small study MR imaging (Fig. 6.25) was at least as good as and maybe superior to CT in the evaluation of ovarian malignancy (Semelka et al 1993). Neither CT nor MRI can exclude microscopic disease (Prayer et al 1993).

Fab '2 fragments of ^{111}In-labelled monoclonal antibody to CA125 gave immunoscintigrams, even with a negative CT and ultrasound, which were highly suggestive of recurrence in the abdomen and pelvis (Peltier et al 1992). ^{111}In CYT103 immunoscintigraphy detected occult disease in 20 of 71 patients with surgically documented ovarian adenocarcinoma (Surwit et al 1993), and this approach may be a valuable addition to presurgical evaluation in patients with suspected, persistent or recurrent pelvic tumour.

SAFETY ISSUES

Although the majority of imaging procedures described are largely non-invasive, some modalities involve exposing the patient to ionizing radiation. This is one of the reasons why techniques such as ultrasound and MR imaging have received so much attention in obstetrics and gynaecology. Nevertheless, ultrasound necessitates irradiation of the patient with sound waves (mechanical vibrations) and MR imaging involves the application of strong and rapidly changing magnetic fields combined with radio waves. Careful studies have failed to reveal harmful effects from the clinical use of ultrasound or MR imaging investigations but each modality has an associated risk, which must be appreciated.

With ultrasound and MR imaging the main biological effect is the conversion of the interrogating source of energy (sound, magnetic flux, radio waves) into heat. The American Institute for Ultrasound in Medicine has issued the following guidelines: 'In the low megahertz frequency range there have been no demonstrated significant biological effects of ultrasound in mammalian tissues exposed in vivo to intensities below 100 mW/cm^2'. Higher powers do damage tissue (mainly by heating, a feature used in physiotherapy) but at diagnostic levels the heating is minimal and continuously removed by the blood circulation. Spectral Doppler delivers the highest intensity and this is compounded by the fact that the beam is trained onto a target for longer periods of time than in imaging. It seems prudent to restrict scanning, especially spectral Doppler, to genuine clinical indications and to use it for the

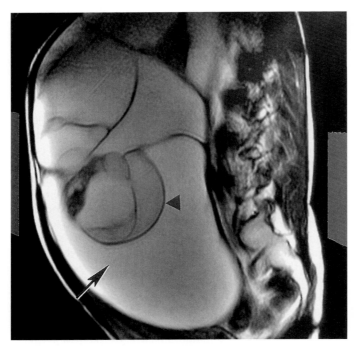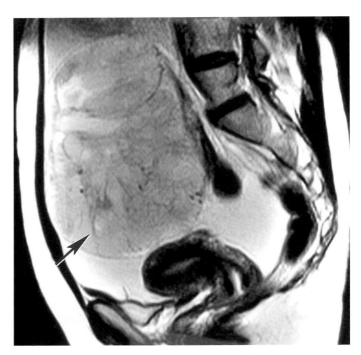

Fig. 6.25 MRI scans (T$_2$) of two patients with ovarian cancer. Sagittal views show a predominantly cystic mass in **a** (arrow) with septations and a polypoid solid component (arrowhead). In **b**, the mass is largely solid (arrow) with a small cystic component.

shortest time and at the lowest intensity needed to make the diagnosis.

As early as 1896 reports were made of a visual sensation of light flashes induced by exposure to changing magnetic fields. However, the main hazards associated with rapidly changing magnetic fields are those from magnetic implants. Patients with cardiac pacemakers or aneurysm clips constitute an absolute exclusion to being scanned. Other metallic implants must be considered on an individual basis. Other hazards arise from electroconvulsion and atrial fibrillation, hence caution should be exercised with epileptic patients and those who have recently suffered from myocardial infarction. Guidelines for the use of MR imaging are laid down by the National British Radiological Protection Board (1984).

Before any imaging investigation is carried out, however, a clinical decision has to be made concerning whether the benefits gained from the results of the investigation outweigh any possible risk to the patient from the procedure to be undertaken.

CONCLUSION

Advances in medical imaging are occurring at a rapid rate, mainly as a result of the development of sophisticated imaging techniques, computer software and display systems. Ultrasound, with its flexibility and relatively low cost, retains an integral diagnostic role in gynaecology with transvaginal sonography a routine adjunct to a bimanual pelvic examination. MR imaging provides superior soft tissue contrast of the pelvic organs and leads to an increase in detection, improved staging and assessment of a range of disease processes, including cancer. The technology needed to overcome the major disadvantages of long scanning times and claustrophobic scanners

is well advanced. Magnetic resonance spectroscopy remains largely unexplored in gynaecology, but is an exciting prospect for the future. The various imaging modalities are complementary to each other and the appropriate choice to produce the greatest diagnostic return while minimizing the risk to the patient should be sought.

KEY POINTS

1. Ultrasound examination is dependent upon both the technical expertise of the ultrasonographer and an understanding of the patient's history and clinical findings.
2. Ultrasound is the technique of choice for imaging the endometrial cavity and the ovaries, but it cannot distinguish reliably between benign and malignant disease.
3. Ultrasound is very valuable in monitoring ovulation induction and is used in directing egg collection for in vitro fertilization.
4. Ultrasound can be valuable in identifying an ectopic gestation.
5. MRI gives the best images of endometrial carcinoma and of adenomyosis. It may identify endometriosis that cannot be visualized in any other way.
6. MRI is the best method for imaging cervical carcinoma, especially when an endovaginal receiver coil is used. Imaging of pelvic lymph nodes is still not reliable.
7. CT scanning is of limited value in assessing the pelvic organs and should probably not be used if MRI is available.
8. Radionuclide imaging can be of value in identifying and locating ovarian carcinoma.
9. Angiographic embolization is probably the treatment of first choice for postoperative pelvic haemorrhage.

REFERENCES

Andolf E, Jorgensen C 1989 Cystic lesions in elderly women, diagnosed by ultrasound. British Journal of Obstetrics and Gynaecology 96:1076–1079

Ascher SM, Arnold LL, Patt RH et al 1994 Adenomyosis: prospective comparison of MR imaging and transvaginal sonography. Radiology 190:803–806

Balfe DM, Heiken JP, McClennan BL 1986 Oncologic imaging of carcinoma of the cervix, ovary and endometrium. In: Bragg DG, Rubin P, Youker JE (eds) Oncologic imaging. Pergamon, Oxford, pp 437–477

Barber RJ, McSweeney MB, Gill RW et al 1988 Transvaginal pulsed Doppler ultrasound assessment of blood flow to the corpus luteum in IVF patients following embryo transfer. British Journal of Obstetrics and Gynaecology 95:1226–1230

Bennett CC, Richards DS 2000 Patient acceptance of endovaginal ultrasound. Ultrasound in Obstetrics and Gynecology 15:52–55

Bourne T, Campbell S, Steer C, Whitehead MI, Collins WP 1989 Transvaginal colour flow imaging: a possible new screening technique for ovarian cancer. British Medical Journal 299:1367–1370

Bourne TH, Campbell S, Steer CV, Royston P, Whitehead MI, Collins WP 1991 Detection of endometrial cancer by transvaginal ultrasonography with colour flow imaging and blood flow analysis: a preliminary report. Gynecologic Oncology 40:253–259

Bourne TH, Campbell S, Reynolds KM et al 1993 Screening for early familial ovarian cancer with transvaginal ultrasonography and colour blood flow imaging. British Medical Journal 306:1025–1029

Bourne TH, Campbell S, Reynolds K et al 1994 The potential role of serum CA 125 in an ultrasound based screening programme for familial ovarian cancer. Gynecologic Oncology 52:379–385

Bradley EA, Reidy JF, Forman RG, Jarosz J, Braude PR 1998 Transcatheter uterine artery embolization to treat large uterine fibroids. British Journal of Obstetrics and Gynaecology 105:235–240

Brinkman JF, Wladimiroff J 2000 A software tool for fetal blood flow analysis. Biomedical Instrumentation and Technology 34:55–60

Brosens IA 1993 Classification of endometriosis revisited. Lancet 341:630

Bryce RL, Shuter B, Sinosich MJ 1982 The value of ultrasound, gonadotrophin and oestradiol measurements for precise ovulation prediction. Fertility and Sterility 37:42–45

Burghardt E, Hofmann HM, Ebner J, Haas J, Tamussino K, Justich E 1989 Magnetic resonance imaging in cervical cancer: a basis for objective classification. Gynecologic Oncology 33:61–67

Burghardt E, Baltzer J, Tulusan AH, Haas J 1992 Results of surgical treatment on 1028 cervical cancers studied with volumetry. Cancer 70:648–655

Byun JY, Kim SE, Choi BG, Ko GY, Jung SE, Choi KH 1999 Diffuse and focal adenomyosis: MR imaging findings. Radiographics 19:S161–170

Campbell S, Bhan V, Royston P, Whitehead MI, Collins WP 1989 Transabdominal ultrasound screening for early ovarian cancer. British Medical Journal 299:1363–1366

Chaudhuri TR, Zinn KR, Morris JS, McDonald GA, Llorens AS, Chaudhuri TK 1994 Detection of ovarian cancer by [198]Au-labelled human monoclonal antibody. Cancer 73:878–883

Choi YL, Kim HS, Ahn G 2000 Immunosuppression of inhibin alpha subunit, inhibin/activin beta A subunit and CD99 in ovarian tumors. Archives of Pathology and Laboratory Medicine 124:563–569

Clark SL, Phelan JP, Yeh SY, Bruce SR, Paul RH 1985 Hypogastric artery ligation for obstetric haemorrhage. Obstetrics and Gynecology 66:353–356

Collins CD, Jackson JE 1995 Pelvic arterial embolization following hysterectomy and bilateral internal iliac artery ligation for intractable primary post partum haemorrhage: case report and review of the literature. Clinical Radiology 50:710–714

deSouza NM, Williams AD 2002 Uterine arterial embolization for leiomyomas: monitoring immediate and late perfusion and volume changes with magnetic resonance imaging and relation to clinical outcome. Radiology (in press)

deSouza NM, Brosens JJ, Schwieso JE, Paraschos T, Winston RML 1995 The potential value of magnetic resonance imaging in infertility. Clinical Radiology 50:75–79

deSouza NM, Scoones DJ, Krausz T, Gilderdale DJ, Soutter WP 1996 High resolution MR imaging of Stage I cervical neoplasia with a dedicated transvaginal coil: MR features and correlation of imaging and pathological findings. American Journal of Roentgenology 166:553–559

deSouza NM, McIndoe GAJ, Hughes C et al 1998 Value of magnetic resonance imaging with an endovaginal receiver coil in the preoperative assessment of Stage I and IIa cervical neoplasia. British Journal of Obstetrics and Gynaecology 105:500–507

Duggan PM, Jamieson MG, Wallie WJ 1991 Intractable postpartum haemorrhage managed by angiographic embolization: case report and review of the literature. Australian and New Zealand Journal of Obstetrics and Gynaecology 31:229–234

Dumontier I, Roseau G, Vincent B et al 2000 Comparison of endoscopic ultrasound and magnetic resonance imaging in severe pelvic endometriosis. Gastroenterologie Clinique et Biologique 24:1197–1204

Ebner F, Kressel HY, Mintz MC et al 1988 Tumour recurrence versus fibrosis in the female pelvis: differentiation with MR imaging at 1.5T. Radiology 166:333–340

Emerson DS, Cartier MS, Altieri LA et al 1992 Diagnostic efficacy of endovaginal color flow Doppler in an ectopic pregnancy screening program. Radiology 183:413–420

Fayers PM, Rustin G, Wood R 1993 The prognostic value of serum CA 125 in patients with advanced ovarian carcinoma: an analysis of 573 patients by the Medical Research Council Working Party on Gynaecological Cancer. International Journal of Gynaecological Cancer 3:285–292

Fedele L, Bianchi S, Dorta M, Arcaini L, Zanotti F, Carinelli S 1992 Transvaginal ultrasonography in the diagnosis of diffuse adenomyosis. Fertility and Sterility 58:94–98

Fleischer AC, Dudley SB, Entman SS, Baxter JW, Kalemeris GE, Everette JA 1987 Myometrial invasion by endometrial carcinoma: sonographic assessment. Radiology 162:307–310

Flueckiger F, Ebner F, Poschauko H, Tamussino K, Einspieler R, Ranner G 1992 Cervical cancer: serial MR imaging before and after primary radiation therapy – a two year follow up study. Radiology 184:89–93

Frei KA, Kinkel K, Bonel HM, Lu Y, Zaloudek C, Hricak H 2000 Prediction of deep myometrial invasion in patients with endometrial cancer: clinical utility of contrast enhanced MR imaging – a meta-analysis and Bayesian analysis. Radiology 216:444–449

Goodwin SC, McLucas B, Lee M et al 1999 Uterine artery embolization for the treatment of uterine leiomyomata midterm results. Journal of Vascular and Interventional Radiology 10:1159–1165

Gordon AN, Fleischer AC, Dudley BS et al 1989 Preoperative assessment of myometrial invasion of endometrial adenocarcinoma by sonography (US) and magnetic resonance imaging (MRI). Gynecologic Oncology 34:175–179

Goto M, Okamura S, Ueki M, Sugimoto O 1990 Evaluation of magnetic resonance imaging in the diagnosis of extension in uterine cervical cancer cases with special attention to imaging planes. Nippon Sanka Fujinka Gakki Zasshi 42:1627–1633

Griffin JW, Parker RG, Taylor WJ 1976 An evaluation of procedures used in staging carcinoma of the cervix. American Journal of Roentgenology 127:825–827

Haag T, Manhes H 1999 Chronic varicose pelvic veins. Journal des Maladies Vasculaise 24: 267–274

Hamlin DJ, Petterson H, Fitzsimmons J, Morgan LS 1985 MR imaging of uterine leiomyomas and their complications. Journal of Computer Assisted Tomography 9:902–907

Hardesty LA, Sumkin JH, Hakim C, Johns C, Nath M 2000 The ability of helical CT to preoperatively stage endometrial carcinoma. American Journal of Roentgenology 176:603–606

Hata K, Hata T, Manabe A, Sugimura K, Kitao M 1992 A critical evaluation of transvaginal doppler studies, transvaginal sonography, magnetic resonance imaging, and CA 125 in detecting ovarian cancer. Obstetrics and Gynecology 80:922–926

Hawighorst H, Knapstein PG, Knopp MV, Vaupel P, van Kaick G 1999 Cervical carcinoma: standard and pharmacokinetic analysis of time-intensity curves for assessment of tumour angiogenesis and patient survival. MAGMA 8:55–62

Hirnle P, Mittman KP, Schmidt B, Pfeiffer KH 1990 Indications for radioisotope bone scanning in staging of cervical cancer. Archives of Gynaecology and Obstetrics 248:21–23

Ho CM, Chien TY, Jeng CM, Tsang YM, Shih BY, Chang SC 1992 Staging of cervical cancer: comparison between magnetic resonance imaging, computed tomography and pelvic examination under anaesthesia. Journal of the Formosan Medical Association 91:982–990

Hobbs JT 1990 The pelvic congestion syndrome. British Journal of Hospital Medicine 43:200–206

Hricak H, Alpers C, Crooks LE, Sheldon PE 1983 Magnetic resonance imaging of the female pelvis: initial experience. American Journal of Roentgenology 141:1119–1128

Hricak H, Fincks S, Honda G, Goransson H 1992 MR imaging in the evaluation of benign uterine masses: value of dimeglumine enhanced T1W images. American Journal of Roentgenology 158:1043–1050

Hubner KF, McDonald TW, Niethammer JG, Smith GT, Gould HE, Buonocore E 1993 Assessment of primary and metastatic ovarian cancer by positron emission tomography (PET) using 2-[18F] deoxyglucose (2-[18F]FDG). Gynecologic Oncology 51:197–204

Hutchins FL Jr, Worthington-Kirsch R, Berkowitz RP 1999 Selective uterine artery embolisation as primary treatment for symptomatic leiomyomata uteri. Journal of the American Association of Gynaecological Laparoscopists 6:279–284

Kang S, Turner DA, Foster GS, Rapoport MI, Spencer SA, Wang JZ 1996 Adenomyosis: specificity of 5mm as the maximum normal uterine junctional zone thickness in MR images. American Journal of Roentgenology 166:1145–1150

Kawai M, Kano T, Kikkawa F, Maeda O, Ogichi H, Tomoda Y 1992 Transvaginal doppler ultrasound with colour flow imaging in the diagnosis of ovarian cancer. Obstetrics and Gynecology 79:163–167

Kim SH, Choi BI, Han JK 1993 Preoperative staging of uterine cervical carcinoma: comparison of CT and MRI in 99 patients. Journal of Computer Assisted Tomography 17:633–640

Kinkel K, Chapron C, Balleyguier C, Fritel X, Dubuisson JB, Moreau JF 1999 Magnetic resonance imaging characteristics of deep endometriosis. Human Reproduction 14:1080–1086

Kunz G, Beil D, Huppert P, Leyendecker G 2000 Structural abnormalities of the uterine wall in women with endometriosis and infertility visualized by vaginal sonography and magnetic resonance imaging. Human Reproduction 15:76–82

Kurjak A 2000 Ultrasound scanning – Prof. Ian Donald (1910–1987). European Journal of Obstetrics, Gynecology and Reproductive Biology 90:187–189

Lam WW, So NM, Yang WT, Metrewli C 2000 Detection of parametrial invasion in cervical carcinoma: role of short tau inversion recovery sequence. Clinical Radiology 55:702–707

Lee MJ, Munk PL, Poon PY, Hassell P 1994 Ovarian cancer: computed tomography findings. Canadian Association of Radiology Journal 45:185–192

Levenback C, Dershaw DD, Rubin SC 1992 Endoluminal ultrasound staging of cervical cancer. Gynecologic Oncology 46:186–190

Lien HH, Blomlie V, Trope C, Kaern J, Abeler VM 1991 Cancer of the endometrium: value of MR imaging in determining depth of invasion into the myometrium. American Journal of Roentgenology 157:1221–1223

Marshall RH, Eliasoph J 1955 The roentgen findings in adenomyosis. Radiology 64:846–851

McCluggage WG 2000 Recent advances in immunohistochemistry in the diagnosis of ovarian neoplasms. Journal of Clinical Pathology 53:327–334

McLucas B, Adler L, Perrella R 2001 Uterine fibroid embolisation: non-surgical treatment for symptomatic fibroids. Journal of the American College of Surgeons 192:95–105

Menon U, Jacobs IJ 2000 Recent developments in ovarian cancer screening. Current Opinion in Obstetrics and Gynecology 12:39–42

National British Radiological Protection Board 1984 Revised guidelines on acceptable limits of exposure during nuclear magnetic clinical imaging. British Journal of Radiology 56:974–977

Noval E, deLima A 1948 A correlative study of adenomyosis and pelvic endometriosis with special reference to the hormonal reaction of eutopic endometrium. American Journal of Obstetrics and Gynecology 56:634–644

Pelage JP, Le Dref O, Soyer P et al 2000 Fibroid-related menorrhagia: treatment with superselective embolization of the uterine arteries and midterm follow-up. Radiology 215:428–431

Peltier P, Wiharto K, Dutin JP 1992 Correlative imaging study in the diagnosis of ovarian cancer recurrences. European Journal of Nuclear Medicine 19:1006–1010

Peppercorn PD, Jeyarajah AR, Woolas R et al 1999 Role of MR imaging in selection of patients with early cervical carcinoma for fertility-preserving surgery: initial experience. Radiology 212:395–399

Popowski Y, Hiltdbrand E, Joliat D, Rouzaud M 2000 Open magnetic resonance imaging using titanium-zirconium needles: improved accuracy for interstitial brachytherapy implants? International Journal of Radiation Oncology, Biology, Physics 47:759–765

Postema S, Pattynama PM, van Rijswijk CS, Trimbos JB 1999 Cervical carcinoma: can dynamic contrast enhanced imaging help predict tumour aggressiveness? Comment in Radiology 213:617–618

Powell MC, Womack C, Buckley JH, Worthington BS, Symonds EM 1986a Pre-operative magnetic resonance imaging of stage I endometrial adenocarcinoma. British Journal of Obstetrics and Gynaecology 93:353–360

Powell MC, Buckley JH, Wasti M, Worthington BS, Sokal M, Symonds EM 1986b The application of magnetic resonance imaging to cervical carcinoma. British Journal of Obstetrics and Gynaecology 93:1276–1285

Prayer L, Kainz C, Kramer J et al 1993 CT and MR accuracy in the detection of tumor recurrence in patients treatment for ovarian cancer. Journal of Computer Assisted Tomography 17:626–632

Randall JM, Fisk NM, McTavish A 1989 Transvaginal ultrasonic assessment of endometrial growth in spontaneous and hyperstimulated menstrual cycles. British Journal of Obstetrics and Gynaecology 96:954–959

Ravina JH, Herbreteau D, Ciraru-Vigneron N et al 1995 Arterial embolization to treat uterine myomata. Lancet 346:671–672

Reinhardt MJ, Ehritt-Braun C, Vogelgesang D et al 2001 Metastatic lymph nodes in patients with cervical cancer: detection with MR imaging and FDG PET. Radiology 218:776–782

Reinhold C, McCarthy S, Bret PM et al 1996 Diffuse adenomyosis: comparison of endovaginal US and MR imaging with histopathological correlation. Radiology 199:151–158

Reinhold C, Tafazoli F, Mehio A et al 1999 Uterine adenomyosis: endovaginal US and MR imaging features with histopathologic correlation. Radiographics 19:S147–160

Rubin SC 1993 Monoclonal antibodies in the management of ovarian cancer. A clinical perspective. Cancer 71:1602–1612

Sato S, Yokoyama Y, Sakamoto T, Futagami M, Saito Y 2000 Usefulness of mass screening for ovarian carcinoma using transvaginal ultrasonography. Cancer 89:582–588

Schatten C, Pateisky N, Vavra N et al 1992 Lymphoscintigraphy with (123) I-marked epidermal growth factor in cervix cancer. Gynakologisch Geburtshilfliche Rundschau 32:17–21

Semelka RC, Lawrence PH, Shoenut JP, Heywood M, Kroeker MA, Lotocki R 1993 Primary ovarian cancer: prospective comparison of contrast enhanced CT and pre- and post-contrast, fat suppressed MR imaging, with histological correlation. Journal of Magnetic Resonance Imaging 3:99–106

Shingawa S 1964 Extraperitoneal ligation of the internal iliac arteries as a life and uterus saving procedure for uncontrollable post partum haemorrhage. American Journal of Obstetrics and Gynecology 88:130–134

Sichlau MJ, Yao JS, Vogelzang RL 1994 Transcatheter embologherapy for the treatment of pelvic congestion syndrome. Obstetrics and Gynecology 83:892–896

Sironi S, Belloni C, Taccagni GL, DelMaschio A 1991 Carcinoma of the cervix: value of MR imaging in detecting parametrial involvement. American Journal of Roentgenology 156:753–756

Sironi S, Taccagni G, Garancini P, Belloni C, DelMaschio A 1992a Myometrial invasion by endometrial carcinoma: assessment by MR imaging. American Journal of Roentgenology 158:565–569

Sironi S, Colombo E, Villa G 1992b Myometrial invasion by endometrial carcinoma: assessment with plain and gadolinium-enhanced MR imaging. Radiology 185:207–212

Smith-Bindman R, Kerlikowske K, Feldstein VA et al 1998 Endovaginal ultrasound to exclude endometrial cancer and other endometrial abnormalities. JAMA 280:1510–1517

Squillaci E, Salzani MC, Grandireth ML et al 1988 Recurrence of ovarian and uterine neoplasms: diagnosis with transrectal US. Radiology 169:355–358

Subak LL, Hricak H, Powell CB, Azizi L, Stern JL 1995 Cervical carcinoma computed tomography and magnetic resonance imaging for preoperative staging. Obstetrics and Gynecology 86:43–50

Surwit EA, Childers JM, Krag DN et al 1993 Clinical assessment of 111In-CYT-103 immunoscintigraphy in ovarian cancer. Gynecologic Oncology 48:283–284

Suzuki M 1989 Role of X-ray, CT and magnetic resonance imaging in the diagnosis of gynecological malignant tumor. Nippon Sanka Fujinka Gakkai Zasshi 41:942–952

Taylor KJ, Schwartz PE 1994 Screening for early ovarian cancer. Radiology 192:1–10

Timmerman D, Bourne TH, Tailor A, Collins WP, Verrelst H, Vandenberghe K, Vergote I 1999 A comparison of methods for preoperative discrimination between malignant and benign adnexal masses: the development of a new logistic regression model. American Journal of Obstetrics and Gynecology 181:57–65.

Timor-Tritsch IE, Bar-Yam Y, Elgali S, Rotlem S 1988 The technique of transvaginal sonography with the use of a 6.5 MHz probe. American Journal of Obstetrics and Gynecology 158:1019–1024

Togashi K, Nishimura K, Itoh K 1987 Uterine cervical cancer: assessment with high field MR imaging. Radiology 160:431–435

Togashi K, Nishimura K, Itoh K et al 1988 Adenomyosis diagnosis with MR imaging. Radiology 166: 111–114

van den Brule FA, Wery O, Huveneers J, Gaspard UJ 1998 Contrast hysterosonography: an efficient means of investigation in gynecology. Review of the literature. Journal de Gynecologie, Obstetrique et Biologie de la Reproduction (Paris) 27:655–664

Vashist A, Studd JW, Carey AH et al 2000 Fibroid embolisation: a technique not without significant complications. British Journal of Obstetrics and Gynaecology 107:1166–1170

Wade R V 1999 Images, imagination and ideas: a perspective on the impact of ultrasonography on the practice of obstetrics and gynecology. Presidential address. American Journal of Obstetrics and Gynecology 181:235–239

Weber G, Merz E, Bahlmann F, Rosch B 1998 Evaluation of different transvaginal sonographic diagnostic parameters in women with postmenopausal bleeding. Ultrasound in Obstetrics and Gynecology 12:265–270

Weiner JL, Chako AC, Merten CW, Gross S, Coffey EL, Stein HL 1986 Breast and axillary tissue MR imaging correlations of signal intensities and relaxation times with pathologic findings. Radiology 160:229–305

Williams AD, Cousins C, Soutter WP et al 2001 Detection of pelvic lymph node metastases in gynaecological malignancy: a comparison of CT, MR imaging and PET. American Journal of Roentgenology 177:343–348.

Yuhara A, Akamatsu N, Sekiba K 1987 Use of transrectal radial scan ultrasonography in evaluating the extent of uterine cervical cancer. Journal of Clinical Ultrasound 15:507–517

7

One-stop gynaecology: the role of ultrasound in the acute gynaecological patient

Karen Jermy   Tom Bourne

INTRODUCTION

The assessment and investigation of the gynaecological patient are rapidly moving away from the operating theatre and ward environment and into the outpatient department. This has been fuelled by the demands of the patient and clinician to provide a rapid, accurate diagnosis, with the minimum of investigations and invasive procedures, and also by the economic constraints of inpatient admission.

Transvaginal ultrasonography has provided a pivotal medium for the assessment of gynaecological patients in almost all areas of the specialty. Transvaginal probes, providing high-resolution images of the pelvic organs, have an established role in the characterization of adnexal masses, providing reliable and reproducible information regarding cyst type and probability of malignancy (Granberg et al 1989, 1990, Tailor et al 1997, Timmerman et al 1999a). They have superiority over transabdominal probes because of the higher resolution of pelvic anatomy. There is also no need for a full bladder, improving patient acceptability.

The assessment of patients with menstrual disorders, post-menopausal bleeding and chronic pelvic pain has been taken out of the constraints of the general gynaecology clinic by the incorporation of transvaginal ultrosonography, along with outpatient endometrial sampling techniques as part of a 'one-stop' approach to diagnosis and management in these areas. When compared with outpatient hysteroscopy in the evaluation of endometrial pathology, transvaginal ultrasonography, with or without the addition of saline as a negative contrast agent, compares favourably (Fedele et al 1991, Indman 1995, Schwarzler et al 1998). It has been shown to be a well-tolerated part of the examination, providing an assessment not only of the uterine cavity and myometrium but also of the adnexa at the same time.

One of the most useful and yet least discussed roles of ultrasonography within the gynaecological setting is the assessment of the acute gynaecological patient, as it provides an effective and rapid means of diagnosis and detection of gynaecological pathology.

The identification of pathology on ultrasound will result in urgent surgery or a more conservative approach. The route taken will depend upon the clinical assessment of the patient. Preoperative ultrasound assessment of the patient will improve patient counselling and allow appropriate staffing levels, to facilitate the use of minimally invasive techniques.

This chapter deals with the initial assessment of the patient presenting acutely, in whom gynaecological pathology is suspected. By adopting a problem-orientated approach to the acute gynaecological patient, we hope to provide a series of reproducible pathways allowing effective investigation of these patients. Transvaginal ultrasonography is central to all these diagnostic pathways and yet it remains an extension of the clinical examination: a normal scan will not exclude all underlying gynaecological conditions.

The main division that exists within the evaluation of a woman presenting with pelvic or abdominal pain and/or per vaginal bleeding is the result of a urinary β-HCG test. The chapter will therefore explore the differentials of pain and/or bleeding in early pregnancy, the role of the early pregnancy assessment unit and the productive use of biochemical assays in diagnosis and management. The second part of the chapter will then give an overview to the role of pelvic ultrasound in the evaluation of acute pelvic pain and vaginal bleeding in those women with a negative pregnancy test.

RESOURCES

Ultrasound machine

Most gynaecology units will already have an ultrasound machine that can be used within a clinic setting. New machines can either be bought outright or leased. Minimum requirements are a transvaginal probe (6–7.5 MHz), a 3.5 MHz abdominal transducer and facilities for capturing images, either as a hard copy or digitally. A portable machine can be a wise investment if it is to be shared, for example, with the delivery suite or to allow for ultrasound-guided procedures in the operating theatre.

Reducing the risk of infection transmission

Transvaginal ultrasonography is a relatively non-invasive procedure. There is, however, a moderate risk of transmission of infection as the probe comes into contact with mucous membranes. The risk of infection is reduced by the use of an appropriate cover for the transducer. It is estimated that up to 7% of covers will sustain perforations and contamination of the probe may also occur on removing the cover after use (Jimenez & Duff 1997). Because of this, appropriate cleaning of the transducer must occur between patients. Sterilization of the probe is not practical and disinfection using a germicidal (e.g. 70% alcohol) cloth or spray, after first wiping off the gel, is effective. The probe is then left to air dry for at least 5 minutes.

Basic hygiene measures, such as washing hands after each case and ensuring that contaminated gloves do not come into contact with the ultrasound machine, must be used to minimize cross-infections.

Ancillary devices

Sonohysterography

A simple technique involving the instillation of sterile saline into the uterine cavity. All the required equipment can be found in a routine gynaecology clinic, except for the catheter used to access the uterine cavity. A number of devices can be used. We use a 5 French paediatric nasogastric feeding tube. Alternatives to this include a modified pipelle du Cornier (its rigidity helps insertion) and thin balloon catheters, either urinary or custom made (e.g. Goldstein sonohysterography catheter, Cook Ob/Gyn, Indiana, USA). The presence of a balloon helps to reduce backflow of saline and maintain uterine distension. However, these devices tend to be more expensive, are not readily available and distension of the balloon at the internal cervical os can cause increased discomfort.

Computer database systems

A number of commercial database systems exist for the storage of data including digital images. This allows a written report to be generated for the referring physician and patient immediately and easy access to previous images for comparison, for example after treatment of conservative management of ovarian cysts.

Resuscitation equipment

All gynaecological clinics should have adequate resuscitation equipment in good order. The clinic staff should have up-to-date training in its appropriate use.

Analgesia and antibiotics

Some units advocate the use of non-steroidal analgesia prior to the appointment. If hysteroscopy is not being performed there is no need. There should be equipment readily available for performing a paracervical block which may be required in some cases of cervical stenosis or at a patient's request.

Transvaginal ultrasonography is a well-tolerated procedure. Even when sonohysterography is performed the routine use of analgesia is not advocated. In one series 98% of patients undergoing transvaginal ultrasound and 87% of patients undergoing saline sonohysterography reported either no, or minimal, discomfort (Schwarzler et al 1998).

Antibiotic use

Sonohysterography (SHS) should not be performed in the presence of overt pelvic infection. The risk of pelvic infection following SHS is very small, if it occurs at all. Despite this, many units advocate the use of prophylactic antibiotics in all potentially fertile women to minimize this risk.

The emergency gynaecological unit

This will comprise a dedicated area for the triage, assessment and initial management of patients presenting with suspected gynaecological disorders. An initial assessment of the clinical condition can be made and recorded on a preformed history sheet. A proforma history provides the best means of collecting demographic and clinical data on the patient, which can be completed by the patient whilst waiting for the scan. Baseline observations are recorded. There should be a separate area where the patient can change. This setting will predispose to a gynaecologist performing the scan, therefore incorporating the procedure into the main clinical examination of the patient. Basic procedures can be performed, such as outpatient endometrial sampling, polypectomy, cryocautery, intrauterine coil insertion and infection screens.

The early pregnancy assessment unit

The early pregnancy unit (EPU) provides an easily accessible, ultrasound-based assessment of pregnancy duration, viability and location, which allows for informed and individualized management and counselling of the patient.

The cost benefits of the EPU are well established (Bigrigg & Read 1991) as admission can be avoided in about 40% of patients, with a further 20% requiring a shorter stay. Ideally, there should be a dedicated unit for the assessment and investigation of those women with suspected complications of early pregnancy. This will be centred around a scan room, run by dedicated ultrasound practitioners. There should be a private area in which the patient can change and also a separate counselling room with access to a counselling service and outside line telephone.

Referral to the EPU may be by prior arrangement with the general practitioner or other consultant or, ideally, a 'walk-in' self-referral system can operate. The latter will provide the patient with the means to contact a unit directly when problems arise, although it will make clinics busy. Again, the history can be collected on a proforma. This will highlight relevant gynaecological and obstetric history for the clinician, including factors predisposing to ectopic pregnancy or those women in whom recurrent miscarriages have been identified, and will also facilitate audit and research. A number of computer databases now exist which aid data collection and facilitate reporting. This means that the patient can leave the clinic with a detailed report and follow-up plan and a report can be distributed to the referring clinician immediately.

Availability of rapid serum β-HCG assays will vary within units, but the judicious use and follow-up of serum changes in β-HCG is essential for a diagnosis where the pregnancy location is not readily identified. This may be achieved in a number of ways but typically will be dependent upon a dedicated staff member to record and interpret results either via a computer database or log book. The patient is either contacted with further follow-up/intervention plans or the patient contacts the unit herself for these results.

Fortunately, the majority of women with pain or bleeding in early pregnancy will present subacutely; in all cases, however, an initial assessment of haemodynamic compromise must be made. Blood pressure, pulse, temperature and pulse oximetry should be recorded. Facilities for obtaining venous access and commencing intravenous volume replacement should be available.

Anti-D immunoglobulin use for rhesus prophylaxis
Current guidelines (RCOG 2000) for the use of rhesus immunoprophylaxis in early pregnancy recommend that anti-D immunoglobulin should be given to all non-sensitized RhD negative women who:

- have an ectopic pregnancy
- have a therapeutic termination of pregnancy (surgical or medical)
- have a threatened or spontaneous miscarriage after 12 weeks gestation*
- have surgical evacuation of retained products of conception prior to 12 weeks gestation.

*Where there is heavy, recurrent or painful bleeding prior to 12 weeks gestation, anti-D Ig prophylaxis is also recommended.

Psychological aspects
Women, and their partners, who are diagnosed with early pregnancy failure should be offered follow-up, to allow for appropriate support and counselling. This will facilitate early referral to formal counselling services when necessary.

ULTRASOUND OVERVIEW
The advantages of transvaginal sonography over the trans-abdominal approach are well documented (Gonzalez et al 1988, Mendelson et al 1988). The placement of the ultrasound probe closer to the pelvic organs means that higher frequency ultrasound transducers (6–7.5 MHz) can be used, which produce high-resolution images. Transvaginal sonographic assessment of ovarian volume and morphology correlates closely with subsequent operative findings at laparotomy (Rodriguez et al 1988).

Transvaginal ultrasonography (TVS) has an established role in the evaluation of adnexal masses. It provides an accurate assessment of ovarian morphology (Granberg et al 1989, 1990, Timmerman et al 1999b) and is a significant contributor to mathematical models being developed to assess ovarian tumours (Tailor et al 1997, Timmerman et al 1999a,c). There are several types of ovarian cyst that can be assessed using the recognition of characteristic morphological patterns (Jermy et al 2001). Endometriomas and benign cystic teratomas are two examples, accounting for over two-thirds of persistent adnexal masses in premenopausal women (Koonings et al 1989). These lesions can be particularly difficult to score using morphological scoring systems and as angiogenesis is ubiquitous throughout the ovarian cycle, colour Doppler is of limited value (Alcazar et al 1997).

Transvaginal ultrasonography is a highly sensitive method for detecting endometrial abnormalities. In the assessment of postmenopausal bleeding, the finding of a regular endometrial echo with a thickness of less than 5 mm has been shown to have a high negative predictive value for the presence of pathology (Granberg et al 1991). However, the premenopausal endometrium is a dynamic structure and wide variations in the endometrial thickness have been associated with pathology (Dijkhuizen et al 1996). The most consistent measurements are taken in the proliferative phase when the endometrium is at its thinnest and most echo-lucent. With all measurements of the endometrial echo, it is important to visualize it as a three-dimensional structure, so as to avoid missing focal irregularities.

The endometrial outline should be regular and un-interrupted, whatever the thickness. A thick, secretory endometrium on unenhanced transvaginal ultrasonography will often disguise endometrial pathology. In contrast, a periovulatory 'triple line' endometrium will offer the best unenhanced views of the uterine cavity. TVS affords good myometrial/endometrial interface definition. This is important in the assessment of suspected endometrial carcinoma. Endometrial polyps tend to be hyperechoic or cystic structures distorting the endometrial echo. Colour Doppler may demonstrate a single feeding blood vessel to the structure.

Transvaginal ultrasound is highly sensitive in the diagnosis of intracavity pathology, but lacks specificity in many cases (Dijkhuizen et al 1996, Granberg et al 1991). The sensitivity and specificity are improved by saline sonohysterography, to equal and in some studies (Timmerman et al 1998) surpass that of outpatient hysteroscopy. When patient preference is considered, TVS with saline SHS is preferred to outpatient hysteroscopy (Timmerman et al 1998), making TVS an ideal first-line investigation for menstrual disorders.

Saline sonohysterography (s-SHS)

This technique involves the introduction of a sonographic negative contrast agent into the uterine cavity, to enhance routine transvaginal ultrasonography in the identification of uterine cavity pathology (Figs 7.1 and 7.2).

A conventional transvaginal scan is performed to assess the uterus and adnexa in coronal and sagittal planes. The examination should ideally be performed in the proliferative phase of the menstrual cycle, once menstruation has ceased. This not only enhances views of the uterine cavity, but also reduces the risk of disturbing an early intrauterine pregnancy. The ultrasound probe is removed and a bivalve/Cusco's speculum inserted. The cervix is identified and cleaned with an antiseptic solution. The procedure should be postponed and an infection screen performed with appropriate antibiotic therapy if there are any signs of pelvic infection. The patient should be warned prior to the procedure that she may experience a dull ache like a period pain. Covering antibiotics may be given for potentially fertile women.

After the cervix has been cleaned, a fine-bore catheter (with or without balloon) is passed through the os using sponge-holding forceps until the uterine fundus is reached. A volsellum may be needed to apply countertraction to the cervix. The catheter should already have been primed with sterile saline solution. The speculum is removed, taking care not to dislodge the catheter, and a 20 ml syringe of sterile saline reattached to the catheter. The ultrasound probe is reintroduced and the saline is slowly infused, causing uterine distension. The uterine cavity is reassessed in both the sagittal and coronal planes once again for focal and global endometrial defects.

When the scan is complete, the catheter is removed and the patient advised to remain supine for 5 minutes to reduce the chance of a vagal reaction after the procedure.

Indications for SHS
- Thickened endometrium.
- Poor views of the endometrium, due to axial position of uterus, large myomas distorting the cavity.
- Preoperative localization, size and relation to the cavity of submucous fibroids/endometrial polyps to plan hysteroscopic surgery.

Complications of the procedure
- Failure – this usually occurs due to cervical stenosis or in the presence of multiple large fibroids. The problems encountered with a patulous cervix may be overcome by using either a balloon catheter or infusing the saline solution faster. Overall failure rates ranging from 1.8% (Bernard et al 1997) to 4.6% (Widrich et al 1996) are quoted.
- There is no evidence to support the theoretical concern that instillation of fluid into the uterine cavity, either at hysteroscopy or s-SHS, may promote dissemination of endometrial carcinoma (De Vare et al 1982).

CLINICAL CONDITIONS

Bleeding and/or pain with a positive pregnancy test

Sensitive urinary pregnancy testing kits, based on immunological assays, are able to detect β-HCG levels of between 20 and 50 iu with 99% accuracy. This has meant that an increasingly large number of women will present with bleeding and/or pain in early pregnancy. It has been estimated that about 30% of women will complain of pain or bleeding during early pregnancy and approximately 15% of clinically recognizable pregnancies will result in miscarriage, the majority before the 13th week (Prendiville 1997). Because of the large volume of work in such a highly sensitive area of gynaecology, an integrated approach to diagnosis and management of women presenting with bleeding and/or pelvic pain during the first trimester is required.

With the judicious use of ultrasound clinicians have the ability to alleviate anxiety concerning early pregnancy complications by accurately dating early pregnancy, confirming viability, diagnosing pregnancy failure and either directly or indirectly confirming extrauterine gestation. To do

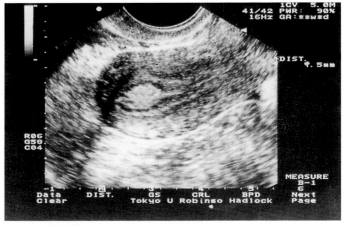

Fig. 7.1 Endometrial polyp. Sagittal view of the uterus, periovulatory, demonstrating a hyperechoic region within the endometrial cavity, which represents an endometrial polyp.

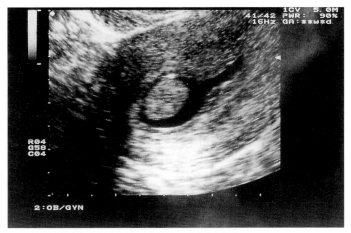

Fig. 7.2 Endometrial polyp. The same image as in Fig. 7.1, with the addition of sterile saline solution (sonohysterography).

this safely, knowledge of early pregnancy development – both ultrasonographically and biochemically – is pivotal.

Normal intrauterine pregnancy

The intrauterine gestation sac can first be visualized from about 4 weeks after the last menstrual period, using a trans-vaginal transducer; about 2 weeks earlier than if using the transabdominal approach (Fossam et al 1988). This is dependent upon a regular 28-day cycle and hence a more accurate approach to confirming pregnancy viability or failure is dependent upon either changes with time or the presence or absence of fetal cardiac activity. The gestational sac grows at approximately 1 mm a day in diameter in early pregnancy (Nyberg et al 1985) and can be differentiated from the 'pseudosac' of ectopic pregnancy by its thick, echogenic rind surrounding the echo-lucent central chorionic sac and eccentric location to the endometrial midline. The presence of a normal intrauterine gestation sac is associated with β-hCG levels of greater than 1000 iu. Detection at levels greater than this is dependent upon a number of factors, including type of probe and ultrasound machine used, the presence of leiomyomas, operator variations and multiple gestations (Bernaschek et al 1988, Nyberg et al 1985). The absence of a gestation sac should prompt the operator to look for an extrauterine gestation (including a close examination of the cornua and cervix as well as the adnexa). The yolk sac can be visualized from 5 weeks gestation (Fig. 7.3) and the early embryonic pole from approximately 6 weeks. First recognized as a thickening along the yolk sac, it is linear to begin with, subsequently becoming curved in nature. Embryonic growth rate is 1 mm/day.

Cardiac activity starts at approximately 5 weeks after the LMP. Cardiac activity not detected in embryos of more than 4 mm is associated with embryonic demise (Brown et al 1990, Goldstein 1992, Levi et al 1990). However, a repeat scan to confirm diagnosis is always indicated. Embryonic bradycardia can be associated with poor outcome (Doubilet et al 1999), and a follow-up scan is warranted to confirm viability.

Miscarriage

Once the diagnosis of intrauterine pregnancy has been established, the potential viability of the pregnancy will need to be addressed. The clinical value of the normal developmental timespan of the early embryonic and extra-embryonic structures is its application in the diagnosis of pregnancy failure. What becomes more relevant is not the earliest point at which a structure can be seen (threshold), but the point at which a structure is always seen in a normally developing intrauterine pregnancy (discriminatory level) and so its absence is diagnostic of pregnancy failure. Once an ectopic pregnancy has been excluded, all intrauterine pregnancies should be given the benefit of the doubt and serial scans performed to confirm a diagnosis. However, cardiac activity should always be visualized in an embryo measuring 6 mm or more (Fig. 7.4).

Knowledge of early pregnancy anatomical landmarks allows us to follow fetal development within a normal pregnancy and to establish safe guidelines in the diagnosis of a pathological pregnancy.

Terminology

- *Missed miscarriage (early fetal demise):* Crown–rump length (CRL) of at least 6 mm with no cardiac activity or no change in size on weekly serial scanning.
- *Blighted ovum (early embryonic demise):* Gestational sac mean diameter of at least 20 mm with no embryonic/extraembryonic structures present.
- *Incomplete miscarriage:* Disrupted endometrial echo, measuring more than 15 mm in the anteroposterior plane (Fig. 7.5).
- *Complete miscarriage:* Endometrial thickness of less than 15 mm measured in the anteroposterior plane associated with the cessation of heavy bleeding and pain.

Trouble shooting

- In practice, the presence of an intrauterine gestation usually excludes an ectopic pregnancy.

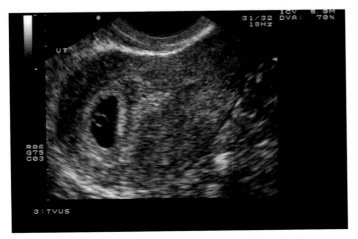

Fig. 7.3 Intrauterine gestation and yolk sac: 5 weeks gestation.

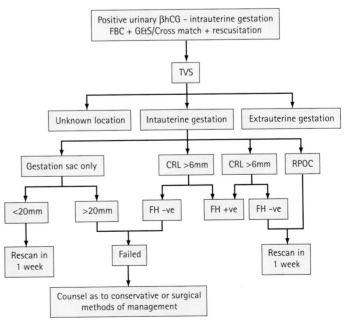

Fig. 7.4 Assessment of viability in early pregnancy.

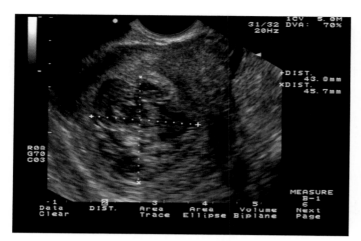

Fig. 7.5 Sagittal view of the uterus demonstrating retained products of conception.

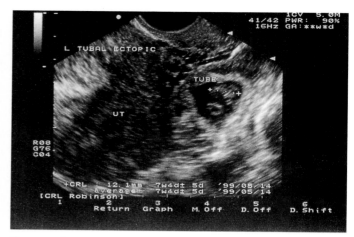

Fig. 7.6 Sagittal section of the left adnexa, demonstrating a tubal ectopic pregnancy. The crown-rump length is marked (12.1 mm).

- Once ectopic pregnancy is excluded, early pregnancies should be given the benefit of the doubt: serial scans are of more value than serial β-HCG values.
- Cardiac activity should be seen with a CRL of 6 mm or greater
- A fetal pole/yolk sac should be seen with a gestation sac mean diameter of 20 mm

Ectopic pregnancy

The exclusion of an ectopic gestation remains a primary goal for the clinician assessing the patient presenting with pain and/or bleeding in early pregnancy. Traditionally, the presence of an empty uterus with a positive urinary pregnancy test has meant hospital admission with either laproscopy of follow-up scans until a diagnosis is made. However, the combined use of high-resolution vaginal probes and serum β-HCG assays has meant that patients with symptoms and clinical findings suggestive of an ectopic gestation will fall into one of three categories.

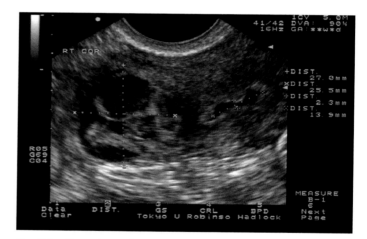

Fig. 7.7 Cornual ectopic pregnancy. The gestation sac is seen separately from the endometrial echo.

1. An intrauterine pregnancy will be diagnosed on scan: to all extents and purposes this will exclude an extrauterine location. The frequency of heterotopic pregnancy in spontaneous conceptions is estimated at between 1:10 000 and 1:50 000, but as high as 1:100 in assisted conceptions (Ludwig et al 1999), and should be suspected if there are persistent symptoms.
2. An extrauterine gestation will be visualized by ultrasound or features highly predictive of one (e.g. haemoperitoneum) (Figs 7.6, 7.7 and 7.8).
3. No evidence of intra- or extrauterine gestation will be found on scan alone: a pregnancy of unknown location.

Further management of the patient will be dependent upon her clinical status. Within our unit we have noted a significant reduction in those patients presenting with acute haemodynamic compromise due to a ruptured ectopic pregnancy since the EPU was established. This has meant that more conservative methods of treatment can be used, whether surgical (laparoscopic salpingectomy, salpingotomy), medical (methotrexate) or expectant (Fig. 7.9).

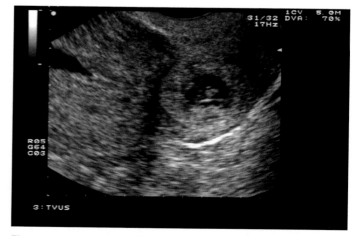

Fig. 7.8 Sagittal view of the cervix containing a gestational sac, fetal pole and yolk sac. The proximal portion of the endometrial cavity contains free fluid and can be seen on the left side of the image.

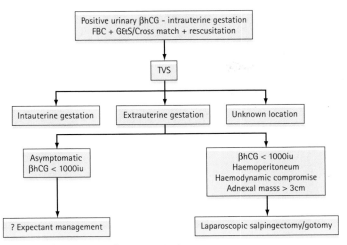

Fig. 7.9   Assessment of an extrauterine pregnancy.

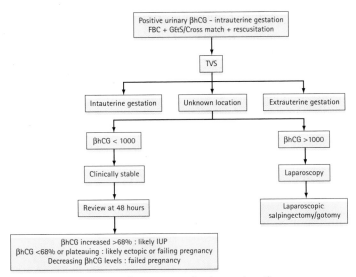

Fig. 7.10   Assessment of pregnancy of unknown location.

Table 7.1   Single-dose intramuscular methotrexate protocol for treatment of unruptured ectopic pregnancy (reproduced with permission from Stovall & Ling 1993)

Day	Therapy
0	β-hCG, FBC, G&S, LFT, U&E
1	β-hCG, intramuscular methotrexate: 50 mg/m²
4	β-hCG
7	β-hCG, FBC, LFT 2nd methotrexate dose if day 7 β-hCG decrease <15% from day 4

β-hCG, human chorionic gonadotrophin
FBC, full blood count
G&S, blood group and serum save
U&E, urea and electrolytes
LFT, liver function tests

All non-surgical methods of treating ectopic gestations will need intensive follow-up to ensure resolution of symptoms and β-HCG values. Table 7.1 demonstrates the follow-up regime for those women receiving methotrexate in use by our unit. Patient compliance is central to these patients being treated on an outpatient basis, along with a dedicated EPU service.

Pregnancy of unknown location

A proportion of women presenting with complications of early pregnancy will have no sonographic features of extra- or intrauterine pregnancy. In this group will be patients who have a very early, continuing, intrauterine pregnancy, those who have an ectopic gestation and those who have a failing pregnancy, whether intra- or extrauterine. Rarely a false-positive result may be due to a placental site tumour, for example of the ovary. Figure 7.10 demonstrates a suggested follow-up regime for those women who fall into this category. Again, a co-ordinated EPU and rapid β-HCG assay service are essential.

Coexistent pathology

The prevalence of ovarian pathology in early pregnancy is high; one advantage of transvaginal ultrasound is the ability to visualize the adnexa clearly in early pregnancy. The majority of adnexal pathology will be functional in nature, typically corpus luteal, and will spontaneously resolve as the pregnancy enters the second trimester. Whether surgical intervention is indicated for persistent, symptomatic cysts will be dictated on an individual basis and the role of cyst aspiration and laparoscopic surgical techniques can be maximized when there is clear ultrasound definition of cyst type.

Those patients managed expectantly should be rescanned 6 weeks postnatally to ensure cyst resolution or to arrange surgical intervention if there is persistence of the cyst.

Postnatal assessment

Few studies have targeted the normal ultrasound parameters of the uterus and ovaries in the postnatal period. The sonographic appearances of retained products of conception are variable (Carlan et al 1997, Hertzberg & Bowie 1991). One study evaluating the appearance of the uterine cavity revealed an echogenic mass in 51% of women with normal postpartum bleeding at 7 days postpartum (Edwards & Ellwood 2000). Sonohysterography has been shown to enhance the ability of transvaginal ultrasound to diagnose retained products of conception (Wolman et al 2000), although in the presence of suspected pelvic infection, this procedure should not be performed. Management should be based primarily on clinical findings with sonographic evaluation of the uterus and endometrium reserved for those cases with persistent symptoms. Rarely, arteriovenous malformations can cause protracted, heavy bleeding in the puerperium. If suspected, colour Doppler assessment of the uterine vasculature will aid their diagnosis, prior to arteriography and embolization. If surgical evacuation of retained products of conception is performed in the immediate postnatal period, the recognized higher morbidity associated with the procedure can be reduced by evacuating the uterus under sonographic guidance (Kohlenberg & Casper 1996).

Pelvic pain and a negative pregnancy test

Transvaginal ultrasound undoubtedly has a pivotal role for the assessment of early pregnancy complications. Its role in those patients who are not pregnant, however, is more subtle and, rather than being central to diagnosis, works in parallel with clinical findings and history, serum analyses, urinalysis and other radiological investigations. We will look at the role of ultrasound in the patient with acute pelvic pain and then in acute vaginal bleeding.

The premenopausal patient

The importance of a complete clinical history and examination cannot be overemphasized, especially with the use of pelvic ultrasound. The premenopausal ovary and endometrium, as visualized with the transvaginal probe, are dynamic structures, exhibiting cyclical changes in morphology and volume throughout the cycle. A knowledge of the normal variations that can be exhibited is important, as the most common ovarian pathology is the functional cyst.

The presence of adnexal pathology in the patient presenting with pelvic pain may be a coincidence and gentle use of the transvaginal probe to map the pain within the pelvis will help indicate the structures giving rise to the pain. The overwhelming advantages of the transvaginal approach in the assessment of pelvic pain are not only the excellent diagnostic capabilities but in the presence of an acute abdomen, especially in those women with pelvic inflammatory disease, this route is tolerated much better than a transabdominal approach with a full bladder.

Pelvic pain in association with pelvic mass   In those patients presenting with pelvic pain in whom there is evidence of a pelvic mass on ultrasound, an assessment needs to be made not only of pain severity and type but also the nature of the mass. Transvaginal ultrasound has a proven track record in experienced hands in the differentiation of uterine myomas from adnexal masses and also in the characterization of adnexal masses.

Ovarian pathology   The prevalence of adnexal pathology among premenopausal women is high and the overwhelming majority of these lesions will be benign in nature. A large proportion of benign ovarian cysts will be functional and, if symptoms settle, may be managed expectantly.

A careful history and a clear knowledge of the day of the menstrual cycle will prompt the sonographer to the most likely cause of the pain. For example, acute onset, midcycle pain may be indicative of a follicular or corpus luteal cyst accident. Haemorrhage into a corpus luteal cyst has characteristic sonographic findings (Fig. 7.11). The condition tends to be self-limiting and often responds to non-steroidal anti-inflammatory analgesia. Surgery should be avoided if possible.

Although usually self-limiting, the cyclical occurrence of haemorrhagic corpus luteal cyst can be a source of persistent morbidity and if there are no contraindications, use of the combined oral contraceptive to suppress ovulation is beneficial. This is also indicated for those women who have clotting factor deficiencies, for example, von Willebrand's disease. They may present with an acute abdomen, secondary to a haemoperitoneum as a result of ovulation or corpus luteal haemorrhage or rupture.

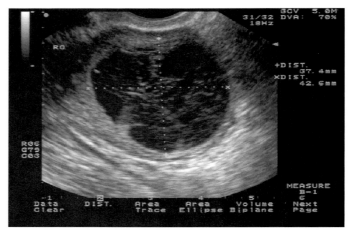

Fig. 7.11   Haemorrhagic corpus luteal cyst. Fine strands of fibrin are seen within the cyst contents.

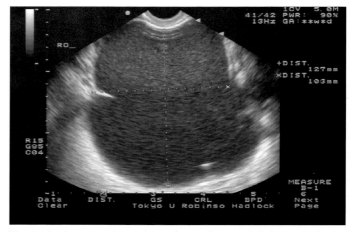

Fig. 7.12   Large ovarian endometrioma: characteristic 'ground-glass' appearance to the cyst contents.

Those women with a history suggestive of endometriosis presenting with acute pain may have sonographic evidence of an endometrioma (Fig. 7.12). These rarely undergo torsion, as they are often fixed within the pelvis, but may undergo rupture or acute haemorrhage within the cyst. Rarely they can become infected. Recent cyst rupture may be suggested by the presence of resolving clinical symptoms, with free fluid present in the pouch of Douglas, often with a collapsing irregular cyst wall.

A suggested follow-up regime for women diagnosed with a pelvic mass is shown in Figure 7.13. Intervention will be dictated by the resolution – or not – of the patient's symptoms. If the symptoms resolve and there are no sonographic features of malignancy on the ultrasound, a repeat scan at 6 weeks should be performed to confirm cyst resolution.

Ovarian torsion is unusual with adnexal masses <5 cm (Nichols & Julian 1985). However, there are no pathognomonic features specific to adnexal torsion and a high degree of clinical suspicion is essential. The clinical history is of acute onset, constant pain not responding to analgesia, often with nausea

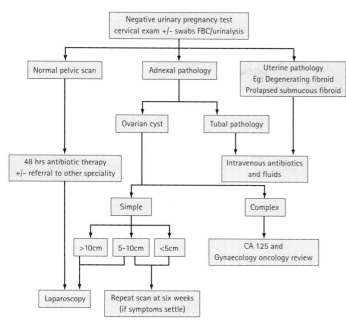

```
Negative urinary pregnancy test
cervical exam +/- swabs FBC/urinalysis
```

```
Normal pelvic scan        Adnexal pathology        Uterine pathology
                                                   Eg: Degenerating fibroid
                                                   Prolapsed submucous fibroid
```

```
                    Ovarian cyst        Tubal pathology
```

```
48 hrs antibiotic therapy              Intravenous antibiotics
+/- referral to other speciality          and fluids
```

```
            Simple                      Complex
```

```
>10cm   5-10cm   <5cm        CA 125 and
                             Gynaecology oncology review
```

```
Laparoscopy    Repeat scan at six weeks
               (if symptoms settle)
```

Fig. 7.13 Assessment of pelvic mass.

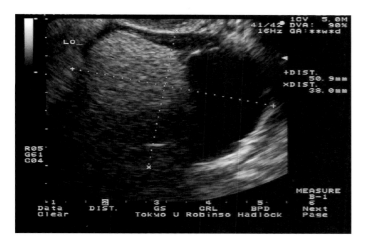

Fig. 7.14 Benign cystic teratoma: acoustic shadowing is demonstrated.

and vomiting and systemic upset. Of the persistent adnexal masses in premenopausal women, benign cystic teratomas (Fig. 7.14) are more likely to undergo torsion than endometriomas. The central feature of ovarian torsion is the cessation of vascular supply. Colour Doppler has therefore been used to interrogate the adnexal mass suspected of undergoing torsion. It is likely, however, that even if flow can be visualized within the mass, despite clinical symptoms and signs of ovarian torsion, ovarian blood flow may still be compromised, as demonstrated by surgically proven ovarian torsion, despite detecting blood flow within the mass (Rosado et al 1992).

Uterine leiomyomas These may undergo torsion if pedunculated in nature, may prolapse through the cervix or

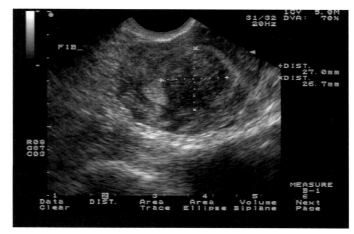

Fig. 7.15 Sagittal view of the uterus, showing a submucous fibroid.

may undergo degeneration, especially during pregnancy. In fibroid degeneration, the patient is often systemically unwell, with a pyrexia, leucocytosis and generalized abdominal tenderness.

The ultrasound characteristics of leiomyomas are well documented and cystic areas can be visualized within the fibroid if it is degenerating. Advances in the management of uterine myomas have resulted in a need to provide accurate pretreatment information concerning their size, quantity and location. This is especially true with the increasing use of minimally invasive techniques of fibroid resection. The ultrasound appearances of myomas are varied. Before the menopause they tend to be a well-defined heterogeneous or hypoechoic uterine mass. TVS is used in conjunction with abdominal scanning to ensure pedunculated subserosal fibroids are not missed. Submucosal fibroids project into the uterine cavity and distort the endometrium (Fig. 7.15). Their accurate classification allows selection for transcervical resection in appropriate cases. Fedele et al (1991) demonstrated the sensitivity of TVS for the diagnosis of submucosal fibroids to be 100%, with a sensitivity of 94%. Hysteroscopy (outpatient) performed on the same population had a sensitivity and specificity of 100% and 96% respectively in their diagnosis. The only criticism of TVS in this study was its apparent inability to differentiate endometrial polyps from submucosal fibroids. All scans were performed in the secretory phase of the cycle. Endometrial polyps tend to be hyperechoic structures, easily masked by a thick secretory endometrium. By performing the scans during the proliferative phase, the distinction between intracavity fibroids and polyps is easier to make (Schwarzler et al 1998).

Tubal pathology Acute pelvic inflammatory disease, with hydrosalpinx, pyosalpinx or frank tubo-ovarian abscesses, tends to present with systemic upset, leucocytosis, unilateral progressing to bilateral pelvic pain, menstrual disturbances and vaginal discharge. The differentials will therefore include adnexal torsion, acute fibroid degeneration, urinary tract infection and appendicitis.

Acute inflammatory processes within the fallopian tubes tend to produce thick-walled, cystic structures, tender to the touch of the probe (Fig. 7.16). However, a chronic hydro-

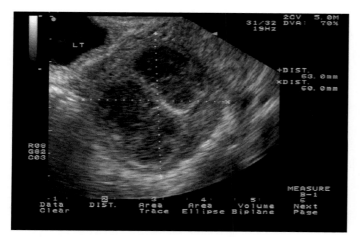

Fig. 7.16 Tubo-ovarian abscess: an irregular, thick-walled multiloculated structure.

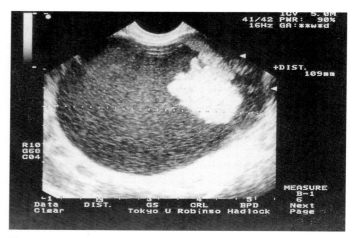

Fig. 7.17 Ovarian endometroid adenocarcinoma: stage Ia. Note the large papillary projection from the cyst wall.

salpinx will have the appearance of a thin-walled structure, not obviously tender on probing and often detected coincidentally (Timor-Tritsch et al 1998).

Acute urinary retention A full bladder may sometimes be confused with an ovarian cyst. If there is any doubt and the patient is unable to void urine, a catheter should be passed to ensure the bladder is empty. Occasionally a blood clot may be visible within the bladder.

Pelvic pain – no mass on scan In the absence of pathology on scan, blood should be taken for leucocytosis and culture. Urinalysis should be performed and a complete infection screen, including endocervical and high vaginal swabs. Contact tracing should be performed via the genitourinary clinic.

Transvaginal scan may reveal evidence of adhesions and loculated fluid, which may be indicative of previous pelvic or abdominal pathology.

Non-gynaecological pathology It is often not possible to make a diagnosis based on clinical, ultrasound and serum findings alone. Medical, surgical and urological opinions should be sought where indicated, with early recourse to laparoscopy in those patients who have persistent or worsening symptoms.

The postmenopausal patient

Characterization of any adnexal mass is important within this age group as the risk of a mass being malignant is high (Fig. 7.17). Unilocular cysts may be found in up to 20% of asymptomatic postmenopausal women. Numerous studies have shown that simple, unilocular cysts measuring less than 5 cm in diameter are associated with a very low risk of malignancy (Kroon & Andolf 1995). Blood should be taken for tumour markers and emergency laparotomy avoided if at all possible, to allow for adequate oncological work-up of the patient if indicated. Urinary retention must be excluded. Other chronic surgical and medical conditions are more predominant in the older age group, such as diverticulitis, constipation and urinary tract infections. Early recourse to advice from other specialties should be considered in those women with pelvic or abdominal pain.

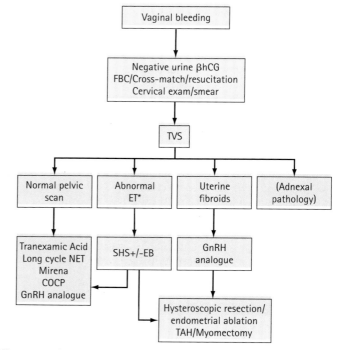

Fig. 7.18 Assessment of acute vaginal bleeding.

Acute bleeding and a negative pregnancy test

This is most effectively divided into problems occurring in the premenopausal and postmenopausal patient, as the aetiology can be very different. A full history and clinical examination is essential, along with resuscitation of the patient.

The investigation of abnormal uterine bleeding will centre on an assessment of the endometrium (Fig. 7.18). Undirected endometrial sampling alone has no role in the evaluation of abnormal uterine bleeding. It will miss focal lesions, such as polyps and fibroids. Whilst transvaginal ultrasound remains a cost-effective, non-invasive, well-tolerated technique for examining the pelvic organs, it is less specific than hysteroscopy when differentiating between endometrial polyps, myomas, carcinoma and hyperplasia. The addition of a negative contrast medium, such as saline, into the uterine cavity addresses this problem. There is an overwhelming quantity of data now which has shown high-resolution transvaginal ultrasound with saline instillation to be as predictive as hysteroscopy in the detection of endometrial pathology.

The premenopausal patient

The main differentials within this group are genital tract disease, systemic disease and iatrogenic causes. When all these have been excluded, a diagnosis of dysfunctional uterine bleeding can be made. History, clinical examination and pelvic ultrasound will help elucidate the cause. Disease of the genital tract in this age group will focus on benign rather than malignant conditions. Benign pelvic conditions will include fibroids, endometrial and cervical polyps, cervicitis, adenomyosis and endometriosis, along with pelvic infection and foreign bodies. Systemic problems contributing to abnormal uterine bleeding will include coagulation disorders, chronic liver and renal disease and thyroid dysfunction. Iatrogenic causes will include anticoagulant therapy, intrauterine contraceptive devices and hormonal preparations. There needs to be heightened suspicion of an underlying systemic disease in younger patients presenting with heavy, vaginal bleeding, as up to 20% (Kadir et al 1998) may have a coagulopathy. Screening for a coagulopathy is also advised in women with abnormal vaginal bleeding who fail medical or surgical therapy. The endometrial thickness on ultrasound will dictate the need for endometrial sampling, as will the patient's history.

The primary goal with acute uterine bleeding will be to ensure cessation of bleeding, usually with a combination of therapies, such as antifibrinolytics, high-dose progestogens, GnRH analogues or the Mirena IUS, until definitive management can be effected. Occasionally, urgent examination under anaesthesia with the introduction of a uterine cavity balloon is indicated to stop the bleeding. Interventional radiology with uterine artery embolization may have a role in the acute management.

The postmenopausal patient

Abnormal vaginal bleeding in this age group should be attributed to malignancy until proven otherwise. Malignant tumours of the endometrium, cervix, vagina and vulva may all present with vaginal bleeding, as can ovarian tumours, such as granulosa cell tumours. It is wise to confirm that the bleeding is genital tract in origin, as occasionally haematuria and rectal bleeding may present as suspected postmenopausal vaginal bleeding.

INTERVENTIONAL ULTRASOUND

Outside the fertility unit, gynaecological interventional ultrasound has its limitations. There is abundant evidence supporting definitive surgery for adnexal pathology, such as ovarian cystectomy, rather than simple cyst puncture. This is not only because cyst recurrence after cyst drainage is higher than if the capsule is removed (Balat et al 1996) but also cyst fluid cytology is not always representative of the cyst wall pathology (Dietrich et al 1999).

With the advent of high-resolution probes, the characterization of adnexal masses has become increasingly accurate and cyst puncture and drainage under ultrasound guidance remains important in those symptomatic patients with adnexal masses which have no sonographic evidence of malignancy, in whom surgery is relatively contraindicated; for example, extensive previous abdominal surgery or during pregnancy.

There has also been a general trend towards treating certain ectopic pregnancies non-surgically. This has been facilitated by the excellent resolution often afforded in early pregnancy, along with serial β-HCG assays, thus allowing diagnosis of ectopic pregnancy without the need for laparoscopy. The use of methotrexate in treating tubal gestations has been variable and appropriate case selection is imperative (Fernandez et al 1998, Sowter et al 2001, Stovall & Ling 1993). Its use in cornual pregnancy management has produced consistent results and an effective route is local administration under ultrasound guidance into the gestation sac (Hafner et al 1999). Although the coexistence of an ectopic gestation and intrauterine pregnancy remains rare outside assisted reproductive technology programmes, the use of transvaginal injection of potassium chloride or hyperosmolar glucose into the ectopic gestation is well documented.

CONCLUSION

The time has come to maximize the role of ultrasound within the routine assessment of the acute gynaecological patient. It complements the clinical examination, affording us a 'view' of the pelvic structures. Its integration into the gynaecology emergency service facilitates a more rapid diagnosis in a number of gynaecological conditions. It also helps to exclude gynaecological pathology, ensuring prompt referral to other specialties. Central to its appropriate use will be training and supervision, with up-to-date protocols and regular audit, and being aware of both personal and the equipment's limitations.

KEY POINTS

1. A normal pelvic scan will not exclude all underlying gynaecological conditions.
2. Visualization of an intrauterine gestation will generally exclude an ectopic pregnancy.
3. Once an ectopic pregnancy has been excluded, early pregnancies should be given the benefit of the doubt.
4. Fetal heart activity should be seen with a crown–rump length of 6 mm or greater.
5. The sonographic appearances of retained products of conception in the immediate postnatal period are variable: management should be based primarily on clinical findings.
6. There are no pathognomonic features specific to adnexal torsion: a high degree of clinical suspicion is paramount.
7. Undirected endometrial sampling alone has no role in the evaluation of abnormal uterine bleeding.
8. Transvaginal saline sonohysterography is as predictive as hysteroscopy in the detection of endometrial pathology.
9. Up to 20% of young women presenting with heavy, vaginal bleeding may have a coagulopathy.

REFERENCES

Alcazar JL, Laparte C, Jurado M, Lopez-Garcia G 1997 The role of transvaginal ultrasonography combined with color velocity imaging and pulsed Doppler in the diagnosis of endometrioma. Fertility and Sterility 67:487–491

Balat O, Sarac K, Sonmez S 1996 Ultrasound guided aspiration of benign ovarian cysts: an alterntive to surgery? European Journal of Radiology 22(2):136–137

Bernard JP, Lecuru F, Darles C, Robin F, de Bievre P, Taurelle R 1997 Saline contrast sonohysterography as first-line investigation for women with uterine bleeding. Ultrasound in Obstetrics and Gynecology 10:121–125

Bernaschek G, Rudelstorfer R, Csascsich P 1988 Vaginal sonography versus serum human chorionic gonadotrophin in early detection of pregnancy. American Journal of Obstetrics and Gynecology 158:608–612

Bigrigg MA, Read MD 1991 Management of women referred to early pregnancy assessment unit: care and cost effectiveness. British Medical Journal 302(6776):577–579

Brown DL, Emerson DS, Felker RE 1990 Diagnosis of embryonic demise by endovaginal sonography. Journal of Ultrasound in Medicine 9:711–716

Carlan SJ, Scott WT, Pollack R, Harris K 1997 Appearance of the uterus by ultrasound immediately after placental delivery with pathologic correlation. Journal of Clinical Ultrasound 25(6):301–308

De Vore G, Schwartz P, Morris J 1982 Hysterography: a five year follow-up in patients with endometrial carcinoma. Obstetrics and Gynecology 60:369–372

Dietrich M, Osmers RG, Grobe G et al 1999 Limitations of the evaluation of adnexal masses by its macroscopic aspects, cystology and biopsy. European Journal of Gynecology and Reproduction Biology 82(1):57–62

Dijkhuizen F, Brolmann H, Potters A, Bongers M, Heintz A 1996 The accuracy of transvaginal ultrasonography in the diagnosis of endometrial abnormalities. Obstetrics and Gynecology 87:345–349

Doubilet PM, Benson CB, Cow JS 1999 Long-term prognosis of pregnancies complicated by slow embryonic heart rates in the early first trimester. Journal of Ultrasound Medicine 18:537–541

Edwards A, Ellwood DA 2000 Ultrasonographic evaluation of the postpartum uterus. Ultrasound in Obstetrics and Gynecology 16(7):640–643

Fedele L, Bianchi S, Dorta M, Biroschi D, Zanotti F, Vercellini P 1991 Transvaginal ultrasonography versus hysteroscopy in the diagnosis of uterine submucosal myomas. Obstetrics and Gynecology 77:745–748

Fernandez H, Yves Vincent SC, Pauthier S, Audibert F, Frydman R 1998 Randomised trial of conservative laparoscopic treatment and methotrexate administration in ectopic pregnancy and subsequent fertility. Human Reproduction 13(11):3239–3243

Fossam GT, Davajan V, Kletzky OA 1988 Early detection of pregnancy with transvaginal ultrasound. Fertility and Sterility 49:788–791

Goldstein SR 1992 Significance of cardiac activity on endovaginal ultrasound in very early embryos. Obstetrics and Gynecology 80:670–672

Gonzalez CJ, Curson R, Parson J 1988 Transabdominal versus transvaginal ultrasound scanning of ovarian follicles: are they comparable? Fertility and Sterility 50:657–659

Granberg S, Norström A, Wikland M 1990 Tumors in the lower pelvis as imaged by transvaginal sonography. Gynecologic Oncology 37:224–229

Granberg S, Wikland M, Jansson I 1989 Macroscopic characterisation of ovarian tumors and the relation to the histological diagnosis: criteria to be used for ultrasound evaluation. Gynecologic Oncology 35:139–144

Granberg S, Wikland M, Karlsson B, Norstrom A, Friberg LG 1991 Endometrial thickness as measured by endovaginal ultrasonography for identifying endometrial abnormality. American Journal of Obstetrics and Gynecology 164:47–52

Hafner T, Aslam N, Ross JA, Zosmer N, Jurkovic D 1999 The effectiveness of non-surgical management of early interstitial pregnancy: a report of ten cases and review of the literature. Ultrasound in Obstetrics and Gynecology 13:131–136

Hertzberg BS, Bowie JD 1991 Ultrasound of the postpartum uterus. Prediction of retained placental tissue. Journal of Ultrasound in Medicine 10(8):451–456

Indman PD 1995 Abnormal uterine bleeding. Accuracy of vaginal probe ultrasound in predicting abnormal hysteroscopic findings. Journal of Reproductive Medicine 40:545–548

Jermy K, Luise C, Bourne T 2001 The characterization of common ovarian cysts in premenopausal women. Ultrasound in Obstetrics and Gynecology 17(2):140–144

Jimenez R, Duff P 1997 Sheathing of the endovaginal probe: is it adequate? Infectious Diseases in Obstetrics and Gynecology 1:37–39

Kadir RA, Economides DL, Sabin CA, Owens D, Lee CA 1998 Frequency of inherited bleeding disorders in women with menorrhagia. Lancet 351:485–489

Kohlenberg CF, Casper GR 1996 The use of intraoperative ultrasound in the management of a perforated uterus with retained products of conception. Australia and New Zealand Journal of Obstetrics and Gynaecology 36(4):482–448

Koonings PP, Campbell K, Mishell D, Grimes D 1989 Relative frequency of ovarian neoplasms: a 10 year review. Obstetrics and Gynecology 74:921–925

Kroon E, Andolf E 1995 Diagnosis and follow-up of simple ovarian cysts detected by ultrasound in postmenopausal women. Obstetrics and Gynecology 85:211–214

Levi CS, Lyons EA, Zheng HX 1990 Endovaginal US: demonstration of cardiac activity in embryos of less than 5 mm in crown rump length. Radiology 176:71–74

Ludwig M, Kaisi M, Bauer O, Diedrich K 1999 Heterotopic pregnancy in a spontaneous cycle: do not forget about it! European Journal of Obstetrics, Gynecology and Reproductive Biology 87(1):91–93

Mendelson EB, Bohm-Velez M, Joseph N, Neiman HL 1988 Endometrial abnormalities: evaluation with transvaginal sonography. American Journal of Radiology 150:139–142

Nicholas D, Julian P 1985 Torsion of the adnexa. Clinical Obstetrics and Gynecology 28:375–380

Nyberg DA, Filly RA, Mahony BS 1985 Early gestation: correlation of hCG levels and sonographic identification. American Journal of Roentgenology 144:951–954

Prendiville WJ 1997 Miscarriage: epidemiological aspects. In: Grudzinskas JG, O'Brian PMS (eds) Problems in early pregnancy: advances in diagnosis and management. RCOG Press, London

Rasado W, Trambert M, Gosink B, Pretorius D 1992 Adnexal torsion: diagnosis by using Doppler sonography American Journal of Radiology 159:1251–1253

Rodriguez MH, Platt LD, Medearis AL, Lacarra M, Lobo RA 1988 The use of transvaginal ultrasonography for evaluation of postmenopausal ovarian size and morphology. American Journal of Obstetrics and Gynecology 159:810–814

Royal College of Obstetricians and Gynaecologists 2000 Clinical guideline number 22. Anti-D immunoglobulin for Rh prophylaxis.

Schwarzler P, Concin H, Bosch H et al 1988 An evaluation of sonohysterography and diagnostic hysteroscopy for the assessment of intrauterine pathology. Ultrasound in Obstetrics and Gynecology 11:337–342

Sowter MC, Farquhar CM, Petrie KJ, Gudex G 2001 A randomized trial comparing single dose methotrexate and laparoscopic surgery for the treatment of unruptured tubal pregnancy. British Journal of Obstetrics and Gynaecology 108(2):192–203

Stovall TG, Ling FW 1993 Single dose methotrexate: an expanded clinical trial. American Journal of Obstetrics and Gynecology 168:1759–1765

Tailor A, Jurkovic D, Bourne T, Collins W, Campbell S 1997 Sonographic prediction of malignancy in adnexal masses using multivariate logistic regression analysis. Ultrasound in Obstetrics and Gynecology 10:41–47

Timmerman D, Bourne TH, Tailor A et al 1999a A comparison of methods for the pre-operative discrimination between benign and malignant adnexal masses: the development of a new logistic regression model. American Journal of Obstetrics and Gynecology 181:57–65

Timmerman D, Deprest J, Bourne T, van den Berghe I, Collins WP, Vergote I 1988 A randomized trial on the use of ultrasound or office hysteroscopy for endometrial assessment in postmenopausal patients with breast cancer who where treated with tomaxifen. American Journal of Obstetrics and Gynecology 1:62–70

Timmerman T, Schwärzler P, Collins W et al 1999b Subjective assessment of adnexal masses using ultrasonography: an analysis of interobserver variability and experience. Ultrasound in Obstetrics Gynecology 13:11–16

Timmerman D, Verrelst H, Bourne T et al 1999c Artificial neural network models for the pre-operative discrimination between malignant and benign adnexal masses. Ultrasound in Obstetrics Gynecology 13:17–25

Timor-Tritsch IE, Lerner JP, Monteagudo A, Murphy KE, Heller DS 1988 Transvaginal sonographic markers of tubal inflammatory disease. Ultrasound Obstetrics Gynecology 12(1):56–66

Widrich T, Bradley LD, Mitchinson AR, Collins RL 1996 Comparison of saline infusion sonography with office hysteroscopy for the evaluation of the endometrium. American Journal of Obstetrics and Gynecology 74:1327–1334

Wolman I, Gordon D, Yaron Y, Kupferminc M, Lessing JB, Jaffa AJ 2000 Transvaginal sonohysterography for the evaluation and treatment of retained products of conception. Gynecology and Obstetrics Investigation 50(2):73–76

8

Preoperative care

Rob J. Gornall

INTRODUCTION

Thorough preoperative assessment of the patient is essential not only for the patient but also for the medical staff and the hospital. It reduces the risks of the procedure for the patient and ensures that the planned procedure is the most appropriate for her. It increases the likelihood of a satisfactory outcome and reduces the risk of delay or cancellation of the procedure.

CHOOSING THE BEST TREATMENT OPTION

Preoperative assessment begins in the outpatient department when the decision is made to undertake surgery. The gynaecologist must weigh up the nature of the disorder and the severity of symptoms and offer advice on the medical and surgical options. A balanced view must be presented of the benefits of the operation and the risks. There are often alternative treatments and it is vital that informed discussion is carried out between the doctor and the patient to determine what is the most appropriate treatment given the wishes of the patient and her condition. Experienced decision making at this stage is essential to the success of the procedure and the patient's satisfaction of the outcome. Subsequent skilled surgery can only rarely correct for a wrongly planned or inappropriate procedure on a poorly prepared patient.

The surgeon will also benefit from accurate documentation of such factors. There is increasing public scrutiny of individual surgical performance. Morbidity and mortality figures are corrected for co-morbidity, such as underlying malignancy or severe medical disease, but such factors will only be taken into account if they have been fully recorded. Cancellation of major procedures on the day of surgery because of inadequate preoperative assessment will be interpreted as poor utilization of expensive theatre sessions lists and may be used in the future as performance indicators.

Fully documented medical assessment is therefore vital to ensure that patients are treated with all the appropriate safeguards in place. Forward planning is essential to ensure that factors that may affect management are identified early and addressed prior to admission. Satisfactory preoperative assessment encompasses evaluation of the surgical risk factors, the obtaining of informed consent and aims to minimize complications.

EXPLANATION AND CONSENT

It is fundamental that the patient should have as clear an understanding as possible about the procedure she is about to undergo so that she may give her consent in the full knowledge of what the risks may be. No surgeon wants to frighten his patient unduly, especially if surgery is unavoidable and the serious risks are rare. One view is that the patient with cancer has more than enough to worry about without being given a detailed account of all the possible complications. Telling her all about what might go wrong puts the surgeon 'in the clear' but increases the patient's fear to almost intolerable levels. On the other hand, most patients are aware that operations can go wrong and find it helpful to have a discussion about the potential hazards that puts these into perspective. It is useful to talk about the problems that are likely to arise, the complications that might happen and those that are unlikely. Ideally, each discussion should be documented although some conversations take place when the notes are not available. The main purpose of the documentation is to ensure that other members of the team know what has already been discussed.

For consent to be valid in law, three conditions must be satisfied:

1. the patient must be competent to give consent
2. appropriate information must be received and understood by the patient
3. the patient's consent must be voluntary and without coercion.

Failure to meet any of these conditions could result in a civil or criminal claim for assault, battery or negligence.

Competence to consent

Adults over 18 years are generally presumed to be competent to make treatment decisions on their own behalf. To demonstrate competence they must be able to understand what is being proposed and to remember the information long enough to make a balanced choice. Mental illness and mental disability do not automatically render an individual incompetent to consent. No adult may give consent on behalf of another. This includes the next of kin.

Young people aged 16–17 are entitled to consent to medical treatment or investigation in the same manner as adults. The only difference is that the refusal of a person aged 16–17 can be over-ridden in certain circumstances by a person with parental responsibility or by the court (Department of Health 2001).

Consent for children under 16 undergoing diagnostic or therapeutic procedures is complex and advice should be sought. In general, the child must give consent if competent to do so. The parents or guardians should usually be consulted and their approval sought. In the case of termination of pregnancy and contraception, the patient's right to confidentiality should be respected if she does not want her parents to be informed and if the doctor is satisfied that she is sufficiently mature to

understand the course of action proposed and its consequences.

Treatment without consent can take place only under special circumstances:

- where the patient is unconscious and unable to provide consent, e.g. the acutely unconscious patient, patients on life support, elective ventilation, permanent vegetative states
- where there are statutory powers requiring examination of a patient, e.g. the Public Health (Control of Disease) Act 1984
- in some cases a court can decide that a minor who is a ward of court should have treatment
- in certain circumstances under the Mental Health Act 1983. This applies only to the treatment of mental conditions.

In these instances the professional should discuss the proposed procedure with the next of kin in case they have substantial objections and make a record of these discussions in the patient's casenotes. The procedure must be carried out in the best interests of the patient.

Consent should always be obtained in an emergency situation wherever possible. If the professional judges that the patient is unable or not competent to provide consent, the procedure may be carried out only in the best interests of the patient, to save life or preserve health. In these instances the professional should discuss the proposed procedure with the next of kin where possible and make a record of these discussions in the patient's casenotes.

Timing of consent

Consent should be sought before the proposed procedure and before sedation is given. It should be discussed when the patient is not unduly stressed and when she has time to consider the information given. Every effort should be made to avoid taking consent immediately before the procedure, e.g. in the anaesthetic room. In cases of elective procedures, consent may be obtained during the outpatient consultation.

If the intended procedure or its impact on the patient changes, consent should be reobtained. Similarly, if a period of time elapses between obtaining consent and admission, it is recommended that the patient's understanding of the procedure and the consent previously given is reconfirmed. A patient can withdraw consent at any time without prejudice.

Who should seek consent?

Consent should always be sought by someone competent to ensure that information on all aspects of the procedure has been given to and understood by the patient. It is preferable that consent be obtained by the person who will carry out the procedure, particularly if the procedure is of a specialist nature.

Providing information

The quality of consent depends on the professional's ability to communicate information simply, accurately and sensitively. Special care should be taken to assess the competence of patients in shock, distress or pain.

If the patient has impaired hearing, sight or speech or has

difficulty in understanding English, appropriate provision must be made, including communication by sign language or through an interpreter. Preferably interpretation should not be provided by the patient's relative, who may have a vested interest.

Consent can be given only on the basis of the information provided. The information discussed with the patient should avoid technical terms and wherever possible be accompanied by written information, diagrams or models where appropriate. It is essential that the patient understand the information given. The process for obtaining consent must include an explanation of:

- the procedure, its purpose and expected outcomes
- any alternatives to the treatment proposed
- an outline of the risks and benefits
- the consequences of refusing treatment.

The professional should ask the patient to confirm that she has understood the discussion and explanation. In every case, a record of the discussion should be entered into the patient's casenotes.

If consent is conditional, the terms of these conditions need to be written down to avoid future misunderstandings. The surgeon must also make clear what will not be done at this procedure – even if it seems obvious that a second laparotomy will be required. The exception to this is when the surgery is urgent and life-saving. Resection of damaged bowel should obviously be undertaken but anterior resection for diverticulosis should not. Removal of malignant ovaries might be correct practice if the surgeon involved is qualified to do so but removal without consent of ovaries apparently affected by endometriosis would not be correct.

Explaining risk

The law states that the material risks of any procedure should be disclosed. Material risks are those to which a reasonable person in the patient's position would be likely to attach significance. However, there is clearly a balance to be struck between warning of risk and deterring a patient from agreeing to a necessary treatment. It is generally agreed that complications that are common or that have a profound effect on the patient's subsequent quality of life should be discussed (Sidaway 1985). It must be remembered that although it is good practice to document discussion of possible complications, this does not absolve the surgeon of any responsibility for complications that occur subsequently.

Jehovah's Witnesses

The Jehovah's Witnesses are a fundamentalist sect formed in the USA in the 1870s. There are now more than 80 000 in the UK. A minor part of their doctrine is taken to imply that blood transfusion should be forbidden as violating God's law. Jehovah's Witnesses accept medical treatment in all other respects and make no attempt to argue against the medical indications for blood transfusion. They are willing to take responsibility for their lives and accept that the constraints they place on their medical attendants may lead to their death.

Special consent forms are required for Jehovah's Witnesses who decline blood transfusion even if this will result in death. It is wise to review the indication for the procedure and to consider possible alternative treatments. It is important to explore fully the patient's beliefs in a variety of clinical scenarios and to determine whether haemodilution or autotransfusion are acceptable. It must be remembered that to administer blood against the wishes of the patient constitutes assault. The situation with regard to children is different by virtue of the Children and Young Persons Act 1933. A doctor may feel that such restrictions place them under undue pressure and most hospitals have protocols for management, including consent procedures involving nominated senior clinicians.

EVALUATION OF PHYSICAL STATUS

The assignment of a physical status category to patients based upon history and examination can act as a useful language when conferring information to the anaesthetists on their preoperative visit. The most widely used system at present is that recommended by the American Society of Anesthesiologists (ASA 1963; Table 8.1). In this system, patients are placed into one of five categories. Although this is a good indicator of the physical status of the patient prior to surgery, because the nature of the intended surgery is not taken into consideration it is not a good prognosticator of postoperative morbidity.

History

It is important in the preoperative preparation to take a detailed history with particular emphasis on those points relevant to the course of surgery and anaesthesia. This should include details of the presenting complaint, current medication, past medical and surgical history. The anaesthetist will be interested in any cardiorespiratory problems as well as any adverse reactions to anaesthesia that the patient may have suffered during previous surgery. Some of the more important questions are outlined in Table 8.2 and their relevance to the course of surgery and anaesthesia is detailed in subsequent sections.

Examination

The importance of a full examination documented in the notes by the house surgeon cannot be overemphasized. The anaesthetist will be interested in signs of respiratory disease,

Table 8.1 Classification of physical status (adapted from ASA 1963)

Status	Definition
ASA 1	Normal healthy patient – no known organic, biochemical or psychiatric disease
ASA 2	Patient with mild to moderate systemic disease
ASA 3	Patient with severe systemic disease that limits normal activity
ASA 4	Patient with severe systemic disease that is a consistent threat to life
ASA 5	Patient who is moribund and unlikely to survive 24 h

The addition of the letter E indicates those patients in whom emergency surgery is undertaken (e.g. ASA 4E).

Table 8.2 Important questions in an anaesthetic preoperative assessment

System or organ	Condition
Cardiovascular	Angina pectoris Myocardial infarction Rheumatic fever Systemic vascular disease
Respiratory	Acute coryza Exercise tolerance Dyspnoea and orthopnoea Asthma and allergic lung disease Bronchitis; cough and sputum production Pulmonary infection Pulmonary surgery Smoking
Nervous system	Epilepsy Neuromuscular disease Neuropathy Psychiatric disease and treatment
Liver	Alcohol consumption Hepatitis
Endocrine	Diabetes mellitus Thyroid disease Adrenal disease
Genitourinary	Renal disease Sexually transmitted disease Menstrual history – ?pregnant
Previous anaesthesia	Nausea and vomiting Adverse reactions Postspinal headache Familial problems with anaesthesia

Table 8.3 Preoperative factors predisposing to the development of postoperative cardiac complications (adapted from Goldman et al 1977)

Factors	Points
Gallop rhythm or elevated jugular venous pressure	11
Myocardial infarction in preceding 6 months	10
Abnormal rhythm other than premature atrial contractions on preoperative ECG	7
>5 premature ventricular contractions per minute	7
Age >70 years	5
Emergency surgery	4
Intraperitoneal, intrathoracic or aortic operation	3
Poor general physical status	3
Significant aortic stenosis	3

including the nature and pattern of respiration, the presence of abnormal breath sounds plus additional signs of respiratory incapacity, e.g. tracheal deviation, cyanosis. Simple bedside tests of respiratory function, such as peak expiratory flow measurements, may be useful indicators of respiratory reserve.

Cardiovascular examination should include assessment of heart rate and rhythm, auscultation for cardiac murmurs with particular emphasis on diastolic murmurs or the presence of a third or fourth heart sound. The measurement of arterial blood pressure is essential and should be repeated at least twice at intervals if it is found to be elevated.

The gynaecologist will obviously be interested in examination pertinent to the presenting complaint. More detailed examination of other systems is dictated by the presence of intercurrent disease. For example, neurological assessment of the patient with multiple sclerosis or assessment of joint mobility in the patient with rheumatoid arthritis is of particular importance if leg stirrups are to be employed.

Cardiovascular disease

The presence of cardiovascular disease is associated with increased morbidity and mortality following anaesthesia (Treasure & van Besouw 1993). Evaluation of the severity of the condition and instigation of measures to reduce the incidence of complications is an essential part of preoperative assessment. A number of attempts have been made to identify perioperative risk factors to try to improve perioperative morbidity. The most widely known is the cardiac risk index score (Goldman et al 1977; Table 8.3). Patients with a score greater than 13 should receive further medical treatment prior to surgery.

Coronary artery disease

The incidence of coronary artery disease in this country is high and patients may present with a spectrum of conditions from angina pectoris to myocardial infarction. The presence of coronary artery disease is associated with a significant increase in perioperative morbidity and mortality, including an increased incident risk of postoperative reinfarction in individuals presenting for surgery within 3 months of myocardial infarction (Mangano 1990, Nettleman et al 1997). In the preoperative assessment of these patients it is essential to determine the nature, frequency and duration of the anginal attacks and the efficacy of current medication. Where control of symptoms is inadequate, a cardiological opinion should be sought. If possible, elective surgery is best postponed for at least 3 months in individuals who have suffered recent myocardial infarction.

Hypertension

Hypertension has been defined by the World Health Organization as a persistently elevated systolic pressure >160 mmHg and/or a diastolic pressure >95 mmHg. Severe hypertension with blood pressure exceeding 180/100 mmHg is found in 11% of patients presenting for surgery. Anaesthesia in the presence of uncontrolled hypertension has a significant morbidity and mortality. Therefore preoperative assessment should determine the adequacy of blood pressure control, the nature of current therapy and assessment of any major organ dysfunction associated with sustained hypertensive disease, notably coronary artery disease, renal disease and cerebrovascular disease. Instigation of appropriate treatment is indicated. Where patients have diastolic blood pressure in excess of 120 mmHg, surgery should be postponed because they have extremely labile blood pressure perioperatively if untreated (Prys-Roberts 1984).

Valvular heart disease

Valvular heart disease may be congenital or acquired. It more commonly affects the left side of the heart, resulting in haemodynamic disturbances in left ventricular function, producing pressure-related disorders secondary to stenotic lesions of the aortic or mitral valves or volume-related disorders secondary to regurgitant lesions of the same valves.

In the preoperative assessment, the degree of cardiac reserve must be ascertained by evaluating exercise tolerance. The degree of compensatory mechanisms, such as increased sympathetic activity and myocardial hypertrophy, in the maintenance of normal cardiac output should be noted. Non-invasive assessment of valvular function by the use of echocardiography is most informative.

At-risk patients (Box 8.1) undergoing high-risk procedures (Box 8.2) should have prophylactic antibiotics before surgery in order to prevent the development of bacterial endocarditis, although proof of the efficacy of such treatment is not available and the risk of endocarditis is low. Recent recommendations for gynaecological surgery in high-risk patients are gentamicin 1.5 mg/kg intravenously and ampicillin 1 g intravenously 30 minutes prior to surgery followed by ampicillin 1 g IV or IM 6 hours later. In those individuals who are penicillin sensitive, vancomycin 1g intravenously is given by infusion over 1–2 hours plus gentamicin 30 minutes before the induction of anaesthesia.

Dysrhythmias

The presence of dysrhythmias may be associated with cardiovascular, renal, pulmonary or metabolic disease or may occur secondary to drug therapy such as digoxin. If untreated, they may result in marked haemodynamic disturbance. The frequency of dysrhythmia is increased by perioperative events, such as hypoxia, hypercarbia, alterations in acid–base balance or potassium homeostasis.

Preoperative assessment should focus on the nature and frequency of the dysrhythmia – whether supraventricular or ventricular – the correction of any exacerbating conditions and the initiation of appropriate therapy. Heart block of any kind is always due to organic damage to the conducting system and, if third-degree or second-degree Mobitz type 2, should be treated with transvenous pacing prior to surgery.

Respiratory disease

Respiratory disease will decrease the efficiency of gas exchange in the lungs. In combination with the respiratory depressant effects of anaesthesia and surgery on pulmonary function, this results in an increase in postoperative morbidity and mortality. Preoperative pulmonary evaluation is mandatory for all patients scheduled for surgery. The tests of respiratory reserve used depend on the severity of the presenting symptoms.

Upper respiratory tract infections

It is seldom necessary for patients with upper respiratory tract infections to undergo elective surgery. The infection, combined with the immunosuppressive effects of anaesthesia, the inhibition of postoperative coughing and the sedative effects of narcotic agents used to relieve postoperative pain, increases the risk of developing postoperative viral pneumonia. It is therefore advisable to delay surgery for at least 2 weeks until recovery is complete.

Obstructive lung disease

This is a heterogeneous group of conditions ranging from bronchitis to asthma which may be chronic or acute, reversible or irreversible and which together constitute the largest single group of respiratory diseases. Preoperative preparation should aim to assess the severity of the condition using a combination of clinical judgement, simple spirometry such as the measurement of vital capacity, forced expiratory volume in 1 second (FEV1) and blood gas analysis where indicated.

From the results of those tests appropriate therapy may be started. This should include advice on stopping smoking, preoperative physiotherapy and breathing exercises. Bronchodilators should be used in those cases where reversibility is demonstrated and antibiotics given for the treatment of any acute exacerbations of chronic bronchitis. It is advisable to repeat these tests following treatment and if necessary to delay surgery until the patient is in an optimum condition. In those patients with severe pulmonary disease where the FEV1, is <25% of that predicted and arterial oxygen tensions are <7.3 kPa in air, the possibility of surgery under regional or local anaesthesia should be considered.

Restrictive lung disease

This group of pulmonary diseases includes fibrosing alveolitis, sarcoidosis, asbestosis and the pulmonary manifestations of systemic disease such as rheumatoid arthritis and systemic lupus erythematosus. They are characterized by a decreased

---

Box 8.1 Cardiac conditions – requirements for antibiotic prophylaxis against endocarditis (adapted from Dajani et al 1997)

High-risk category
  Prosthetic cardiac valves
  Previous bacterial endocarditis
  Complex cyanotic congenital heart disease
  Surgically constructed systemic pulmonary shunts or conduits

Moderate-risk category
  Most other congenital cardiac malformations
  Acquired valvular dysfunction
  Hypertrophic cardiomyopathy
  Mitral valve prolapse with regurgitation or thickened leaflets

---

Box 8.2 Recommendations for antibiotic prophylaxis against endocarditis in gynaecological procedures (adapted from Dajani et al 1997)

- Cystoscopy
- Urethral dilatation
- Drainage of perineal infection

In the presence of infection during the following procedures:
- urethral catheterization
- urinary tract surgery

Prophylaxis optional in high-risk patients:
- vaginal hysterectomy
- vaginal delivery

---

transfer capacity with a restrictive lung volume. The clinical features are of dyspnoea and hypoxia on mild exertion with a normal sensitivity to carbon dioxide. Patients are frequently on steroid therapy. Most cases will not be a problem to the anaesthetist; however, any chest infection should be treated before surgery and postoperative oxygen therapy may be necessary.

Haematological disorders

Anaemia

Anaemia is an acute or chronic reduction in the number of circulating erythrocytes manifest by a decrease in the concentration of haemoglobin and a concomitant reduction in the oxygen-carrying capacity of the blood. In most cases the cause may be known, for example menorrhagia. However, where this is unclear, relevant investigations to elucidate the cause are essential before surgery. In patients with chronic anaemia (for example, chronic renal failure) compensatory changes include a shift to the right of the oxyhaemoglobin dissociation curve (thus increasing oxygen release at tissue level) and an increase in cardiac output to maintain oxygen availability.

The need for a minimum preoperative haemoglobin of 10 g/dl is based on a physiological requirement for at least 250 ml of oxygen per minute. Oxygen availability is the product of the cardiac output, the haemoglobin concentration, the haemoglobin saturation and ability to carry oxygen. Therefore in patients with a normal cardiac output and a normal haemoglobin, around 1000 ml of oxygen per minute is available. A reduction of the haemoglobin to 10 g/dl decreases this to around 650 ml of oxygen per minute. If during the course of surgery, hypovolaemia or myocardial depression occurs because of anaesthesia, oxygen availability will fall further and could approach a level where tissue hypoxia results.

If it is not possible to delay surgery until anaemia is corrected or if there is no other practicable means of increasing the haemoglobin concentration, blood transfusion 48 hours before surgery may be required.

Sickle cell disease

Described by Herrick in 1910, sickle cell disease is an inherited group of disorders ranging from benign sickle cell trait to a severe form of sickle cell anaemia characterized by the substitution of normal haemoglobin A by abnormal haemoglobin S. The symptoms of the disease are related to haemoglobin S forming tactoids when oxygen levels fall. These cause disruption and eventual rupture of the red cell. This leads to microvascular occlusion with infarction and organ damage. Sickle cell trait, the heterozygous form of the condition, generally presents few problems as far as surgery and anaesthesia are concerned. It is prevalent in patients of Afro-Carribbean origin who are often unaware of their condition.

Surgery in such patients should be undertaken with care, avoiding hypoxia and ensuring excellent pain relief postoperatively to minimize the risk of a sickle cell crisis. Sickle cell anaemia presents a grave threat to the patient in the perioperative period and preoperative exchange transfusion is indicated in those individuals with a haemoglobin of <8 g/dl, preferably with freshly donated blood. It is desirable to achieve >70% normal red cells in a peripheral blood film.

Thalassaemia

This is a collective term for a group of inherited disorders associated with a reduction in β-globulin production (β-thalassaemia) or of α-globulin production (α-thalassaemia). Patients should be treated in a similar way to those who have sickle cell disease.

Bleeding disorders

Coagulation defects leading to a bleeding tendency may be divided into the rare hereditary conditions, those iatrogenically acquired by treatment with warfarin and those arising from intercurrent disease, typically chronic liver disease.

Haemophilia B (Christmas disease, factor IX deficiency) causes failure of the intrinsic coagulation pathway and can be diagnosed by a prolonged activated partial thromboplastin time (APTT) and by direct assay of the individual factors. The opinion of the haemophilia team is essential before undertaking any surgical intervention. The patient may need to be transferred to the regional centre for her surgery. No patients with haemophilia should receive intramuscular injections and NSAIDS are contraindicated in view of the risk of peptic ulceration. Von Willibrand's disease is inherited as an autosomal dominant trait resulting in a deficiency of a platelet adhesion factor. Patients may present with menorrhagia and exhibit a prolonged skin bleeding time. Preoperatively this may be corrected by fresh frozen plasma or infusion of desmopressin in combination with an antifibrinolytic agent such as tranexamic acid to counteract the release of plasminogen activator caused by desmopressin.

Warfarin may be administered long term because of the presence of a prosthetic heart valve or increased risk of recurrent thromboembolism. It antagonizes vitamin K function in the activation of factors II, VII, IX and X. Close collaboration is required with the haematological team. Warfarin should be stopped 2–3 days before surgery and the INR monitored. A heparin infusion may be needed to cover the immediate postoperative period in those at high risk such as women with prosthetic valve replacements. Warfarin-induced coagulation defects can be corrected with fresh frozen plasma and vitamin K injection. Drugs such as metronidazole, erythromycin or cimetidine that increase the activity of warfarin should be avoided.

Thrombophilia

These comprise a group of rare disorders predisposing to venous thrombosis especially after surgery but also during pregnancy and when on the combined contraceptive pill. These include deficiency of antithrombin III which can be familial and affects 1:4000 of the population. Deficiency of the liver-derived vitamin K-dependent factors protein C and protein S is another cause of thrombophilia. Protein C inhibits factor V and VIIIc while protein S serves as a regulatory factor for protein C but also has a direct regulatory effect. Direct measurement is usually incorporated as part of a thrombophilia screen in patients with a characteristic history but interpretation of the result is difficult during pregnancy or when on anticoagulant medication.

Diseases of the nervous system

Although there are many neurological diseases, few are of consequence to the course of surgery and anaesthesia. However, problems may be encountered with the following.

Epilepsy

Patients who have epileptic seizures who lead normal lives and are satisfactorily controlled on medication are at low risk of peri- or postoperative complications. It is advisable for patients to continue with anticonvulsant therapy in the perioperative period and for the anaesthetist to be informed of the epilepsy, as a number of anaesthetic agents predispose to seizure activity.

Degenerative, progressive diseases

For those with degenerative progressive diseases such as multiple sclerosis or those complicated by spasticity and contraction, further assessment is required. Respiratory function tests may be required to assess ventilatory reserve caused by weakened respiratory muscles, which would be further compromised by increased abdominal pressure during laparoscopic procedures. Access needs to be planned when contemplating vaginal procedures in those who have severe adductor contractions, making Lloyd Davies or lithotomy positioning impractical. Likewise care of the bladder should be discussed as an indwelling catheter may be required until the patient is fully recovered. In those with progressive neurological disorders there is no evidence to suggest that regional anaesthesia will precipitate a deterioration in their condition. Indeed, it may be of benefit in reducing the risk of postoperative chest infection.

Renal disease

The most important feature in the preoperative preparation of patients with renal disease is the assessment of the biochemical abnormality relative to the therapeutic manoeuvres taken to correct it. Patients on dialysis with established renal failure presenting for elective surgery should be dialysed 12–24 hours prior to surgery to correct any hyperkalaemia or acid–base abnormality. The position of a renal transplant may influence port site placement for laparoscopic surgery.

In patients with chronic anaemia, correction by preoperative transfusion is generally unnecessary. However, it is worth remembering that it will be difficult to detect cyanosis when the patient is anaemic. Drugs excreted by routes other than the kidneys should be used where possible. Infusions of morphine should be used cautiously as its active metabolite, morphine-6-glucuronide, is excreted by the kidneys and may accumulate in sufficient concentrations to produce respiratory depression.

Hepatic disease

Patients with moderate-to-severe hepatic disease are at considerable risk of developing perioperative problems. Hepatic failure is associated with alterations of renal, pulmonary and cardiovascular physiology, impaired metabolic and haematological homeostasis and altered pharmacokinetics.

Preoperative assessment is aimed at identifying the severity of the hepatic disease both clinically and biochemically.

In the preoperative preparation it is necessary to give prophylactic antibiotics, vitamin K and possibly diuretics for ascites. Clotting abnormalities should be corrected with the appropriate blood products. There is a high risk of developing renal failure postoperatively. This is frequently fatal.

Endocrine disease

Perioperative problems in patients with endocrine diseases tend to arise as a result of mismanagement of replacement therapy. As such they are dealt with in the section on the influence of pre-existing medication.

SURGICAL RISK FACTORS

Obesity

Obesity can be defined as a ratio of weight over height^2 greater than $30 \, kg/m^2$. Patients in this category are at considerable risk from anaesthesia because of abnormalities of respiratory and cardiovascular physiology. There are also technical problems with access for surgery and problems with postoperative mobilization. Obesity is very often associated with other medical conditions such as diabetes, hypertension, respiratory and heart disease.

When surgery for a benign condition is being considered, preoperative weight loss should be encouraged. When surgery is required for malignancy, radical surgery may still be appropriate because of the difficulties of administering radiotherapy to such women. Early mobilization is very important. Prophylaxis against thromboembolism and infection will be needed.

Previous surgery

Previous open abdominal procedures may result in loops of bowel stuck under the scar, increasing the risk of bowel damage when entry is attempted at the same site either by laparoscopy or laparotomy (Krebs 1986). Laparoscopic incisions should therefore be made away from the scar where possible or open rather than blind entry methods employed.

The division of intra-abdominal adhesions following previous surgery will often add an extra hour to the length of an operation. Recovery may be delayed by postoperative ileus when the bowel is handled extensively. It can be very difficult indeed to identify the ovaries in women who have dense pelvic adhesions – especially after previous hysterectomy.

It is important to obtain consent for an open laparotomy prior to laparoscopic sterilization when difficulty identifying the fallopian tubes is anticipated because of adhesions following previous surgery or pelvic inflammatory disease.

Smoking

The ill effects of smoking should not be underestimated. Cigarettes have a number of deleterious effects, including:

- reduction in oxygen availability secondary to carbon monoxide binding to haemoglobin
- impairment of mucociliary clearance and hyper-reactivity

of small airways, increasing the predisposition to post-operative chest infections

- reduction in neutrophil chemotaxis and immunoglobin concentration
- increase in platelet aggregatibility.

In addition to an association with chronic medical conditions, smoking increases 10-fold the rate of postoperative respiratory tract infections, depresses the immune response and has adverse affects on tissue oxygen delivery. At least 3 months abstinence is required to show any improvement in small airway vessel disease, increased viscid secretions and the depressed cough response that result in postoperative chest infections (Grass & Olsen 1986). Patients should be encouraged to stop smoking at least 6 weeks before surgery in order to improve pulmonary function. They should at the very least stop 48 hours prior to surgery in order to eliminate carbon monoxide and thereby improve oxygen availability.

INFLUENCE OF PRE-EXISTING MEDICATION

Corticosteroids

Patients treated with systemic corticosteroids may develop suppression of the hypothalamic-pituitary-adrenal axis. The degree of suppression is dependent on the dose and duration of treatment but some adrenal suppression can occur within 1 week of starting corticosteroids. Following the cessation of corticosteroid therapy it may be some months before complete recovery in the hypothalamic-pituitary axis occurs.

It has been estimated that a major surgical operation results in an increased secretion of around 200–400 mg cortisol. Therefore additional corticosteroids should be given to avoid the risk of adrenal cortical insufficiency. Patients undergoing minor surgery can be managed by a small increase in the daily dose of corticosteroids or by monitoring vital signs and treating with incremental hydrocortisone if features suggestive of adrenal cortical insufficiency arise.

For major surgery it is usual to give increased cover in the form of hydrocortisone 100–200 mg intramuscularly with the premedication and then 50–100 mg four times daily, reducing to a daily maintenance dose after several days. Patients treated with topical steroids (e.g. to the skin or rectum) occasionally absorb sufficient quantities to cause adrenal suppression and those patients who use high-dose beclomethasone inhalers to treat their asthma may have a degree of adrenocortical insufficiency.

Oral contraceptives and hormone replacement therapy

Women taking the older formulations of the combined oral contraceptive pill have a higher incidence of deep venous thrombosis than non-pill users. This risk is increased by anaesthesia and surgery with its accompanying immobilization. It was estimated that among pill takers undergoing major surgery, the relative risk of deep vein thrombosis was twice that of non-users (0.96% vs 0.5%; Vessey et al 1986). With the reduction in the dosage of the oestrogen component of modern pills, that risk may now be less. Six weeks after stopping the pill, changes

in the coagulation and fibrinolytic systems have reverted to normal but epidemiological evidence suggests that the excess risk of deep vein thrombosis reverts to normal in less than a month.

The risk of deep vein thrombosis following minor surgery, including laparoscopy, is extremely small and any risk from the oral contraceptive pill is more than outweighed by the risk of pregnancy. In the absence of other risk factors, there is insufficient evidence to support a policy of routinely stopping the oral contraceptive pill prior to major surgery (RCOG 1995). When patients continue to take the pill up until the time of surgery, prophylactic low-dose heparin should be considered if there are other risk factors such as obesity and smoking.

These recommendations do not apply to those individuals taking the progestogen-only pill because there is no evidence of any increased risk of thrombosis with this method of contraception. Similarly, hormone replacement therapy (HRT) is associated with only a small increased risk of thrombo-embolic disease that seems to be confined to the first year of use (Gutthann et al 1997). Thus there is no indication to stop HRT prior to surgery (RCOG 1995).

Insulin and oral hypoglycaemic agents

Anaesthesia and surgery lead to a stress reaction resulting in an outpouring of catabolic hormones such as catecholamines, corticosteroids, glucagon and thyroxin. One of the metabolic effects of these is to stimulate glycogenolysis and glyconeogenesis, resulting in increased glucose liberation. These hormones also increase lipolysis which under normal circumstances is offset by the antilipolytic effect of the increased secretion of insulin stimulated by hypoglycaemia. The resultant effect is a depletion of liver glycogen and protein catabolism. In patients with untreated type 1 insulin-dependent diabetes, hyperglycaemia and ketoacidosis result. In the type 2 diabetic where some residual insulin secretion is retained, these effects may be less profound and the tendency to ketoacidosis is less marked. The perioperative management of the diabetic patient aims to avoid these problems by control of glucose homeostasis.

Type 1 diabetics
For all surgery involving general anaesthesia insulin-dependent diabetic patients should be admitted prior to the operation and stabilized on short-acting insulins. Numerous different regimes for perioperative management have been advocated; however, the simplest consists of omission of the insulin dose on the day of operation and administration of an infusion of 10% glucose with potassium and soluble insulin. Alternatively an infusion of glucose and potassium may be supplemented by soluble insulin administered separately intravenously by a pump or by regular small subcutaneous injections. These are continued until the patient is re-established on her normal diet and insulin regimen. All such regimens require regular and careful monitoring of glucose and potassium.

Type 2 diabetics
For minor surgery it is often insufficient to omit the oral hypoglycaemic agent on the morning of the operation with perioperative measurement of the blood sugar using Dextro-sticks.

The hyperglycaemic effect of the operation is usually counter-acted by the residual effect of the previous day's dose of hypo-glycaemic agents. If there are problems or the operation becomes prolonged, the patient may be managed as for type 1 diabetes.

For major surgery patients should be treated as type 1 diabetics.

Drugs acting on the cardiovascular system

Patients whose cardiovascular disease is controlled with drugs should in general continue on their medication in the peri-operative period. Many patients with cardiovascular disease will be on various permutations of β-adrenergic blocking drugs, calcium channel blocking agents and nitrates. In general, all cardiac medication should be continued through the peri-operative period as abrupt withdrawal may precipitate myo-cardial infarction. The myocardial depressant nature of these agents is of importance to the anaesthetist as some volatile anaesthetic agents may synergize with these drugs with adverse effects on cardiovascular haemodynamics. Patients with coronary artery disease and those with a recent history of myocardial infarction in particular will be on low-dose aspirin therapy to reduce platelet coagulability. Although these patients are at increased risk of perioperative bleeding this is less than the risk of perioperative myocardial infarction.

Patients on potassium-losing diuretics, whether or not being given potassium supplements, should have their plasma potassium estimated and hypokalaemia corrected pre-operatively, particularly if they are also taking digoxin.

Drugs acting on the nervous system

Monoamine oxidase inhibitors

These drugs are used in the treatment of resistant depression. Their therapeutic effects are believed to result from the inhibition of monoamine oxidase in the brain, leading to an increase in the concentrations of catecholamine and 5-hydroxytriptamine. Their peripheral effects include monoamine oxidase inhibition, inhibition of hepatic drug oxygenation and a variable degree of sympathetic blockade. Sympathomimetic agents may promote a hypertensive crisis, opiates (in particular pethidine) may cause profound hypotension and barbiturates are metabolized at a variable and unpredictable rate. Although these problems can be overcome by withdrawing the drug at least 2 weeks before surgery, this can only be done in liaison with the pre-scribing psychiatrist.

Tricyclic, quadricyclic antidepressants and major tranquillizers

It is generally safe for patients to continue on these drugs provided that the anaesthetist is made aware that they are being given so that the anaesthetic may be varied appropriately. The sudden cessation of administration of these agents may result in an acute exacerbation of the psychiatric illness. In the case of patients suffering from a psychotic illness stabilized on an oral major tranquillizer, it may be worth considering giving it parenterally over the operative period.

Lithium

It is the usual practice to withdraw lithium 1 week before major surgery because of the risk of toxicity should there be an electrolyte imbalance or a deterioration in renal function. This risk, however, must be balanced against the possible relapse of the affective disorder for which the drug is being prescribed and again, liaison with the psychiatrist is important.

Anticonvulsants

It is vital that patients continue to receive anticonvulsant medication over the operative period. It is usual to give the dose orally on the day of surgery and then parenterally until such time as the patient is able once again to take oral tablets.

Sodium valproate deserves particular mention because in addition to its anticonvulsant properties it interferes with haemostasis. This drug causes depression of platelet count, including frank thrombocytopenia, in a dose-related fashion and it has been reported on occasions to cause impairment of platelet aggregation and minor defects of coagulation, including hypofibrinogenaemia. It is therefore recommended that patients taking this agent who require surgery should have a platelet and coagulation screen beforehand.

Alcohol

The heavy drinker is at greater risk because of diminution of the stress response, an impaired immunity and abnormalities of electrolyte control. The development of the withdrawal symptoms can occur within 8 hours of abstention and treat-ment with infusions of alcohol is sometimes necessary. In the alcoholic with symptoms of severe hepatic disease (e.g. bleeding diathesis), pretreatment with parenteral vitamins and the correction of clotting abnormalities are essential. The preoperative administration of steroids in alcoholics with severe impairment of the stress response may also be necessary.

RELEVANT INVESTIGATIONS PRIOR TO SURGERY

All patients scheduled for major surgery should have basic haematological and biochemical screening beforehand. In ASA grade 1 patients without evidence of intercurrent disease under-going minor surgery, the value of such tests is contentious.

Haematological tests

A full blood count is a minimum requirement prior to surgery, supplemented in patients of negroid or Mediterranean extrac-tion by a sickle cell test and, if necessary, haemoglobin elec-trophoresis. Where perioperative transfusion is envisaged, blood should be sent for grouping, including rhesus group and crossmatch, preferably 24 hours before surgery. In patients with abnormalities of clotting, such as those on anticoagulant therapy or with liver disease, full clotting profiles should be sent and appropriate corrective therapy instituted prior to surgery.

Biochemical tests

Biochemical analysis of a patient's urine is generally per-formed by the nursing staff on admission or in the outpatient clinic using one of the many multitest dipstick kits. These can detect glycosuria, proteinuria, etc. and if results are abnormal, further investigation is warranted.

Serum analysis for abnormalities of urea, electrolytes and liver function is indicated in the following circumstances.

- If renal function is impaired by virtue of the primary gynaecological pathology, such as late-stage carcinoma of the cervix, or secondary to systemic disease.
- If current medication includes drugs likely to affect serum electrolytes, e.g. diuretic therapy or corticosteroids.
- If hepatic or bony secondaries are suspected.
- If postoperative nephrotoxic cytotoxic therapy is contemplated.
- If postoperative enteral or parenteral nutrition is envisaged.

Microbiology

A midstream urine specimen should be sent for microscopic examination and culture to exclude urinary tract infection before any gynaecological procedure is carried out. In those patients in whom pelvic inflammatory disease is suspected or where tubal surgery is to be undertaken with a known previous history of pelvic inflammatory disease, swabs from the vagina, cervix and urethra should be sent for microscopic culture and sensitivity studies.

Virology

Testing for hepatitis surface antigen is necessary in individuals such as drug abusers or those with a previous history of hepatitis where hepatitis B virus infection is suspected.

Human immunodeficiency virus (HIV) is a lente virus and the aetiologic agent responsible for causing the acquired immune deficiency syndrome. The screening of at-risk individuals for HIV infection, e.g. prostitutes, intravenous drug abusers and partners of bisexual males, can only be undertaken with a patient's permission and following counselling.

At-risk individuals should be managed according to local hospital policy following the Department of Health guidelines (DHSS 1985a,b, 1986, HMSO Circular 1990).

Imaging and electrocardiography

Many of these procedures are indicated by the nature of the presenting complaint and the anticipated surgery: for example, lymphangiography and pelvic carcinoma; ultrasound of the liver where hepatic secondaries are suspected. Preoperative chest X-ray is only necessary in those patients where underlying pulmonary or cardiac disease is present or in those individuals such as immigrants where exposure to chest diseases such as tuberculosis is suspected. Routine electrocardiographic examination is only necessary in the elderly or if cardiovascular disease is present. An abnormal electrocardiogram is associated with an increased perioperative risk.

PREOPERATIVE PREPARATION

Thromboembolism prophylaxis

Most gynaecological surgery is associated with a moderate risk of thromboembolism: 10–40% risk of DVT and 0.1–1% risk of fatal pulmonary embolism. In major pelvic surgery this rises to a 40–80% risk of DVT and a 1–10% risk of fatal pulmonary embolism. These risks increase with age, obesity, malignancy and the complexity and duration of the procedure. The Thromboembolic Risk Factors Consensus Group (THRIFT 1992) and the RCOG Working Party on Prophylaxis against Thromboembolism (1995) both recommended that all patients be individually assessed as to risk of thromboembolism and treated appropriately (Table 8.4). Beginning heparin at least 12 hours before the operation is suggested for high-risk women (Box 8.3) (Clarke-Pearson et al 1990). These regimens will reduce the incidence of thromboembolic events by two-thirds.

Table 8.4 Risk assessment and prophylaxis for thromboembolism in gynaecological surgery (adapted from RCOG 1995)

Degree of risk	Risk factors	Prophylactic measures
Low risk	Minor surgery (<30 min) with no other risk factors Major surgery (>30 min) less than 40 years old and no other risk factors	Early mobilization and hydration
Moderate risk	Minor surgery (<30 min) in patients with a personal or family history of thromboembolic disease or thrombophilia Major surgery (>30 min) Extended laparoscopic surgery Obesity Immobility prior to surgery for more than 4 days Major intercurrent illness Non-gynaecological malignancy	Unfractionated heparin 5000 iu bd (sc) or Low molecular weight heparin (e.g. enoxaparin 20 mg daily) (To begin 2–8 hours prior to surgery) plus Graduated elastic compression stockings
High risk	Three or more of moderate risk factors Major pelvic or abdominal surgery for gynaecological malignancy Major surgery (>30 min) in patients with a personal or family history of thromboembolic disease or thrombophilia	Unfractionated heparin 5000 iu tds (sc) or Low molecular weight heparin (e.g. enoxaparin 40 mg daily) (To begin 12 hours prior to surgery) plus Graduated elastic compression stockings

Box 8.3   Administration of prophylactic subcutaneous heparin

1. Begin 2–24 hours before surgery, depending on degree of risk.
2. Administer at a site well away from the wound – flank or thigh.
3. Introduce full length of needle vertically into a skinfold which should be held throughout the procedure.
4. Continue heparin for 5 days or until fully mobilized.
5. Check platelet count daily if continued more than 5 days.

Low molecular weight or fractionated heparins (LMWH) are now in widespread use and have practical and theoretical advantages. Unfractionated heparin contains a mixture of aminoglycosans, which non-specifically block the actions of antithrombin III acting via factors II and X across the intrinsic and extrinsic pathway. This produces both an anticoagulant and anticlotting effect. By contrast, LMWH target factor X only, producing an anticlotting reaction without unwanted anticoagulant side-effects. In addition, LMWH do not interact with von Willebrand factor and do not produce thrombocytopenia, which can exacerbate any bleeding tendency. This is coupled with their once-daily regime and the ability to achieve true anticoagulation in the treatment of established thromboembolic disease without the need for intravenous infusion (Hull et al 1992).

Pneumatic compression boots are comparable to heparin in preventing deep vein thrombosis but this necessitates continued use postoperatively until mobile, which may be impractical. Thus it would seem sensible to restrict their use to those thought to be at very high risk in conjunction with LMWH.

A filter may be inserted transcutaneously into the inferior vena cava to prevent pulmonary embolism in women at particularly high risk (see Chapter 6). Such patients might include those who already have lower limb or pelvic thrombosis distal to a pelvic mass due to be removed surgically.

There is evidence that low-dose aspirin is effective in reducing the rates of postoperative deep vein thrombosis and pulmonary embolism (Sors & Meyer 2000). It probably adds nothing to inpatient LMWH treatment but may be beneficial in preventing thromboembolic complications after discharge from hospital. It remains to be seen whether prolonging prophylaxis with low-dose aspirin when the patient has returned home is as effective as continuing LMWH prophylaxis at home.

Antibiotic prophylaxis

Good surgical technique with scrupulous sterile technique in theatre and on the ward is the cornerstone of reducing post-operative infections. All major gynaecological surgery, either vaginal or abdominal, carries a significant risk of infectious morbidity (20%) and the prophylactic use of antibiotics is strongly recommended since they will reduce the incidence by 50% (Mittendorf et al 1993). For those women who are not allergic to penicillin, augmentin and metronidazole or a cefuroxime/metronidazole combination is recommended. A single dose at the time of induction gives optimum tissue levels during surgery when bacteraemia is likely to occur and is as effective as therapy for 24 hours or 5 days. A single dose will provide cover for surgery that lasts for up to 1 hour but if surgery takes longer it is advisable to give two further doses postoperatively. In prolonged surgical cases where there is a high risk of bacterial infection, a second intravenous dose may be repeated after 2 hours.

Antibiotic prophylaxis is recommended for high-risk groups when instruments are inserted into the uterus. This includes termination of pregnancy where 10% chlamydia carriage rates are found and risk of upper tract disease is increased. Those who are immunocompromised and those at risk of bacterial endocarditis may require prophylactic antibiotics.

The risk of postoperative respiratory infections can be reduced by optimization of lung function by medication and physiotherapy, cessation of smoking and early mobilization with good pain control. Attention to the indications for the use and duration of indwelling catheters may influence the frequency of urinary tract infections.

Bowel preparation

Most gynaecological procedures do not require a rigorous bowel preparation unless bowel surgery is expected. However, it is useful in pelvic surgery to try to ensure that a loaded colon does not limit access. A disposable enema or two suppositories given the night before surgery help to avoid this in most patients. More radical measures may be required for patients known to be constipated!

The need for systematic bowel preparation in patients undergoing gynaecological surgery is rare but necessary in those who may require a large bowel resection. Patients with extensive ovarian cancer presenting with a change in bowel habit, those undergoing resection of endometriosis in the rectovaginal septum and those where a pelvic mass is present and the diagnosis is in doubt may benefit. Current methods rely on osmotic oral purgation using polyethylene glycol solutions such as Kleanprep or Golytely. The patient is required to drink up to 4 litres of such mixtures and elderly patients require intravenous fluids to avoid dehydration. Satisfactory bowel preparation for those undergoing bowel anastomosis may mean that this can be safely accomplished without the need for a defunctioning colostomy or ileostomy.

DAY-CARE SURGERY

Day surgery represents an important facet of modern gynae-cological practice. Both patients and hospitals benefit from the provision of a properly run service. With the ever-increasing demands for improvement in patient care and the financial restraints that now affect all healthcare provision, expansion of day care will continue. In the report *Guidelines for day case surgery* (1985) the Royal College of Surgeons suggested that about 50% of all elective procedures could be performed as day surgery. This figure has already been achieved in North America and is likely to increase further. In the UK only 20% of elective surgery is performed on a day-care basis.

Selection of procedures and patients

The nature and the extent of day surgery offered should be agreed by both surgical and anaesthetic staff. Operations

Box 8.4   Gynaecological procedures suitable for day surgery

Examination under anaesthesia
Dilatation and curettage
Hysteroscopy
Loop or laser conization
Cystoscopy
Excision or ablation of small vulval lesions
Marsupialization of Bartholin's gland cysts
Termination of pregnancy
ERPC
Laparoscopic procedures:
   diagnostic including dye insufflation
   division of adhesions
   treatment of endometriosis by laser
   ovarian diathermy
   ovarian surgery
   sterilization
Transcervical resection or ablation of endometrium of fibroids

should not be unduly complex and last less than an hour; postoperative analgesia should be achievable with simple analgesics (Box 8.4).

The nature of modern gynaecological practice, with increasing demand and use of hysteroscopy and laparoscopy, requires the presence of more senior surgeons in day-care theatres. Such a strategy should achieve a higher turnover of patients and a reduced complication rate. Correct selection of patients is essential and local guidelines should be established. In general, patients need to be of ASA 1 or 2 status, non-obese and have an appropriate carer to support and help in the first 24 hours after surgery. Where social support is inadequate, an on-site patient hotel facility may be used. Assessment of suitability for day-case surgery is similar to that for inpatients. The majority of modern units have a preadmission clinic where patients are seen, assessed, relevant investigations ordered, consent taken and information pertaining to the perioperative course of the proposed surgery discussed. Such clinics are run by a combination of medical and nursing staff conforming to local policies as dictated by individual circumstances. After the operation, patients should be seen by both surgeon and anaesthetist. Prior to discharge future plans for treatment, analgesia and emergency procedures should be communicated to the patient. It is essential that the patient's family doctor is informed.

KEY POINTS

1. Preoperative assessment and identification of risk factors are essential to minimize postoperative complications.
2. Optimization of intercurrent medical conditions should be attempted prior to elective surgery.
3. Consent should be gained by the operating surgeon or a deputy who is competent to explain the benefits and possible complications that may arise.
4. Ideally, estimation of risk should be undertaken jointly by the surgeon and anaesthetist prior to a decision regarding suitability for surgery in cases of high risk.

KEY POINTS (CONTINUED)

5. Thromboprophylaxis reduces the incidence of postoperative deep vein thrombosis and pulmonary embolus.
6. Prophylactic antibiotic therapy reduces the incidence of postoperative febrile episodes by 50%.
7. Day-care surgery should be undertaken within dedicated units with agreed protocols for procedures undertaken.
8. Day-care surgical management should be performed by experienced gynaecological and anaesthetic staff.

REFERENCES

American Society of Anesthesiologists 1963 New classification of physical status. Anesthesiology 24:111

Clarke-Pearson DL, DeLong ER, Synan IS et al 1990 A controlled trial of two low-dose heparin regimens for the prevention of deep vein thrombosus. Obstetrics and Gynecology 75:684–689

Dajani AS, Taubert KA, Wilson W et al 1997 Prevention of bacterial endocarditis. JAMA 277(22):1794–1801

Department of Health 2001 Reference guide to consent for examination or treatment. DoH, London

DHSS 1985a Acquired immune deficiency syndrome. Booklet 1: AIDS general information for doctors. DHSS, London

DHSS 1985b Booklet 2: information for doctors concerning the introduction of HTLV III antibody tests. DHSS, London

DHSS 1986 Booklet 3: guidance for surgeons, anaesthetists, dentists and their teams in dealing with patients infected with HTLV 111. DHSS, London

Gass GD, Olsen GN 1986 Preoperative pulmonary function testing to predict postoperative morbidity and mortality. Chest 89:127–129

Goldman L, Caldera D, Nussbaum SR et al 1977 Multifactorial index of cardiac risk in non cardiac surgical procedures. New England Journal of Medicine 297:845–850

Gutthann SP, Rodriguez LAG, Castellsague J, Oliart AD 1997 Hormone replacement therapy and risk of venous thromboembolism: population-based case control study. British Medical Journal 314:796

HMSO Circular 1990 Guidance for clinical health care workers: protection against infection with HIV and hepatitis viruses. HMSO, London

Hull RD, Raskob GE, Pineo GF et al 1992 Subcutaneous low molecular weight heparin compared with continuous heparin intravenous proximal vein thrombosis. New England Journal of Medicine 326:975–982

Krebs HB 1986 Intestinal injury in gynecologic surgery: a ten year experience. American Journal of Obstetrics and Gynecology 155:505–514

Mangano DT 1990 Perioperative cardiac morbidity. Anesthesiology 72:153–184

Mittendorf R, Aronson MP, Berry RE et al 1993 Avoiding serious infections associated with abdominal hysterectomy. A meta-analysis of antibiotic prophylaxis. American Journal of Obstetrics and Gynecology 169:1119–1124

Nettleman MD, Banitt L, Awan I, Gordon EE 1997 Predictors of survival and the role of gender in postoperative myocardial infarction. American Journal of Medicine 103(5):357–362

Prys-Roberts C 1984 Anaesthesia and hypertension. British Journal of Anaesthesia 56:711–724

Royal College of Obstetricians and Gynaecologists 1995 Report of the Working Party on prophylaxis against Thromboembolism in Obstetrics and Gynaecology. RCOG, London

Royal College of Surgeons 1985 Commission on the provision of surgical services. Guidelines for day case surgery. RCS, London

Sidaway v Board of Governors of Bethlem Royal and Maudsley Hospital 1985. Weekly Law Report 2:480

Sors H, Meyer G 2000 Place of aspirin in prophylaxis of venous thromboembolism. Lancet 355:1288–1289

Thromboembolic Risk Factors (THRIFT) Consensus Group 1992 Risk of and prophylaxis for venous thromboembolism in hospital patients. British Medical Journal 305:567–574

Treasure T, van Besouw JP 1993 The surgical patient with cardiac disease. In: Hobsley M, Johnson A, Treasure T (eds) Current surgical practice. Edward Arnold, London, pp 39–55

Vessey MP, Mant D, Smith A, Yeates D 1986 Oral contraceptives and venous thromboembolism: findings in a large prospective study. British Medical Journal 292:526–528

9

Principles of surgery and management of intraoperative complications

G. Angus McIndoe

INTRODUCTION

In major surgery, occasional damage to vital structures is unavoidable but with good training, appropriate experience and careful application, such damage should be rare. Timely recognition of potential problems has a major impact on the long-term outcome for patients. The request for appropriate assistance from a more experienced colleague, either within the specialty or from another specialty, and early repair, preferably during the original operation, can make the difference between complete and rapid recovery and long-term morbidity and further surgery.

To minimize complications, a surgical technique should be developed that involves careful and accurate identification of tissue planes, preferably with sharp dissection, with the aim of causing the minimum of damage to tissues and structures that are to be preserved. A gentle approach should be used and tissues handled in such a way as to maintain optimum viability.

Operate under direct vision at all times. Avoid the temptation to push an instrument deep into a plane of dissection since inadvertent damage may be caused and bleeding down a deep hole is more difficult to control. Allow enough time for each operation and do not hurry surgery. Particularly when in training, greater speed will develop by a methodical attention to detail of technique rather than by hurrying individual cases, and outcome is always more important than operative time.

Every case undertaken should be seen as an opportunity to improve technique. Straightforward cases are particularly useful for the practice of sharp dissection to the correct tissue planes. When tissue planes are more difficult to identify, this practice will be invaluable.

Aim to keep the operation under control at all times; it is much better to spend a little time controlling bleeding, so that the operation can proceed unhurriedly and with good visibility, than to rush on hoping to stop the bleeding as the operation progresses.

In this chapter I will discuss the common intraoperative complications and the aspects of technique that reduce the likelihood of these complications occurring. I will also highlight the range of methods used to repair damage, although for the most part, detailed descriptions are not appropriate in a textbook of this type.

THE ROUTE

The provisional decision whether to use an abdominal or a vaginal approach for hysterectomy should be made before theatre but the final assessment of suitability for vaginal

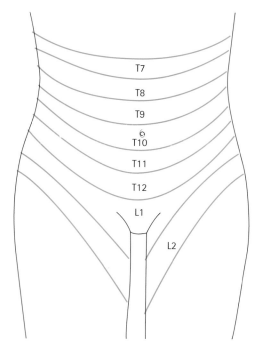

Fig. 9.1   Dermatomes.

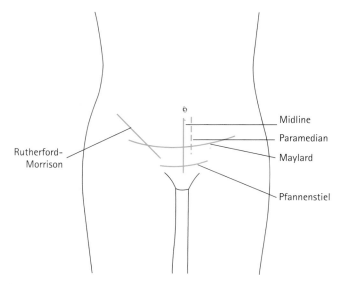

Fig. 9.2   Abdominal incisions.

hysterectomy is performed under anaesthesia. Each surgeon has personal criteria for attempting vaginal hysterectomy that are based upon training and experience. While some advocate the vaginal removal of large fibroid uteri, most gynaecologists adopt a more cautious approach. Some also described the removal of normal-sized ovaries, with or without the fallopian tubes, by a vaginal approach but this requires both special training and instruments. In the event of difficulty, the surgeon should not hesitate to change to an abdominal approach.

OPENING AND CLOSING THE ABDOMEN

The layers of the anterior abdominal wall include skin, subcutaneous fat, rectus sheath and oblique abdominal muscles, transversalis fascia and peritoneum. Within these structures lie segmental arteries, veins and nerves that supply the dermatomes and myotomes and also the epigastric vessels (Fig. 9.1). Abdominal incisions have been developed that preserve function as well as possible and which heal rapidly with good strength. Commonly used incisions are shown in Figure 9.2.

It should not be forgotten that inappropriate wound closure technique can increase the risk of pulmonary complications and death (Niggebrugge et al 1999). While some surgeons prefer to use electrocautery rather than a cold scalpel to open the wound, there seems to be no difference in the early or late complications in midline incisions (Franchi et al 2001).

Incisions

The vertical midline incision avoids all major nerves, vessels and muscles by dividing the rectus sheath. It gives good access to the whole of the abdomen except the subdiaphragmatic areas and is a very fast incision to make. Its principal drawback

is that it heals slowly and suffers from a high incidence of wound dehiscence and incisional hernia. The development of improved sutures and technique has dramatically reduced these complications. A midline incision should always be closed using the 'mass closure' technique. This involves 1 cm deep bites of the rectus muscle and peritoneum in a continuous closure with sutures placed 1 cm apart. The suture material used does not affect the rates of dehiscence or infection, but incisional hernia is more common if braided absorbable material is used (Rucinski et al 2001). The same meta-analysis showed that incision pain and suture sinus formation are more common after non-absorbable material is inserted. Absorbable monofilament used in a continuous mass closure gave the best results.

The paramedian incision is included only for historical interest. The layered closure that was used improved strength when catgut sutures were employed and reduced the incidence of dehiscence. It is inferior to the mass closure technique described above and does not provide improved access to either side of the abdomen.

The majority of gynaecological surgery is performed through a transverse incision, usually a Pfannenstiel incision. By dividing each layer in a different direction, the function is well preserved. Even the muscle-cutting variants of the transverse incision heal more rapidly than vertical incisions. The cosmetic result is superior and, if correctly placed, access to the pelvis is good although access to the pelvic brim is limited. This incision is difficult to extend if improved abdominal access is required.

The Maylard incision involves dividing all layers in the line of the skin incision and also divides the inferior epigastric vessels. The rectus sheath is not separated from the muscle and closure is in layers, leaving the muscle to be drawn together by the sheath. This incision provides improved access to the pelvic side wall when compared with Pfannenstiel and is useful for oncological surgery. Many centres now use this incision or a Pfannenstiel incision for radical hysterectomy (Orr et al 1995, Scribner et al 2001).

The Cherney incision is similar to the Pfannenstiel but the

rectus muscles are divided 1 cm from their insertion into the symphysis pubis. The incision is closed in layers, but the muscle is repaired using a continuous suture in the membranous distal portion of the muscle. This incision can also be useful in oncological surgery or, if placed lower, is useful for complex urogynaecological procedures.

The Rutherford-Morrison incision involves dividing all layers in the line of the incision and is particularly useful for approaching ovarian masses in the second half of pregnancy. The incision is closed in layers and heals well.

Drains

Drains are used either therapeutically, to remove pus, infected material and products from an abscess, or to prevent an accumulation of blood, pus, urine, lymph, bile or intestinal secretions. There is little evidence to support the use of prophylactic drains. In abdominal incisions, drains have been used in an attempt to reduce the incidence of haematoma and wound infection. Unfortunately, they tend to introduce organisms into an otherwise clean area and increase the incidence of wound infection (Cruise & Foord 1973). Nor do pelvic drains reduce infection following radical pelvic surgery (Orr et al 1987). Careful attention to haemostasis is preferable and drains should be avoided in most closures.

Closure of peritoneum

Recently this practice has been questioned. Research in animal models has suggested that closure of the peritoneum increases rather than decreases peritoneal adhesions. Human studies support this finding, showing that closure of the pelvic peritoneum does not reduce the incidence of postoperative adhesions or obstruction (Table 9.1; Tulandi et al 1988). The Peritoneum rapidly spreads across any raw areas left after surgery, although devascularized tissue, such as pedicles, is a focus for adhesion formation. Practice still varies with regard to peritoneal closure although it probably results in increased adhesion formation (RCOG 1998). However, if a suction drain is used in the wound, the peritoneum must be closed to avoid drawing the bowel into the wound.

URETERIC DAMAGE

Ureters are the organs most respected by gynaecologists. They lie close to the genital tract and repair of a damaged ureter is technically demanding, with results that are not always satisfactory. By recognizing when and where the ureters are most

Table 9.1   The effect of peritoneal closure on wound infection and adhesion formation (after Tulandi et al 1988)

	Closed	Not closed
Wound infection	3.6%	2.4%
Adhesions	22.2%	15.8%
Obstruction	1.6%	0%

at risk and by adopting a safe technique, the risk of damage to the ureter should be minimized.

Anatomical relations

The urinary and genital tracts are closely related in embryological development and their anatomy and physiology, not surprisingly, are intertwined. The ureter develops from a bud on the posterolateral border of the mesonephric duct near the cloaca, which elongates and eventually fuses with the developing kidney. The ventral portion of the cloaca develops into the urethra, bladder and lower portion of the vagina.

The ureters enter the pelvis by crossing the common iliac arteries in the region of their bifurcation. They descend on the pelvic side wall, medial to the branches of the internal iliac arteries and lateral to the ovarian fossae. From there, they run on the anterior surface of the levator ani muscles lateral to the uterosacral ligaments to pass beneath the uterine arteries, 1–1.5 cm lateral to the cervix and vagina. The ureters then swing medially around the vagina, to enter the bladder 2–3 cm below the anterior vaginal fornix.

The ureter is accompanied by a plexus of freely anastomosing fine vessels running in the loose tissue surrrounding it. The blood supply in the upper portion is derived from the renal and ovarian vessels, in the middle third from branches of the aorta, common iliac and internal iliac arteries, and in the lower part from branches of the uterine, vaginal, middle haemorrhoidal and vesical arteries. The ureter may be mobilized extensively provided this plexus of vessels is preserved.

The ureter is at risk during gynaecological surgery in four regions: at the pelvic brim where it can be confused with the infundibulopelvic ligament; lateral to the ovarian fossa where it can be adherent to an ovarian mass; in the ureteric tunnel beneath the uterine artery; and anterior to the vagina where it runs into the bladder.

The ureter at the pelvic brim and ovarian fossa

At the pelvic brim, the infundibulopelvic ligament with the ovarian vessels also crosses the iliac vascular bundle, usually 1–2 cm distal to the bifurcation of the common iliac artery and the ureter (Fig. 9.3). At this point the ureter and the ovarian vessels are running in parallel in a similar plane and may be confused if care is not taken. Occasionally the ureter may be duplex. Where the ureter runs lateral to the ovary, it will almost inevitably be associated with any inflammatory or malignant mass. Happily, it will lie on the lateral aspect of the mass where it can be identified and dissected free, usually without difficulty, although in patients with endometriosis the ureter may be fixed in dense fibrosis.

The key to the safe identification of the ureter on the pelvic side wall is to open the peritoneum and dissect in the retroperitoneal space. This is most easily done by dividing the round ligament between two clips, dividing the peritoneum in a cranial direction 1.5 cm lateral to the ovarian vessels and in a caudal direction down towards the uterovesical fold. The loose areolar tissue then encountered should be separated by blunt dissection with careful diathermy of any small vessels. The ureter will lie on the lateral aspect of the leaf of peritoneum reflected by

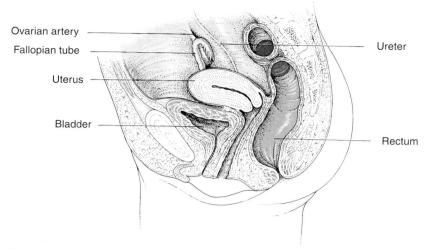

Fig. 9.3   Relationship of ureter to ovarian vessels in the infundibulopelvic ligament. Note how close the ureter lies to the ovarian vessels at the pelvic brim.

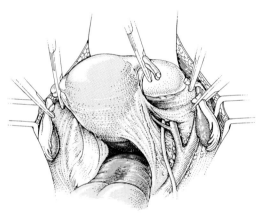

Fig. 9.4   Relationship of ureter to the uterine artery. This diagram shows the dissection performed for a radical hysterectomy, but illustrates the close relationship between the ureter and the uterine artery.

this manoeuvre. At this stage the infundibulopelvic ligament can be safely divided with the ureter under direct vision. If the anatomy of the pelvic side wall has been distorted, this technique will almost always allow the ureter to be identified and followed within the pelvis. If an ovarian mass is present the ureter may be dissected free from the mass in this retroperitoneal plane.

The lower ureter

The third position where the ureter is at risk is in the ureteric tunnel, where the ureter crosses beneath the uterine artery but superior to the cardinal ligament and about 1–1.5 cm lateral to the angle of the vagina (Fig. 9.4). It is possible to palpate the ureter in this position by gripping the paracervical tissue between one finger in the pouch of Douglas and the thumb placed laterally in front of the uterine pedicle. The ureter, which is felt as a firm cord running across the cardinal ligament, is surprisingly far lateral to the cervix if the bladder

has been properly reflected and the anatomy is normal. However, adhesions, fibrosis or inadequate dissection may disrupt these relationships, causing the ureter to remain fixed near the lateral margin of the cervix.

Damage to the ureter in this site is prevented by carefully reflecting the bladder and by not taking a large pedicle that includes both the uterine artery and the paracervical tissue. I prefer to take the uterine artery relatively high, at the level of the internal os, which allows the parametrium to fall laterally, taking the ureter with it. The ureter can then be palpated again and a second pedicle taken medial to the first, to include the cardinal ligament.

In most cases, damage to the ureter occurs at this site because the pedicle slips or the original ligature is not adequate. Avoid this by preparing the pedicle carefully before clamping it. Use modern clamps, such as Roget's or Zeppelin's parametrial clamps which rarely slip, and place ties accurately. If bleeding does occur, palpate the ureter again after replacing the clamp to ensure that it has not been included.

The ureter is occasionally damaged in its course across the anterior surface of the vagina. This may occur when taking a cuff of vagina, during a vaginal hysterectomy or colpo-suspension. When dissecting the upper vagina it is important to keep in the correct plane close to the vaginal wall. Stitches placed either vaginally or abdominally in this area must be in tissue that has been accurately identified.

Repairing ureteric damage

If a ureter is damaged, the presence of the contralateral kidney should be checked. If the ureter has not been cut across but merely crushed or ligated in error, and this is recognized on the table, it is acceptable to remove the ligature and insert a stent into the ureter in the hope that a stenosis will not result. If the ureter is divided, repair will be necessary. In the past, gynae-cologists have resorted to simply tying off the divided ureter but this is rarely justifiable now.

Repair of the ureter is technically demanding and may lead to long-term complications. It is not appropriate for a gynae-

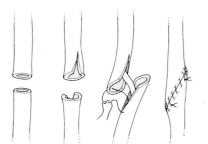

Fig. 9.5 Reanastomosis of a divided ureter. A cleanly cut ureter may be reanastomosed by spatulating the ends and repairing it with fine sutures over a suitable splint. The splint is withdrawn from the bladder at a later date. Reproduced with permission from Blandey J 1986 Operative Urology, 2nd edn. Blackwell Science, Oxford.

cologist without urological training or extensive urological experience to undertake this. In principle, an end-to-end anastomosis can be performed for ureteric damage at the pelvic brim or above. The ureter is mobilized so that the ends can be brought together without tension. They are spatulated and the anastomosis performed using fine interrupted sutures over a Silastic stent (Fig. 9.5). This is removed several weeks later. An alternative for damage at this level is to perform a uretero-ureteric anastomosis.

If the damage has occurred at the level of the ureteric tunnel or lower, the safest method of repair is to reimplant the ureter into the bladder. The bladder is opened between stay sutures. A submucosal tunnel is fashioned, taking care to avoid the other ureter. The distal end of the ureter is brought through the tunnel and, after spatulating the end, it is sutured to the bladder mucosa. A couple of sutures into the serosal surface anchor the ureter to the outer layer of the bladder (Fig. 9.6).

When damage has occurred higher on the pelvic side wall, the bladder can be elevated to the cut end of the ureter to allow reimplantation without tension, using either a psoas hitch or a Boari flap. In the former, an appropriate part of the bladder is elevated towards the end of the ureter. To facilitate this, the cystotomy is performed across the direction of elevation and is closed in the opposite direction to elongate the bladder. In addition, the contralateral superior vesical pedicle may be divided. The ureter is reimplanted as previously described and the bladder is fixed to the psoas muscle to relieve any tension. This technique will allow a ureter divided at any level in the pelvis up to the pelvic brim to be safely reimplanted (Fig. 9.7).

The Boari flap is an alternative to the psoas hitch. A flap of bladder is elevated, the ureter is reimplanted into this and the flap is closed as a tube (Fig. 9.8). This allows good elevation of the bladder at the expense of a reduced bladder capacity.

Alternatively a uretero-ureteric anastomosis to the opposite ureter can be performed. This has the disadvantage that both ureters may be compromised but may be the only method if access to the bladder is difficult.

BLADDER DAMAGE

Anatomical relations

The bladder, like the ureters, is intimately related to the genital

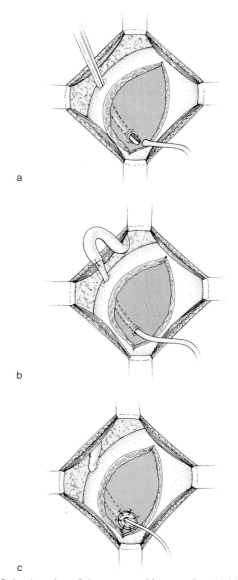

Fig. 9.6 Reimplanation of the ureter. **a** After opening the bladder, a submucosal tunnel is made along the lateral posterior wall of the bladder. A thin rubber tube is slipped over the ends of the scissors. **b** The ureter is drawn through the tunnel with the rubber tube. **c** The end of the ureter is spatulated and sutured to the bladder mucosa with fine sutures. An indwelling stent may be left in place, although this is not usually necessary. Reproduced with permission from Blandey J 1986 Operative Urology, 2nd edn. Blackwell Science, Oxford.

tract by virtue of its embryological development. Repair of the bladder, however, is more straightforward and the results are very good. It is an extraperitoneal organ that is located behind the symphysis pubis and rests on the anterior part of the levator diaphragm, the anterior vaginal wall and the cervix. The trigone is at the level of the upper vagina, with the base of the bladder related to the anterior vaginal fornix and cervix. When full, the bladder rises out of the pelvis towards the level of the umbilicus and presents a hazard during abdominal incision. The bladder is also at risk in this position if it is adherent after previous surgery or during caesarean section in labour,

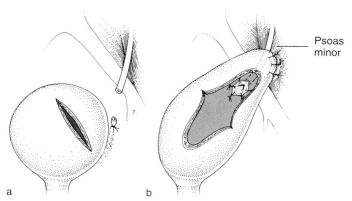

Fig. 9.7 The psoas hitch procedure. **a** The bladder is incised in the transverse axis. **b** The bladder is fixed to the psoas minor tendon to relieve tension and the ureter is reimplanted as described. The bladder is closed in the longitudinal axis. Reproduced with permission from Blandey J 1986 Operative Urology, 2nd edn. Blackwell Science, Oxford.

when the lower segment of the uterus is lifted out of the pelvis, elevating the bladder with it.

Avoiding damage

The bladder must always be emptied prior to pelvic surgery

and the peritoneum should be opened superiorly, away from the bladder, when making a transverse incision. It can be palpated as a thickening in the peritoneum and if there is any doubt about its position, careful dissection should allow the detrusor muscle to be recognized before the mucosa is opened. Opening the peritoneum by blunt dissection with fingers will not necessarily protect the bladder, as it is possible to dissect bluntly into it. Similarly, the technique of tearing the parietal peritoneum open by 'stretching' the wound once the abdominal cavity has been opened can lead to damage to the top of the bladder, particularly after previous surgery.

An essential part of any hysterectomy is separation of the bladder from the cervix and upper vagina. This plane can be found after division of the uterovesical fold of peritoneum merely by pushing caudally with a swab applied firmly to the anterior surface of the cervix cranial to the bladder. This is very quick but inevitably leaves a few small bleeding points on the back of the bladder that may be difficult to find. In addition, the bladder is occasionally damaged by this manoeuvre, particularly after previous surgery.

An alternative approach is to use a combination of sharp and blunt dissection. After dividing the uterovesical fold of peritoneum, the scissors are held slightly opened to begin separation in this plane by pushing the bladder off the cervix. Small blood vessels can be recognized and diathermied before cutting, to maintain haemostasis at all times. Once the correct

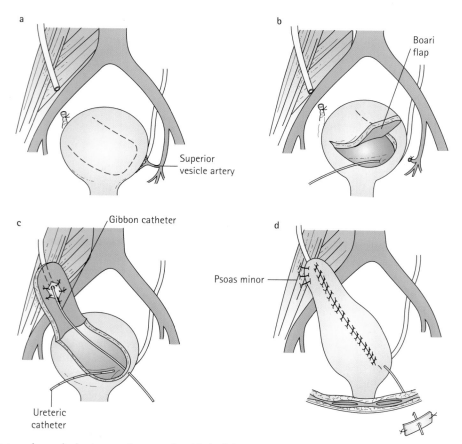

Fig. 9.8 Boari flap. **a** The superior vesical artery on the opposite side is divided. **b** The Boari flap is fashioned. A stent in the contralateral ureter may be helpful. **c** The ureter is reimplanted through a submucosal tunnel in the flap. **d** The Boari flap is closed and fixed to the psoas muscle to relieve tension. Reproduced with permission from Blandey J 1986 Operative Urology, 2nd edn. Blackwell Science, Oxford.

plane has been identified in the midline, the dissection is extended laterally to mobilize the ureters and can be continued as far as necessary down the vagina. Although a little more time consuming, this technique is safe and can be used on simple cases to gain experience for more difficult situations.

When performing the operation vaginally, the same plane needs to be defined and dissected. If the plane does not develop easily, it is important to use sharp dissection, as merely pushing on the bladder may tear a hole. A sound in the bladder may help to define the correct plane. Alternatively, a finger over the fundus of the uterus or over the broad ligament to the side, once the pouch of Douglas is opened, can define the uterovesical fold of peritoneum and clarify the correct plane for dissection.

The bladder can also be damaged during closure of the vaginal vault, particularly if it has not been sufficiently mobilized. Sutures may be placed through the detrusor muscle or even into the bladder itself, although this rarely causes problems (Meeks et al 1997). However, if this is recognized at the time of surgery, such stitches should be removed and the bladder mobilized to allow closure of the vault without including the bladder. If damage to the bladder has occurred, this should be repaired and the bladder drained as discussed below.

Repair of the bladder

Should a hole be made in the bladder, this can be repaired after the dissection of the bladder is complete. A stay stitch is usually placed at either end of the hole and the incision is repaired in two layers using either chromic catgut or Vicryl. Care is taken that the ureters are well away from the sutures and if there is any doubt, ureteral stents should be inserted. After repair, the bladder is drained with an indwelling catheter for 7–10 days. Provided the bladder is well mobilized and repaired without tension, an excellent result should be achieved.

Repair of the bladder is less likely to be successful after radical radiotherapy and a high incidence of fistulae is seen in this situation. An additional blood supply is provided by interposing a flap of omentum.

BOWEL DAMAGE

Inadvertent damage to the bowel should be unusual, unless adhesions are present. The occasions when damage is most likely to occur are during opening of the peritoneal cavity or when dissecting dense intra-abdominal adhesions. In addition, the rectum lies close to the uterosacral ligaments and posterior wall of the vagina and may be at risk during extensive pelvic dissection for cervical or vaginal carcinoma.

When reopening a previous incision, it is preferable to enter the peritoneal cavity away from the previous closure. If that is not possible, great caution should be used when approaching the peritoneum. Very occasionally, the peritoneal cavity is almost obliterated and it may be neccessary to dissect extraperitoneally around the adhesions to enter the peritoneal cavity.

When dense intraperitoneal adhesions are encountered, with care and patience the adhesions can usually be divided safely. Occasionally, the bowel is so matted together that resection of a small portion may be necessary. Particular care must be used in a patient who has been treated with radiotherapy, as the bowel is more friable and often densely adherent.

When dividing the uterosacral ligaments close to the pelvic side wall during a radical hysterectomy, the rectum is at risk of being included in the clamps. The rectovaginal space must be opened widely and the retum dissected free. Care is neccessary when entering this space to avoid direct damage to the rectum.

Repair of bowel

Repair of damaged bowel either may involve primary closure of a small hole or may be facilitated by the excision of a portion of unhealthy bowel and reanastomosis (Fig. 9.9). Consideration should be given to a defunctioning colostomy proximal to anastomosis of large bowel, particularly if the blood supply to the bowel wall is compromised in any way. Factors that have bearing on this decision are previous radiotherapy, bowel obstruction, gross infection of the operative field or other medical factors such as diabetes, steroid therapy, malignancy and advanced age. If no adverse factors are present, a colostomy may not be necessary. Small bowel usually heals without the need for defunctioning. If there is any doubt about the safety of a repair, a surgeon who specializes in bowel should be involved to help with the repair.

VASCULAR DAMAGE

Bleeding may occur at any stage of gynaecological surgery, especially if the anatomy is distorted or small tributaries are increased in size, providing collateral supply to fibroids or tumours. Careful and accurate surgical technique will avoid most but not all haemorrhagic complications.

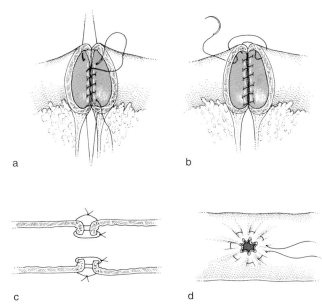

Fig. 9.9 Small bowel repair. a Suture of small intestine with continuous all-layers suture. b Connell inverting suture. c Full-thickness sutures reinforced with inverting Lembert suture. d Purse-string suture of small intestinal perforation.

Careful, gentle packing of the bowel out of the pelvis reduces the risk of haemorrhage by maximizing exposure of the operative field. While the bowel must be kept out of the pelvis as much as possible, the packs should not compress the inferior vena cava and obstruct the flow of blood out of the pelvis. Excessively tight packing results in distended pelvic veins and excessive venous bleeding. In the same way, a modest head-down tilt lowers the venous pressure in the pelvis and reduces blood loss.

Bleeding may occur from the main uterine or ovarian vessels while they are being identified, clamped and ligated. Using the technique of pelvic dissection described previously, the ovarian vessels can usually be identified and ligated without difficulty. However, the ovarian vein is particularly delicate and easily torn. A tie around the whole pedicle is preferable to transfixion, as the latter risks haematoma formation proximal to the tie. The proximity of the ureter to these vessels at the pelvic brim is an added problem when endometriosis, inflammatory disease, adhesions or tumours distort the anatomy. In contrast, the uterine artery is divided lateral to the uterus as a plexus of vessels in relatively tough tissue and sutures must be inserted. Care must be taken to include all branches in the ligature. The paracervical tissue and vaginal angle are also rich with arterial tributaries and similar considerations apply. A figure-of-eight suture in the angle of the vagina is useful to ensure that the heel of the pedicle that contains these vessels does not slip out of the ligature. These pedicles should be adjacent to each other with no space between as haemorrhage can occur later, even if the area looks dry at the completion of the procedure.

Small bleeding points on peritoneum or bladder can be diathermied but slight oozing from a pedicle signals inaccurate technique and should be corrected by oversewing the pedicle and the adjacent pedicle if necessary. The position of the ureter can be identified by palpation of the cardinal ligament lateral to the pedicle prior to the insertion of further sutures.

If bleeding from these vessels occurs, it will usually be controlled temporarily with pressure while appropriate instruments and ligatures are readied. The swab can then be removed gradually, exposing more of the field bit by bit until the bleeding point is revealed. Suction may be needed to keep the operative field clear. The location of the ureter must be determined by palpation or inspection before attending to the bleeding vessel. It is usually best to stop the bleeding by grasping the vessel gently with fine, long-handled artery forceps. A suture may then be inserted.

Damage to the large iliac vessels usually occurs only during surgery for cancer when lymph nodes or tumour are being removed from the surface of the vessels. However, deeply infiltrating endometriosis may become adherent to the internal iliac vessels and any retroperitoneal tumour or postoperative adhesions may distort the anatomy so that the iliac vessels are exposed to trauma.

If the blood supply to the leg is compromised by damage to the external or common iliac vessels, serious morbidity can result and it is vital that repair is carried out to the highest standard. Usually a vascular surgeon should be involved.

The internal iliac vessels may be safely ligated if damage occurs but bleeding from the thin-walled veins on the pelvic side wall can be very difficult to control. Initially bleeding should be controlled by direct pressure, either by a well-placed finger or using a swab. This allows time to assemble the necessary instruments, a fine sucker and fine sutures on small needles to repair the laceration or ligate the vessel and also a chance to take a deep breath so that the subsequent suturing is not carried out in a panic. Great care should be taken, as rough handling of the vessels can make the situation worse. If in doubt, more experienced help should be obtained.

In most cases, tears in the common and external iliac veins can be repaired by suturing with fine Vicryl. Damage to the arteries is usually less of a problem because the muscular vessel wall constricts and contains the haemorrhage. Local pressure, sometimes supplemented by sutures, usually gives a very satisfactory result. The real danger comes from damage to the internal iliac veins and their branches or ragged tears removing parts of the wall of the external or common iliac veins. The deeply placed veins retract into the muscle on the pelvic side wall where they become relatively inaccessible. Deeply placed mattress sutures are required to control the haemorrhage. Unfortunately, such sutures may involve one of the large pelvic nerves. This will only become apparent after the operation when the patient wakes up. It may prove impossible to control bleeding from these veins completely. The often-quoted technique of tying off the internal iliac artery in cases of troublesome bleeding is not without its own hazards. The origin of the artery lies over the bifurcation of the common iliac vein and great care is needed to avoid damaging the internal iliac vein while dissecting behind the artery to pass the ligature. This technique is often less effective than might be hoped in controlling pelvic haemorrhage because such bleeding is often venous. Firm packing may prove to be the only alternative.

More common than either of the two dramatic scenarios above but equally dangerous is a steady ooze from many small venules and arterioles. This usually follows an extensive dissection such as may be required to remove an endometrioma or to mobilize an adherent bladder. This often happens at the end of a long operation during which there has been a slow but steady blood loss that, because it has not been particularly dramatic, has not been replaced fully. A consumptive coagulopathy results as the clotting factors are exhausted. The first step therefore is to hold a hot pack firmly on the bleeding area for 10 minutes. The second is to commence the prompt replacement of blood and clotting factors. When the pack is removed gently, all may be well or no more than two or three bleeders may persist. These may be controlled with judicious use of diathermy. If there is still significant generalized blood loss not obviously coming from a single significant vessel, a hot pack should be reinserted and kept firmly in place until the blood volume and clotting factors have been replaced adequately. This may take more than an hour during which it is often helpful for the surgical team to take a break. If necessary, the abdomen may be closed with the packs in place. Antibiotics are given and the packs removed gently the following day.

UTERINE PERFORATION AND FALSE PASSAGE

During dilatation of the cervix, pushing an instrument through the substance of the cervix rather than following the canal may create a false passage. Instruments may also be pushed through the fundus of the uterus into the peritoneal cavity.

When learning to dilate the cervix one must develop a gentleness of touch that combines pressure with sensitivity or 'feel' for the tissues. It is important to avoid using force with instruments but rather to feel for the path of least resistance. Because of the barrel-shaped contour of the endocervical canal, an exploring instrument can deviate from the axis of the cervix and not engage the internal os. The size of instrument chosen for this exploration is important, as a fine probe will more easily create its own passage and therefore less pressure should be used. It is said that right-handed people are more likely to perforate towards the right side of the cervical canal although a false passage can be created in any direction. It then becomes very difficult to identify the true cervical canal and gain access to the uterine cavity.

If a false passage is suspected, one helpful manoeuvre is to perform a bimanual examination with the vulsellum attached and sound still within the passage. It is often possible to feel where the sound is in relation to the axis of the cervix and in which direction the true passage is likely to be found.

When a false passage has been created, provided damage to other organs is not suspected and the patient is not pregnant, the situation can usually be managed conservatively. In most cases it is best to desist from further attempts at dilatation. In the pregnant patient, however, significant haemorrhage may occur, particularly following lateral perforation into the broad ligament and damage to the uterine vessels. If vaginal bleeding continues or the patient's general condition deteriorates, laparotomy will be necessary. The broad ligament will be full of blood if the uterine vessels have been damaged and hysterectomy may be necessary to control the blood loss, although ligation of the uterine artery and repair of the perforation may be an option. In some cases, bleeding into the retroperitoneal space may not become apparent for several hours. Careful postoperative observation is necessary to detect this at an early stage.

The consequences of fundal perforation depend on whether the patient is pregnant and what instrument has created the perforation. In a non-pregnant uterus, a dilator through the fundus is very unlikely to cause any problems. Probably most perforations are not recognized by the surgeon at all. The patient should be observed for a period after recovery but is unlikely to need further intervention. In a pregnant patient, perforation is said to be more likely to cause haemorrhage but in general, a simple perforation can be managed conservatively. Avoid the temptation to 'confirm' the perforation by repeatedly reintroducing instruments into the uterus as this may make matters worse.

If there is significant risk of damage to intra-abdominal organs, a laparotomy is indicated because laparoscopy cannot be relied upon to exclude damage to bowel. For example, if a suction catheter has been inserted through a perforation with suction connected, laparotomy and careful examination of the bowel are mandatory.

LAPAROSCOPY

This incidence of complications in laparoscopic surgery relates very closely to the experience of the surgeon and the training they have received. Gynaecologists have built up an extensive experience in the specialty with simple procedures over the last generation. Most SHOs and junior registrars are trained in diagnostic laparoscopy as one of their earliest procedures. Nevertheless, the adoption of the more advanced operative techniques has been slow and experience in these areas is still very limited. If a high incidence of complications is to be avoided, it is essential that individual surgeons are well trained in the procedures they undertake. General complications of laparoscopy will be discussed but consideration of complications encountered in advanced laparoscopic surgery is outside the scope of this chapter (see Chapter 4, Laparoscopy, for more information).

Damage to bowel

Blind insertion of the Veress needle and first trocar may lead to perforation of intra-abdominal and retroperitoneal structures. Bowel is rarely damaged unless it is adherent to the anterior abdominal wall but great care must be taken if the patient has had a previous operation or intra-abdominal sepsis. In these cases, the initial trocar may be placed away from the site of the previous incision in an attempt to avoid fixed bowel. Alternatively, the abdomen may be entered using an open minilaparotomy technique and then the incision sealed around a blunt-ended trocar. Difficulty may be encountered in maintaining a good seal using this technique but specially designed trocars reduce this problem. A new device is available now that incises the tissue in front of a blunt-ended trocar 1 mm at a time and allows visualization of the end of the instrument as it is being inserted. This may prove to be useful in the small number of cases where difficulty is anticipated.

A surgeon experienced in laparoscopic suturing may repair minor damage to the bowel endoscopically. In most cases it is much safer to perform a laparotomy to allow careful inspection of the whole bowel and open repair of any damage. Because it can be difficult to find the hole in the bowel subsequently, it is wise to leave the offending instrument in place until the abdomen is open.

Damage to blood vessels

When inserting the Veress needle and the first trocar it is vital that these instruments are kept away from the major vessels. The position of the sacral promontory can be palpated and the instruments angled in such a way that they pass below the promontory and into the free space in the midline of the pelvis. While damage to a major blood vessel may be all too obvious, the bleeding may be predominantly retroperitoneal and difficult to see laparoscopically. If the patient's blood presure has dropped and pulse rate risen sufficiently to suggest the possibility of vascular damage, a laparotomy should be performed immediately. If the abdomen has to be opened in a hurry, one technique is to lift the laparoscope up to the anterior abdominal wall and cut down onto it, allowing immediate access.

Blood vessels in the abdominal wall may also be damaged. To reduce this risk, the abdominal wall is usually trans-illuminated to visualize vessels prior to insertion of secondary trocars. The location of the inferior epigastric vessels should be recognized, as they will bleed profusely and this may be difficult to control. Minor bleeding around a trocar may be controlled either by leaving the trocar in place to tamponade the vessel or by inserting a Foley catheter through the trocar, inflating the balloon with 30–50 ml of saline and withdrawing the trocar and balloon to apply pressure to the bleeding point. If the vessel requires suturing, this is facilitated by a long J-shaped needle.

Diathermy damage

Problems with laparoscopic use of diathermy stem either from the heat generated at the site of tissue destruction or from current finding an alternative path to earth through an adjacent organ. Tissue coagulated by diathermy becomes very hot and may retain its heat for several minutes. This heat will spread to underlying structures and adjacent organs and may cause damage. Diathermied tissue must be allowed to cool before coming in contact with adjacent structures. A further problem is the rising impedance in desiccated, diathermied tissue. This may result in the current arcing to a nearby organ that offers a low-resistence path to earth. In a similar way, current may arc to nearby organs if the current is activated before the electrode is in contact with the tissue to be treated.

KEY POINTS

1. Accurate identification of tissue planes and careful dissection will reduce intraoperative complications.
2. The ureter should always be identified on the pelvic side wall before the infundibulopelvic ligament is divided.
3. Identify and free the ureter from ovarian masses by opening the retroperitoneal space.
4. If the ureter is damaged, repair should usually be undertaken by a urologist.
5. The bladder may be repaired using two layers of absorbable sutures. Ensure that the ureters are not included in this repair.
6. Repair of bowel or great vessels, apart from minor damage, should usually be undertaken by a specialist surgeon.
7. Uterine perforation may often be managed conservatively.
8. Repair of laparoscopic damage to bowel will usually require a laparotomy.
9. If laparoscopic damage to major pelvic vessels is suspected, a laparotomy must be performed without delay.
10. Diathermy should be applied only when the electrodes are securely applied to the target tissue and the target and surrounding tissues are in clear view.

REFERENCES

Cruise PJE, Foord R 1973 A 5 year prospective study of 23,649 surgical wounds. Archives of Surgery 107:206

Franchi M, Ghezzi F, Benedetti-Panici PL et al 2001 A multicentre collaborative study on the use of cold scalpel and electrocautery for midline abdominal incision. Amerian Journal of Surgery 181:128–132

Meeks GR, Sams JO 4th, Field KW, Fulp KW, Margolis MT 1997 Formation of vesicovaginal fistula: the role of suture placement into the bladder during closure of the vaginal cuff after transabdominal hysterectomy. American Journal of Obstetrics and Gynecology 177:1298–1303

Niggebrugge AHP, Trimbos JB, Hermans J, Steup W-H, Van De Velde CJH 1999 Influence of abdominal-wound closure technique on complications after surgery: a randomised study. Lancet 353:1563–1567

Orr JW Jr, Garter JF, Kilgore LC et al 1987 Closed suction pelvic drainage following radical pelvic surgery. American Journal of Obstetrics and Gynecology 155:867

Orr JW Jr, Orr PJ, Bolen DD, Holimon JL 1995 Radical hysterectomy: does the type of incision matter? American Journal of Obstetric and Gynecology 173:399–405

Royal College of Obstetrics and Gynaecologists 1998 Peritoneal closure. Guideline no. 15. RCOG, London

Rucinski J, Margolis M, Panagopoulos G, Wise L 2001 Closure of the abdominal midline fascia: met-analysis delineates the optimal technique. American Surgeon 67:421–462

Scribner DR Jr, Kamelle SA, Gould N et al 2001 A retrospective analysis of radical hysterectomies done for cervical cancer: is there a role for the Pfannenstiel incision? Gynecological Oncology 81:481–484

Tulandi T, Hum HS, Gelfand MM 1988 Closure of laparotomy incisions with or without peritoneal suturing and second look laparoscopy. American Journal of Obstetrics and Gynecology 158:536

10

Postoperative care

Rob J. Gornall

INTRODUCTION

The postoperative management of women undergoing surgery is an area of care that sometimes receives less attention than the preoperative and operative management. This is unfortunate since, if performed well, there should be an associated reduction in morbidity leading to shorter and less costly hospital admissions and an increase in patient satisfaction. Getting the obvious wrong is much worse than overlooking a rare condition and it is paramount that we consistently apply the fundamentals of patient care to achieve the highest safety standards.

The prevention or early recognition of postoperative complications should be our goal. The use of prophylactic drugs such as those for thromboembolic disease will reduce the morbidity and mortality from deep vein thrombosis and pulmonary embolism but early mobilization and skilled physiotherapy play a vital role in preventing complications and speeding recovery. Known risk factors such as obesity and smoking should be identified at the time of preoperative assessment and the postoperative care planned so as to minimize the potential complications (Gass & Olsen 1986). The development of local audit will help to identify problem areas and lead to reduced mobidity.

POSTOPERATIVE CARE

Correct environment

Patients should be cared for in an environment where they can have privacy but still be observed closely when necessary by skilled nursing staff. The nursing staff should have received the specialist training necessary to care for gynaecological patients and there should be sufficient staff to provide that care 24 hours a day.

Physiotherapists, dieticians and pharmacists should be available on the ward every day. Some surgical procedures need specialist postoperative management such as wound care following radical vulval surgery and therefore it is best that such women are cared for in specialist centres. An elderly patient may require periods of convalescence and rehabilitation that can be provided by local hospitals near to the patient's home or by community teams that care for her in her own home. These needs should be determined by preoperative nursing assessment so that discharge plans can be put in place at an early stage.

Fluid replacement

For most minor and intermediate procedures peri- and postoperative intravenous fluid replacement is not required. Intravenous access is used only for the induction and safe maintenance of general anaesthesia and may be removed soon after the patient returns from theatre. Patients undergoing day-case procedures recommence oral fluids soon after recovery from anaesthesia.

For patients undergoing major abdominal or vaginal surgery, intravenous fluid replacement is required to replace blood and fluid loss and to allow for a period of decreased intake postoperatively as a result of recovery from anaesthesia. The average patient requires 2.5–3 litres of fluid per 24 hours and at least 75–100 mEq of sodium per day and 60 mEq of potassium per day. Potassium supplementation is required only after 24 hours because cell death and a mild renal acidosis will maintain potassium levels during the acute postoperative phase. Potassium loss may be increased by persistent vomiting and replacement should be planned to take this into account.

When planning postoperative fluid replacement it is worth remembering that some patients approach surgery depleted of fluids and electrolytes. An obvious example is

Box 10.1 Circumstances in which additional fluid supplementation will be needed

High fluid loss through a drain

A long abdominal operation – 1l lost per hour

Pyrexia – 15% extra per 1°C rise in body temperature

Loss into the "Third space", e.g. ascites or pleural effusion

Box 10.2 Effects of inadequate analgesia

Impairs oxygenation

Reduces deep breathing

Increases risk of atelectasis

Prolongs hospitalization

reduced intravascular volume because of haemorrhage from a ruptured ectopic pregnancy. Less obviously, patients presenting with prolonged vomiting and decreased fluid intake over a number of days may be fluid and electrolyte depleted. Likewise oral, osmotically active bowel preparation will lead to substantially increased fluid loss. While this may not upset young women, older patients may benefit from intravenous fluid replacement.

There are certain situations where additional replacement will be required to replace increased losses (Box 10.1). These include long open abdominal operations when the small bowel is exteriorized. Fluid loss may occur via pelvic drains following surgery or inguinal drains following block dissection of the inguinal lymph glands. Marked fluid shifts can occur into the so-called 'third space' which includes dilated bowel, pleural or peritoneal cavity following drainage of ascites and debulking of ovarian tumours. Extensive removal of the pelvic peritoneum leads to increased fluid loss and rapid accumulation of ascites can occur in the presence of residual disease. Drains are rarely used in such cases and therefore the gynaecologist should be aware of fluid shifts even if there is no outward sign. There is some debate about the speed of drainage of ascites in elective situations but, in practice, rapid drainage of ascites secondary to malignancy rarely leads to complications. This contrasts with those patients who have ascites as a result of undiagnosed cirrhosis where unavoidable surgical drainage at laparotomy may precipitate profound fluid shifts and subsequent decompensation leads to hepatorenal failure. Rapid reaccumulation of ascites postoperatively in patients with ovarian cancer suggests progressive residual disease which may respond to early commencement of chemotherapy. Other common situations leading to increased fluid requirements include pyrexia and 15% more fluid should be given for each degree C rise in temperature. Patients with newly formed ileostomies or colostomies may experience significant outputs of 3–4 litres over 24 hours which may not be appreciated unless formal measurement is requested. This may be exacerbated by peri- or postoperative antibiotic therapy that alters the gut flora.

Postoperative analgesia

The management of postoperative pain is often a neglected area of care. This was highlighted by a joint commission of the Royal College of Surgeons of England and College of Anaesthetists (1990) which found that postoperative pain was often inadequately recognized, monitored and treated. This situation is changing with the increasing recognition of the ill effects of ineffective analgesia (Box 10.2). The effect of pain in reducing deep breathing impairs oxygenation and compounds the process of atelectasis which starts as a result of general anaesthesia.

Patient mobility is reduced and hospitalization may be prolonged. Effective management of postoperative pain will reduce these complications and reduce postoperative morbidity and mortality.

The degree of discomfort experienced following surgery is very subjective and although guidelines estimating the degree of analgesia required are available, the aim should be to individualize pain control. Explanation of the procedure and the likely postoperative course with an assurance that postoperative discomfort will be minimized is effective in reducing anxiety and postoperative analgesia requirements (Karanikolas & Swarm 2000). Simple techniques such as infiltration of laparoscopy incision sites with marcaine may be of benefit.

Patients who undergo day-case surgery should be given suitable analgesia to use at home following discharge and be aware of the type and extent of discomfort that they may experience before seeking medical advice. Contact with the patient by telephone the following day provides reassurance, can help auditing of practice and pain control and may also alert staff to possible complications developing.

Patient-controlled analgesia (PCA) systems have been introduced to individualize pain control and minimize the delay in assessing pain and administering analgesia. These allow the patient to control the rate and level of analgesia. The patient is instructed how to use the 'trigger' to release a bolus of drug but, by presetting the minimum delay between boluses, overdosage is prevented. The patient must be totally pain free before they take over control of their own analgesia if this method is to be effective. A constant background infusion may be used but this does not proportionately reduce the number of boluses required and increases the risk of respiratory depression. The major side-effects are nausea and vomiting. This problem may be reduced by regular antiemetic injections or inclusion of the antiemetic in the infusion. Because the maximum delivery rate of the opioids is limited, the risk of respiratory depression is reduced and so this technique may be used on wards with less intensive nursing levels. When the patient is mobilizing on day 2 or 3 following surgery, she is transferred to oral analgesia.

In patients undergoing extended surgery, epidural analgesia may be employed. This reduces the depth of anaesthesia required and improves pain relief after surgery. Hypotension can occur but should respond to volume replacement. It may be difficult in such circumstances to differentiate this from postoperative haemorrhage, particularly as volume replacement may lead to haemodilution and a low hemoglobin concentration.

Non-steroidal analgesics are useful once the acute pain has started to subside. Long-acting agents or preparations such as diclofenac and ketoprofen given as a suppository provide effective analgesia and are less traumatic than repeated intramuscular injection. Breakthrough pain can be controlled with agents such as co-proxamol. The use of these agents after minor gynaecological procedures reduces the need for intramuscular injections of opioids. These drugs should not be used in women with a history of asthma or upper gastrointestinal haemorrhage or ulceration.

Management of drains

Drains inserted because of the risk of haemorrhage can be safely removed after 24 hours if loss is minimal. Small suction drains such as Redivac can be unreliable in the identification of intraperitoneal haemorrhage as they often become blocked by surrounding tissue and a larger gravity drain such as Robinson type is preferred. It may be appropriate to leave drains in place for a longer period of 3–5 days if placed in an abscess cavity or near a bowel anastomosis and a large-bore drain without suction is more appropriate to allow drainage of viscid material and minimize trauma to surrounding tissues as a result of suction.

Suction drains are useful in removing lymphatic fluid from the groins after lymphadenectomy. They may need to remain in place for up to 10 days. Thereafter, they are unlikely to offer any further value, may become infected and are better removed. For the majority of routine gynaecological procedures routine drain placement should not be required and they should not be seen as a substitute for conscientious haemostatic technique.

Management of urinary catheters

Indwelling urinary catheters are routinely used by the majority of gynaecologists at the time of major pelvic surgery (Hilton 1988). This is done to reduce the risk of bladder damage at the time of surgery and for patient comfort in the acute recovery phase. However, catheters predispose to urinary tract infection and may hinder mobilization. Therefore, following uncomplicated pelvic surgery, catheters should be removed once the patient is able to get out of bed. Extended bladder drainage for 7–10 days should be employed when the bladder has been opened during surgery.

Suprapubic catheters are preferred following bladder neck surgery or radical hysterectomy. This allows residual urine volumes to be measured after spontaneous voiding. Regimes may vary between units but the suprapubic catheter should not be removed until the volume of residual urine in the bladder is consistently less than 100 ml after spontaneous voiding. If high residual volumes persist, the patient may be allowed home with the suprapubic catheter in situ after being taught catheter care. The patient measures residual volumes and telephones a nominated member of the ward team for advice about clamping. She can then return to the ward to have the catheter removed. Radical hysterectomy may impair the sensation of bladder distension and contractility and result in a poor urinary stream and persistently high residuals. In some cases despite prolonged catheterization, adequate spontaneous voiding fails to resume and patients need to use intermittent urethral self-catheterization until bladder function has recovered.

Mobilization and physiotherapy

Early mobilization reduces muscle loss through inactivity and enables the woman to return to normal activity more quickly. The rate of muscle loss associated with bedrest is dramatic. Even a reduction of 12 hours in the onset of mobilization will make a substantial difference. In addition, the risk of thromboembolic disease and respiratory infection is reduced by early mobilization.

Skilled physiotherapists are essential to facilitate early mobilization and to deal with the problems that inevitably accompany a more prolonged postoperative recovery. They play a pivotal role in the prevention and treatment of respiratory infection.

Wound care

Wound care begins in theatre with careful haemostasis, the minimum pressure on the wound with self-retaining retractors and carefull closure of the wound, avoiding excessive tension and ensuring good apposition of the skin edges. While a dressing is usually applied to surgical wounds, it does nothing to prevent infection. Its primary purpose is to protect the patient's clothing from any seepage of blood or serum and to prevent the sutures catching on other objects. While no harm can result from a shower, soaking in a bath with bath gels or other products containing strong detergents is best avoided in the first week because of the possible effect on the newly formed coagulum on the wound. Sutures and staples can be removed from transverse wounds after 4–5 days. Vertical wounds usually require 7–10 days to heal but longer may be required in some cases.

Wound infections present on about the fifth postoperative day and are usually preceded by induration and erythema around the incision. Sutures should be removed and the wound opened in the infected area if there are signs of a collection. The wound should be probed to break down any loculations of pus and necrotic material should be removed. A moist pack soaked in honey helps to clean the wound and reduce the oedema. The defect should be allowed to heal by secondary intention. Antibiotic therapy is only indicated if there is significant cellulitis, systemic signs of bacteraemia or evidence of necrotizing infection. A swab should be taken before starting antibiotic treatment. Flucloxacillin or erythromycin are suitable antibiotics while sensitivities are awaited.

Necrotizing fasciitis is a rare, rapidly progressive and often fatal infection of the superficial fascia and subcutaneous tissues (Addison et al 1984). Diabetic patients are especially vulnerable but any chronic illness may predispose to this condition. It is seen most commonly on the vulva or perineum and it is often not related to surgery, but it can be seen in the region of a recent surgical wound. There is extensive tissue necrosis and a moderate or severe systemic toxic reaction. Very radical excision is essential with antibiotics and supportive therapy.

RECOGNITION AND TREATMENT OF COMPLICATIONS

Surgery performed for those appropriately selected by those appropriately trained may minimize the risk of complications but they nevertheless occur. Different operations may result in general complications, which may lead to the clinical picture of shock, but also predispose to particular complications. The surgeon should be aware of these and have counselled the patient appropriately when gaining informed preoperative consent.

Haemorrhage

Detection

Primary haemorrhage occurs in the immediate postoperative period; secondary haemorrhage is delayed. The distinction between primary and delayed haemorrhage is rarely clear. The rate of haemorrhage will normally determine when the patient exhibits signs. Fit patients can compensate for decreased intravascular volume and can maintain blood pressure by tachycardia and peripheral vasoconstriction. This may conceal the severity of their condition until their ability to continue compensating is exhausted and the blood pressure falls suddenly and precipitously. Those with intercurrent cardiovascular disease cope poorly with much smaller degrees of haemorrhage and decompensate much earlier and in an unpredictable fashion.

The normal clinical monitoring of postoperative patients with pulse and blood pressure recordings is adequate for most gynaecological patients. In high-risk cases, the hourly urine output is a sensitive measure of peripheral circulation. However, a fall in urine volume may occur because of relative dehydration and the volume will increase in the diuretic phase of recovery from renal failure. Measurement of the difference between the core temperature, measured rectally, and the peripheral temperature, measured on the toe, is a very sensitive indication of peripheral perfusion and, by inference, blood volume and cardiac output. It is widely used in intensive care units and deserves more frequent use in monitoring high-risk patients. Oximetry, measuring the oxygenated haemoglobin content in peripheral vessels, is also dependent in part on peripheral perfusion. The central venous pressure is a less useful measurement than the above, is invasive, requires constant supervision and is much more prone to measurement errors. However, it is particularly valuable in warming of fluid over-load during resuscitation. This is more important in older women or patients with cardiac or renal disease whose ability to cope with excess fluid is limited.

The early signs of haemorrhage are a rising pulse rate, vasoconstriction, manifest by cold hands and feet, and reduced urinary output. If the early signs are not detected or if major haemorrhage occurs rapidly the blood pressure will fall and the patient may be restless, confused and complain of severe thirst.

Abdominal signs may be absent, particularly if the bleeding is retroperitoneal and little weight should be placed on lack of output from a small suction drain which often becomes blocked. Assessment may be further compromised by the use of epidural pain relief and medication for concurrent conditions such as β-blockers which may mask early signs.

When massive blood loss occurs, a consumptive co-agulophathy may develop as all the coagulation factors are exhausted. It is therefore important to monitor the coagulation status of the patient repeatedly during resuscitation and if an abnormality develops expert advice from a haematologist should be sought.

Volume replacement

There is much debate over the value of colloid preparations compared with crystalloids when a patient requires volume replacement because of haemorrhage (Cochrane Injuries Group Albumin Reviewers 1998, Hanken & Beez 1998, Offringa 1998, Schierhout & Roberts 1998, Webb 2000, Wilkes & Navickis 2001). In the immediate management, crystalloids will maintain the cardiac output and renal function as effectively as colloids although twice the volume is required. Crystalloids are more effective than colloids in replacing the deficit in the extracellular fluid compartment but may cause fluid overload. The mobilization of this extra fluid during the recovery phase leads to a diuresis which may protect against renal failure (Shires et al 1983, Virgilio et al 1979). However, if more than 1000 ml of fluid are required, synthetic colloid replacement fluids such as Haemacell are generally recommended until blood becomes available (Lowe et al 1977). It is wise not to use more than 1000–1500 ml of Haemacell in 24 hours. It may cause clotting in giving sets if mixed with citrated blood or fresh frozen plasma (FFP). There is controversy about the value of 4.5% human albumin solution (HAS) in this situation (Cochrane Injuries Group Albumin Reviewers 1998, Wilkes & Navickis 2001).

Red blood cell products are required to correct the loss of oxygen-carrying capacity. It should be noted, however, that oxygen-carrying capacity is not compromised until the haematocrit falls below 22% (Hb < 7 g/l). Whole blood is seldom available now because transfusion centres remove the plasma and other components to prepare products required for other purposes. Supplemented red cell concentrate (SAG-M) is generally supplied in the UK. All the plasma has been removed from these cells and replaced by a supplement of adenine, glucose and mannitol. This product flows just as well as whole blood. If more than three units of SAG-M are given to patients with a previously normal serum albumin, the plasma deficit should be made up with crystalloid.

In patients with pre-existing coagulation defects or in those who have undergone lengthy procedures with high recorded blood loss, coagulopathies should be considered and a platelet count and coagulation screen performed to aid replacement with appropriate blood products. FFP contains all the protein constituents of plasma, including the coagulation factors. It should be used to replace coagulation factors and not used for plasma expansion. Cryoprecipitate contains a high concentration of fibrinogen that may be required in massive blood transfusion. After 5–6 units of rapidly transfused red cells, two units of FFP should be given without waiting for the results of coagulation tests. Platelet transfusion will be required if the platelet count is less than $50 \times 10^9/l$.

Re-exploration

Deciding when to re-explore a patient who is bleeding post-operatively can be one of the most difficult decisions a gynaecologist has to face. The advice and help of the most experienced person available should be sought. If at all possible, the patient should be stabilized by transfusion first. The sooner after surgery the bleeding presents, the more likely it is that re-exploration will identify a single obvious bleeding vessel. If the patient presents with an obvious haematoma more than 24 hours after surgery, it can be very difficult to identify a single bleeding vessel. More often, a generalized ooze is encountered and adequate haemostasis is difficult to achieve. In this situation, it may be better to continue the transfusion and correct any coagulation defect rather than to re-explore. Angiographic embolization is probably the management of choice if it is available (Mann et al 1980) (see below and Chapter 6).

It is important to avoid hypothermia in any patient who requires further surgery because this will tend to worsen any coagulation abnormalities. If the patient is bleeding vaginally after a hysterectomy, it is often worth examining her vaginally under anaesthesia in the hope of identifying a bleeding point that can be sutured from below. The vaginal branch of the uterine artery is often the culprit. If re-laparotomy is required, clot must be removed gently to avoid provoking more bleeding and the operation site explored carefully. Do not close up without examining all the pedicles even after a bleeding vessel has been identified – there are often multiple bleeding sites! Intra-abdominal bleeding frequently originates from the ovarian vessels. These must be clearly identified and separated from the ureter which lies very close at this point. Bleeding in the pelvis is often difficult to localize and may be venous rather than arterial. It is often necessary to extend the dissection substantially in order to visualize the source of the problem. Sutures can be placed medial to the uterine pedicles without fear of ureteric damage but, if in doubt after careful palpation, dissect out the ureter so that it can be seen or ask for help.

Ligation of the internal iliac artery is often advocated when bleeding cannot be controlled by other means. The effect of this is often disappointing. The technique is simple if the surgeon has experience of the method but there is the potential for damaging the underlying vein and compounding the problem. If in doubt – do not do it! Large, hot packs pressed firmly into the pelvis for a full 5 minutes will often be effective or will at least reduce the general ooze so that the main bleeding sites can be seen. If it proves impossible to achieve satisfactory haemostasis, the omentum may be brought into the pelvis and several large packs placed firmly over it. The abdomen is then closed loosely over the packs with the tapes gathered together and brought through the wound. These may be removed under general anaesthesia 24–48 hours later.

Angiographic embolization of bleeding vessels in the pelvis

Embolization of actively bleeding blood vessels using interventional radiological techniques is a highly effective alternative to surgery in the management of surgical haemorrhage in the pelvis. It requires a skilled team of intervention radiologists who are able to provide an emergency service. Percutaneous angiography is performed via the femoral artery to identify the source of the bleeding and then the offending arteries are selectively embolized using materials such as gelatin sponge or metal coils or adhesive agents such as iso-butyl-2-cyanocrylate (Allison et al 1992; see Chapter 6). This avoids what is often very difficult surgery in very sick patients and is often the more reliable and faster method of controlling the bleeding.

Pelvic haematoma

Vault haematoma are a common complication of hysterectomy, particularly by the vaginal route. It has been reported that one-third of patients undergoing hysterectomy will have a haematoma identified by ultrasound and two-thirds of these will develop a postoperative pyrexia (Toglia & Pearlman 1994). Generally these are self-limiting and will either resolve or more commonly discharge via the vaginal vault in the second week following surgery. Haematomas are normally walled off from the general peritoneal cavity and therefore generalized contamination of the peritoneal cavity is rare unless there has been associated bowel perforation. Surgical drainage may be required, however, in the event of persisting pelvic pain or systemic upset with pyrexia. This can be accompanied by ultrasound-guided placement of a drain or more commonly under general anaesthetic with separation of loculations and wide reopening of the vaginal vault to allow complete drainage of often viscid secretions. Such patients often demonstrate a striking thrombocythaemia which will slowly resolve following discharge.

Abdominal wound haematoma are also common and tend to be self-limiting. They may cause discomfort on mobilizing and the spreading bruising that develops in the days following surgery may prove alarming for the patient. She should be reassured that this represents old bruising that will improve with time. Such bruising from the lateral port sites for laparoscopic surgery can also be severe, especially if the port incisions have been widened to remove samples contained in retrieval bags.

Infection

Postoperative pyrexia is common after gynaecological surgery but the incidence can be reduced from 20% to 10% with the routine use of prophylactic antibiotics (Mittendorf et al 1993). Many patients with fever in the first 48 hours do not have an identifiable infection and the temperature settles without active treatment (Box 10.3).

Pyrexia within the first 48–72 hours is usually caused by pulmonary atelectasis developing during general anaesthesia. The risk of atelectasis is increased by age, obesity, a history of smoking, poor postoperative analgesia and upper abdominal surgery. Patients may be asymptomatic but crepitations and reduced air entry will be found. This condition is best treated with physiotherapy, incentive spirometry and adequate

Box 10.3 Common causes of postoperative pyrexia

Early pyrexia <36 hr	Late pyrexia >36 hr
Unexplained fever	Any of the early causes
Atelectasis	Urinary tract infection
Peritoneal soiling: occult bowel injury anastomotic leak	Pneumonia
	Haematoma: pelvic
Urinoma: occult ureteric or bladder injury	wound
	Deep venous thrombosis
Ureteric obstruction	Septic thrombophlebitis
Wound infection: streptococcal clostridial	

analgesia. Antibiotic therapy may be required if atelectasis persists.

After 72 hours the most likely cause of a pyrexia is a urinary tract infection, especially if the patient has been catheterized. Many patients are asymptomatic so urine should be sent for microscopy and culture in any suspected cases. Antibiotic therapy may be started empirically if the patient is unwell. The routine use of prophylactic antibiotics at the time of surgery does not reduce the incidence of urinary tract infection but may alter the pattern of bacterial isolates (Brown et al 1988).

Wound infections present on about the fifth postoperative day and are usually preceded by induration and erythema around the incision. The wound should be inspected and a wound swab taken if an infection is suspected. However, such swabs often grow commensal skin organisms which are non-pathogenic and lead to inappropriate choice of antibiotic therapy.

A pelvic ultrasound should be undertaken if the pyrexia persists despite broad-spectrum intravenous antibiotics. This may demonstrate the presence of an infected pelvic haematoma post hysterectomy. Small abscesses, especially loculated collections lying between small bowel loops, can be missed by both ultrasound and CT.

In overwhelming sepsis, shock can supervene manifested by hypotension and multisystem failure (Iverson 1988). In the initial phase peripheral vasodilatation is seen with normal or increased cardiac output, tachycardia, oliguria, fever and often mental changes. Prompt resuscitation and antibiotic therapy are required to reduce the mortality rate.

Thromboembolic disease

Deep vein thrombosis

The development of a deep vein thrombosis (DVT) is a common postoperative event with 30% of patients developing a DVT after moderate and major surgical procedures. The most common site for the thrombosis is the calf (Kakkar et al 1969). The level of risk is dependent on various factors, some patient related, some disease related and some procedure related. The summation of these factors allows each patient to be assigned a risk level for developing a DVT (THRIFT 1992). Although less well studied than general surgery, there is no evidence to suggest that the incidence of DVT is lower after gynaecological surgery. It is therefore prudent to offer appropriate prophylaxis against thromboembolic disease to all gynaecology patients undergoing surgery (see Chapter 8).

Unfortunately the majority of patients with acute deep venous thrombosis are asymptomatic and in patients with fatal pulmonary embolism the preceding DVT goes unrecognized (Karwinski & Svendsen 1989). It is the extension of the clot into the proximal veins that causes the majority of significant pulmonary embolisms and most of the fatal ones. The symptoms associated with DVT are pain, swelling and erythema of the affected calf. On examination, there may be a low-grade pyrexia, the leg may be warmer and larger in circumference, the peripheral veins distal to the occlusion may be dilated and the calf may be tender to palpation over the site of the thrombosis. Eliciting Homan's sign, pain on forced dorsiflexion of the foot, should be avoided as it may inadvertently lead to embolization of clot. In symptomatic patients the investigation of choice is compression ultrasonography. The vein is visualized using B-mode ultrasound and the vein compressed with the transducer. If the vein fails to collapse an intraluminal clot is present even if it cannot be visualized. Venography is occasionally necessary but it is associated with the risk of embolism.

Once the diagnosis has been made the patient must receive anticoagulation therapy to prevent pulmonary embolism and to restore venous patency. Heparin is equally effective intravenously (28–40 000 units/24 h by continuous infusion) or subcutaneously (15–17 500 units 12 hourly) (Drug and Therapeutics Bulletin 1992). It should be administered with the goal of achieving full anticoagulation within 24 hours and the treatment should be continued at a level to maintain the activated partial thromboplastin time (APTT) at 1.5–2.5 times the control. Low molecular weight heparin given subcutaneously once daily is as effective as standard heparin regimens in preventing further thromboembolic events without increasing the risk of major bleeding (Hull et al 1992). Although more expensive, it may well be cost effective because it can be given as an outpatient without monitoring coagulation and there are savings in labour and disposables.

Conversion to oral anticoagulation therapy with warfarin should commence after 5 days of heparin therapy and the heparin discontinued once oral anticoagulation is within the therapeutic range. The dosage of warfarin should be adjusted to maintain the international normalized ratio (INR) at between 2.0 and 3.0 (Hyers et al 1993). The duration of warfarin therapy has been the subject of a randomized trial, comparing 4 weeks against 3 months of treatment. Four weeks' anticoagulation appears adequate for postoperative DVT (Research Committee of the British Thoracic Society 1992). Although this treatment is very effective it should be remembered that the risk of pulmonary embolism or further DVT is not zero.

Pulmonary embolism

The true incidence of pulmonary embolism after surgery is unknown. In patients not receiving prophylactic treatment the incidence of recognized pulmonary embolism is about 4% with about 25–50% of these being fatal (Kakkar et al 1969). Despite previous calls for routine prophylaxis against thromboembolic disease, pulmonary embolism accounted for 20% of fatalities after hysterectomy in 1991–92 (National Confidential Enquiry into Perioperative Deaths 1993). The low usage of perfusion/ventilation scanning and postmortems suggests that this figure is probably an underestimation. While most pulmonary emboli become apparent while the patient is in hospital, a substantial number occur after discharge (Sors & Meyer 2000).

Minor pulmonary embolism is associated with a history of pleuritic chest pain, haemoptysis, a pleural rub and fine crepitations at the base of the lungs. At least 50% of the pulmonary tree must be involved to cause any haemodynamic disturbance. In this situation the patient may complain of central chest pain or dyspnoea or have collapsed. The ECG may show signs of right-sided strain with an S wave in lead 1, a Q wave in lead 3 and T wave inversion in lead 3 (S_1, Q_3, T_3). The chest X-ray after a massive pulmonary embolism may show areas of reduced vascular shadowing due to oligaemia, enlarged pulmonary arteries and abrupt ending of pulmonary arteries. Arterial blood gas analysis may show a reduced oxygen tension in the presence of a normal carbon dioxide tension. A ventilation/perfusion scan is probably the investigation of choice, an area of hypoperfusion in the presence of normal ventilation confirming the diagnosis. In an emergency, a perfusion scan alone with a chest X-ray will also aid diagnosis. Pulmonary angiography may be required in cases of uncertainty, but requires a degree of expertise not always available.

Thromboprophylaxis with heparin does not exclude a pulmonary embolus, particularly in high-risk patients such as those with disseminated malignancy. Treatment with heparin therapy should start immediately rather than await confirmatory tests. There may be a delay prior to performing a ventilation/perfusion scan and such tests may give equivocal results, especially post surgery when there may be coexistent basal atelectasis and infection. Therefore when interpreting the results, the clinical impression should be borne in mind. Treatment is based on anticoagulant therapy incorporating heparin and warfarin. Thrombolytic therapy can be instituted with streptokinase or urokinase but is contraindicated in patients who have undergone major surgery within 10 days, are pregnant or who have a history of gastrointestinal bleeding. In those patients with persisting risk factors and who clinically have recurrent pulmonary emboli despite high-dose anticoagulation a vena caval umbrella filter may need to be fitted. This may be temporary prior to surgery, if the predisposing factors can be corrected, or permanent. Anticoagulation following pulmonary embolism may need to be lifelong if there are strong predisposing factors but in uncomplicated postsurgical cases, it may be needed for 3–6 months.

Cardiac complications

Preoperative assessment will often identify those patients at risk of cardiovascular events during surgery and the decision to proceed needs to be based on the severity of the disease and the likely benefit of surgery (Nettleman et al 1997). Any patient receiving a general anaesthetic is at increased risk of myocardial ischaemia but this is greatly increased when there is pre-existing cardiac disease. Eliciting a good preoperative history of cardiac disease is generally more predictive than screening tests such as ECG stress testing which are associated with a high false-positive rate. Elective surgery should be delayed in patients with a history of myocardial infarction within the preceding 6 months.

Patients with chest pain postoperatively should be investigated with serial cardiac enzymes and ECG. If patients have received postoperative analgesia, pain may not be a profound symptom. In a patient with tachycardia and hypotension, myocardial infarction must come into the differential diagnosis once haemorrhage has been excluded. Women with pulmonary oedema or a new heart murmur should also be investigated for evidence of myocardial infarction. The association of acute pulmonary oedema and myocardial infarction implies a poor prognosis. Referral to a cardiologist is warranted but thrombolytic therapy is contraindicated within 5 days of surgery. Unexpected arrhythmias or myocardial infarction can present in the immediate postoperative period. Prolonged arrhythmias may lead to hypotension and exacerbate the effects of hypovolaemia secondary to surgery, resulting in further compromised tissue perfusion. Cardiac function may be further compromised by acidosis, hypoxaemia and fluid overload as a consequence of enthusiastic fluid replacement to correct hypotension and oliguria.

Wound dehiscence and incisional hernias

This complication may range from a small defect in the skin to a burst abdomen. A small dehiscence does not require active management and will heal by secondary intention. Provided any infection has been adequately treated and the edges can be brought together easily, without tension, larger skin defects can be closed using sutures or skin tapes under local or general anaesthesia. Any necrotic tissue should be debrided before this is undertaken. If the wound is not clean or cannot be closed easily, it is better to pack it with gauze soaked in honey and allow it to heal by secondary intention. It is surprising how rapidly this can occur.

Complete wound dehiscence is a rare event. It is very exceptional after a Pfannenstiel incision and can be largely prevented in vertical incisions by mass closure (Bucknall et al 1982). There may be problems with the surgical technique or the use of incorrect suture material but factors such as wound infection, abdominal distension and postoperative coughing are also contributory. Dehiscence is more common in patients who are infected, malnourished or have an underlying malignancy. The first line of management is replacement of the bowel and resuturing of the wound. The high mortality (15–24%) associated with this condition is largely due to the coexisting medical problems.

Incisional herniation occurs in 7–8% of patients with midline incisions and the incidence after lower transverse incisions is believed to be much lower (Bucknall et al 1982). Several studies have reported a high incidence (16–22%) of incisional hernias following gynaecological surgery (Devlin & Nicholson 1994). Many hernias do not present until 1 year after surgery. Primary closure of the defect may be feasible but the use of synthetic Prolene grafts will aid repair of larger hernias. It is advisable that the repair should be undertaken by a surgeon experienced with the technique.

Urinary complications

Many patients undergoing gynaecological surgery have pre-existing urinary dysfunction such as stress or urge incontinence, frequency, poor stream or incomplete bladder emptying. These symptoms may be transiently made worse in the short term by any pelvic surgery. The most common complications of the urinary system are urinary tract infection related to drainage of the bladder with a temporary or indwelling urinary catheter.

The incidence of ureteric injury in gynaecological surgery is between 0.5% and 2.5%. Damage which is recognized at the time of surgery and repaired correctly will have low morbidity. Damage to the urinary tract occurs at three sites. The most common injury is to the bladder, particularly if there has been previous surgery. The other sites of injury are the ureter at the angle of the vagina and near the pelvic brim close to the ovarian blood supply. Conditions such as endometriosis and ovarian cancer are associated with distortion of the normal course of the ureter which increases the likelihood of damage. A higher-incidence of injury and fistula formation is associated with surgery following pelvic radiotherapy because the dissection is more difficult and irradiated tissue does not heal well. Preoperative intravenous urography (IVU) is very unlikely to reduce the risk of ureteric injury.

Most primary injuries to the bladder are noted at the time of surgery and occur during dissection from the cervix and upper vagina. This is more common in those who have previously undergone caesarean section or anterior myomectomy and occur in the midline near the bladder dome. A vesicovaginal fistula may result from ischaemia of the bladder wall.

Damage to the urinary tract may become apparent within a few days of surgery or may not present for several weeks. Sometimes, postoperative ureteric obstruction is only discovered many years later as an incidental finding. A vesicovaginal fistula developing in the first postoperative week is more likely to be due to trauma to the bladder at surgery. The aetiology of fistulae presenting later is shrouded in uncertainty but often may be the end-result of a pelvic haematoma.

The signs and symptoms will result from extravasation of urine or ureteric obstruction. Urine may leak from the abdominal or vaginal incision or collect in a pelvic drain. A collection of urine may develop in the pelvis, causing discomfort and pyrexia. Loin pain and pyrexia may occur following ureteric obstruction. Delayed ureteric injury may present with persistent vaginal discharge from a fistula or abdominal wound.

If a fistula is suspected in the immediate postoperative phase, the patient should be catheterized to assess urine output. This will often reduce the amount of urine leaking through a bladder fistula. Fluid from any abdominal drain may be analysed for urea or creatinine content. It is often difficult to see a small fistula in the vagina and the 'three swab test' is helpful to confirm the presence of such a fistula. Three swabs are placed in the vagina and the patient is given a preparation which colours the urine. Pyridium (phenazopyridine) 100 mg orally was often used as it gives a strong orange colour to the urine. However, it is now difficult to obtain and intravenous indigo carmine may be used instead. When the urine in the bladder is strongly coloured, the swabs are removed. The lower swab is often coloured by urine from the urethra, but staining of the upper two swabs indicates a fistula. The same strategy can be used to confirm the nature of fluid leaking from abdominal wounds or drains. Alternatively, dilute methylene blue can be instilled into the bladder. However, this will not help to identify a ureteric fistula.

Imaging of the renal tract by intravenous urography (IVU) will help in locating the site of damage but small fistulae may be difficult to see. Percutaneous nephrostomy should be performed when there is evidence of hydronephrosis. This relieves the obstruction and allows antegrade pyeloureterography to locate the site of injury. Cystoscopy and retrograde insertion of ureteric stents is an alternative but often less satisfactory approach.

Repair of the damaged bladder is dependent upon the extent of urinary leakage. Women who are voiding spontaneously and troubled only by a small-volume leak may be managed satisfactorily by catheterization for 7–10 days. If this fails or if the leakage is more significant, surgical repair of the defect will be required. The fistula must be fully mobilized and the edges debrided (see Chapter 9 for details). The repair should be performed using absorbable sutures in one or two layers. An omental flap should be placed between the suture lines in the bladder and the vault of the vagina to improve the blood supply and to prevent apposition of the suture lines. The patient should remain catheterized for 7–10 days. Repair of the ureter should only be undertaken by a urologist with expertise in the area. Injury near the brim of the pelvis is managed by end-to-end anastomosis or, more commonly, by end-to-side anastomosis to the opposite ureter. Damage near to the bladder is better repaired with ureteric reimplantation into the bladder using either a psoas hitch or bladder flap to relieve tension on the repair.

Complications related to the gastrointestinal tract

Most complications affecting the bowel are minor and transient and not only occur as a result of surgery but may also be due to the effects of analgesia, anaesthetic agents or simply change in diet and routine. Cases of ileus following surgery can normally be anticipated by the degree of handling and dissection required near the bowel.

Postoperative feeding and nasogastric drainage

Different regimes for the initiation of fluid and diet are employed but early feeding seems to reduce the risk of infection and the average length of stay (Lewis et al 2001). The presence or absence of bowel signs is unreliable as a basis for the commencement of diet as activity returns at different sites in the gastrointestinal tract at different rates. Nasogastric drainage need only be performed if vomiting occurs, even in those cases where bowel resection has been undertaken. Nasogastric tubes are uncomfortable and may provoke vomiting by enhancing reflux.

Paralytic ileus

After manipulation of the bowel during surgery, normal peristaltic activity of the small bowel will return within 16 hours. Failure of this to recommence will result in the development of paralytic ileus. Patients with paralytic ileus are intolerant of oral fluids and clinically have abdominal distension with quiet or absent bowel sounds and delayed passage of flatus or stool. The majority of such cases will settle with conservative management by resting the bowel and employing intravenous fluid replacement and nasogastric drainage once an ileus has been confirmed.

However, cases that do not settle require further investigation to ensure that there are no potentiating factors. Intraperitoneal abscess formation or retroperitoneal haematoma may need to be drained under radiological control (Gerzof et al 1981). Electrolyte imbalance – typically hypokalaemia – should be corrected. It is rare for further laparotomy to be required in the abscence of any localizing signs.

Table 10.1 The effect of peritoneal closure on wound infection and adhesion formation (% incidence)

	Closed	Not Closed
Wound infection	3.6	2.4
Adhesions	22.2	15.8
Obstruction	1.6	0

Bowel obstruction

Bowel obstruction in the immediate postoperative period is rare following gynaecological surgery and usually does not become apparent before the fifth postoperative day. In parenthesis, it is worth noting that closure of the pelvic peritoneum does not reduce the incidence of postoperative adhesions or obstruction (Table 10.1; Tulandi et al 1988).

In the absence of peritonism, the initial treatment should be conservative with nasogastric suction and intravenous fluids. This will usually resolve the problem within 48–72 hours. Persistent vomiting or pain or high volumes of nasogastric aspirate and minimal passage of flatus after this length of time will usually mean that surgery will be required. Large amounts of aspirate from a woman who otherwise appears to have improved may be due to the end of the catheter having migrated into the duodenum! If abdominal tenderness increases or if pyrexia or tachycardia develop, suggesting peritonitis, immediate surgery is required.

Surgical damage

Damage to the bowel is an uncommon event. The incidence is reported to be between 0.3% and 0.8%, with the majority (70%) being minor lacerations. The small bowel is the site for injury in approximately 75% of cases. Abdominal surgery, rather than vaginal or laparoscopic surgery, is associated with a higher rate of damage and the majority (72%) follow uncomplicated gynaecological procedures. Risk factors for bowel damage include the presence of abdominal adhesions from malignancy, endometriosis or sepsis (Krebs 1986). Women who have received abdominal or pelvic radiotherapy are also at increased risk of bowel damage at the time of surgery. The incidence of bowel damage after laparoscopy is reported to be under 0.3% (Chamberlain & Brown 1978, Franks et al 1987). The risk of bowel perforation increases 10–20 fold after previous abdominal or pelvic surgery. Obesity or a history of pelvic inflammatory disease may increase the risk twofold (Brill et al 1975, Franks et al 1987).

The presentation, management and outcome of any injury to the bowel are dependent on the site and extent of the injury and the delay between injury and repair. Injuries that are recognized and repaired at the time of damage are associated with good outcomes; high morbidity and occasional mortality occur in the group presenting late with peritonitis.

Timing of presentation. Most cases of inadvertent enterotomy are noticed at the time of primary operation and should be managed as described in the preceding chapter. Those cases that present in the postoperative period can therefore be divided into those where inadvertent opening of the bowel has not been appreciated or, more commonly, when the bowel has been damaged and partially devascularized during the dissection and perforation subsequently takes place as a later event. This later event may occur when there is co-existent bowel pathology such as diverticular disease or bowel adhesions following previous surgery.

Damage recognized during the operation. It is often the case that bowel and sigmoid mesentery damage is only fully assessed when the gynaecological procedure has been completed. Rather than just hoping for the best, the safest course of action is to seek the opinion of a colorectal surgeon as to the likely outcome. Considerable experience is required to decide whether simply oversewing a partial or full-thickness injury is appropriate or whether the safest course of action is a local resection and reanastomosis. Although primary anastomosis is usually feasible, a temporary defunctioning stoma may be required in the presence of other bowel pathology such as diverticular disease or where the patient has not undergone bowel preparation. Early involvement of a colorectal surgeon may also be useful in the subsequent management of the patient and any complications that arise can then be jointly managed.

Perforation recognized after the operation. Patients who have received more than a minor laceration, such as puncture with a Veress needle at the time of laparoscopy, will normally present after 48–72 hours. The site of the leak will determine the clinical presentation. Postoperative intraperitoneal large bowel leak is a serious complication which carries a high mortality rate. The true diagnosis may not be apparent until septic shock and collapse supervene as intra-abdominal symptoms and signs may be attributed to recent surgery. Peritonitis may be generalized giving widespread peritonism and guarding with absent bowel sounds and severe systemic upset. Leakage may, however, be localized with abscess formation, resulting in a swinging pyrexia which does not settle with appropriate antibiotics and recurrent gastrointestinal symptoms of vomiting, abdominal distension and intolerance of recommencement of fluids. Abdominal X-ray may show signs of gas under the diaphragm or distended loops of small bowel but, in general, plain films are not helpful.

Small bowel perforation. Small bowel leaks often produce less dramatic signs initially and bowel sounds may still be present with flatus and stool per rectum. Investigation by contrast CT scan may aid in the localization of collections, although these are often not visible on either ultrasound or CT scans. It is important to constantly assess the clinical progress of the patient as localizing signs of tenderness and a pelvic mass may develop within the first week.

In the absence of a large leak and no evidence of obstruction distally, consideration should be given to radiological guided placement of a large-bore drain into any collection. Periodic irrigation may be used to remove viscid material (Gerzof et al 1981). When there are large leaks or signs of generalized peritonitis, laparotomy should be undertaken via a midline incision after resuscitation with fluids and antibiotics. Diversion proximal to a leak arising from large bowel or a complex inflammatory mass may be required. If the area of ischaemia or leakage is limited to the small bowel, limited resection with primary anastomosis can be performed. Copious washout of the peritoneal cavity, including around the liver, is undertaken with placement of drains to minimize persistent collections.

Such patients often have an unstable cardiac output and require volume replacement with invasive arterial and central venous monitoring. They are best managed in a high-dependency or intensive care setting. Fortunately, such scenarios are rare but the gynaecologist should be aware of the possibility, especially when covering patients under the care of the gynaecological oncology service.

Faecal fistula. As mentioned previously, the most common site of bowel injury is likely to be at the level of the sigmoid and rectum, typically at the time of performing a difficult hysterectomy with scarring or obliteration of the pouch of Douglas (Krebs 1986). If the leak is localized, the proximity of the vaginal vault closure often results in spontaneous discharge through the vault some days later, resulting in a rectovaginal fistula. Once the patient has complained of faecal incontinence, the diagnosis is normally straightforward if a vaginal speculum examination is performed. A one-shot soluble Gastrograffin enema may show the site of a large rectal or sigmoid fistula. Small fistulae may be hard to demonstrate and a formal barium enema may be required if the gynaecologist is confident that there is no intraperitoneal extension. Although small fistulae can be managed conservatively with a proximal defunctioning colostomy, the majority require surgical correction with resection of the affected bowel segment either as part of a Hartmann's procedure or, if performed as a delayed procedure, primary anastomosis with covering ileostomy/colostomy may be possible.

KEY POINTS

1. Careful preoperative assessment and medical optimization prior to surgery improve postoperative care.
2. Appropriate choice of operation performed by those appropriately trained is the most important factor in minimizing postoperative complications.
3. Effective postoperative analgesia using patient-based methods allows early mobilization and reduces respiratory complications.
4. Atelectasis and urinary tract infection are the commonest causes of postoperative pyrexia.
5. Pelvic haematomas are common after hysterectomy and may be the cause of postoperative pyrexia or unexpected anaemia.
6. There is a significant risk of DVT after major gynaecological procedures.
7. The majority of DVTs which precede pulmonary embolism are not recognized clinically.
8. If postoperative complications occur it is the responsibility of the operating gynaecologist to liase with the appropriate specialty and ensure that the patient is investigated and treated promptly.
9. Early recognition of bowel and urinary tract damage reduces the risk of serious morbidity.
10. Damage to bowel and urinary tract should be repaired only by experienced practitioners.
11. Local audit will identify areas of concern in surgical technique and infection control.

REFERENCES

Addison WA, Livengood CH, Hill GB, Sutton GP, Fortier KJ 1984 Necrotizing fasciitis of vulvar origin in diabetic patients. Obstetrics and Gynecology 63:473–479

Allison D, Wallace S, Machan LS 1992 Interventional radiology. In: Grainger RG, Allison DJ (Eds) Diagnostic radiology, 2nd edn. Churchill Livingstone, Edinburgh, pp 2329–2390

Brill AI, Nezhat F, Nezhat CH, Nezhat C 1995 The incidence of adhesions after prior laparotomy, a laparoscopic appraisal. Obstetrics and Gynecology 85:269–272

Brown EM, Depares J, Robertson AA et al 1988 Amoxycillin – clavulanic acid (Augmentin) versus metronidazole as prophylaxis in hysterectomy: a prospective, randomised clinical trial. British Journal of Obstetrics and Gynaecology 95:286–293

Bucknall TE, Cox PJ, Ellis H 1982 Burst abdomen and incisional hernia: a prospective study of 1129 major laparotomies. British Medical Journal 284:931–933

Chamberlain G, Brown JC (eds) 1978 Gynaecological laparoscopy: report on the Confidential Enquiry into Gynaecological Laparoscopy. Royal College of Obstetrics and Gynaecologists, London

Cochrane Injuries Group Albumin Reviewers 1998 Human albumin administration in critically ill patients: systematic review of randomised controlled trials. British Medical Journal 317:235–240

Devlin HB Nicholson S 1994 Hernias of the abdominal wall and pelvis, incisional hernias and parastomal hernias. In: Keen G, Farndon J (eds) Operative surgery and management. Butterworth Heinemann, Oxford, pp 41–54

Drug and Therapeutics Bulletin 1992 How to anticoagulate. 30:77–80

Franks AL, Kendrick JS, Peterson HB 1987 Unintended laparotomy associated with laparoscopic tubal sterilisation. American Journal of Obstetrics and Gynecology 157:1102–1105

Gass GD Olsen GN 1986 Preoperative pulmonary function testing to predict postoperative morbidity and mortality. Chest 89:127–129

Gerzof SG, Robbins AH, Johnson WC 1981 Percutaneous catheter drainage of abdominal abscesses. New England Journal of Medicine 305:193–197

Hankeln KB, Beez M 1998 Haemodynamic and oxygen transport correlates of various volume substitutes in critically ill patients with various aetiologies of haemo-dynamic instability. International Journal of Intensive Care 5:8–14

Hilton P 1988 Bladder drainage: a survey of practices among gynaecologists in the British Isles. British Journal of Obstetrics and Gynaecology 95:1178–1189

Hull RD, Raskob GE, Pineo GF et al 1992 Subcutaneous low molecular weight heparin compared with continuous heparin intravenous proximal vein thrombosis. New England Journal of Medicine 326:975–982

Hyers TM, Hull RD, Weg J G 1993 Antithrombotic therapy for venous thromboembolic disease. Chest 102 (suppl): 408S–425S

Iverson R L 1988 Septic shock: A clinical perspective. Critical Care Clinic 4:215

Kakkar VV, Hower CT, Flanc C, Clarke MB 1969 Natural history of postoperative deep vein thrombosis. Lancet 2:230–232

Karanikolas M, Swarm RA 2000 Current trends in perioperative pain management. Anesthesiology Clinics of North America 18/3:575–599

Karwinski B, Svendsen E 1989 Comparisons of clinical and post mortem diagnosis of pulmonary embolism. Journal of Clinical Pathology 42:135–139

Krebs HB 1986 Intestinal injury in gynecologic surgery: a ten year experience. American Journal of Obstetrics and Gynecology 155:505–514

Lewis S J, Egger M, Sylvester PA, Thomas S 2001 Early enteral feeding vesus "nil by mouth" after gastrointestinal surgery: systemic review and meta-analysis of controlled trials. British Medical Journal 323:733–736

Lowe RJ, Moss GS, Jilak J, Levine HD 1977 Crystalloid vs colloid in the etiology of patient failure after trauma: a randomised controlled trial in man. Surgery 81:676

Mann WJ, Jander HP, Partridge EE et al 1980 Selective arterial embolisation for control of bleeding in gynaecologic malignancy. Gynecological Oncology 10:279–283

Mittendorf R, Aronson MP, Berry RE et al 1993 Avoiding serious infections associated with abdominal hysterectomy. A meta-analysis of antibiotic prophylaxis. American Journal of Obstetrics and Gynecology 169:1119–1124

National Confidential Enquiry into Perioperative Deaths 1991–2 (1993) NCEPD, London

Nettleman MD, Banitt L, Awan I, Gordon EE. Predictors of survival and the role of gender in postoperative myocardial inarction. American Journal of Medicine 1997 103(5) 357–62

Offringa M 1998 Excess mortality after human albumin administration in critically ill patients. Clinical and pathophysiological evidence suggests albumin is harmful. British Medical Journal 317:223–234

Research Committee of the British Thoracic Society 1992 Optimum duration of anticoagulation for deep vein thrombosis and pulmonary embolism. Lancet 340:873–876

Royal College of Surgeons in England 1990 Pain after surgery. Report of the Working Party of the Commission on the Provision of Surgical Services. Royal College of Surgeons in England and the College of Anaesthetists, London

Schierhout G, Roberts I 1998 Fluid resuscitation with colloid or crystalloid solutions in critically ill patients: a systematic review of randomised trials. British Medical Journal 316:961–964

Shires GT III, Pettzman AB, Albert SA et al 1983 Response of extravascular lung water to intraoperative fluids. Annals of Surgery 197:515–518

Sors H, Meyer G 2000 Place of aspirin in prophylaxis of venous thromboembolism. Lancet 355:1288–1289

Thromboembolic Risk Factors (THRIFT) Consensus Group 1992 Risk of and prophylaxis for venous thromboembolism in hospital patients. British Medical Journal 305:567–574

Toglia MR, Pearlman MD 1994 Pelvic fluid collections following hysterectomy and their relation to febrile morbidity. Obstetrics and Gynecology 83:766–770

Tulandi T, Hum HS, Gelfand MM 1988 Closure of laparotomy incisions with or without peritoneal suturing and second-look laparoscopy. American Journal of Obstetrics and Gynecology 158:536

Virgilio RW, Rice CL, Smith DE et al 1979 Crystalloid vs. colloid resuscitation: is one better? Surgery 85:129–139

Webb AR 2000 The appropriate role of colloids in managing fluid imbalance: a critical review of recent meta-analytic findings Critical Care 4:S26–32

Wilkes MM, Navickis, RJ 2001 Patient survival after human albumin administration. A meta-analysis of randomised, controlled trials. Annals of Internal Medicine 135:149–164

11

Hormones: their action and measurement in gynaecological practice

Jurgis Geddes Grudzinskas

INTRODUCTION

Hormones are one of the important means by which cells communicate with each other. They ensure that the body's physiological systems are co-ordinated appropriately. Impaired communication leads to abnormal function. Classically, hormones are secreted by a gland and transported through the circulation to a distant site of action. However, as cellular communication also occurs at a local level, it is evident that several factors can combine to modulate and co-ordinate function. The types of communication to be considered are endocrine, paracrine and autocrine.

- *Endocrine* – intergland or structure communication involves secretion from a gland into the circulatory system (blood or lymph) of a regulatory substance that has a specific effect on another gland or structure, e.g. pituitary secretion of follicle-stimulating hormone (FSH) stimulating ovarian activity (Fig. 11.1).
- *Paracrine* – intercellular communication involves the local diffusion of regulating substances from a cell to contiguous cells, e.g. insulin-like growth factor (IGF-1) secretions by granulosa cells in the ovary (Fig. 11.1).
- *Autocrine* – intracellular communication involves the production of regulating substances by a single cell which binds to receptors on or within the same cell, e.g. oestradiol, modulating granulosa cell action (Fig. 11.1).

Hormones comprise two chemical groups – steroid hormones and trophic hormones. Steroid hormones include oestrogens, progestogens and androgens. Trophic hormones include the releasing hormones originating in the hypothalamus and a variety of hormones released by the pituitary gland and tropho-blast. The composition of these substances is summarized here.

Steroids

Steroids are a group of lipids composed of four linked carbon rings (hydrogenated cyclopentophenanthrene ring system). Steroid hormones, which are derived from cholesterol, can be classified according to the number of carbon atoms they possess: C-21 (progestogens, cortisol, aldosterone), C-19 (androgens) and C-18 (oestrogens).

Peptides

Peptides are compounds which yield two or more amino acids on hydrolysis. Linked together, they form polypeptide hormones, e.g. gonadotrophin-releasing hormone (GnRH).

Glycoproteins

Glycoproteins consist of a protein (combination of amino acids in peptide linkages) to which carbohydrate groups (CHO-1) are bound, e.g. luteinizing hormone (LH).

Hormones often circulate in extremely low concentration and, in order to respond in a specific manner, target cells require specific receptors which recognize and bind the hormone and thereby alter cell function. Hormones act at the cellular level in two ways. Steroid hormones enter the cell and mediate action via receptors within the nucleus (Beato & Klug 2000).

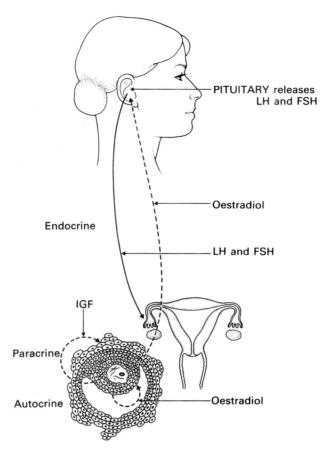

Fig. 11.1   Examples of endocrine, paracrine and autocrine hormonal communication. LH, luteinizing hormone: FSH, follicle-stimulating hormone: IGF, insulin-like growth factor.

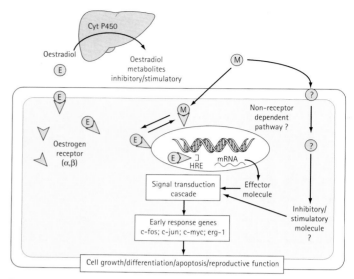

Fig. 11.2   Schematic representation of the various mechanisms via which oestrogen (oestradiol) can induce its biological effects. E, oestradiol; M, metabolite of oestradiol; Cyt P450, cytochrome P450 (drug-metabolizing enzymes); HRE, hormone response element; mRNA, messenger RNA.

By contrast, trophic hormones bind to receptors on the cell membranes which then activate 'second messengers' via coupling to G-proteins within the cell (Wheatley & Hawtin 1999). It is the affinity, specificity and concentration of receptors for a particular hormone which allow a small amount of hormone to produce a biological response.

MECHANISM OF ACTION OF STEROID HORMONES

The specificity of the tissue reaction to steroid hormones is due to the presence of specific intracellular receptor proteins for each hormone. The mechanisms, illustrated in Figure 11.2, are common to the five main classes of steroid hormone: oestrogens, progestogens, androgens, glucocorticoids and mineralocorticoids.

Circulating free (unbound) hormone passes across cell membranes by simple diffusion. However, most steroid hormone is bound with low affinity to albumin or with high affinity to a specific binding globulin: sex hormone-binding globulin (SHBG) or cortisol-binding globulin (CBG). The concentration of free (unbound) hormone in the bloodstream seems to be an important determinant of the rate of diffusion but there may be specific membrane-bound receptors which transport the hormone into the cell.

Once in the cell, the hormone dissociates from the binding globulin and is transported across the nuclear membrane. The hormone binds with its receptor, in the case of oestrogen being ERα. Receptors are complexed to chaperones, e.g. heatshock protein 90, to help other proteins to fold and prevent aggregation.

After dissociation from the chaperones, the hormone–reception complex can bind to DNA sequences in the vicinity of target genes called hormone response elements (HRE) or, in the case of oestrogen, oestrogen response elements (ERE). These hormone–receptor bound complexes activate to repress signals to the target genes' 'transcription machinery'. The mRNA is synthesized and then transported to the ribosome.

Transfer of mRNA to the cytoplasmic ribosome results in the synthesis of protein (translation). The proteins produced, e.g. enzymes, have specific intracellular effects, the endpoint of the hormone action. For example, high midcycle levels of oestradiol from the ovary lead to the increase in LH synthesis and secretion by the anterior pituitary that results in ovulation (Hillier 1994).

Regulation of steroid hormone action

Regulation of hormone action is required to enhance or reduce target tissue response and is used in clinical therapy. There are six major components.

1. Availability of hormone to cell
2. Hormone specificity of receptor
3. Availability of receptor
4. Binding of hormone-receptor complex
5. Protein synthesis
6. Agonism/antagonism

Availability of hormone to cell

Even if a cell has multiple receptors it will not be active in the absence of its specific hormone. For example, uterine epithelial cells have receptors for oestrogen, androgen, glucocorticoid and progestogen but because progesterone is not produced in the first half of the menstrual cycle, there is no progestational response.

In addition, a hormone can be present in the bloodstream but unavailable to the target cell. A hormone circulating in the bloodstream, not attached to a binding protein, readily enters cells by simple diffusion. However, most of the circulating hormone is bound to protein carriers, such as SHBG, and therefore unavailable (King 1988). Consequently, alterations in the amount of circulating binding globulins can modulate the biological activities of each of their respective hormones. For example, about 40% of circulating oestrogen is bound to SHBG and the remainder to albumin and membrane proteins (Hovarth 1992). As testosterone is largely (80%) bound to SHBG and is 19% loosely bound to albumin, its androgenicity is mainly dependent upon the unbound fraction and partly upon the fraction associated with albumin. SHBG production in the liver is decreased by androgens so the binding capacity in men is lower than in normal women. In a hirsute woman, the SHBG level is depressed by the excess androgen and the percentage of free and therefore active testosterone is elevated (Nestler et al 1991).

Hormone specificity of receptor

This is the most important factor which determines specificity of action and occurs at two levels (King 1988). Presence or absence of a given receptor determines whether a cell will respond to a given class of steroids whilst hormone specificity controls which particular compound is active. For example, the oestrogen receptor which has the greatest specificity binds oestradiol 10 times more efficiently than oestrone and about 1000 times more than the androgen, testosterone; progesterone and cortisol are not recognized at all (Garcia & Rochefort 1977). This recognition specificity is a reflection of the different affinities the receptor has for the different hormone structures (Fig. 11.3). In biological terms, this means that oestradiol is more active than oestrone whilst testosterone can have oestrogenic effects but only at pharmacological concentration (Fig. 11.4).

It is notable that the oestrogen receptor is not a single entity and also that it is not restricted to the reproductive system. There are at least two oestrogen receptors (ER), the best defined being ERα and ERβ. Binding to the receptor, ER is dependent on the molecule having an aromatic ring corresponding to the

A ring of oestrogen. The β receptor is smaller than ERα and they differ in their distribution throughout the body and their affinity for oestrogens. ERα has been identified in the central nervous system, the ovary, the breast, the liver and the uterus whilst ERβ has been identified in the central nervous system, the ovary, blood vessels, bone, lungs and urogenital tract. The binding of oestradiol or selective oestrogen receptor modulators such as raloxifene (see below) to the receptor leads to oestrogen agonism and antagonism according to which receptor the ligand has bound to (see below) (Kearney & Purdie 2000). The domain structure and structured functional relationship of the steroid hormone receptor are illustrated in Figure 11.5. The human steroid hormone receptor family and its isoforms are shown in Figure 11.6.

Androgen, glucocorticoid, progestogen and mineralocorticoid receptors are less precise in their binding requirements than the oestrogen receptor (Beato & Klug 2000). For example, many progestogens, especially the synthetic ones, bind to both progestogen and androgen receptors when present in pharmacological concentrations. This dual specificity is reflected in the biological activities of the compounds. For example, the practice of giving synthetic progestogens to pregnant women to prevent miscarriage resulted in some of their offspring having clinical features associated with androgen exposure (Aarskog 1970). The androgenic side-effects of the synthetic progestogens used in the oral contraceptive pill are another example.

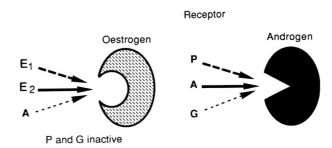

Fig. 11.3 Specificity determined by structural specificity of receptor. The oestradiol receptor has a higher affinity for oestradiol (E_2) than oestrogen (E_1); androgens (A) such as testosterone have a very low affinity while progestogens (P) and glucocorticoids (G) are inactive. The androgen receptor has less precise specificity, recognizing both P and G, albeit with less affinity than androgens.

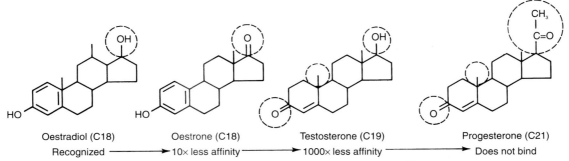

Fig. 11.4 Oestrogen receptor recognition is influenced by the differing side chains of hormones, e.g. oestrogens, testosterone and progesterone.

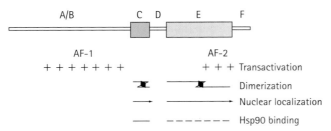

Fig. 11.5 Steroid hormone receptor (SHR) domain structure and structure–function relationships. Domains are numbered A to F, originally based on the comparison of human oestrogen and glucocorticoid receptor sequences. Domain C (dark green box) is the DNA-binding domain (DBD) and domain E (light green box) is the ligand-binding domain (LBD), AF-1 and -2 are the transcription activation functions 1 and 2. Indicated regions are required for receptor dimerization (symbolized by hooked lines), nuclear localization (arrows) and heat shock protein (Hsp) 90 binding (dashed lines).

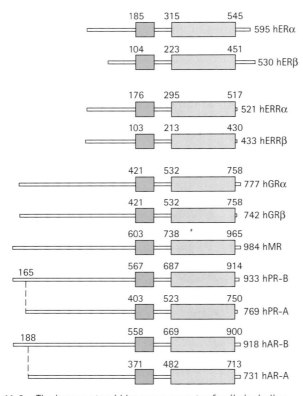

Fig. 11.6 The human steroid hormone receptor family including isoforms and variants. The numbers refer to amino acid positions. Highlighted are the DNA-binding domain (dark green box) and the ligand-binding domain (light green box). The A/B and F domains are drawn to scale. The name of each receptor is indicated: h, human; ER, oestrogen receptor; ERR, oestrogen-related receptor; GR, glucocorticoid receptor; MR, mineralocorticoid receptor; PR-A/PR-B, progesterone receptor form A and B; AR-A/AR-B, androgen receptor form A and B.

Availability of receptor

A hormone can modify its own and/or another steroid hormone's activity by regulating the concentration of receptors in a cell. This has the biological effect of increasing tissue response to the hormone if the receptor number is increased and vice versa if the receptor number is decreased. Oestrogen, for example, increases target tissue responsiveness to itself by increasing the concentration of FSH receptors in granulosa cells (Hillier 1994). This process is important in the selection and maintenance of the dominant ovarian follicle in the menstrual cycle. In order to respond to the ovulatory surge and become a 'successful' corpus luteum, the granulosa cells must acquire LH receptors. FSH induces LH receptor development on the granulosa cells of large antral follicles with oestrogen acting as chief co-ordinator.

Progesterone, on the other hand, limits the tissue response to oestrogen by reducing over time the concentration of oestrogen receptors; hence its use in the prevention of endometrial hyperplasia and carcinoma (Studd & Wadsworth 2000).

Binding of hormone–receptor complex

Biological activity is maintained only while the nuclear site is occupied with the hormone–receptor complex at the HRE, receptors for progesterone, glucocorticoids, mineralocorticoids and androgens binding to the same HREs (Beato & Klug 2000). The dissociation rate of the hormone and its receptor is therefore an important component of the biological response. Only low circulating levels of oestrogen are necessary for biological activity because of the long half-life of the oestrogen hormone–receptor complex (Sutherland et al 1988). As a consequence of lower affinity for the oestrogen receptor, the less potent oestrogens (oestrone, oestriol) also have higher rates of dissociation from the receptor and therefore the oestrogen–receptor complex occupies the nucleus for a short period of time (Katsenellenbogen 1984).

The higher rate of dissociation with a weak oestrogen can be compensated for by continuous application to allow prolonged nuclear-binding activity. Cortisol and progesterone circulate in higher concentrations because their receptor complexes have short half-lives in the nucleus. This regulatory mechanism is used clinically in the induction of ovulation with clomiphene citrate (Adashi 1996). The structural similarity between clomiphene citrate and oestrogen is sufficient to achieve uptake and binding of clomiphene citrate by oestrogen receptors. It has a very weak oestrogen effect but occupies the nuclear receptor for long periods of time – weeks rather than hours.

Protein synthesis

The limited ability of the receptors for progestogens, gluco-corticoids and mineralocorticoids to discriminate between these hormones reduces their biological specificity. However, this effect could be counteracted if a gene's response to a hormone could be determined by specificity requirements in the DNA. Multiple regulatory units are present in the DNA proximal to the site when RNA transcription is initiated and interactions between these units and hormone–receptor complexes occur (Yamamoto 1985). It is generally agreed that these interactions are involved in the regulation of protein synthesis by steroids.

Agonism/antagonism

When a compound binds to a receptor, such as the oestrogen

receptor, it may act as an agonist, for example oestrogen when it binds to the β receptor (ERβ), or as an antagonist when raloxifene binds to the α receptor in the breast. An agonist is a substance that has affinity for cell receptors of a naturally occurring substance and stimulates the same type of physiological activity, e.g. oestradiol. An antagonist tends to nullify the action of another substance, binding to its receptor without eliciting a biological response, e.g. raloxifene. Raloxifene was the first compound to be classified as a selective oestrogen receptor modulator (SERM) and other substances, older and more recently developed, have also been shown to behave as SERMs. In the case of the steroid hormones these activities do not necessarily require the compound to have the four-ring steroid structure. Binding to the receptor is dependent on having an aromatic ring equivalent to the A ring of oestrogen such as raloxifene. Other examples include diethylstilboestrol which is a non-steroidal oestrogen agonist, whilst tamoxifen is a non-steroidal oestrogen antagonist (Fig. 11.7). Cyproterone acetate and RU486 (mifepristone) are the steroidal antagonists of testosterone and progesterone respectively (Fig. 11.8). In these cases the conversion of agonists to antagonists is achieved by the addition of side chains. Each of these compounds blocks hormone action at the receptor level. Some clinical uses of steroid antagonists are listed in Table 11.1.

There are problems, however, in the clinical application of antagonists, related to the regulatory mechanisms described above. First, because of the relative lack of receptor specificity, an antagonist for one class of hormone can have antagonistic effects on another class of hormone (Wakeling 1988). For example, the progesterone antagonistic RU486 has affinity for the glucocorticoid receptor as well as the progesterone receptor and therefore is a potent antiglucorticoid. Second, hormones have central and peripheral actions, mediated by specific receptors. Therefore an antagonist may have adverse effects apart from the intended use. Cyproterone acetate, for example, an androgen antagonist, illustrates this diversity. It has effects as diverse as suppression of libido and regression of the prostate gland. In addition, it may act as agonist for other chemically related hormones. It acts as a potent progestogen having agonist effects on the progesterone receptor. Hence it is used as a contraceptive agent in combination with ethinyl oestradiol.

MECHANISM OF ACTION OF TROPHIC HORMONES

As trophic hormones cannot enter the cell, they stimulate physiological events by uniting with a receptor on the surface of the cell and activating a sequence of communications using a second messenger system within the cell. The most widely studied and best understood of these systems is adenylate cyclase/cyclic adenosine monophosphate (cAMP) (Fig. 11.10; Rodbell 1980).

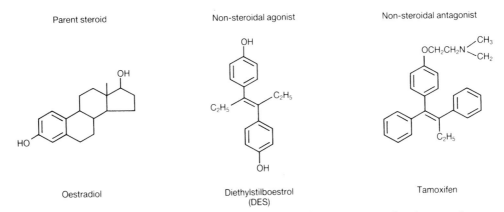

Fig. 11.7   Oestradiol with examples of non-steroidal agonist (diethylstilboestrol) and antagonist (tamoxifen).

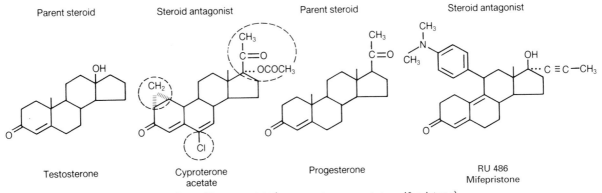

Fig. 11.8   Steroids with examples of steroid antagonists (e.g. cyproterone acetate, mifepristone).

Table 11.1 Clinical uses of steroid hormone antagonists

Drug	Clinical use
Antiprogestogens	Contraception Termination of pregnancy
Antiandrogens	Acne Benign prostatic hypertrophy Hirsutism Prostate cancer
Anti-oestrogens	Breast cancer Benign breast disease Endometriosis Uterine disease
Antiglucocorticoids	Adrenocortical carcinoma Cushing's syndrome
Antimineralocorticoids	Essential hypertension Oedema/ascites

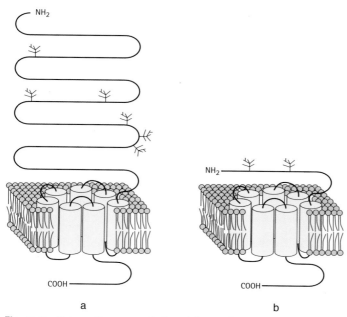

Fig. 11.9 Schematic representation of G-protein coupled receptors (GPCR) assembled in a plasma membrane. **a** A glycohormone receptor and **b** a 'classic' GPCR. In each case the seven α-helical transmembrane domains are represented as cylinders traversing the lipid bilayer. Glycosylation is indicated by the branched structures attached to the main polypeptide chain. The amino and carboxy termini are labelled.

Stage 1 Binding to the cell membrane
The hormone, sometimes called the 'first messenger', binds to a receptor on the cell surface.

Stage 2 Activation of adenyl cyclase in the cell membrane
Binding of the hormone to the receptor activates the enzyme, adenylate cyclase, within the membrane wall which catalyses the conversion of adenosine 5'-triphosphate (ATP) within the cell to cyclic AMP, the second messenger. Some hormones, such as GnRH, use other second messengers, such as calcium.

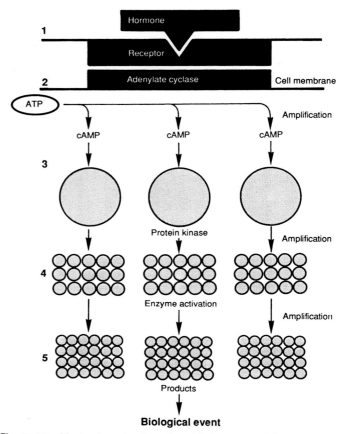

Fig. 11.10 Mechanism of action of trophic hormones. ATP, adenosine triphosphate; cAMP, cyclic adenosine monophosphate. See text for details of stages 1–5.

Stage 3 Activation of protein kinase
The cAMP is bound to a cytoplasmic receptor protein which activates a protein kinase.

Stages 4 and 5 Activation of enzymes
The protein kinase causes phosphorylation and thereby activation of specific enzymes. These enzymes catalyse specific intracellular processes which give rise to the observed physiological effect of the hormone. The cAMP system provides a method for amplification of the hormonal signal in the circulation. Each cyclase molecule produces a lot of cAMP; the protein kinases activate a large number of molecules which in turn lead to the production of an even greater number of cellular products.

Regulation of trophic hormone action

Regulation of hormone action is required for enhancing or reducing target tissue response and is used in clinical therapy. There are five major components.

1. Availability of the hormone to the cell
2. Hormone specificity of the receptor
3. Availability of the receptor (up- and downregulation)
4. Regulation of second messengers
5. Agonism/antagonism

Availability of hormone to cell

An effect can only occur if a cell carries a receptor for that hormone and the hormone is available to the cell receptor.

Hormone specificity of receptor

The specificity of a hormone's action and/or its intensity of stimulation are dependent upon the configuration of the cell membranes receptor (Wheatley & Hawtin 1999). It can be altered by changes in the structure or concentration of the receptor in the cell membrane. Similarly, changes in the molecular structure of a trophic hormone can interfere with cellular binding and therefore physiological action. Hormones that are structurally similar may have some overlap in biological activity. For example, the similarity in structure between growth hormone and prolactin means that growth hormone has a lactogenic action whilst prolactin has some growth-promoting activity and stimulates somatomedin production.

The glycoprotein hormones (LH, FSH, thyroid-stimulating hormone (TSH) and human chorionic gonadotrophin (hCG) share an identical α-chain and require another portion, the β-chain, to confer the specificity inherent in the relationship between hormones and their receptors. The β subunits differ in both amino acid and carbohydrate content and the chemical composition may be altered under certain conditions, thereby affecting the affinity of the hormone and its receptor (Willey 1999).

Availability of the receptor (up- and downregulation)

The cell's mechanism for sensing the low concentration of circulating trophic hormone is to have an extremely large number of receptors but to require only a very small percentage (as little as 1%) to be occupied by the hormone for its action to be evident (Sairam & Bhargavi 1985). Positive and negative modulation of receptor numbers by hormones is known as up- and downregulation. The mechanism of upregulation is unclear but prolactin and GnRH, for example, can increase the concentration of their own receptors in the cell membrane (Katt et al 1985).

In downregulation, an excess concentration of a trophic hormone such as LH or GnRH results in a loss of receptors on the cell membranes and therefore a decrease in biological response. This process occurs by internalization of the receptors and is the main biological mechanism by which the activity of polypeptide hormones is limited (Ron-El et al 2000). Thus the formation of the hormone–receptor complex on the cell surface initiates the cellular response and the internalization of the complex (with eventual degradation of the hormone) terminates the response. It therefore appears that the principal reason for the pulsatile secretion of trophic hormones is to avoid downregulation and to maintain adequate receptor numbers. The pulse frequency, therefore, is a key factor in regulating receptor number.

It is believed that receptors are randomly inserted into the cell membrane after intracellular synthesis. They have two important sites – an external binding site which is specific for a polypeptide hormone and an internal site which plays a role in the process of internalization (Kaplan 1981). When a hormone binds to the receptor and high concentrations of the hormone

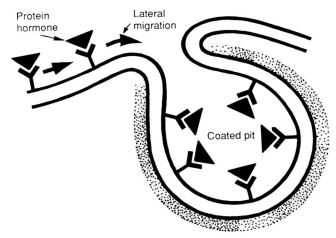

Fig. 11.11 Structure of a coated pit, illustrating lateral migration.

are present in the circulation, the hormone–receptor complex moves laterally in the cell membrane, in a process called lateral migration, to a specialized area, the coated pit, the internal margin of which has a brush border (Goldstein et al 1979). Lateral migration, which takes minutes rather than seconds, thus concentrates hormone–receptor complexes in the coated pit, a process referred to a 'clustering' (Fig. 11.11). When fully occupied, the coated pit invaginates, pinches off and enters the cell as a vesicle. The coated vesicle is delivered to the lysosomes where it undergoes degradation, releasing the hormone and receptors. The receptors may be recycled to the cell membranes and used again or the receptor and hormone may be metabolized, thus decreasing the hormone's biological activity. This process is called receptor-mediated endocytosis (Goldstein et al 1979; Fig. 11.12).

Besides downregulation of polypeptide hormone receptors, the process of internalization can be utilized for other cellular metabolic events, including the transfer into the cell of vital substances such as iron and vitamins. Hence, cell membrane receptors can be separated into two classes. The class I receptors are distributed in the cell membrane and transmit information to modify cell behaviour for these receptors. Internalization is a method for downregulation and recycling is not usually a feature. Hormones which utilize this category of receptor induce FSH, LH, hCG, GnRH, TSH and insulin (Kaplan 1981). The class II receptors are located in the coated pits. Binding leads to internalization which provides the cell with required factors or removes noxious agents from the biological fluid bathing the cell. These receptors are spared from degradation and can be recycled. Examples of this category include low-density lipoproteins which supply cholesterol to steroid-producing cells (Parinaud et al 1987) and transfer of immunoglobulins across the placenta to provide fetal immunity.

Regulation of second messengers

The second messenger system provides amplification of a small hormone signal in the bloodstream and only a small percentage of the cell membrane receptors need to be occupied in order to generate a response. The regulation of adenylate

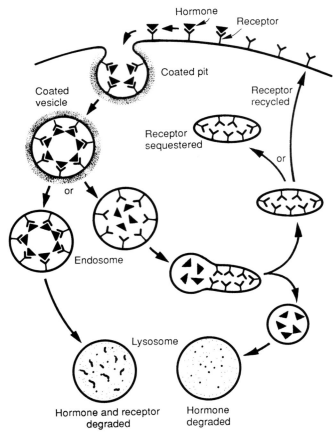

Fig. 11.12 Possible routes of receptor and hormone during receptor-mediated endocytosis.

cyclase and cyclic AMP production is important for intracellular metabolic activity (Gilman 1984). Prostaglandins, guanine nucleotides, calmodulin and calcium all appear to participate in controlling the second messenger cascade (Rasmussen 1986). The ability of the hormone–receptor complex to work through a common messenger (cAMP) and produce contrasting actions (stimulation and inhibition) is thought to be due to the presence of both stimulatory and inhibitory regulatory units (Gilman 1984, Rodbell 1980). For example, LH stimulates steroidogenesis in the corpus luteum through the coupling of stimulatory regulatory units to adenylate cyclase, stimulating the production of cAMP. Prostagladin $F2_a$ is directly luteolytic, inhibiting luteal steroidogenesis, and this action may be exerted via inhibitory units that lock the production of cAMP (Rojas & Asch 1985).

Increasing concentrations of trophic hormones, such as gonadotrophins, are directly associated with desensitization of adenylate cyclase. There are some exceptions, namely the trophic hormones, which do not utilize the adenylate cyclase mechanisms (oxytocin, insulin, growth hormone, prolactin and human placental lactogen). The message of these hormones is passed directly to nuclear and cytoplasmic metabolic sites (Rasmussen 1986). The receptors are coupled to phospho-inositidase C via G protein Gq/11, thereby increasing intracellular calcium and regulating gonadotrophin exocytosis (Wheatley & Hawtin 1999).

Agonism/antagonism

In common with the steroid hormones, these compounds can have agonist and antagonist effects, synthetic peptide agonists such as analogues to GnRH being the most commonly used for both these effects.

The potency of the analogues is up to 200 times greater than GnRH, due to an increased affinity for pituitary GnRH receptors and a prolonged association with the receptor compared to GnRH. Though the analogues act as agonists, chronic administration stops the normal pulsatile pattern of GnRH, leading to a loss of pituitary GnRH receptors and, therefore, downregulation. This has profound effects on the pituitary, leading to a fall in serum LH and FSH and consequently gonadal steroid secretion.

The mode of action of GnRH antagonists at the GnRH receptor is quite different from that of the agonists. Although the antagonists bind to the receptor, the downregulation characteristic of agonist action does not occur (Ron-El et al 2000). Rather, there is continuous occupancy of a large proportion of the receptors. There is now increasing usage of antagonists in clinical practice, predominantly in women undergoing controlled ovarian hyperstimulation for IVF or related procedures.

CLINICAL ASSAYS

This section considers assay methodology for the endocrinological investigations commonly used in gynaecological practice. An understanding of basic methodology permits the clinician to have confidence in selection of specific laboratory tests and leads to a greater understanding of the assay for better interpretation of results (Chard 1987).

An assay determines the amount of a particular constituent of a mixture. The three types of analytical procedure commonly available in clinical practice are physicochemical assays, bioassays and binding assays.

Physicochemical assays

Some aspect of the physicochemical properties of a compound is utilized for its quantification. These are the assays used to measure electrolytes.

Bioassays

Detection or quantification is dependent on the biological actions of the compound. This was the original method of hormone assay. For example, human pregnancy could be diagnosed by the injection of the maternal urine into the black African toad. If a high concentration of hCG was present in the urine, the toad would lay eggs.

Very recently, bioassays have stimulated interest in the development of very sensitive systems. For example, in the bioassay of prolactin, when neural tumour cells grown in culture are exposed to prolactin, they replicate.

Binding assays

These assays involve the combination of the compound, for example an antigen, with a binding substance, for example an antibody, which is added in a fixed amount to the solution. The distribution of the antigen between the bound and free phases

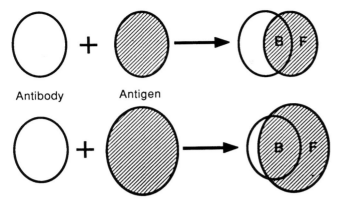

Fig. 11.13 Distribution of free (F) and bound (B) antigen in the presence of a fixed amount of antibody.

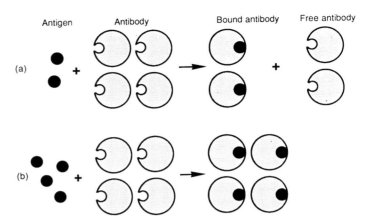

Fig. 11.14 Immunometric assay with an 'excess' of antibody. Increasing concentrations of antigen give rise to a corresponding increase in bound antibody.

is directly related to the total amount of antigen present and provides a means for quantifying the latter (Fig. 11.13). Binding assays can be further subdivided into three groups: receptor assays, competitive protein-binding assays and immunoassays.

Receptor assays

A specific site on the surface of a tissue acts as the binding agent for a particular hormone, for example oestrogen receptors in breast tissue.

Competitive protein-binding assay

A naturally occurring binding protein, for example SHBG, is used as the binder to quantify the amount of hormone present.

Immunoassays

A reaction which reaches equilibrium occurs between the hormone to be measured (antigen) and an antibody to monitor the reaction. A 'tracer' is attached to either the antigen or antibody. Non-isotopic tracers have superseded isotopic (radioactive) ones, e.g. ^{125}I, and typically are based on enzymatic action.

The basic principle of an immunometric assay and how a result is obtained is described below. The basic binding reaction can be subdivided into two categories, based on whether the antibody is present in a limited concentration or in excess.

If varying concentrations of the labelled antigen react with a constant but excess amount of antibody (Fig. 11.14) it is termed an 'immunometric assay'. This is the type of assay used when labelled antibody, rather than antigen, acts as the tracer. As the concentration of antigen increases, so does the amount of complexed labelled antibody (Fig. 11.15). Many factors can influence the construction of the standard curve; hence every time a sample analysis is performed, a standard curve is also constructed. The acceptance of the results on the patient sample is dictated by quality control specimens containing known amounts of the antigen to be measured.

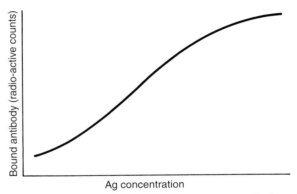

Fig. 11.15 Relationship between bound radiolabelled antibody and concentration of antigen in the immunoradiometric assay.

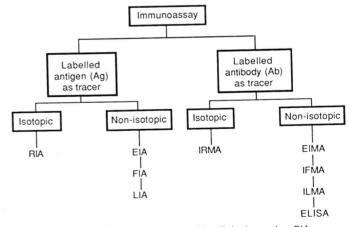

Fig. 11.16 Types of immunoassay used in clinical practice. RIA, radioimmunoassay; EIA, enzymoimmunoassay; FIA, fluoroimmunoassay; LIA, luminoimmunoassay; JRMA, immunometric assay; EMA, enzymoimmunometric assay; IFMA, ILMA, immunofluorometric assay; ELISA, enzyme-labelled immunosorbent assay.

IMMUNOASSAYS

Non-isotopic assays

The most commonly used assays use a non radio-active label (non-isotopic assays). They can also be divided on the basis of whether the tracer or label is on the antigen or the antibody, as indicated in Figure 11.16.

The second marker antibody has an enzyme, fluorescent or chemiluminescent tag. Assay systems that require separation of bound and free phases after incubation are referred to as heterogeneous and are more sensitive than those that do not require separation (homogeneous). The most commonly used assays are based on enzyme action.

Enzyme

Enzymoimmunoassay (EIA), enzymoimmunometric assay (EIMA) and enzyme-labelled immunosorbent assay (ELISA) are currently the most widely used non-isotopic labels. Small quantities of antigen can be quantified by studying enzymatic substrate conversion that leads to a colour change. The colour formation can be a simple yes/no answer (Fig. 11.17), as in a rapid pregnancy test, or the intensity of colour can be used to quantify the patient sample. The second marker antibody will not be bound, so following the wash-step will not be present to react with its substrate.

Fluorescence

Fluoroimmunoassay (FIA) and immunofluorometric assay (IFMA) use fluorescence, which is the property of certain molecules to absorb light at one wavelength and emit light at a longer wavelength. The incident light excites the molecule to a higher level of vibrational energy: as the molecule returns to the ground state it emits a photon which is the fluorescence emission.

The potential sensitivity of fluorescence is very high, but in practice it is often limited by background noise. As with EIA, FIA can be divided, according to whether a separation step is required, into heterogeneous and homogeneous assays.

Chemiluminescence

Luminoimmunoassay (LIA) and immunofluorometric assay (ILMA) use luminescence, which is a very similar phenomenon to fluorescence. Whereas the exciting energy in fluorescence is in the form of light, in luminescence it is provided by a chemical reaction. Chemiluminescent reactions produce light from simple chemical reactions, involving the action of oxygen or a peroxide on certain oxidation organic substances. Because there is high sensitivity inherent in the techniques and the instrumentation is potentially simple, the application of luminescent labels in immunoassays should increase dramatically.

Agglutination assays

Agglutination assays are another type of immunoassay, using

Porous white cellulose with coupled Ab against hCG
↓
Urine/blood containing hCG from patient
↓
2nd Ab coupled to an enzyme
↓
Cellulose solid-phase reagent washed
↓
Add enzyme substrate to generate colour on white background

Fig. 11.17 Principle of rapid pregnancy test (tube test) using non-isotopic reagents: hCG, human chorionic gonadotrophin.

---

the principle that if the antigen–antibody reaction is coupled with visible compounds, such as red blood cells (haemagglutination) or latex particles (latex particle immunoassay), the presence or absence of a specific antigen or antibody can be detected in a patient sample by the presence or absence of agglutination of the cells or particles. As these assays lack the sensitivity of those described above, they have been largely superseded but they can be used without any sophisticated instrumentation. The results are evaluated by eye, although the endpoint is subjective.

ACTION OF INDIVIDUAL HORMONES

Anterior pituitary hormones

Follicle-stimulating hormone

Because of the marked fluctuations in FSH levels in a normal ovulatory cycle, timing of the blood sample in relation to ovulation is required to interpret results (Fig. 11.18). The level can be as low as 0.5 iu/l at the luteal phase nadir and as high as 20 iu/l at the midcycle peak. However, values below

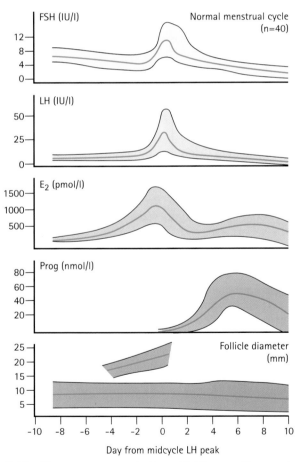

Fig. 11.18 Mean serum concentration with 95 percentiles are given for LH, FSH, oestradiol and progesterone from 8 days prior to the midcycle LH peak until 10 days thereafter. The bottom panel shows the emergence and growth of the dominant follicle in relation to the time of the midcycle LH peak. Data obtained from regularly cycling women (n = 40) (Macklon & Fauser 2000).

1 iu/l are associated with hypothalamic pituitary failure and values of 20 iu/l or above indicate ovarian failure, as in the menopause.

In addition, FSH values within the wide range of normal can be associated with absent ovarian function if the production is below the threshold of follicular development for that patient, i.e. a normal result does not guarantee a normal endocrinological pattern in an individual patient. Fluctuating FSH levels mean the investigation needs to be performed in the early follicular phase, in particular in a perimenopausal patient.

Luteinizing hormone

As for FSH, timing the sample in relation to the phase of the ovulatory cycle is vital (Fig. 11.18). For example, the ovulatory surge is taken as above 20 iu/l. However, in polycystic ovarian disease, a raised LH (13–25 iu/l) with normal FSH values is characteristic. Therefore, a raised LH in the early to midfollicular phase is of more significance than a midcycle raised LH. The LH level is within the normal range in a significant number of women with polycystic ovarian disease (PCOD) and the diagnosis requires the use of other tests. Immunologically anomalous forms of LH (v-LH) due to two point LHβ gene have been described and their role is currently under investigation (Lamminen & Huhtaniemi 2001). This is also the case with other glycoproteins.

As the prospective timing of ovulation using the LH peak presents the difficulty that the peak cannot be identified until the next value significantly lower than the peak is observed, clinical action is taken on the basis of the first definite rise in LH values (LH surge) rather than on the peak, which usually occurs a day later. This measurement is typically performed on urine rather than blood samples.

Prolactin

Prolactin levels are influenced by the time of day when blood is collected and are increased by stress (including venepuncture). Transient rises can occur at ovulation. Therefore a small elevation above the normal range can occur in normal women. Such a rise should be judged in the clinical setting. If a woman has a normal menstrual cycle, the result is unlikely to be significant. However, if she is amenorrhoeic she should be investigated further.

Growth hormone

Growth hormone is secreted in short bursts, most of which occur in the first part of the night. These bursts are more frequent in children, so the results vary depending upon timing and age. Secretion is also stimulated by stress and hypoglycaemia and is inhibited by glucose and corticosteroids.

Thyrotrophin-stimulating hormone

Normal levels of TSH range from 0.4 to 5 mmol/l. The measurement of tetra-iodothyronine (T4) and TSH provides the most accurate assessment of thyroid functions. When using thyroid hormone replacement therapy, both TSH and T4 should be measured because TSH alone cannot detect overdosage.

Thyroid hormones

Deficiency of thyroid hormones tri-iodothyronine (T3) and T4 leads to anovulation associated with increased gonadotrophin levels. Therefore, it is important to assess thyroid function prior to diagnosing premature ovarian failure.

Normal levels are as follows: free T4, 10–25 pmol/l; T3, 1.1–2.3 nmol/l (non-pregnant, no OCP), 1.4–4.3 nmol/l (pregnant/OCP) (OCP = oral contraceptive pill).

Circulating thyroid hormone is tightly bound to a group of proteins, chiefly thyroxine globulin. Oestrogen produces a rise in thyroxine-binding capacity and, therefore, thyroid function tests are affected by pregnancy and oestrogen-containing medications such as the contraceptive pill. Consequently, a raised thyroxine level does not mean that the free thyroxine concentration (the unbound and metabolically active hormone) is above the normal range.

Because of the peripheral source of T3, its levels are not a direct reflection of thyroid secretion. In addition, T3 levels may be normal despite the presence of goitre with elevated TSH and depressed T4 concentrations, as T4 plays the instrumental role in TSH regulation. Therefore, measurement of free T4 and SH provides the most accurate assessment of thyroid function. RIA of T3 is important for the occasional case of hyperthyroidism due to excessive production of T3 with normal T4 levels (T3 toxicosis). Drugs taken orally for cholecystograms inhibit the peripheral conversion of T4 to T3 and can disrupt normal thyroid levels (giving elevated T4) for up to 30 days after administration.

Adrenal hormones

The adrenal cortex comprises three morphologically and functionally distinct regions. The outermost region (zona glomerulosa) secrets aldosterone. The zona fasciculata is the intermediate region and produces cortisol, which will be dealt with here. The zona reticularis encircles the medulla and synthesizes oestrogens and androgens.

Cortisol

Normal levels of cortisol in adults at 09.00 hours range from 300 to 700 nmol/l.

If a 24-hour urine collection is used, it is necessary to ensure that a complete collection has been obtained. The measurement of creatinine excretion will identify whether a collection is incomplete. As blood levels of cortisol vary greatly throughout a 24-hour period, sample timing is important. Blood levels are highest in the morning and lowest in the evening. Most laboratories' normal values are based on sampling at 09.00 hours.

Ovarian hormones

Oestradiol

Serum levels of oestradiol in spontaneous ovulation in relation to changes in FSH, LH and progesterone and the size of the dominant follicle are shown in Figure 11.18 (Macklon & Fauser 2000). There is a variation in oestradiol levels throughout the menstrual cycle so results need to be interpreted in relation to the timing of the sample in the cycle. Serum oestradiol levels in pregnancy range from 2–10 nmol/l in the first trimester to 20–80 nmol/l in the third trimester. The major oestrogen in pregnancy is oestriol.

Progesterone

Variations throughout the menstrual cycle can lead to difficulties in interpretation if the result is taken at an unidentified time in the cycle, particularly if a single progesterone level is taken as a marker of ovulation (Fig. 11.18). Normally results taken 5–8 days prior to the next menstruation are suitable for the detection of ovulation, so the patient should be asked to keep a record of the timing of the blood sample and her next menstrual period. A result >30 nmol/l indicated ovulation, even if timing is not known.

Levels in the mother during pregnancy increase in parallel with the growth of the placenta, being 30–45, 70–150 and 150–600 nmol/l in the first, second and third trimesters respectively. Maternal progesterone levels are related to the weight of the fetus and placenta at term.

Inhibin

In the female, inhibin is synthesized predominantly by ovarian granulosa cells. Inhibin levels increase in the late follicular phase, acting synergistically with oestradiol to inhibit FSH synthesis and release, though this is predominantly over-ridden by the preovulatory LH and FSH surge (Bevan & Scanlan 1998). Inhibin A and B are dimeric proteins capable of suppressing FSH, inhibin B being the principal form produced by the Sertoli cells in the testis which inhibits pituitary FSH secretion. Activin A and B and AB are dimeric proteins which share β subunits with inhibin but stimulate FSH (Groome et al 2001).

Testosterone

Testosterone levels are lower in females than in males (females 0.5–3.0 nmol/l, males 9–35 nmol/l). The reverse is the case for SHBG (females 39–103 nmol/l, males 17–50 nmol/l). Testosterone arises from a variety of sources in the female. Approximately 50% is derived from peripheral conversion of androstenedione (secreted by the adrenal cortex), while the adrenal gland and ovary contribute approximately equal amounts (25%) to the circulating levels of testosterone, except at midcycle when the ovarian contribution increases by 10–15%. About 80% of circulating testosterone is bound to SHBG.

Placenta

Human chorionic gonadotrophin (hCG)

This is secreted by the blastocyst and appears in maternal blood shortly after implantation and then rises rapidly until 8 weeks' gestation. Levels show little change at 8–12 weeks, then decline to 18 weeks and remain fairly constant until term. There is some short-term variation in blood hCG levels but no circadian rhythm. At term, the levels in the female fetus are substantially higher than those in the male (Obiekwe &

Chard 1983). The mechanisms which determine the levels of hCG in maternal blood are unknown.

A patient can continue to have a positive pregnancy test for at least a week after a miscarriage or therapeutic abortion due to the prolonged half-life of hCG; hCG may be detected up to 20 weeks later if sensitive assays are used.

The range of serum hCG levels in ectopic pregnancy is very wide (Grudzinskas & O'Brien 1997) so that a negative result does not rule out an ectopic pregnancy or distinguish it from a missed miscarriage. Quantification of hCG is used to monitor postoperative progress in trophoblastic and medical management of miscarriage and ectopic pregnancy. Measurement of free β hCG and its subunits is used for maternal serum screening for Down's syndrome in the first and second trimesters (Grudzinskas & Ward 1997).

Pregnancy-associated plasma protein A (PAPP-A)

This large glycoprotein can be detected in the maternal blood at 6–8 weeks gestation, concentrations rising steadily throughout the pregnancy. The mechanisms which regulate the synthesis of PAPP-A are not as yet determined but depressed levels of PAPP-A are seen in association with some fetal chromosomal abnormalities (trisomy 21, trisomy 18 and trisomy 13, Cornelia de Lange syndrome) and ectopic pregnancy (El-Farra & Grudzinskas 1995).

Maternal serum screening in the first trimester of pregnancy (10–13 weeks) in conjunction with the ultrasound assessment of nuchal translucency, together with maternal age, will detect up to 85% of pregnancies affected by Down's syndrome and some other aneuploidies (Grudzinskas & Ward 1997, Wald & Hackshaw 2000).

Fetus

α-Fetoprotein (AFP)

AFP is synthesized by the yolk sac, fetal liver and gastrointestinal tract. Its function is unknown. It is used as a marker in clinical practice for the identification of congenital abnormalities.

Neural tube defects are associated with raised midtrimester levels of AFP while Down's syndrome is associated with reduced midtrimester AFP levels.

The value of AFP varies with gestation and number of fetuses present. The concentration of AFP in fetal serum rises rapidly to reach a peak at 12–14 weeks' gestation, at which time the levels are 2–3 g/l. Thereafter it falls until term with a sharp drop at 32–34 weeks. In the mother, circulating AFP levels rise progressively to reach a peak at 32 weeks, then decrease towards term.

The interpretation of normality of levels depends upon gestation. Therefore incorrect assessment of gestation could lead to an erroneous conclusion on the normality of the fetus. Levels are also raised in obstetric problems (threatened miscarriage, intrauterine growth restriction, perinatal death and antepartum haemorrhage) and some congenital abnormalities (exomphalos, nephrosis, Turner's syndrome, trisomy 13), but depressed in trisomy 21 (Grudzinskas & Ward 1997).

KEY POINTS

1. Steroids exert their action through intracellular receptors whereas trophic hormones act through receptors located on the cell membrane, then through a second messenger system within the cell.

2. Androgen, progesterone and glucocorticoid receptors are less precise than oestrogen receptors in their binding affinity.

3. Synthetic progestogens can bind to both androgen and progesterone receptors, reflecting the dual biological activities of progestogens.

4. Hormone potency is directly related to the length of time the hormone–receptor complex occupies the nucleus.

5. Due to structural similarities with oestrogen, clomiphene citrate binds to oestrogen receptors and occupies the nucleus for long periods.

6. Agonists are substances that occupy cell receptors and stimulate natural physiological activities.

7. Antagonists are substances that can occupy receptors without being internalized, hence blocking the cell function.

8. An antagonist may block different classes of hormones due to the lack of receptor specificity.

9. Selective oestrogen receptor modulators (SERMS) are structurally diverse non-steroidal molecules that bind to oestrogen receptors and produce agonist effects in some tissues and antagonist effects in others.

10. Due to amplification of hormone signals by the second messenger system, only 1% of the cell receptors need to be occupied by the hormone for its action to be evident.

11. Downregulation by internalization of hormone receptors is a unique mechanism for limiting polypeptide hormone activity.

12. Endocrine investigations of ovarian function should be timed early in the follicular phase to guard against false results.

13. The use of TSH estimation only cannot detect overdosage and T4 should also be measured in women receiving thyroxine replacement therapy.

14. T3 measurement is necessary only in patients suspected to be thyrotoxic yet with normal T4 values.

15. Due to its long half-life, hCG can be detected in blood or urine for a few weeks after a miscarriage using a sensitive assay method.

16. Oestrogen increases target tissue responsiveness to itself by increasing FSH receptors in granulosa cells whereas progesterone limits the tissue response to oestrogen by reducing the concentration of oestrogen receptors.

REFERENCES

Aarskog D 1970 Maternal progestin as a possible cause of hypospadias. New England Journal of Medicine 300:75

Adashi FY 1996 Ovulation induction: clomiphene citrate. In: Adashi EY, Rock JA, Rozenwaks Z (eds) Reproductive endocrinology, surgery and technology. JB Lippincott, Philadelphia

Beato M, Klug J 2000 Steroid hormone receptors: an update. Human Reproduction 6:225–236

Bevan JS, Scanlan MF 1998 Regulation of the hypothalamus and pituitary. In: Grossman A (ed) Clinical endocrinology. Blackwell Science, Oxford

Chard T 1987 An introduction to radioimmunoassay and related techniques. Elsevier, Amsterdam

El-Farra K, Grudzinskas JG 1995 Will PAPP-A be a biochemical marker for screening of Down's syndrome in the first trimester? Early Pregnancy 1:4–12

Garcia M, Rochefort H 1977 Androgens on the oestrogen receptor. II. Correlation between nuclear translocation and uterine protein synthesis. Steroids 29:11

Gilman AG 1984 Guanine nucleotide-binding regulatory proteins and dual control of adenylate cyclase. Journal of Clinical Investigation 73:1

Goldstein JL, Anderson RGW, Brown MS 1979 Coated pits, coated vesicles, and recepto-mediated endocytosis. Nature 279:679

Groome NP, Tsigou A, Cranfield M, Knight PG, Robertson DM 2001 Enzyme immunoassays for inhibin, activen and follistatin. Molecular and Cellular Endocrinology 180:73–77

Grudzinskas JG, O'Brien PMS 1997 Recommendations arising from the 33rd RCOG Study Group: Problems in Early Pregnancy. In: Grudzinskas, JG, O'Brien PMS (eds) Problems in early pregnancy: advances in diagnosis and treatment. RCOG Press, London

Grudzinskas JG, Ward RHT 1977 Screening for Down's syndrome in the first trimester. RCOG Press, London

Hillier SG 1994 Current concepts in the roles of follicle stimulating hormones and luteinising hormone in folliculogenesis. Human Reproduction 9:188–191

Hovarth PM 1992 Sex steroids: physiology and metabolism. In: Swarz DP (ed) Hormone replacement therapy. Williams and Wilkins, Baltimore

Kaplan J 1981 Polypeptide-binding membrane receptors: analysis and classification. Science 212:14

Katt JA, Duncan JA, Herbon L et al 1985 The frequency of gonadotrophin-releasing hormone stimulation determines the number of pituitary gonadotrophin-releasing hormone receptors. Endocrinology 116:2113

Katzenellenbogen GS 1984 Biology and receptor interactions of estriol and estriol derivatives in vitro and in vivo. Journal of Steroid Biochemistry 20:1033

Kearney CE, Purdie DW 2000 Selective oestrogen receptor modulators (SERMs). Obstetrician and Gynaecologist 2:6–10

King RJB 1988 An overview of molecular aspects of steroid hormone action. In: Cooke BA, King RB, van der Molen JGJ (eds) Hormones and their actions. Elsevier Science, Amsterdam

Lamminen T, Hutaniemi 2001 A common genetic variant of luteinising hormone: relation to normal and aberrant pituitary-gonadal function. European Journal of Pharmacology 414:1–7

Macklon NS, Fauser BCJM 2000 Regulation of follicle development and novel approaches to ovarian stimulation for IVF. Human Reproduction 6:307–312

Nestler JE, Powers LP, Matt DW 1991 A direct effect of hyperinsulinaemia on serum SHBG in obese women with PCOS. Journal of Clinical Endocrinology and Metabolism 72:83–89

Obiekwe BC, Chard T 1983 Placental proteins in late pregnancy: relation to fetal sex. Journal of Obstetrics and Gynaecology 3:163

Parinaud J, Perret B, Ribbes H et al 1987 High density lipoprotein and low density lipoprotein utilization by human granulosa cells for progesterone synthesis in serum-free culture: respective contributions of free and esterified cholesterol. Journal of Clinical Endocrinology and Metabolism 64:409

Rasmussen H 1986 The calcium messenger system. New England Journal of Medicine 314:1094

Rodbell M 1980 The role of hormone receptors and GTP-regulatory protein in membrane transduction. Nature 284:17

Rojas RJ, Asch RH 1985 Effects of luteinizing hormone-releasing hormone agonist and calcium upon adenyl cyclase activity of human corpus luteum membranes. Life Sciences 36:841

Ron-EL R, Raziel A, Schachter M et al 2000 Induction and ovulation with an RH antagonist. Human Reproduction 6:318–321

Sairam MR, Bhargavi GN 1985 A role for glycosylation of the alpha subunit in transduction of biological signal in glycoprotein hormone. Science 229:65

Studd J, Wadsworth F 2000 Hormone replacement therapy. In: O'Brien PMS (ed) The yearbook of obstetrics and gynaecology. RCOG Press, London

Sutherland RL, Watt CKW, Clarke CL 1988 Oestrogen actions. In: Cooke BA, King RJB, van der Molen HJ (eds) Hormones and their actions. Elsevier Science, Amsterdam

Wakeling AE 1988 Physiological aspects of luteinizing hormone releasing factor and sex steroid actions: the interrelationship of agonists and antagonist activities. In: Cooke BA, King RJB, van der Molen HJ (eds) Hormones and their actions. Elsevier Science, Amsterdam

Wald NJ, Hackshaw AK 2000 Advances in antenatal screening for Down's syndrome. Baillière's Clinical Obstetrics and Gynaecology 14:565–580

Wheatley M, Hawtin SR 1999 Glycosylation of G-protein-coupled receptors or hormones central to normal reproductive functioning: its occurrence and role. Human Reproduction 4:356–364

Willey KP 1999 An elusive role for glycosylation in the structure and function of reproductive hormones. Human Reproduction 5:330–355

Yamamoto KR 1985 Steroid receptor regulated transcription of specific genes and gene networks. Annual Review of Genetics 19:209

12

Biosynthesis of steroid hormones

Anthony E. Michael   D. Robert E. Abayasekara

INTRODUCTION

Steroid hormones are lipid molecules synthesized within the ovary, testis, placenta and adrenal cortex. Striking parallels exist in the organization of the biosynthetic pathways and in the hormonal control of steroid production in each of these four steroidogenic tissues. In this chapter, we outline the general principles of steroid hormone formation as regulated by trophic hormones, before considering detailed aspects of ovarian and adrenal biochemistry in health and disease. The chapter opens with a consideration of the general structures of steroid hormones since relatively minor differences in steroid structures have a profound impact on the biological and clinical actions of each steroid hormone.

PHYSIOLOGY

The classification of steroid hormones

Steroid hormones are all derived from the 27 carbon substrate cholesterol and so share the same cyclohexaphenanthrene ring structure (Figs. 12.1, 12.2). Steroid hormones are classified into five families dependent upon the number of carbon (C)

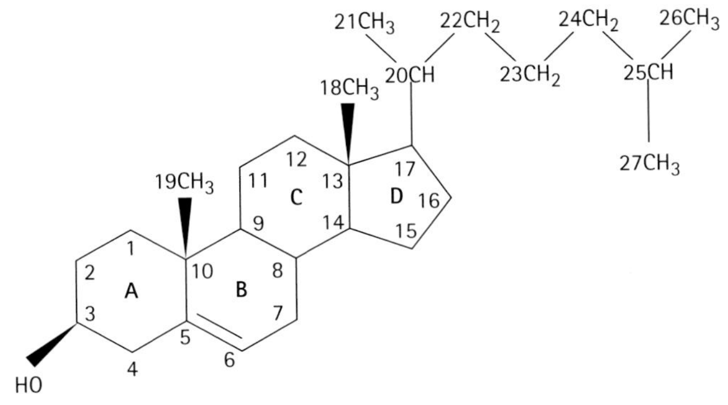

Fig. 12.1   The cyclohexphenanthrene ring structure of cholesterol – the steroidogenic substrate.

atoms and the chemical groups present at key carbon residues (Table 12.1). All steroid hormones with 21 carbon atoms are collectively termed pregnenes. This category of steroid hormones can be subdivided into three steroid families: the progestins (e.g. progesterone), glucocorticoids (e.g. cortisol) and mineralocorticoids (e.g. aldosterone). While the progestins are secreted predominantly from the ovary, the glucocorticoids and mineralocorticoids are collectively termed corticosteroids, reflecting their origin in the cortex of the adrenal gland. The major structural difference between the three pregnene families is that while progestins possess a methyl group (CH_3) at position C21, both glucocorticoids and mineralocorticoids possess a hydroxyl group (CH_2OH) at the same position (see Table 12.1 and Fig. 12.2).

Progestins can be metabolized to generate 19 carbon steroids, termed androgens (dehydroepiandrosterone, androstenedione and testosterone), which are secreted from both the testis and the adrenal cortex. Within the ovary, androgens are usually metabolized to generate the oestrogens (e.g. oestradiol-17β) with their characteristic 18 carbon structure (see Table 12.1 and Fig. 12.2).

Within this classification scheme, there is a distinction to be made between Δ^5 and Δ^4 steroid hormones. Progestins and androgens of the Δ^5 series are characterized by possessing a hydroxyl group at position C3 and a C=C double bond between positions C5 and C6 in the steroid B-ring, as in cholesterol (Fig. 12.1). In contrast, progestins and androgens of the Δ^4 series possess a ketone (C=O) at position C3 and have a C=C double bond which lies between positions C4 and C5 in the A-ring of the steroid molecule (Fig. 12.2). While this difference may seem a trivial biochemical detail, nothing could be further from the truth. The nature of the chemical group at position C3, together with the position of the C=C double bond, profoundly alters the conformation of the steroid molecule and, in so doing, influences the ability of a steroid hormone to activate intracellular receptors. Hence, Δ^5 steroids, such as pregnenolone and dehydroepiandrosterone (DHEA), have low affinities for steroid receptors and so exert limited biological actions. In contrast, the Δ^4 steroid hormones, such as

167

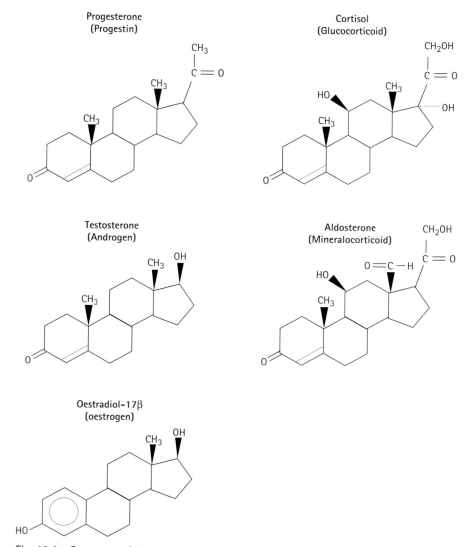

Fig. 12.2   Structures of the major physiological steroid in each steroid family.

Table 12.1   Definitive structural features of the five major families of steroid hormones

		Steroid family				
		Progestins	Glucocorticoids	Mineralocorticoids	Androgens	Oestrogens
No. of carbon atoms		21	21	21	19	18
Chemical group present at position:	C21	CH_3	CH_2OH	CH_2OH	Absent	Absent
	C18	CH_3	CH_3	H–C=O (aldehyde)	CH_3	CH_3
	C17	D-ring side chain	D-ring side chain	D-ring side chain	17β-hydroxyl or ketone	17β-hydroxyl or ketone
	C11	Nil	11β-hydroxyl	11β-hydroxyl		
	C3	Ketone or 3β-hydroxyl	Ketone	Ketone	Ketone or 3β-hydroxyl	Planar hydroxyl group attached to aromatic A-ring

Essentially there are three potential causes of ovarian hyperandrogenism:

- a disturbance in the LH:FSH ratio
- stimulation of ovarian androgen synthesis by an agent other than a gonadotrophin
- decreased aromatase activity.

In accordance with the two cell–two gonadotrophin model of oestradiol biosynthesis, alterations to the LH:FSH ratio, as reported in patients with PCOS and in menopausal women, can cause an imbalance between LH-stimulated androgen synthesis in the theca cells and the FSH-dependent aromatization of androstenedione in the granulosa cells. When LH is inappropriately elevated and/or FSH is suppressed, the synthesis of androstenedione in the theca can exceed the capacity of aromatase to metabolize the thecal androgen substrate, such that there is net secretion of androgen from the ovary into the general circulation.

As noted earlier in this chapter, insulin and IGFs can also stimulate thecal androgen production, significantly enhancing the steroidogenic response of theca cells to LH (Nahum et al 1995). By definition, PCOS is characterized by elevated plasma concentrations of insulin (hyperinsulinaemia) accompanied by clinical signs of hyperandrogenism (see Ch. 19). A number of studies have indicated that the hyperinsulinaemia reported in women with PCOS reflects resistance to the cellular actions of insulin in peripheral tissues (muscle and adipose tissue) (Dunaif et al 1989). However, recent studies have revealed that the ability of insulin to act on ovarian cells is uncompromised in PCOS patients (Willis et al 1996). Hence, in this syndrome, the elevated concentrations of insulin may act in concert with LH to hyperstimulate ovarian androgen production.

A final mechanism for disturbing the delicate biochemical balance between the theca and granulosa cell compartments of the ovarian follicle is to decrease the capacity of the granulosa cells to metabolize thecal androstenedione substrate. The simplest mechanism to explain such a distortion in the steroidogenic pathway would be a complete loss-of-function mutation in the CYP19 gene that encodes aromatase. Due to the requirements for oestradiol and oestriol in pregnancy, fetuses affected by complete loss of function in P450$_{AROM}$ are usually miscarried. However, a few patients with severely limited aromatase activity have been reported. In such patients, failure of the granulosa cells to metabolize any androgen precursor results in profound ovarian hyperandrogenism with progressive clitoromegaly and accelerated linear growth (Morishima et al 1995). Interestingly, affected girls do not show the usual cessation of linear growth at puberty, despite having plasma testosterone concentrations far in excess of the reference range for normal adolescent boys. These patients have revealed the crucial role for the aromatase enzyme in the fusion of the epiphyses in the long bones. It would appear that in both sexes, closure of the epiphyseal plates requires testosterone to be metabolized within the bone to oestradiol since women with negligible aromatase activity require administration of exogenous oestrogen to halt their linear growth (MacGillivray et al 1998, Simpson 2000).

Although mutations in P450$_{AROM}$ are rare, there are other disease states in which the capacity of granulosa cells to aromatize androgens is limited to the extent that ovarian hyperandrogenism ensues. For example, loss-of-function mutations in the FSH receptor, which have been associated with hypergonadotrophic ovarian dysgenesis, can prevent FSH from upregulating aromatase expression in the granulosa cells despite a normal plasma LH:FSH ratio (Chan 1998, Tapanainen et al 1998). Alternatively, glucocorticoids can inhibit the expression and activity of P450$_{AROM}$ in cultured granulosa cells (Ben-Rafael et al 1988, Fitzpatrick & Richard 1991, Hsueh & Erickson 1978): an observation that explains, in part, the association between adrenal hyperactivity and dysregulation of ovarian steroid synthesis in conditions such as anorexia nervosa and other chronic stress syndromes.

KEY POINTS

1. Steroid hormones are all synthesized from cholesterol, derived predominantly from plasma lipoproteins.
2. Steroid hormones can all be classified into just five families, the names of which reflect their biological functions.
3. The biosynthesis of steroid hormones involves just two families of steroidogenic enzymes: cytochrome P450 enzymes and hydroxysteroid dehydrogenase (HSD) enzymes.
4. Steroid synthesis is controlled by trophic hormones which increase the expression and activities of steroidogenic enzymes.
5. The endocrine actions of the gonadotrophins and of ACTH are moderated by paracrine agents arising within the ovary and adrenal cortex, respectively.
6. In addition to compromising fertility, defects in the synthesis of ovarian and adrenal steroid hormones can dramatically alter the development of the external genitalia and the secondary sexual characteristics of a patient.

REFERENCES

Abayasekara DRE, Michael AE, Webley GE, Flint APF 1993 Mode of action of prostaglandin F2α in human luteinized granulosa cells: role of protein kinase C. Molecular and Cellular Endocrinology 97:81–91

Auletta FJ, Flint APF 1988 Mechanisms controlling corpus luteum function in sheep, cows, non-human primates and women especially in relation to the time of luteolysis. Endocrine Reviews 9:88–105

Balasubramanian K, Lavoie HA, Garmey JC, Stocco DM 1997 Regulation of porcine granulosa cell steroidogenic acute regulatory protein (StAR) by insulin-like growth factor I: synergism with follicle-stimulating hormone or protein kinase A agonist. Endocrinology 138:433–439

Begeot M, Shetty U, Kilgore M, Waterman MR, Simpson ER 1993 Regulation of expression of the CYP11A (P450scc) gene in bovine ovarian luteal cells by forskolin and phorbol esters. Journal of Biological Chemistry 268:17317–17325

Ben-Rafael Z, Benadiva CA, Garcia CJ, Flickinger GL 1988 Cortisol stimulation of estradiol and progesterone secretion by human granulosa cells is independent of follicle-stimulating hormone effects. Fertility and Sterility 9:813–816

Benyo DF, Zelezink AJ 1997 Cyclic adenosine monophosphate signalling in the primate corpus luteum: maintenance of protein kinase A activity throughout the luteal phase of the menstrual cycle. Endocrinology 138:3452–3458

Bergh C, Carlsson B, Olsson JH, Selleskog U, Hillensjo T 1993 Regulation of androgen production in cultured human thecal cells by insulin-like growth factor I and insulin. Fertility and Sterility 59:323–331

Bramley TA, Stirling D, Swanston IA, Menzies GS, McNeilly AS, Baird DT 1987 Specific binding sites for gonadotropin-releasing hormone, LH/chrionic gonadotropin, low density lipoprotein, prolactin and FSH in homogenates of the human corpus luteum II. Concentrations throughout the luteal phase of the menstrual cycle and early pregnancy. Journal of Endocrinology 113:317–327

Casper RC, Chatterton Jr RT, Davis JM 1979 Alterations in serum cortisol and its binding characteristics in anorexia nervosa. Journal of Clinical Endocrinology and Metabolism 49:406–411

Chan WY 1998 Molecular, genetic, biochemical, and clinical implications of gonadotrophin receptor mutations. Molecular Genetics and Metabolism 63:75–84

Chryssikopoulos A 1997 The relationship between the immune and endocrine systems. Annals of the New York Academy of Sciences 816:83–93

Clark BJ, Ranganathan V, Combs R 2001 Steroidogenic acute regulatory protein expression is dependent upon post-translational effects of cAMP-dependent protein kinase A. Molecular and Cellular Endocrinology 173:183–192

Cooke BA 1999 Signal transduction involving cyclic AMP-dependent and cyclic AMP-independent mechanisms in the control of steroidogenesis. Molecular and Cellular Endocrinology 151:25–35

Culty M, Li H, Boujrad N et al 1999 In vitro studies on the role of the peripheral-type benzodiazepine receptor in steroidogenesis. Journal of Steroid Biochemistry and Molecular Biology 69:123–130

Curnow KM, Tusie-Luna M-T, Pascoe L et al 1991 The product of the CYP11B2 gene is required for aldosterone biosynthesis in the human adrenal cortex. Molecular Endocrinology 5:1513–1522

De Kretser DM, Robertson DM 1989 The isolation and physiology of inhibin and related proteins. Biology of Reproduction 40:33–47

Dennefors BL, Sjörgen A, Hamberger L 1982 Progesterone and adenosine 3′,5′-monophosphate formation by isolated human corpora lutea of different ages: influences of human chorionic gonadotropin and prostaglandins. Journal of Clinical Endocrinology and Metabolism 55:102–107

Dunaif A, Segal KR, Futterweit W, Dobrjansky A 1989 Profound peripheral insulin resistance, independent of obesity, in polycystic ovary syndrome. Diabetes 38:1165–1174

Endoh A, Kristiansen SB, Casson PR, Buster JE, Hornsby PJ 1996 The zona reticularis is the site of dehydroepiandrosterone and dehydroepiandrosterone sulfate in the adult human adrenal cortex resulting from its low expression of 3β-hydroxysteroid dehydrogenase. Journal of Clinical Endocrinology and Metabolism 81:3558–3565

Farookhi R, Desjardins J 1986 Luteinizing hormone receptor induction in dispersed granulosa cells requires estrogen. Molecular and Cellular Endocrinology 47:13–24

Felderbaum RE, Ludwig M, Diedrich K 2000 Clinical application of GnRH-antagonists. Molecular and Cellular Endocrinology 166:9–14

Filicori M, Butler JP, Crowley Jr WF 1984 Neuroendocrine regulation of the corpus luteum in the human. Journal of Clinical Investigations 73:1638–1647

Findlay JK, Clarke IJ, Luck MR et al 1991 Peripheral and intragonadal actions of inhibin-related peptides. Journal of Reproduction and Fertility 43 (suppl):139–150

Fisch B, Margara RA, Winston RML, Hillier SG 1989 Cellular basis of luteal steroidogenesis in the human ovary. Journal of Endocrinology 122:303–311

Fitzpatrick SL, Richards JS 1991 Regulation of cytochrome P450 aromatase messenger ribonucleic acid and activity by steroids and gonadotropins in rat granulosa cells. Endocrinology 129:1452–1462

Flint APF, Hearn JP, Michael AE 1990 The maternal recognition of pregnancy in mammals. Journal of Zoology (London) 221:327–341

Franks S (1998) Growth hormone and ovarian function. Baillière's Clinics in Endocrinology and Metabolism 12:331–340

Franks S, Mason H, Willis D (2000) Follicular dynamics in the polycystic ovary syndrome. Molecular and Cellular Endocrinology 163:49–52

Geva E, Jaffe RB 2000 Role of vascular endothelial growth factor in ovarian physiology and pathology. Fertility and Sterility 74:429–438

Giudice LC, van Dessel HJ, Cataldo NA, Chandrasekher YA, Yap O, Fauser BC 1995 Circulating and ovarian IGF binding proteins: potential role in normo-ovulatory cycles and in polycystic ovarian syndrome. Progress in Growth Factor Research 6:397–408

Golos TG, August AM, Strauss III JF 1986 Expression of low density lipoprotein receptor in cultured human granuloca cells: regulation by human chorionic gonadotropin, cyclic AMP and sterol. Journal of Lipid Research 27:1089–1096

Gwynne GT, Strauss III 1982 The role of lipoproteins in steroidogenesis and cholesterol metabolism in steroidogenic glands. Endocrine Reviews 3:299–329

Hearn JP, Webley GE, Gidley-Baird AA 1991 Chorionic gonadotrophin and embryo-maternal recognition during the peri-implantation period in primates. Journal of Reproduction and Fertility 92:497–509

Hillier SG 1991 Regulatory functions for inhibin and activin in human ovaries. Journal of Endocrinology 131:171–175

Hillier SG, Miro F 1993 Inhibin, activin and follistatin. Potential roles in ovarian physiology. Annals of the New York Academy of Sciences 687:29–38

Hillier SG, Whitelaw PF, Smyth CD 1994 Follicular oestrogen synthesis: the 'two-cell, two-gonadotrophin' model revisited. Molecular and Cellular Endocrinology 100:51–54

Hsueh AJW, Erickson GF 1978 Glucocorticoid inhibition of FSH-induced estrogen production in cultured rat granulosa cells. Steroids 32:639–648

Hsueh AJW, Dahl KD, Vaughan J et al 1987 Heterodimers and homodimers of inhibin subunits have different paracrine action in the modulation of luteinizing hormone-stimulated androgen biosynthesis. Proceedings of the National Academy of Sciences USA 84:5082–5086

Hurwitz A, Payne DW, Packman JN et al 1991 Cytokine-mediated regulation of ovarian function: interleukin-1 inhibits gonadotropin-induced androgen biosynthesis. Endocrinology 129:1250–1256

Jia X-C, Oikawa M, Bo M et al 1991 Expression of human luteinizing hormone (LH) receptor: interaction with LH and chorionic gonadotropin from human but not equine, rat and ovine species. Molecular Endocrinology 5:759–768

Kessel B, Liu YX, Jia XC, Hsueh AJW 1985 Autocrine role for estrogens in the augmentation of luteinizing hormone receptor formation in cultured rat granulosa cells. Biology of Reproduction 32:1038–1050

Knecht M, Tsai-Morris C-H, Catt KJ 1985 Estrogen dependence of luteinizing hormone receptors expression in cultured rat granulosa cells. Inhibition of granulosa cell development by the antiestrogens tamoxifen and keoxifene. Endocrinology 116:1771–1777

Knobil E 1980 The neuroendocrine control of the menstrual cycle. Recent Progress in Hormone Research 36:53–88

Lado-Abeal J, Rodriguez-Arnao J, Newell-Price JDC et al 1998 Menstrual abnormalities in women with Cushing's disease are correlated with hypercortisolemia rather than raised circulating androgen levels. Journal of Clinical Endocrinology and Metabolism 83:3083–3088

Lauber ME, Bengston T, Watermann MR, Simpson ER 1991 Regulation of CYP11A (P450scc) and CYP17 (P450$_{17\alpha}$) gene expression in bovine luteal cells in primary culture. Journal of Biological Chemistry 266:11170–11175

Levine LS, Rauh W, Gottesdiener K et al 1980 New studies of the 11β-hydroxylase and 18-hydroxylase enzymes in the hypertensive form of congenital adrenal hyperplasia. Journal of Clinical Endocrinology and Metabolism 50:258–263

Lund J, Bakke M, Mellgren G, Morohashi K-I, Doskeland S-O 1997 Transcriptional regulation of the bovine CYP17 gene by cAMP. Steroids 62:43–45

MacGillivray MH, Morishima A, Conte F, Grumbach M, Smith EP 1998 Pediatric endocrinology update: an overview. The essential roles of estrogens in pubertal growth, epiphyseal fusion and bone turnover: lessons from mutations in genes for aromatase and estrogen receptor. Hormone Research 49(suppl 1):2–8

McFarland KC, Sprengel R, Phillips HS et al 1989 Lutropin-choriogonadotrophin receptor: an unusual member of the G-protein-coupled receptor family. Science 25:494–499

Michael AE, Cooke BA 1994 A working hypothesis for the regulation of steroidogenesis and germ cell development in the gonads by glucocorticoids and 11β-hydroxysteroid dehydrogenase (11βHSD). Molecular and Cellular Endocrinology 100:55–63

Prenatal diagnosis. If the parents are heterozygous carriers of 21-hydroxylase deficiency, the fetus has a 1 in 4 chance of being affected. Thus, prenatal diagnosis is important, either by amniocentesis to measure amniotic fluid 17-hydroxyprogesterone levels, HLA typing of amniotic cells or chorionic villus sampling and the use of specific DNA probes. Once the diagnosis has been made, the option is available to treat the pregnant woman with oral dexamethasone, which crosses the placenta and suppresses the secretion of ACTH and thus the circulating androgen levels.

11-Hydroxylase deficiency

This is the hypertensive form of congenital adrenal hyperplasia which accounts for about 5–8% of all cases (Zachmann et al 1983). The absence of 11-hydroxylase leads to elevated levels of 11-deoxycorticosterone (DOC) and although this means a decreased amount of aldosterone, DOC has salt-retaining properties, leading to hypertension. Androstenedione levels are also elevated and this can result in ambiguous genitalia.

The diagnosis is made by measuring elevated levels of urinary 17-hydroxycorticosteroids and raised serum androstenedione. Treatment is similar to 21-hydroxylase deficiency, with glucocorticoid replacement therapy.

The genetics, however, are rather different. There is no HLA association with 11-hydroxylase deficiency, but the use of a DNA probe has located the gene on the long arm of chromosome 8 (White et al 1985).

3β-Dehydrogenase deficiency

This rare form of congenital adrenal hyperplasia results in a block of steroidogenesis very early in the pathway, giving rise to a severe salt-losing adrenal hyperplasia. The androgen most elevated is dehydroepiandrosterone, an androgen which causes mild virilization. The diagnosis rests on the measurement of elevated dehydroepiandrosterone. The gene encoding 3β-dehydrogenase has not yet been cloned but it is not linked to HLA.

Androgen-secreting tumours

Androgen-secreting tumours are rare in pregnancy, but may arise in the ovary or the adrenal. They cause fetal virilization. When they occur in the non-pregnant woman, annovulation is induced.

Ovary

A number of androgen-secreting tumours have been reported including luteoma (Cohen et al 1982, Hensleigh & Woodruff 1978), polycystic ovaries (Fayez et al 1974), mucinous cystadenoma (Novak et al 1970, Post et al 1978), arrhenoblastoma (Barkan et al 1984) and Krukenberg tumours (Connor et al 1968, Forest et al 1978). Not all female fetuses will be affected and there is no association with gestation and exposure. The fetus may be partly protected by the conversion of the maternally derived androgen to oestrogen in the placenta and thus the degree of virilization is variable.

Adrenal

There are only two reports of adrenal adenomas causing fetal masculinization (Fuller et al 1983, Murset et al 1970). These tumours may be hCG responsive and thus levels of androgen may be higher in pregnancy than in the non-pregnant state, leading to androgenization of the fetus.

Drugs

The association between the use of progestogens and masculinization of the female fetus has received much publicity, but the only progestogen proven to have such an effect is 17-ethinyl testosterone (Ishizuka et al 1962). These infants had clitoromegaly and in some cases labioscrotal fusion, but the risk is very small (1/50). Gestogens which are derived from testosterone should be avoided in the pregnant woman. There have been two case reports of androgenization of female fetuses from exposure to danazol during pregnancy (Castro-Magana et al 1981, Duck & Katamaya 1981) and both babies were born with external genitalia similar to those with adrenogenital syndrome.

Associated multiple congenital abnormalities

Female intersex has been described in association with a number of multiple abnormality states, most commonly those in association with the urinary and gastrointestinal tracts. It has also been described in association with VATER syndrome (Say & Carpentier 1979).

The management of these children with masculinized genitalia is to ensure the assignation of a sex of rearing and modify the genitalia appropriately. In all of these rare cases, the female role has been chosen and reduction clitoroplasty performed.

XY FEMALE

The normal differentiation of the gonad to become a testis has been described above and its subsequent secretion of testosterone leads to development of the wolffian duct and the urogenital sinus to produce the normal male internal and external genitalia. Testosterone is the predominant male sex hormone secreted by the testis but two other processes are necessary for normal development: the conversion of testosterone to DHT by 5α-reductase, and the presence of androgen receptors in the target cell which bind with the DHT or testosterone and produce appropriate nuclear function. Thus, normal male genotype, i.e. XY, with a female phenotype will occur if there is:

- failure of testicular development
- error(s) in testosterone biosynthesis, or
- androgen insensitivity at the target site.

Failure of testicular development

This group of disorders includes true gonadal dysgenesis, Leydig cell hypoplasia and the persistent müllerian duct syndrome.

True gonadal dysgenesis

True gonadal dysgenesis is characterized by streak gonads, normal müllerian structures and normal external female genitalia. It has been suggested that the streak gonads in these individuals were originally ovaries which contained oogonia which then subsequently underwent massive atresia, in a similar fashion to Turner's syndrome. The karyotype is either 46XY or 46XX and these patients usually present in teenage years, with failure of pubertal development (see Chapter 1).

46XY partial gonadal dysgenesis

In this condition, the infants are born with ambiguous genitalia, which results from the partially dysgenetic development of the testis. The dysgenetic gonads have various histological arrangements, with poor seminiferous tubules. However, some androgen can be produced by these testes, which results in partial androgenization of the external genitalia, leading to the genital ambiguity. These children have a high risk of gonadal tumours, especially gonadoblastoma, and in these circumstances, the gonads should be removed early to prevent this development.

Leydig cell hypoplasia

Leydig cell hypoplasia is an uncommon condition, of which the aetiology remains speculative. The role of fetal luteinizing hormone in normal testicular development is unknown, but it may be necessary for maturation of the interstitial cells into Leydig cells. Failure of luteinizing hormone production in the first trimester will result in Leydig cell hypoplasia and male pseudohermaphroditism (or an autosomal recessive disorder resulting in absent luteinizing hormone receptors will cause absence of Leydig cells). This manifests as ambiguous genitalia, in both circumstances due to some androgen production by Sertoli cells. Clinically, Leydig cell hypoplasia usually presents as a phenotypical female with primary amenorrhoea and sexual infantilism (see Chapter 1) but ambiguity at birth may result in diagnosis in infancy.

46XY true hermaphroditism

These individuals have the presence of both testicular and ovarian tissue with a 46XY karyotype. It has been suggested that mutation of the SRY gene may be the aetiology of this (Berkovitz & Seeherunvong 1998).

46XX sex reversal

This nomenclature is used to describe the situation in which testicular tissue develops in someone with a 46XX karyotype. If testicular development is normal, they are referred to as 46XX males but when testicular determination is incomplete, they are referred to as 46XX true hermaphrodites. In 46XX males, the external genitalia are usually normal or a small percentage may have hypospadias. Clinically, they do not present until puberty, when this is delayed due to failure to be able to produce testosterone and due to the degeneration of seminiferous tubules and Leydig cell hyperplasia, which seems to occur just prior to puberty. It seems that in the majority of these individuals, the sex reversal is related to the translocation of Y chromosome sequences, including the SRY gene from the paternal Y chromosome to the paternal X chromosome (Tomomasa et al 1999). However, one-third of individuals are not found to have Y chromosome sequences in their DNA and this means there must be a mutation in the genomic DNA which permits testicular determination to occur in the absence of TDF. These gene defects remain to be explained.

Errors in testosterone biosynthesis

This type of disorder accounts for only 4% of XY females and results from deficiency of an enzyme involved in testosterone synthesis (see Fig. 14.4).

20–22 Desmolase deficiency

Absence of this enzyme results in failure to convert cholesterol to pregnenolone and a failure of subsequent steroid production. Most of the reported cases have died in early chilhood due to adrenal insufficiency, but the XY individuals are all partially virilized with a small blind vaginal pouch. It is considered to be an autosomal recessive disorder.

3β-Hydroxysteroid dehydrogenase deficiency

This is a rare disorder which affects both adrenal and gonadal function and is again autosomally recessive. The deficiency may be complete or incomplete and thus the degree of virilization is variable, with various degrees of hypospadias or a small blind vagina with normal internal male genitalia and absent müllerian structures. Those individuals who have survived and reached puberty have developed gynaecomastia, presumably because the absence of testosterone during fetal life has allowed breast bud development. The diagnosis is made by elevated levels of pregnenolone and 17-hydroxypregnenolone and low levels of corticosteroids and testosterone.

17α-Hydroxylase deficiency

This syndrome produces a phenotype in XY individuals varying from normal female external genitalia and a blind vaginal pouch to hypospadias with a small phallus. The diagnosis is usually only made in adulthood with failure to develop secondary sexual characteristics. The impaired adrenal production of cortisol is not associated with clinical symptoms as the elevated levels of corticosterone compensate. The gonads should be removed if the patient is assigned a female gender and hormone replacement therapy instituted.

17–20 Desmolase deficiency

This enzyme defect primarily affects testosterone production and there is no adrenal insufficiency. The clinical findings range from normal female to undervirilized male genitalia and the endocrine findings are of very low serum levels of testosterone with normal corticosteroids. Again, diagnosis may not be made until failure of pubertal development.

17-Ketosteroid reductase deficiency

This enzyme is responsible for the reversible conversion of androstenedione to testosterone and oestrone to oestradiol. These patients almost always present at birth with female external genitalia and testes in the inguinal canal, and undergo masculinization at puberty. Those individuals to be raised as females should have their gonads removed before puberty and oestrogen therapy begun at puberty.

Androgen insensitivity at the target site (Table 14.1)

In this group of patients testicular function is normal and circulating levels of androgen are consistent with normal

Table 14.1 Types of androgen insensitivity and their abnormalities

Defect	External genitalia	Internal genitalia	Gonad	Phenotype at puberty
5α-Reductase deficiency	Female or ambiguous	Male	Testis	Masculine
Complete androgen insensitivity	Female	Male	Testis	Infantile and breast growth
Partial androgen insensitivity	Ambiguous	Male	Testis	Partial masculine and breast growth

male development. The majority of patients present at puberty with primary amenorrhoea, but some will present with ambiguous genitalia. The defect may be 5α-reductase deficiency or complete or partial androgen insensitivity.

5α-Reductase deficiency

This results in the failure of the conversion of testosterone to DHT in target tissues and thus a failure of masculinization of the site. In infancy, there is usually a small phallus, some degree of hypospadias, a bifid scrotum and a blind vaginal pouch. The testes are found either in the inguinal canal or in the labioscrotal folds and müllerian structures are absent. At puberty, elevated levels of androgen lead to masculinization, including an increase in phallic growth, although this remains smaller than normal. Seminal production has been reported (Petersen et al 1977).

It is an autosomal recessive trait and the resulting enzyme defect gives predictable hormone profiles with normal levels of testosterone, but low levels of DHT. The diagnosis is important in individuals born with ambiguous genitalia in order to assign the sex of rearing and this should be based on the potential for normal sexual function in adult life. The gonads should be removed if the sex of rearing is to be female and at puberty oestrogen replacement therapy instituted.

Complete androgen insensitivity

This is an X-linked recessive disorder characterized by the clinical features of normal female external genitalia, a blind vaginal pouch and absent müllerian and wolffian structures. The testes are found either in the labial folds or inguinal canal or they may be intra-abdominal.

These patients may lack the androgen receptor and may be shown to lack the gene located on the X chromosome between Xp11 and Xq13. Work by Brown et al (1982), however, suggests that there may be a variety of defects, ranging from absence of receptors to presence of a normal number of receptors which are inactive. The exact mechanism of the defects in patients with androgen receptors awaits definition.

The hormonal levels of testosterone which are elevated above normal due to increased luteinizing hormone production and the associated increase in testicular oestradiol and peripheral conversion of androgens to oestradiol promotes some breast development. Pubic hair growth depends on the degree of insensitivity but is usually rather scanty.

Patients either present with a hernial mass or with primary amenorrhoea despite secondary sexual characteristics; karyotyping makes the diagnosis. The gonads should be removed because of the malignant potential. The vagina may be of variable length and may be adequate, but those with a short vaginal pouch may need manual dilatation.

Partial androgen insensitivity

This is a complex condition which has been found to be due to a reduced binding affinity of DHT to the receptor or because the receptor binds the DHT but there are defects in the transcription to the nucleus. It is an X-linked recessive disorder and the partial expression means inevitable ambiguous genitalia with a blind vaginal pouch and phallic enlargement. The penis can be normal. The wolffian ducts can be rudimentary or normal, but the testes are azoospermic. The most common presentation in infancy is hypospadias, with the urethra opening at the base of the phallus, and there may be cryptorchidism. At puberty, male secondary sexual characteristics develop poorly, but there is usually gynaecomastia. The management is dependent on the degree of ambiguity and subsequent choice of sex of rearing, with gonadectomy and hormone replacement therapy for those assigned the female role.

ANOMALOUS VAGINAL DEVELOPMENT

When the vagina does not develop normally, a number of abnormalities have been described. The vagina may be partially maldeveloped, leading to a vaginal obstruction which may be complete or incomplete, or there may be total maldevelopment of the müllerian ducts leading to various disorders.

Classification

Vaginal anomalies may be categorized as follows:

- congenital absence of the müllerian ducts (the Mayer–Rokitansky–Kuster-Hauser syndrome)
- disorders of vertical fusion
- failure of lateral fusion.

Aetiology

There are three mechanisms which may explain most vaginal anomalies. They may be familial, for example XY females who have a hereditary disorder as described previously. Congenital absence of the vagina has been very rarely reported in XX siblings (Jones & Mermut 1974) and also in monozygotic twins with only one child affected (Lischke et al 1973).

The case of a female limited autosomal dominant trait was first reported by Shokeir (1978) who studied 16 Saskatchewan families in which there was a proband with vaginal agenesis. However, Carson et al (1983), in a study of 23 probands, disputed the Shokeir theory. The previous evidence with regard to monozygotic twins also makes this mode of inheritance unlikely. Polygenic or multifactorial inheritance does, however, offer some explanation that families may exhibit the trait as

195

reported. The recurrent risk of a polygenic multifactorial trait in first-degree relatives is reported to be between 1% and 5%.

Finally, it is possible that müllerian duct defects could be secondary to teratogens or other environmental factors but no definite association has been demonstrated.

Epidemiology

The incidence of vaginal malformations has been variously estimated at between 1/4000 and 1/10 000 female births (Evans et al 1981). The infrequency of this anomaly makes accurate estimates of the true incidence very difficult to obtain but when considered as a cause of primary amenorrhoea, vaginal malformation ranks second to gonadal dysgenesis.

Pathophysiology

The pathophysiology of vaginal absence may be either as a result of failure of the vaginal plate to form or failure of cavitation. Absence of the uterus and fallopian tubes indicates total failure of müllerian duct development but in the Rokitansky syndrome, the uterus is often present, although rudimentary, and therefore it must be failure of vaginal plate formation and subsequent vaginal development which leads to the absent vagina. Vertical fusion defects (Fig. 14.5) may result from failure of fusion of the müllerian system with the urogenital sinus or may be due to incomplete canalization of the vagina. Disorders of lateral fusion are due to the failure of the müllerian ducts to unite and may create a duplicated uterovaginal septum which may be obstructive or non-obstructive, depending on the mode of development (Fig. 14.6).

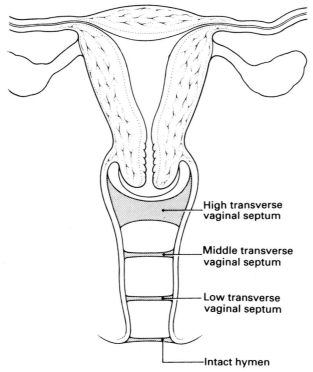

High transverse vaginal septum

Middle transverse vaginal septum

Low transverse vaginal septum

Intact hymen

Fig. 14.5 Disorders of vertical fusion.

Presentation

Vaginal atresia
Vaginal atresia presents at puberty with complicated or uncomplicated primary amenorrhoea. In the majority who have an absent or rudimentary uterus, uncomplicated primary amenorrhoea is the presenting symptom, but those women who have a functional uterus may develop an associated haematometra and present with cyclical abdominal pain. If a haematometra does develop, there will be uterine distension and an abdominal mass may be palpable but more commonly it is felt on rectal examination.

Vertical fusion defects
Here, the transverse vaginal septum prevents loss of menstrual blood and therefore cryptomenorrhoea results. Most patients present as teenagers with cyclical abdominal pain and a haematocolpos will be palpable within the pelvis on rectal examination. The patient may also present with associated pressure symptoms of urinary frequency and/or retention. The incidence of vertical fusion defects is reported as 46% high, 35% mid and 19% low septae in the vagina (Rock et al 1982).

Disorders of lateral fusion
These patients usually present with the incidental finding of a vaginal septum which is usually asymptomatic. It may first be diagnosed during pregnancy at which time excision will be necessary to ensure a vaginal delivery. However, these patients may present with dyspareunia cause by the septum and in most cases one vagina is larger than the other and intercourse may have occurred partially successfully in the larger side. In the unilateral vaginal obstruction group, presentation is usually with abdominal pain and the associated symptoms of a haematometra and haematocolpos. The confusing clinical sign is the associated menstruation from the other side and the diagnosis may be missed if careful examination is not performed in these teenagers.

Investigation

Vaginal atresia
A patient presenting with a clinically absent vagina and no cyclical abdominal pain requires an ultrasound examination of the pelvis to determine the presence or absence of a uterus and/or a haematometra. Laparoscopy in these patients is unnecessary. Some 15% of patients with the Rokitansky syndrome suffer major defects of the urinary system, including congenital absence of a kidney; 40% of patients also have trivial urinary abnormalities (d'Alberton et al 1981). It is therefore important to perform an intravenous urogram in order to establish any abnormalities in the renal system or the presence of a pelvic kidney which may alert the surgeon to take extra care if abdominal operation becomes necessary.

Anomalies of the bony skeleton occur in about 12% of patients. These include abnormalities of the lumbar spine, the cervical vertebrae and also limb abnormalities. However, it may be that the incidence of bony abnormalities is higher than this, as investigation of the skeletal system is rarely performed.

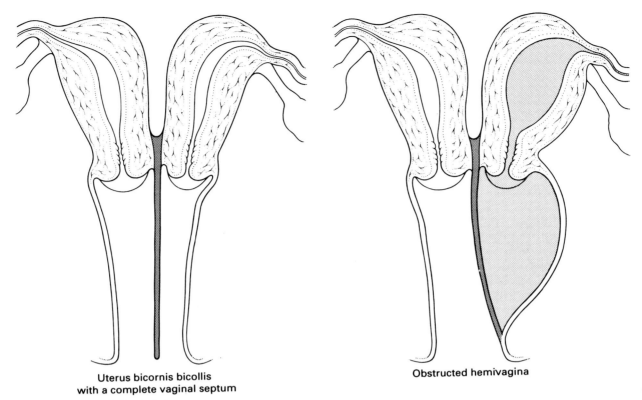

**Uterus bicornis bicollis
with a complete vaginal septum**

Obstructed hemivagina

Fig. 14.6   Lateral fusion defects.

Transverse vaginal septum

Investigations in these patients are limited to ultrasound assessment of the uterus for the detection of a haematometra and haematocolpos and this may also be used to assess the level of the septal defect. Again, investigation of the urinary tract is pertinent.

Lateral fusion defects

Investigations in this group are only important if there is an obstructed outflow problem and should follow those outlined for vertical fusion defects.

Treatment

Vaginal atresia

The patient with müllerian agenesis requires careful psychological counselling and associated therapy. The psychological impact of being informed of the absent vagina comes as an immense shock to both patient and parents. It is almost always followed by a period of depression in which many patients question their femininity and look upon themselves as abnormal females. They very much doubt their ability to enter a heterosexual relationship which will be lasting and feel worthless both sexually and certainly as regards being a reproductive partner. In some patients the depression can be very profound and suicide may be threatened. There is also great maternal anxiety over the aetiology as most mothers feel that they are responsible for the abnormality. Reassurance of the mother is as important as that of the daughter in the management of the patient.

Occasionally cultural problems arise which make management much more difficult, especially in ethnic groups where the ability to procreate is fundamental to marriage and social acceptance. These patients and their parents can be very difficult to console and often refuse to accept the situation, questioning the diagnosis of their sterility over a number of years. The immediate reaction of most patients is to request surgical correction of the abnormality to return them to 'normal'. Unfortunately, opting for surgical treatment without adequate psychological and physical preparation inevitably leads to disaster. We recommend a minimum of 6 months of preparation before any surgical procedure is performed and during this time psychological support can be implemented for the patient and her parents. There are two major areas of support required: first, the correction of the loss of esteem and inevitable depression and repeated counselling sessions by trained personnel are required if these symptoms are to be overcome. The second problem involves the psychological aspect and again prolonged counselling sessions will be required if an adequate and fulfilling sex life is going to be possible in the future. The sexual life achieved by well-managed patients can be excellent and has been reported as comparable to that of the normal population (Poland & Evans 1985, Raboch & Horejsi 1982).

Management of the absent vagina with a non-functioning uterus

In a patient with an absent or rudimentary uterus, the creation of a vaginal passage may be non-surgical or surgical. The non-surgical technique involves the repeated use of graduated vaginal dilators over a period of 6–12 months. A minimum of 1 cm of vaginal dimple is necessary for this technique to succeed and patients require support and encouragement during this time. Patients are instructed to begin with a small vaginal dilator which is pressed firmly against the vaginal dimple for a period of some 20 minutes twice a day. Pressure is exerted but pain should be avoided and repeated use of these vaginal dilators will meet with success in about 90% of cases with appropriate selection (Broadbent et al 1984). This technique was first described by Frank in 1938 and in view of its undoubted success, with no complications, this method must be attempted in all girls with an absent vagina and a 1 cm dimple before any surgical procedure is considered.

In those girls with a vagina of less than 1 cm or those in whom Frank's procedure fails, vaginoplasty will be required. There are currently three techniques in popular usage: the McIndoe–Reed operation, the amnion vaginoplasty and the Williams vulvovaginoplasty.

The *McIndoe–Reed procedure* was first described in 1938 (McIndoe & Banister 1938) and involved the use of a split-thickness skin graft over a solid mould; this mould is placed in a surgically created space between the urethra and the rectum. This space is created digitally following a transverse incision in the vaginal dimple. Digital exploration of the space must be performed with great care as damage to the bladder or the rectum may occur. The space created must reach the peritoneum of the pouch of Douglas if an adequate length of a vagina is to be created. A split-thickness skin graft is then taken from a donor site and an appropriately sized mould is chosen. The skin graft is then fashioned over the mould with the external skin surface in apposition to the mould. The skin-covered mould is then placed in the neovaginal space and the labia are sutured together to hold the mould in situ. McIndoe reported his own series of 105 patients in 1959 and had a satisfactory outcome in 80% of patients. Cali & Pratt (1968) reported on their series of 123 patients; 90% had good sexual function but 6% had major complications which were primarily fistulae and subsequent reconstructive surgery was necessary in 8%. These complications resulted in modifications of the technique and the use of a soft material for the mould to prevent fistula formation due to pressure necrosis.

The search for an alternative material to line the neovagina and avoid the scarring of the donor skin site led to the use of *amnion* for the vaginoplasty procedure (Ashworth et al 1986). The technique involves the creation of a neovaginal space in the same way as described for the McIndoe–Reed procedure but amnion obtained at the time of elective caesarean section is used to line the neovagina. The mesenchymal surface of the amnion is placed against the new vaginal surface to promote epithelialization and the mould is kept in situ for 7 days and then replaced with a new amnion graft for a further 7 days. Subsequently, patients are encouraged in the frequent use of dilators to maintain the vaginal passage. Again, reported success of around 90% has been achieved by these authors.

The *Williams vulvovaginoplasty* (Williams 1976) still has an important place in the management of these disorders, but is much less frequently used than in the past. In patients in whom dissection of a neovagina is impossible but the labia majora are normal, this technique is invaluable. The principle of the operation is to create a vaginal pouch from the full-thickness skin flaps created from the labia majora, which are united in the midline. Following surgery and adequate healing, the patient is taught to use vaginal dilators in the same way as described in the Frank technique. There is no doubt that this does allow the patient and her partner to enjoy a sex life with mutual orgasm but the angle of the vagina is unnatural and unsatisfactory for some patients. Although the operation is simple to perform, the psychological problems of the distorted external genitalia can be considerable.

The absent vagina with a coexistent functional uterus

This situation presents major problems as the release of menstrual blood and the relief of associated pain are the primary aims; the creation of a normal vagina is an equally important yet secondary role. The functional uterus may be normal and a cervix may be present or absent. This situation is very rare; an operation to create a neovagina in an attempt to reanastomose a uterus which has been drained of its haematometra is highly specialized and will not be discussed further.

Complications

Some 25% of women will have some degree of dyspareunia following a vaginoplasty (Smith 1983). This is most commonly due to scarring at the upper margin of the vagina, involving the peritoneum. Similar incidences of dyspareunia occur in nearly all series and it is difficult to know how best to avoid this. It seems to occur regardless of technique, but contraction of the upper part of the vagina is difficult to avoid. The artificial vagina created in these ways acquires all the characteristics of normal vaginal epithelium and the exposure of the grafted epithelium to a new environment means that care has to be taken to ensure it remains healthy. Four cases of intraepithelial neoplasia in neovaginas have been reported (Ducker 1972, Imrie et al 1986, Jackson 1959, Rotmensch et al 1983).

Management of disorders of vertical fusion

In these abnormalities, the type of procedure is governed by the type of abnormality. In the obstructed hymen the procedure is extremely simple and a cruciate incision through the hymen will release the accumulated menstrual blood and resolve the problem. In obstructing transverse vaginal septae in the lower and middle thirds, surgical removal of the septum can almost always be performed transvaginally and a reanastomosis of the upper and lower vaginal segments may be performed. Great care must be taken to ensure that the excision is adequate or a vaginal stenosis at the site of the septum will remain a problem. The high vaginal septum is the most difficult abnormality to manage and it is almost always necessary to perform a laparotomy in order to expose the haematometra. The passage of a probe through the uterine cavity and cervix into the short upper vagina allows a second vaginal surgeon to explore the vagina from below and excise the septum. The absent portion of vagina is usually so great that reanastomosis of the vaginal mucosa cannot be achieved and either a soft mould is inserted and granulation allowed to occur or an amnion-covered soft mould should be inserted to promote epithelialization. Vaginal dilatation following removal of the mould must be encouraged in order to prevent constriction of the new vaginal area.

Results. The results of surgery are extremely good when judged by sexual satisfaction. However, Rock et al (1982) reported pregnancy success following surgical correction of transverse vaginal septa and noted that patients with a transverse vaginal septum had only a 47% pregnancy rate when the site of the septum was taken into account. If the obstruction was in the lower third, then all patients achieved a pregnancy; in the middle third 43% and in the upper third 25% of patients became pregnant. It is suggested that the difficulties in conceiving may be secondary to the development of endometriosis and the higher the site of the septum, the more likely the development of this disorder may be. Thus prompt diagnosis and surgical correction are important in an attempt to preserve the maximum reproductive capacity in these patients.

Complications. Complications are primarily those of dyspareunia and failure of pregnancy, as described above.

Disorders of lateral fusion

The treatment of this condition depends on the abnormality. In patients with a midline septum and no other abnormality, excision of the septum should be performed and care must be taken as these septa can be very thick and removal can be rather difficult. When resecting the septum, generous pedicles should be taken to ensure haemostatis and the results are extremely good as the remaining tissue usually retracts and causes no problem. In patients in whom there is an incomplete vaginal obstruction, again the septum needs to be removed and care must be taken to remove as much of it as possible. Failure to do this will result in healing of an ostium and repeat obstruction of the hemivagina. The results and outlook for these patients are extremely good.

MALFORMATIONS OF THE UTERUS

Classification and pathophysiology

There have been numerous classification systems for uterine malformations, varying from those based on embryological development to those based on obstetric performance. However, the most widely used classification is that of Buttram & Gibbons (1979) which is based upon the degree of failure of normal development. Six categories are described.

Class I: Müllerian agenesis or hypoplasia
Class II: Unicornuate uterus
Class III: Uterus didelphis
Class IV: Uterus bicornuate
Class V: Septate uterus
Class VI: Diethylstilboestrol (DES) anomalies

A separate class of uterine malformations has been identified in the presence of communication between two separate uterocervical cavities.

The pathophysiology of failure of normal union of the müllerian ducts is not clear. As proposed in the section on vaginal agenesis, the hypothesis of teratogens has been suggested but unsupported by evidence. It is most likely that this is a polygenic or multifactorial inheritance which slightly increases the risk of a uterovaginal abnormality arising in a family with no anomalies.

Incidence

The incidence of uterine anomalies is difficult to define as it depends entirely upon the interest of the investigator and the diligence with which investigation is pursued. Obstetric series show an incidence of uterine abnormalities ranging from 1/100 to 1/1000 (Semmens 1962). In an infertile population, the incidence increases to around 3% (Sanfillippo et al 1978). It is likely that incidence of uterine malformations is greatly overestimated, as in the vast majority of patients no gynaecological or reproductive problems are ever experienced.

Presentation

Abnormal uterine development may be symptomatic or asymptomatic. The most common clinical situations that will lead to a diagnosis of malformation of the uterus are recurrent pregnancy loss, primary infertility, urological abnormalities, menstrual disorders and DES exposure.

Recurrent pregnancy loss

Recurrent pregnancy wastage in the form of abortion or premature labour is a common way in which uterine anomalies will be discovered. The role of uterine anomalies in pregnancy wastage is discussed in Chapter 20.

Primary infertility

Uterine abnormalities may be discovered during investigation of an infertile woman. However, the relationship between infertility and uterine abnormalities remains controversial.

Urological abnormalities

Not uncommonly, urologists who discover malformations of the urinary system investigate the genital system and find abnormalities. Thompson & Lynn (1966) reported that 66% of patients with a maldevelopment of the renal tract had an associated müllerian duct abnormality. However, only 13.5% of women with anomalous renal development had anomalous uterine development. In patients with a single kidney, the most common uterine abnormality is uterus didelphis with a vaginal septum which is associated with unilateral occlusion.

Menstrual disorders

Uterine abnormalities may be responsible for a number of menstrual disorders including oligomenorrhoea, dysmenorrhoea and menorrhagia. The specific menstrual symptoms will depend on the anomaly. In an interesting study by Sorensen (1981), investigating infertile women with oligomenorrhoea, 56% of patients were found to have mild uterine abnormalities. The author suggested that this oligomenorrhoea might be due to poor vascularization or steroid receptor development in the malformed uterus. With regard to dysmenorrhoea, uterine abnormalities seem to be associated with a higher incidence of primary dysmenorrhoea, although this may also be associated with obstructed outflow problems.

Rudimentary hemiuteri may be also the cause of dysmenorrhoea in some women.

DES exposure

The malformations associated with DES exposure have been well described (Kaufman et al 1980). These abnormalities include the classic T-shaped uterus with a widening of the interstitial and isthmic portions of the fallopian tubes and narrowing of the lower two-thirds of the uterus, as well as non-specific uterine abnormalities with changes of cavity seen on hysterosalpingography. These patients may present with impaired reproductive function and pregnancy wastage may be as high as 50–60%.

Investigations

It is obvious that investigation of patients with suspected uterine abnormalities must be done with the aid of hysterosalpingography. This radiographic demonstration of the intrauterine shape is the most appropriate procedure, although care must be taken to ensure that if a double cervix is present, both cervical canals are cannulated and contrast medium is injected.

Treatment

A number of uterine malformations are suitable for surgical repair and the types of treatment and results are described in Chapter 24.

KEY POINTS

1. Gonadal differentiation into a testicle or ovary depends on the presence or absence of a Y chromosome.
2. The testis develops from the medulla whereas the ovary originates from the cortex or the primitive gonad.
3. Development of normal ovaries depends on the presence of two X chromosomes.
4. Deletion of either the short or long arms of the X chromosome may result in variable ovarian development or dysgenesis.
5. Development of the testis depends on the testicular determining factor which controls the expression of the H-Y antigen, but other autosomally located genes are also involved.
6. Female intersex disorders denote external genital masculinization in patients with 46XX karyotype.
7. Differentiation of internal female sexual organs is not androgen dependent and unlike the clitoris, the labia are adversely affected only if exposed to androgens before the 12th week of intrauterine life.
8. 21-Hydroxylase deficiency is an autosomal recessive disorder and accounts for 90% of cases of congenital adrenal hyperplasia (CAH).
9. 21-Hydroxylase deficiency is the only adrenal enzymatic deficiency associated with the HLA gene located in chromosome 6.
10. Female fetus defeminization may follow maternal use of testosterone-related progestogens.

KEY POINTS (CONTINUED)

11. Prenatal diagnosis of CAH in heterozygous carriers is necessary and treatment with dexamethasone prevents fetal infliction.
12. Successful pregnancy following resection of vaginal septum is inversely related to the level of the septum in the vagina.
13. Intrauterine diethylstilboestrol (DES) exposure may lead to T-shaped uterus with impaired reproductive function.

REFERENCES

Ashworth MF, Morton KE, Dewhurst CJ et al 1986 Vaginoplasty using amnion. Obstetrics and Gynecology 67:443–444

Barkan A, Cassorla F, Loriaux D, Marshall JC 1984 Pregnancy in a patient with virilising arrhenoblastoma. American Journal of Obstetrics and Gynecology 149:909–910

Behlke MA, Bogan JS, Beer-Romero P, Page DC 1993 Evidence that the SRY protein is encoded by a single exon on the human Y chromosome. Genomics 17:736–739

Berkovitz GD, Seeherunvong T 1998 Abnormalities of gonadal differentiation. Baillière's Clinical Endocrinology and Metabolism 12:133–142

Broadbent RT, Woolf RM, Herbertson R 1984 Non-operative construction of the vagina. Plastic and Reconstructive Surgery 73:117–122

Brown TR, Maes M, Rothwell SW, Migeon CJ 1982 Human complete androgen insensitivity with normal dihydrotestosterone receptor binding capacity in cultured genital skin biopsies. Journal of Clinical Endocrinology and Metabolism 55:61–69

Buttram VS, Gibbons WE 1979 Mullerian anomalies – a proposed classification. Fertility and Sterility 32:40–48

Cacciari E, Balsamo A, Cassio A et al 1983 Neonatal screening for congenital adrenal hyperplasia. Archives of Disease in Childhood 58:803–806

Cali RW, Pratt JH 1968 Congenital absence of the vagina. American Journal of Obstetrics and Gynecology 100:752–754

Carson SA, Simpson JL, Malinak LR et al 1983 Heritable aspects of uterine anomalies II. Genetic analysis of mullerian aplasia. Fertility and Sterility 40:86–91

Castro-Magana M, Chervanky T, Collipp PJ, Ghavami-Maibadi Z, Angulo M, Stewart C 1981 Transient adrenogenital syndrome due to exposure to danazol in utero. American Journal of Diseases of Childhood 135:1032–1034

Cohen VA, Daughaday WH, Weldon V 1982 Fetal and maternal virilization association with pregnancy. American Journal of Diseases of Childhood 136:353–356

Connor TB, Ganis FM, Levin HS, Migeon CJ, Martin LG 1968 Gonadotrophin dependent Krukenberg tumour causing virilization during pregnancy. Journal of Clinical Endocrinology and Metabolism 28:198–201

D'Alberton A, Reschini E, Ferrari N, Candiani P 1981 Prevalence of urinary tract abnormalities in a large series of patients with uterovaginal atresia. Journal of Urology 126:623–627

Dong WF, Heng HH, Lowsky R 1997 Cloning, expression and chromosomal localisation to 11p12-13 of a human LIM homeobox gene, hLIM-1. DNA and Cell Biology 16:671–78

Donohoue PA, van Dop C, McLean RH et al 1986 Gene conversion in salt-losing congenital adrenal hyperplasia with absent complement C4B protein. Journal of Clinical Endocrinology and Metabolism 62:995–1002

Duck SC, Katamaya KP 1981 Danazol may cause female pseudohermaphroditism. Fertility and Sterility 35:230–231

Duckler L 1972 Squamous cell carcinoma developing in an artificial vagina. Obstetrics and Gynecology 40:35

Dupont B, Oberfield SE, Smithwick EM et al 1977 Close genetic linkage between HLA and congenital adrenal hyperplasia. Lancet ii:1309–1312

Edmonds DK 1989 Intersexuality. In: Dewhurst's practical paediatric and adolescent gynaecology, 2nd edn. Butterworths, London

Evans TN, Poland ML, Boving RL 1981 Vaginal malformations. American Journal of Obstetrics and Gynecology 141:910–916

Fayez JA, Bunch TR, Miller GL 1974 Virilization in pregnancy associated with polycystic ovary disease. Obstetrics and Gynecology 44:511–521

Forest MG, Orgiazzi J, Tranchant D, Mornex R, Bertrand J 1978 Approach to the mechanism of androgen production in a case of Krukenberg tumor responsible for virilization during pregnancy. Journal of Clinical Endocrinology and Metabolism 47:428–434

Frank RT 1938 The formation of an artificial vagina without operation. American Journal of Obstetrics and Gynecology 35:1053–1055

Fuller PJ, Pettigrew IG, Pike JW, Stockigt JR 1983 An adrenal adenoma causing virilization of mother and infant. Clinical Endocrinology 18:143–153

Guellaen G, Casanova M, Bishop C 1984 Human XX males with Y single copy DNA fragments. Nature 307:172–173

Hastie ND 1994 The genetics of Wilm's tumour. Annual Review of Genetics 28:523–558

Hensleigh PA, Woodruff DA 1978 Differential maternal fetal response to androgenizing luteoma or hyperreactio luteinalis. Obstetrical and Gynaecological Surgery 33:262–271

Hughes IA, Wilton A, Lole CA, Glay OP 1979 Continuing need for mineralocorticoid therapy in salt-losing congenital adrenal hyperplasia. Archives of Disease in Childhood 54:350–358

Imrie JEA, Kennedy JH, Holmes JD et al 1986 Intraepithelial neoplasia arising in an artificial vagina. British Journal of Obstetrics and Gynaecology 93:886–887

Ishizuka SC, Kawashima Y, Nakanishi T et al 1962 Statistical observations on genital anomalies of newborns following the administration of progestins to their mothers. Journal of the Japanese Obstetrical and Gynaecological Society 9:271–282

Jackson GW 1959 Primary carcinoma of an artificial vagina. Obstetrics and Gynaecology 14:534

Jones HW, Mermut S 1974 Familial occurrence of congenital absence of the vagina. Obstetrics and Gynecology 42:38–40

Kaufman RH, Adam E, Binder GL, Gerthoffer E 1980 Upper genital tract changes and pregnancy outcome in offspring exposed in utero to DES. American Journal of Obstetrics and Gynecology 137:299–306

Lefebvre V, Huang W, Harley VR 1997 SOX9 is a potent activator of the chondrocyte-specific enhancer of the proα1(II) collagen gene. Molecular Cellular and Biology 17:2336–2246

Lischke JH, Curtis CH, Lamb EJ 1973 Discordance of vaginal agenesis in monozygotic twins. Obstetrics and Gynecology 41:902–922

McIndoe AH 1959 Discussion on treatment of congenital absence of the vagina with emphasis on long term results. Proceedings of the Royal Society of Medicine 52:952–953

McIndoe AH, Banister JB 1938 An operation for the cure of congenital absence of the vagina. Journal of Obstetrics and Gynaecology of British Commonwealth 45:490–495

Mulaikal RM, Migeon CJ, Rock JA 1987 Fertility rates in female patients with congenital adrenal hyperplasia due to 21-hydroxylase deficiency. New England Journal of Medicine 315:178–181

Murset G, Zachmann M, Prader A, Fischer J, Labhart A 1970 Male external genitalia of a girl caused by a virilizing adrenal tumour in the mother. Acta Endocrinologica 65:627–638

Newns GH 1974 Congenital adrenal hyperplasia. Archives of Disease in Childhood 49:716–724

Novak DJ, Lauchlan SC, McCauley JC 1970 Virilization during pregnancy: case report and review of literature. American Journal of Medicine 49:281–286

Pang S, Murphey W, Levine LS et al 1982 A pilot newborn screening for congenital adrenal hyperplasia in Alaska. Journal of Clinical Endocrinology and Metabolism 55:413–420

Pang SY, Wallace MA, Hofman L et al 1988 Worldwide experience in newborn screening for congenital adrenal hyperplasia. Pediatrics 81:866–874

Petersen RE, Imperato-McGinley J, Gautier T, Sturla E 1977 Male pseudohermaphroditism due to 5a reductase deficiency. American Journal of Medicine 62:170–191

Poland ML, Evans TN 1985 Psychologic aspects of vaginal agenesis. Journal of Reproductive Medicine 30:340–348

Post WD, Steele HD, Gorwill H 1978 Mucinous cystadenoma and virilization during pregnancy. Canadian Medical Association Journal 118:948–953

Prader A 1958 Vollkommen männliche aussere Genitalentwicklung und Salzverlustsyndrom bei Mädchen mit kongenitalem adrenogenitalem Syndrom. Helvetica Paediatrica Acta 13:5–14

Raboch J, Horejsi J 1982 Sexual life of women with Kuster–Rokitansky syndrome. Archives of Sexual Behavior 11:215–219

Rock JA, Zacur HA, Dlugi AM et al 1982 Pregnancy success following surgical correction of imperforate hymen and complete transverse vaginal septum. Obstetrics and Gynecology 59:448–454

Rotmensch J, Rosenheim N, Dillon M et al 1983 Carcinoma arising in a neovagina. Obstetrics and Gynecology 61:534

Sanfillippo JS, Yussman MA, Smith O 1978 Hysterosalpingography in the evaluation of infertility. Fertility and Sterility 30:636–639

Say B, Carpentier NJ 1979 Genital malformations in a child with VATER association. American Journal of Diseases of Childhood 133:438–439

Semmens JP 1962 Congenital anomalies of the female genital tract. Obstetrics and Gynecology 19:328–333

Shokeir MHK 1978 Aplasia of the mullerian system. Evidence of probable sex limited autosomal dominant inheritance. Birth Defects 14:147–151

Smith MR 1983 Vaginal aplasia: therapeutic options. American Journal of Obstetrics and Gynecoloy 146:534–538

Sorensen SS 1981 Minor mullerian anomalies and oligomenorrhoea in infertile women. American Journal of Obstetrics and Gynecology 140:636–640

Swain A, Narvaez V, Burgoyne P 1998 Dax 1 antagonises SRY action in mammalian sex determination. Nature 391:761–767

Thompson DP, Lynn HB 1966 Genital abnormalities associated with solitary kidney. Mayo Clinic Proceedings 41:438–442

Tomomasa H, Adachi Y, Iwabuchi M 1999 XX-male syndrome bearing the sex-determining region Y. Archives of Andrology 42:89–96

White R, Leppert M, Bishop DT et al 1985 Construction of linkage maps with DNA markers for human chromosomes. Nature 313:101–105

Williams EA 1976 Uterovaginal agenesis. Annals of the Royal College of Surgeons of England 58:266–277

Zachmann M, Tassinari D, Prader A 1983 Clinical and biochemical variability of congenital adrenal hyperplasia due to 11-hydroxylase deficiency. Journal of Clinical Endocrinology and Metabolism 56:222–229

15

Control of hypothalamic–pituitary ovarian function

Robert W. Shaw

INTRODUCTION

Over the last 50 years it has become increasingly apparent that a major component of endocrine regulation is a function of the brain and of the hypothalamus in particular (Hohlweg & Junkmann 1932, Moore & Price 1932).

The hypothalamus lies at the base of the brain between the anterior margin of the optic chiasma anteriorly and the posterior margin of the mammillary bodies posteriorly. Precise boundaries are difficult to define but it extends from the hypothalamic sulcus above to the tuber cinereum below, which itself connects the hypothalamus with the pituitary gland via its extension distally into the pituitary stalk.

The hypothalamus is the important final pathway between the brain and the pituitary gland. Secretion of hormones from the anterior pituitary is under the control of hypothalamic-releasing or -inhibiting factors. In turn, the pituitary hormones regulate cellular growth and differentiation and functional activity in their separate target organs. Internal environmental maintenance results in multiple biochemical signals converging upon neurones within the hypothalamus whose response in turn leads to the release of the pituitary hormones which co-ordinate appropriate metabolic responses.

ANATOMY OF THE HYPOTHALAMIC-PITUITARY AXIS

The portion of the hypothalamus of special interest in the control of reproductive function is the neurohypophysis, which can be divided into three regions:

1. the infundibulum, which constitutes the floor of the third ventricle (often termed the median eminence) and parts of the wall of the third ventricle, which is continuous with
2. the infundibular stem or pituitary stalk, which is continuous distally with
3. the infundibular process or posterior pituitary gland (Fig. 15.1).

The adenohypophysis consists of:

1. the pars distalis or anterior lobe of the pituitary
2. the pars intermedia, the intermediate lobe
3. the pars tuberalis, which is a thin layer of adenohypophyseal cells lying on the surface of the infundibular stem and infundibulum.

The anterior pituitary does not normally receive an arterial vasculature but it receives blood through portal vessels. The

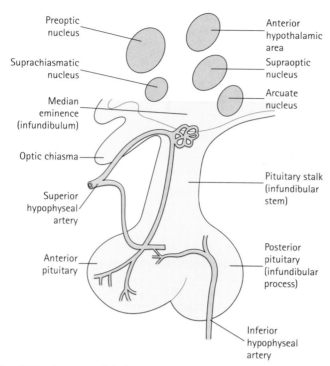

Fig. 15.1   Anatomy of the hypothalamus and pituitary.

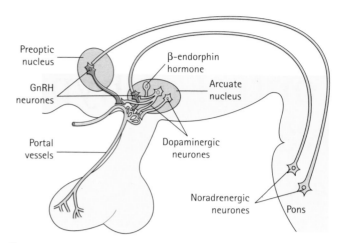

Fig. 15.2   Representation of neurochemical interactions which are important in the control of gonadotrophin-releasing hormone (GnRH) secretion.

arteries supplying the median eminence and infundibular stalk empty into a dense network of capillaries, which are heavily innervated and drain into the portal venous plexus. In the human these are present on all sides of the infundibular stalk, particularly posteriorly. These lead to the anterior pituitary formed by vessels from the median eminence and upper stalk joined ventrally by the short portal vessels arising in the lower infundibular stalk. Some 80–90% of the blood supply to the anterior pituitary is provided by the long portal vessels; the remainder comes from the short portal veins. The sinusoids of the adenohypophysis thus receive blood that has first traversed capillaries residing in the neurohypophyseal complex and this unique relationship provides the basis for the view that the hypothalamus regulates the secretion of adenohypophyseal hormones through neurohormonal mechanisms involving hypothalamic-releasing and -inhibiting factors.

Neural connections

There are numerous and extensive neural pathways connecting the hypothalamus with the rest of the brain. The majority of afferent hypothalamic nerve fibres run in the lateral hypothalamic areas whilst efferent pathways are more medially placed. One important efferent connection is the supraopticohypophyseal nerve tract carrying fibres from the supraoptic and paraventricular nuclei to the infundibular process of the pituitary, whilst other fibres carry hypothalamic-releasing or -inhibiting factors from the medial and basal parts of the hypothalamus to the anterior pituitary (Fig. 15.2).

The gonadotrophin-releasing hormone (GnRH) secreting neurones appear in the medial olfactory placode and enter the brain with the nervus terminalis, a cranial nerve that projects from the nose to the septal preoptic nuclei in the brain. The cells that produce GnRH thus originate from the olfactory area and migrate to their final positions. Failure of this migration has now been shown to occur in Kallmann's syndrome, resulting in a failure of both GnRH secretions and of smell, i.e. anosmia (Schwanzel-Fukunda et al 1989).

HYPOTHALAMIC REGULATION OF PITUITARY SECRETION

Considerable efforts have been made in the past 25 years to identify, characterize and synthesize the substances thought to be produced in the neural elements of the infundibulum. Several substances which can either stimulate or suppress the rate of release of one or more hormones from the pituitary gland have been found in the infundibular complex. These can be classified into hypophysiotrophic, neurohypophyseal and pituitary peptide hormones and are listed in Box 15.1. Other substances will probably be added to this list in the future.

Further discussion in this chapter will be restricted to the roles played by GnRH, dopamine and other neurotransmitters controlling the rates of release and synthesis of the gonadotrophins.

GnRH

In 1971 Schally and co-workers isolated pure preparations of porcine luteinizing hormone-releasing hormone (LHRH) from hypothalamic extracts and subsequently its structure was discovered and synthesis was achieved (Matsuo et al 1971a,b). The finding of follicle-stimulating hormone (FSH)-releasing activity of this LHRH led to the hypothesis of a single hypothalamic releasing hormone, gonadotrophin-releasing hormone (GnRH), controlling secretion of both luteinizing hormone (LH) and FSH from the pituitary gland, with the suggestion that sex steroids might play a role in modulating the proportions of LH and FSH released. The amino acid sequence of GnRH is shown in Figure 15.3.

Box 15.1   Hypothalamic and pituitary hormones

Hypophysiotrophic hormones
Gonadotrophin-releasing hormone   GnRH
Thyrotrophin-releasing hormone   TRH
Corticotrophin-releasing hormone   CRH
Growth hormone-releasing hormone   GHRH
Somatostatin
Prolactin-inhibiting factor   PIF

Neurohypophyseal products
Vasopressin
Oxytocin
Neurophysin I and II

Pituitary peptide hormones
Adrenocorticotrophic hormone   ACTH
β-Endorphin
α-Melanocyte-stimulating hormone
Prolactin   PRL
Luteinizing hormone   LH
Follicle-stimulating hormone   FSH
Growth hormone   GH
Thyroid-stimulating hormone   TSH

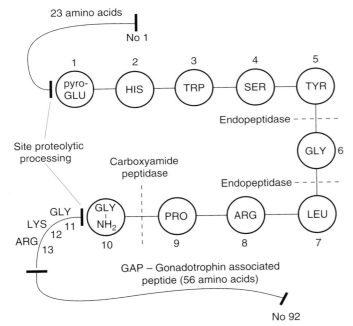

Fig. 15.3   The structure of pre-pro-GnRH. Highlighted is the decapeptide of the active molecule GnRH (mol wt. 1181). Sites of cleavage from the gonadotrophin-associated peptide (GAP) are shown, as well as the main sites of enzymatic degradation of GnRH by endo- and carboxyamide-peptidases in the pituitary.

GnRH neurone system

The GnRH neurone system has been mapped in detail, using primarily immunocytochemical methods. The GnRH neurones are not grouped into specific nuclei but form a loose network in several anatomical divisions. However, GnRH neurone bodies are found principally in two areas: the preoptic anterior hypothalamic area and the tuberal hypothalamus, particularly the arcuate nucleus and periventricular nucleus. Axons from GnRH neurones project to many sites in the brain; the most distinct tract is from the medial basal hypothalamus to the median eminence where extensive plexuses of boutons are found on the primary portal vessels. GnRH, then, has ready and direct access to the anterior pituitary gonadotroph cells via the portal capillary plexus (see Fig. 15.2). There are also numerous projections of GnRH-secreting neurones to the limbic system and the circumventricular organ, other than the median eminence. The role of these connections is currently unknown, but they may connect with other cells or GnRH may bind to different receptors (type II) which may modulate sexual behaviour or arousal.

The GnRH terminals in the median eminence remain outside the blood–brain barrier and thus can be exposed to chemical agents within the general circulation. The GnRH neurones have themselves receptors for a number of neuro-transmitters, in common with other neurones, and release them also in their contacts with other neurones. In addition, their activity and release of GnRH can be influenced by GnRH agonists and antagonists. Exposure to GnRH agonist causes a greater release of GnRH but at less frequent pulse intervals. Exposure to GnRH antagonists induces a slower and non-pulsatile release of GnRH. Hence GnRH neurones have an internal feedback loop for control of GnRH release through receptors for their own secretory product.

It has been estimated that there may be as few as 1500 GnRH neurones dispersed within the hypothalamus, located pre-dominantly in the preoptic and mediobasal areas. Con-siderable reduction in number can occur without affecting pulsatile release of gonadotrophins. The pulsatile nature of gonadotrophin release is dependent upon small numbers of GnRH neurones working in synergy – the so-called 'pulse generators'.

Regulation of gonadotrophin secretion by GnRH

The GnRH gene sequence was first isolated by Seeburg & Adelman in 1984. The GnRH decapeptide is derived from the post-translational processing of a larger precursor molecule that has been termed pre-pro-GnRH. This appears to be a tripartite structure with a preceding 23-amino acid sequence, joined to the decapeptide GnRH, which is then attached via a 3-amino acid sequence, glycine (GLY)-lycine (LYS)-arginine (ARG), to a 56-amino acid terminal peptide, which is termed the gonadotrophin-associated peptide (GAP). The post-GnRH-decapeptide GLY-LYS-ARG 3-amino acid section is an important site for proteolytic processing. GAP itself is thought to have some prolactin-inhibiting properties (Fig. 15.3). GnRH genes are encoded from a single gene located on the shorter arm of chromosome 8.

Using radio-immunoassays, GnRH has been demonstrated in the hypophyseal portal blood from a number of animal species (Carmel et al 1976). Electrical stimulation of the preoptic area of the brain in female rats on the day of pro-oestrus increases the GnRH concentration in portal blood and the stimulus induces a marked release of LH from the anterior pituitary. In contrast, administration of antibodies against

GnRH prevents this electrically stimulated LH release. These data provide evidence favouring a cause-and-effect relationship between GnRH release by the hypothalamus and LH release by the anterior pituitary.

It is now firmly established that GnRH can stimulate the secretion of both LH and FSH in animals and humans. Following intravenous administration of synthetic GnRH a significant rise in serum LH will be seen within 5 minutes, and sometimes of FSH, reaching a peak within about 30 minutes, but FSH peaks are often delayed further. LH release has a linear log-dose relationship up to doses of 250 mg but no such relationship can be found for FSH.

In the female the magnitude of gonadotrophin release, particularly LH, in individuals varies with the stage of the menstrual cycle, being greatest in the preovulatory phase, less marked in the luteal phase and least in the follicular phase of any individual cycle (Shaw et al 1974, Yen et al 1972) (Fig. 15.4).

GnRH is thus the humoral link between the neural and endocrine components controlling LH and FSH release.

Mechanism of action of GnRH on pituitary cells

The first step in the action of GnRH on the pituitary gonadotroph is recognition of a specific receptor. The GnRH receptor complexes often form clusters and become internalized, then undergo degradation in the lysosomes. The receptor fragments then pass back rapidly to the surface of the cell. This recycling process is causally related to *upregulation* of the receptor by GnRH. GnRH receptors tend to be of 60 kDa, to be a glycoprotein and to have a transmembrane character of a complex nature with seven transmembrane domains. A negatively charged domain interacts predominantly with arginine (ARG) in position 8 of the GnRH molecule.

The transmembrane domains have many formats which are common to humans and other species and ligand-binding sites are fairly superficial within the receptor. In the human the C-terminal tail is lost on the type 1 receptor (as found in the pituitary) and thus once GnRH binds to the receptor, decoupling does not occur rapidly. This may be beneficial in allowing protracted LH release to occur.

Various GnRH agonists and antagonists have different binding ligands. An understanding of the site and mechanisms of binding to the GnRH receptor have allowed specific structural changes to be made to GnRH analogues to produce more potent pharmacological agents and to attempt to develop non-peptide antagonists.

Prolonged exposure to GnRH produces suppression of LH release, which is called *downregulation*, which is associated with reduced numbers of GnRH receptors. This phenomenon is vitally important in understanding the mechanism of action of the gonadotrophin-releasing hormone analogues.

The current generation of GnRH analogues in clinical use are agonistic analogues and initially produce supraphysiological levels of LH and FSH from multiple receptor activation. The analogues are predominantly modified in position 6, with replacement of the glycine with a number of D-amino acids. The structures of some of the more common analogues are shown in Table 15.1. The replacement of glycine in position 6 introduces a foreign amino acid which the endopeptidases in the pituitary are less able to degrade. In addition, many current GnRH agonistic analogues have a substitution in amino acid position 10 (GLY-NH$_2$) or the replacement of amino acid 10 by an NH-ethylamide group, thus interrupting the action of the carboxyaminopeptidase in degradation. Such changes result in an increased 'half-life' of the GnRH agonists to between 2 and 6 hours.

A number of GnRH antagonists (Table 15.1), with multiple amino acid substitution to the GnRH amino acid sequence have been produced. Two have entered clinical practice, particularly within the field of assisted reproduction treatments. They have a long half-life, are relatively hydrophobic and need to be given by daily or alternate day injections, but have a rapid and profound effect of suppressing gonadotrophin secretion within hours of administration. As better formulations and potentially orally active non-peptide antagonists become available, GnRH antagonists may replace agonistic analogues in long-term treatment indications, e.g. endometriosis, fibroids and, in the male, prostate cancer.

The binding of GnRH to its receptor induces a complex series of intracellular responses, which result in hormone secretion and biosynthesis of the α and β subunits of LH and FSH. In addition, dimerization of α and β subunits and the glycosylation processes are induced. The mechanism of action of GnRH is depicted in Figure 15.5. Within seconds of GnRH binding to and activating GnRH receptors on the pituitary gonadotrophs, intracellular free Ca2+ concentrations increase.

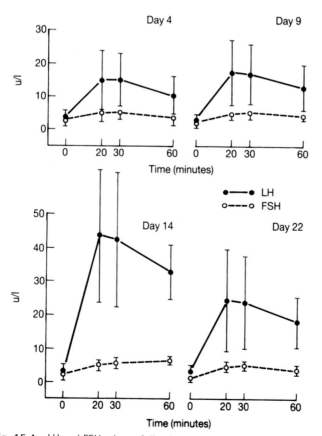

Fig. 15.4 LH and FSH release following 100 mg GnRH at different phases of the same menstrual cycle in six normal women (mean ± SD). From Shaw et al (1974).

Table 15.1   Some of the more common GnRH agonists now used in clinical practice and their amino acid sequence compared to native GnRH

	Amino acid position number									
	1	2	3	4	5	6	7	8	9	10
Native GnRH	pGlu	His	Trp	Ser	Tyr	Gly	Leu	Arg	Pro	Gly-NH₂
Decapeptide analogues										
Nafarelin						(D-Nal)₂				
Tryptorelin						D-Trp				
Goserelin						D-Ser (BUᵗ)			AzaGly-NH₂	
Nonapeptide analogues										
Buserelin						D-Ser (BUᵗ)			Pro-N-Et	
Leuprorelin						D-Leu			Pro-NEt	
Histrelin						D-His (Imbzl)			Pro-NEt	

B. Structure of GnRH and two GnRH antagonists

pGlu^1, His^2, Trp^3, Ser^4, Trp^5, Gly^6, Leu^7, Arg^8, Pro^9, Gly^{10}-NH₂

[N-Ac-D-Nal(2)^1, D-pCl-Phe^2, D-Trp^3, D-hArg(ET₂)^6, D-Ala^{10}] LHRH

[N-Ac-D-Nal(2)^1, D-pCl-Phe^2, D-Pal^3, Lys(Nic)^5, D-Lys(Nic)^6, Lys(iPr)^8, D-Ala^{10}]

GnRH
Deitirelix (Syntex)

This Ca2+ is initially mobilized from intracellular stores (e.g. endoplasmic reticulum) but also, to maintain sustained LH release, extracellular Ca2+ enters the gonadotroph through receptor-regulated voltage-dependent Ca2+ channels.

The initial mobilization of intracellular Ca2+ is induced by inositol triphosphate, released as a consequence of receptor activation of the membrane-bound phospholipase-C enzyme. Diacylglycerol is also released by the action of phospholipase-C and in turn activates the phosphorylating enzyme protein kinase C. The adenyl cyclase complex is also stimulated and cyclic adenosine monophosphate (cAMP) is generated. Ca2+, protein kinase C and cAMP all then interact to stimulate release of stored LH and FSH and subsequent biosynthesis (for review, see Clayton 1989).

MODULATORY ROLE OF MONOAMINES, OTHER NEUROTRANSMITTERS AND SECOND MESSENGERS ON GnRH SECRETION

Past studies indicated that LH release and ovulation were dependent upon drug-affected neural stimuli of both cholinergic and adrenergic origins. The infundibulum contains large stores of noradrenaline (norepinephrine), a lesser quantity of dopamine and a small amount of adrenaline (epinephrine) (Fig. 15.6).

Dopamine and norepinephrine are synthesized in nerve terminals by decarboxylation of dihydroxyphenylalanine (DOPA), itself derived from hydroxylation from tyrosine.

Dopamine

The hypothalamic tuberoinfundibular dopaminergic pathway is formed by neurones, with cell bodies located in the arcuate nucleus and axons which project to the external layer of the median eminence in close juxtaposition to portal vessels. The coexistence of dopamine- and GnRH-containing axons in the same region of the median eminence suggests the possibility of dopaminergic involvement in the control of gonadotrophin secretion.

The addition of dopamine to pituitaries coincubated with hypothalamic fragments increases the release of LH, while the addition of phentolamine, an α-receptor blocker, prevents dopamine-induced LH release. These early in vitro experiments suggested that the hormonal background was capable of

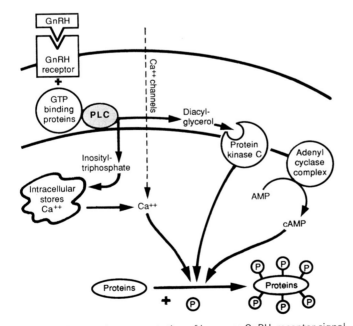

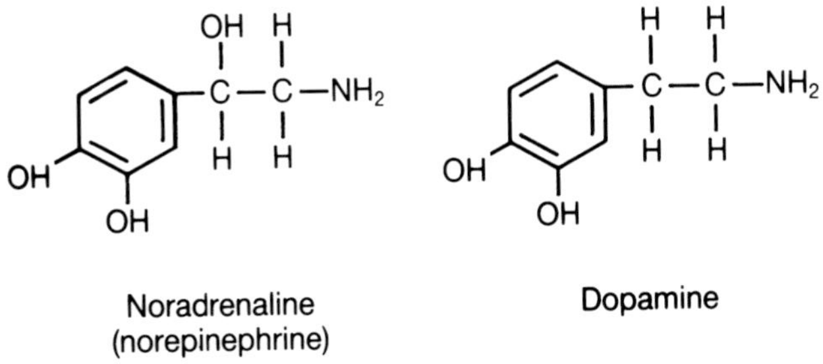

Fig. 15.5   Schematic representation of hormone GnRH–receptor signal activation. GTP, guanosine triphosphate; PLC, phospholipase-C enzyme; AMP, adenosine monophosphate; cAMP, cyclic AMP; P, phosphate group.

Noradrenaline
(norepinephrine)

Dopamine

Fig. 15.6   Chemical structure of biogenic amines.

modifying the response to dopamine, since it seemed ineffective in ovariectomized animals or during oestrus or dioestrus day 1 of the oestrous cycle. Dopamine was more effective at pro-oestrus or in oestrogen- and progesterone-primed rats (McCann et al 1974, Ojeda & McCann 1978).

In humans the inhibitory role of dopamine and its agonists on LH, as well as that of prolactin release, has been demonstrated (Lachelin et al 1977, LeBlanc et al 1976). Elevated levels of prolactin can also stimulate dopamine turnover in the hypothalamus and it is postulated that the stimulated dopamine secretion in turn alters GnRH secretion and hence reduces FSH and LH release. Hence dopamine in the human may principally have an inhibitory effect on GnRH secretion.

The contradictory roles played by dopamine in GnRH release are, in all likelihood, the consequence of more than one action of dopamine on the GnRH-secreting neurone. The steroid environment appears to modify the components involved in the dopaminergic control of GnRH secretion, with oestrogen appearing to affect the population of excitatory or inhibitory dopamine receptors and suggesting that the feedback control of GnRH output by oestrogen is partly exerted at a hypothalamic level by reducing dopamine neuronal activity.

Noradrenaline (norepinephrine)

Most experimental evidence supports a stimulatory role for noradrenaline in the control of gonadotrophin release. Turnover of hypothalamic noradrenaline is increased during the preovulatory surge of gonadotrophins at pro-oestrus and noradrenaline synthesis in the anterior hypothalamus is enhanced in ovariectomized rats. These effects on GnRH secretion appear to be mediated by α receptors, since phenoxybenzamine, an α blocker, suppresses the postcastration rise in gonadotrophins in male rats and phentolamine blocks the pulsatile release of LH in ovariectomized monkeys (for review, see McCann & Ojeda 1976).

Selective blockade of noradrenaline synthesis prevents the preovulatory LH surge and that induced by gonadal steroids; the above data suggest that noradrenergic terminals in the preoptic or anterior hypothalamic area synapse with GnRH neurones involved in the control of the preovulatory surge of gonadotrophins.

Serotonin

High concentrations of serotonin are found in the median eminence, with most of the serotonin-containing neurones originating from the raphe nucleus in the midbrain–pons area. Present evidence shows that serotonin plays a predominantly inhibitory role in gonadotrophin release (see McCann & Ojeda 1976).

Endogenous opioids

Endogenous opioids play a central role in the neural control of gonadotrophin secretion, by way of an inhibitory effect on hypothalamic GnRH secretion. These are a fascinating group of peptides, endorphins being the name coined to denote a substance with morphine-like action, of endogenous origin, in the brain. Endorphin production is regulated by gene transcription and since these are precursor peptides, all opioids are derived from three precursor peptides.

- pro-opiomelanocortin (POMC) is the source of endorphins
- pro-enkephalin A and B are the source of enkephalins
- pro-dynorphin yields dynorphins.

A single injection of morphine, administered to oophorectomized monkeys, brings about immediate cessation of GnRH pulse generation (Yen et al 1985). Hypothalamic opioidergic neurones are found in the actuate nucleus of the medial basal hypothalamus, in close contact with GnRH neurones. The administration of an opioid antagonist, naloxone, produces an increased frequency and amplitude of GnRH and LH secretion. These changes are most marked in the luteal phase of the cycle and it is thought that the negative feedback of oestrogen may partly be effected through opioid-induced inhibition of GnRH secretion (Ropert et al 1981).

OTHER NEUROTRANSMITTERS AND SECOND MESSENGERS

Other neurotransmitters may play a less important role in the regulation of GnRH neurones. Acetylcholine and γ-aminobutyric acid stimulate LH release. Both these agents are far more common as neurotransmitting agents than dopamine or noradrenaline (norepinephrine) in central nervous system nerve terminals in general, but their importance in GnRH neuronal activity seems to be less than that of dopamine and noradrenaline.

Prostaglandins

The role of prostaglandins in brain function is not clear, but the brain can synthesize and release prostaglandins and they do modify the adenyl cyclase-AMP system in central and peripheral neurones. Prostaglandins, particularly those of the E series, can induce gonadotrophin release in several species and prostaglandin synthetase inhibitors, e.g. indomethacin, block steroid-induced LH release (Ojeda & McCann 1978). Prostaglandin E is found in the median eminence in greater quantity than the rest of the medial basal hypothalamus; this distribution is consistent with the concept of its physiological role in the neural control of pituitary function.

The role played by prostaglandin E in GnRH release from hypothalamic secretory neurones appears to be an intracellular one. Activation of noradrenaline (norepinephrine) release from nerve terminals synapsing with GnRH neurones stimulates postsynaptic production of prostaglandin E which in turn enhances the release of GnRH. The prostaglandin E effect may either be a direct one or be mediated by a cyclic nucleotide.

Inhibins and activins

A group of compounds isolated from developing follicles, termed inhibins and activins, are now thought to be important in the control of FSH secretion from the pituitary. In addition, they play an important role in the paracrine regulation of androgen production in the ovary, with activins having an

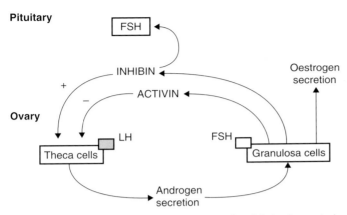

Fig. 15.7 Presumed interactions of inhibin and activin in the control of pituitary and ovarian hormone production.

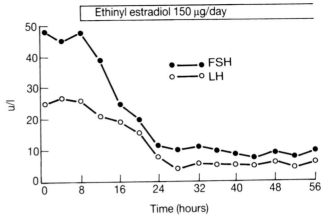

Fig. 15.8 The negative feedback effect of oestrogen on serum LH and FSH in a postmenopausal woman (Shaw 1975, unpublished data).

effect on granulosa cells. The nature of these gonadal inhibins has recently been clarified and they are shown to be composed of α and β subunits derived from separate genes. FSH secretion is suppressed by the α-β heterodimer and stimulated by the β homodimer, activin (Vale et al 1990). The molecular weight of the α subunit is approximately 18 000 Da, and that of the beta A and beta B subunits is 14 000 Da. The secretory patterns and the role of inhibins and activins throughout the menstrual cycle in the human have yet to be precisely elucidated (Fig. 15.7).

The control of GnRH secretion is thus highly complex and dependent upon a number of inhibitory and excitatory pathways involving various neurotransmitters. The control mechanisms are further complicated by the role of ovarian steroids in altering GnRH release and in modifying pituitary responsiveness to GnRH.

MODULATORY EFFECT OF OVARIAN STEROIDS

Negative feedback

Negative feedback control or inhibition of pituitary LH and FSH release has been postulated since 1932, when Moore & Price considered that the ovary and adenohypophysis were linked in a rigid system of hormonal interactions. The quantitative relationship between ovarian steroids and gonadotrophin release can be demonstrated by disturbing the negative feedback loop by oophorectomy which produces, over a period of days, an increase in circulating LH and FSH; this reaches a plateau at about 3 weeks with levels which are some 10 times preoperative values. Alternatively the administration of exogenous oestrogens to oophorectomized or postmenopausal women will result in rapid suppression of elevated circulating gonadotrophin levels (Fig. 15.8).

The negative feedback changes result from both a direct pituitary site of action of oestradiol, with a decrease in sensitivity of the gonadotroph to GnRH (McCann et al 1974), and an action within the hypothalamus and a decrease in GnRH secretion, possibly via increased inhibitory dopaminergic and opiate activity.

The threshold for the negative feedback action of oestrogen is set to bring about suppression of gonadotrophin release with

relatively small increases in oestradiol-17β in the normal female. This negative feedback loop is the main factor which maintains the relatively low basal concentrations of plasma LH and FSH in the normal female. Circulating levels of oestradiol-17β within the range of 100–200 pmol/l will suppress the early follicular phase gonadotrophin rise which initiates follicular development.

A negative feedback effect of progesterone on gonadotrophin secretion is now well established. Whilst progesterone, even in large doses, has little effect on baseline LH release, it can suppress the ovulatory surge of LH, as demonstrated in human females administered synthetic progestogens (Larsson-Cohn et al 1972), and oestrogen-induced positive feedback surges cannot be produced during the luteal phase in women (Shaw 1975). The principal negative feedback action of progesterone is thus upon the midcycle gonadotrophin surge and it may be responsible for its short 24-hour duration. It also seems likely that progesterone is an important factor in the reduced frequency of gonadotrophin pulses observed during the luteal phase of the cycle when compared to their frequency in the follicular phase (see below).

Positive feedback

The fact that under certain circumstances oestrogen may stimulate (positive feedback) rather than inhibit gonadotrophin release was first proposed by Hohlweg & Junkmann (1932). Their proposal has since been substantiated by numerous experimental reports in animals and humans. Under physiological conditions the positive feedback operates only in females; it is brought about by oestrogen and appears to be an essential component in producing the midcycle ovulatory surge of gonadotrophins. Administration of estradiol-17β to females during the early or midfollicular phase of the cycle will induce a surge of gonadotrophins (Shaw 1975, Yen et al 1974) (Fig. 15.9), but treatment with the same doses of oestrogen during the midfollicular phase induces a far greater release of LH than during the early follicular phase (Yen et al 1974). Studies on the dynamics of this positive feedback response to oestrogen, observed in greatest detail in the rhesus

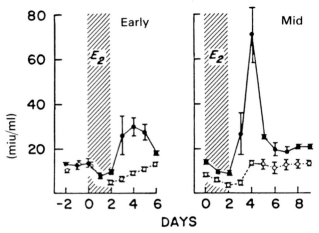

Fig. 15.9 The positive feedback effect of exogenous oestrogen (E_2 = 200 μg ethinyl estradiol/day) on gonadotrophin release; qualitative differences in the early and midfollicular phase of the cycle. •, LH; ○, FSH. From Yen et al (1974) with permission.

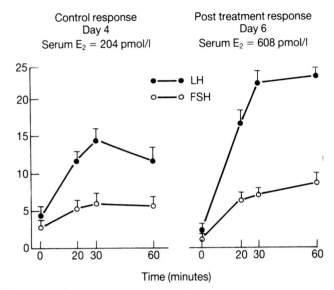

Fig. 15.10 Oestrogen augmentation of pituitary response to 100 mg GnRH bolus in four women receiving 2.5 mg estradiol benzoate IM, 2 hours after initial control response on day 4 of cycle and retested 48 hours later on day 6 of cycle. From Shaw (1975).

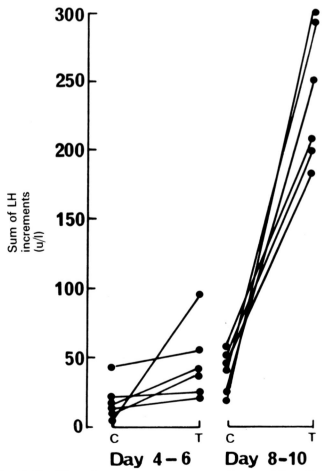

Fig. 15.11 Effect of progesterone pretreatment (12.5 mg IM) on LH response to 100 mg GnRH IV during the early and midfollicular phases of the cycle, showing the increased priming effect of oestrogen. C, control; T, after progesterone. Modified from Shaw et al (1975b).

monkey, demonstrate an activation delay of some 32–48 hours from the commencement of oestrogen administration until the onset of the positive feedback-induced gonadotrophin surge; a minimum threshold level to be exceeded and a strength–duration aspect of the stimulus (Karsch et al 1973).

Oestrogen elicits gonadotrophin release by increasing pituitary responsiveness to GnRH and possibly by stimulating increased GnRH secretion by the hypothalamus. In the normally menstruating female, oestrogen pretreatment produces an initial suppressive action on pituitary responsiveness (Shaw et al 1975a) followed by a later augmenting action which is both concentration and duration dependent (Shaw et al 1975a, Young & Jaffe 1976). The augmenting effect of oestrogen on GnRH pituitary responsiveness is demonstrated in Figure 15.10.

These data and others suggest that the midcycle oestrogen-induced surge of gonadotrophins may occur without any increased output of hypothalamic GnRH being necessary and indeed, this occurs in patients with endogenous GnRH deficiency receiving pulsatile GnRH treatment at a constant rate.

Progesterone by itself does not appear to exert a positive feedback effect. However, when administered to females in whom the pituitary has undergone either endogenously induced or exogenously administered oestrogen priming, progesterone can induce increased pituitary responsiveness to GnRH (Shaw et al 1975b, Fig. 15.11). Since circulating progesterone levels are increasing significantly during the periovulatory period, this action may be of importance in determining the magnitude and duration of the midcycle gonadotrophin surge.

SELF-PRIMING OF THE PITUITARY GONADOTROPH BY GnRH

Results from in vitro experiments with pituitary cells in culture indicate that GnRH is not only involved in the release of stored

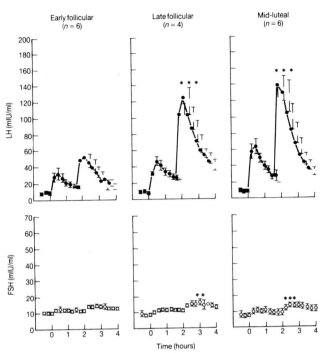

Fig. 15.12 Self-priming effect of bolus injection of GnRH: differing responses at different phases of the menstrual cycle. From Wang et al (1976), with permssion.

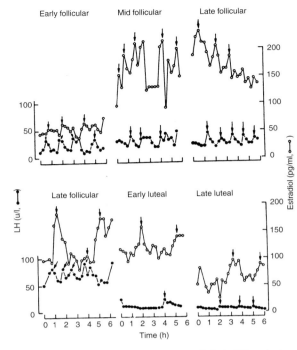

Fig. 15.13 Concentrations of LH and estradiol at different phases of the menstrual cycle, demonstrating different pulse frequency and amplitude. From Backstrom et al (1982), with permission.

LH and FSH but is of importance in maintaining the synthesis of gonadotrophins within the gonadotroph. Hence repeated exposure to GnRH of the gonadotrophin-producing cells seems essential for the maintenance of adequate pituitary stores.

Rommler & Hammerstein (1974) first demonstrated that the response to a second injection of GnRH was greater than the initial response in females, when they were retested 1–4 hours following the first exposure. This response has been termed 'self-priming'.

Wang and co-workers (1976) published more intensive studies, carried out throughout the menstrual cycle, and were able to demonstrate that self-priming had a definite cycle relationship which was greatest in the late follicular phase and around midcycle, i.e. at times of increased circulating oestrogen levels, and that oestrogen preferentially induces LH rather than FSH release (Fig. 15.12).

This self-priming effect of GnRH is of importance in understanding the physiological control mechanism of gonadotrophin release. It suggests that there are two pools of gonadotrophins, one readily releasable by initial exposure to GnRH and a second reserve pool. The exposure of this larger reserve pool to GnRH allows it to be more readily released by a subsequent exposure to GnRH and is suggestive of a transfer of gonadotrophins from one pool to the other. The stage of the cycle, i.e. the prevailing environment of endogenous sex steroids, which are the modulators, and the degree of GnRH stimulation which is the prime controller, together influence these transfer capabilities and sensitivity of the pituitary in its response to GnRH.

PULSATILE NATURE OF GONADOTROPHIN RELEASE

The pulsatile nature of hypothalamic GnRH release is now known to determine episodic pituitary gonadotrophin secretion.

This pulsatile pattern of GnRH concentration has been reported in the pituitary stalk effluent of the rhesus monkey (Carmel et al 1976). This suggests that the pulsatile pattern of gonadotrophin release from the anterior pituitary is probably causally related to the periodic increase in the hypothalamic GnRH system.

Further support for this hypothesis is obtained from the facts that antisera to GnRH abolish the pulsatile release of gonadotrophins and that pulsatile LH release can only be reinstated by pulsed delivery of GnRH and not by constant infusion.

Comparison of the pulsatile pattern of gonadotrophin release at different phases of the menstrual cycle demonstrates profound modulation by ovarian steroids (Fig. 15.13).

In hypogonadal subjects, pulses exhibit high amplitude and high frequency with reversal of the LH:FSH ratio. However, the higher circulating level of FSH is probably not due to a higher FSH secretory rate but rather to an accumulation related to its slower clearance rate (longer half-life).

In females with normal cycles, a characteristic low-amplitude, high-frequency pulse pattern is observed during the follicular phase. This suggests that oestrogen appears to be most effective in reducing the amplitude of gonadotrophin pulses, more markedly in FSH and LH. In contrast, the pulse pattern during the luteal phase is one of high amplitude and low frequency, probably modified by progesterone effects,

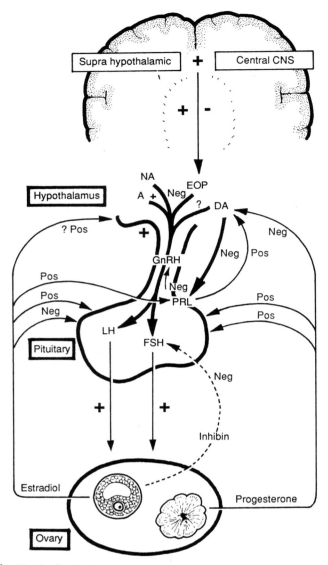

Fig. 15.14 Feedback control mechanisms in the hypothalamic-pituitary-ovarian axis. CNS, central nervous system; NA, noradrenaline (norepinephrine); A, adrenaline (epinephrine); EOP, endogenous opioids; PRL, prolactin; DA, dopamine; GnRH, gonadotrophin-releasing hormone; LH, luteinizing hormone; FSH, follicle-stimulating hormone.

on the catecholaminergic and GnRH neurone systems (Fig. 15.13).

INTEGRATIVE CONTROL OF THE HYPOTHALAMIC-PITUITARY UNIT DURING THE MENSTRUAL CYCLE

How can the complex interrelated changes in ovarian steroids and pituitary gonadotrophins that occur within each menstrual cycle be explained on the basis of our present understanding of the control of the hypothalamic pituitary unit (Fig. 15.14)?

LH and FSH are released from the anterior pituitary in an episodic, pulsatile manner and the available evidence supports a hypothalamic mechanism for this pulsatile release. Both estradiol-17β and progesterone can induce a positive feedback

release of gonadotrophins, in many respects comparable to that seen at midcycle, but progesterone can only produce its effect on a previously oestrogen-primed pituitary gland. There is presumptive evidence that these positive feedback stimuli also involve a direct pituitary action, with alteration in sensitivity to GnRH preceding an induced increase in hypothalamic release of GnRH.

The pattern of gonadotrophin release from the pituitary in response to repeated pulses of submaximal dose of GnRH or constant low-dose infusion over several hours suggests the presence of two functionally related pools of gonadotrophins. The first primary pool is immediately releasable, while the secondary pool requires a continued stimulus input and represents the effect of GnRH on synthesis and storage of gonadotrophins within the pituitary cell. The sizes or activity of these two pools represent pituitary sensitivity and reserve respectively which vary throughout the cycle and are regulated by the feedback action of ovarian steroids and by the self-priming action of GnRH itself. Oestradiol preferentially induces the augmentation of reserve and impedes sensitivity to GnRH, with a differential effect apparent for LH release. This estradiol effect is both dose and time related.

Follicular phase

In the early follicular phase, both the immediately releasable and the reserve pool of gonadotrophins are at a minimum. The increased FSH release, responsible for initiating follicle development, must indicate an increased output of GnRH, with the lowering of negative feedback action in the presence of low levels of oestrogen and progestogen. As follicles develop, oestrogen levels rise and the negative feedback action of oestrogen on GnRH increases, suppressing FSH levels.

With these progressive increases in estradiol throughout the midfollicular phase, the quantitative estimates of the primary, immediately releasable, pool of gonadotrophins increase slightly, whilst the reserve pool increases greatly, thus demonstrating the augmentation action of estradiol primarily upon the reserve pool. Since there is no marked increase in circulating gonadotrophin levels during this phase, secretion of GnRH must be minimal or else there is evidence of impedance of GnRH sensitivity by oestrogen.

Mechanism for preovulatory gonadotrophin surge

During the late follicular phase there is an increase in the amount of oestradiol secreted by the ovary. Under this influence, the sensitivity of the gonadotroph to GnRH eventually reaches a phase when GnRH can exert its full self-priming action. The consequence is the transference of gonadotrophins from the secondary reserve pool to the releasable pool. The increased pituitary responsiveness to GnRH may be further enhanced by the slight progesterone rise which can affect its action on a fully oestrogen-primed anterior pituitary. These changes culminate in the production of the ovulatory gonadotrophin surge. It is possible that these events could occur even if the gonadotrophs were exposed to a constant level of GnRH. However, an increased secretion of GnRH, as reported in rhesus monkeys and rats (Sarker et al 1976), at midcycle, which would act synergistically with the changes in pituitary sensitivity, seems likely also in the human.

The LH and FSH surges begin abruptly (LH levels doubling over 2 hours) and are temporarily associated with attainment of peak oestradiol-17β levels. The mean duration of the LH surge is 48 hours, with an ascending limb of 14 hours which is accompanied by a decline in estradiol-17β and 17-hydroxyprogesterone concentrations but a sustained rise in inhibin levels.

The ascending limb of LH is followed by a peak plateau of gonadotrophin levels lasting some 14 hours and a transient levelling of progesterone concentrations. The descending limb is long, lasting about 20 hours, and accompanying this is a second rise in progesterone, a further decline in estradiol-17β and 17-hydroxyprogesterone and a rise in inhibin levels.

The concentration of inhibin during the periovulatory interval is not correlated with estradiol-17β or progesterone changes. It may merely reflect the release from follicular fluid of stored inhibin.

Ovulation occurs 1–2 hours before the final phase of progesterone rise or 35–44 hours from the onset of the LH surge.

Luteal phase

The significantly lower basal gonadotrophin secretion in the face of high pituitary capacity during the midluteal phase suggests that endogenous GnRH should be very low.

A progressive decrease in sensitivity and reserve characterizes pituitary function during the late luteal phase and into the early follicular phase of the next cycle. This is probably due to a progressive decline in oestrogen and progesterone on which sensitivity and reserve are dependent. The role played by the proposed ovarian inhibin on preferentially controlling FSH secretion has still to be determined.

It is therefore apparent that the functional state of the pituitary gonadotroph as a target cell is ultimately determined by the modulating effect of ovarian steroid hormones via their influence on the gonadotroph's sensitivity and reserves and upon the hypophysiotrophic effect of GnRH.

With such a complex interrelated control mechanism, it is perhaps not surprising that many drugs which affect neurotransmitters or ill health or associated endocrine disorders can disrupt normal hypothalamic-pituitary-ovarian function, resulting in disordered follicular growth and suppression of ovulation.

KEY POINTS

1. The unique portal blood supply to the pituitary gland provides the basis of hypothalamic regulation of the pituitary secretion. It also explains the vulnerability of the gland to hypotension.
2. GnRH, secreted by neurones of the hypothalamus into the portal system, controls the release of both FSH and LH, with ovarian sex steroids playing the role in modulating the proportions of each hormone secreted.

KEY POINTS (CONTINUED)

3. The final step in the release of stored LH and FSH, and subsequent induction of further biosynthesis of both hormones following GnRH stimulation, involves Ca2+, protein kinase C and cAMP.
4. The control of GnRH secretion is highly complex and depends upon a number of inhibitory (dopamine, endorphins) and excitatory (noradrenaline (norepinephrine), prostaglandins) neurotransmitters, modulated by stimulation.
5. The response of the pituitary gland to exogenous GnRH depends upon the ovarian sex steroid environment prevailing and the degree of GnRH stimulation. Prolonged exposure to GnRH produces downregulation of LH release.

REFERENCES

Backstrom CT, McNeilly AS, Leak RM, Baird DT 1982 Pulsatile secretion of LH, FSH, prolactin, oestradiol and progesterone during the human menstrual cycle. Clinical Endocrinology 17:29–42

Carmel PD, Araki S, Ferin M 1976 Prolonged stalk portal blood collection in rhesus monkeys. Pulsatile release of gonadotrophin-releasing hormone (GnRH). Endocrinology 99:243–248

Clayton RN 1989 Cellular actions of gonadotrophin-releasing hormone: the receptor and beyond. In: Shaw RW, Marshall JC (eds) LHRH and its analogues – their use in gynaecological practice. Wright, London, pp19–34

Hohlweg W, Junkmann K 1932 Die hormonal-nervosae Regulierung der Funktion des Hypophysenvorderlappens. Klinische Wochenschrift 11:321–323

Karsch FJ, Weick RF, Butler WR et al 1973 Induced LH surges in the rhesus monkey: strength–duration characteristics of the oestrogen stimulus. Endocrinology 92:1740–1747

Lachelin GCL, LeBlanc H, Yen SSC 1977 The inhibitory effect of dopamine agonists on LH release in women. Journal of Clinical Endocrinology and Metabolism 44:728–732

Larsson-Cohn V, Johansson EDB, Wide L, Gemzell C 1972 Effects of continuous daily administration of 0.1mg of norethindrone on the plasma levels of progesterone and on the urinary excretion of luteinizing hormone and total oestrogens. Acta Endocrinologica (Copenhagen) 71:551–556

LeBlanc H, Lachelin GCL, Abu-Fadil S, Yen SSC 1976 Effects of dopamine infusion on pituitary hormone secretion in humans. Journal of Clinical Endocrinology and Metabolism 43:668–674.

Matsuo H, Arimura A, Nair RMG, Schally AV 1971a Synthesis of the porcine LH- and FSH-releasing hormone by the solid phase method. Biochemical and Biophysical Research Communications 45:822–827

Matsuo H, Baba Y, Nair RMG, Anmura A, Schally AV 1971b Structure of porcine LH- and FSH-releasing hormone. I The proposed amino acid sequence. Biochemical and Biophysical Research Communications 43:1334–1339

McCann SM, Ojeda SR 1976 Synaptic transmitters involved in the release of hypothalamic releasing and inhibiting hormones. In: Ehrenpreis S, Kopin I J (eds) Reviews of neuroscience, vol 2. Raven Press, New York, pp 91–110

McCann SM, Ojeda SR, Fawcett CP, Krulich L 1974 Catecholaminergic control of gonadotrophin and prolactin secretion with particular reference to the possible participation of dopamine. Advances in Neurology 5:435

Moore CR, Price D 1932 Gonad hormone function and the reciprocal influence between gonads and hypophysis. American Journal of Anatomy 50:13–72

Ojeda SR, McCann SM 1978 Control of LH and FSH release by LHRH: influence of putative neurotransmitters. Clinics in Obstetrics and Gynaecology 5:283–303

Rommler A, Hammerstein J 1974 Time-dependent alterations in

pituitary responsiveness caused by LH-RH stimulations in man. Acta Endocrinologica (Copenhagen) 21 (suppl):184

Ropert JR, Quigley ME, Yen SSC 1981 Endogenous opiates modulate pulsatile LH release in humans. Journal of Clinical Endocrinology and Metabolism 52:584–585

Sarker DK, Chiappa SA, Fink G 1976 Gonadotrophin releasing hormone surge in proestrus rats. Nature 264:461–463

Schally AV, Arimura A, Kastin A 1971 Gonadotrophin releasing hormone – one polypeptide regulates secretion of LH and FSH. Science 173:1036–1038

Schwanzel-Fukunda M, Bick D, Pfaff DW 1989 Luteinizing hormone-releasing hormone (LHRH) – expressing cells do not migrate normally in an inherited hypogonadal (Kallmann) syndrome. Molecular Brain Research 6:311–315

Seeburg PH, Adelman JP 1984 Characterisation of CDNA for precursor of human luteinizing hormone-releasing hormone. Nature 311:611

Shaw RW 1975 A study of hypothalamic-pituitary-gonadal relationships in the female. MD thesis, Birmingham University, Birmingham, UK.

Shaw RW, Butt WR, London DR, Marshall JC 1974 Variation in response to synthetic luteinizing hormone-releasing hormone (LHRH) at different phases of the same menstrual cycle in normal women. Journal of Obstetrics and Gynaecology of the British Commonwealth 81:632–639

Shaw RW, Butt WR, London DR 1975a Effect of oestrogen pretreatment on subsequent response to luteinizing hormone-releasing hormone (LH-RH) in normal women. Clinical Endocrinology 4:297–304

Shaw RW, Butt WR, London DR 1975b The effect of progesterone on FSH and LH response to LH-RH in normal women. Clinical Endocrinology 4:543–550

Vale W, Hsueh A, Rivier C, Yu J 1990 The inhibin, activin family of hormones and growth factors. In: Sporn MB, Roberts AB (eds) Peptide growth factors and their receptors II. New York, Springer-Verlag, pp 211–248

Wang CF, Lusley BL, Lein A, Yen SSC 1976 The functional changes of the pituitary gonadotrophs during the menstrual cycle. Journal of Clinical Endocrinology and Metabolism 42:718–724

Yen SSC, van den Berg G, Rebar R, Ehara Y 1972 Variations of pituitary responsiveness to synthetic LRF during different phases of the menstrual cycle. Journal of Clinical Endocrinology and Metabolism 35:931–934

Yen SSC, van den Berg G, Tsai CC, Siler T 1974 Causal relationship between the hormonal variables in the menstrual cycle. In: Ferin M et al (eds) Biorhythms and human reproduction. John Wiley, New York, pp 219–238

Yen SSC, Quigley ME, Reid RL, Cetel NS 1985 Neuroendocrinology of opioid peptides and their role in the control of gonadotrophin and prolactin secretion. American Journal of Obstetrics and Gynecology 152: 485–493

Young JR, Jaffe RB 1976 Strength duration characteristics of estrogen effects on gonadotrophin response to gonadotrophin-releasing hormone in women. II Effects of varying concentrations of estradiol. Journal of Clinical Endocrinology and Metabolism 42:432–442

16

Disorders of puberty

Adam Balen

INTRODUCTION

Puberty and adolescence are recognized as periods involving marked endocrine changes which regulate growth and sexual development. Normal pubertal development is known to be centrally driven and dependent upon appropriate gonadotrophin and growth hormone (GH) secretion and normal functioning of the hypothalamic-pituitary-gonadal axis. The mechanisms which control the precise timing of the onset of puberty, however, are still not clearly understood but are influenced by many factors including general health, nutrition, exercise, genetic influences and socio-economic conditions (Rees 1993). Most of the changes during puberty are gradual, although menarche is a single event that can be dated in girls. Normal puberty involves a fairly regular sequence of events between the ages of 10 and 16 years and abnormal puberty can be defined as any disturbance in this. This chapter will provide an overview of the endocrine changes observed during normal pubertal development and will describe the factors believed to influence the tempo of puberty and ovarian maturation before discussing some of the conditions that result in disordered pubertal development.

In broad terms once a girl has passed menarche, she is potentially fertile and should be considered as a young woman. The degree of sexual and reproductive maturity is not always mirrored by emotional and psychological maturity and so consideration must be given to the particular needs of adolescent girls when they attend clinics and hospital with gynaecological problems.

It is recognized that adolescents have special needs. Adolescents with gynaecological problems also have additional needs and often require a degree of privacy and sensitive handling. Many of the gynaecological problems encountered relate to intimate bodily functions at a time when the individual is maturing sexually and having to deal with issues that are embarrassing and may be considered taboo. Furthermore, consideration should be given to ethnic and cultural differences and potential problems with communication, particularly as amongst the parents from ethnic minorities it is often the father and not the mother who can speak English. And so the need for interpreters and information written in different languages should be borne in mind.

During puberty and adolescence, the reasons why young women attend for consultation may be broadly subdivided as follows.

1. *Sexual health*: contraception, family planning, sexually transmitted disease.
2. *Pregnancy*: wanted and unwanted teenage pregnancy.
3. *Gynaecological complaints*: menstrual cycle dysfunction, pelvic pain, ovarian cysts and gynaecological pathology, which may occur at any stage during the reproductive years.
4. *Disorders of sexual development*: complex and rare endocrine and developmental disorders of sexual differentiation and puberty, including intersex conditions.

This chapter will deal largely with the fourth group, apart from when there is overlap with other chapters (see Chapters 14, 17 and 32).

PUBERTAL DEVELOPMENT

Puberty represents a period of significant growth, hormonal change and the attainment of reproductive capacity. Its onset is marked by a significant increase in the amplitude of pulsatile release of gonadotrophin-releasing hormone (GnRH) by the hypothalamus (Mauras et al 1996). This usually occurs between the ages of 8 and 13.5 years in girls and stimulates an increase in pituitary release of LH and FSH, which initially occurs as high-amplitude nocturnal pulses, though eventually both daytime and nocturnal pulsatile release are established (Delemarve et al 1991). FSH and LH in turn act upon the ovary to promote follicular development and sex steroid synthesis. Because endocrine activity is initially nocturnal there is no point in measuring gonadotrophin or sex steroid levels during the day.

In the female this period is characterized clinically by accelerated linear growth, the development of breasts and pubic hair and the eventual onset of menstruation (menarche) which occurs between the ages of 11 and 16 years in most women in the UK (Stark et al 1989). Menarche is often used as a marker of pubertal development as it is an easily identifiable event which can usually be dated with some accuracy. Adrenarche – the growth of pubic hair – is due to the secretion of adrenal androgens and precedes gonadarche by about 3 years. Thus prepubertal children often have pubic hair, although if pronounced this should be investigated to exclude pathological causes (see below). Whilst androgen secretion is essential, oestrogen secretion facilitates pubic hair growth.

In tandem with the onset of pulsatile GnRH secretion, there is an increase in the amplitude of GH pulses released by the pituitary. Evidence suggests that this amplification of GH secretion may be regulated by the pubertal increase in levels of both androgenic and oestrogenic hormones (Caufriez 1997, Mauras et al 1996). In addition to this action, sex steroids have been shown to stimulate skeletal growth directly and thus augment the role of GH in promoting somatic growth and development (Giustina et al 1997). During the adolescent growth spurt there is a greater gain in sitting height (mean 13.5 cm for girls and 15.4 cm for boys) than leg length (mean 11.5 cm for girls and 12.1 cm for boys) as the spurt for sitting height lasts longer (and is longer in boys). At this time there is a minimum rate of fat gain and maximum attainment of muscle bulk, with differential and opposite changes in boys and girls. Ossification of the skeleton, as measured in terms of 'bone age', is helpful in determining a child's progress through puberty and as a determinant of final stature.

Rising concentrations of GH are also believed to exert some effects on circulating insulin levels although precise mechanisms are unclear. Some authors believe that GH induces peripheral insulin resistance which leads to compensatory increases in insulin secretion (Nobles & Dewailly 1992, Smith et al 1988). Increased levels of insulin during puberty may directly stimulate protein anabolism (Amiel et al 1991). Insulin also acts as a regulator of insulin-like growth factor-1 (IGF-1) through its effects on insulin-like binding protein 1 (IGFBP-1). IGF-1 is produced by hepatic cells under the influence of GH and has actions which stimulate cellular growth and maturation. IGFBP-1 competes with IGF receptors

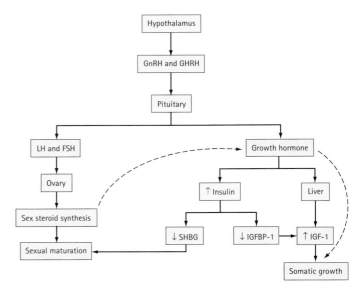

Fig. 16.1 Schematic representation of the endocrine changes which regulate pubertal development.

to bind IGF-1, thus inhibiting cellular action of IGF-1. Studies have indicated that insulin acts to suppress production of IGFBP-1 and therefore increases circulating IGF-1 bio-availability (Holly et al 1989, Nobles & Dewailly 1992). Insulin has also been shown to be a regulator of free sex steroids through the control of sex hormone-binding globulin (SHBG) production by the liver. Studies have shown that levels of SHBG decrease during puberty and that this fall parallels the rising levels of insulin (Holly et al 1989, Nobles & Dewailly 1992). The endocrine interactions involved in normal pubertal development are represented in a simplified diagram in Figure 16.1.

Tempo of pubertal development

Although the endocrine changes during puberty have become better understood, the exact 'trigger' which determines onset of pulsatile GnRH release, and thus the initiation of puberty, is still unclear. The question of which factors might regulate the onset of puberty and control the rate of pubertal development has prompted extensive research. The majority of studies examining young women have used age at menarche as the key marker of sexual maturity and have attempted to elucidate which factors are involved in the timing of this event.

The first physical sign of puberty in girls is breast development which occurs at an average age of 10–12.5 years old (Fig. 16.2). Age at onset of puberty is influenced by family history, race (earlier in Afro-Caribbeans) and nutrition (earlier in obese girls, with a secular trend to younger ages). Fifty per cent of girls show signs of breast development by the age of 11 years and investigations should be performed if there is no sign of breast development by the age of 14. In girls, the adolescent growth spurt occurs around 1 year after pubertal onset, while menarche occurs in the later stages of puberty at an average age of 12–15 years, at breast and pubic hair stage 4 (Figs 16.3, 16.4; Marshall & Tanner 1969). Oestradiol concentration affects both the uterus and skeletal maturity. Most girls begin to menstruate when their bone age is between 13

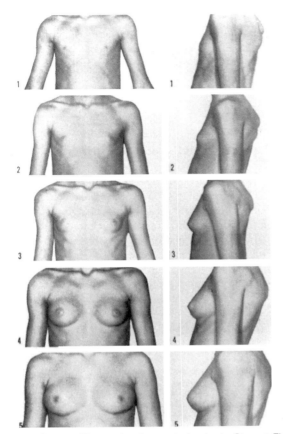

Fig. 16.2 Stages of breast development at puberty. **Stage 1** This is the infantile stage, which persists from the time the effect of maternal oestrogen on the breasts disappears, shortly after birth, until the changes of puberty begin. **Stage 2** The bud stage. The breasts and papillae are elevated as a small mound and there is an increase in the diameter of the areola. This stage represents the first indication of pubertal change in the breast. **Stage 3** The breasts and areola are further enlarged to create an appearance similar to that of a small adult breast, with a continuous rounded contour. **Stage 4** The areola and papilla enlarge further to form a secondary mound projecting above the contour of the remainder of the breast. **Stage 5** The typical adult breast with smooth rounded contour. The secondary mound present in stage 4 has disappeared.

and 14 years and fewer than 20% are outside these limits. The appearance of axillary hair may antedate the rest of puberty by a few years and does not bear a constant relationship to the development of breasts as, again, it is androgens and not oestrogens that are most significant. The apocrine glands of the axilla and vulva begin to function at the time when axillary and pubic hair is appearing.

It has long been recognized that early maturing women have a tendency to be heavier for their heights than their later maturing counterparts and, in contrast, that malnutrition and anorexia nervosa are associated with delayed menarche and amenorrhoea. These observed relationships between body weight and menarche led to the 'critical weight hypothesis' of Frisch & Revelle (1970) which hypothesized that attainment of a critical body weight led to metabolic changes which in turn triggered menarche. In further work, the

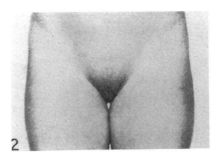

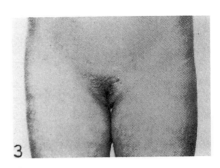

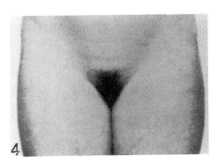

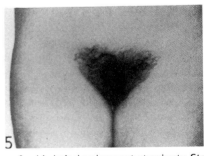

Fig. 16.3 Stages of pubic hair development at puberty. **Stage 2** Sparse growth of slightly pigmented hairs on either the labia or the mons pubis. **Stage 3** The hair is darker and coarser and spreads sparsely over and on either side of the midline of the mons pubis. **Stage 4** The hair is adult in character but covers a smaller area than in most adults and has not spread to the medial surface of the thighs. **Stage 5** Hair distributed as an inverse triangle and spreading to the medial surfaces of the thighs. It does not spread to the linea alba or elsewhere above the base of the triangle.

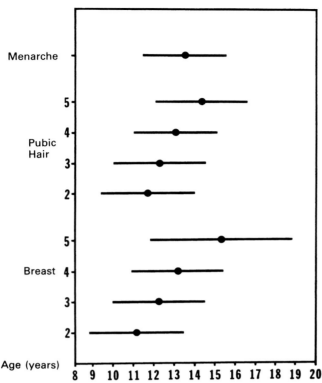

Fig. 16.4 Timing of pubic hair and breast changes and menarche. Horizontal line represents mean ±2 SD.

Breast stage	2 (9.2 – 13.2)	3 (10.2 – 14.2)	4 (10.8 – 15.6)	5 (11.8 – 18.6)
Pubic hair stage	2 (9.3 – 13.7)	3 (10.0 – 14.4)	4 (10.7 – 15.1)	5 (12.2 – 16.5)
Menarche		(11.2 – 14.8)		
Peak height velocity	(10.2 – 13.6)			

Age 10 ....11 ....12 ....13 ....14 15

Fig. 16.5 Timing of events in female puberty (95 percentiles for age in years).

investigators demonstrated that the ratio of lean body weight to fat decreased during the adolescent growth spurt in females from 5:1 to 3:1 at menarche, when the proportion of body fat was approximately 22% (Frisch 1990). They suggested that adipose tissue specifically was responsible for the development and maintenance of reproductive function, through its action as an extragonadal site for the conversion of androgens to oestrogens.

While few authors will dispute that nutrition and body weight play a role in pubertal development, the 'critical weight hypothesis' for menarche has not been supported by other studies. Cameron (1976) studied 36 British girls longitudinally, measuring weight and skinfold thickness at 3-month intervals for the 2 years premenarche to 2 years postmenarche. He postulated that if a 'critical body fatness' was the true explanation for onset of menarche, he should expect to detect

a reduction in the variability of his measurements at menarche compared with measurements taken before and after menarche and this was not demonstrated in his study. In a much larger study, Garn et al (1983) analysed the triceps skinfold distributions of 2251 girls collected during three national surveys in the United States. Comparing premenarcheal and postmenarcheal girls, they confirmed that those who had attained menarche were on average fatter than premenarcheal girls. However, there was a marked overlap in skinfold thickness for both groups and there was no evidence of a threshold level of fatness below which menarche did not occur. In a more recent study, de Ridder et al (1992) performed a longitudinal assessment of 68 premenarcheal schoolgirls, including pubertal staging, skinfold measurements, waist–hip ratios and blood samples for the monitoring of gonadotrophins. They did not demonstrate a relationship between body fat mass and the age at onset of puberty or age at menarche, but did find that a greater body fat mass was related to a faster rate of pubertal development.

Although the studies above dispute the association of age at menarche with the achievement of a threshold weight or body fat percentage, the association of earlier maturation in heavier girls still exists. Stark et al (1989) reported on data from 4427 girls who were part of the National Child Development Study cohort. Data relating to birth weight, age at menarche and weights and heights measured at 7, 11 and 16 years were available. The authors reported that a larger proportion of girls with early menarche (before the age of 11 years) were heavier for their height at all ages when compared with those with late menarche (after 14 years). Interestingly, however, changes in relative weight in the years preceding menarche (ages 7–11 years) were not strongly associated with age at menarche, whereas being overweight at the age of 7 years was much more strongly associated with an early age at menarche. Birth weight was not related to age at menarche. The authors concluded that the increase in weight for height associated with early maturation actually begins well before the onset of puberty. These findings were replicated by Cooper et al (1996) who examined 1471 girls in the MRC National Survey of Health and Development. They found that girls who were heavier at age 7 experienced an earlier menarche; however, contrary to Stark et al, they found that birth weight was related to age at menarche and that girls with heavier birthweights experienced menarche at a later age.

Intense exercise, such as long-distance running, ballet, rowing, long-distance cycling and gymnastics, is associated with delayed menarche in young girls and with amenorrhoea in older women (Baxter-Jones et al 1994, Frisch et al 1981, Malina et al 1976, 1978). These 'endurance' sports are associated with lower body weight and percentage fat. The extent to which menarche is 'delayed' has been shown to be related to the age at which participation in the sport begins and to the intensity of training (Frisch et al 1981). In view of the association between body weight and menarche described above, it is perhaps not surprising that girls participating in intense sporting activity experience a later age of menarche.

The influence of genetic factors on age at menarche is evident in the correlation demonstrated between mother–daughter and sister–sister pairs. Garn & Bailey (1978) analysed data from 550 mother–daughter pairs and reported a correlation of 0.25, which was adjusted to 0.23 once a correction was made for fatness. Similar correlation coefficients have been reported in other studies of mother–daughter pairs from European, African, and American populations (Benso et al 1989, Cameron & Nagdee 1996, Flug et al 1994, Malina et al 1994). The strength of this 'genetic effect', however, must be interpreted carefully as in most of these studies the mothers' age at menarche was based on recall, and the accuracy of the estimation is therefore questionable. In addition, we must consider the effect of similarity in socio-economic status (and hence nutrition and fatness) that is likely to exist between mothers and daughters and this in itself may contribute to similarity in menarcheal age.

The association between body weight and age at menarche has formed part of the basis for the explanation of the secular trend towards earlier menarche noted in the UK and other industrialized countries over the last century (Ostersehlt & Danker Hopf 1991, Roberts et al 1971). It has been generally accepted that this trend has reflected improvements in nutrition, health and environmental conditions. However, a recent plateau in this trend has been observed and even reversal in some countries, which is at present unexplained (Dann & Roberts 1993, Tryggvadottir et al 1994, Veronesi & Gueresi 1994). It has been suggested that the recent decrease in menarcheal age is related to changes in social conditioning in developed countries. Promotion of very thin women as 'ideal' role models through media and fashion has contributed to an increase in dieting in adolescent girls. Increasing participation of women in endurance sports which have intense training regimens may also be a factor related to lower body weight in young girls.

These studies all indicate that pubertal development and body weight are intrinsically linked. However, the mechanism for this relationship has not been conclusively defined. Insulin has been suggested as a modulator of the tempo of pubertal development through regulation of IGFBP-1 and SHBG (Holly et al 1989, Nobles & Dewailly 1992, Smith et al 1988). States of overnutrition and obesity are associated with increased serum concentrations of insulin (Parra et al 1971, Rosenbaum et al 1997). Therefore if excessive nutritional intake persists during childhood, it is possible that hyperinsulinaemia may lead to lower levels of IGFBP-1 and reduced SHBG concentrations, thus enhancing IGF-1 and sex steroid bioavailability. The converse would be true in states of malnutrition, where low levels of insulin would allow for the development of increased IGFBP-1 and SHBG levels.

However, it is still unclear whether hyperinsulinaemia in childhood is a result of obesity or if it is the cause of obesity. The role of genetic factors, which may determine insulin production and obesity risk in childhood, have also yet to be clearly explained. Recently there has been much interest in the actions of the newly identified hormone leptin which is produced by adipose tissue (Sorensen et al 1996). Serum concentrations of leptin – a 167 amino acid product of white fat – have been shown to be related to body fat mass and it is believed that leptin exerts its action on the hypothalamus to control calorie intake, decrease thermogenesis, increase levels of serum insulin and increase pulsatility of GnRH (Considine

et al 1996, Sorensen et al 1996). With these actions, leptin may potentially have a role in the hormonal control of pubertal development and some studies have shown that leptin levels do increase before the onset of puberty (Clayton et al 1997, Mantzoros et al 1997). It has been postulated that changes in circulating leptin levels may act as an initiator for the onset of puberty and that this may explain the relationships between body fat and maturation observed by Frisch & Revelle (1970). This hypothesis is supported by the recent work of Clement et al (1998) who identified a homozygous mutation of the leptin receptor gene which results in early-onset morbid obesity and the absence of pubertal development in association with reduced GH secretion. These findings suggest that increased leptin levels associated with gains in fat mass may signal the hypothalamus to act as an important regulator of sexual maturation. It is possible that future research may clarify the role of leptin and leptin receptors in pubertal development and may explain the variation in the timing of the onset of puberty between individuals.

Ovarian and uterine development

Development of primordial follicles and secretion of oestrogens may be regarded as the final common path in the hormonal activity of puberty and there is a close correlation between oestrogen levels and sexual maturation. The uterus grows in concordance with somatic growth, with differential increased growth of the corpus starting from about the age of 7 years. However, the main differential increase of uterine size compared with somatic growth is obvious only after oestradiol secretion is measurably increased and tends to occur between breast stages 3 and 4. Awareness of this comparatively late relative increase in uterine size has clinical relevance in the differentiation of arrested puberty and müllerian agenesis and also in the diagnosis of causes of precocious puberty. Blood oestrogen levels rise before and during puberty and continue to do so for about 3 years after menarche before the normal adult follicular levels of oestrogen are seen. This gradual maturation is a reflection of the finding that many of the early cycles are anovulatory and of the observation that the early postmenarcheal years are relatively infertile.

Ultrasound is the most suitable imaging technique for the examination of the internal genitalia of girls as it is free from the risks of radiation and involves a quick, quiet and non-invasive procedure. Whilst higher resolution images can be obtained of the ovaries and uterus using transvaginal ultrasonography, we can only use the transabdominal approach in young girls and it may not always be possible to visualize both ovaries; furthermore, a full bladder is required. None the less transabdominal ultrasonography is an invaluable tool for the delineation of normal changes before and through puberty and also the evaluation of paediatric disorders, such as pelvic masses and abnormal pubertal development. Ultrasonography can also be used in postmenarcheal girls to detect abnormal ovarian morphology and hence increase our understanding of common conditions such as the polycystic ovary syndrome (PCOS).

There are relatively few normal data on the maturation of the internal genitalia in girls and a paper by Holm et al (1995) provides cross-sectional data of a large cohort of 166 school girls and medical students. It was demonstrated that uterine and ovarian volumes increase in size prepubertally, from as early as the age of 6 years. Griffin et al (1995) have demonstrated similar changes from the age of 4 years and, in their study of 153 girls, included subjects as young as 3 days. It was found that uterine shape changes constantly throughout childhood from a pear to a cylindrical and finally to the adult heart shape.

As girls go through puberty the ovaries have been described as characteristically becoming multicystic due to low levels of FSH stimulating only partial folliculogenesis (Stanhope et al 1985). The multicystic appearance is also seen during resumption of ovarian activity after periods of quiescence, for example, in women who are recovering from weight-related amenorrhoea or those with hypogonadotrophic hypogonadism who are treated with pulsatile GnRH. The multicystic ovary differs from the polycystic ovary in that the cysts are larger (6–10 mm) and the stroma is of normal echogenicity. The morphological appearance of the polycystic ovary, on the other hand, requires the presence of at least 10 cysts (2–8 mm) per ovary in the presence of an echodense stroma (see Chapter 19).

Menarche

The first period occurs because there has been sufficient endometrial stimulation to result in a withdrawal bleed when there is a temporary fall in the oestrogen level. It can be associated with an ovulatory/corpus luteum sequence but this is not usual. The first menstruation simply indicates that a particular threshold has been reached in an already oscillating system but is an obvious outward sign and of significance: menarche denotes an intact hypothalamic–pituitary–ovarian axis, functioning ovaries, the presence of a uterus and patency of the genital tract.

Menarche generally occurs within 2 years of the earliest sign of breast development and within 1 year of peak growth velocity and close to breast stage 4, usually between the ages of 10 and 16 years.

PRECOCIOUS PUBERTY

Precocious onset of puberty is defined as occurring younger than 2 SD before the average age, i.e. <8 years old in females (compared with <9 years in males). Thus, in many girls early onset of puberty merely represents one end of the normal distribution. However, a number of pathological conditions may prematurely activate the GnRH-LH/FSH axis, resulting in the precocious onset of puberty. Furthermore, certain physical secondary sexual features (e.g. virilization without breast development) may occur in the absence of 'true puberty' (i.e. absent hypothalamic-pituitary activation) due to abnormal peripheral secretion of sex steroids.

True precocious puberty

The appearance of pubertal physical features follows the normal sequence ('consonance'), beginning with breast development. The diagnosis is made by the finding of elevated basal gonadotrophin levels and after stimulation with i.v.

Box 16.1   Causes of precocious puberty

Gonadotrophin dependent ('true' or 'central' precocious puberty)
- Idiopathic (family history, overweight/obese)
- Intracranial lesions (tumours, hydrocephalus, irradiation, trauma, encephalitis)
- Gonadotrophin-secreting tumours
- Congenital brain defects, third ventricle cysts, neurofibromatosis, hamartomas
- Hypothyroidism (autoimmune)
- Sexual abuse (rare)

Variants
- Premature thelarche (and thelarche variant)
- Adrenarche

Gonadotrophin independent
- Congenital adrenal hyperplasia (CAH)
- Cushing's disease
- Sex steroid-secreting tumours (adrenal or ovarian), chorion epithelioma
- McCune–Albright syndrome
- Exogenous oestrogen ingestion/administration

GnRH, the serum LH concentration is higher than FSH. It is important to consider intracranial pathology and arrange imaging if indicated. Pelvic ultrasound will reveal the presence of multicystic ovaries and a uterus that is developing adult proportions. Bone age will be advanced.

Premature thelarche

Premature breast development in the absence of other signs of puberty may present at any age from infancy. Breast size may fluctuate and is often asymmetrical. Bone maturation, growth rate and final height are unaffected. The cause is unknown. The diagnosis is made by the finding of elevated FSH levels (but not LH), both basal and post-GnRH stimulation. Ovarian ultrasound often reveals a single large, functional ovarian cyst. Serum oestradiol concentrations are usually low and bone age is unaffected. It is important to monitor carefully in order to exclude the onset of true precocious puberty.

Autoimmune hypothyroidism may also result in isolated breast development although this is rarely seen before the age of 5 years.

Thelarche variants

There appears to be a whole spectrum of presentations between premature thelarche and true precocious puberty. Thus, some girls with early breast development also demonstrate increased height velocity, bone maturation and ovarian ultrasound reveals a multicystic appearance (as distinct from polycystic – see Chapter 19).

Premature adrenarche

The normal onset of adrenal androgen secretion ('adrenarche') occurs 1–2 years prior to the onset of puberty. 'Premature' or 'exaggerated' adrenarche results in mild virilization (e.g. pubic hair and acne, but not clitoromegaly). The cause is unknown. The diagnosis is made by the finding of low serum gonadotrophin levels and mildly elevated adrenal androgen levels (DHEAS, androstenedione). It is important to exclude late-onset CAH and androgen-secreting tumours.

Congenital adrenal hyperplasia

Congenital adrenal hyperplasia (CAH) due to deficiency of the enzyme 21-hydroxylase leads to cortisol deficiency, ACTH oversecretion due to loss of feedback inhibition and excessive production of adrenal androgens (see also Chapter 12). Inheritance is autosomal recessive. Classic CAH usually presents in the neonate with ambiguous genitalia and a salt-losing crisis (see Chapter 15) whilst non-classic or late-onset CAH presents in adolescence with moderate to severe virilization (pubic hair, hirsutism, acne and clitoromegaly) and rapid growth.

The diagnosis is made by the finding of raised levels of cortisol precursors, particularly 17-OH progesterone, both at baseline and post i.v. ACTH stimulation, in both plasma and urine. Gonadotrophin levels are suppressed. Bilateral adrenal hyperplasia may be seen on abdominal US. Management of CAH is by hydrocortisone replacement therapy, which suppresses ACTH and adrenal androgen secretion (the classic presentation may also require fludrocortisone to replace aldosterone secretion).

Androgenization of the female external genitalia may lead not only to clitoromegaly but also fusion of the labioscrotal folds. There may in addition be a urethral fistula which may require careful repair at the time of an introitoplasty. Clitoral reduction should be undertaken with care to preserve the neurovascular bundle and sensation. Surgery may be undertaken during the neonatal period and may be required again during adolescence. As with all surgery for intersex disorders, the precise timing is open to debate as is the degree to which the patient – rather than her parents and physicians – is involved in the decision-making process.

Peripheral tumours

Sex steroid-secreting tumours
Abnormal production of androgens ± oestrogens may arise from tumours of the adrenal glands (adenomas or carcinomas), ovaries (granulosa cell or theca cell neoplasia) or teratomas. Androgen-secreting tumours are usually associated with severe virilization in young girls (<6 years old). The diagnosis is made by the finding of excessively raised circulating plasma sex hormone levels. A 24-hour urine collection for steroid profile often demonstrates excess levels of sex steroid metabolites. Gonadotrophin levels are suppressed and α-fetoprotein levels may be raised. These tumours are often palpable and an abdominal ultrasound scan will confirm the diagnosis.

Gonadotrophin-secreting tumours
Very rarely, an hCG-secreting hepatoblastoma, choriocarcinoma or dysgerminoma causes precocious puberty. Circulating levels of hCG are usually extremely high.

McCune-Albright syndrome

This sporadic condition results in spontaneous activation of gonadotrophin receptors and excessive sex steroid secretion independent of normal ligand binding. It is due to a somatic activating mutation of the G-protein α subunit which also affects bones (polyostotic fibrous dysplasia), skin (café au lait spots) and potentially multiple other endocrinopathies (hyperthyroidism or hyperparathyroidism). All cells descended from the mutated embryonic cell line are affected, while cells descended from non-mutated cells develop into normal tissues. Thus, the phenotype is highly variable in physical distribution and severity. The diagnosis is made by clinical assessment, based on the presence of skin, bone and other lesions. Biopsy of affected skin may allow identification of the genetic mutation. Gonadotrophin levels are suppressed.

Management of precocious puberty

It is important to exclude severe diseases (e.g. CAH, cranial or peripheral tumours) which will require specific therapy. Following reduction in peripheral sex steroid levels, due to CAH or sex steroid-secreting tumours, central precocious puberty may occur due to hypothalamic maturation (especially if the girl's bone age is already >11 years). Premature thelarche and thelarche variant need no treatment as there are no long-term consequences and, furthermore, treatment appears to be without effect.

Inhibition of puberty
Pituitary gonadotrophin secretion can be suppressed by constant high levels of a GnRH agonist, given by subcutaneous depot injection (e.g. leuprorelin acetate 3.5 mg monthly). Circulating sex steroid levels should become undetectable and LH and FSH levels post i.v. LHRH should return to prepubertal levels. The dose interval may need to be shortened to 3 weeks to fully suppress puberty.

Following investigation and reassurance, however, many older girls and their parents are happy to avoid treatment. The aims of stopping puberty are:

- to avoid psychosocial problems arising from early sexual maturation
- to prevent reduction in final adult height due to premature bone maturation and early epiphyseal fusion. A wrist X-ray for estimation of bone age is essential in the investigation of precocious puberty and may be used to predict final height when considering the need for treatment.

Androgen receptor blockade
Androgen receptor blocking agents, such as cyproterone acetate, finasteride or flutamide, may be used for symptomatic treatment of excess androgen production in girls with premature adrenarche.

DELAYED PUBERTY

Delayed puberty is defined as absence of onset of puberty by >2 SDs later than the average age, i.e. >14 years in females (compared to >16 years in males). Delayed puberty may be

Box 16.2   Causes of delayed puberty

General
- Constitutional delay of growth and puberty
- Malabsorption (e.g. coeliac disease, inflammatory bowel disease)
- Underweight (due to severe dieting/anorexia nervosa, overexercise or competitive sports)
- Other chronic disease (asthma, cystic fibrosis, renal failure)

Gonadal failure (hypergonadotrophic hypogonadism; see also Chapter 17)
- Turner's syndrome, gonadal dysgenesis and premature ovarian failure
- Post malignancy (following chemotherapy, local radiotherapy or surgical removal)
- Polyglandular autoimmune syndromes

Gonadotrophin deficiency
- Congenital hypogonadotrophic hypogonadism (±anosmia)
- Hypothalamic/pituitary lesions (tumours, post radiotherapy or surgery)
- Haemochromatosis/iron overload
- Rare inactivating mutations of genes encoding LH, FSH or their receptors

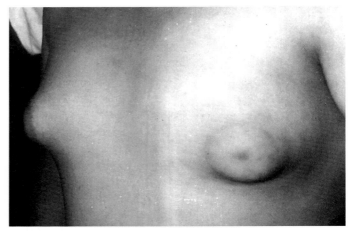

Fig. 16.6   Breast development in Turner's syndrome following oestrogen administration. There is good areolar development but little breast tissue after several years of hormone replacement.

idiopathic/familial or due to a number of general conditions resulting in undernutrition. Absence of puberty may also be due to gonadal failure (elevated gonadotrophin levels) or impairment of gonadotrophin secretion. Occasionally, some girls enter puberty spontaneously but then fail to progress normally through puberty.

Constitutional delay of growth and puberty

Rates of skeletal and sexual maturation are closely linked, but vary widely between individuals and are influenced by family history and rate of early childhood weight gain. Although constitutional delay presents more commonly in males, this may merely reflect their higher level of concern. These girls are otherwise healthy. The diagnosis is made by exclusion, but often can only be confirmed retrospectively following spontaneous initiation of the hypothalamic-pituitary axis. It can be very difficult to distinguish hypogonadotrophic hypogonadism from constitutional delay in puberty and therefore it is better to provide treatment and revisit the diagnosis at a later date. Appropriate investigations, after physical examination and measurement of weight and height, include assessment of serum concentrations of gonadotrophins, prolactin and thyroid function and an assessment of bone age (radial X-ray). Pelvic ultrasonography may be helpful as is a karyotype if features of Turner's syndrome are suspected.

Turner's syndrome

Characteristic features of Turner's syndrome may not be obvious, particularly if due to chromosomal mosaicism, and karyotype should be investigated in all girls presenting with pubertal delay. Up to 25% of girls with Turner's syndrome enter puberty spontaneously; however, only 10% progress through puberty and only 1% develop ovulatory cycles. Thus, the chromosomal abnormality seems to result in premature

ovarian exhaustion rather than a primary failure of ovarian development. Turner's syndrome is the commonest cause of gonadal dysgenesis. In its most severe form the XO genotype is associated with the classic Turner's features including short stature, webbing of the neck, cubitus valgus, widely spaced nipples, cardiac and renal abnormalities and often autoimmune hypothyroidism. Spontaneous menstruation may occur (particularly when there is mosaicism), but premature ovarian failure usually ensues.

The clinical diagnosis is confirmed by the finding of a 45XO karyotype (at least 30 cells should be examined due to the possibility of mosaicism). Cytogenetic analysis should also be performed looking for the presence of Y fragments, which indicate an increased risk of gonadoblastoma, and thus the 'streak' gonads should be removed (usually laparoscopically). Serum gonadotrophin concentrations are elevated compared with adolescents of the same age and may approach the menopausal range.

Management includes low-dose oestrogen therapy to promote breast development without further disturbing linear growth (Fig. 16.6). Treatment with growth hormone has also benefited some individuals. Cyclical oestrogen plus progestogen may be used as maintenance therapy. A regular withdrawal bleed is essential in order to prevent endometrial hyperplasia. Spontaneous conception has been reported in patients with Turner's syndrome, but is rare. However, the possibility of assisted conception and oocyte donation should be discussed at an early age.

Other causes of premature ovarian failure

Premature ovarian failure (POF), by definition, is the cessation of periods accompanied by raised gonadotrophin concentration prior to the age of 40 years. It may occur at any age. The exact incidence of this condition is unknown as many cases go unrecognized, but estimates vary between 1% and 5% of the female population (Coulam et al 1986). In approximately two-thirds of cases, the cause of ovarian failure cannot be identified (Conway et al 1996). It is unknown whether these cases are truly 'idiopathic' or due to as yet undiscovered genetic, immunological or environmental factors. A series of 323 women with POF attending an endocrinology clinic in London identified 23% with Turner's syndrome, 6% after chemotherapy, 4% with familial POF and 2% each who had pelvic surgery, pelvic irradiation, galactosaemia and 46XY gonadal dysgenesis (Conway et al 1996). Viral and bacterial infection may also lead to ovarian failure; thus infections such as mumps, CMV or HIV in adult life can adversely affect long-term ovarian function, as can severe pelvic inflammatory disease.

Ovarian failure occurring before puberty is usually due to a chromosomal abnormality or a childhood malignancy that required chemotherapy or radiotherapy, from which, parenthetically, there are increasing numbers of survivors into adulthood with POF. The likelihood of developing ovarian failure after therapy for cancer is difficult to predict but the age of the patient is a significant factor; the younger the patient, the greater the follicle pool and the better her chances of retaining ovarian function.

Adolescents who lose ovarian function soon after menarche are often found to have a Turner's mosaic (46XX/45X) or an X-chromosome trisomy (47XXX). There are many genes on the X chromosome that are essential for normal ovarian function. It would appear that two active X chromosomes are required during fetal life in order to lay down a normal follicle store. In fetuses with Turner's syndrome normal numbers of oocytes appear on the genital ridge but accelerated atresia takes place during late fetal life. Thus streak gonads occur and it is only the mosaic form of Turner's syndrome that permits any possibility of ovarian function. X mosaicisms are the commonest chromosomal abnormality in reported series of POF, ranging from 5% to 40% (Anasti 1998). Other X chromosome anomalies may result in ovarian failure; for example, balanced translocations in the long arm of chromosome X between Xq13 and q26, which is a critical region for ovarian function.

There are a number of syndromes that are associated with premature ovarian failure, such as familial blepharophimosis, in which the abnormality is on chromosome 3. Galactosaemia is another rare example, in which a metabolic defect has a direct inhibitory effect on ovarian function, probably due to a build-up of galactose within the ovary that decreases the initial number of oogonia.

Polyglandular autoimmune syndromes

Antiovarian antibodies are occasionally detected in both type 1 (hypoparathyroidism, Addison's disease, mucocutaneous candidiasis) and type 2 (Addison's disease, hypothyroidism, type 1 diabetes) polyglandular autoimmune syndromes. Autoimmune ovarian failure may also occur in the absence of positive antibodies due to poor sensitivity of current assays.

Congenital hypogonadotrophic hypogonadism

Congenital hypogonadotrophic deficiency associated with complete or partial anosmia ± other midline defects and mental retardation (Kallman or DeMorsier syndrome) may be inherited in autosomal dominant, recessive or X-linked recessive patterns, suggesting that a number of mutated genes

may be causative. Congenital hypogonadotrophism may also occur without anosmia in isolation or in pan-hypopituitarism. The diagnosis is made by a family history or related features of Kallman syndrome. Absent LH and FSH response to i.v. GnRH stimulation may be indistinguishable from constitutional delay of puberty and retesting may be required after completing pubertal development with exogenous oestrogen.

Management of delayed puberty

Following exclusion of other diagnoses, many patients are happy to await spontaneous pubertal development. However, severe delay in pubertal onset may be a risk factor for decreased bone mineral density and osteoporosis. In subjects with hypergonadotrophic hypogonadism puberty may be induced from any age; however, in Turner's syndrome delay in induction to around 14 years old possibly permits maximal response to growth hormone therapy.

Pubertal development

Oral oestrogen therapy should be commenced at a very low dose (e.g. ethinyloestradiol 2 µg daily) and gradually increased according to breast response and age. Oral progesterone should be added if breakthrough bleeding occurs or when ethinyloestradiol dose reaches 20 µg/day. Eventually maintenance therapy is provided either with a combined oral contraceptive pill or a conventional, cyclical postmenopausal hormone replacement preparation.

Fertility

In gonadotrophin deficiency, ovulation and fertility may be achieved by ovulation induction using either pulsatile GnRH (for hypothalamic problems) or gonadotrophin therapy (for pituitary or hypothalamic disease). If the patient with hypogonadotrophic hypogonadism is particularly anxious about future fertility a non-therapeutic trial of exogenous pulsatile GnRH administration, via a miniature portable infusion pump, confirms pituitary responsiveness. However, induction of ovulation can be achieved, bypassing the pituitary, by direct administration of human menopausal gonadotrophin (hMG). hMG is a more suitable choice than the more recently developed recombinant FSH preparations as it also contains LH which is necessary to stimulate oestrogen biosynthesis. Patients with premature ovarian failure may choose assisted conception with donated oocytes.

Box 16.3 Induction of puberty for girls with ovarian failure

Ethinyloestradiol	2 µg daily for 6 months
	5 µg daily for 6 months
	10 µg daily for 6 months
	15 µg daily for 6 months
	20 µg daily for 6 months
	30 µg daily for 6 months

Menstruation may occur once a 15 µg preparation is being used. Once bleeding occurs a cyclical oestrogen/progestogen preparation should be prescribed, usually in the form of the contraceptive pill.

PRESENTATION OF CONGENITAL ANOMALIES OF THE GENITAL TRACT (see also Chapter 14)

Disorders of sexual development may result in ambiguous genitalia or anomalies of the internal genital tract and may be due to genetic defects, abnormalities of steroidogenesis and dysynchrony during organogenesis. Age of presentation will depend upon the degree of dysfunction caused. Ambiguous genitalia occur in approximately 1:30 000 newborns. The rate with which other congenital anomalies present varies depending upon the population studied and the age at which the problem is likely to be noticed. Population-based statistics are still lacking for many conditions, largely because patients present to different specialists (e.g. gynaecologists, paediatric endocrinologists, urologists, etc.) and there are rarely clear pathways for communication between the different professional groups from which to create a comprehensive service for both provision of treatment and collection of data.

Patients require sensitive care by an expert multidisciplinary group that includes: gynaecologists, paediatric endocrinologists, paediatric surgeons and urologists, plastic surgeons, psychologists, specialist nurses, geneticists and urologists. A network of support should be provided to both the patient and her parents and family. The adolescent period is a particularly sensitive time as the individual becomes aware of her diagnosis and its impact on her sexuality, sexual function and fertility. It is particularly important to provide a seamless handover from paediatric to adult services at this time and dedicated adolescent clinics may have an important role.

Müllerian duct abnormalities

In the absence of a Y chromosome, testis and testosterone, the wolffian duct regresses after the 6th week of embryonic life. The müllerian ducts then develop into the uterus and fallopian tubes and fuse caudally with the urogenital sinus to form the vagina. Abnormalities in the process of fusion may be either medial or vertical and result in primary amenorrhoea; complete or partial müllerian agenesis may also occur. Renal developmental abnormalities are commonly seen in association with abnormalities of the genital tract so assessment by intravenous urography is advisable before attempting corrective surgery.

Congenital absence of the vagina

Women with Mayer-Rokitansky-Kuster-Hauser syndrome (MRKH or Rokitansky syndrome) have a 46XX genotype and a normal female phenotype with spontaneous development of secondary sexual characteristics, as ovarian tissue is present and functions normally. The müllerian ducts have failed to fuse and so there is vaginal agenesis. The incidence is about 1:5000 female births and may be associated with renal tract anomalies (15–40%) or anomalies of the skeletal system (10–20%). The external genitalia have a normal appearance but the vagina is short and blind ending, such that either surgery or gradual dilatation is necessary to achieve a capacity appropriate for normal sexual function. Hormone treatment is not required as ovarian oestrogen output is normal. Indeed, ovulation occurs and ovarian stimulation followed by oocyte retrieval can be performed in order to achieve a 'biological' pregnancy through the services of a surrogate mother.

The vaginal dimple can vary in length from just a slight depression between the labia to up to 5–6 cm. Vaginal dilators, made of plastic or glass, are used first to stretch the vaginal skin and the patient is encouraged to apply pressure for 15 minutes twice daily with successive sizes of dilator. An adequately sized vagina is usually formed by 6 months but this may take longer and long-term use of dilators may be required, depending upon the frequency of sexual intercourse.

A number of surgical approaches have been employed to create a neovagina. The Vecchetti procedure uses the same principle of progressive dilatation with the application of pressure from a plastic sphere in the vagina which is attached to two wires that have been passed from the top of the vagina through to the anterior wall of the abdomen where they are attached to a traction device that is tightened daily. Plastic surgical techniques include:

- the McIndoe vaginoplasty in which a split skin graft is placed over a mould which has been inserted into a space created where the vagina should be
- tissue expansion vaginoplasty in which expansion balloons are inserted into the labia and inflated with water over a period of 2 weeks in order to stretch the labial skinfolds sufficiently to be used to fashion a vagina
- an artificial vagina created from bowel, a technique less favoured nowadays because of problems with persistent discharge
- the Williams vaginoplasty in which the labia are used to create a pouch, also rarely used nowadays because of problems with a poor anatomical result and an awkward angle for intercourse.

The diagnosis of Rokitansky syndrome can usually be made without the need for a laparoscopy. Sometimes, however, an ultrasound scan will reveal the presence of a uterine remnant (anlagan) which is usually small and hardly ever of sufficient size to function normally. If there is active endometrial tissue within the uterine anlagan the patient may experience cyclical pain and the anlagan should be excised (usually laparoscopically).

Fusion abnormalities of the vagina

Longitudinal fusion abnormalities may lead to a complete septum that may be associated with two complete uterine horns with two cervices or a partial septum causing a unilateral obstruction. Excision is required to both prevent retention of uterine secretions and permit sexual intercourse.

Transverse fusion abnormalities usually present with primary amenorrhoea and require careful assessment before surgery. The commonest problem is an imperforate hymen in which cyclical lower abdominal pain combines with a visible haematocolpos and a bulging purple/blue hymen with menstrual secretions stretching the thin hymen. The surgery required is a simple incision which should be performed when the diagnosis is made to prevent too big a build-up of menstrual blood, which may lead to a haematometra and consequent increased risk of endometriosis (secondary to retrograde menstruation). A transverse vaginal septum due to failure of fusion or canalization between the müllerian tubercle and sinovaginal bulb may present like an imperforate hymen but is associated with a pink bulge at the introitus as the septum is thicker than the hymen. Greater care must be taken during surgery to prevent annular constriction rings and the procedure should only be performed in dedicated centres by experienced surgeons. When there is a transverse septum it has been found to be high in 46% of patients, in the middle of the vagina in 40% and low in the remaining 14%. It is the patients in the last two groups who have higher pregnancy rates after surgery.

Müllerian/uterine anomalies

Uterine anomalies occur in between 3% and 10% of the fertile female population and can be subdivided according to the nature of the abnormality and have been usefully classified by the American Society for Reproductive Medicine into six groups.

1. Segmental agenesis or hypoplasia, which may involve vagina, cervix, uterine corpus or fallopian tubes. Mayer-Rokitansky-Kuster-Hauser syndrome is included here.
2. Unicornuate uterus, with or without a rudimentary horn that may or may not contain endometrium and be connected to the main uterine cavity. On the affected side the kidney and ureter are generally absent.
3. Uterus didelphis: due to partial or complete failure of lateral müllerian duct fusion leading to partial or complete duplication of the vagina, cervix and uterus.
4. Bicornuate uterus, with a single vagina and cervix and two uterine bodies, that may be completely separated or fused centrally with a partial septum.
5. Septate or arcuate uterus, with a septum that may be partial or complete.
6. Diethylstilboestrol-related anomalies, which might demonstrate various shapes due to the effect of diethylstilboestrol.

These anomalies are often discovered by chance during coincidental investigations for infertility. The diagnosis is made by a combination of ultrasound, magnetic resonance imaging and X-ray hysterosalpingography (the latter during the course of an infertility work-up). Women with uterine anomalies are usually asymptomatic, unless there is obstruction to menstrual flow, when cyclical pain may be experienced. Whilst infertility per se is rarely caused by uterine anomalies, they may be associated with endometriosis if there is retrograde menstruation secondary to obstruction. Furthermore, recurrent miscarriage may be experienced by some women with uterine malformations.

Surgery is reserved for those cases where there is obstruction; for example, the removal of a rudimentary uterine horn or excision of a vaginal septum. The excision of a uterine septum has been shown to improve pregnancy outcome and should be performed by an experienced hysteroscopist. On the other hand, metroplasty (Strassman procedure) of the horns of a bicornuate uterus is seldom performed nowadays as its benefit has been questioned.

Androgen insensitivity syndrome

Girls who are phenotypically normal but have absent pubic and axillary hair in the presence of normal breast development are likely to have complete androgen insensitivity syndrome (CAIS, formerly known as testicular feminization syndrome, a term that is no longer favoured). In this condition, the karyotype is 46XY and, whilst testes are present, there is an insensitivity to secreted androgens because of abnormalities in the androgen receptor. The incidence is approximately 1:60 000 'male' births and it is inherited as an X-linked trait (the androgen receptor is on the short arm of the X chromosome). Anti-müllerian factors prevent the development of internal müllerian structures and the wolffian structures also fail to develop because of the insensitivity to testosterone. The external genitalia appear female. In about 10% the defect is incomplete (PAIS – partial androgen insensitivity syndrome); the external genitalia may be ambiguous at birth, with labioscrotal fusion, and virilization may sometimes occur before puberty.

After puberty gonadal tissue should be removed to prevent malignant transformation (dysgerminoma), which occurs in about 5% of cases. Exogenous oestrogen should then be prescribed: cyclical treatment is not required because the uterus is absent. The syndrome may be diagnosed in infancy if a testis is found in either the labia or an inguinal hernia, in which case both testes should be removed at this time because of the potential risk of malignancy. Some cases, however, only present at puberty with primary amenorrhoea and removal of abdominal/inguinal testes should then be performed.

Careful psychological assessment and counselling are obligatory to allow an understanding of the gonadal dysfunction and necessity for hormone treatment. It may be helpful to describe the gonads as internal sexual organs that have been incompletely formed and which are therefore prone to develop cancer if they are not removed. In general, a completely honest approach is favoured so that the individual is provided with full information about her condition, its origins and management. It is certainly our experience that the vast majority of patients desire a full explanation of their condition and respond better to treatment if they are included in the decision-making processes. Patients with these problems should be referred to centres where there are specialists experienced in their management so that a comprehensive team approach can be provided.

There are several uncommon intersex disorders which result in primary amenorrhoea and while their management must be individualized, it will often broadly follow the above outline. Examples are male pseudohermaphroditism, caused by 5α-reductase deficiency, and female pseudohermaphroditism, caused by congenital adrenal hyperplsia (see above). In contrast to the androgen insensitivity syndrome, in these conditions there is deficient or absent breast development, yet normal or increased pubic and axillary hair. 5α-reductase deficiency is an autosomal recessive condition, diagnosed by the presence of undervirilization (which may change at puberty) and an elevated testosterone to dihydrotestosterone ratio.

Cloacal anomalies

Cloacal anomalies may take a variety of forms depending upon the relative contribution of gastrointestinal, genital and renal tracts. The cloaca should be divided anteriorly into the urogenital sinus and posteriorly into the rectum. Major surgery is often required during the neonatal period to provide anterior abdominal wall integrity and continence of faeces and urine. Several operations may be required and the uterus and genitalia, if present, may be adversely affected such that at puberty there is obstruction to menstrual flow and also an increased rate of ovarian cyst formation, presumably due to ovarian entrapment restricting normal follicular growth and ovulation.

GYNAECOLOGICAL COMPLAINTS

Disorders of the menstrual cycle are common and often normal in adolescence and will rarely require secondary level care unless there is underlying pathology. Most conditions will be dealt with in an outpatient setting and will seldom require a hospital stay. The adolescent female will require careful explanation of what is normal, what can be expected and how things may change. Provision should be made to see her either alone, with her mother or, as is often the case, with a close female friend. Adolescents need to be given autonomy and ownership of their condition in order to encourage attendance for follow-up appointments.

Menorrhagia

In a young woman with intractable menorrhagia, an assessment of blood clotting may be beneficial. Disorders of haemostasis such as von Willebrand's disease and deficiencies of factors V, VII, X, and XI and idiopathic thrombocytopenic purpura are thought to increase menstrual loss. Young girls with heavy periods in the years after the menarche are very unlikely to have any pelvic pathology. There are a very few young girls with persistent heavy irregular periods associated with anovular cycles – particularly those with PCOS (see Chapter 19). In these cases sustained unopposed oestrogen levels lead to endometrial hyperplasia which may ultimately progress in later years to carcinoma.

Primary dysmenorrhoea

In general primary dysmenorrhoea appears 6–12 months after the menarche when ovulatory cycles have become established. The early cycles after the menarche are usually anovular and tend to be painless. The pain usually consists of lower abdominal cramps and backache and there may be associated gastrointestinal disturbances such as diarrhoea and vomiting. Symptoms occur predominantly during the first 2 days of menstruation. Primary dysmenorrhoea tends not to be associated with excessive menstrual bleeding. Although excessive levels of prostaglandins, leukotrienes and vasopressin have been found in primary dysmenorrhoea, the primary stimulus for their production remains unknown. The clear involvement of prostaglandins in primary dysmenorrhoea has led to the use of prostaglandin synthetase inhibitors such as mefenamic acid, naproxen, ibuprofen and aspririn to treat the disorder. Ibuprofen is the preferred analgesic because of its favourable efficacy and safety profiles.

SUMMARY

The endocrine changes during puberty are regulated by the hypothalamic-pituitary-ovarian axis which controls growth and gonadotrophin pulsatility. Insulin plays a pivotal role by its influence on insulin-like growth factor binding protein (IGFBP-1) and sex hormone-binding globulin (SHBG) levels. Recent studies also indicate that the hormone leptin, which is secreted by fat cells and which acts on the hypothalamus to induce satiety, may influence energy metabolism and GnRH pulsatility. Body weight, nutrition, genetic and socio-economic factors may all play a role in the initiation and timing of puberty, but as yet the precise mechanisms remain unclear.

Anomalous pubertal development requires careful evaluation to exclude sinister causes. Once initial investigations have been performed it is often reasonable to hold off medical therapies and observe the rate of change. Treatments are available to both suppress precocious puberty and initiate breast development and menstruation for girls with delayed puberty or ovarian failure.

Management of all intersex conditions requires the skills of a multidisciplinary team that includes paediatric surgeons, urologists (often paediatric and adult), plastic surgeons, endocrinologists, specialist nurses, psychologists and also the gynaecologist, whose role is to help co-ordinate the transition from childhood through adolescence and then womanhood and help with issues relating to sexual function and sexual identity, endocrinology and fertility. It is during the difficult time of adolescence that the patient usually first realizes that there are serious problems and it is often the specialist gynaecologist who helps her to understand the diagnosis and requirements for management. The support of a skilled nurse and clinical psychologist is invaluable at this time.

Acknowledgements

I am grateful to Dr Kathy Michelmore DPhil, Department of General Practice, Royal Victoria Hospital, Newcastle and Dr Ken Ong DPhil, Department of Paediatrics, Addenbrookes Hospital, Cambridge for help in preparing this chapter.

KEY POINTS

1. Puberty is a coherent process involving oestrogen production, increased somatic growth and the development of secondary sexual characteristics.
2. The essential hormonal event of puberty is the augmentation of pulsatile gonadotrophin secretion, which is affected by endocrine, nutritional and psychological factors.
3. Menarche occurs after sufficient endometrium has developed to result in a withdrawal bleed when the oestrogen level temporarily falls. It usually occurs within 2 years of the earliest sign of breast development.
4. Appropriate investigation of abnormal events surrounding puberty must be based upon detailed history and examination of the patient.

KEY POINTS (*CONTINUED*)

5. The commonest cause of delayed puberty is ovarian failure. More than half of the girls with delayed puberty have chromosome anomalies.

6. Serum gonadotrophin levels are important in distinguishing hypo- and hypergonadotrophic causes of delayed puberty.

7. Oestrogen and progesterone replacement are used in primary ovarian failure to induce pubertal growth and secondary sexual characteristics.

8. Precocious puberty, where breast development occurs before the age of 8 years, is most commonly due to constitutional early development.

9. Precocious puberty requires prompt investigation and treatment in order to avoid short stature from premature closure of the epiphyses.

10. Anorexia nervosa and acute weight loss are associated with amenorrhoea.

11. The psychological stress of pubertal disorders must be recognized and dealt with sympathetically in order to avoid excessive undermining of the patient's self-confidence.

12. Oocyte donation has been successfully used to allow patients with primary ovarian failure to achieve pregnancy and have their own children.

REFERENCES

Amiel SA, Caprio S, Sherwin RS, Plewe G, Hymond MW, Tamborlane WV 1991 Insulin resistance of puberty: a defect restricted to peripheral glucose metabolism. Journal of Clinical Endocrinology and Metabolism 72:277–282

Anasti JN 1998 Premature ovarian failure: an update. Fertility and Sterility 70:1–15

Baxter Jones AD, Helms P, Baines Preece J, Preece M 1994 Menarche in intensively trained gymnasts, swimmers and tennis players. Annals of Human Biology 21:407–415

Benso L, Lorenzino C, Pastorin L, Barotto M, Signorile F, Mostert M 1989 The distribution of age at menarche in a random series of Turin girls followed longitudinally. Annals of Human Biology 16:549–552

Cameron N, Nagdee I 1996 Menarcheal age in two generations of South African Indians. Annals of Human Biology 23:113–119

Cameron N 1976 Weight and skinfold variation at menarche and the critical body weight hypothesis. Annals of Human Biology 3:279–282

Caufriez A 1997 The pubertal spurt: effects of sex steroids on growth hormone and insulin-like growth factor I. European Journal of Obstetrics, Gynecology and Reproductive Biology 71:215–217

Clayton PE, Gill MS, Hall CM, Tillmann V, Whatmore AJ, Price DA 1997 Serum leptin through childhood and adolescence. Clinical Endocrinology 46:727–733

Clement K, Vaisse C, Lahlou N et al 1998 A mutation in the human leptin receptor gene causes obesity and pituitary dysfunction. Nature 392:398–401

Considine RV, Sinha MK, Heiman ML et al 1996 Serum immunoreactive-leptin concentrations in normal-weight and obese humans. New England Journal of Medicine 334:292–295

Conway GS, Kaltas G, Patel A, Davies MC, Jacobs HS 1996 Characterization of idiopathic premature ovarian failure. Fertility and Sterility 65:337–341

Cooper C, Kuh D, Egger P, Wadsworth M, Barker D 1996 Childhood growth and age at menarche. British Journal of Obstetrics and Gynaecology 103:814–817

Coulam CB, Adamson SC, Annegers JF 1986 Incidence of premature ovarian failure. Obstetrics and Gynecology 67:604–606

Dann TC, Roberts DF 1993 Menarcheal age in University of Warwick young women. Journal of Biosocial Science 25:531–538

Delemarre HA, Wennink JM, Odink RJ 1991 Gonadotrophin and growth hormone secretion throughout puberty. Acta Paediatrica Scandinavica 372(suppl):26–31

de Ridder CM, Thijssen JH, Bruning PF, van den Brande JL, Zonderland ML, Erich WB 1992 Body fat mass, body fat distribution, and pubertal development: a longitudinal study of physical and hormonal sexual maturation of girls. Journal of Clinical Endocrinology and Metabolism 75:442–446

Flug D, Largo RH, Prader A 1984 Menstrual patterns in adolescent Swiss girls: a longitudinal study. Annals of Human Biology 11:495–508

Frisch RE, Revelle R 1970 Height and weight at menarche and a hypothesis of critical body weights and adolescent events. Science 169:397–399

Frisch RE 1990 The right weight: body fat, menarche and ovulation Baillière's Clinical Obstetrics and Gynaecology 4:419–439

Frisch RE, Gotz Welbergen AV, McArthur JW et al 1981 Delayed menarche and amenorhea of college athletes in relation to age of onset of training. JAMA 246:1559–1563

Garn SM, LaVelle M, Pilkington JJ 1983 Comparisons of fatness in premenarcheal and postmenarcheal girls of the same age. Journal of Pediatrics 103:328–331

Garn SM, Bailey SM 1978 Genetics of maturational processes. In: Falkner F, Tanner J (eds) Human Growth. Baillière Tindall, London

Giustina A, Scalvini T, Tassi C et al 1997 Maturation of the regulation of growth hormone secretion in young males with hypogonadotropic hypogonadism pharmacologically exposed to progressive increments in serum testosterone. Journal of Clinical Endocrinology and Metabolism 82:1210–1219

Griffin IJ, Cole TJ, Duncan KA, Hollman AS, Donaldson MDC 1995 Pelvic ultrasound measurements in normal girls. Acta Paediatrica 84:536–543

Holly JM, Smith CP, Dunger DB et al 1989 Relationship between the pubertal fall in sex hormone binding globulin and insulin-like growth factor binding protein-I. A synchronized approach to pubertal development? Clinical Endocrinology 31:277–284

Holm K, Mosfeldt Laursen E, Brocks V, Muller J 1995 Pubertal maturation of the internal genitalia: an ultrasound evaluation of 166 healthy girls. Ultrasound in Obstetrics and Gynecology 6:175–181

Malina RM, Bouchard C, Shoup RF, Demirjian A, Lariviere G 1979 Age at menarche, family size, and birth order in athletes at the Montreal Olympic Games, 1976. Medicine and Science in Sports 11:354–358

Malina RM, Spirduso WW, Tate C, Baylor AM 1978 Age at menarche and selected menstrual characteristics in athletes at different competitive levels and in different sports. Medicine and Science in Sports 10:218–222

Malina RM, Ryan RC, Bonci CM 1994 Age at menarche in athletes and their mothers and sisters. Annals of Human Biology 21:417–422

Mantzoros CS, Flier JS, Rogol AD 1997 A longitudinal assessment of hormonal and physical alterations during normal puberty in boys. V. Rising leptin levels may signal the onset of puberty. Journal of Clinical Endocrinology and Metabolism 82:1066–1070

Mauras N, Rogol AD, Haymond MW, Veldhuis JD 1996 Sex steroids, growth hormone, insulin-like growth factor-1: neuroendocrine and metabolic regulation in puberty. Hormone Research 45:74–80

Marshall WA, Tanner JM 1969 Variations in the pattern of pubertal changes in girls. Archives of Disease in Childhood 44:291–303

Nobels F, Dewailly D 1992 Puberty and polycystic ovarian syndrome: the insulin/insulin-like growth factor I hypothesis. Fertility and Sterility 58:655–666

Ostersehlt D, Danker Hopf E 1991 Changes in age at menarche in Germany: evidence for a continuing decline. American Journal of Human Biology 3(6):647–654

Parra A, Schultz RB, Graystone JE, Cheek DB 1971 Correlative studies in obese children and adolescents concerning body composition and plasma insulin and growth hormone levels. Pediatric Research 5:603–613

Rees M 1993 Menarche when and why? Lancet 342:1375–1376

Roberts DF, Rozner LM, Swan AV 1971 Age at menarche, physique and environment in industrial north east England. Acta Paediatrica Scandinavica 60:158–164

Rosenbaum M, Leibel RL, Hirsch J 1997 Obesity. New England Journal of Medicine 337:396–407

Stanhope R, Adams J, Jacobs HS, Brook CGD 1985 Ovarian ultrasound assessment in normal children, idiopathic precocious puberty and during low dose pulsatile GnRH therapy of hypogonadotrophic hypogonadism. Archives of Diseases in Childhood 60:116–119

Stark O, Peckham CS, Moynihan C 1989 Weight and age at menarche. Archives of Diseases in Childhood 64:383–387

Smith CP, Archibald HR, Thomas JM et al 1988 Basal and stimulated insulin levels rise with advancing puberty. Clinical Endocrinology 28:7–14

Sorensen TI, Echwald S, Holm JC 1996 Leptin in obesity. British Medical Journal 313:953–954

Tryggvadottir L, Tulinius H, Larusdottir M 1994 A decline and a halt in mean age at menarche in Iceland. Annals of Human Biology 21:179–186

Veronesi FM, Gueresi P 1994 Trend in menarcheal age and socioeconomic influence in Bologna (northern Italy). Annals of Human Biology 21:187–196

FURTHER READING

Balen A, Creighton S, Davies M et al (Eds) 2002 The multidisciplinary approach to paediatric and adolescent gynaecology. Cambridge University Press, Cambridge

Sanfilippo JS 1994 Pediatric and adolescent gynaecology. WB Saunders, Philadelphia

17

Amenorrhoea and oligomenorrhoea, and hypothalamic–pituitary dysfunction

Hilary O.D. Critchley

INTRODUCTION

Amenorrhoea and oligomenorrhoea are symptoms of ovarian and reproductive dysfunction. Patients thus commonly present to the gynaecologist with complaints of problematic menstruation or fertility delay. This chapter provides an overview of the current understanding and general management of the associated disorders of the hypothalamic-pituitary-ovarian (HPO) axis which result in amenorrhoea and oligomenorrhoea. These symptoms are also features of the polycystic ovarian syndrome (PCOS) and a detailed description of the symptoms, diagnosis and management of PCOS is provided in Chapter 19.

DEFINITIONS

Normal menstruation

Regular monthly menstruation is a phenomenon of modern society. The availability of effective contraception has enabled couples to choose both the size and timing of their desired family. The classic data (derived from 22 754 calendar years of experience) from the studies of Treloar et al (1967) demonstrated that each woman has her own central trend and variation in menstrual cycle length, both of which change with age (Fig. 17.1). The first (and last) few years of menstrual life are marked by a variable pattern of mixed short and long intervals with a characteristic transition into and out of the more regular pattern of middle life (Fig. 17.2). The length, regularity and frequency of normal menstrual cycles have been described in both population and observational studies (Fraser & Inceboz 2000, Harlow & Ephross 1995). Mean menstrual cycle length between the ages of 20 and 34 years varies between 28 and 30.7 days (range 19.7 to 43.5 between the 5th and 95th centiles). Physiologically regular menses indicate cyclical ovarian activity, in turn dependent upon an

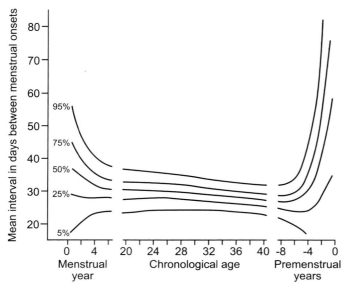

Fig. 17.1 Distribution of menstrual intervals during three zones of experience: post mencheal, age 20–40 years and premenopausal. Reproduced with permission from Treloar et al (1967).

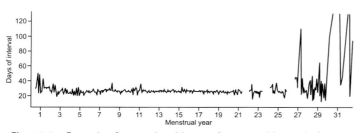

Fig. 17.2 Example of a complete history of menstrual intervals from menarche to menopause. Reproduced with permission from Treloar et al (1967).

Box 17.1 Classification of causes of amenorrhoea (adapted from Baird 1997)

Physiological
Prepuberty
Pregnancy
Lactation
Postmenopause

Pathological
Local genital causes
Congenital – testicular feminization, congenital absence of the uterus, imperforate hymen
Acquired – Asherman's syndrome

Hypothalamic
Congenital – Kallman's syndrome
Acquired – weight loss, extreme exercise, craniopharyngioma

Pituitary
Tumour – prolactinoma
Infarction – Sheehan's syndrome
Iatrogenic damage – surgery, radiotherapy

Ovarian
Congenital – gonadotrophin receptor defect, resistant ovary syndrome, ovarian dysgenesis
Acquired – irradiation, chemotherapy, surgical, autoimmune disease, PCOS

intact HPO axis. Aberrations in menstrual pattern are thus an indication of disorder of ovarian function.

Amenorrhoea

Amenorrhoea is complete absence or cessation of menstrual bleeding for greater than 6 months (not due to pregnancy). Primary amenorrhoea is defined as no spontaneous onset of menstruation by the age of 16 years. Secondary amenorrhoea is defined as the absence of menstruation for 6 months or longer if the patient has previously experienced regular menses and for 12 months or more when a patient has oligomenorrhoea. The usual age limits are 16 and 40 years, for menarche and menopause respectively.

Oligomenorrhoea

Oligomenorrhoea is the reduction is frequency of menstruation where menstrual intervals may vary between 6 weeks and 6 months. It is important to note, however, that regular menstrual cycles every 6 weeks are usually indistinguishable from normal shorter interval cycles (described above) in terms of follicular growth and hormone production. Oligo-

menorrhoea may therefore include a spectrum of conditions ranging from virtual normality at one end to the same causes as amenorrhoea at the other. The main difference appears to be in the frequency of polycystic ovaries, which ultrasound and endocrine studies show to account for about 90% of cases of oligomenorrhoea and 33% of amenorrhoea (although often without the classic syndrome, including hirsutism and obesity (Adams et al 1986, Hull 1987).

CAUSES OF AMENORRHOEA

Causes of amenorrhoea are classified according to a systematic endocrine approach and are listed in Box 17.1 (Baird 1997). Disorders in other endocrine systems, for example thyroid disease and adrenal disease, may result in amenorrhoea.

Physiological amenorrhoea

Amenorrhoea is physiological at certain critical times in a woman's life, these being prepuberty, during pregnancy and lactation and in the postmenopause period. Amenorrhoea, if not physiological, has an estimated prevalence in the female population of reproductive age of 1.8–3% (Pettersson et al 1973). Amenorrhoea may be either primary or secondary. The prevalence of secondary amenorrhoea is in the order of 2–5% (Pettersson et al 1973, Singh 1981). The aetiology of primary and secondary amenorrhoea may be similar.

Causes of primary amenorrhoea are listed in Box 17.2. In practice investigation of primary amenorrhoea is usually initiated by the age of 14 years if there is evidence of delayed puberty (absent secondary sexual characteristics and absent menses) or no menstruation within 4 years of the onset of

Box 17.2   Causes of primary amenorrhoea

Delayed puberty
Familial
Nutritional
Delayed adrenarche

Structural congenital abnormalities
Imperforate hymen (crytomenorrhoea)
Absent uterus ± vagina

Chromosomal obnormalities
XO (Turner's syndrome)
XO/XY mosaics
XY (Testicular feminization)

Endocrine causes
Hyperprolactinaemia
Ovarian failure
Gonadotrophin deficiency (hypogonadotrophic hypogonadism)
Polycystic ovarian syndrome (hyperandrogenism)
Thyroid dysfunction (hypothyroidism)
Tumours

Box 17.3   Anatomical causes of amenorrhoea

Developmental defects
Absent ovaries (extremely rare)
Absent uterus (with or without absent vagina)
Imperforate hymen (lower vaginal aplasia)

Developmental defects of endocrine origin
Androgen-resistant syndrome (testicular feminization) in male pseudohermaphrodites (genetic and gonadal males) including inhibition of uterovaginal development

Acquired conditions
Endometrial fibrosis – traumatic (Asherman's syndrome), infective (pelvic tuberculosis)
Cervical stenosis (extremely rare) – surgical trauma, infective
Vaginal stenosis (extremely rare) – chemical inflammation

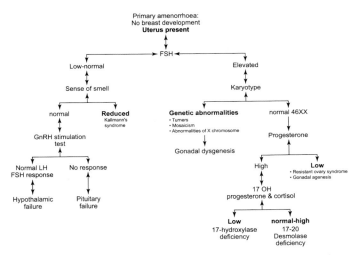

Fig. 17.3   The investigation of primary amenorrhoea. Reproduced from Zreik & Olive (1998), with permission from Oxford University Press.

adrenarche and thelarche (Zreik & Olive 1998). The diagnosis of cause of primary amenorrhoea may be categorized depending on whether the uterus is present and whether or not there is breast development. Zreik & Olive (1998) have described a very useful scheme to aid diagnosis of primary amenorrhoea (Fig. 17.3).

Anatomical causes

Anatomical abnormalities of the genital tract account for about 1% of cases of amenorrhoea. The anatomical causes of amenorrhoea are summarized in Box 17.3. In girls with breast development but evidence of an absent uterus two disorders need to be considered. First, congenital absence of the uterus (Müllerian agenesis, Mayer-Rokitansky-Kuster-Hauser syndrome) is due to an early development failure of the Müllerian system. Affected girls have a normal XX

karyotype, normal ovaries and secondary sex characteristics. The vagina is absent or hypoplastic. Magnetic resonance imaging is a useful adjunct diagnostic test for establishment of the diagnosis (thereby avoiding laparoscopy). Since anomalies of the wolffian duct system may be present in these patients an intravenous urogram is an important investigation for this condition.

The second disorder to consider is testicular feminization or androgen insensitivity, an X-linked inherited disorder. Patients have a 46XY karyotype, a female phenotype and undescended testes. The uterus is absent and there is a short, blind vaginal pouch. The X-linked androgen receptor (AR) is essential for androgen action, leading to normal primary male sexual development prior to birth (masculinization). Thus AR dysfunction in XY individuals results in androgen insensitivity syndromes (AIS)

Diagnosis of AIS is established on clinical findings, endocrine investigations and, if possible, family history. There are three phenotypes: complete androgen insensitivity syndrome (CAIS), partial androgen insensitivity syndrome (PAIS) and mixed androgen insensitivity syndrome (MAIS). CAIS is most often diagnosed on clinical findings and laboratory investigations and PAIS and MAIS usually require a family history consistent with X-linked inheritance (Gottlieb et al 1999). Androgen insensitivity may be caused by several mutations of the androgen receptor (Gottlieb et al 1999), resulting in a lack of androgenization during sexual differentiation (Imperato-McGinley 1995). Development of the uterus and upper vagina is inhibited, as the secretion of müllerian duct inhibitory hormone by the testes is normal in these patients.

Recently, due to nationwide co-operation between paediatric endocrinologists in the United Kingdom, an extensive database (278 cases) of phenotypic features, AR binding and mutational analysis of cases of intersex and ambiguous genitalia has been established (Ahmed et al 2000). All cases of PAIS presented within the first month of life. The median age for presentation of individuals with CAIS was 1 year. The gonads were removed prepuberty in 66% cases with CAIS and in 29% postpuberty. The indication for gonadal removal is the high incidence of neoplasia (5%).

A further anatomical cause of primary amenorrhoea is the presence of an imperforate hymen that obstructs the outflow

Box 17.4 Disorders of the HPO axis

Hypothalamic
Kallman's syndrome
Compression by tumours (for example, craniopharyngioma)
Weight loss
Extreme exercise
Psychological disturbances

Pituitary
Hyperprolactinaemia
Compression by tumours
Damage by surgery, irradiation
Infarction (Sheehan's syndrome)
Functional failure, secondary to hypothalamic failure

Ovarian
Dysgenesis due to chromosome anomaly, e.g. Turner's syndrome
Damage by surgery, chemotherapy, radiotherapy
Autoimmune disease
Idiopathic premature menopause
Resistant ovary syndrome
Functional failure, secondary to hypothalamic-pituitary failure
Polycystic ovarian syndrome

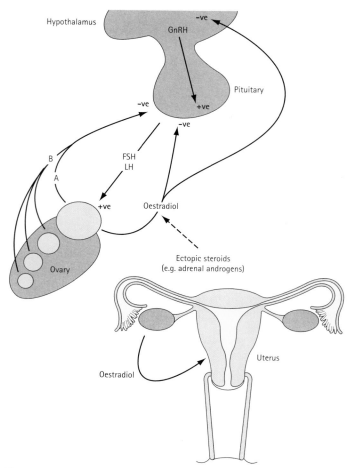

Fig. 17.4 The hypothalamic-pituitary-ovarian-uteric axis. GnRH, gonadotrophin-releasing hormone; FSH, follicle-stimulating hormone; LH, luteinizing hormone. Adapted with permission from Baird, Amenorrhoea. Lancet 350:275–279. ©The Lancet Ltd 1997.

of menses. Girls commonly present with cyclical pelvic pain and a delayed menarche.

An anatomical cause of secondary amenorrhoea is destruction of the endometrial lining of the uterine cavity as a result of infection (pelvic tuberculosis), an endometrial ablation procedure or as a complication of uterine curettage (Asherman's syndrome: Asherman 1948). Amenorrhoea may be achieved in 15–40% of women depending upon method of endometrial ablation (Parkin 2000). Uterine balloon ablation has been reported to result in amenorrhoea in 15% of women and 40% amenorrhoea rates for women treated with microwave endometrial ablation or transcervical resection of the endometrium.

HYPOTHALAMIC–PITUITARY DYSFUNCTION (ENDOCRINE CAUSES)

The hypothalamic-pituitary axis is regulated at two levels. At a higher level, GnRH neurones within the hypothalamus are stimulated by afferent inputs from the central nervous system. Further, there is endocrine control of GnRH synthesis and secretion by means of gonadal feedback mechanisms and GnRH itself. At the lower level, the output of FSH and LH by the gonadotropes in the anterior pituitary reflects GnRH activity. Gonadotrophin synthesis and secretion are in turn influenced by endocrine feedback from the ovaries as well as paracrine mechanisms and other extrinsic factors. Endocrine causes of amenorrhoea/oligomenorrhoea include disorders of the HPO axis that are summarized in Box 17.4. Disturbances in menstrual pattern will be the consequence of either a structural or functional defect in the tightly controlled feedback system involving the hypothalamus, anterior pituitary and ovary (Baird 1997; Fig 17.4). If the uterus is present and there is no breast development, absence of menstruation may be due to failure of secretion of GnRH or to

failure of pituitary or gonadal function (see Figs 17.3 and 17.4). Hypothalamic amenorrhoea suggests an intact HPO axis.

Kallman's syndrome

Kallman's syndrome, occurring in one in 50 000 girls (Kallman et al 1944), has the associated symptom of anosmia and is an inherited autosomal dominant or X-linked autosomal recessive anomaly. The impairment of olfactory sensation is often subtle. The gonadotrophin deficiency is due to an inability to activate pulsatile GnRH secretion (Leiblich et al 1982). Many cases are due to a mutation in the gene (KAL gene) situated on the p22.3 region (tip of the short arm) of the X chromosome that codes for an adhesion molecule-like X chromosome (AD-MLX; Ballabio et al 1989, Legouis et al 1991). This protein has homology with fibronectin and plays a role in the migration of GnRH-like neurones from the nasal pit to the hypothalamus (Rugarli & Ballabio, Schwanzel-Fukuda et al 1989). Ovulation induction can achieve pregnancy for these women.

Hypogonadotrophic hypogonadism

Hypogonadotrophic hypogonadism is characterized by reduced secretion of FSH and LH. There is a consequent failure of follicular development and oestradiol production by the ovaries. A hypo-oestrogenic state thus prevails. If the situation is present prepuberty the girl will present with primary amenorrhoea and a lack of secondary sexual features. Usually no organic lesion is identified in the hypothalamus or anterior pituitary and the situation is then considered to be idiopathic.

In an impressive gene transfer experiment in mice the transgenic insertion of a normal GnRH gene or hypothalamic implants of GT-1 GnRH neuronal cells into hypogonadotrophic hypogonadal mouse (hpg mouse) restored reproductive function. This is strong evidence for GnRH gene deletion as a cause of hypogonadism in the mouse. In the human, however, no evidence exists for an analogous deletion of the GnRH gene (Nakayama et al 1990, Weiss et al 1989). The underlying cause for idiopathic hypogonadotrophic hypogonadism is still unknown and a further candidate is the GnRH receptor gene, although to date there are no data in this context.

Severe weight loss, psychological stress and chronic debilitating disease are all associated with a cessation of hypothalamic function and are conditions that will be addressed later.

Hypothalamic and pituitary lesions

The most likely hypothalamic lesion to present to a gynaecologist is a craniopharyhgioma. Compression of the hypothalamus will suppress GnRH secretion and interrupt portal flow of GnRH in the pituitary stalk. The peripubertal period is the commonest age for presentation. The lesions are cystic and often calcified and readily recognizable on a lateral skull radiograph or with more modern imaging techniques, such as magnetic resonance imaging. Other tumours which may affect hypothalamic-pituitary function are gliomas (which may arise from the optic tract), meningiomas, endodermal sinus tumour (yolk sac carcinoma), which secretes α-fetoprotein, and congenital hamartomas composed of GnRH neurosecretory cells which can lead to precocious puberty (Yen 1999).

Congenital absence of the anterior pituitary gland along with other midline structural defects is extremely rare. Primary deficiency of pituitary hormone secretion is also very uncommon. Growth hormone deficiency may occur in isolation or with panhypopituitary dwarfism. Pituitary failure may be secondary to other organic disease, such as pituitary adenoma, mumps, encephalitis, infarction (Sheehan's syndrome) and irradiation. Sheehan's syndrome is the consequence of severe and prolonged hypotension on the pituitary gland that enlarges during pregnancy. It is usually associated with a history of major obstetric haemorrhage (Sheehan 1939). Pituitary cells are relatively resistant to irradiation, compared to other brain tissues that are more radiosensitive. Disturbance of pituitary function may therefore be indirectly due to hypothalamic damage.

Subjects with gonadal failure are oestrogen deficient and have elevated gonadotrophins (hypergonadotrophic hypogonadism). Causes of gonadal failure are listed in Box 17.5 and will be addressed in detail later. One of the commonest chromosomal causes of primary amenorrhoea is Turner's syndrome. Enzyme deficiency states associated with primary

---

Box 17.5 Aetiological classification of premature ovarian failure

Genetic
Gonadal dysgenesis – with X chromosome deletion (XO; Turner's syndrome); with normal XX complement (pure gonadal dysgenesis)

Metabolic disorders, e.g. galactosaemia; 17-hydroxylase deficiency

Immunological deficiency

Autoimmune diseases

Infectiions – pelvic tuberculosis, mumps

Environmental causes – cigarette smoking

Iatrogenic – surgery, chemotherapy, irradiation

Idiopathic

---

amenorrhoea are galactosaemia and 17-hydroxylase deficiency. In rare circumstances ovarian failure is due to the 'resistant ovary syndrome' (see later).

CNS-HYPOTHALAMIC DISTURBANCE

The modulating influence of extrahypothalamic brain centres on the pulsatile nature of hypothalamic GnRH secretion is addressed in Chapter 15. Psychological disorders account for approximately one-third of cases of CNS-hypothalamic derived amenorrhoea. Functional disorders of the hypothalamic-pituitary axis that cause amenorrhoea result from weight loss, extreme exercise and psychological stress. In each of these situations there is a decrease in GnRH neuronal activity in the hypothalamus with a subsequent decrease in gonadotrophin secretion (FSH and LH). Ovarian follicular development and ovulation fail to occur if LH pulsatility is less frequent than every 2 hours (Baird 1997, Leyendecker & Wildt 1983).

Weight-related amenorrhaoea

Marked weight loss may result in amenorrhoea. The amount of weight loss that may result in cessation of menstruation varies from a few kilograms in an adolescent who is dieting to a loss of up to 50% of body weight in women with anorexia nervosa (Warren 1995). Regular menses are unlikely to occur in subjects whose body mass index is under 19 kg/m^2 (Balen et al 1995). It has been reported that nearly one-fifth of the body mass should be adipose tissue for ovulatory cycles to be sustained (Frisch 1976, 1984). The rate of loss of weight seems to be important and rapid loss is frequently associated with psychological disturbance. Adipose tissue is an important extragonadal source of oestrogen by peripheral conversion from androgen precurors, for example, androstenedione. The chronic hypo-oestrogenic state that becomes established in long-standing amenorrhoea carries significant risk of premature osteoporosis and cardiovascular disease.

Exercise-related amenorrhoea

Excess exercise may be detrimental to reproductive function. Irregularities of menstrual pattern are reported in association with many competitive sporting activities. There is typically a progressive failure of regular menses with anovulatory cycles and amenorrhoea and, in prepubertal girls, a delayed menarche. Usually the degree of menstrual aberration reflects the intensity and length of sporting activity (Cumming & Wheeler 1990, Yen 1999). Women with hypothalamic amenorrhoea associated with an excessive exercise habit, weight loss and stress have hypercortisolism (on account of raised corticotrophin-releasing hormone (CRH) and ACTH. Consequently there is likely to be disruption of reproductive function as CRH directly inhibits GnRH secretion, possibly via increased endogenous opioid secretion (Barbarino et al 1989, Speroff et al 1999a).

A detailed study was reported by Laughlin & Yen (1996), in which the interactions between energy balance and regulators of metabolic fuel and the association with reduced LH pulsatility in women with exercise-induced menstrual dysfunction were addressed. Notable differences were observed in nutritional intake, insulin/glucose dynamics, the somatotrophic axis and LH pulsatility with both degree of exercise and menstrual pattern. Those athletes who were amenorrhoeic demonstrated an increase in insulin sensitivity and a reduced hypoglycaemic effect of IGF-1 along with raised growth hormone and cortisol concentrations. The authors suggest that there is a cascade of glucoregulatory adaptations designed to redistribute metabolic fuel and thereby conserve protein. Furthermore, the reduced GnRH/LH pulse generator activity is in response to both a reduced stimulatory effect of IGF-1 (due to increased IGFBP-1) and central negative effects of CRF.

Secondary amenorrhoea and oligomenorrhoea are recognized as also being common in professional dancers (Warren et al 1986).

The discovery of leptin in 1994 (Bray & York 1997, Zhang et al 1994), using molecular cloning techniques, has made a considerable contribution to the understanding of obesity. Leptin is the primary product of the *ob* gene and is a 167 amino acid peptide made exclusively in adipose tissue. It is likely that leptin plays a central role in energy production and reproduction. Leptin has been proposed as a mediator between adipose tissue and the gonads (Matkovic et al 1997). A critical blood leptin level has been reported as necessary to trigger reproductive function in women, suggesting a threshold effect. In this context severe weight loss is known to result in subnormal gonadotrophin concentrations. Leptin receptors have been identified in the hypothalamus and leptin inhibits neuropeptide Y (NPY) synthesis and release. A link between leptin and GnRH neurones is in part mediated by NPY. Secondary leptin deficiency is represented by weight-related amenorrhoea in women (Conway & Jacobs 1997). Speroff et al (1999a) have noted that CRH is elevated in stress and particularly weight loss amenorrhoea. It has been proposed that the decrease in leptin concentrations and increase in NPY described in stress-related weight loss are inadequate to suppress the stress-induced increase in CRH. Moreover, the increase in CRH and resulting hypercortisolism exacerbate further the increase in metabolism and weight loss.

The outlook for women with stress/exercise-related amenorrhoea is very good if recognized early. Most women see a return of ovulatory cycles with weight gain or reduction in levels of stress or exercise habit (Speroff et al 1999a, Stager

et al 1984). Hormone replacement may be indicated for women with long-standing hypothalamic amenorrhoea as there will be a risk of bone loss and cardiovascular changes.

IDIOPATHIC DELAYED PUBERTY

The limiting factor for increasing amounts of gonadotrophin secretion as normal puberty approaches is hypothalamic GnRH release (Apter et al 1993, Yen 1999). Delayed puberty may be recognized by the age of 14 years if breast development is still absent. Most cases are due to idiopathic hypothalamic failure and usually resolve spontaneously. There may often be a family history of late puberty. Enquiry should seek any history of impaired olfaction, marked weight loss, extremes of exercise and ill health. Other causes of amenorrhoea with oestrogen deficiency should be excluded with a lateral skull radiograph/hypothalamic-pituitary imaging (non-endocrine tumours, e.g. craniopharyngioma) and serum prolactin (prolactinoma) and FSH measurements (ovarian dysgenesis). If the diagnosis is idiopathic delayed puberty it remains difficult to distinguish whether the failure is purely delayed or permanent and thus treatment should commence without delay. Once the patient's secondary sexual characteristics are mature, treatment may be periodically interrupted to establish whether there is spontaneous HPO activity.

HYPERPROLACTINAEMIA

In girls with primary amenorrhoea with normal breast development and a uterus, hyperprolactinaemia must be considered. Approximately 15–20% of women with secondary amenorrhoea have elevated serum prolactin concentrations (Jacobs et al 1976). Unlike the other trophic hormones secreted by the anterior pituitary, prolactin secretion is regulated primarily by inhibition from the hypothalamus, by dopamine. Prolactin secretion is not subject directly or indirectly to negative feedback by peripheral hormones. Regulation of secretion is via a short-loop feedback on hypothalamic dopamine by means of a countercurrent flow in the hypophyseal portal system (as well as inhibition of GnRH pulsatile secretion). Prolactin secretion is stimulated by peripheral oestrogen and in pregnancy this is derived from the placenta. During pregnancy, circulating concentrations of prolactin rise to reach values by term that are 4–20 times those in non-pregnant women. After delivery, prolactin levels decline in non-lactating women over a 15–20 day period.

In lactating women circulating levels of prolactin are maintained by suckling and hyperprolactinaemia may last for up to 2 years. During breastfeeding there is an increase in the sensitivity of the HPO axis to the negative feedback effect of oestradiol (Illingworth et al 1995, McNeily 1984). The duration and causes of this period of hypersensitivity to oestrogen are unknown. Recent data are available to support the concept that the suckling-induced suppression of the GnRH system during lactation is associated with an enhancement of the negative effects of oestradiol on the hypothalamic GnRH system (Perheentupa et al 2000). Pathological hyperprolactinaemia is associated with amenorrhoea. There is no ovarian function, reduced or absent pulsatility of LH secretion and an absence of

Box 17.6 Pharmacological agents associated with hyperprolactinaemia

Phenothiazines
Perphenazine (Fentazin)
Chlorpromazine (Largactil)
Thioridazine (Melleril)
Trifluoperazine (Stelazine)
Prochlorperazine (Stemetil)

Butyrophenones
Haloperidol (Haldol, Serenace)

Pimozide (Orap)

Bezamides
Metoclopramide (Maxalon)
Clebopride (Cleboril)

Cimetidine (Tagamet)

Rauwolfia alkaloids
Reserpine (Serpasil)

Methyldopa (Aldomet)

positive feedback response to oestrogen. Treatment of raised prolactin concentrations restores ovulation in 80–90% of women (Randeva et al 2000) and normal cyclical activity returns once prolactin levels are reduced.

Pathological hyperprolactinaemia may be induced by drugs that inhibit dopamine action or production. A list of potential compounds is given in Box 17.6. Pharmacological agents account for 1–2% of cases (see Box 17.6). The commonest causes of hyperprolactinaemia are pituitary prolactinomas (40–50% of cases) and idiopathic hypersecretion. Primary hypothyroidism will be the coincident diagnosis in 3–5% cases. Rare causes are ectopic production from a distant extrapituitary tumour and chronic renal failure may be associated with hyperprolactinaemia, due to both decreased excretion of the hormone and central mechanisms affecting dopamine secretion.

Only about half of the patients who present with hyper-prolactinaemia describe galactorrhoea. Moreover, only about half of the women who report galactorrhoea have raised prolactin levels (Baird 1997, Kleinberg et al 1977). Serum prolactin measurements are essential. Usually a second sample is required if the first is raised. A common problem is the misinterpretation of the upper normal limit of a geometric (skewed) distribution of normal values. The upper limit is taken at about 800 milli units/l. The functional relevance of borderline hyperprolactinaemia is unclear. It is most important to consider the prolactin concentration in the context of the associated ovulatory disorder. Significant hyperprolactinaemia is usually associated with oligomenorrhoea or amenorrhoea. Mild hyperprolactinaemia is identified with some cases of PCOS. The phenomenon is likely to be the consequence of excess oestrogenic stimulation. Conversely, prolactin levels are low in hypothalamic amenorrhoea and are likely to be due to lack of oestrogenic stimulation.

The mechanism by which hyperprolactinaemia interferes with ovarian function is not clearly defined. It has been suggested that in hyperprolactinaemia, endogenous opioids may have an inhibitory effect on hypothalamic GnRH-secreting neurones (Grossman et al 1982, Ropert et al 1981). This is not, however, a consistent observation and prolactin may in fact have a direct effect on hypothalamic activity.

Although serum levels of prolactin in women with idiopathic hyperprolactinaemia or with pituitary tumours may normalize after treatment with a dopamine agonist (or after pituitary surgery), there are many issues about treatment and long-term follow-up that remain unresolved. The natural history of hyperprolactinaemia is not yet known. Interestingly, as many as 10% of patients may have a spontaneous remission (Glasier et al 1987). In a longitudinal prospective 3–7 year study of 30 women with untreated hyperprolactinaemia, with annual clinical, radiographic and hormonal evaluation, progression of the disease was observed to be unlikely and some in fact had clinical and radiographic improvement (Schlechte et al 1989).

OVARIAN FAILURE

It is well established that the number of follicles in the human ovary declines steadily from midlife onward. The onset of menopause is prompted by the number of ovarian follicles falling below a critical number as the consequence of the programmed disappearance of a limited store of follicles. The process is irreversible as oogonal stem cells disappear after birth. The loss of follicles is age dependent and the rate of disappearance increases with age. There is a reported acceleration of loss from the age of 37.5 years (Faddy et al 1992). In this context, Richardson et al (1987) have observed that the entry into the perimenopause phase of life was associated with a marked decline in follicle reserve and that the reserve of follicles was nearly exhausted as menopause approached.

Premature ovarian failure (POF) is defined as the triad of amenorrhoea, oestrogen deficiency and elevated concentrations of FSH and LH in women less than 40 years old. It also includes women with primary amenorrhoea; that is, those who have no known prior ovarian function. Secondary ovarian failure occurs in women who have previously menstruated. The causes of both are similar.

The age that best separates 'premature' from 'normal' menopause is arbitrary. The definition of POF assumes that those patients with the disorder constitute a group with specific characteristics that distinguish them from patients with normal menopause (Alper et al 1986). Forty is the preferred age for definition for practical purposes. Many women with POF at 40 or younger are concerned with fertility. If one were to define abnormality as those values greater than or less than two standard deviations (SD) from the mean (where 95% of the observations of a normally distributed variable are found), then 40 is also an appropriate age. If the age of menopause is assumed to be a normally distributed variable, Walsh (1978) reported the mean age of menopause as 50.4 years, with an SD of 3.72 years, and 2.5% of women reach menopause at age 43 or younger.

There are no unique features that unequivocally establish the diagnosis of POF. However, ovarian failure itself is an irreversible pathological process with major implications for the patient and thus its diagnosis is an important responsibility for the gynaecologist. The incidence of POF is not precisely known. Calculations based on the incidence of permanent secondary amenorrhoea suggest 2–3% (Bachmann & Kemmann 1982, Pettersson et al 1973). Coulam et al (1986) reported POF in 1–3% of the general population. These latter authors conducted a detailed assessment of age-specific incidence rates of natural menopause for a cohort of 1858 women during a 4-year period and identified a 1% risk at age 40 years. The incidence at 30 years is 0.1% and decreases as age decreases (Anasti 1998). The condition is thus not rare. Advances in modern molecular biology have enabled major contributions to be made to the understanding of the aetiology of POF but despite this still only one-third of women have an identifiable pathology (Conway 1997).

POF indicates absent ovarian function; it is not a disease but a clinical state. Ovarian failure may be primary or secondary and the chromosomes of the patient normal or abnormal. Common causes of premature ovarian failure are summarized in Box 17.5. Genetic disorders are the most common identifiable causes.

Chromosomal anomalies are found in women with primary amenorrhoea and ovarian dysgenesis. In Turner's syndrome there is an X chromosome deletion. Typically these patients have streak ovaries, are of short stature and have a characteristic phenotype, including one or some of the following features: neck webbing, widely spaced nipples and increased carrying angle. Approximately two-thirds of Turner's patients have the total loss of one X chromosome and the rest either exhibit a structural abnormality in one X chromosome or display mosaicism with an abnormal X chromosome (Speroff et al 1999b). Menstrual function and pregnancy are possible among patients with XO mosaicism. In Turner girls, 10–20% experience spontaneous puberty and 2–5% spontaneous menstruation (Pasquino et al 1997).

Girls with ovarian dysgenesis may be grouped according to their karyotype (Speroff et al 1999c). Fifty per cent of girls will have Turner's syndrome and 25% will be mosaics (45X/46XX). Patients may have gonadal dysgenesis and a normal XX chromosome complement (25%). This is pure gonadal dysgenesis and the girls invariably have streak ovaries (Sohval 1965), diagnosis of the latter only being made after direct visualization, usually at laparoscopy. In X-Y gonadal dysgenesis, the testis fails to develop due to loss or mutation of the sex-determining region of the Y chromosome (Tdy or SRY). The testis-determining gene, Tdy, is situated on the short arm of the Y chromosome and the gene responsible for the H-Y antigen is on the long arm (Goodfellow & Lovell-Badge 1993). If an XY karyotype is detected the gonadal streaks should be removed since there is a risk of neoplastic transformation.

Recent attention has focused on other genetic determinants of POF. Gonadotrophin resistance as a consequence of an FSH receptor mutation has been described (Aittomaki et al 1995). Fragile X syndrome is the commonest inherited form of mental retardation. Women who carry one X chromosome with a fragile X premutation display an increased prevalence of POF (Conway et al 1995). Preliminary data from an international collaborative group indicate a significant association between fragile X premutation carrier status and POF (Allingham-

Hawkins et al 1999). The causal link with this association is not yet defined. Family history remains a predictor of early menopause. In a case control study of 344 cases of early menopause a family history of earlier menopause (before 46 years) was associated with an increased risk of early menopause, with the link being strongest in women with a history of menopause before 40 years (Cramer et al 1995). Very recently, a mutation in the FOXL2 gene, located on chromosome 3, has been implicated in POF (Crisponi et al 2001). The authors indicate that this is the first human gene to be identified that may play a role in the maintenance of ovarian follicles. FOXL2 mutations will only account for a small fraction of cases of POF but the identification of genes regulated by FOXL2 will contribute to the understanding of the biochemical pathways that may be aberrant in POF.

Patients with galactosaemia treated in early life with a galactose-free diet exhibit a high frequency of ovarian failure. Affected individuals have mutations of the galactose 1-phosphate uridyltransferase gene (Kaufman et al 1981). The associated feature of ovarian failure is considered to be a consequence of accumulated galactose disturbing the migration of the germ cells from the urogenital ridge to the gonad in fetal life.

There is an association between autoimmune disease and ovarian failure and between 10% and 20% of women with POF have intercurrent autoimmune conditions (Conway et al 1996). These include Addison's disease, hypothyroidism, pernicious anaemia, Hashimoto's disease, idiopathic thrombocytopenia, rheumatoid arthritis with vitiligo, alopecia areata, Cushing's disease, autoimmune haemolytic anaemia and myaesthenia gravis. Among patients in whom the aetiology of POF is obscure there are other lines of evidence to suggest autoimmune mechanisms. Circulating antibodies to ovarian tissue have been demonstrated in the sera of women with POF. Organ-specific autoimmunity may be directed against the intracellular enzymes involved in hormone production. 3-β-Hydroxysteroid dehydrogenase (3-β-HSD) has been identified as an autoantigen in a fifth of women with POF. This observation now offers a potential marker for autoimmune ovarian damage although the presence of anti-3-β-HSD antibodies may be the consequence of ovarian inflammation rather than the causal antigen (Arif et al 1996). Infections associated with loss of ovarian function are mumps and pelvic tuberculosis. Environmental factors contributing to an early menopause include cigarette smoking.

As a consequence of the improved survival for patients with certain neoplastic conditions treated with radiotherapy and chemotherapy, an increasing number of survivors are facing the absence of ovarian function. Irradiation is known to induce POF and was indeed once a method of castration. The reproductive system is one of the major sites of secondary effects of anticancer treatment (Ogilvy-Stuart & Shalet 1993). Different therapeutic insults will be associated with different risks for early menopause. For survivors of treatment for cancer, treatment with radiotherapy below the diaphragm and alkylating agent chemotherapy, the average age at menopause was about 31 years. Other modes of treatment conferred an excess risk of ovarian failure, although not as great (Byrne 1999; Fig. 17.5).

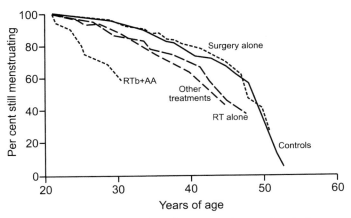

Fig. 17.5 Menopause in childhood cancer survivors and controls expressed as the proportion still menstruating. RTB+AA = radiation therapy below the diaphragm plus alkylating agents; other, all other types of treatment. Reproduced with permission from Byrne et al (1992).

Adverse effects on female reproductive function may be mediated through effects at one or more levels of the HPO axis (Wallace et al 1989a) or at the uterus (Bath et al 1999, Critchley et al 1992a). Commonly anticancer treatment (chemotherapy, particularly alkylating agents, and scatter radiation to the ovary) affects the ovary as a consequence of depletion of the stock of primordial follicles, thereby advancing or inducing menopause (Wallace et al 1989b)

Effects on the hypothalamus and pituitary may be subtle. High-dose cranial irradiation is known to have direct damaging effects but the effects of the lower doses used in the management of childhood leukaemia are as yet uncertain. Data concerning ovarian function after treatment of standard risk leukaemia have been reassuring (Wallace et al 1993). However, with the recent advances in treatment and improved survival as yet few patients are beyond their 30th birthday. A recent study by Bath and colleagues (2001) examined HPO function in 12 women in first remission from childhood acute lympho-blastic leukaemia. This study revealed a high prevalence of short luteal phases (<11 days) among these women compared with a normal control group. A reduced LH excretion (probably secondary to cranial irradiation) and ovarian oestrogen production (probably reflecting a reduction in gonadotrophic stimulus) were observed in the women with acute lympho-blastic leukaemia. Such disturbances in LH secrection may have an effect on reproductive potential.

Resistant ovary syndrome

The resistant ovary syndrome is similar to and may represent an early stage of POF. Goldenberg et al (1973) claimed that raised FSH reliably predicted the absence of ovarian follicles. Earlier, however, Jones & de Moraes-Ruehsen (1969) had described three patients with raised gonadotrophins who presented with primary amenorrhoea and normally developed secondary sexual characteristics and in whom follicles could be detected in the ovaries at laparoscopy. This condition was termed the 'resistant ovary syndrome' to distinguish it from premature menopause where follicles are not detected, but it is unclear whether there is really such a clear distinction.

A single mutation in the FSH-B subunit gene has now been described in women with primary amenorrhoea and infertility (Matthews et al 1993). In these patients there is absent FSH activity but normal follicular development and ovulation can be restored following the administration of exogenous FSH. Mutations in the FSH receptor have also been described in some women with this diagnosis (Huhtaniemi et al 1996). Furthermore, it has been reported that the problem lies in recruitment from primordial to primary follicle (a gonadotrophin-independent step). Hence the defect may be due to a genetic defect in a vital growth factor, for example GDF9, normally involved in the recruitment of primordial follicles (Dong et al 1996).

ENDOCRINE DISORDERS ARISING OUTSIDE THE HPO AXIS LEADING TO CHRONIC ANOVULATION

Other endocrine disorders may interfere with the normal feedback loops of the HPO axis, thereby causing a disturbance in cyclical ovarian activity and manifesting as amenorrhoea or oligomenorrhoea. Thyroid disease may cause amenorrhoea and oligomenorrhoea. There is an increase in circulating concentrations of oestrogen and testosterone in hyper-thyroidism as levels of sex hormone-binding globulin increase. In hypothyroidism there may be associated raised levels of prolactin due to stimulation with thyrotrophic-releasing hormone. In adrenal disease the excessive secretion of sex steroids leads to amenorrhoea, as gonadotrophin secretion will be suppressed.

DIAGNOSIS AND MANAGEMENT OF OLIGO/AMENORRHOEA

The successful management of amenorrhoea/oligomenorrhoea is dependent upon the correct diagnosis and an assessment of the requirements of the patient. Patients will articulate different needs, which may include advice about future fertility prospects, fertility control, symptoms of hirsutism, delayed secondary sexual development, protection from oesteoporosis and endometrial protection from unopposed oestrogen action. A thorough history and clinical examination (as appropriate) are of paramount importance in establishing the diagnosis of an endocrine disorder, complemented with an appropriate examination and conduct of straightforward endocrine investigations. Since the withdrawal of sex steroids results in endometrial bleeding, a detailed menstrual history will be extremely valuable in the determination of endogenous ovarian activity. As long as the patient has not been administered exogenous hormone preparations, a report of only light menstrual bleeding will indicate sufficient ovarian production of oestrogen to produce endometrial proliferation. Hence if a history is given of oligomenorrhoea there must be some capacity for ovarian activity.

It is essential to exclude an anatomical cause of amen-orrhoea. The bimanual assessment of a young woman who has never been sexually active is inappropriate. The examination

237

of secondary sexual characteristics (breast development) and the external genitalia of an adolescent should be performed in the presence of the patient's parent. Indeed, a deferred examination separate from the initial consultation may be most appropriate, thereby providing an opportunity for confidence to be established in the subsequenct doctor–patient relationship. Modern imaging techniques, particularly trans-abdominal ultrasound, are valuable non-invasive modes of establishing information about reproductive anatomy.

In the context of a history of amenorrhoea an enquiry about experience of hot flushes may elicit a diagnosis of ovarian failure. A detailed drug history (see Box 17.6) and information about diet, exercise habit and weight change are essential. Furthermore, enquiry about life events producing psychological stress should be made. Signs of hyperandrogenism may be evident, such as hirsutism, acne and balding. Enquiry about presence of galactorrhoea should be made. A distinction is required between hyperandrogenism and virilization and acanthosis nigricans is a feature of severe insulin resistance. An assessment of the development of secondary sexual characteristics and body mass index is important.

Baseline endocrine investigations should include the exclusion of pregnancy (commonest cause of secondary amenorrhoea), measurement of serum gonadotrophin (FSH and LH), oestradiol and prolactin concentrations and markers of thyroid function – thyroxine and/or TSH – if there are clinical signs of thyroid disease. It is also possible to assess endogenous ovarian activity over the cycle with once- or twice-weekly serial measurements of oestradiol and progesterone concentrations in serum (or plasma) or their metabolites in urine. Serum androgens (testosterone) should be measured in subjects with hirsutism or androgenization. The possible use of transabdominal (and, where appropriate, transvaginal) ultrasound as mentioned above may be a useful adjunct to clinical examination. These baseline endocrine investigations will permit the categorization of patients into essentially one of four diagnostic groups: hypergonadotrophic hypogonadism; hyperprolactinaemia; hypogonadotrophic hypogonadism and normogonadotrophic anovulation (Baird 1997; Fig. 17.6).

Hypergonadotrophic hypogonadism

The endocrine status in ovarian failure (or, rarely, resistant ovary syndrome) is identified by the demonstration a raised serum FSH concentration (>30 iu/l) and a low serum oestradiol level (<60 pmol/l). In cases of primary amenorrhoea and thus primary ovarian failure, a chromosomal analysis will permit identification of women with testicular dysgenesis. It is important that women have their residual gonadal tissue removed on account of the risk of neoplastic change. Sex steroid replacement therapy with cyclic oestrogen and progestogen should be started without delay, particularly in girls with primary ovarian failure, in the latter group to induce secondary sexual characteristics and among all affected patients in order to prevent premature bone loss.

Hyperprolactinaemia

Hyperprolactinaemia (raised serum prolactin) is diagnosed when concentrations of prolactin are outwith the normal range (up to 500 milliunits/l). It should be noted that serum prolactin levels may be transiently and moderately raised (levels above 700 milliunits/l) at times of stress. A persistent, albeit moderate elevation of prolactin will be recorded in the presence of hypothyroidism and is a common feature among women with PCOS. in the latter group, levels as high as 2500 milliunits/l have been reported (Baird 1997, Balen 2000). Thyroid disease may be excluded with estimation of serum thyrotrophin concentrations. Patients with PCOS-related hyperprolactinaemia may be distinguished from women with unrelated hyperprolactinaemia and polycystic ovaries on ultra-sound by means of a progestogen challenge test (Lunenfeld & Insler 1974) which will induce a withdrawal bleed from an oestrogen-primed endometrium.

Serum prolactin measurements greater than 1500 milli-units/l will require more detailed investigations. Imaging of the pituitary fossa is best undertaken with either magnetic resonance imaging (MRI) or computed tomography (CT). Serum prolactin concentrations over 5000 milliunits/l are associated with macroprolactinomas (greater than 1 cm diameter). Diagnostic imaging will detect the presence of a hypothalamic tumour or a non-functioning pituitary tumour causing compression of the hypothalamus or a pituitary microadenoma (Figs 17.7, 17.8).

Hypogonadotrophic hypogonadism

Hypogonadotrophic hypogonadism is characterized by reduced FSH and LH secretion and consequent absence of follicular development and oestradiol production. Prepuberty the situation will manifest as primary amenorrhoea and lack of development of secondary sexual charcteristics. Usually, however, no organic disease is identified in the hypothalamus or anterior pituitary gland. On rare occasions it may be necessary to distinguish hypothalamic causes from pituitary causes with a GnRH stimulation test (100 µg SC) following a week of ethinyl oestradiol orally at a dose of 5–10 µg/day. The administration of this supraphysiological dose of GnRH assesses the responsiveness and capacity of the pituitary to secrete gonadotrophins (Yen et al 1973).

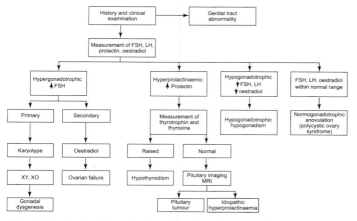

Fig. 17.6 An algorithm for the evaluation of women with amenorrhoea. FSH, follicle-stimulating hormone; LH, luteinizing hormone; MRI, magnetic resonance imaging. Reproduced with permission from Baird, Amenorrhoea. Lancet 350:275–279. ©The Lancet Ltd 1997.

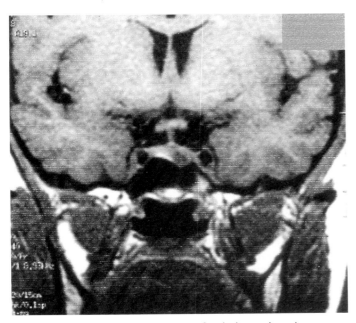

Fig. 17.7 Magnetic resonance image of a pituitary microadenoma (coronal T1 non-contrast image) demonstrating a focal rounded area of low signal in the left half of the gland measuring 7 mm. The lesion distorts both the superior and inferior margins of the pituitary gland. The pituitary infundibulum is midline with no evidence of extension into the suprasellar cistern. Picture kindly provided by Dr Dilip Patel, Edinburgh Royal Infirmary.

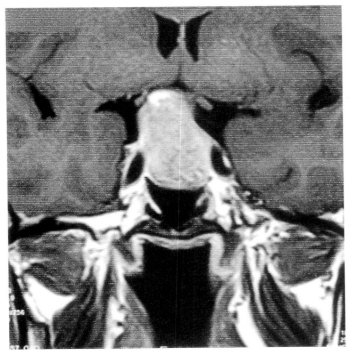

Fig. 17.8 Magnetic resonance image of a pituitary macroadenoma (coronal T1 post-contrast image) demonstrating a large contrast-enhancing mass arising from the pituitary fossa (which is enlarged) and extending into the suprasellar cistern and compressing the optic chiasm. Picture kindly provided by Dr Dilip Patel, Edinburgh Royal Infirmary.

A better index of 'pituitary reserve' is provided by assessment of the response to repeated physiological doses of GnRH (5–10 µg) at 2–3 hour intervals (rather than a single supra-physiological injection). This assessment of pituitary secretory capacity correlates better with the degree of spontaneous secretion, as indicated by the amplitude and frequency of LH pulses. Raised FSH and LH concentrations in response to GnRH stimulation may indicate hypothalamic failure. Such patients require imaging to exclude a craniopharyngioma and consideration of Kallman's syndrome.

Normogonadotrophic anovulation

Normogonadotrophic anovulation occurs in a third of women with secondary amenorrhoea who display normal gonado-trophin concentrations. Women with polycystic ovarian syndrome should be considered in this category and their diagnosis and treatment are discussed in depth in Chapter 19.

THERAPEUTIC ISSUES

Oestrogen deficiency

Women with ovarian failure require sex steroid replacement therapy with cyclic oestrogen and progestogen. Lack of oestrogen after the normal age of menopause has an adverse effect on bone and blood vessel health. Premenopausal levels of oestradiol in women with normal ovarian function protect the female skeleton from demineralization (Howell & Shalet 1999). The cardiovascular protective effects of oestrogen are well documented in older women who have had endogenous protection for many years before the menopause (Mendelsohn & Karas 1999). In Turner's syndrome, there is evidence to suggest that women do not achieve peak bone mass and have a higher rate of fractures (Davies et al 1995). In girls with Turner's syndrome the rate of bone mineral acquisition on the oral contraceptive pill is less than is seen in normal adolescents, with a 25% reduction in bone mineral content from that predicted for age, height, weight and bone size. It is possible that this may be a reflection of suboptimal oestrogen replacement.

Research to date has delivered well-evaluated hormone replacement regimens for older women designed to mitigate the adverse effects of lack of oestrogen and taken for somewhere in the order of 10 years. Currently younger women with a premature menopause are offered combined sex steroid replacement in the convenient form of the combined oral contraceptive pill or hormone replacement regimens designed for older women after menopause. These preparations are not designed to achieve physiological replacement of oestrogen or progesterone, either in dosage or biochemical structure. The optimal mode and formulation of sex steroid replacement have not yet been established for young women with ovarian failure (Conway 2001, Guttman et al 2001).

Management of hyperprolactinaemia

The management of women with hyperprolactinaemia has to take into account the individual's desire or otherwise for pregnancy, her oestrogen status and the presence/absence and size of a pituitary tumour. Women who describe regular menses and who are found to have raised prolactin concentrations do not require treatment unless their menstrual cycles are anovulatory and they wish for pregnancy (Soule & Jacobs 1995). Dopaminergic agents are recommended as the primary therapy for prolactin-secreting adenomas and idiopathic hyperprolactinaemia (Crosignani & Ferrari 1990, Webster et al 1994). Surgery (trans-sphenoidal adenectomy) is usually reserved for dopamine-resistant conditions, intolerable side-effects of therapy and where there is failure to adequately shrink a macroadenoma (Balen 2000). Bromocriptine remains the most widely used dopamine agonist in this condition administered at a dose range between 2.5 and 15 mg daily. Long-acting dopaminergic agents are also now available; an example is cabergoline (administered twice weekly as opposed to daily).

The fall in circulating prolactin concentrations with therapy is accompanied by an increase in frequency of LH pulses. The return of menstruation is usually associated with anovulatory cycles. Since normal ovarian cycles have usually returned by 6 months it may be necessary to provide contraception unless immediate fertility is desired. A tumour of greater than 1 cm in diameter should be surgically removed or reduced in size by dopaminergic therapy prior to pregnancy since there is a small risk of tumour enlargement during pregnancy. Once pregnancy is diagnosed dopaminergic therapy should be discontinued. There is no evidence to indicate that bromocriptine is teratogenic. Bromocriptine therapy should be recommenced if there was evidence during the pregnancy of tumour enlargement.

Should the hyperprolactinaemia be the consequence of drug administration itself (see Box 17.6), cessation of the offending preparation should be recommended after due consultation with other health professionals involved in the patient's care. If continuation of a psychotrophic preparation is essential for the patient's good health (for example, in the case of schizophrenia) then administration of a low-dose oral contraceptive preparation, in addition to continuation of the required dopaminergic therapy, will provide protection against co-incident symptoms of oestrogen deficiency. Serum concentrations of prolactin should continue to be monitored.

Surgical intervention is necessary for non-functioning tumours. These tumours are detected by a combination of imaging and a serum prolactin concentration below 3000 milliunits/l (Balen 2000). A suprasellar extension of the tumour will also be an indication for surgery when dopaminergic therapy has failed to produce regression or there is a wish for pregnancy. Surgery may carry a risk of hypopituitarism and, if present, usually manifests promptly following surgery. Pituitary irradiation (although not common) has a risk of incipient hypopituitarism and therefore necessitates long-term surveillance (Soule & Jacobs 1995).

Fertility issues

There may be reasonable optimism about future fertility prospects for women with amenorrhoea, so long as they do not have POF. Women with oligomenorrhoea, however, have a slightly reduced chance overall (Hull et al 1982). In women with normal gonadotrophin concentrations it is relatively easy to restore fertility with induction of ovulation with an anti-oestrogen preparation such as clomiphene citrate. Some women will also require administration of hCG to induce ovulation, despite a response to clomiphene in terms of follicular development.

Patients with low gonadotrophin concentrations will require ovulation induction with gonadotrophins or pulsatile GnRH therapy. Detail about ovulation induction regimes is addressed in Chapter 18. The assessment of oestrogen status is a useful index of likely responsiveness to ovulation induction agents, such as clomiphene citrate. Furthermore, it identifies the requirement for long-term hormone replacement, where there is a risk of osteoporosis due to oestrogen deficiency, or for endometrial protection with a progestogen, where there is continuous unopposed oestrogen stimulation. The progestogen challenge test utilizes the endometrial response to administration and withdrawal of progestogen. The oestrogen-primed endometrium will exhibit a withdrawal bleed some 24–48 hours following cessation of progestogen administration. An alternative mode of assessment of oestrogen status is the measurement of double endometrial thickness with ultrasound.

The restoration of fertility may be possible in young women with ovarian failure with hormone replacement therapy and assisted reproduction which includes the use of donor oocytes and embryo transfer (Critchely et al 1992b). More controversial is the use of assisted reproductive technology and surrogacy for the fulfilment of family desires among women who have congenital absence of the uterus or who have undergone hysterectomy for cancer at a young age (Brinsden et al 2000).

Contraceptive advice

It is inevitable that young women with ameno/oligomenorrhoea will have concerns about contraceptive requirements and perceived influences on future fertility potential. Furthermore, contraception may be required after ovulation induction therapy. The usual range of contraceptive options should be considered. Copper intrauterine contraceptive devices (IUCD) are usually avoided in nulliparous patients. Women with ameno/oligomenorrhoea are likely to have a degree of oestrogen deficiency with a small uterus. In these women, even those who are parous, insertion and containment of the IUCD may be problematic.

There is no evidence that combined oestrogen/progestogen contraceptive preparations contribute to subsequent amenorrhoea or subfertility. Indeed, there are positive benefits for the use of such preparations. Protection against unopposed oestrogen stimulation of the endometrium in women with chronic anovulation is provided by use of the combined pill or administration of cyclic progestogens.

Acknowledgements

Material in this chapter contains contributions from the previous edition and I am grateful to the previous authors for the work done. I wish to thank Mr Ted Pinner for his assistance with the preparation of the illustrations, Miss Natasha Mallion for secretarial support and Mrs Janet Khindria for help with the references.

KEY POINTS

1. Physiologically regular menses are an indication of cyclical ovarian activity, in turn dependent upon an intact HPO axis. Amenorrhoea and oligomenorrhoea are symptoms of ovarian and reproductive dysfunction.

2. Amenorrhoea is physiological at certain critical times in a woman's life, these being prepuberty, during pregnancy and lactation and in the postmenopausal period. Pathological amenorrhoea may be primary or secondary and there may be common aetiology.

3. The hypothalamic-pituitary axis is regulated at two levels. At a higher level, GnRH neurones within the hypothalamus are stimulated by afferent inputs from the CNS. At a lower level, the output of FSH and LH from the anterior pituitary reflects GnRH activity. Gonadotrophin synthesis in turn is influenced by endocrine feedback from the ovaries as well as paracrine mechanisms and other extrinsic factors. Disturbances in menstrual pattern will be the consequence of either a structural or a functional defect in the tightly controlled feedback system involving the hypothalamus, pituitary and ovary.

4. Baseline endocrine investigations will permit the categorization of patients into essentially one of four diagnostic groups: hypergonadotrophic hypogonadism; hyperprolactinaemia; hypogonadotrophic hypogonadism and normogonadotrophic anovulation.

5. The number of follicles in the human ovary declines steadily from midlife onward. Premature ovarian failure (POF) is the triad of amenorrhoea, elevated FSH and LH in women less than 40 years of age (hypergonadotrophic hypogonadism). Subjects with gonadal failure are oestrogen deficient. One of the commonest chromosomal causes of primary ovarian failure (and primary amenorrhoea) is Turner's syndrome. Women with ovarian failure require sex steroid replacement therapy with cyclic oestrogen and progestogen. Oestrogen deficiency has an adverse effect on bone (osteoporosis) and blood vessel health.

6. Hyperprolactinaemia is diagnosed when prolactin concentrations are outwith the normal range. Serum levels may be transiently raised at times of stress. Serum prolactin measurements greater than 1500 milliunits/l require diagnostic imaging of the pituitary fossa. Approximately 15–20% of women with secondary amenorrhoea display elevated serum prolactin concentrations. In 1–2% of cases the hyperprolactinaemia is induced by drugs that inhibit dopamine action or production. Only half the women who present with hyperprolactinaemia describe galactorrhoea. It is most important to consider the prolactin concentration in the context of the associated ovulatory disorder. Significant hyperprolactinaemia is usually associated with oligomenorrhoea or amenorrhoea.

7. Hypothalamic hypogonadism is characterized by reduced FSH and LH secretion and an absence of follicular development and oestradiol production. As a rule no organic disease is identified in the hypothalamus or anterior pituitary gland.

KEY POINTS (CONTINUED)

8. Severe weight loss, stress and excessive exercise habit are all associated with cessation of hypothalamic function. In each of these situations there is a decrease in GnRH neuronal activity in the hypothalamus with a consequent decrease in gonadotrophin secretion. Thus ovarian follicular development and ovulation fail to occur and a hypo-oestrogenic state develops. A chronic hypo-oestrogenic state will carry significant risk of premature osteoporosis and cardiovascular disease.

9. Other endocrine disorders, such as thyroid and adrenal disease, may interfere with the normal feedback loops of the HPO axis and cause disturbance of cyclical ovarian activity and thus oligomenorrhoea or amenorrhoea.

10. Successful management of amenorrhoea and oligomenorrhoea is dependent upon the correct diagnosis and assessment of the needs of the patient. Each woman will have different requirements, which may include advice on future fertility prospects, fertility control, symptoms of hirsutism, delayed secondary sexual development, risk of osteoporosis and endometrial protection from unopposed oestrogen action.

11. There may be reasonable optimism about future fertility prospects for women with amenorrhoea, so long as they do not have POF. Women with oligomenorrhoea have a slightly reduced chance overall. The mainstay of management is ovulation induction. The restoration of fertility is possible in young women with POF with hormone replacement and assisted reproductive technology that includes the use of donor oocytes and embryo transfer.

REFERENCES

Adams J, Polson DW, Franks S 1986 Prevalence of polycystic ovaries in women with anovulation and idiopathic hirsutism. British Medical Journal (clinical research edition) 293:355–359

Amed SF, Cheng A, Dovey L et al 2000 Phenotypic features, androgen receptor binding, and mutational analysis in 278 clinical cases reported as androgen insensitivity syndrome. Journal of Clinical Endocrinology and Metabolism 85:658–665

Aittomaki K, Lucena JLD, Pakarinen P et al 1995 Mutation in the follicle-stimulating hormone receptor gene causes hereditary hypergonadotrophic ovarian failure. Cell 82:959–968

Allingham-Hawkins DJ, Babul-Hirji R, Chitayat D et al 1999. Fragile X premutation is a significant risk factor for premature ovarian failure. American Journal of Medical Genetics 83:322–325

Alper MM, Garner PR, Seibel MM 1986 Premature ovarian failure: current concepts. Journal of Reproductive Medicine 31: 699–708

Anasti JN 1998 Premature ovarian failure: an update. Fertility and Sterility 70: 1–15

Apter D, Bhtzow T, Laughlin GA, Yen SS 1993 Gonadotropin-releasing hormone pulse generator activity during pubertal transition in girls: pulsatile and diurnal patterns of circulating gonadotropins. Journal of Clinical Endocrinology and Metabolism 76: 940–949

Arif S, Vallian S, Farazneh F et al 1996 Identification of 3 beta-hydroxysteroid dehydrogenase as novel target of steroid cell autoantibodies: association of autoantibodies with endocrine autoimmune disease. Journal of Clinical Endocrinology and Metabolism 81: 4439–4445

Asherman JG 1948 Amenorrhoea traumatica (atretica). Journal of Obstetrics and Gynaecology of the British Empire 55:23–30

Bachmann GA, Kemmann E 1982 Prevalence of oligomenorrhoea and amenorrhoea in a college population. American Journal of Obstetrics and Gynecology 144: 98–102

Baird DT 1997 Amenorrhoea. Lancet 350:275–279

Balen AH 2000 Amenorrhoea, oligomenorrhoea and polycystic ovarian sydnrome. In: O'Brien S, Cameron I, Maclean A (Eds) Disorders of the menstrual cycle. RCOG Press, London

Balen AH, Conway GS, Kaltsas G, Techatraisak K, Manning PJ, West C 1995 Polycystic ovary syndrome: the spectrum of the disorder in 1741 patients. Human Reproduction 10:2017–2111

Ballabio A, Bardoni B, Carrozzo R et al 1989 Contiguous gene syndromes due to deletions in the distal short arm of the human X-chromosome. Proceedings of the National Academy of Science USA 86:10001–10005

Barbarino A, de Marinis L, Tofani A et al 1989 Corticotropin-releasing hormone inhibition of gonadotropin release and the effect of opioid blockade. Journal of Clinical Endocrinology and Metabolism 68:523–528

Bath LE, Critchley HOD, Chambers SE, Anderson RA, Kelnar CJH, Wallace WHB 1999 Ovarian and uterine characteristics after total body irradiation in childhood and adolescence: response to sex steroid replacement. British Journal of Obstetrics and Gynaecology 106: 1265–1272

Bath LE, Anderson RA, Critchley HOD, Kelnar CJH, Wallace WHB 2001 Hypothalamic-pituitary-ovarian dysfunction after pre-pubertal chemotherapy and cranial irradiation for acute leukaemia. Human Reproduction 16: 1838–1844

Bray GA, York DA 1997 Leptin and clinical medicine: a new piece in the puzzle of obesity. Journal of Clinical Endocrinology and Metabolism 82:2771–2776

Brinsden PR, Appleton TC, Murray E, Hussein M, Akagbosu F, Marcus SF 2000 Treatment by in vitro fertilisation with surrogacy: experience of one British centre. British Medical Journal 320:924–928

Byrne 1999 Infertility and premature menopause in childhood cancer survivors. Medical and Pediatric Oncology 33:24–28

Byrne J, Fears TR, Gail MH et al 1992 Early menopause in long-term survivors of cancer during adolescence. American Journal of Obstetrics and Gynecology 166:788–793

Conway GS 1997 Premature ovarian failure. Current Opinion in Obstetrics and Gynecology 9:202–206

Conway GS 2001 Oestrogen replacement in young women with Turner's syndrome. Clinical Endocrinology 54:157–158

Conway GS, Jacobs HS 1997 Leptin: a hormone of reproduction. Human Reproduction 12:633–635

Conway GS, Hettiarachi S, Murray A, Jacobs PA 1995 Fragile X permutations in familial premature ovarian failure. Lancet 346:309–310

Conway GS, Kaltsas G, Patel A, Davies MC, Jacobs HS 1996 Characteristics of idiopathic premature ovarian failure. Fertility and Sterility 65:337–341

Coulam CB, Adamson SC, Annegers JF 1986 Incidence of premature ovarian failure. Obstetrics and Gynecology 67:604–606

Cramer DW, Xu H, Harlow BL 1995 Family history as predictor of early menopause. Fertility and Sterility 64:740–745

Crisponi L, Deiana M, Loi A et al 2001 The putative forkhead transcription factor FOXL2 is mutated in blepharophimosis/ptosis/epicanthus inversus syndrome. Nature Genetics 27:159–166

Critchley HOD, Wallace WHB, Shalet SM et al 1992a Abdominal irradiation in childhood: the potential for pregnancy. British Journal of Obstetrics and Gynaecology 99:392–394

Critchley HOD, Healy DL, King CM, Leeton JF 1992b Practical aspects of oocyte donation. Reproduction, Fertility and Development 4:739–748

Crosignani PG, Ferrari C 1990 Dopaminergic treatments for hyperprolactinaemia. Baillière's Clinical Obstetrics and Gynaecology 4:441–455

Cumming DC, Wheeler GD 1990 Exercise-associated changes in reproduction: a problem common to women and men. In: Reisch RE (Ed) Adipose tissue and reproduction. Karger, Basel

Davies MC, Gulekli B, Jacobs HS 1995 Osteoporosis in Turner's syndrome and other forms of primary amenorrhoea. Clinical Endocrinology (Oxford) 43:741–746

Dong J, Albertini DF, Nishimori K, Kamur TR, Lu N, Matzuk MM 1996 Growth differentiation factor-9 is required during early ovarian folliculogenesis. Nature 383:531–535

Faddy MJ, Gosden RG, Gougeon A, Richarson SJ, Nelson JF 1992 Accelerated disappearance of ovarian follicles in mid-life: implications for forecasting menopause. Human Reproduction 7:1342–1346

Fraser IS, Inceboz US 2000 Defining disturbances of the menstrual cycle In: O'Brien S, Cameron I, Maclean A (Eds) Disorders of the menstrual cycle. RCOG Press, London

Frisch RE 1976 Fatness of girls from menarche to age 18 years, with a nomogram. Human Biology 48:353–359

Frisch RE 1984 Body fat, puberty and fertility. Biological Reviews of the Cambridge Philosophical Society 59:161–188

Glasier AF, Hendry RA, Seth J et al 1987 Does treatment with bromocriptine influence the course of hyperprolactinaemia? Clinical Reproduction and Fertility 5:359–366

Goldenberg RL, Grodin JM, Rodbard D, Ross GT 1973 Gonadotrophins in women with amenorrhoea. The use of plasma FSH to differentiate women with and without ovarian follicles. American Journal of Obstetrics and Gynecology 116:1003–1012

Goodfellow PN, Lovell-Badge R 1993 SRY and sex determination in mammals. Annual Review of Genetics 27:71–92

Gottlieb B, Pinsky L, Beitel LK, Trifiro M 1999 Androgen insensitivity. American Journal of Medical Genetics 89:210–217

Grossman A, Moult PJA, McIntyre H et al 1982 Opiate mediation of amenorrhoea in hyperprolactinaemia and in weight loss related amenorrhoea. Clinical Endocrinology (Oxford) 17:379–388

Guttman H, Weiner Z, Wikolski E et al 2001 Choosing an oestrogen replacement therapy in young adult women with Turner syndrome. Clincial Endocrinology 54:159–164

Harlow SD, Ephross SA 1995 Epidemiology of menstruation and its relevance to women's health. Epidemiologic Reviews 17:265–286

Howell SJ, Shalet SM 1999 Aetiology-specific effect of premature ovarian failure on bone mass – is residual ovarian function important? Clinical Endocrinology (Oxford) 51:531–534

Huhtaniemi I, Pakarinen P, Nilsson C, Pettersson K, Tapanainen J, Aittomaki K 1996 Polymorphisms and mutations of gonadotropin and gonadotropin receptor genes. In: Filicori M, Flamigni C (eds) The ovary: regulation, dysfunction and treatment. Elsevier Science Amsterdam

Hull MGR 1987 Epidemiology of infertility and polycystic ovarian disease: endocrinological and demographic studies. Gynecological Endocrinology 1:235–245

Hull MGR, Savage PE, Bromham DR 1982 Anovulatory and ovulatory infertility: results with simplied management. British Medical Journal (clinical research edition) 284:1681–1685

Illingworth PJ, Seaton JEV, McKinlay C, Reid-Thomas V, McNeilly AS 1995 Low dose transdermal oestradiol suppresses gonadotrophin secretion in breast feeding women. Human Reproduction 10:1671–1677

Imperato-McGinley J 1995 Male pseudohermaphroditism. In: Adashi EY, Rock JA, Rosenwalks Z (eds) Reproductive endocrinology, surgery and technology, vol 1. Philadelphia

Jacobs HS, Franks S, Murray MAF, Hull MGR, Steele SJ, Nabarro JDN 1976 Clinical and endocrine features of hyperprolactinemic amenorrhoea. Clinical Endocrinology (Oxford) 5:439–454

Jones GS, de Moraes-Ruehsen M 1969 A new syndrome of amenorrhea in association with hypergonadotropism and apparently normal ovarian follicular apparatus. American Journal of Obstetrics and Gynecology 104:597–600

Kallman F, Schonfield WA, Barrera SE 1944 The genetic aspects of primary eunuchoidism. American Journal of Mental Deficiency 48:203–236

Kaufman FR, Kogut MD, Donnel GN 1981 Hypergonadotropic hypogonadism in female patients with galactosemia. New England Journal of Medicine 304:994–998

Kleinberg DL, Noel GL, Frantz AG 1977 Galactorrhoea: a study of 235 cases including 48 with pituitary tumours. New England Journal of Medicine 296:589–600

Laughlin GA, Yen SSC 1996 Nutritional and endocrine-metabolic aberrations in amenorrheic athletes. Journal of Clinical Endocrinology and Metabolism 81:4301–4309

Legouis R, Hardelin JP, Levilliers J et al 1991 The candidate gene for the X-linked Kallman syndrome encodes a protein related to adhesion molecules. Cell 67: 423–435

Leiblich JM, Rogol AD, White BJ, Rosen SW 1982 Syndrome of anosmia with hypogonadotropic hypogonadism (Kallman's syndrome). American Journal of Medicine 73:506–519

Lunenfeld B, Insler V 1974 Classification of amenorrhoea states and their treatment by ovulation induction. Clinical Endocrinology (Oxford) 3:223–237

Leyendecker G, Wildt L 1983 Induction of ovulation with chronic intermittent (pulsatile) administration of GnRH in women with hypothalamic amenorrhoea. Journal of Reproduction and Fertility 69:397–409

Matkovic V, Ilich JZ, Skugor M et al 1997 Leptin is inversely related to age at menarche in human females. Journal of Clinical Endocrinology and Metabolism 82:3239–3245

Matthews CH, Borgato S, Beck-Peccoz P et al 1993 Primary amenorrhoea and infertility due to a mutation in the beta-subunit of follicle stimulating hormone. Nature Genetics 5:83–86

McNeilly AS 1984 Prolactin and ovarian function. In: Muller EE, MacLeod RM (eds) Neuroendocrine perspectives, vol. 3. Elsevier Science, Amsterdam

Mendelsohn ME, Karas RH. 1999 The protective effects of estrogen on the cardiovascular system. New England Journal of Medicine 340:1801–1811

Nakayama Y, Wondisford FE, Lash RW et al 1990 Analysis of gonadotropin-releasing hormone gene structure in families with familial central precocious puberty and idiopathic hypogonadotropic hypogonadism. Journal of Clinical Endocrinology and Metabolism 70:1233–1238

Ogilvy-Stuart A, Shalet SM 1993 Effect of radiation on the human reproductive system. Environmental Health Perspectives 101(suppl 12):109–116

Parkin DE 2000 Surgical techniques for the treatment of dysfunctional uterine bleeding. In: O'Brien S, Cameron I, Maclean A (Eds) Disorders of the menstrual cycle. RCOG Press, London

Pasquino AM, Passeri F, Pucarelli I, Segni M, Municchi G 1997 Spontaneous pubertal development in Turner's syndrome. Italian Study Group for Turner's Syndrome. Journal of Clinical Endocrinology and Metabolism 82:1810–1813

Perheentupa A, Critchley HOD, Illingworth PJ, McNeilly AS 2000 Enhanced sensitivity to steroid-negative feedback during breast feeding: low dose estradiol (transdermal estradiol supplementation) suppresses gonadotropins and ovarian activity assessed by inhibin B. Journal of Clinical Endocrinology and Metabolism 85:4280–4286

Pettersson F, Fries H, Nillius SJ 1973 Epidemiology of secondary amenorrhoea. I. Incidence and prevalence rates. American Journal of Obstetrics and Gynecology 117:80–86

Randeva HS, Davis M, Prelevic GM 2000 Prolactinoma and pregnancy. British Journal of Obstetrics and Gynaecology 107:1064–1068

Richarson SJ, Senikas V, Nelson JF 1987 Follicular depletion during the menopausal transition: evidence for accelerated loss and ultimate exhaustion. Journal of Clinical Endocrinology and Metabolism 65:1231–1237

Ropert JF, Quigley ME, Yen SCC 1981 Endogenous opiates modulate pulsatile luteinising hormone release in humans. Journal of Clinical Endocrinology and Metabolism 52: 583–585

Rugarli EI, Ballabio A 1993 Kallman syndrome from genetics to neurobiology. Journal of the American Medical Association 270:2713–2716

Schlechte J, Dolan K, Sherman B, Chapler F, Luciano A 1989 The natural history of untreated hyperprolactinemia: a prospective analysis. Journal of Clinical Endocrinology and Metabolism 68:412–418

Schwanzel-Fukuda M, Bick D, Pfaff DN 1989 Luteinising-hormone-releasing hormone (LHRH) - expressing cells do not migrate normally in an inherited hypogonadal (Kallman) syndrome. Molecular Brain Research 6:311–326

Sheehan HL 1939 Simmond's disease due to postpartum necrosis of the anterior pituitary. Quarterly Journal of Medicine 8(32):277–309

Singh KB 1981 Menstrual disorders in college students. American Journal of Obstetrics and Gynecology 140:299–302

Sohval AR 1965 The syndrome of pure gonadal dysgenesis. American Journal of Medicine 38:615–625

Soule SG, Jacobs HS 1995 Prolactinomas: present day management. British Journal of Obstetrics and Gynaecology 102:178–181

Speroff L, Glass RH, Kase NG 1999a Amenorrhoea. In: Speroff L, Glass RH, Kase NG (Eds) Clinical gynecologic endocrinology and infertility 6th edn. Lippincott, Williams and Wilkins, Baltimore

Speroff L, Glass RH, Kase NG 1999b Amenorrhoea. In: Speroff L, Glass RH, Kase NG (Eds) Clinical gynecologic endocrinology and infertility 6th edn. Lippincott, Williams and Wilkins, Baltimore

Speroff L, Glass RH, Kase NG 1999c Normal and abnormal sexual development. In: Speroff L, Glass RH, Kase NG (Eds) Clinical gynecologic endocrinology and infertility 6th edn. Lippincott, Williams and Wilkins, Baltimore

Stager JM, Ritchie-Flanagan RB, Robertshaw D 1984 Reversibility of amenorrhoea in athletes. New England Journal of Medicine. 310:51–52

Treloar Ae, Boynton RE, Behn BG, Brown BW 1967 Variation of the human menstrual cycle through reproductive life. International Journal of Fertility 12:77–126

Wallace WHB, Shalet SM, Crowne EC et al 1989a Ovarian failure following abdominal irradiation in childhood: natural history and prognosis. Clinical Oncology (Royal College of Radiologists) 1:75–79

Wallace WHB, Shalet SM, Hendry JH, Morris-Jones PH, Gattameneni HR 1989b Ovarian failure following abdominal irradiation in childhood: the radiosensitivity of the human oocyte. British Journal of Radiology 62:995–998

Wallace WHB, Shalet SM, Tetlow LJ, Morris-Jones PH 1993 Ovarian function following the treatment of childhood acute lymphoblastic leukaemia. Medical and Pediatric Oncology 21:333–339

Walsh RJ 1978 The age of the menopause of Australian women. Medical Journal of Australia 2:181–182, 215

Warren MP 1995 Anorexia nervosa. In: de Groot LJ (ed) Endocrinology, 3rd edn. WB Saunders, Philadelphia

Warren MP, Brooks-Gunn J, Hamilton LH, Warren LF, Hamilton WG 1986 Scoliosis and fractures in young ballet dancers: relation to delayed menarche and secondary amenorrhoea. New England Journal of Medicine 314:1348–1353

Webster J, Pistitelli G, Poli A et al 1994 A comparison of cabergoline and bromocriptine in the treatment of hyperprolactinaemic amenorrhoea. New England Journal of Medicine 331:904–909

Weiss J, Crowley WF Jr, Jameson JL 1989 Normal structure of the gonadotropin–releasing hormone (GnRH) gene in patients with GnRH deficiency and idiopathic hypogonadotropic hypogonadism. Journal of Clinical Endocrinology and Metabolism 69:299–303

Yen SCC 1999 Chronic anovulation due to CNS-hypothalamic-pituitary dysfunction. In: Yen SSC, Jaffe RB, Barbieri RL (Eds) Reproductive endocrinology, physiology, pathophysiology, and clinical management, 4th edn. WB Saunders, Philadelphia

Yen SCC, Rebar R, van den Berg G et al 1973 Pituitary gonadotrophin responsiveness to synthetic LRF in subjects with normal and abnormal hypothalamic-pituitary-axis. Journal of Reproduction and Fertility 20(Suppl):137–161

Zhang Y, Proenca R, Maffei M, Barone M, Leopold L, Friedman JM 1994 Positional cloning of the mouse obese gene and its human homologue. Nature 372:425–432

Zreik TG, Olive D 1998 Amenorrhoea. In: O'Brien S, Cameron I, Maclean A (Eds) Disorders of the menstrual cycle. RCOG Press, London

replacement therapy to protect their skeleton and cardio-vascular systems from the deleterious effects of hypo-oestrogenism. Although there have been case reports of spontaneous pregnancies or successful ovulation induction treatment with various methods in patients with ovarian failure, any form of ovulation induction is not advisable in these women. There is also no advantage in performing laparoscopy and ovarian biopsy to detect the presence of follicles in the resistant ovary syndrome because of the invasive nature and the doubtful value of the procedure.

Hypogonadotrophic hypogonadism

These patients present with primary or secondary amenorrhoea. They have very low serum oestradiol concentration due to low FSH and LH secretion from the pituitary gland (hypo-gonadotrophic hypogonadism). It can be due to either congenital causes such as Kallmann's syndrome (isolated gonadotrophin deficiency and anosmia) or acquired causes such as pituitary tumour, pituitary necrosis (Sheehan's syndrome), stress and excessive weight loss (anorexia nervosa). Computed tomography of the skull should be performed to exclude any space-occupying lesion around the hypothalamus and pituitary region, which can disturb gonadotrophin secretion. The commonest tumour of the pituitary region in childhood and adolescence is craniopharyngioma, a tumour of the Rathke's pouch. Detailed neurological and visual field examinations are required. Patients who have undergone a hypophysectomy may also present with hypogonadotrophic hypogonadism.

Surgery is clearly indicated in patients with central nervous system tumours. Patients with anorexia nervosa may benefit from psychotherapy and weight gain after extensive counselling but achieving sufficient weight gain to re-establish ovulatory cycles is notoriously difficult in such patients. Pulsatile GnRH or gonadotrophins are offered to patients with other hypo-gonadotrophic causes or with persisting anovulation despite weight gain.

Normogonadotrophic hypogonadism

This includes a heterogeneous group of patients who can present either with regular cycles, oligomenorrhoea or even amenorrhoea. The midluteal serum progesterone is low, FSH and LH levels are in the normal range and prolactin is normal. Most of these patients are likely to have polycystic ovary syndrome (PCOS), which is discussed in much more detail in Chapter 19. Other causes include congenital adrenal hyperplasia, adrenal tumours and androgen-producing ovarian tumours. In these conditions, the patient may have clinical symptoms or signs of hyperandrogenism such as hirsutism, which should require more detailed investigations such as measurement of serum testosterone, dehydroepiandrosterone sulphate and 17-OH progesterone.

Obese PCOS women will benefit from weight loss, as this will not only improve their response to ovulation induction but also might lead to resumption of spontaneous ovulation. They usually respond well to clomiphene citrate or, failing that, to gonadotrophins for induction of ovulation. Insulin-sensitizing agents or laparoscopic ovarian drilling may be considered in those not responding to clomiphene citrate (see Chapter 19). Specific causes, such as adrenal or ovarian tumours, should be treated by removing the cause and congenital adrenal hyper-plasia benefits from appropriate corticosteroid replacement therapy.

WEIGHT REDUCTION

Overweight women have a higher incidence of menstrual disturbance, ovulation disorders and infertility. If ovulation induction is required, they have lower success rates. The dose of clomiphene citrate required to achieve ovulation is positively correlated with body weight and non-responders are more likely to be obese. Obese PCOS women respond poorly to pulsatile GnRH therapy. Women with a BMI of 25–28 need a gonadotrophin dose 50% higher than normal-weight women (Galtier-Dereure et al 1997). Moreover, obese women are more prone to pregnancy complications such as miscarriage, gestational diabetes, hypertension, macrosomia and difficult delivery.

Excessive body fat is associated with insulin resistance, hyperinsulinaemia, high insulin-like growth factors and LH concentrations. An increased waist:hip ratio indicating body fat deposition appears to have a more important effect than body weight alone. Obese women should be encouraged to lose weight before active treatment is contemplated. Even moderate weight loss (<5%) may restore regular menstruation, improve ovulation, achieve spontaneous pregnancy and ameliorate the abnormal endocrine parameters. Reproductive outcomes for all forms of infertility treatment and psychological assessment of self-esteem, anxiety and depression were significantly improved after weight reduction (Clark et al 1998).

Achieving successful weight reduction is, however, extremely difficult. A multidisciplinary approach is advisable. Behavioural therapy was more successful than the use of drugs such as appetite suppressants, which should be reserved for extremely obese women and given under close medical supervision. Weight loss is more likely to be maintained when the weight-reducing programme is run in a group situation rather than in a one-to-one format. It is certainly more cost effective and involves fewer risks to run a weight-reducing programme than to start medical or surgical methods of ovulation induction.

MEDICAL INDUCTION OF OVULATION

Effective use of ovulation induction agents requires under-standing of their mechanism of action, appropriate indications, different regimens, monitoring methods and potential complications.

Dopamine agonists

Mechanism of action

The secretion of prolactin from the lactotroph cells in the anterior pituitary gland is mainly regulated by the tonic inhibitory control of a prolactin-inhibiting factor, which in humans is predominantly dopamine. Drugs with dopaminomimetic activity lower prolactin secretion, restore gonadal function and shrink a prolactinoma, if present.

Regimen and monitoring

Bromocriptine is by far the most commonly used drug and is given at a daily dosage of 2.5–20 mg in divided doses 2–3 times a day. Serum prolactin concentrations are regularly measured and ovulation is checked by midluteal progesterone concentrations. Other forms of monitoring for ovarian response are not required as its use is not associated with multiple pregnancy or ovarian hyperstimulation syndrome. In patients who do not ovulate even when prolactin concentrations are within normal range, dopamine agonists can be combined with anti-oestrogen, pulsatile GnRH or gonadotrophin as appropriate.

New oral dopamine agonists such as cabergoline and quinagolide are licensed for hyperprolactinaemia and have longer biological half-lives than bromocriptine. Cabergoline can be taken once or twice weekly and quinagolide once daily. Two large, multicentre randomized controlled trials (Pascal Vigneron et al 1995, Webster et al 1994) comparing cabergoline and bromocriptine in the treatment of hyper-prolactinaemia found that cabergoline was significantly more effective than bromocriptine in restoring normal prolactin concentrations and ovulatory cycles.

Results

Serum prolactin concentrations are normalized in about 80% of patients with microprolactinoma or idiopathic disease after taking bromocriptine and ovarian function is restored in about 85%. Prolactin concentrations return to normal in about 65% of patients with macroprolactinoma, with restored gonadal function in over 50%. A decrease in tumour size is reported in about 70% of patients with a prolactinoma. Long-term treatment with bromocriptine achieves pregnancy rates of 35–70%.

Side-effects

Side-effects with bromocriptine are common. Although they are usually transient and mild, around 5% of patients discontinue the treatment for this reason. Gastrointestinal side-effects such as nausea, vomiting and abdominal cramps may be caused by a local effect on the gastric mucosa. Other side-effects such as vertigo, postural hypotension, headaches and drowsiness are likely to be due to smooth muscle relaxation in the splanchnic beds and inhibition of the sympathetic activity. The side-effects can be minimized by increasing the dose gradually from a low starting dose given with a meal in the evening or by administering vaginal bromocriptine. A depot injection or a slow-release preparation may also reduce the incidence of side-effects. Significantly fewer gastrointestinal side-effects such as nausea and vomiting were noted in patients taking cabergoline.

There is no increase in the incidence of multiple pregnancy, ovarian hyperstimulation syndrome (OHSS) and spontaneous abortion in patients treated with dopamine agonists.

Anti-oestrogens

Clomiphene citrate

Mechanism of action   Clomiphene citrate (CC) has been used for induction of ovulation since 1962. It is usually indicated as the first-line drug in women with ovulatory disorders who have withdrawal bleeding after progestogen, i.e. normally oestrogenized. CC, an orally active non-steroidal compound structurally related to diethylstilboestrol, has both oestrogenic and anti-oestrogenic properties. Its primary mechanism of action is not fully understood. Acting as anti-oestrogen, CC displaces endogenous oestrogen from oestrogen receptors in the hypothalamic-pituitary axis. This diminishes the negative feedback and increases the secretion of GnRH and thus gonadotrophins. The use of CC may result in a 50% increase in endogenous FSH and LH concentrations.

Regimen and monitoring   CC should be started with a daily dose of 50 mg for 5 days, taken from day 5 to day 9 of the cycle. Alternatively, starting the treatment on day 2, 3 or 4 of the cycle gives the same results in terms of ovulation and pregnancy (Wu & Winkel 1989). Ovulation usually occurs within 5–10 days after the last tablet. If there is no ovulation, the dose is increased to 100 mg daily for 5 days and further increments of 50 mg are used until ovulation occurs or a maximum dose of 250 mg daily is reached. The same dose should be continued in those patients showing ovulation for at least 12 cycles or until pregnancy occurs. Polson et al (1989) found that patients who fail to respond to CC 100 mg daily will not ovulate when given higher doses. Extended CC therapy or continuous administration of CC >5 days may provide a more potent stimulant to ovulation and has been reported in some studies (Kelly & Jewelewicz 1990). However, gonadotrophin changes show a peculiar pattern when CC is given to normal women for 15 instead of 5 days (Messinis & Templeton 1988). If the patient fails to ovulate on higher doses, other appropriate treatments should be offered.

Because of the variable response of patients to CC, it is important to monitor the response at least during treatment until ovulation is confirmed to ensure that each patient receives an appropriate dose. Serum progesterone concentrations are usually measured in the midluteal phase to check for ovulation. It is recommended that ultrasound examination should be performed as well to look for development of multiple follicles in some patients, particularly those with polycystic ovary syndrome, in whom the dose of CC should be decreased in the next cycle in order to reduce the risk of multiple pregnancy (RCOG 1998).

Results   The effectiveness of CC for ovulation induction in normally oestrogenized women is well established. Studies have shown an ovulation rate of 60–85% and a pregnancy rate of 30–40%. A recent meta-analysis (Hughes et al 2000a) of four randomized, double-blind, placebo-controlled crossover studies showed that the odds ratio for ovulation using standard doses (50–250 mg daily) was 6.82 (95% confidence interval 3.92–11.85), compared with placebo. This dropped to a non-significant odds ratio of 1.29 (95% confidence interval 0.48–3.49) with low dose (10 mg daily). Two of the studies reported pregnancy and the odds ratio for pregnancy rate per treatment cycle was 3.41 (95% confidence interval 4.23–9.48). There is no increase in spontaneous abortion or congenital abnormalities in CC pregnancies. The rate of multiple pregnancy is 5–10%, with the great majority being twins, although higher order multiple pregnancies have been reported (Levene et al 1992).

Absence of follicular development despite an appropriate

rise in serum FSH concentrations appears the main reason for anovulation. Non-responders to CC are more likely to be obese and have greater ovarian volumes and greater numbers of small follicles on ultrasound than responders. Concentrations of serum LH or androgens have not consistently differed between responders and non-responders.

The two commonest causes of failure to conceive in response to CC are the presence of other infertility factors and the failure to persist with repeated attempts. CC treatment can be given up to 12 cycles in women who ovulate with CC and have no other infertility factors as the cumulative conception rates continue to rise after six cycles but begin to plateau by 12 cycles (RCOG 1998).

Side-effects   Due to its combined oestrogenic and anti-oestrogenic properties, CC can lead to hot flushes, breast discomfort, abdominal distension, nausea and vomiting, nervousness, sleeplessness, headache, mood swings, dizziness, hair loss and disturbed vision. These side-effects are dose dependent and are usually completely reversible once CC is stopped. Ovarian enlargement can also occur, sometimes to a significant extent, but usually disappears by the end of the cycle. Severe OHSS is very rare with CC unless hCG is also administered as a 'surrogate LH' ovulatory surge.

Tamoxifen

Tamoxifen is a triphenylethylene derivative with a structure similar to CC. The suggested dose in ovulation induction is 20–40 mg daily, beginning on cycle day 3 for 5 days. It appears to be as effective as CC in terms of ovulation and pregnancy rates and may have less anti-oestrogenic effect on the cervical mucus. Tamoxifen has been used much less often than CC for ovulation induction and is not licensed for this use in the United Kingdom.

Insulin–sensitizing agents

Insulin resistance and compensatory hyperinsulinaemia are prominent features of PCOS. Increased insulin concentrations lead to hyperandrogenism because of increased production of ovarian androgen and decreased synthesis of sex hormone-binding globulin. As hyperinsulinaemia plays a significant role in anovulation in women with PCOS, clinical improvement can be anticipated by reducing serum insulin concentrations. Weight loss in obese women with PCOS may lead to reduction of hyperinsulinaemia. Insulin-sensitizing agents have been tried in the management of patients with PCOS, as the initial treatment or when these patients remain anovulatory while on CC.

A number of studies have shown significant improvements in insulin sensitivity and hyperinsulinaemia in obese PCOS women after taking metformin (Sattar et al 1998). These improvemens were associated with reduction in serum androgen concentrations and an increase in sex hormone-binding globulin concentrations. Metformin treatment seemed to have no effect on ovarian function in women with normal testosterone concentrations whereas patients with elevated pretreatment testosterone concentrations showed the most marked increase in ovulation rate. Troglitazone, another insulin-sensitizing agent, has been shown to induce ovulation

in 15 of 18 (83%) women with CC-resistant PCOS (Mitwally et al 1999) but this drug has been withdrawn from the market because of hepatotoxicity caused by an idiosyncratic reaction.

Gonadotrophin-releasing hormone

Mechanism of action

Pulsatile gonadotrophin-releasing hormone (GnRH) has been used since 1980 for ovulation induction in anovulatory women. In patients with intact hypothalamic-pituitary-ovarian function, GnRH administered in a pulsatile fashion will fully restore the normal pattern of gonadotrophin and gonadal steroid secretion of a spontaneous menstrual cycle, leading to the development of a single dominant follicle.

Regimen and monitoring

In general, GnRH is given via a small battery-operated pump, delivering $2.5–20.0\,\mu g$ per bolus at 60–90-minute intervals. It can be administered either subcutaneously ($15–20\,\mu g$ starting dose) or intravenously ($2.5–5.0\,\mu g$) through a small butterfly cannula which may be maintained in situ for the duration of the treatment. The intravenous route is preferred by some because more physiological LH profiles and higher ovulatory rates result when GnRH is administered intravenously. A lower GnRH dose is required as well in the intravenous route. Treatment can be monitored by regular serum oestradiol measurements and pelvic ultrasound at 3–4-day intervals. Couples are advised to have regular intercourse during the treatment cycle. The luteal phase has to be supported, either by continuing with the same regimen of pulsatile GnRH administration or using exogenous hCG injections.

Ovulation may also be induced by the concomitant use of CC (100 mg daily for 5 days) or gonadotrophin during the pulsatile GnRH treatment in PCOS patients who are resistant to pulsatile GnRH alone. Administration of a GnRH agonist for a period of 4–6 weeks immediately prior to pulsatile GnRH treatment causes a remarkable improvement of endocrine profile and ovulation rates of these unresponsive PCOS patients (Filicori et al 1994).

Results

The ovulation rates and pregnancy rates per treatment cycle are 70–93% and 18–29% respectively (Table 18.1). Hypogonadotrophic patients of normal or low weight are the best candidates for this treatment and PCOS patients or patients with excessive weight, elevated serum LH and insulin concentrations have lower success rates. Multiple pregnancy rates ranged between 3.8% and 13.5% and are increased in less severe forms of hypogonadotrophic hypogonadism (not primary amenorrhoea) and higher GnRH starting doses.

Side-effects

When compared to gonadotrophin treatment in a retrospective analysis (Martin et al 1993), pulsatile GnRH results in higher rates of ovulation and conception and a decreased risk of multiple follicular development, higher order multiple pregnancies, ovarian enlargement and cycle cancellation. Pulsatile GnRH treatment is likely to be less expensive than gonadotrophin treatment because of a decreased need for

Table 18.1   Results on the use of pulsatile GnRH for ovulation induction

	Homburg et al (1989)	Braat et al (1989)	Martin et al (1993)	Filicori et al (1994)
Patients	118	NA	41	292
Cycles	434	NA	118	600
Ovulation rate (%)	70	NA	93	75
PR per treatment cycle (%)	23	NA	29	18
Multiple pregnancy rate (%)	7.0	13.5	8.3	3.8
Abortion rate (%)	28.0	10.3	23.8	29.5

NA, not available

Table 18.2   Different gonadotrophin preparations

Preparation	Source of FSH	FSH activity (iu/ampoule)	LH activity (iu/ampoule)	FSH specific activity (iu/mg protein)	Non-FSH urinary proteins
HMG	Urine	75	75	75–150	95%
Urinary FSH	Urine	75	<0.7	150–150	95%
Urinary FSH-high purity	Urine	75	<0.001	10 000	>1%
Recombinant FSH	Chinese hamster ovary	50, 75, 100, 150, 200	None	10 000	None

intensive monitoring and a lower risk of multiple pregnancies. However, patients may be reluctant to use the pump because of worry about pump failure and the problems of the needle being left in situ for such a long time (e.g. displacement, local reaction, infection) and inconvenience. As a result, it is used in very few patients for whom alternatives such as gonadotrophin treatment are available.

Gonadotrophins

Preparations (Table 18.2)
Human menopausal gonadotrophins are extracted from the urine of postmenopausal women. They are available mainly in three preparations: an FSH and LH mixture with a 1:1 ratio (e.g. hMG: Pergonal from Serono or Humegon from Organon); a 3:1 ratio (e.g. Normegon from Organon), and a purified FSH preparation (e.g. Metrodin or Metrodin HP from Serono). Besides the difficulty in collecting urine, urinary gonadotrophins have many disadvantages including the presence of LH, contamination with >95% non-FSH urinary proteins, a higher incidence of local allergic reactions and batch-to-batch inconsistency.

The increasing demand for treatment with assisted reproduction leads to the shortage problem of urinary gonadotrophins. Recombinant human FSH (Gonal-F from Serono or Puregon from Organon) is produced by a Chinese hamster ovary cell line, transfected with the genes encoding for the two FSH subunits. This results in an almost totally pure FSH preparation, devoid of the disadvantages associated with urinary gonadotrophins.

Mechanism of action
FSH is the key gonadotrophic hormone during the follicular phase and only minute amounts of LH are needed in different stages of follicular development and function. Excessive levels of LH in the early or late follicular phase have adverse effects on fertilization, implantation, pregnancy rates and early embryonic development. The classic indications for gonadotrophin treatment are patients with hypogonadotrophic hypogonadism and with normogonadotrophic anovulation who failed to ovulate on CC.

Hypogonadotrophic hypogonadal women who have very low serum LH concentrations (0.5 iu/l) should be given a preparation containing both FSH and LH because of the fundamental role of LH in ovarian steroidogenesis. When recombinant FSH is offered to these women, follicular development is satisfactory but serum oestradiol concentration remains low and the endometrial lining is thin.

Regimens of administration (Fig. 18.4)
Regular-dose step-up protocol   In this protocol, gonadotrophin injection is started on day 2–3 of the cycle or following an induced withdrawal bleed, at a dose of FSH 150 iu/day. The injection is continued daily and the dose is increased by 75 iu every 4–5 days according to the ovarian response assessed by serum oestradiol concentration or ultrasound follicular measurement. The same dose will be maintained when an ovarian response is seen. Once 1–2 dominant follicles reach 18 mm in mean diameter, human chorionic gonadotrophin (hCG) is administered at a dose of 5000–10 000 iu to induce ovulation. The couple is advised to have intercourse on the day of hCG injection and on the following day. This protocol is associated with a high incidence of multiple pregnancy and ovarian hyperstimulation syndrome, especially in patients with PCOS.

Chronic low-dose, step-up protocol   The principle of this protocol is to reach the FSH threshold gradually, avoiding excessive stimulation and development of multiple follicles. The patient is given a low starting dose of FSH (37.5–75 iu/day) for at least 10–14 days and the daily dose is

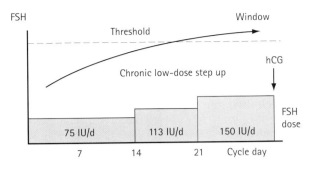

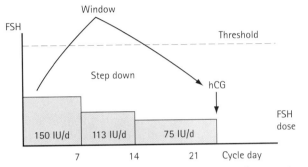

Fig. 18.4 Chronic low-dose step-up protocol vs step-down protocol.

increased by 37.5 iu at weekly intervals up to a maximum of 225 iu/day if there is no evidence of follicular development. The same dose is maintained once an ovarian response is present. The criteria for administering hCG are similar to those in the regular-dose step-up protocol.

As it may take several weeks to achieve an ovarian response in those with a high FSH threshold, patients should be counselled about the timescale prior to the first treatment cycle. In subsequent cycles, the patient can then be started at a dose that gives rise to ovarian response in the first cycle and this will shorten the duration required.

Step-down protocol The aim of this protocol is to mimic the physiological changes of normal cycles. Development of a single dominant follicle is achieved by decreasing serum FSH levels and limiting the duration of FSH levels above the threshold (FSH window theory). In this protocol, patients are usually given gonadotrophin injection 150 iu FSH/day starting on day 2–3 of the cycle and the ovarian response is monitored by transvaginal scanning every 2–3 days. The same dose is continued until dominant follicle ≥ 10 mm is seen on scanning. The dose is then reduced to 112.5 iu/day followed by a further decrease to 75 iu/day 3 days later, which is continued until hCG is administered to induce ovulation.

Monitoring The purpose of monitoring ovarian response during gonadotrophin treatment is to time the hCG injection for inducing ovulation and to reduce the risk of multiple pregnancy and ovarian hyperstimulation. Cycles with excessive response can be cancelled by withholding the ovulatory hCG injection. Both serum oestradiol levels and ultrasound examination are commonly used for monitoring purposes. Serum oestradiol level reflects the total amount of oestradiol secreted from growing follicles and thus cannot differentiate between single dominant follicle and multiple intermediate-

sized follicles. Ultrasound examination gives an immediate result of the number of dominant follicles and their sizes. Shoham et al (1991) have shown that oestradiol levels did not add any additional information to the monitoring solely based on ultrasound.

Concomitant use of gonadotrophin–releasing hormone agonists (GnRH-a) High LH levels commonly found in the follicular phase of patients with PCOS are associated with an increased rate of spontaneous abortion. LH levels may be elevated inappropriately in some patients before the dominant follicle reaches 16–18 mm in mean diameter, causing premature luteinization. The use of GnRH-a prior to gonadotrophin administration will lower the tonic high LH levels during the follicular phase and prevent the occurrence of premature LH surges. This may improve the results of ovulation induction in patients with CC-resistant PCOS and reduce the associated high abortion rate.

A recent meta-analysis (Hughes et al 2000b) of three randomized trials shows that there is no clear advantage in the routine use of GnRH-a in conjunction with gonadotrophin for ovulation induction in patients with CC-resistant PCOS. Common odds ratios for pregnancy per treatment cycle and moderate to severe OHSS are 1.5 (95% CI: 0.72–3.12) and 1.40 (95% CI: 0.5–3.92) respectively. Moreover, the use of GnRH-a will further increase the cost of gonadotrophin treatment because of the GnRH-a and the increased amount of gonadotrophins used after using GnRH-a. Therefore, routine administration of GnRH-a with gonadotrophin is not indicated. It is more appropriate to use GnRH-a in women who show evidence of premature luteinization in previous gonadotrophin treatment cycles.

Concomitant use with CC Some programmes use a combination of CC and gonadotrophin, to lessen the overall cost by reducing the amount of gonadotrophin needed. CC is used initially (100 mg daily on days 2–6) for follicular recruitment, followed by gonadotrophin (150 iu daily or on alternate days) to promote follicular growth, thus reducing the gonadotrophin requirement by up to 50%. This regimen is only of use in anovulatory patients who have reasonable endogenous gonadotrophin secretion.

Results

Gonadotrophin treatment is very effective in inducing ovulation and the results may depend on the indication, the regimen employed and the preparation used. The 6-month cumulative conception rate (CCR) in non-PCOS patients is around 90% with an abortion rate of 25% whereas the corresponding results in PCOS are only 50–60% 6-month CCR with an abortion rate of 30–40%. Regular-dose step-up protocol in PCOS patients leads to 5% severe OHSS rate and 34% multiple pregnancy rate. When chronic low-dose step-up protocol is used in these women, similar pregnancy rates are achieved but the rates of severe OHSS and multiple pregnancy can be reduced to <0.1% and 6% respectively. A randomized study (van Stantbrink & Fauser 1997) comparing low-dose step-up and step-down protocols in PCOS patients showed a reduction of the duration of the treatment and total gonadotrophin dosage. Monofollicular development is more common in those receiving the step-down protocol. This may further reduce the risk of severe OHSS and multiple pregnancy during gonado-trophin treatment.

It was previously thought that the use of purified urinary FSH or recombinant FSH preparations in PCOS patients who had high endogenous LH levels might improve the results of ovulation induction because of low or no LH activity in these products. Daya et al (1995), in a meta-analysis of eight randomized trials on in vitro fertilization cycles, demonstrated that the use of urinary FSH or recombinant FSH was associated with a significantly higher clinical pregnancy rate than hMG. No such advantage in the pregnancy rate was demonstrated when urinary FSH and hMG were compared in the treatment of CC-resistant PCOS (Hughes et al 2000c). However, the use of FSH appeared to be associated with a reduction in moderate to severe OHSS with a common odds ratio of 0.2 (95% CI: 0.09–0.46), although the reason for this reduction was un-explained. Purified urinary FSH and recombinant FSH are equally efficient for inducing ovulation in women with CC-resistant PCOS but significantly more single follicle development was noted in the recombinant group (Yarali et al 1999).

Given similar costs, purified urinary or recombinant FSH may be preferable to hMG in treating these women because of purity and a possible reduction in OHSS. However, the purified urinary and recombinant FSH are more expensive than hMG in developing countries and their benefits should be balanced against the increased cost when choosing the gonadotrophin preparation.

Side-effects

Serious complications of gonadotrophin therapy include ovarian hyperstimulation syndrome and multiple pregnancy, which will be discussed in detail in the next section of this chapter. Other complications include local reaction at the site of the injection or, rarely, anaphylactic reaction, perhaps due to the protein content of the urinary products. Such patients should be switched to recombinant FSH preparations.

Risks of medical induction of ovulation

Ovarian hyperstimulation syndrome

Ovarian hyperstimulation syndrome (OHSS) is a serious and potentially life-threatening complication of ovulation induction, usually arising from excessive ovarian stimulation. Only a few cases have been reported in spontaneous cycles. Before offering ovulation induction, every patient should be properly counselled about the risk associated with the method used and educated on the presenting symptoms. Patients at risk of the syndrome are identified and different measures can be taken to prevent the syndrome or reduce the risk. Clear guidelines on the management should be available.

Pathophysiology The hallmark of this syndrome is abnormal fluid accumulation in the third space such as the peritoneal, pleural and, rarely, the pericardial space, resulting in intravascular volume depletion and haemoconcentration. The exact mechanism of this remains unclear. Excessive gonadotrophin stimulation on the ovary leads to development of multiple follicles and accounts for ovarian enlargement commonly encountered in OHSS (Fig. 18.5). Many ovarian factors and mediators have been proposed, among which are

oestradiol, the renin-angiotensin cascade, histamine, serotonin, prolactin and prostaglandins. However, there is no significant evidence to prove that these ovarian regulators have any role in the pathogenesis of this syndrome. Recent evidence strongly suggests the role of vascular endothelial growth factor in the increase of capillary permeability and leakage of protein-rich fluid into the third space, mainly the peritoneal cavity (Rizk et al 1997). Interleukins (especially IL-2) may also be implicated.

In more severe conditions there is also hypotension, increased coagulability, reduced renal perfusion and oliguria because of hypovolaemia and haemoconcentration. Deranged liver function tests, venous and arterial thrombosis, renal failure and adult respiratory distress syndrome have all been reported in severe cases and some fatalities have occurred.

Classification Various classifications for OHSS have been proposed. The classification by Jenkins & Mathur (1998) divides OHSS into four grades: mild, moderate, severe and critical (Box 18.2).

Risk factors It is essential to appreciate that any patient undergoing ovulation induction is at risk, although some more than others. Significant (moderate to critical) OHSS is very rare with CC and GnRH but this is an important complication of cycles using gonadotrophins. The incidences of mild, moderate and severe OHSS following gonadotrophins are approximately 20%, 6–7% and 1–2%, respectively (Rizk 1993). This risk is further increased by combined use of GnRH agonists (Nugent et al 2000), which extend the period of ovarian stimulation by blocking the natural LH surge. The combination leads to development of more follicles and higher

---

Box 18.2 Classification of severity of ovarian hyperstimulation syndrome

Mild
Abdominal bloating, mild pain
Ovarian size usually <8 cm diameter

Moderate
Increased abdominal discomfort accompanied by nausea, vomiting and/or diarrhoea
Ultrasound evidence of ascites
Ovarian size usually 8–12 cm diameter

Severe
Clinical ascites
Sometimes hydrothorax
Haemoconcentration (Hct >45%. WBC >15 000/ml)
Oliguria with normal serum creatinine
Liver dysfunction
Anasarca
Ovarian size usually >12 cm diameter

Critical
Tense ascites
Hct >55%
WBC >25 000/ml
Oliguria with elevated serum creatinine
Renal failure
Thromboembolic phenomena
Ovarian size usually >12 cm diameter

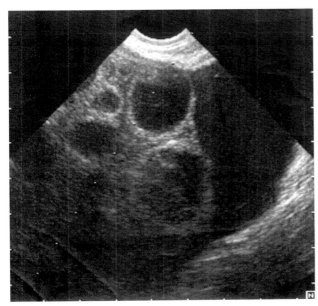

Fig. 18.5 Vaginal scan of a patient with moderate ovarian hyperstimulation syndrome (OHSS). Note the enlarged ovaries, luteal cysts and ascites.

serum oestradiol concentrations. A wide variation among different studies and units may be explained by differences in patients' characteristics, stimulation regimens, classification to grade the severity and the use of preventive strategies.

Patients with polycystic ovaries are at a particularly higher risk of developing OHSS. The increased ovarian stromal blood flow velocity and higher serum vascular endothelial growth factor concentrations in women with polycystic ovaries may help to explain the excessive response commonly seen during gonadotrophin administration (Agrawal et al 1998). Younger patients and those who are lean are also more prone to develop OHSS. Pregnancy is a well-recognized risk factor; OHSS is four times more common in conception cycles and pregnancy is three times more likely in cycles where OHSS develops. This is thought to be due to the effect of embryonic hCG. This also explains a much higher incidence of OHSS when exogenous hCG is given for luteal support.

Prevention   Prevention of OHSS is based upon detecting those patients with high-risk factors and implementing preventive measures, i.e. starting with a lower starting dose of gonadotrophin, more frequent monitoring, reducing the dose of gonadotrophin in those with excessive response or cancelling the cycle by withholding the ovulating hCG injection. The couples are advised to refrain from intercourse or to use contraception for a week. The cycles with excessive response can also be converted to in vitro fertilization treatment, in which the aspiration of follicles may have a protective effect against OHSS. Whatever methods are used, OHSS is never totally predictable nor preventable. This is especially true for late-onset OHSS, which is induced by the rising serum hCG secreted by the early pregnancy (Lyons et al 1994).

Treatment   Treatment of OHSS is supportive while waiting for spontaneous resolution. The main principles of management are to:

- provide reassurance and symptomatic relief to the patient
- maintain circulatory and renal function
- prevent thromboembolism (RCOG 1995).

Protocols for the management of significant OHSS should be established in units providing ovulation induction and specialists in reproductive medicine should be involved early in management decisions. Initially a comprehensive assessment of the patient's symptoms and hydration state should be made, including a full blood picture, clotting profile, renal and liver function tests and ultrasound examination for ovarian size, ascites and pleural effusion.

Symptomatic relief should be given: paracetamol or even opiates for pain and metoclopramide or prochlorperazine for nausea. Non-steroidal anti-inflammatory agents are not recommended as a routine treatment for pain relief as they may cause further renal impairment. The intravascular volume is maintained by encouraging oral fluid intake or intravenous replacement in those with significant hypovolaemia or severe vomiting. Colloids are preferred to crystalloids and, in the presence of hypoproteinaemia and oliguria, albumin is the volume expander of choice. Diuretics are avoided in these cases as they induce further contraction of the intravascular compartment.

Drainage of ascitic fluid provides rapid symptomatic relief of the pain caused by severe abdominal distension and dyspnoea. Urine production is significantly improved following abdominal paracentesis, which should be performed under ultrasound guidance. Ascitic fluid can also be drained transvaginally under transvaginal ultrasound guidance to avoid the enlarged ovaries and distended bowels. Repeated paracentesis may result in significant loss of serum albumin, accelerating the fluid shift from the intravascular compartment. Full-length elastic stockings reduce the risk of venous thrombosis and prophylactic subcutaneous heparin is indicated in severe forms.

Multiple pregnancy

Multiple pregnancies carry extra risks for both the mother and fetuses. Obstetric complications include an increased incidence of pre-eclampsia and eclampsia, antepartum haemorrhage, preterm labour and surgical or assisted delivery. The high incidence of prematurity and low birth weight in high-order multiple pregnancies results in marked increase in the perinatal mortality associated with multiple births. There is also increased risk for infant and childhood morbidity such as cerebral palsy and mental retardation. The rate of multiple pregnancies, particularly high-order multiple pregnancies, has increased enormously since the availability of gonadotrophin for ovulation induction and ovarian stimulation. The rise in the rate of triplet and other higher order births in the United Kingdom was much steeper than that for all multiple births, increasing from 0.13 sets of triplets per thousand maternities in 1975 to 0.41 in 1994 (Dunn & Macfarlane 1998). Levene et al (1992) found that more triplet, quadruplet and quintuplet pregnancies followed ovulation induction than IVF.

Patients at risk of multiple follicular development, e.g. patients with PCOS, are identified. A lower starting dose of the ovulation drug is preferred and careful monitoring by ultrasound examination provides good assessment of ovarian response in terms of the number of developing follicles. Cycles with more than two dominant follicles should be cancelled in order to reduce the risk of multiple pregnancies and the starting dose of the drug should be reduced in the next cycle. Other options such as converting ovulation induction cycles to IVF treatment with replacement of two embryos only (Bergh et al 1998), aspirating supernumerary follicles (de Geyter et al 1998) and selective fetal reduction can also help the reduction of multiple pregnancies. However, selective fetal reduction is not without complications and it should never be considered a substitute for careful monitoring.

Ovarian cancer

Recently, there has been increasing concern about a possible link between drugs given for ovulation induction or ovarian stimulation and development of ovarian cancer, which accounts for 5–6% of cancer deaths in women in the UK. Because of late presentation and lack of an effective screening method, it is the fourth leading cause of cancer-related deaths in British women. Repeated and multiple ovulations increasing trauma on the ovarian epithelium (Fathalla's incessant ovulation hypothesis), a hypergonadotrophic state causing malignant transformation and production of intra-ovarian chemical carcinogens after ovarian stimulation are possible explanations for an increased risk of ovarian cancer in infertile women receiving these agents.

A number of case reports first raised the association between the fertility drugs and ovarian cancer. The results of a collaborative analysis of 12 US case control studies (Whittemore et al 1992) then caused much concern and attention in this area. The study showed that infertile women who had used fertility drugs had an increased risk of invasive ovarian cancer compared with women who were not infertile (OR 2.8; 95% CI 1.3–6.1), while infertile women without fertility drug use had no such increase in risk (OR; 0.91 95% CI 0.66–1.3). Furthermore, this risk was only present among nulligravid women (OR 27.0; 95% CI 2.3–315.6). The association is further strengthened by another large case cohort study (Rossing et al 1994), which found a significantly higher risk of ovarian cancer in women using clomiphene citrate for 12 or more cycles (RR 7.2; 95% CI 1.2–43.9).

The available evidence does not lead to the conclusion of a firm link between fertility drugs and ovarian cancer (Nugent et al 1998). Infertility is an independent risk factor of ovarian cancer, separate from any effects of nulliparity, which in itself doubles the risk of ovarian cancer. More than half of the tumours discussed in the case reports are serous borderline tumours and no correlation between the drugs and tumour histological type has been demonstrated. Case control studies suffer from methodological flaws and had weakness in estimating the risks (Whittemore 1994). Moreover, other studies (Mosgaard et al 1997, Parazzini et al 1997, Ron et al 1987, Shu et al 1989), reported no increase in the incidence of ovarian cancer after using fertility drugs.

Although firm evidence is still lacking, patients should be counselled about the possible risk of ovarian cancer prior to the ovulation induction treatment. The available evidence with its incumbent limitations is discussed. The Committee on Safety of Medicines in the UK has recommended that clomiphene citrate should not be used for >6 cycles because of an increased risk of ovarian cancer with >12 cycles. If patients are to continue beyond the 6-month limit, then further counselling is mandatory and a risk-benefit analysis advisable. The relationship between gonadotrophin use and ovarian cancer risk is less clear but it seems prudent that gonadotrophins are given at the lowest effective doses and limited to the least number of cycles.

SURGICAL INDUCTION OF OVULATION

Laparoscopic ovarian drilling

Surgical treatment for anovulation in PCOS patients was restricted in the past to ovarian wedge resection performed via laparotomy. This is thought to work by removing part of the hormone-producing ovarian tissue, thus reducing androgen and inhibin levels. This is usually followed by a rise in FSH, a drop in LH and resumption of spontaneous ovulation. However, the response is variable and the operation may lead to significant periadnexal adhesions, thus reducing the chance of conception. The availability of effective medical induction of ovulation made the classic wedge resection obsolete.

Gjonnaess (1984) first reported that laparoscopic ovarian drilling resulted in ovulation in 90% and pregnancy in 70% of the 62 women treated. Ovarian drilling involves the formation of multiple holes on the surface of the ovary with diathermy or laser. Various mechanisms have been put forward, including reducing the size of enlarged ovaries, reducing abnormal hormone secretion, reducing secretion of inhibitory factors and augmenting the effect of FSH on folliculogenesis by release of growth factors in response to injury. The exact mechanism for stimulating ovulation, however, is uncertain.

Laparoscopic ovarian drilling has now replaced open ovarian wedge resection as the surgical treatment for women with CC-resistant PCOS and appears to be as effective as gonadotrophin treatment in these women (Farquhar et al 2000). In general, laparoscopic ovarian drilling in patients with PCOS resulted in 55–93% spontaneous ovulation and 0–84% pregnancy rates (RCOG 1998). Patients with high basal LH concentrations have a better response but pretreatment testosterone concentration, body mass index or ovarian volume did not affect the outcome. Patients who do not ovulate spontaneously following the procedure become more responsive to CC. However, the value of laparoscopic ovarian drilling as a primary treatment for anovulatory infertility in patients with PCOS is undetermined.

This treatment should only be carried out by practitioners with appropriate laparoscopic training as there are potential risks to pelvic structures. The advantages of ovarian drilling over gonadotrophin are that it is a one-step treatment, no intensive monitoring is required and the risk of multiple pregnancy and ovarian hyperstimulation is eliminated. The disadvantages are that it requires an operative procedure with general anaesthesia and postoperative adhesions can still occur, albeit at a lower rate than with laparotomy. Cases of ovarian failure have been reported after ovarian drilling. An additional concern is the possibility of premature menopause later because of ovarian destruction.

KEY POINTS

1. The cohort of growing follicles undergo a process of recruitment, selection, dominance and growth which takes about 85 days.
2. Understanding of the concept of FSH threshold and window is essential to achieve the goal of ovulation induction, i.e. development of a single follicle and subsequent ovulation in anovulatory women.
3. In developed countries, 20–25% of patients who present with infertility suffer from ovulation disorders.
4. Appropriate investigation of the hypothalamic-pituitary-ovarian axis, thyroid and adrenal function are necessary to accurately categorize patients and choose an appropriate method of ovulation induction.
5. Anovulatory patients should be fully informed of the success of each method, the monitoring required and the possible risks associated prior to initiating the treatment. Simple treatment associated with low complication rates and less cost should be tried first.
6. Each unit offering ovulation induction treatment should be equipped with skilful ultrasonography and specialist endocrine laboratory service. Local protocols should be available to reduce or prevent the risk of multiple pregnancy and ovarian hyperstimulation syndrome.
7. Pulsatile GnRH treatment should be the treatment of choice for anovulatory patients suffering from hypogonadotrophic hypogonadism with low levels of endogenous oestradiol because of reduced risks, when compared with gonadotrophin treatment.
8. Treatment of anovulatory patients with polycystic ovary syndrome remains a challenge. These patients should be counselled about the pros and cons of various options available.
9. The association between ovarian cancer risk and gonadotrophins or prolonged clomiphene use remains uncertain.

REFERENCES

Adams J, Polson DW, Franks S 1986 Prevalence of polycystic ovaries in women with anovulation and idiopathic hirsutism. British Medical Journal 293:355–359

Agrawal R, Sladkevicius P, Engmann et al 1998 Serum vascular endothelial growth factor concentrations and ovarian stromal blood flow are increased in women with polycystic ovaries. Human Reproduction 13:651–658

Bergh C, Bryman I, Nilsson L, Janson PO 1998 Results of gonadotrophin stimulation with the option to convert cycles to in vitro fertilisation in cases of multifollicular development. Acta Obstetrica et Gynaecologica Scandinavica 77:68–73

Braat DD, Ayalon D, Blunt SM et al 1989 Pregnancy outcome in luteinizing hormone-releasing hormone induced cycles: a multicentre study. Journal of Gynecological Endocrinology 3:35–44

Brown JB 1978 Pituitary control of ovarian function-concepts derived from gonadotrophin therapy. Australian and New Zealand Journal of Obstetrics and Gynaecology 18:46–54

Clark AM, Thornley B, Tomlinson L, Galletley C, Norman RJ 1998 Weight loss in obese infertile women results in improvement in reproductive outcome for all forms of fertility treatment. Human Reproduction 13:1502–1505

Daya S, Gunby J, Hughes EG et al 1995 Follicle-stimulating hormone versus human menopausal gonadotrophin for in vitro fertilization cycles: a meta-analysis. Fertility and Sterility 64:347–354

De Geyter C, De Geyter M, Nieschlag E 1998 Low multiple pregnancy rates and reduced frequency of cancellation after ovulation induction with gonadotrophins, if eventual supernumerary follicles are aspirated to prevent polyovulation. Journal of Assisted Reproduction and Genetics 15:111–116

Dunn A, Macfarlane J 1998 Recent trends in the incidence of multiple births and associated mortality in England and Wales. Archives of Diseases in Childhood 75:10–19

Farquhar C, Vandekerckhove P, Arnot M, Lilford R 2000 Laparoscopic 'drilling' by diathermy or laser for ovulation induction in anovulatory polycystic ovary syndrome. Cochrane Database Systematic Review. Issue 2. Update Software, Oxford

Filicori M, Flamigni C, Dellai P et al 1994 Treatment of anovulation with pulsatile gonadotropin-releasing hormone: prognostic factors and clinical results in 600 cycles. Journal of Clinical Endocrinology and Metabolism 79: 1215–1220

Galtier-Dereure F, Pujol P, Devailly D, Bringer J 1997 Choice of stimulation in polycystic ovarian syndrome: the influence of obesity. Human Reproduction 12 (suppl 1): 88–96

Gjonnaess H 1984 Polycystic ovarian syndrome treated by ovarian electrocautery through the laparoscope. Fertility and Sterility 41:20–25

Homburg R, Eshel A, Armar NA et al 1989 One hundred pregnancies after treatment with pulsatile luteinsing hormone releasing hormone to induce ovulation. British Medical Journal 298:809–812

Hughes E, Collins J, Vandekerckhove P 2000a Clomiphene citrate for ovulation induction in women with oligo-amenorrhea. Cochrane Database Systematic Review. Issue 2. Update Software, Oxford

Hughes E, Collins J, Vandekerckhove P 2000b Gonadotrophin-releasing hormone analogue as an adjunct to gonadotrophin therapy for clomiphene-resistant polycystic ovarian syndrome. Cochrane Database Systematic Review. Issue 2. Update Software, Oxford

Hughes E, Collins J, Vandekerckhove P 2000c Ovulation induction with urinary follicle stimulating hormone versus human menopausal gonadotrophin for clomiphene-resistant polycystic ovary syndrome. cochrane Database Systematic Review. Issue 2. Update Software, Oxford

Hull MGR 1992 The causes of infertility and relative effectiveness of treatment. In: Templeton AA, Drife JO (eds) Infertility, Springer-Verlag, London

Jenkins J, Mathur R 1998 PACE review: ovarian hyperstimulation syndrome, RCOG, London

Kelly AC, Jewelewicz R 1990 Alternate regimens for ovulation induction in polycystic ovarian disease. Fertility and Sterility 54: 195–202

Levene MI, Wild J, Steer P 1992 Higher multiple births and the modern management of infertility in Britain. British Journal of Obstetrics and Gynaecology 99:607–613

Lyons CAD, Wheeler CA, Frishman GN, Hackett RJ, Seifer DB, Haning RV Jr 1994 Early and late presentation of the ovarian hyperstimulation syndrome: two distinct entities with different risk factors. Human Reproduction 9:792–799

Martin KA, Hall JE, Adams JM, Crowley WF Jr 1993 Comparison of exogenous gonadotropins and pulsatile gonadotropin-releasing hormone for induction of ovulation in hypogonadotropic amenorrhea. Journal of Clinical Endocrinology and Metabolism 77:125–129

Messinis IE, Templeton A 1988 Blockage of the positive feedback effect of oestradiol during prolonged administration of clomiphene citrate to normal women. Clinical Endocrinology 29:509–516

Mitwally MFM, Kuscu NK, Yalcinkaya TM 1999 High ovulatory rates with the use of troglitazone in clomiphene-resistant women with polycystic ovary syndrome. Human Reproduction 14:2700–2703

Mosgaard BJ, Lidegaard O, Kjaer SK, Schou G, Andersen AN 1997 Infertility, fertility drugs, and invasive ovarian cancer: a case-control study. Fertility and Sterility 67:1005–1012

Nugent D, Salha O, Balen AH, Rutherford AJ 1998 Ovarian neoplasia and subfertility treatment. British Journal of Obstetrics and Gynaecology 105:584–591

Nugent D, Vandekerckhove P, Hughes E, Arnot M, Lilford R 2000 Gonadotrophin therapy for ovulation induction in subfertility associated with polycystic ovary syndrome. Cochrane Database Systematic Review. Issue 4. Update Software, Oxford

Parazzini F, Negri E, La Vecchia C, Moroni S, Franceschi S, Crosignani PG 1997 Treatment of infertility and risk of invasive epithelial ovarian cancer. Human Reproduction 12:2159–2161

Pascal Vigneron V, Weryha G, Bosc M, Leclere J 1995 Hyperprolactinemic amenorrhea: treatment with cabergoline versus bromocriptine. Results of a national multicenter randomised double-blind study. Presse Medicale 24:753–757

Polson DW, Kiddy DS, Mason HD, Franks S 1989 Induction of ovulation with clomiphene citrate in women with polycystic ovary syndrome: the difference between responders and non-responders. Fertility and Sterility, 51:30–34

Rizk B 1993 Ovarian hyperstimulation syndrome. In Studd J (ed) Progress in obstetrics and gynaecology. Churchill Livingstone, Edinburgh

Rizk B, Aboulghar M, Smitz J, Ron-El R 1997 The role of vascular endothelial growth factor and interleukins in the pathogenesis of severe ovarian hyperstimulation syndrome. Human Reproduction Update 3:255–266

Ron E, Lunenfield B, Menczer J et al 1987 Cancer incidence in a cohort of infertile women. American Journal of Epidemiology 125:780–790

Rossing RA, Daling JR, Weiss NS. Moore DE, Self SG 1994 Ovarian tumours in a cohort of infertile women. New England Journal of Medicine 331:771–776

Royal College of Obstetricians and Gynaecologists 1995 Green-top guidelines no. 5. Management and prevention of ovarian hyperstimulation syndrome (OHSS). RCOG, London

Royal College of Obstetricians and Gynaecologists 1998 Evidence-based clinical guidelines no. 3. The management of infertility in secondary care. RCOG, London

Sattar N, Hopkinson ZEC, Greer IA 1998 Insulin-sensitising agents in polycystic ovary syndrome. Lancet 351:305–307

Shoham Z, di Carlo C, Patel A, Conway GS, Jacobs HS 1991 Is it possible to run a successful ovulation induction program based solely on ultrasound monitoring? The importance of endometrial measurements. Fertility and Sterility 56:836–841

Shu XO, Brinton LA, Gao YT, Yuan JM 1989 Population-based case control study of ovarian cancer in Shanghai. Cancer Research 49:3670–3674

van Santbrink EJP, Fauser BCJM 1997 Urinary follicle-stimulating hormone for normogonadotropic clomiphene-resistant infertility: prospective, randomised comparison between low-dose step-up and step-down regimens. Journal of Clinical Endocrinology and Metabolism 82:3597–3602

Webster J, Piscitelli G, Polli A, Ferrari CI, Ismail I, Scanlon MF 1994 A comparison of cabergoline and bromocriptine in the treatment of hyperprolactinaemic amenorrhea. New England Journal of Medicine 331:904–909

Whittemore AS 1994 The risk of ovarian cancer after treatment for infertility. New England Journal of Medicine 331:805–806

Whittemore AS, Harris R, Itnyre J for the Collaborative Ovarian Cancer Group 1992 Characteristics relating to ovarian cancer risk: collaborative analysis of 12 US case-control studies II. Invasive epithelial ovarian cancers in white women. American Journal of Epidemiology 136:1184–1203

Wu CH, Winkel CA 1989 The effect of therapy initiation day on clomiphene citrate therapy. Fertility and Sterility 52:564–568

Yarali H, Bukulmez O, Gurgan T 1999 Urinary follicle-stimulating hormone (FSH) versus recombinant FSH in clomiphene citrate-resistant, normogonadotrophic. chronic anovulation: a prospective randomised study. Fertility and Sterility 72:276–281

19

The polycystic ovary syndrome

Adam Balen

INTRODUCTION

The polycystic ovary syndrome (PCOS) is the commonest endocrine disturbance affecting women yet it is only in the last decade that we have begun to piece together a clearer idea of its pathogenesis (Balen 1999). It has long been recognized that the presence of enlarged ovaries with multiple small cysts (2–8 mm) and a hypervascularized, androgen-secreting stroma are associated with signs of androgen excess (hirsutism, alopecia, acne), obesity and menstrual cycle disturbance (oligomenorrhoea or amenorrhoea). There is considerable heterogeneity of symptoms and signs amongst women with PCOS (Table 19.1) and for an individual these may change over time (Balen et al 1995). The PCOS is familial (Franks et al 1997) and various aspects of the syndrome may be differentially inherited. Polycystic ovaries can exist without clinical signs of the syndrome, which may then become expressed over time.

There are a number of interlinking factors that affect expression of PCOS. A gain in weight is associated with a worsening of symptoms whilst weight loss will ameliorate the endocrine and metabolic profile and symptomatology (Clark et al 1995). Normal ovarian function relies upon the selection of a follicle, which responds to an appropriate signal (follicle-stimulating hormone) in order to grow, become 'dominant' and ovulate. This mechanism is disturbed in women with PCOS, resulting in multiple small cysts, most of which contain potentially viable oocytes but within dysfunctional follicles.

Elevations in serum concentrations of insulin are common in both lean and obese women with PCOS, even when allowance is made for differences in weight or body composition (Conway et al 1992). Indeed, it is hyperinsulinaemia that many feel is the key to the pathogenesis of the syndrome (Dunaif 1997) as insulin stimulates androgen secretion by the ovarian stroma and appears to affect the normal development of ovarian follicles, both by the adverse effects of androgens on follicular growth and possibly also by suppressing apoptosis and permitting the survival of follicles otherwise destined to disappear. Insulin stimulates androgen secretion by the ovarian stroma, thus restricting folicular growth, and leads to suppression of liver production of sex hormone-binding globulin (SHBG), an important determinant of the free androgen index. The prevalence of diabetes in obese women with PCOS is 11% (Conway 1990) and so a measurement of impaired glucose tolerance is important and long-term

Table 19.1 The spectrum of clinical manifestations of the polycystic ovary syndrome

Symptoms	Serum endocrinology	Possible late sequelae
Obesity	↑ Androgens (testosterone and androstenedione)	Diabetes mellitus Dyslipidaemia
Menstrual disturbance	↑ Luteinizing hormone	Hypertension
Infertility	↑ Fasting insulin ↑ Prolactin	Cardiovascular disease
Hyperandrogenism	↓ Sex hormone-binding globulin	Endometrial carcinoma Breast cancer
Asymptomatic	↑ Oestradiol, oestrone	

screening advisable. An underlying insulin resistance, promoting compensatory hyperinsulinaemia, could explain links with type 2 diabetes and risk of gestational diabetes.

PATHOGENESIS

High-resolution ultrasound scanning has made an accurate estimate of the prevalence of polycystic ovaries possible. Several studies have estimated the prevalence of polycystic ovaries in 'normal adult' women and have found rates of 22–33% (Clayton et al 1992, Farquhar et al 1994, Michelmore et al 1999, Polson et al 1988) but it is not known at what age they first appear.

PCOS appears to have its origins during adolescence and is thought to be associated with increased weight gain during puberty (Balen & Dunger 1995). However, the polycystic ovary gene(s) has not yet been identified and the effect of environmental influences such as weight changes and circulating hormone concentrations and the age at which these occur are still being unravelled. Detecting polycystic ovaries in girls relies upon transabdominal scanning, which in a study by Fox et al (1991) in adults failed to detect 30% of polycystic ovaries compared to 100% detection rate with a transvaginal scan. Bridges et al (1993) performed 428 ovarian scans in girls aged between 3 and 18 years and found polycystic ovaries in 101 girls (24% of the total). The rate of detection of polycystic ovaries was 6% in 6-year-old girls rising to 18% in those aged 10 years and 26% in those aged 15 years. The implication of this study is that polycystic ovaries are present before puberty and are more easy to detect in older girls as the ovaries increase in size.

Prior to puberty, there appear to be two periods of increased ovarian growth. The first is at adrenarche in response to increased concentrations of circulating androgens and the second just before and during puberty due to rising gonadotrophin levels, the actions of growth hormone and insulin-like growth factor-1 (IGF-1) and insulin on the ovary. Sampaolo et al (1994) reported a study of 49 obese girls at different stages of puberty, comparing their pelvic ultrasound features and endocrine profiles with 35 age- and pubertal stage-matched controls. They found that obesity was associated with a significant increase in uterine and ovarian volume. They also found that obese postmenarchal girls with polycystic ovaries had larger uterine and ovarian volumes than obese postmenarchal girls with normal ovaries. Sampaolo concludes that obesity leads to hyperinsulinism, which causes both hyperandrogenaemia and raised IGF-1 levels, which augments the ovarian response to gonadotrophins. This implies that obesity may be important in the pathogenesis of polycystic ovaries, but further study is required to evaluate this. It is known that obesity is not a prerequisite for the polycystic ovary syndrome. Indeed, in a series of 1741 women with polycystic ovaries in a study by Balen et al (1995), only 38.4% of patients were overweight (BMI >25 kg/m^2).

Many women with polycystic ovaries detected by ultrasound do not have overt symptoms of the PCOS, although symptoms may develop later, after a gain in weight, for example. Ovarian morphology using the ultrasound criteria described by Adams et al (1985) (10 or more cysts, 2–8 mm in diameter,

arranged around an echo-dense stroma, as seen by transabdominal scan) appears to be the most sensitive diagnostic marker for polycystic ovaries.

Genetics of PCOS

Genetic study of PCOS has identified links with insulin secretion and insulin action. Association has been reported with common allelic variation at the variable number of tandem repeat locus (VNTR) in the promoter region of the insulin gene (Waterworth et al 1997). This locus has been variably associated with the risk of obesity, insulin resistance and type 2 diabetes. The identified association has been with the class III/III genotype, particularly in women who have anovulatory cycles and are hyperinsulinaemic (Waterworth et al 1997). These associations are particularly evident where the III allele has been inherited from the father. Recent systematic screens of 37 candidate genes for PCOS have demonstrated linkage with follistatin, an activin-binding neutralizing protein (Urbanek et al 1999). Amongst the actions of activin are included promotion of follicular development, increased FSH production and pancreatic β-cell secretion of insulin.

A recently completed population study of 224 women randomly recruited from GP surgeries and local universities revealed a prevalence of PCO of around 33%, but only 26% of the total fulfilled the European criteria for PCOS and 4% the American criteria (Michelmore et al 1999). Polycystic ovaries were associated with irregular menstrual cycles and significantly higher serum testosterone concentrations when compared with women with normal ovaries. However, only a small proportion of women with polycystic ovaries (15%) had 'elevated' serum testosterone concentrations outside the normal range.

This study reflected the rather benign characteristics of PCO, detected by routine screening in young women with only marginal elevation of testosterone and few significant differences with respect to features of hyperandrogenism and menstrual cycle disturbance. There were no differences in *INS*

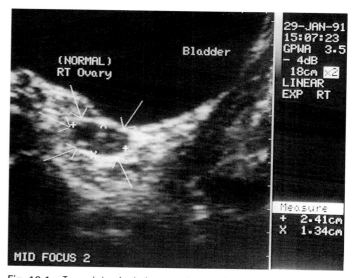

Fig. 19.1   Transabdominal ultrasound scan of a normal ovary.

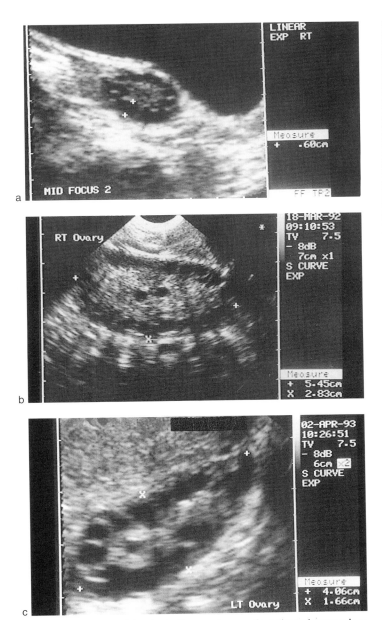

Fig. 19.2   a Transabdominal ultrasound scan of a polycystic ovary. b, c Transabdominal ultrasound scans of a polycystic ovary.

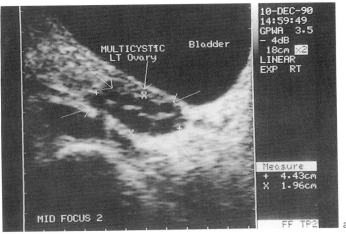

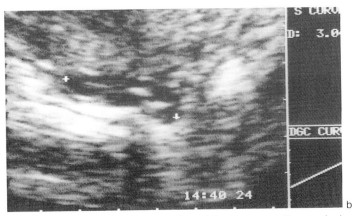

Fig. 19.3   a Transabdominal scan of a multicystic ovary. b Transvaginal ultrasound scan of a multicystic ovary.

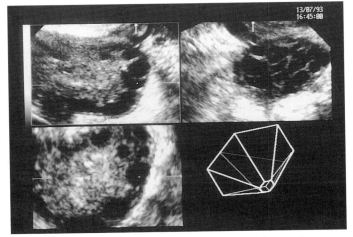

Fig. 19.4   Three-dimensional transvaginal ultrasound scan of a polycystic ovary. Courtesy of Dr A. Kyei-Mensah.

VNTR genotype between those with and without PCO but the association between PCO and larger size at birth was highly significant ($p = 0.004$). The study did, however, confirm the profound heterogeneity of association between PCO, birth weight and insulin sensitivity.

Heterogeneity of PCOS

The findings of a large series of more than 1800 women with polycystic ovaries detected by ultrasound scan have been reported (Balen et al 1995). All patients had at least one symptom of the polycystic ovary syndrome. Thirty-eight per cent of the women were overweight (BMI >25 kg/m²). Obesity was significantly associated with an increased risk of hirsutism, menstrual cycle disturbance and an elevated serum testosterone concentration and with an increased rate of infertility and menstrual cycle disturbance. Twenty-six per cent of patients with primary infertility and 14% of patients with secondary infertility had a BMI of more than 30 kg/m².

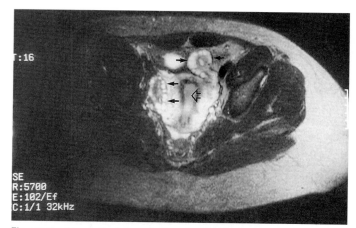

Fig. 19.5 Magnetic resonance imaging (MRI) of a pelvis, demonstrating two polycystic ovaries (closed arrows) and a hyperplastic endometrium (open arrow).

Approximately 30% of the patients had a regular menstrual cycle, 50% had oligomenorrhoea and 20% amenorrhoea. A rising serum concentration of testosterone was associated with an increased risk of hirsutism, infertility and cycle disturbance. The rates of infertility and menstrual cycle disturbance also increased with increasing serum luteinizing hormone concentrations greater than 10 iu/l. The serum LH concentration of those with primary infertility was significantly higher than that of women with secondary infertility and both were higher than the LH concentration of those with proven fertility. Ovarian morphology appears to be the most sensitive marker of the PCOS, compared with the classic endocrine features of raised serum LH and testosterone, which were found in only 39.8% and 28.9% of patients respectively in this series (Balen et al 1995).

Hypersecretion of LH

Hypersecretion of LH occurs in approximately 40% of women who have polycystic ovaries. The risk of infertility and miscarriage is raised in these patients. Several hypotheses have been suggested to explain this oversecretion of LH, including increased pulse frequency of gonadotrophin-releasing hormone (GnRH), increased pituitary sensitivity to GnRH, hyperinsulinaemic stimulation of the pituitary gland and disturbance of the ovarian steroid–pituitary feedback mechanism. However, none of these fully explains hypersecretion of LH and it may be that leptin also has a role to play here.

Leptin

Leptin is a 167 amino acid peptide that is secreted by fat cells in response to insulin and glucocorticoids. Leptin is transported by a protein which appears to be the extracellular domain of the leptin receptor itself. Leptin receptors are found in the choroid plexus, on the hypothalamus and ovary and at many other sites. Leptin decreases the intake of food and stimulates thermogenesis. It also appears to inhibit the hypothalamic peptide neuropeptide-Y, which is an inhibitor of GnRH pulsatility. Leptin appears to serve as the signal from the body

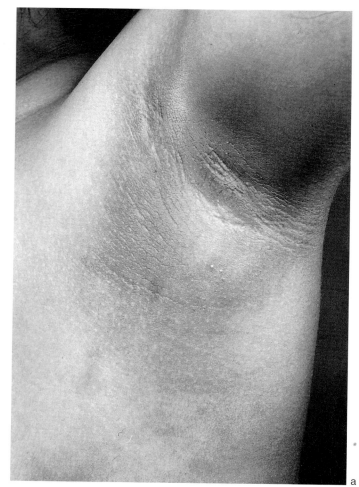

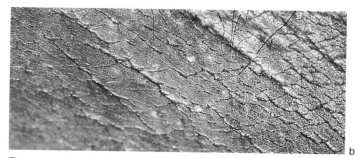

Fig. 19.6 Acanthosis nigricans, as seen typically in the axilla or skin of the neck. a Axilla. b Close-up, demonstrating hypertrophic and pigmented skin.

fat to the brain about the adequacy of fat stores for reproduction. Thus menstruation will only occur if fat stores are adequate. Obesity, on the other hand, is associated with high circulating concentrations of leptin and this in turn might be a mechanism for hypersecretion of LH in women with PCOS.

To date, most studies have been in the leptin-deficient and consequently obese *Ob/Ob* mouse. Starvation of the *Ob/Ob* mouse leads to weight loss, yet fertility is only restored after the administration of leptin. Leptin administration to overweight, infertile women may not be as straightforward as it might initially seem because of the complex nature of leptin transport into the brain. None the less, the role of leptin in human reproduction is an exciting area of ongoing research.

MANAGEMENT OF THE POLYCYSTIC OVARY SYNDROME

Obesity

The clinical management of a woman with PCOS should be focused on her individual problems. Obesity worsens both symptomatology and the endocrine profile and so obese women (BMI >30 kg/m²) should therefore be encouraged to lose weight. Weight loss improves the endocrine profile (Kiddy et al 1992), the likelihood of ovulation and a healthy pregnancy. A recent study by Clark et al (1995) looked at the effect of a weight loss programme on women with at least a 2-year history of anovulatory infertility, clomiphene resistance and a BMI >30 kg/m². Weight loss had a significant effect on endocrine function, ovulation and subsequent pregnancy. Twelve of the 13 subjects resumed ovulation, 11 becoming pregnant (five spontaneously). Fasting insulin and serum testosterone concentrations also fell.

Menstrual irregularity

The easiest way to control the menstrual cycle is the use of a low-dose combined oral contraceptive preparation. This will result in an artificial cycle and regular shedding of the endometrium. An alternative is a progestogen (such as medroxyprogesterone acetate [Provera] or dydrogesterone [Duphaston]) for 12 days every 1–3 months to induce a withdrawal bleed. It is also important once again to encourage weight loss. As women with PCOS are thought to be at increased risk of cardiovascular disease, a 'lipid-friendly' combined contraceptive pill should be used.

In women with anovulatory cycles the action of oestradiol on the endometrium is unopposed because of the lack of cyclical progesterone secretion. This may result in episodes of irregular uterine bleeding and in the long term endometrial hyperplasia and even endometrial cancer. An ultrasound assessment of endometrial thickness provides a bio-assay for oestradiol production by the ovaries and conversion of androgens in the peripheral fat. If the endometrium is thicker than 15 mm a withdrawal bleed should be induced and if the endometrium fails to shed then endometrial sampling is required to exclude endometrial hyperplasia or malignancy. The only young women to get endometrial carcinoma at less than 35 years of age, which otherwise has a mean age of occurrence of 61 years in the UK, are those with anovulation secondary to PCOS or oestrogen-secreting tumours.

Infertility

Ovulation can be induced with the anti-oestrogens clomiphene citrate (50–100 mg) or tamoxifen (20–40 mg), days 2–6 of a natural or artificially induced bleed. Whilst clomiphene is successful in inducing ovulation in over 80% of women, pregnancy only occurs in about 40%. Clomiphene citrate should only be prescribed in a setting where ultrasound

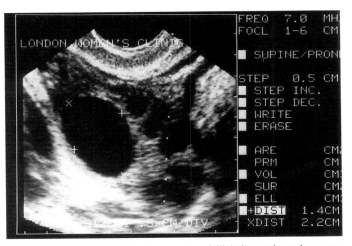

Fig. 19.7 Stimulation of a single mature follicle in a polycystic ovary (transvaginal ultrasound scan).

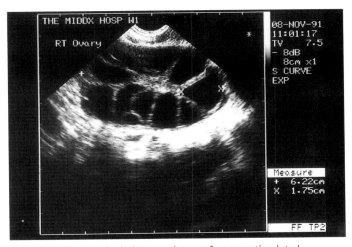

Fig. 19.8 Transvaginal ultrasound scan of an overstimulated polycystic ovary. Both ovaries are likely to have this appearance and the treatment must be discontinued to minimize the risk of multiple pregnancy and ovarian hyperstimulation syndrome.

monitoring is available (and performed) in order to minimize the 10% risk of multiple pregnancy and to ensure that ovulation is taking place (RCOG 1998). A daily dose of more than 100 mg rarely confers any benefit and can cause thickening of the cervical mucus, which can impede passage of sperm through the cervix. Once an ovulatory dose has been reached, the cumulative conception rate continues to increase for up to 10–12 cycles (Kousta et al 1997). Clomiphene is only licensed for 6 months use in the UK and so we would advise careful counselling of patients if clomiphene citrate therapy is continued beyond 6 months.

The therapeutic options for patients with anovulatory infertility who are resistant to anti-oestrogens are either parenteral gonadotrophin therapy or laparoscopic ovarian diathermy. Because the polycystic ovary is very sensitive to stimulation by exogenous hormones, it is very important to start with very low doses of gonadotrophins and follicular development must be carefully monitored by ultrasound scans. The advent of transvaginal ultrasonography has enabled the multiple pregnancy rate to be reduced to approximately 7% because of its higher resolution and clearer view of the developing follicles. Cumulative conception and livebirth rates after 6 months may be 62% and 54% respectively and after 12 months 73% and 62% respectively (Balen et al 1994). Close monitoring should enable treatment to be suspended if three or more mature follicles develop, as the risk of multiple pregnancy obviously increases.

Ovarian hyperstimulation syndrome

Women with the polycystic ovary syndrome are also at increased risk of developing the ovarian hyperstimulation syndrome (OHSS). This occurs if too many follicles (>10 mm) are stimulated and results in abdominal distension, discomfort, nausea, vomiting and sometimes difficulty in breathing. The mechanism for OHSS is thought to be secondary to activation of the ovarian renin–angiotensin pathway and excessive secretion of vascular epidermal growth factor (VEGF). The ascites, pleural and pericardial effusions exacerbate this serious condition and the resultant haemoconcentration can lead to thromboembolism. The situation worsens if a pregnancy has resulted from the treatment as hCG from the placenta further stimulates the ovaries. Hospitalization is sometimes necessary in order for intravenous fluids and heparin to be given to prevent dehydration and thromboembolism. Although the OHSS is rare it is potentially fatal and should be avoidable with appropriate monitoring of gonadotrophin therapy.

Ovarian Diathermy

Ovarian diathermy is free of the risks of multiple pregnancy and ovarian hyperstimulation and does not require intensive ultrasound monitoring. Laparoscopic ovarian diathermy has taken the place of wedge resection of the ovaries (which resulted in extensive periovarian and tubal adhesions) and it appears to be as effective as routine gonadotrophin therapy in the treatment of clomiphene-insensitive PCOS (Abdel Gadir et al 1990). An appropriately powered RCT is yet to be performed.

Altering insulin sensitivity

A number of pharmacological agents have been used to amplify the physiological effect of weight loss, notably metformin. This biguanide inhibits the production of hepatic glucose and enhances the sensitivity of peripheral tissue to insulin, thereby decreasing insulin secretion. It has been shown that metformin ameliorates hyperandrogenism and abnormalities of gonadotrophin secretion in women with PCOS (Nestler & Jakubowicz 1996) and can restore menstrual cyclicity and fertility (Velazquez et al 1997). Not all authors agree with these findings, particularly if there is no concurrent weight loss (Ehrmann et al 1997). The insulin-sensitizing agent troglitazone also appears to significantly improve the metabolic and reproductive abnormalties in PCOS although this product has been withdrawn recently because of reports of deaths from hepatotoxicity. Newer insulin-sensitizing agents are currently being evaluated as is the phosphoglycan-containing drug D-chiro-inositol.

Metformin is the most promising and safest sensitizer to insulin available in the UK at the present time and may have benefits for short- and long-term health, by improving obesity, hyperandrogenism, fertility, insulin sensitivity and lipid profile. There has been much publicity about its use and data are still being accumulated. Further reseach is required with adequately powered clinical studies. Insulin-sensitizing agents such as metformin might also play a role in the longer term management of some of the other features and long-term health risk of PCOS.

Hyperandrogenism and hirsutism

The bioavailability of testosterone is affected by the serum concentration of SHBG. High levels of insulin lower the production of SHBG and so increase the free fraction of androgen. Elevated serum androgen concentrations stimulate peripheral androgen receptors, resulting in an increase in 5α-reductase activity and directly increasing the conversion of testosterone to the more potent metabolite, dihydrotestosterone. Symptoms of hyperandrogenism include hirsutism, which can be a distressing condition. Hirsutism is characterized by terminal hair growth in a male pattern of distribution, including chin, upper lip, chest, upper and lower back, upper and lower abdomen, upper arm, thigh and buttocks. A standardized scoring system, such as the modified Ferriman and Gallwey score (Fig. 19.9), should be used to evaluate the degree of hirsutism before and during treatments.

Treatment options include cosmetic and medical therapies. Medical regimens stop further progression of hirsutism and decrease the rate of hair growth. However, drug therapies may take 6–9 months or longer before any benefit is perceived and so physical treatments including electrolysis, waxing and bleaching may be helpful whilst waiting for medical treatments to work.

Symptoms of hyperandrogenism can be treated by a combination of an oestrogen (such as ethinyloestradiol or a combined contraceptive pill) and the antiandrogen cyproterone acetate (50–100 mg). Oestrogens lower circulating androgens by a combination of a slight inhibition of gonadotrophin secretion and gonadotrophin-sensitive ovarian steroid production and by an increase in hepatic production of SHBG resulting in lower free testosterone. The cyproterone is taken for the first 10 days of a cycle (the 'reversed sequential' method) and the oestrogen for the first 21 days. After a gap of exactly 7 days, during which menstruation usually occurs, the regimen is repeated. As an alternative, the preparation Dianette (Schering Healthcare Ltd) contains ethinyloestradiol in combination with cyproterone, although at a lower dose (2 mg). Cyproterone acetate acts as a competitive inhibitor at the androgen receptor. Serum levels of LH, FSH, oestradiol, androstenedione, total and free testosterone are lowered whilst SHBG increases. However, there is an increase in triglycerides, apolipoprotein A1, A2 and B. Cyproterone acetate can cause liver damage and liver function should be checked regularly. Other antiandrogens such as spironolactone, ketoconazole and flutamide have been tried, but are not widely used due to their adverse side-effects.

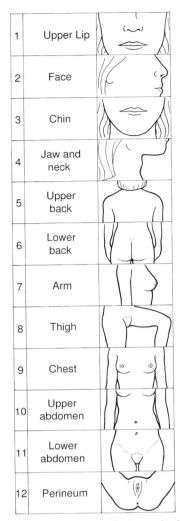

1	Upper Lip	
2	Face	
3	Chin	
4	Jaw and neck	
5	Upper back	
6	Lower back	
7	Arm	
8	Thigh	
9	Chest	
10	Upper abdomen	
11	Lower abdomen	
12	Perineum	

Fig. 19.9 Ferriman and Gallwey score. Each area is given a score from 1 to 4 (1 = mild, 2 = moderate, 3 = complete light coverage, 4 = heavy coverage).

LONG-TERM CONSEQUENCES OF PCOS

The long-term risk of endometrial hyperplasia and endometrial carcinoma due to chronic anovulation and unopposed oestrogen has long been recognized. With increasing awareness of the metabolic abnormalities associated with the syndrome there is concern regarding cardiovascular risk and other long-term health implications in these women.

Obesity and metabolic abnormalities are recognized risk factors for the development of ischaemic heart disease (IHD) in the general population and these are also recognized features of PCOS. The basis for the idea that women with PCOS are at greater risk for cardiovascular disease is that:

- these women are more insulin resistant than weight-matched controls
- the metabolic disturbances associated with insulin resistance are known to increase cardiovascular risk in other populations.

Insulin resistance

Insulin resistance is defined as a diminution in the biological responses to a given level of insulin. In the presence of an adequate pancreatic reserve, normal circulating glucose levels are maintained at higher serum insulin concentrations. In the general population cardiovascular risk factors include insulin resistance, obesity, glucose intolerance, hypertension and dyslipidaemia. Central obesity (i.e. an increased waist:hip ratio) is a more important risk factor than obesity itself.

Burghen and colleagues (1980) made the first suggestion of a relationship between the hyperandrogenism of PCOS and hyperinsulinaemia. There was a significant correlation between basal insulin measurements with both serum testosterone and androstenedione concentrations and between insulin response during the OGTT to serum testosterone concentrations. Since then there have been a large number of studies demonstrating the presence of insulin resistance and corresponding hyper-insulinaemia in both obese and non-obese women with PCOS. Obese women with PCOS have consistently been shown to be insulin resistant to a greater degree than their weight-matched controls. It appears that obesity and PCOS have a synergistic effect on the degree and severity of the insulin resistance and subsequent hyperinsulinaemia in this group of women. Conway (1990) found that 30% of non-obese women with PCOS have a mild degree of insulin resistance and that the degree of insulin resistance was positively correlated with intermenstrual interval.

Impaired glucose tolerance and diabetes

These are known risk factors for cardiovascular disease. It is reported that 18–20% of obese women with PCOS domonstrate impaired glucose tolerance. Dahlgren et al (1992) noted the prevalence of type 2 diabetes was 15% in women with PCOS compared with 2% in the controls. Dunaif (1997) suggested that up to 20% of obese women with PCOS have impaired glucose tolerance or frank diabetes mellitus by their third decade, making PCOS a common risk factor for non-insulin dependent diabetes (NIDDM). Gjonnaess (1989) found an 8% incidence of gestational diabetes amongst 36 obese women with PCOS who conceived after ovarian diathermy compared with the rate of 0.25% for the general pregnant population in Norway. Insulin resistance combined with abdominal obesity is thought to account for the higher prevalence of NIDDM in PCOS. This is probably modified by genetic or environmental factors, as not all women with PCOS develop diabetes.

Hypertension

The prevalence of treated hypertension has been found to be three times higher in women with PCOS between the age of 40 and 59 years compared with controls (Dahlgren et al 1992). In their series, Gjonnaess (1989) reported the incidence of pre-eclampsia in obese women with PCOS conceiving after ovarian electrocautery to be 12.9% compared with 3.8% in the general pregnant population.

Dyslipidaemia

Abnormalities in lipid metabolism in PCOS were reported by Wild et al (1985) who demonstrated that women with PCOS had twice as high concentrations of serum triglyceride and the mean HDL was 26% lower in women with PCOS compared with controls. Others have also shown that lean women with PCOS have a lower HDL_2 subfraction compared with weight-matched controls. Others have failed to demonstrate any difference between PCOS and controls and submitted that the observed changes in triglycerides and HDL cholesterol were secondary to obesity.

HDLs play an important role in lipid metabolism and are the most important lipid parameter in predicting cardiovascular risk in women. They remove excess lipids from the circulation and tissues to transport them to the liver for excretion or transfer them to other lipoprotein particles. Cholesterol is only one component of HDL, a particle with a constantly changing composition forming HDL3 then HDL2, as unesterified cholesterol is taken from tissue, esterified and exchanged for triglyceride with other lipoprotein species. Consequently measurement of a single constituent in a particle involved in a dynamic process gives an incomplete picture.

In a recent detailed study of HDL composition it was found that obesity was the most important factor associated with elevated serum total triglyceride, cholesterol and phospholipid concentrations in both PCOS subjects and controls (Rajkhowa et al 1997). In addition, obese women with PCOS had lower HDL cholesterol and phospholipid concentrations in all subfractions compared with obese controls. This was in the presence of normal quantities of the protein component of HDL – apolipoprotein A1. These findings imply that the number of HDL particles were the same in obese PCOS subjects compared with obese controls, but the HDL particles were lipid depleted, hence less effective in function. The only factor which appeared to have an independent influence on the HDL composition was the presence of PCOS, rather than obesity, or raised serum androgen or insulin concentrations.

Plasminogen activator inhibitor-1 (PAI-1) is a potent inhibitor of fibrinolysis and has been found to be elevated in both obese women and non-obese women with PCOS. Plasma levels of PAI-1 correlate directly with serum insulin concentrations and have been shown to be an important predictor of myocardial infarction.

Thus, in summary, examining the risk factors, there is evidence that insulin resistance, central obesity and hyperandrogenaemia are features of PCOS and have an adverse effect on lipid metabolism. Women with PCOS have been shown to have dyslipidaemia, with reduced HDL cholesterol and elevated serum triglyceride concentrations, along with elevated serum PAI-1 concentrations. The evidence is thus mounting that women with PCOS may have an increased risk of developing cardiovascular disease and diabetes later in life, which has important implications for their management.

Long-term follow-up in PCOS

In a follow-up study it has been shown that women with PCOS have a 7.4-fold greater risk of myocardial infarction than age-matched controls (Dahlgren et al 1992). However, in another study Pierpoint et al (1998) reported the mortality rate in 1028 women diagnosed as having polycystic ovary syndrome between 1930 and 1979. All the women were older than 45 years and 770 women had been treated by wedge resection of the ovaries. Seven hundred and eighty-six women were traced; the mean age at diagnosis was 26.4 years and average duration of follow-up was 30 years. There were 59 deaths, of which 15 were from circulatory disease. Of these 15 deaths, 13 were from ischaemic heart disease. There were six deaths from diabetes as an underlying or contributory cause compared with the expected 1.7 deaths. The standard mortality rate both overall and for cardiovascular disease was not higher in the women with PCOS compared with the national mortality rates in women, although the observed proportion of women with diabetes as a contributory or underlying factor leading to death was significantly higher than expected (odds ratio 3.6, 95% CI 1.5–8.4). Thus despite surrogate markers for cardiovascular disease, in this study, no increased rate of death from CVS disease could be demonstrated.

Ischaemic heart disease

Wild et al (1990) reported that in 102 women undergoing coronary angiography to evaluate the significance of chest pain, hirsutism and acne were found to be twice as common in those with coronary artery disease than those without. In addition, an increased waist:hip ratio was associated with both hirsutism and coronary artery disease. They concluded that altered fat distribution (android pattern) associated with classic manifestations of androgen excess (hirsutism and/or acne) may be an indicator of a greater risk of IHD. Birdsall and colleagues (1997) reported the association between polycystic ovaries and extent of coronary artery disease in 143 women aged 60 years or younger, undergoing cardiac catheterization. Polycystic ovaries were detected in 42% of the subjects and these women showed a trend towards greater severity of IHD than women with normal ovaries. By multivariate regression analysis the extent of coronary artery disease was found to be independently associated with polycystic ovaries ($p = 0.032$) as was family history of heart disease ($p = 0.022$).

The incidence of coronary artery disease is strongly correlated with carotid atherosclerosis. Early carotid atherosclerosis as assessed by ultrasonography has been reported to be associated with cardiovascular risk factors, especially abnormal lipid profiles, in middle-aged and post-menopausal women. It has been shown that women with PCOS are more likely to have subclinical atherosclerosis of the carotid vessels. Although definitive evidence of a progression of carotid lesions from intima-media thickness to plaque formation and to clinical events is lacking, increase in intima-media thickness has been viewed as early subclinical atherosclerosis before the occurrence of gross atheromatous plaque formation and blood flow alteration.

THERAPEUTIC OPTIONS

Obesity and insulin resistance together and in isolation do play a major role in increasing the risk of cardiovascular disease in women. Exercise and weight loss have so far been the most physiological way to improve insulin sensitivity and improve the metabolic abnormalities associated with the syndrome. In women with PCOS it has been demonstrated that even partial weight loss improves the hormonal profile and improvement in the reproductive outcome for all forms of fertility treatment. Since the association between insulin resistance and BMI is stronger in obese women with PCOS than in weight-matched controls, the benefits of weight loss should be even greater in these women than in women without PCOS.

There have been reports in the literature regarding the use of insulin-sensitizing agents such as metformin and troglitazone in women with PCOS to reduce insulin resistance and improve the metabolic profile (Velazquez et al 1997). Studies to date have demonstrated improvements in endocrine profiles, menstrual cyclicity and also a reduction in PAI-1, along with an improvement in lipid profile, with varying degrees of, and sometimes no, weight loss. Thus there may be a decrease in the risk for atherosclerosis following metformin therapy although long-term follow-up studies are required.

POLYCYSTIC OVARY SYNDROME AND CANCER

The long-term risk of endometrial hyperplasia and endometrial carcinoma due to chronic anovulation and unopposed oestrogen has long been recognized; similarly there may be an increased risk of breast carcinoma. The multifactorial nature of the syndrome combined with its heterogeneous presentation makes it difficult to ascertain which factors (i.e. hyperinsulinaemia, elevated serum concentrations of growth factors, obesity or genetic predisposition) cause the most significant risk with respect to the development of cancer.

Endometrial cancer

While endometrial adenocarcinoma is the second most common female genital malignancy, only 4% of cases occur in women less than 40 years of age. The risk of developing endometrial cancer has been shown to be adversely influenced by a number of factors including obesity, long-term use of unopposed oestrogens, nulliparity and infertility. In fact, the relative risk of endometrial cancer is 1.6 in women with a menarche before the age of 12 years and 2.4 in women with their menopause after the age of 52 years (Elwood et al 1977). Women with endometrial carcinoma have fewer births compared with controls and it has also been demonstrated that infertility per se gives a relative risk of 2. Hypertension and type 2 diabetes mellitus have long been linked to endometrial cancer, with relative risks of 2.1 and 2.8 respectively (Elwood et al 1997), conditions that are now known also to be associated with PCOS.

A study by Coulam et al (1983) examined the risk of developing endometrial carcinoma in a group of 1270 patients who were diagnosed as having 'chronic anovulation syndrome'. The defining characteristics of this group included pathological or macroscopic evidence of the Stein–Leventhal syndrome or a clinical diagnosis of chronic anovulation. This study identified the excess risk of endometrial cancer to be 3.1 (95% CI 1.1–7.3) and proposed that this might be due to abnormal levels of unopposed oestrogen. Other authors have expanded this theory by suggesting that hyperandrogenism and hyperinsulinaemia may further increase the potential for neoplastic change in the endometrium through their effects on levels of SHBG, IGF-1 and circulating oestrogens. The true risk of endometrial carcinoma in women with PCOS, however, is difficult to ascertain. Studies to date have been limited by the relatively small numbers of cases of endometrial carcinoma identified specifically in women with PCOS and thus the confidence limits for relative risks are very wide.

Endometrial hyperplasia may be a precursor to adenocarcinoma, with cystic glandular hyperplasia progressing in maybe 0.4% of cases and adenomatous hyperplasia in up to 18% of cases over a time period of 2–10 years, although a precise estimate of progression rate is impossible to determine. In a study of 97 women under the age of 36 years with adenomatous or atypical adenomatous hyperplasia, 25% were found to have typical polycystic ovaries confirmed by biopsy. The mean age of the 24 women in this group was 25.7 years and all were nulliparous (23 were married). In 12 patients the diagnosis of polycystic ovaries was made at the time of hysterectomy (at which time two were found to have carcinoma). Treatment was by wedge resection of the ovaries in the other 12 patients, of whom eight had follow-up endometrial curettage and only three had persistent hyperplasia (one of which progressed to adnocarcinoma). One patient was found on initial curettage to have focal adenocarcinoma, which regressed after wedge biopsy, following which a normal pregnancy resulted from clomiphene citrate treatment. The other patients all had problems with infertility; some were treated with clomiphene citrate although results were poor (Chamlian & Taylor 1970).

Other authors have also reported conservative management of endometrial adenocarcinoma in women with PCOS with a combination of curettage and high-dose progestogens. The rationale is that cancer of the endometrium often presents at an early stage, is well differentiated, at low risk of metastasis and therefore is not perceived as being life-threatening, whilst poorly differentiated adenocarcinoma in a young woman has a worse prognosis and warrants hysterectomy. In general, however, the literature on women with PCOS and endometrial hyperplasia or adenocarcinoma suggests that this group of patients have a poor progonosis for fertility. This may be because of the factors that predisposed to the endometrial pathology – chronic anovulation combined often with severe obesity – or secondary to the endometrial pathology disrupting potential embryonic implantation. Case studies and small series of cases treated successfully without recourse to hysterectomy may be subject to publication bias and may not represent widespread medical opinion. Thus a more traditional and radical surgical approach (i.e. hysterectomy) is suggested as the safest way to prevent progression of the cancer. Early-stage disease may permit ovarian conservation and the possibility of pregnancy by surrogacy.

Although the degree of risk has not been clearly defined, it is generally accepted that for women with PCOS who experience symptoms of amenorrhoea or oligomenorrhoea, the induction of artificial withdrawal bleeds to prevent endometrial hyperplasia is prudent management. Indeed, we consider it important that women with PCOS shed their endometrium at least every 3 months. For those with oligo/amenorrhoea who do not wish to use cyclical hormone therapy we recommend an ultrasound scan to measure endometrial thickness and morphology every 6–12 months (depending upon menstrual history). An endometrial thickness greater than 10 mm in an amenorrhoeic woman warrants an artificially induced bleed, which should be followed by a repeat ultrasound scan and endometrial biopsy if the endometrium has not been shed.

Breast cancer

Obesity, hyperandrogenism and infertility occur frequently in PCOS and are features known to be associated with the development of breast cancer. However, studies examining the relationship between PCOS and breast carcinoma have not always identified a significantly increased risk. A study by Coulam et al (1983) calculated a relative risk of 1.5 (95% CI 0.75–2.55) for breast cancer in their group of women with chronic anovulation which was not statistically significant. After stratification by age, however, the relative risk was found to be 3.6 (95% CI 1.2–8.3) in the postmenopausal age group. Anderson et al (1997) designed a large prospective study to examine the development of breast carcinoma in postmenopausal women. The prevalence of PCOS in their cohort of 34 835 women was found to be only 1.35% and they determined that PCOS was not associated with an increased risk of breast carcinoma in this cohort. In this series, although women with PCOS were 1.8 times as likely to report benign breast disease as control women (p<0.01), they were not more likely to develop breast carcinoma (relative risk [RR] = 1.2; 95% CI 0.7–2). Adjustment for age at menarche, age at menopause, parity, oral contraceptive use, BMI, waist:hip ratio and family history of breast carcinoma lowered the RR to 1 (95% CI 0.6–1.9.) Thus despite the high-risk profiles of some women with PCOS, these results do not suggest that the syndrome per se is associated with an increased risk of postmenopausal breast carcinoma (Anderson et al 1997).

More recently, Pierpoint et al (1998) reported a series of 786 women with PCOS in the UK who were traced from hospital records after histological diagnosis of polycystic ovaries between 1930 and 1979. Mortality was assessed from the national registry of deaths and standardized mortality rates (SMR) calculated for patients with PCOS compared with the normal population. The average follow-up period was 30 years. The SMR for all neoplasms was 0.91 (95% CI 0.60–1.32) and for breast cancer 1.48 (95% CI 0.79–2.54). In fact, breast cancer was the leading cause of death in this cohort.

Ovarian cancer

In recent years there has been much debate about the risk of ovarian cancer in women with infertility, particularly in relation to the use of drugs to induce superovulation for assisted conception procedures. Inherently the risk of ovarian cancer appears to be increased in women who have multiple ovulations; that is, those who are nulliparous (possibly because of infertility) with an early menarche and late menopause. Thus it may be that inducing multiple ovulations in women with infertility will increase their risk (see review by Nugent et al 1998), a notion that is by no means proven. Women with PCOS who are oligo/anovulatory might therefore be expected to be at low risk of developing ovarian cancer if it is lifetime number of ovulations rather than pregnancies that is critical. Ovulation induction to correct anovulatory infertility aims to induce unifollicular ovulation and so in theory should raise the risk of

a woman with PCOS to that of a normal ovulating woman. The polycystic ovary, however, is notoriously sensitive to stimulation and it is only in recent years, with the development of high-resolution transvaginal ultrasonography, that the rate of unifollicular ovulation has attained acceptable levels. The use of clomiphene citrate and gonadotrophin therapy for ovulation induction in the 1960s, 1970s and 1980s resulted in many more multiple ovulations (and indeed multiple pregnancies) than in more recent times and might therefore present with an increased rate of ovarian cancer when these women reach the age of greatest risk.

There are a few studies which have addressed the possibility of an association between polycystic ovaries and ovarian cancer. The results are conflicting and generalizability is limited due to problems with the study designs. Coulam et al (1983) showed no increased risk of ovarian carcinoma in their group of anovulatory women. Schildkraut et al (1996), however, suggested that PCOS conferred a relative risk of 2.5 (95% CI 1.1–5.9) for epithelial ovarian cancer in their case control study. The prevalence of PCOS as determined by questionnaire was found to be 1.5% in cases and 0.6% in controls. The authors acknowledge that the small number of women with PCOS (31) limits the interpretation of their findings and that consideration must be given to the possibility of recall bias in subjects affected with ovarian cancer. In the large UK study of Pierpoint et al (1998), the SMR for ovarian cancer was 0.39 (95% CI 0.01–2.17).

CONCLUSION

The polycystic ovary syndrome is one of the most common endocrine disorders, although its aetiology remains unknown. This heterogeneous disorder may present, at one end of the spectrum, with the single finding of polycystic ovarian morphology as detected by pelvic ultrasound. At the other end of the spectrum symptoms such as obesity, hyperandrogenism, menstrual cycle disturbance and infertility may occur either singly or in combination. Metabolic disturbances (elevated serum concentrations of luteinizing hormone, testosterone, insulin and prolactin) are common and may have profound implications on the long-term health of women with PCOS.

The polycystic ovary syndrome is a familial condition and appears to have its origins during adolescence when it is thought to be associated with increased weight gain during puberty. At the other end of reproductive life it has been shown recently that women with oligo/amenorrhoeic PCOS appear to gain regular menstrual cycles as they get older. In a study of 205 women aged 30 years or older there was a highly significant linear trend for a shorter menstrual cycle length with age (Elting et al 2000). The hypothesis is that this phenomenon is due to both the decline in follicle cohort with age and a new balance between inhibin B and FSH in the early follicular phase of the cycle. The findings of this study have implications for the continued use of agents such as the oral contraceptive pill, which carries increased cardiovascular risks for women over the age of 35 years. It is prudent, therefore, to consider stopping artificial methods of cycle control for short periods to see if there has been a natural resolution of the problem.

upward such that they can be found in the fallopian tube within 5 minutes of intracervical insemination. Sperm have been shown to be released from storage in the cervix over a period up to 72 hours but do not appear to be stored in the fallopian tubes. Within the fallopian tube the sperm begin to display a new pattern of motility, i.e. hyperactivated motility, which has characteristics of greater speed and more positive direction. This change may result from an interaction between spermatozoa and tubal mucosa and/or secretions.

Cervical mucus is a complex structure which is not homogeneous. It is secreted in granular form and a networked structure of the mucus is formed within the cervical canal. Not all areas of the mucus appear to be equally penetrable. (For review, see Harper 1988.)

Capacitation and activation

Immediately following ejaculation spermatozoa are unable to achieve fertilization. They only gain this capacity after a delay of several hours as they pass through the female genital tract.

The initial change of *capacitation* appears to involve the stripping from the spermatozoa of the surface coat of glycoprotein molecules, which have been adsorbed in the epididymis and from the seminal plasma. The loss of this protein coat is effected by proteolytic enzymes and the high ionic concentration found in the secretions of an oestrogen-dominated uterus.

Despite completing this process of capacitation, the sperm are still not fully ready to fertilize oocytes until the final process of *activation* has occurred. This process is calcium dependent and involves changes throughout the spermatozoon. Before sperm are activated three accomplishments are required. They must:

1. undergo the acrosome reaction
2. acquire the ability to bind to the zona pellucida
3. acquired appropriate motility patterns, i.e. hyperactivated motility.

The first process or 'acrosome reaction' is one in which the acrosome swells and its membrane fuses at a number of points, with the overlying plasma membrane acquiring a vesiculated appearance (Fig. 20.3). As a result of this process, the contents of the acrosomal vesicle and the inner acrosomal membrane are exposed to the exterior. At the same time there is a change in the movement pattern of the spermatozoon. The tail movements of the spermatozoon, which previously demonstrated regular wave-like flagellar beats, now exhibit more episodic wide-amplitude whiplash movements which carry it forward.

The other apparent change occurs in the surface membrane overlying the middle and posterior half of the spermatozoon head. This membrane, previously incapable of fusion, now becomes capable of fusing with the surface membrane of the oocyte.

The exact mechanisms involved in this process of activation are not fully determined. However, activated spermatozoa tend only to be found in close association with the oocyte and cumulus mass. This suggests that a constituent of follicular fluid, a secretion from the cumulus mass or a product in the zone pellucida itself may be responsible for this activation

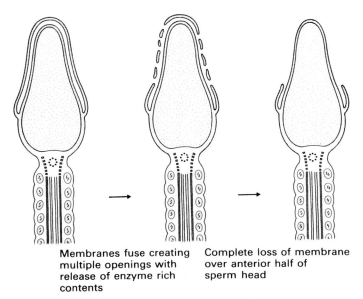

Membranes fuse creating multiple openings with release of enzyme rich contents

Complete loss of membrane over anterior half of sperm head

Fig. 20.3   Acrosome reaction.

which facilitates the binding of the spermatozoa to the oocyte membrane.

THE OOCYTE

Structure of the ovary

The ovary consists of stromal tissue, which contains the primordial follicles, and glandular tissue consisting of interstitial cells. It is the primordial follicle, consisting of the primordial germ cell surrounded by a layer of flattened mesenchymal cells, which is the fundamental functional unit within the ovary. The process of gamete production in the female consists of cell proliferation by mitosis, genetic reshuffling and reduction, i.e. meiosis, and finally the reduction to the haploid number of chromosomes during oocyte maturation. One major difference between the female and the male is the need for proliferation by mitosis, essential in the male to maintain a massive sperm output from the testes but less essential in the female since only one or at most a few eggs are released during each menstrual cycle.

The primordial germ cells which enter the gonad continue mitotic proliferation well after ovarian morphology is established in utero. However, unlike the situation in the male, the mitotic phase of the primordial germ cells, or oogonia, terminates finally before birth when all oogonia enter into their first meiotic division and hence become the primary oocytes. One major consequence of this early meiosis is that by the time of birth the woman has within her ovary all the oocytes that she will ever have. In the progress through the first meiotic phase, oocytes become surrounded by ovarian mesenchymal cells to form the primordial follicles. The follicles form the oocytes which become arrested in the diplotene stage of their first meiotic phase. The chromosomes remain enclosed by a nuclear membrane in the nucleus, known as the germinal vesicle. The primordial follicle remains in this arrested state within the ovary until it receives the appropriate signals to resume development.

Selection and maturation of follicles

Regular recruitment of primordial follicles to a pool of subsequently growing developing follicles occurs first at puberty. Thereafter follicles recommence growth daily so that there is a continuing supply of developing follicles being formed. During the late luteal phase, the largest healthy follicles are between 2 and 5 millimetres in diameter. Their number and quality rise in response to the rising FSH levels during the late luteal phase and early follicular phase of the cycle. It is from amongst these follicles that the follicle destined to ovulate in a subsequent cycle will be selected (di Zerega & Hodgen 1981, Erickson 1986).

Morphological changes

Once the primordial follicle is recruited to begin maturational changes (Fig. 20.4), the granulosa cells surrounding the oocytes start to change from squamous to cuboidal in appearance. An increase in follicular diameter occurs in the major part of growth, resulting from an increase in diameter in the primordial oocyte from 20 microns to between 60 and 100 microns. During this critical growth phase a massive synthetic activity is occurring, particularly with the synthesis of large amounts of RNA; this activity loads the oocytes' cytoplasm with essential materials for the later stages of egg maturation. During this increase in size of the oocyte an acellular glycoprotein matrix, termed the zona pellucida, is secreted by the granulosa cells and forms an envelope surrounding the oocyte. Contact with the oocyte and the granulosa cells is maintained by cytoplasmic processes which penetrate the zona and form gap junctions at the oocyte surface. Gap junctions are also formed between adjacent granulosa cells, thus providing a basis for intracellular communication. Through this network, low molecular weight substrates, some amino acids and nucletides can be passed to the growing oocyte. Concurrently spindle-like stromal cells come into close proximity with the basal lamina of the granulosa cells. These theca cells and cells most proximal to the basal membrane are termed theca interna cells.

Towards the end of this critical growth and reorganization phase of the follicle, cells of the granulosa layer develop receptors for oestrogen and follicle-stimulating hormone (FSH) and the theca cells develop luteinizing hormone (LH) receptors. These are essential to gain entry into the next phase of follicular development which becomes greatly dependent upon gonadotrophin secretion patterns.

This gonadotrophin stimulation converts preantral follicles to antral follicles and encourages further proliferation of granulosa and theca cells. However, there is little addition or increase in size of the oocyte itself; its chromosomes remain in the dictyate stage while RNA synthesis and protein production continue.

At the start of the follicular phase, the largest healthy follicles appear to be the selected follicles with diameters between 5.5 and 8 millimetres. Apart from size and granulosa cell mitotic index, there are no morphlogical differences apparent between the selected and other non-selected healthy follicles. Responsive follicles contain granulosa cells with high numbers of FSH receptors which lead to an increase in aromatase activity (in response to FSH stimulation). There may also be selected activation of the insulin-like growth factor 1 (IGF-1) system in the chosen follicle. As a follicle matures granulosa cells become able to bind FSH and the theca cells increase their facility to synthesize 3β-hydroxysteroid dehydrogenase which also appears in granulosa cells following ovulation.

Steroid hormone production – two-cell theory

During this second phase of growth, follicles show a steady increase in the synthesis of androgens and oestrogens.

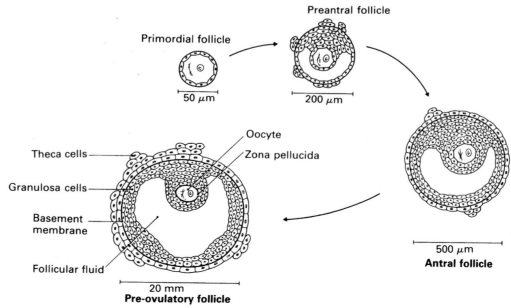

Fig. 20.4   Follicular development from primordial follicle to preovulatory stage.

Production of these steroids is under the control of gonadotrophins which appear to facilitate effects at different locations within the follicle. Only the granulosa cells bind FSH and only the theca cells LH. LH primarily stimulates the cells of the theca interna to synthesize androgens from acetate and cholesterol. Oestrogen synthesis by these cells is possible to only a limited degree, particularly in the early stages of growth. In contrast, the granulosa cells are unable to form androgens. However, androgen supplied to the granulosa cells from the theca cells is readily aromatized to oestrogens (Fig. 20.5). Thus androgens are produced by developing follicles from the theca cells whilst oestrogens arise via two routes: primarily from thecal androgens aromatized by granulosa cells and to a lesser degree by de novo synthesis from acetate in thecal cells.

Both the production of steroids and the increase in follicular size are interlinked. Oestrogen in conjunction with FSH plays a crucial role within the follicle towards the end of the second phase of growth. Oestrogen and FSH together stimulate the appearance of LH-binding sites in the outer layers of the granulosa cells. These LH-binding sites are crucial for the antral follicle to enter the final phase of development: the conversion to the preovulatory follicle.

Regulation of oocyte maturation

There are complex interactions between the oocyte and the follicular somatic cells (granulosa and theca cells) which are essential for the development and function of both cell types. The oocyte nucleus is called the germinal vesicle. The most obvious manifestation of reinitiation of meiosis is the disappearance or breakdown of the germinal vesicle. This appears to be initiated by the preovulatory surge of gonadotrophins. The gonadotrophins do not directly act on the oocyte since the oocyte does not contain gonadotrophin receptors. Germinal vesicle breakdown is a multistep process

and the apparently LH-induced germinal vesicle breakdown occurs by an indirect action mediated by follicular somatic cells. LH may induce a positive germinal vesicle breakdown susbtance in granulosa cells and this is passed to the oocyte. The process is thought to involve alterations in calcium ions and may also result in alterations in the level of cyclic AMP within the oocyte.

With the completion of the final stage of meiosis and extrusion of the first polar body, the oocyte is then capable of undergoing fertilization.

THE FALLOPIAN TUBE

Structure of the fallopian tube

The ovulated oocyte plus attached cumulus cells is picked up from the peritoneal cavity by the fimbriated ostium of the oviduct (fallopian tube) and swept by oviductal cilia along the ampulla towards the junction with the isthmus. The fallopian tube serves a number of essential functions in the reproductive process. First, it is responsible for transferring the ovum into its lumen when discharged from the rupturing follicle. Second, it provides an environment for the ovum and spermatozoa in which fertilization can occur, and finally it transfers the fertilized, cleaving embryo into the uterus after a timed interval of 3–4 days (Diaz et al 1980). At the distal end of the tube are the delicate finger-like projections or fimbriae. These are lined with cilia which beat in the direction of the tubal lumen. The fimbrial cilia are capable of cyclic regeneration which occurs under the influence of oestrogen. The entire length of the fallopian tube contains cilia; ciliary beat creates a current within the tubal lumen to transport the oocyte from the peritoneal cavity into the uterus (Fig. 20.6).

Oocyte transport is affected adversely if cumulus cells are lacking and/or if oviductal cilia are malfunctional. There is no evidence that muscular activity in the tube is essential for transport of the oocyte along its course, but pharmacological doses of ovarian steroids and prostaglandin may adversely affect ooctye transport (Coutinho & Mala 1971). Oocytes and spermatozoa come together in the ampulla and it is here that the final events of spermatozoal activation become clear as the first phase of fertilization commences.

Tubal secretory proteins in the human oviduct

During the reproductive events in the oviduct, the male gametes and the resultant embryo are antigenically different from the female host but appear not to be affected by the maternal immune system. The mechanism of protection is unknown and at present, our ability to test tubal function is limited to a simple patency test or the more recent development of visualization of the fallopian tubal mucosa with falloposcopy, the value of which is yet to be proven.

The secretory elements of the tubal mucosa are modified during a normal menstrual cycle but as ovulation approaches, under the influence of oestrogen, the secretory cells become tall and columnar and project beyond the cilial ends, discharging secretions into the tubal lumen. The production of fluid in the fallopian tube is greatest immediately before ovulation but still

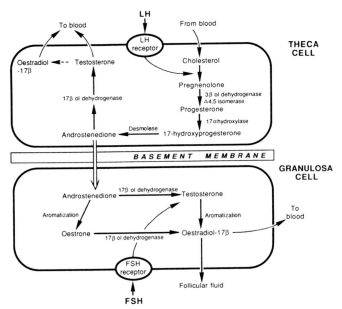

Fig. 20.5 Two-cell theory of follicular oestrogen production. LH, luteinizing hormone; FSH, follicle-stimulating hormone.

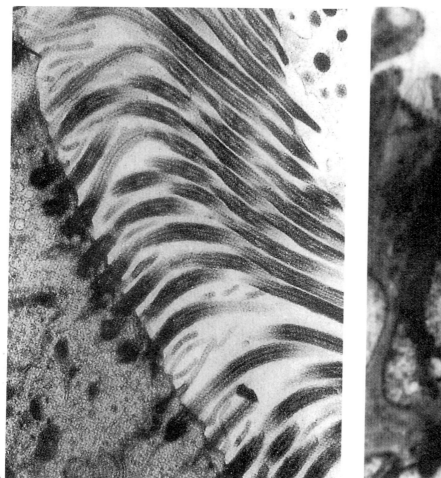
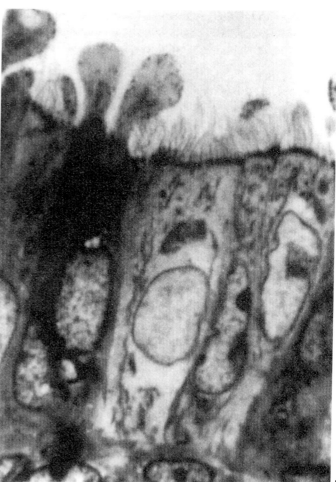

Fig. 20.6 Electron microscopy pictures of **a** fimbrial cilia and **b** the postovulatory tubal mucosa demonstrating secretory and ciliated cells. Reproduced with permission from Mastroianni & Coutifaris (1990).

remains a poorly investigated area (Lippes et al 1973). What is known is that the total concentration of many constituents in oviductal fluid is lower than in serum and that there is selected passage of macromolecules, such that lactate is 50% and complement component C3 is 17% of serum concentrations (Oliphant et al 1978). Immunoelectrophoresis of oviduct fluid has suggested the presence of unique proteins which may be synthesized and secreted by the oviduct: a specific β-glycoprotein of molecular weight 54 000 daltons capable of binding to spermatozoa heads, PAPP-A and placental protein 5 (PP5) have been reported (Butzow 1989). Thus the oviduct synthesizes and secretes both specific proteins and proteins of general müllerian origin. There are few results from human studies to determine the relevance or importance of these specific components to date, but further knowledge may lead to improved in vitro fertilization culture media and our increased understanding of the important role of the fallopian tubes in the process of fertilization and early development.

FERTILIZATION

Fertilization is not a single event but a continuum. The fertilization process begins when the capacitated spermatozoa

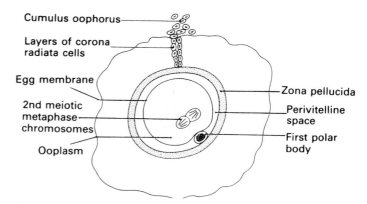

Fig. 20.7 Schematic representation of freshly ovulated oocyte.

come in contact with the ovum and its cellular coverings. Before a spermatazoon can achieve fertilization it must first penetrate the cellular covering of the oocyte, the cumulus oophorus, the corona radiata and the zona pellucida (Fig. 20.7). The cumulus cells are embedded in a matrix rich in hyaluronic acid and the acrosome located at the end of the spermatozoon contains the enzyme hyaluronidase. This may well be important in the dispersion of the cumulus cells. This process of dispersion is further completed by the action of the cilia of the fallopian tube.

The zona pellucida

The zona pellucida is a dense translucent protein layer immediately surrounding the oocyte. This acellular layer remains in place until implantation. It appears to have two functions. First, it contains receptors for sperm which are species specific and second, it undergoes a zonal reaction in which the zona becomes impervious to other sperm once the fertilizing sperm has penetrated the oolema, thus providing a bar to polyspermia.

Zona–sperm binding

Initial contact between sperm and oocyte is a receptor-mediated process. A number of glycoproteins have been identified in the zona, termed ZP1, ZP2, and ZP3, of which ZP3 is the most abundant and expressed only in growing oocytes (Shabonowitz & O'Rand 1988).

Initial binding of sperm to the zona requires the sperm to recognize the carbohydrate component of the species-specific glycoprotein receptor molecules. Once binding is accomplished (Fig. 20.8), the acrosome reaction is triggered by the peptide chain component of the receptor glycoprotein. Formation of the enzyme–ZP3 complex therefore not only produces binding but also induces the acrosome reaction.

During the acrosome reaction, there is a release of acrosomal contents which include hyaluronidase. Granulosa cells are held together by an intracellular matrix of hyaluronic acid. This is digested by the enzyme hyaluronidase, thus allowing sperm to pass through the corona radiata cells towards the zona pellucida. Thus the sperm binds to the glycoprotein receptor on the zona and the proteolytic proenzyme proacrosin on the exposed acrosomal membranes is activated to form acrosin. This digests through the zona, aided by the whiplash forward propulsion of the sperm. The spermatozoon, both the head and tail, is then incorporated into the cytoplasm of the oocyte, completing the penetration process. The first phase of fertilization from entry of the cumulus mass to fusion lasts between 10 and 20 minutes. The assumed process of fertilization lasts some 20 hours or so and results in the return of the

diploid genetic constitution of the embryo and the initiation of the latter's development programme.

Initiation of the block to further penetration of spermatozoa is mediated by the cortical reaction. This is a release of materials from the cortical granules, lysosome-like organelles which are found just below the egg surface (Barros & Yamagimachi 1971). The lysosomes include hydrolytic enzymes which induce the zona reaction, producing a hardening of the extracellular layers by crosslinking of proteins and inactivation of sperm receptors. As the sperm enter the periviteline space at an angle, the postacrosomal region of the sperm makes initial contact with the vitelline membrane. First the egg membrane engulfs the sperm head and subsequently there is fusion of the egg and sperm membranes. This fusion is mediated by specific proteins, of which two have been sequenced: PH20, which is important for binding, and PH30, which is important for fusion (Blobel et al 1992). The fusion triggers the cortical reaction, metabolic activation of the oocyte and completion of meiosis, such that the second polar body is released.

Conception

Within 2 or 3 hours of oocyte–sperm fusion, the second polar body has been expelled and the remaining haploid set of female chromosomes lies in the ooplasm. When the sperm head enters the ooplasm its chromosome material is tightly packed. During the next 2–3 hours these chromosomes uncoil under the influence of cytoplasm of the oocyte and the sperm head is transformed into the male pronucleus. The male and female pronuclei increase somewhat in size and then migrate towards the centre of the egg; with the formation of the metaphase spindle, the chromosomes assume their position at its equator. This occurs 18–21 hours after gamete fusion. The coming together of the gametic chromosomes, syngamy, is the final phase of fertilization. Immediately anaphase and telophase are completed, the cleavage furrow forms and the one-cell zygote becomes a two-cell embryo.

IMPLANTATION

Changes in the endometrium

The endometrium has undergone extensive proliferation under the influence of oestrogen in the days prior to ovulation. Its cells exhibit marked mitotic activity. Under the combined influence of oestrogen and progesterone following ovulation, with the increasing quantities of these hormones secreted by the corpus luteum, the endometrial stroma and glands change rapidly. The glands display a secretory pattern and the products of their secretion are discharged into the uterine lumen (for further details, see Ch. 28).

The differentiation of endometrium prior to implantation is controlled by a large variety of growth factor interactions in which epidermal growth factor (EGF) and IGF-1 are thought to be important. Receptors for both of these are expressed in the endometrium and regulated by receptor number or specific binding proteins throughout the menstrual cycle. In vitro progesterone downregulates IGF-1 binding sites in intact stromal cell culture layers. In the uterus, messages of the

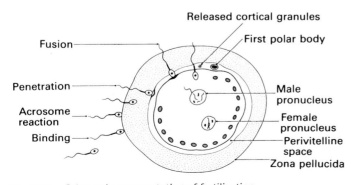

Fig. 20.8 Schematic representation of fertilization.

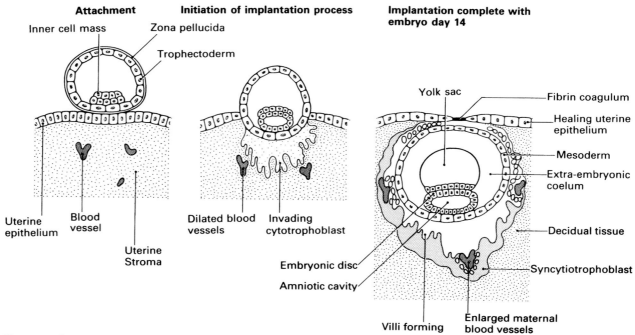

Fig. 20.9 Stages of implantation.

oestrogenic signal between the different cellular compartments have been postulated. A combination of EGF and progesterone seems necessary to fully decidualize endometrial stromal cells, thus modulating the secretion of IGF-binding proteins (Guidice et al 1992).

The implantation process

The embryo remains in the fallopian tube, the site of fertilization, for approximately 3–4 days (Diaz et al 1980). It is suspended in the tubal fluid and continues to develop into the morula. It is then transferred through the isthmus of the tube into the uterine cavity. This transfer is facilitated by the change in endocrine environment of the early luteal phase. Within the uterine cavity the embryo establishes nutritional and physical contact with the maternal tissue at the site of implantation (Fig. 20.9).

After hatching and attachment the penetration process starts.

Human implantation occurs during a period of endometrial change, preceded by intense tissue remodelling by growth factors such as cytokines and proteases, induced by embryo–maternal interactions and endocrine events. Implantation involves extensive modification of the embryo and the endometrium. This is induced by contacts between the embryo and uterus and by extracellular signals which affect both blastocyst and uterine epithelium (for review, see Denker 1983, Glasser 1986). These include:

- the binding of invading cells to glycoproteins within the basement membranes (laminin, fibronectin) through their specific receptors (integrins)
- activation of proteases and pericellular degregation of matrix components (matrix metalloproteinases)

- migration of the cells into the matrix, i.e. cells progressing through the endometrial epithelium towards basement membrane, recognizing laminin and collagen type IV through their integrins.

These processes activate the expression of the gene for gelatinases A and B, which degregate the basement membrane. This allows the cytotrophoblastic cells to migrate through the basement membrane and make contact in the extracellular matrix through their fibronectin receptors. During the invasion process, the collagenolytic activity of cytotrophoblast is modulated by endometrial factors such as cytokines that inhibit trophoblastic proteolytic activity, thus controlling the depth of invasion (Liotta et al 1984). Within 3–5 days of attachment, the whole embryo is completely embedded within the uterine epithelium in the endometrial stroma. By 14–21 days after fertilization, the trophoblastic structure at the periphery of the blast cells resembles the villi of the mature placenta and the area of the inner cells mass has started to organize itself into the embryo proper.

The details of the further development undergone by the embryo are beyond the scope of this book and readers are referred to relevant chapters in the textbook of *Obstetrics* (Turnbull & Chamberlain 2001).

KEY POINTS

1. The process of fertilization and implantation is highly complex. It entails the completion and co-ordination of a number of highly organized events which involve the gametes, the male and female genital tracts and the various components of the endocrine system.

KEY POINTS (*CONTINUED*)

2. A mature spermatozoon contains the haploid number of chromosomes. It possesses a head which includes the acrosome, a midpiece that contains the mitochondria, the residual body and a tail which is essential for propulsion.

3. Abnormally developed spermatozoa comprise up to 40% of the total contained in a fertile semen sample.

4. During its passage through the vasa efferentia and the epididymis, the spermatozoon gains the capability of movement and the potential to fertilize an oocyte.

5. Following entry into and storage within the cervical crypts, the intermittent release of sperm (over a period of up to 72 hours after coitus) is dependent on uterine contraction and intrinsic sperm motility.

6. In order to gain full ability to fertilize, the spermatozoon undergoes the processes of capacitation and activation. The latter occurs within the fallopian tube and consist of three components: acrosome reaction, binding to the zona pellucida and attainment of hyperactivated motility.

7. The number of oocytes a woman possesses is predetermined by the number of oogonia entering into the first meiotic division which is arrested in the diplotene stage, during fetal life.

8. Following recruitment to the pool of maturing follicles, the primordial oocyte undergoes development that includes acquisition of the acellular zona pellucida which is secreted by the granulosa cells.

9. The theca cells, with specific receptors for LH, synthesize androgens in response to LH stimulation. Oestrogen synthesis is brought on by the availability of androgens to the granulosa cells which, in response to FSH stimulation, increase their aromatase activity responsible for the conversion of androgen to oestrogen. This is the 'two-cell two-gonadotrophin' hypothesis.

10. The preovulatory surge of gonadotrophins induces the breakdown of the germinal vesicle which is followed by the completion of the final stage of meiosis, such that the oocyte is capable of undergoing fertilization.

REFERENCES

Barros C, Yamagimachi R 1971 Induction of zona reaction in golden hamster eggs by cortical granule material. Nature 233:2368

Blobdel CP, Wolfsberg TG, Turck CW, Myles DG, Primakoff P, White JM 1992 A potential fusion peptide and an integrin ligand domain in a protein active in sperm–egg fusion. Nature 356:248

Butzow R 1989 The human fallopian tube contains placental protein 5. Human Reproduction 1:17–20

Chamberlain G (ed) 1995 Turnbull's obstetrics, 2nd edn. Churchill Livingstone, New York

Coutinho EM, Mala HS 1971 The contractile response of the human uterus, fallopian tubes and ovary to prostaglandins in vivo. Fertility and Sterility 22:539–543

Denker HW 1983 Basic aspects of ova implantation. Obstetrical and Gynaecological Annual Reviews 12:15–42

Diaz S, Ortiz ME, Crozatto HB 1980 Studies on the duration of ovum transport by the human oviduct. The time interval between the luteinizing hormone peak and recovery of ova by transcervical flushing of the uterus in normal women. American Journal of Obstetrics and Gynecology 137:116

Di Zerega GS, Hodgen GD 1981 Folliculogenesis in the primate ovarian cycle. Endocrine Reviews 2:27

Erickson GF 1986 An analysis of follicle development in ovum maturation. Seminars in Reproductive Endocrinology 4:233–254

Glasser SR 1986 Current concepts of implantation and decidualization. In: Hoszar G (ed) The physiology and biochemistry of the uterus in pregnancy and labor. CRC Press, Boca Raton, Florida

Guidice LC, Dsupin BA, Irwin JC 1992 Steroid and peptide regulation of insulin-like growth factor binding proteins secreted by human endometrial stromal cells is dependent on stromal differentiation. Journal of Clinical Endocrinology and Metabolism 75:1235–1241

Harper NJK 1988 Gamete and zygote transport. In: Knobil E, Neill J (eds) The physiology of reproduction. Raven Press, New York

Liotta LA, Rao CN, Terranova VP, Barksy S, Thorgeirsson U 1984 Tumour cell attachment and degradation of basement membrane. In: Nicholson GL, Milas L (eds) Cancer invasion and metastasis, biologic and therapeutic aspects. Raven Press, New York

Lippes J, Enders RG, Pragay DA, Bartholomew WR 1973 The collection and analysis of human fallopian tube fluid. Contraception 5:85–93

Mastroianni L, Coutifaris C (eds) 1990 Reproductive physiology, vol I. Parthenon, Carnforth, Lancashire

Oliphant G, Bowling A, Eng LA, Keen S 1978 The permeability of the rabbit oviduct to proteins present in the serum. Biology of Reproduction 18:516–520

Shabonowitz RB, O'Rand MG 1988 Characterisation of the human zona pellucida from fertilized and unfertilized eggs. Journal of Reproductive Medicine 82:151–161

Wang C, Baker HWG, Jennings MG, Burger HG, Lutjen P 1985 Interaction between human cervical mucus and sperm surface antibodies. Fertility and Sterility 44:484–488

21

Investigation of the infertile couple

Neil McClure

INTRODUCTION

This chapter presents a simple, logical and evidence-based account of the investigation of the infertile couple. Therefore, the emphasis is on clinical practice through an ordered scheme of basic investigations. In some instances descriptions of more complex investigations are included even though they may only be required occasionally. It is more important to perform relevant tests in their proper order and at an appropriate time interval than to subject the couple to a large range of investigations, many of which bear little relevance to the day-to-day management of their problem.

Using life table analysis, it has been calculated that the chances of conception for a given couple having regular, unprotected intercourse are 80% after 12 and 90% after 18 months (Cooke et al 1981). It is usual, therefore, to wait for at least 1 year of appropriate, unprotected intercourse before beginning investigations for infertility. However, where the woman is known not to be ovulating or the man has had chemotherapy or the couple are in their early 40s the situation is different and the timescale and range of investigation should be dictated by the couple and their individual situation. Medically, in an ideal world free of the limitations of waiting lists, etc. it should be easily possible to complete a programme of basic tests within 6 months. However, it would be inappropriate to proceed with laparoscopy to evaluate tubal status if a significant, uncorrected male factor or a disorder of ovulation exists. Throughout the work-up a clear explanation of the indication and nature of the tests must be given to both partners. This is facilitated if they are seen together in a dedicated infertility clinic where adequate time is available for counselling and facilities exist to permit a proper assessment of the situation.

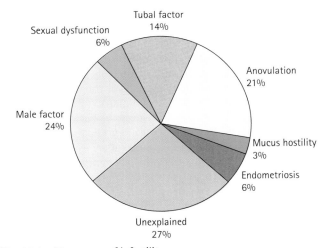

Fig. 21.1   The causes of infertility.

The causes of infertility and their relative frequency are shown in Figure 21.1. However, all incidence figures are suspect since most are derived from specialist units. Many couples are dealt with successfully by their general practitioners or in district general hospitals and never reach a specialized clinic. Further, unexplained infertility is an ill-defined entity and the categorization clearly depends on identifying no other cause and that depends both on how hard the doctor looks for a cause and on the degree of significance attached to any positive finding. For example, stage 1 endometriosis may be ignored by some and identified as 'the cause' by others; similarly, views on the postcoital test vary considerably between units. This explains, in part, the variation from 6% to 60% in the reported incidence of unexplained infertility in various publications (Templeton & Penney 1982).

The approach to the infertile couple should begin with detailed medical, sexual and social histories followed by physical examination of both partners. The sequence of investigations should be ordered such that the simplest, least invasive and most productive tests are completed first. Therefore, at the initial consultation (or preferably in primary care before referral), semen analysis and a test of ovulation are arranged. At the second consultation the results are reviewed with the couple. If the results are normal and the couple so wish, they should proceed to assessment of tubal patency. However, the couple should not be forced into this and within the confines of waiting lists and service funding, the range of investigations should be determined by the doctor but the pace and nature of the investigations should be controlled by the patients.

HISTORY AND EXAMINATION

The female history

There are three main disorders of female fertility: anovulation, tubal disease and endometriosis. All will have historical pointers. Initially, though, the duration of infertility should be established: use of contraception, incidents of separation through work, social activities or marital breakdown should be identified and a detailed sexual history obtained. What is the frequency of coitus? Is dyspareunia a significant factor? Do both partners achieve orgasm? Is sexual intercourse limited to the so-called 'best time' of the month and if so, how is this determined? Often even the most apparently informed couples have the fertile time of the month completely mixed up.

Abnormalities of ovulation are likely if the menstrual cycle is irregular. Traditionally the normal menstrual cycle is taken as between 25 and 35 days. However, at either end of this range the chances of ovulation are significantly decreased. Mittelschmerz and a midcycle 'cascade' of cervical mucus both suggest ovulation. If the periods are irregular, historical factors associated with polycystic ovarian syndrome (acne, oily skin, hirsutism), hyperprolactinaemia (galactorrhoea), hypothalamic-pituitary axis failure (excessive weight loss or an aggressive training schedule, anorexia or bulimia nervosa) or thyroid dysfunction may be present.

Tubal disease is the commonest cause of secondary infertility. All patients should be asked about pelvic inflammatory disease, vaginal discharge and deep dyspareunia. With parous patients a history of puerperal sepsis and secondary postpartum haemorrhage is relevant. A general medical history is also necessary: a ruptured appendix, for instance, may result in tubal damage as may tuberculosis if it affected the pelvic organs.

Endometriosis can be asymptomatic even when quite advanced. However, it more often presents with secondary (worsening) dysmenorrhoea or deep dyspareunia.

The points to be elicited in the female history are summarized in Box 21.1.

The male history

The male should be asked about episodes of testicular pain, swelling or trauma and about testicular or groin surgery,

Box 21.1   Investigation of infertility: the female history

Sexual dysfunction	Dyspareunia and vaginismus Coital frequency Orgasm
Endocrine	Menstrual pattern Hirsutism/acne/oily skin Weight changes and eating disorders Galactorrhoea Thyroid symptoms
Uterine and tubal	Pelvic/abdominal surgery Pelvic infection/sexually transmitted diseases Pelvic pain Dysmenorrhoea
Cervical factor	Mucus secretion (ovulation cascade) Conization/cautery Incompetence
Previous obstetric history	Pregnancy loss Puerperal sepsis
Contraception	Hormonal Intrauterine contraceptive device

particularly for maldescent of the testes or hernia repair, as a child. Severe head injury, meningitis and encephalitis can affect the function of the hypothalamic-pituitary axis. Chronic general illnesses may be associated with infertility: cystic fibrosis, for example, is associated with bilateral absence of the vas deferens and some drugs, such as sulphasalazine, given for the treatment of inflammatory bowel disease, adversely affect seminal parameters. An acute pyrexial illness can alter sperm counts for several weeks. There is also evidence to suggest that the testes function most efficiently if their temperature is approximately 1° below normal body temperature. However, the importance of sedentary jobs or tight-fitting underwear in affecting sperm quality is highly debatable. Excessive use of tobacco, alcohol or cannabis can lower sperm counts. With cannabis the changes are largely anecdotal but with alcohol and tobacco there are large supportive population studies although any changes are relatively small. The role of environmental pollutants has never been properly answered in male fertility although specific problems like aniline dyes have been demonstrated. The UK-based CHAPS Study should provide answers to the question of environmental pollutants and sperm quality once completed and published.

The points to be elicited in the male history are summarized in Box 21.2.

Examination

Once the history is taken both partners should be examined. In the female, height and weight are recorded and the body mass index (kg/m^2) calculated. Breasts are checked for development and secondary sexual characteristics are noted. Abdominal palpation and a pelvic examination should check for gross normality of the pelvic organs. Tenderness or nodularity of the uterosacral ligaments often indicates endometriosis. Vaginal

Box 21.2 Investigation of infertility: the male history

Occupation	Sedentary Toxin/irradiation
Illnesses/operations	Febrile conditions Bladder neck surgery Cryptorchidism
Infection	Venereal Orchitis/epididymitis Tuberculosis
Drugs	Sulphasalazine Chemotherapy Antimicrobials Antihypertensives Alcohol/nicotine/cannabis
Sexual function	Coital frequency Erection/orgasm Ejaculation
Trauma/stress	

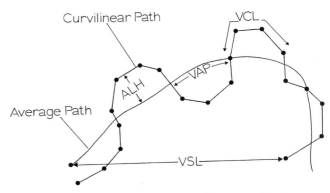

Fig. 21.2 Terminology of measurements of sperm motility in computer-assisted semen analysis. ALH, amplitude of lateral head displacement; VAP, average path velocity; VCL, curvilinear velocity; VSL, straight-line velocity. Reproduced with permission of Cambridge University Press from WHO (1992).

ultrasound may be performed at this stage to identify a polycystic ovary appearance and to exclude ovarian cysts, endometriomas and uterine fibroids.

In the male, weight and general appearance are recorded. Abdominal palpation is followed by examination of the external genitalia. The penis is inspected for hypospadias and the testes are assessed for size (with reference to an orchidometer), consistency and tenderness. The epididymis should be examined for tenderness and fullness: if flaccid, it is more likely that the man has non-obstructive azoospermia. The vasa deferentia must be identified (characteristically they feel like 'whipcord') and varicoceles and inguinal herniae excluded with the patient standing, performing a Valsalva manoeuvre. If the presence of varicocoele is questioned, Doppler or ultrasound examination may be of help in confirming the suspected clinical diagnosis. Finally, rectal examination should be performed for prostatic enlargement or tenderness which might indicate prostatitis.

INVESTIGATION OF MALE FACTORS

The standard basic investigation of male infertility is the semen analysis. What constitutes a normal semen analysis remains controversial which is not surprising as no one knows the number of motile, normal sperm above which there is no increase in fertility. In effect, this is probably different for every couple and depends on a whole range of defined and undefined variables. However, the WHO criteria are now broadly accepted (WHO 1999). The issue is further confounded by within- and between-laboratory variation which can be up to 80%. Therefore, it is essential that semen laboratories are subject to quality control and, in the UK, the National External Quality Assessment Scheme (NEQAS) has been introduced.

Proponents of computer-aided sperm analysis (CASA) have suggested that much of the variability can be eliminated by this approach. However, for example, the presence of contaminating cells and debris in the sample can confuse the computer. Therefore, whilst counts appear to be reproducible, the analysis of morphology is often unsatisfactory (Boyers et al 1989). By contrast, a number of new motility parameters have been developed including the curvilinear velocity, the straight-line velocity and the average path velocity (Fig. 21.2). Agreement between different laboratories in the analysis of these parameters is good (Davis & Katz 1992), but their relationship with fertility in vivo is unclear although a clear association has been demonstrated between good sperm progression and the ability of sperm to penetrate cervical mucus (Mortimer et al 1986), and between good sperm progression and zona-free hamster egg penetration (Aitken et al 1985).

In vitro fertilization has allowed a crude assessment of fertilization potential. In an attempt to rationalize and standardize the investigation of these problems, tests for the attachment and penetration by sperm for both the zona pellucida and the oolemma have been developed. However, these tests are only relevant where fertilization has failed to occur during in vitro fertilization with adequate, normal sperm.

Routine semen analysis

All semen samples should be obtained by masturbation into a clean, wide-mouthed, non-toxic plastic container. It is preferable for the sample to be produced within the hospital and a dedicated facility should be identified for this in order that conditions during the liquefaction process can be optimized. However, some patients will be unable to produce a sample under this 'pressure' and they should be given written and verbal instructions about the importance of delivering the sample at body temperature and within 1 hour of collection. For some masturbation is offensive. Non-toxic condoms exist and the couple can be supplied with these in order to obtain the sample during coitus. Coitus interruptus is not recommended as the first part of the ejaculate is likely to be lost. This part usually contains the greatest density of sperm.

Different clinics recommend different intervals of abstinence prior to the production of semen for analysis. It is common

Box 21.3 Routine semen analysis

Volume	2–6 ml
Liquefaction	Complete in 30 min
Count	20 million/ml or more
Motility	60% (forward progressive)
Morphology	70% or more normal forms

practice to advise the male to have ejaculated at least once within the week prior to the test but not within the previous 2 days. Many clinics also record the most recent ejaculation prior to the test sample. Because of the known variability in semen quality from the same individual, at least two specimens should be examined during the course of the fertility investigations.

The basic semen analysis should provide the information given in Box 21.3, as well as an analysis of the presence of antisperm antibodies. This can be done using either the mixed antiglobulin reaction test (MAR test) or, more usually now, the Immunobead test (see below).

Semen liquefaction and viscosity

Human semen forms a gel-like clot soon after ejaculation due to a fibrinogen-like substrate from the seminal vesicles. Liquefaction, which is necessary for microscopic examination, usually occurs within 30 minutes and depends on the liquefying enzyme, vesiculase, produced by the prostate gland. During this process the semen sample should be stored at 37°C and analysis performed as soon as possible after this. A complete absence of the coagulum indicates an obstruction of the ejaculatory duct or congenital absence of the seminal vesicles.

The relevance of increased viscosity is unclear. It may be associated with chronic infection in the accessory glands. Sperm from hyperviscid semen usually show no difficulty in entering cervical mucus at microscopy. Further, the viscosity of the ejaculate may vary considerably between different patients and also between samples from the same individual. If the specimen of semen is excessively viscid it should be repeatedly forced through a narrow-gauge hypodermic needle (no. 19) prior to microscopic examination.

A prolonged liquefaction time (more than 1–2 hours can be caused by a deficiency of vesiculase from reduced prostatic secretion. This situation, particularly if found in association with a negative postcoital test, may be a cause of infertility. Several methods can be used to liquefy the ejaculate prior to microscopic examination, for example the addition of bromelin 1 g/l, plasmin 0.35–0.50 casein units/ml or chymotrypsin 150 USP/ml.

Semen volume

The volume of the ejaculate should be measured either with a graduated cylinder or by aspirating the whole sample into a pipette. The average range is 2–5 ml. The commonest cause of low volume is spillage of the sample either at production or during transport. This should be excluded by questioning the patient and the test repeated.

A persistently low semen volume (<0.5 ml) may be due to an obstruction of the ejaculatory ducts or congenital absence of the seminal vesicles. In both cases, the low volumes are

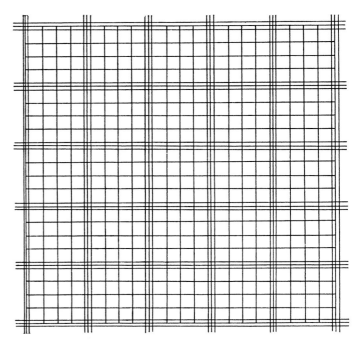

Fig. 21.3 Neubauer haemocytometer grid with 25 large squares each containing 16 small squares.

associated with reduced seminal plasma fructose levels. Absence of ejaculatory fluid, but with the sensation of orgasm, suggests retrograde ejaculation and such men will sometimes have noted a 'cloudy' urine after coitus. To confirm this diagnosis a urine sample is obtained as soon as possible after masturbation and centrifuged for 10 minutes at 3000 rpm. The residue is then resuspended in a small volume of buffer and examined for the presence of motile sperm.

An abnormally large semen volume (greater than 6 ml) may be associated with a reduced sperm concentration but this is not usually a problem. Alternatively, if the motility of the sperm is poor it may be a long time since the man's previous ejaculation: understandably, some couples believe that if the man abstains from ejaculation for a long period of time then at timed intercourse there will be so many sperm the woman is bound to conceive. Of course, what actually happens is that the sperm are too old and are largely dead or dying.

Semen pH

A drop of semen is spread over litmus paper and the colour change read from the scale on the litmus paper dispenser. If pH is <7.0, with azoospermia, there may be dysgenesis of the vas deferens, epididymis or seminal vesicles.

Sperm count and concentration

The haemocytometer (improved Neubauer) counting chamber is the method most frequently used to assess sperm concentration (Fig. 21.3). The ejaculate is diluted (usually 20-fold) with a spermicidal solution and both chambers are loaded with the sample. After counting, if there is a discrepancy of >10% between the two chambers the sample should be remixed and assessed again.

Other techniques for counting sperm include the Makler chamber (Makler 1980) or a similar device such as the Howell fertility counting chamber. These chambers have a depth of 10 mm and permit direct estimation of the sperm concentration without dilution. However, they are less accurate than the Neubauer chamber.

Oligozoospermia The WHO defines oligozoospermia as a sperm concentration <20 million per ml. However, the sperm count should not be taken in isolation. It is obvious that a high count of dead sperm is of little value whilst a low count of highly progressively motile sperm may result in normal fertility. Various motility parameters have been produced to allow for this (see section on motility below).

Azoospermia The diagnosis of azoospermia should be regarded with some suspicion if made in non-specialized laboratories. Further, it should only be made where two samples, separated by at least 4 weeks, have been spun and examined under oil emersion microscopy. The majority of cases are obstructive in origin, most commonly from infection or cystic fibrosis. All men with obstructive azoospermia should have their cystic fibrosis (CF) gene status determined as this is often positive. However, over 300 mutations are recognized in CF: most laboratories only test for the 15 or so commonest in their region. If the man tests positive then his partner must also be tested as if they are both carriers they have a 25% chance of having a child with the condition.

Non-obstructive causes include Sertoli cell only syndrome (SCOS) and maturation arrest. Absence of the germinal epithelium may be congenital or acquired, as in radio- or chemotherapy. Maturation arrest is diagnosed histologically and is usually at the round cell spermatid stage.

If azoospermia is confirmed, serum follicle-stimulating hormone (FSH) and testosterone should be estimated. A high serum FSH almost certainly confirms a non-obstructive aetiology for the absence of sperm. By contrast, azoospermia in the presence of testes of normal size and consistency and with a normal serum FSH level indicates that the lesion is likely to be obstructive. In a very low percentage of cases FSH levels are low (hypogonadotrophic hypogonadism). Here the outlook is optimistic and fertility can be restored in more than 50% of cases by the use of exogenous gonadotrophins, typically human chorionic gonadotrophin (Finkel et al 1985).

Azoospermia in association with eunuchoid features suggests Klinefelter's syndrome. This can be confirmed by chromosomal analysis. Other rare non-disjunctions and translocation abnormalities may also be associated with azoospermia or profound oligoasthenoteratozoospermia.

A testicular biopsy should be performed to determine whether normal sperm maturation is occurring. Open biopsy requires a general anaesthetic and postoperatively is extremely painful. It also disrupts the subcapsular arcade of blood vessels which supply the testicular substance. By contrast, fine needle or Trucut needle biopsy can easily be performed under local anaesthetic which is injected around the spermatic cord and into the skin over the biopsy site. Fine needle biopsy will provide significantly less sperm than the Trucut needle technique which, if sperm are present, usually provides sufficient for several straws to be frozen away for subsequent therapeutic use. Steele et al (2001) have followed up a series of men who have had the Trucut procedure performed. They have reported high acceptability, low complication rates and in the longer term no alteration in testicular Doppler flow patterns or antisperm antibody status. The success of testicular sperm in ICSI is now well established since the original report by Tournaye et al (1994). Alternatively, sperm may be obtained by fine needle aspiration from the epididymis or by open microscopic epididymal sperm aspiration (MESA). However, Steele et al (2000) demonstrated that sperm in the obstructed epididymis show a significantly increased degree of DNA damage and, therefore, the use of testicular sperm is recommended (Steele et al 2000).

Sperm morphology

In its simplest form, morphology is analysed by direct visualization of the sperm. To assess morphology properly semen should be smeared onto a slide, air dried and stained. A variety of stains exists. The Giemsa stain is better for leucocyte than sperm morphology. The Papanicolaou is the most commonly used and, in its modified form, gives good definition to the acrosomal and postacrosomal regions of the head, the midpiece and the tail. The Bryan–Leishman stain is useful for differentiating immature sperm cells from leucocytes. However, the Shorr stain is the simplest to perform and gives good overall definition of sperm morphology.

The WHO (1992) recommends that at least 100 and preferably 200 sperm are examined. Each one is assessed for normality of its head, neck and midpiece and tail and for the presence of cytoplasmic droplets of more than one-third the area of a normal sperm head. Using these strict criteria at least 30% of all sperm should be of normal morphology. Others have suggested even stricter definitions of normality showing that where <15% of sperm fail to meet their criteria, fertilization rates in assisted reproduction are significantly decreased (Kruger et al 1988).

Debilitating illnesses, including viral and bacterial infections, will produce an increase in the number of abnormal sperm, as will some drugs. The increase in abnormal sperm cells usually starts within 30 days of an acute illness and may be present for up to 2–3 months, even though the clinical condition of the patient has markedly improved. The presence of a large number of sperm containing cytoplasmic droplets may suggest incomplete maturation and thus epididymal pathology. Scanning and transmission electron microscopy may also be employed to identify specific structural abnormalities of the sperm but routine evaluation of the ultrastructure is neither practical nor necessary.

Sperm motility

Traditionally, motility has been expressed as the percentage of moving sperm in the sample. The accepted normal value is at least 60% at 1 hour. However, a more detailed analysis of the percentages showing each of the different degrees of forward progression is of more value. Using the scoring system in Box 21.4, a motility index can be calculated using the equation from Pandaya et al (1986):

Motility index = (% progressive × progression ratings × 2.5) + % non-progressive

Box 21.4   Sperm progression ratings

0	None = absence of forward progression
1	Poor = weak or sluggish forward progression
2	Moderate = definite forward progression
3	Good = good forward progression
4	Excellent = vigorous, rapid forward progression

Poor motility, particularly in the presence of normal sperm numbers, suggests that the sample may have become cold and a further specimen should be sought. Other causes of reduced motility include seminal infection and sperm autoantibodies. Sperm motility is totally dependent on mitochondrial function. Abnormalities of mitochondrial function have been reported in association with poor motility (O'Connell et al 2000). Most often, however, asthenozoospermia is merely one aspect of generally poor semen quality including reduced count and increased numbers of abnormal sperm.

If sperm motility is virtually non-existent the possibility of a severe intrinsic defect in sperm movement is raised, as occurs with Kartagener's syndrome. Alternatively, the sperm may all be dead. Therefore, tests for sperm vitality may be applied. These include the eosin Y (or eosin-nigrosin) test where sperm with physically intact membranes appear bluish-white, whilst dead sperm are coloured reddish-yellow. Alternatively, the H33258 fluorochrome test or the hypo-osmotic swelling tests may be used. A sample is considered abnormal if more than 50% of the sperm stain 'dead'. The hypo-osmotic swelling test has been shown to be reasonably predictive of semen fertilizing capacity. However, its correlation with the zona-free hamster egg penetration test (van der Ven et al 1986) has not been confirmed.

Sperm aggregation and agglutination
Aggregation refers specifically to the situation where sperm are clumped with other particulate debris or cells. Often, in normal samples there are small aggregates but large aggregates are abnormal. Agglutination refers to the sticking together of sperm by antibodies. The pattern should be recorded: head to head, midpiece to midpiece, tail to tail or tail tip to tail tip. Sometimes the patterns are mixed. Agglutination, whilst indicating the presence of antisperm antibodies, is not confirmatory for antibodies and further tests are required (Fig. 21.4).

Antisperm antibodies
Sperm antibodies are typically IgA or IgG in type. Depending on the individual laboratory's set-up, these tests may be reserved for samples exhibiting marked agglutination or for those couples with an abnormal cervical mucus-sperm interaction. Alternatively, some laboratories offer these tests on all semen samples. The two most commonly used tests are the Immunobead and the MAR test (Fig. 21.5). However, results from these two tests do not always agree (Hellstrom et al 1989). Immunobeads are polyacrylamide spheres with covalently bound rabbit antihuman immunoglobulins directed against IgG, IgA and IgM. Sperm are washed, resuspended and mixed with the beads. If the sperm has antibodies on its membrane, the Immunobeads will bind to it. If more than 20% of sperm show binding the test is positive, although

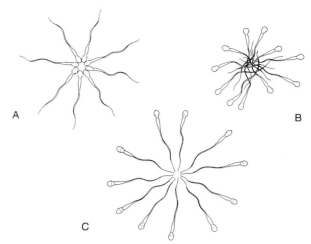

Fig. 21.4   Human sperm agglutination patterns: **a** head to head; **b** tail to tail; **c** tail tip to tail tip.

usually 50% of sperm should show binding before the test is thought clinically significant as only at this level of binding is cervical mucus penetration impeded (Ayvaliotis et al 1985). Immunobead binding to the tail tip is irrelevant.

The MAR test can be performed by mixing washed sperm with either sheep red blood cells or with latex particles coated with human IgG. Antihuman IgG antiserum is then added. If the particles, or red blood cells, agglutinate with more than 50% of the sperm, IgG antisperm antibodies are said to be present in clinically significant amounts. The major disadvantages of this test are that it requires a ready supply of sensitized sheep erythrocytes and it is only sensitive to the IgG class of antibody. The Immunobead test has the additional advantage of being able to detect the presence of antisperm antibodies in serum or in cervical mucus if used as an indirect test.

Further tests of sperm function

If the routine semen analysis is normal it is not usually necessary to proceed with any further investigation of sperm function. However, if it is not, then some of the additional tests listed in this section may be of use.

Semen culture
Pyospermia is not necessarily an indicator of infection of the accessory glands. However, it has been associated with significant adverse effects on seminal parameters (Wolff et al 1990). Furthermore, infection of the accessory glands is often asymptomatic. In the prostate, infection may cause enlargement which, in turn, may produce an obstructive oligo- or azoospermia. In these cases the semen volume will be slightly lowered and the zinc content will be significantly decreased. Infection of the seminal vesicles results in a substantial reduction in ejaculate volume and a low seminal fructose concentration. Therefore, both fructose and zinc content may be measured. If culture of semen is indicated, the sample should be collected aseptically after the patient has urinated and washed both hands and penis in soap and water.

A

RBC coated with anti D

RBC coated with anti D
and IgG oTr IgA

Mixed agglutinate of
RBC and spermatozoa

Sperm coated with antisperm
antibodies

B

a

b

c

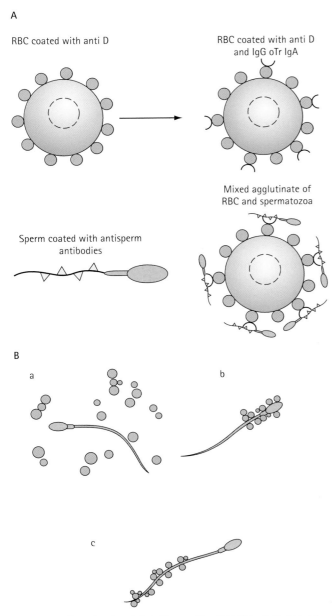

Fig 21.5   a The mixed antiglobulin reaction (MAR) test. Red blood cells (RBC), coated with IgA or sensitized with IgG, are mixed with a non-specific anti-IgA or an anti-IgG and then incubated with sperm under test. Sperm with antisperm antibodies will adhere to the red blood cells. b The Immunobead test: a negative test; b and c positive tests showing beads attached to sperm head and tail, respectively.

Chlamydia cannot be cultured from semen as it is toxic to the cell line used to culture this organism. Thus, urethral swabs should be used. Where epididymitis is suspected, L-carnitine has been used as a specific marker of epididymal function. However, this has been replaced by the measurement of the neutral isoform of α-glucosidase.

Tests of fertilization potential
With the introduction of in vitro fertilization techniques for the treatment of infertility, it has become obvious that sperm

from some infertile couples may not have the ability to fertilize oocytes. Although several tests have been developed to investigate this further they are rarely used in clinical practice now as intracytoplasmic injection bypasses any clinical problems with fertilization and the sensitivity and specificity of the tests are so poor. For fertilization to occur, the sperm first undergoes capacitation. This process results from a variety of influences including the release of the sperm from the inhibition of the seminal plasma and exposure to the various endocrine and anatomical environments of the female reproductive tract. Once capacitated, the sperm is seen in a state of hyperactivation; that is, its movement becomes highly vigorous but non-progressive. This hyperactivation appears to be necessary for both penetration of the cumulus cells and the acrosome reaction. Previously it was thought that the acrosome reaction was essential for penetration of the cumulus. It would now appear that it occurs only once the sperm has come into contact with the zona pellucida. Having passed through the zona, the sperm then fuses with the oolemma, is absorbed into the oocyte and fertilization occurs.

The zona-free hamster egg penetration test is a measure of the absorption of the sperm into the oocyte. It depends on the fact that the hamster egg is not species specific for sperm. However, as the zona has been removed, the acrosome reaction must occur spontaneously. This is aided by washing and incubating the sperm. It is a major drawback of the test that the acrosome reaction is left to chance. Aitken et al (1991) have described a method for inducing the acrosome reaction with the divalent cation ionophore A23187 which has improved the sensitivity of the test.

As the major weakness of the above test is the absence of an effective zona, tests have been developed to assess the zona-sperm interaction. Oocytes are obtained from IVF programmes or from ovaries at oophorectomy. They are then either frozen or stored in high salt solutions. In order to have an effective control, either the zona is split and one half exposed to test and the other to control sperm, or the test and control samples are labelled with different fluorochromes and the ratios of the two sperm populations in the zona counted. In this way an assessment of the ability of the sperm to penetrate the zona can be obtained. This test has the advantage that the acrosome reaction occurs naturally.

FEMALE FACTORS

Ovulation detection

Symptoms and signs
Ovulation pain (mittelschmerz) and midcycle staining occur regularly in some women. Observation of midcycle mucus is the best clinical marker of ovulation and is useful in the timing of procedures such as donor insemination, although anovulatory oestrogen-dominant states, such as polycystic ovarian syndrome, may produce an apparently ovulatory mucus. Therefore, none of these symptoms or signs should be considered proof of ovulation.

Basal body temperature recording
This technique has been used for ovulation detection in infertility and natural family planning. It has also been used to

diagnose luteal phase deficiency. The test depends on the midcycle rise of 0.5–1.0°C, due to the thermogenic effect of progesterone, and is best detected, using a fertility thermometer, first thing in the morning. The oral route is most popular although vaginal or rectal readings approximate better to core temperature. A comparison of this technique with endocrine markers of ovulation has shown a poor correlation (Paulson et al 1986). In addition, it can be confusing and undoubtedly introduces another layer of stress and inconvenience for the couple. However, from a practical point of view, it may be of some value for timing luteal-phase progesterone estimation or as an adjunct to monitoring the response to clomiphene in anovulatory women.

Hormone assays

In women with regular periods the simplest and most reliable method of confirming ovulation is to measure the midluteal-phase serum progesterone level. Those patients with oligomenorrhoea or amenorrhoea may have their progesterone measured weekly from day 21 of the cycle until menstruation. Where the progesterone is anovulatory the serum FSH, both as a ratio with LH for polycystic ovaries and alone for premature menopause and hypothalamic hypogonadism, should be determined as well as serum prolactin for hyperprolactinaemia and TSH and possibly thyroxine for thyroid dysfunction. Serum progesterone should be measured in at least two cycles to confirm the regularity of ovulation. The minimum level of serum progesterone taken to indicate ovulation (within 95% confidence limits) is 30 nmol/l (Hull et al 1982).

Detection of the preovulatory surge of LH may also be used to predict ovulation. The LH peak occurs between 8 and 20 hours before ovulation. Whilst levels are usually elevated for 24 hours, they may be detectable for only 12 hours. Therefore, accurate detection requires twice-daily blood or urine sampling. There are now several commercially available kits allowing women to undertake this test at home but they are inconvenient and expensive and, as with basal body temperature charts, they focus the couple's attention onto their infertility and away from their marriage and relationship.

Ovarian ultrasonography

Ultrasonographic visualization of developing follicles is useful in tracking follicle development in ovulation induction. However, it is also of use in detecting the luteinized, unruptured follicle syndrome (Daly et al 1985). In this condition the follicular diameter increases but the typical rupture of the follicle does not occur, even though serum progesterone levels rise into the ovulatory range. The significance of this is questionable, though, and in the UK follicular tracking is no longer commonly performed.

Endometrial biopsy

Using the criteria of Noyes et al (1950), the luteal-phase endometrium can be dated histologically. Biopsies are obtained from high in the uterus, as an outpatient procedure using a disposable curette (Thompson 1995). This method is probably best for assessing inadequate luteal function. However, the Noyes criteria for endometrial dating were determined using cycle length and basal body temperature charts for cycle

timing. When the LH peak was used as a reference point, the method was shown to be imprecise (Tredway et al 1973). Further, there is considerable interobserver variation in the interpretation of the histology results. Whilst this is still popular in parts of the USA it has largely been abandoned in the UK.

Tubal, uterine and pelvic factors

Hysterosalpingography was the traditional way to assess the uterine cavity, tubal structure and tubal patency. No anaesthetic is required and the procedure is simple. However, it has now been largely superseded by hysteroscopy and laparoscopy. Salpingoscopy and falloposcopy to assess internal tubal architecture were developed in the 1980s and 1990s but have not really been absorbed into routine clinical practice.

Hysterosalpingography (HSG)

In this investigation a cannula is inserted into the cervical canal. A radio-opaque dye is then injected through the uterine cavity into the fallopian tubes and out into the peritoneal cavity under fluoroscopic control. The procedure can be painful, though this is minimized if the dye is injected slowly and under low pressure. Tubal spasm may occur and is often misinterpreted as uni- or bilateral cornual blockage. An intravenous glucagon injection can help relax this spasm. With HSG there is also a risk of reactivation of previous salpingitis and, if tubal disease is discovered, the patient should receive prophylactic antibiotics after the procedure.

In terms of the information given, an HSG is a very limited investigation: correlation with hysteroscopy in the identification of uterine cavity pathology is poor (Golan et al 1996, Wang et al 1996). Further, whilst HSG will identify if the tubes are patent it does not identify the presence of peritubal adhesions. Clearly, these may significantly compromise tubal function despite patency of the tube. Therefore, HSG should be considered a test for hydrosalpinx, not tubal patency. Under one other circumstance HSG may be useful: in the presence of severe tubal disease where salpingitis isthmica nodosa (SIN) is suspected, hysterosalpingography is the only readily accessible method of diagnosis (Fig. 21.6). This condition cannot be diagnosed by visualization of the exterior aspects of the tubes.

Laparoscopy

Over the last 10 years, there has been an explosion in gynaecological endoscopic surgery but the role of diagnostic laparoscopy in the assessment of the infertile couple has been challenged. Some say that if the tubes are damaged or there is severe endometriosis, or indeed if there is no abnormality, then the couple will proceed to assisted reproduction. Therefore, what is the indication for performing a potentially life-threatening procedure? On the other hand, some argue that treatment of peritubal adhesions and even minimal endometriosis significantly increases the chances of spontaneous pregnancy and, therefore, laparoscopy should be performed on all couples. Some would even argue that laparoscopy should be performed even where a clearly identifiable cause for the infertility has already been found, such as a profound

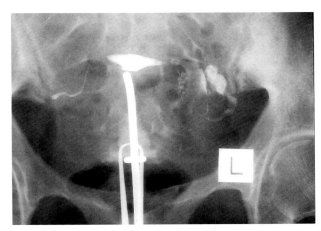

Fig. 21.6 Hysterosalpingogram showing no flow from the distal end of the right tube, a left hydrosalpinx and salpingitis isthmica nodosa (SIN), with its typical cottonwool appearance, around the isthmic portion of the left tube.

malefactor or anovulation.

If a laparoscopy is to be performed it is important to emphasize that a thorough examination of the pelvic organs cannot be performed unless a double-puncture technique is employed. This permits the introduction of a probe or grasper to manipulate the fallopian tubes and ovaries and to determine the presence of adhesions or endometriosis. A third or even fourth puncture site can be used for the introduction of scissors to divide adhesions and for diathermy or laser tools, graspers and suction/irrigation apparatus. Thus a diagnostic procedure can be readily converted to an operative one.

At the end of the laparoscopic examination, a detailed description of all the findings (including negative ones) should be made with the aid of simple diagrams (Fig. 21.7). The presence of a lead follicle or of a corpus luteum should also be recorded as useful information about ovulation. Accurate records ensure that others gain an accurate impression of the problems that may be present and of the prognosis for fertility. Some units now routinely provide their patients with a video-recording of their surgery. Whilst this is expensive it is particularly useful for any surgeon who is subsequently considering surgery.

Over the last decade laparoscopic equipment has been refined to such an extent that, particularly in the USA, office laparoscopy is performed under light sedation and local anaesthetic. It is the author's experience, though, that manipulation of the pelvic organs is more difficult, the degree of abdominal distension is not so great and, therefore, the view is at least partially compromised. More recently, transvaginal hydrolaparoscopy has been reported with apparently good diagnostic views of the pelvic organs (Campo et al 1999).

Hysteroscopy

Although hysteroscopy can be easily performed as an outpatient procedure, it is sensible to perform it, in infertile women, at the same time as laparoscopy. Whilst liquid can be used to distend the uterine cavity, carbon dioxide is the preferred medium. However, it is essential that the insufflators for the abdominal and uterine cavities are not confused: the former delivers gas at 10 times the rate of the latter and deaths have been reported from insufflation with the wrong machine. Uterine malformations, endometrial polyps, intrauterine adhesions, fibroids and other conditions can be detected and these conditions are now relatively easily treated by operative hysteroscopy.

Salpingoscopy and falloposcopy

These techniques have been introduced and reported on extensively over the last 15 years (de Bruyne et al 2000, Kerin et al 1990). However, they have not gained widespread popularity. Those in support argue that where external tubal disease is identified at laparoscopy it is important to assess the state of the lining of the tube if the patient is to be advised whether tubal surgery or in vitro fertilization would be of greater benefit. Those against argue that the additional cost and time involved are of little practical advantage in the management of the couple.

Salpingoscopy is the passage of a very fine rigid endoscope through the fimbriated end of the tube. Whilst it is performed at laparoscopy, it only allows direct visualization of the tubal lining to the isthmoampullary junction (Fig. 21.8). Falloposcopy is a more complicated and much more expensive procedure, involving the passage of an extremely fine flexible fibreoptic device from the uterine cavity distally to the fimbriae (Kerin et al 1990). In order to pass the device, a balloon surrounding the endoscope is inflated along the tube and the scope advanced, bit by bit, to minimize tubal damage. The tube is then assessed as the scope is withdrawn (Fig. 21.9). Neither of these procedures is ideal but both provide a much more detailed assessment of tubal status than was previously available.

Contrast hystero–ultrasonography

This new technique of examination of the uterus and tubal patency is being evaluated. The injection of a small amount of fluid within the uterine cavity at the time of ultrasound aids definition and the technique may prove valuable.

Cervical factor

Around the time of ovulation, cervical mucus becomes both watery and stretchy. This is due to the predominance of oestrogen and the lack of progesterone. The stretchiness of the mucus, known as *spinnbarkeit*, can be determined either whilst removing mucus from the cervix or by using two glass slides to pull the sample apart: at ovulation it should stretch at least 8 cm. Ovulatory mucus can be further identified by microscopic examination of a dried sample to identify the characteristic ferning pattern. If satisfactory mucus is not seen, previous cervical surgery and chlamydial infection should be excluded. Oral oestrogen may be given to improve cervical mucus quality. If the mucus fails to improve, intrauterine insemination of washed sperm may be of therapeutic value.

The role of the cervical mucus tests has decreased significantly in importance in recent years. First, reliable direct and indirect tests are now readily available for antisperm antibodies. Second, the replicability and interobserver variation of the tests suggests that they are not reliable. Third, and most

R.B.U. LAPAROSCOPY REPORT

UR

Surname

Given Names

Date of Birth   Age   Religion   Sex   Marital Status

Medical Officer

Date   Surgeon   Assistant

Anaesthetist   Theatre   Scrub Nurse

Procedure

Findings

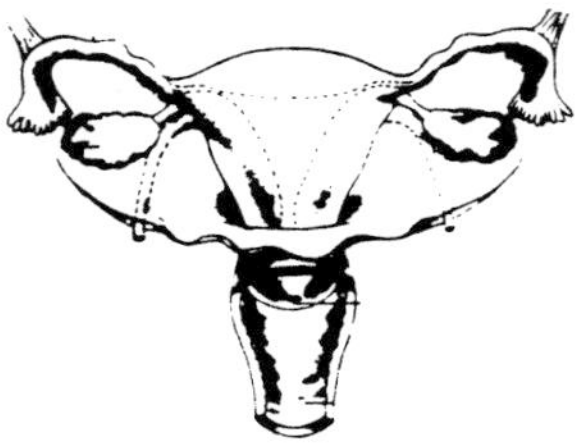

Left Tube

Normal / Abnormal

Right Tube

Normal / Abnormal

For anastomosis demonstrate tubal segments and lengths on diagram.

Left Ovary

Normal / Abnormal   GRAF. FOL. /CORP. LUT. /PCOS

Right Ovary

Normal / Abnormal   GRAF. FOL. /CORP. LUT. /PCOS

Uterus

Normal / Abnormal

Anterior Pouch

Normal / Abnormal

Pouch of Douglas

Normal / Abnormal

Upper Abdomen / Appendix

Normal / Abnormal

Other Findings

Summary

Management

Doctor's Signature

Fig. 21.7 An example of a standard laparoscopy report form.

practically, if the test is normal in the absence of any other abnormality the couple will proceed either to ovulation induction and intrauterine insemination (hMG/IUI) or IVF. If the test is abnormal, whether any other abnormality is present or not, the couple will also proceed to hMG/IUI or IVF. Therefore, what is the reason for performing the test?

The postcoital test

After ejaculation, sperm pass very quickly into the cervical mucus, escaping the seminal plasma. However, if antisperm antibodies are present in the mucus the sperm may be killed. The most common test of the sperm–mucus interaction is the postcoital test (PCT). This test can only be performed at the time of ovulation when the mucus is showing spinnbarkeit and therefore is penetrable to sperm. Perversely, in patients with anovulation due to polycystic ovarian syndrome where oestrogen is always dominant, it can be performed at virtually any time. If there is difficulty in pinpointing the correct time, it is important to be certain that ovulation is occurring. Alternatively, the test may be performed on alternate days near

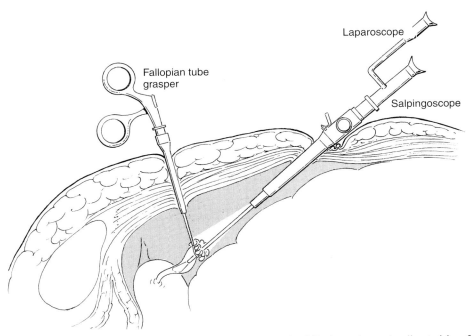

Fig. 21.8 Salpingoscopy: the salpingoscope is guided into the fallopian tube, under direct vision, from the operating channel of the laparoscope.

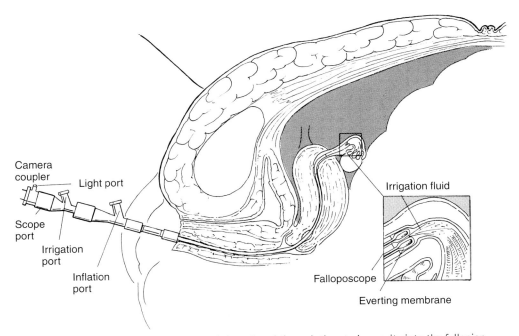

Fig. 21.9 Falloposcopy: the falloposcope is introduced through the uterine cavity into the fallopian tube. The tube is flushed, lubricated and distended by the irrigation fluid. The flexible fibreoptic scope is introduced along the tube, using the inflated membrane to protect and open the tube in advance of the scope.

midcycle until adequate cervical mucus is observed. Some units use home test kits to identify the LH surge to time the PCT. There are no firm rules about a period of abstinence prior to the test though a period of 2 or 3 days is usually recommended. There has also been disagreement about the optimum timing of the PCT in relation to coitus: intervals of 2–24 hours have been reported. A 2-hour interval usually means having intercourse in the early morning which can, through 'pressure to perform', lead to temporary impotence. A more reliable approach is to perform the test 8–12 hours after coitus so that intercourse can take place the previous evening.

Mucus is collected from the cervix using either a tuberculin syringe or a fine plastic tube (Rocket, UK) and its amount, viscosity and cellularity recorded. The mucus is then placed on a slide, a coverslip applied and high-power microscopic examination performed. The test is best scored on the presence or absence of progressively motile sperm. This correlates reasonably with the final outcome in terms of pregnancy rates (Hull et al 1982). The actual number of progressively motile sperm per high-power field which constitutes a normal test is, however, unclear. Usually 5 is taken as the lower limit of normality. However, Collins et al (1984) found no difference in pregnancy rates between groups with no sperm, no motile sperm, 1–5, 6–10 or >10 motile sperm per high-power field. In a study of couples with normal fertility, 20% had 0 or 1 sperm per high-power field (Kovacs et al 1978). By contrast, Hull et al (1982) found significantly higher pregnancy rates in those couples with progressively motile sperm compared with those with no motile sperm. Hull & Evers (1998) also reported that the PCT is useful in identifying those couples with otherwise unexplained infertility who will go on to conceive a pregnancy spontaneously.

If sperm are not present in repeated PCTs despite a normal semen analysis, a coital problem should be suspected. Gross asthenozoospermia, profound oligozoospermia or aspermia may also result in a negative test. The presence of sperm which are immotile or which exhibit the 'shaking phenomenon' (non-progressive motility) suggests the presence of antisperm antibodies. In a few instances non-progressive motility may simply be due to thick, sticky cervical mucus, despite proper timing of the test. A negative test in the presence of poor cervical mucus should be repeated in a subsequent cycle.

In vitro mucus penetration tests

If the PCT is repeatedly negative despite good cervical mucus and sperm counts, an in vitro mucus penetration test should be performed. This permits a more detailed assessment of sperm–mucus interaction and allows crossover tests with donor sperm and donor mucus to be undertaken. The two commonly used techniques are the sperm penetration test (SPT) and the sperm–cervical mucus contact test (SCMCT). The former is usually performed on a microscope slide although tube methods have also been reported. A drop of semen is placed adjacent to an equivalent amount of preovulatory mucus and a coverslip applied to form an interface (Fig. 21.10a). The donor mucus may be obtained, for example, from another patient attending the clinic or from a patient attending for artificial insemination. Bovine mucus and synthetic gels are both commercially available as alternatives, but the results are unsatisfactory. Penetration of the mucus by sperm is assessed by microscopic examination over the course of the next hour. A negative test is indicated by complete failure of penetration or immobilization of those sperm which have penetrated. The shaking phenomenon (see below) may also be observed. This test is simple to perform but is less specific for the presence of sperm antibodies than the SCMCT, since non-immunological factors may lead to a negative test.

The SCMCT, devised by Kremer & Jager (1976), is reported to correlate well with the presence of antisperm antibodies in either semen or cervical mucus. It can therefore be used as the primary diagnostic method for local immunological factors if more complex antibody tests are not available. The test is performed by mixing a drop of cervical mucus with a similar

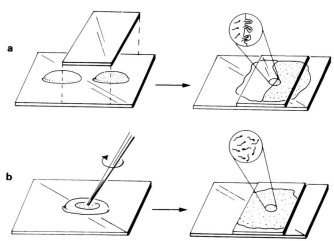

Fig. 21.10 a The sperm penetration test. Here an interface is produced between the sperm and the cervical mucus. b The sperm–cervical mucus contact test (SCMCT), where there is mixing of the components.

volume of semen at one end of a microscope slide and placing a drop of semen at the other end. Both drops are covered with a coverslip. After 30 minutes the drops are observed (Fig. 21.10b). If more than 25% of sperm are exhibiting jerking or shaking movements rather than forward motility in the sample mixed with mucus but not in the pure sample, the presence of antibodies is presumed. In strongly positive tests the proportion of such sperm equates to the antibody titre. Crossover testing with donor sperm and donor mucus permits an accurate assessment of whether antibodies are present in the semen or the mucus.

UNEXPLAINED INFERTILITY

If the basic investigations are normal yet there is a persistent failure to conceive, couples are said to have unexplained (idiopathic) infertility. This poorly defined entity is usually reported in 10–20% of cases although a range of 6–60% has been cited (Templeton & Penney 1982). It has been clearly demonstrated that the chance of conception in such couples is most closely related to the duration of their infertility, the age of the female partner and whether the infertility is primary or secondary (Hull et al 1985, Lenton et al 1977). These authors all agree that an eventual pregnancy rate of 60–70% will be achieved after 3 years of follow-up with no specific treatment. In view of this, counselling is an appropriate basis of management. However, this is incredibly frustrating for the couple who usually want action.

Despite the presence of these solid epidemiological data, in some clinics couples with unexplained infertility may undergo a range of more detailed investigations in an effort to find a cause for their failure to conceive. There is no evidence that this approach is superior to waiting for spontaneous conception to occur (Haxton et al 1987). Furthermore, if treatment is undertaken on the basis of results of these tests its apparent success may be wrongfully attributed to the therapy, rather than to natural conception.

CONCLUSION

Infertility is a distressing problem for the couple. Often they are entering their 30s by the time they present for investigation, both may have demanding jobs and both are certainly aware that the biological clock is ticking away. Therefore, the pressure is to investigate quickly and efficiently and offer a simple therapy which will guarantee pregnancy. Of course, this is not possible. Couples find it hard to accept that in any 4 weeks of a normal menstrual cycle, there are only 2 or 3 days, at most, when the woman can conceive. Therefore, as clinicians it is our duty not only to ensure maximum efficiency in investigation but also targeted, appropriate therapies. However, options only should be presented to the couple: they must decide, within the options you offer, which is for them. Not everyone wants to have every investigation and proceed to IVF immediately. Further, management must take place against the background of what is available and feasible in your unit and the confines of funding for health in your community.

KEY POINTS

1. It is more important to perform the relevant investigations in a logical order at the correct time than to perform a battery of tests blindly.
2. Investigations should be performed only if there is at least a 1-year history of infertility, as the chances of pregnancy occurring for a given couple having regular unprotected intercourse are 80% after 1 year and 90% after 18 months.
3. The simplest, least invasive and most productive investigations should be performed first.
4. Irregular cycles are suggestive of ovulatory dysfunction; polycystic ovaries are the commonest pathology found.
5. Men with an obstructive cause for azoospermia now have a relatively good prognosis with the advent of intracytoplasmic sperm injection (ICSI). The success rates are similar to those obtained with severe oligospermia using standard in vitro fertilization procedures.
6. Hypogonadotrophic hypogonadism is manifested by a low FSH and low testosterone level and is amenable to treatment with gonadotrophins.
7. At least two semen analyses should be carried out, because of known variability within an individual, before consistency of abnormality can be determined.
8. Midluteal progesterone is the simplest and most reliable method of ovulation assessment (progesterone measurements in excess of 30 nmol/l confirming ovulation).
9. Laparoscopy is the most useful method of assessment of the patency of fallopian tubes and gives other information concerning pathology/normality of the pelvis. It is essential to use a double-puncture technique for adequate inspection of the pelvis, with careful inspection of all areas, especially the ovarian fossae.
10. A hysterosalpingogram is indicated if salpingitis isthmica nodosa is suspected, but it may be superseded by salpingoscopy and falloposcopy in the future.

KEY POINTS (CONTINUED)

11. A negative postcoital test may be due to poor semen quality, coital difficulty, failure to produce adequate cervical mucus or immunological factors in either partner, but is most often due to inappropriate timing. LH monitoring kits may overcome this problem.
12. Of couples with unexplained infertility, 60–70% will conceive within 3 years without any intervention. Beyond that time a number of empirical treatments have been shown to be beneficial.

REFERENCES

Aitken RJ, Sutton M, Warner P, Richardson DW 1985 The relationship between the movement characteristics of human spermatozoa and their ability to penetrate cervical mucus and zona-free oocytes. Journal of Reproduction and Fertility 73:411–449

Aitken RJ, Irvine DS, Wu FSW 1991 Prospective analysis of sperm oocyte fusion and reactive oxygen species generation as criteria for the diagnosis of infertility. American Journal of Obstetrics and Gynecology 164:542

Ayvaliotis B, Bronson R, Rosenfeld D, Cooper G 1985 Conception rates in couples where autoimmunity to sperm is detected. Fertility and Sterility 43:739–742

Boyers SP, Davis RO, Katz DF 1989 Automated semen analysis. Current Problems in Obstetrics, Gynaecology and Fertility XII:173–200

Campo R, Gordts S, Rombauts L, Brosens I 1999 Diagnostic accuracy of transvaginal hydrolaparoscopy in infertility. Fertility and Sterility 71:1157–1160

Collins JA, So Y, Wilson EH, Wrixon W, Casper RF 1984 The post coital test as a predictor of pregnancy among 355 infertile couples. Fertility and Sterility 41:703

Cooke ID, Sulaiman RA, Lenton EA, Parsons RJ 1981 Fertility and infertility statistics: their importance and application. Clinics in Obstetrics and Gynaecology 8:3

Daly DC, Soto-Albors C, Walters C, Ying Y, Riddick DH 1985 Ultrasonic evidence of luteinised unruptured follicle syndrome in unexplained infertility. Fertility and Sterility 43:62–67

Davis RO, Katz DF 1992 Standardisation and comparability of CASA instruments. Journal of Andrology 13:81–86

de Bruyne F, Balan P, Hucke J 2000 Indications and possibilities of tubal endoscopy: salpingoscopy and falloscopy. Gynakologe 33:303–308

Finkel DM, Phillips JL, Snider PJ 1985 Stimulation of spermatogenesis by gonadotrophins in men with hypogonadotrophic hypogonadism. New England Journal of Medicine 313:651

Golan A, Eilat E, Ron-El R, Herman A, Soffer Y, Bukovsky I 1996 Hysteroscopy is superior to hysterosalpingography in infertility investigations. Acta Obstetrica et Gynaecologica Scandinavica 75:654–656

Haxton MJ, Fleming R, Hamilton MPR, Yates RW, Black WP, Coutts JRT 1987 Unexplained infertility – results of secondary investigations in 95 couples. British Journal of Obstetrics and Gynaecology 94:539–542

Hellstrom WJG, Samuels SJ, Waits AB, Overstreet JW 1989 A comparison of the usefulness of the sperm-MAR and immunobead tests for the detection of antisperm antibodies. Fertility and Sterility 36:219–221

Hull MGR, Evers JLH 1998 Postcoital testing: criterion for positive test was not given. British Medical Journal 317:1007

Hull MGR, Savage PE, Bromham DR 1982 Prognostic value of the postcoital test: prospective test based on time specific conception rates. Fertility and Sterility 38:384

Hull MGR, Glazener CMA, Kelly NJ 1985 Population study of causes, treatment and outcome of infertility. British Medical Journal 291:1693–1697

Kerin J, Daykhovsky L, Segalowitz J et al 1990 Falloposcopy: a microendoscopic technique for visual exploration of the human fallopian tube from the uterotubal ostium to the fimbria using a transvaginal approach. Fertility and Sterility 54:390–400

Kovacs GT, Newman GB, Henson GL 1978 The postcoital test: what is normal? British Medical Journal 1:818

Kremer J, Jager S 1976 The sperm-cervical mucus contact test: a preliminary report. Fertility and Sterility 27:335–340

Kruger TF, Acosta AA, Simmons KF, Swanson RJ, Matta JF, Oehninger S 1988 Predictive value of abnormal sperm morphology in in vitro fertilization. Fertility and Sterility 48:112–117

Lenton EA, Weston GA, Coke ID 1977 Long term follow-up of the apparently normal couple with a complaint of infertility. Fertility and Sterility 28:913–919

Makler A 1980 The improved 10-micrometer chamber for rapid sperm count and motility evaluation. Fertility and Sterility 33:337–338

Mortimer D, Pandaya IJ, Sawers RS 1986 Relation between human sperm motility characteristics and sperm penetration into cervical mucus in vitro. Journal of Reproduction and Fertility 78:93

Noyes RW, Hertig AT, Rock J 1950 Dating the endometrial biopsy. Fertility and Sterility 1:3

O'Connell M, St John JC, McClure N, Lewis SEM 2000 A comparison of mitochondrial DNA deletions in proximal epididymal and testicular spermatozoa in males with obstructive azoospermia. Human Reproduction 15:114–115

Pandaya IJ, Mortimer D, Sawers RS 1986 A standardized approach for evaluating the penetration of human spermatozoa into cervical mucus in vitro. Fertility and Sterility 45:357

Paulson JD, Negro-Vilar A, Lucena E, Martini L 1986 The prediction and detection of ovulation in artificial insemination. In: Heasley RN, Thompson W 1986 Andrology, Male fertility and sterility. Academic Press, Florida

Steele EK, Kelly JD, Lewis SEM, McNally JA, Sloan JM, McClure N 2000 Testicular sperm extraction by Trucut needle and milking of seminiferous tubules: a technique with high yield and patient acceptability. Fertility and Sterility 74:380–383

Steele EK, Ellis PK, Lewis SEM, McClure N 2001 Ultrasound, antisperm antibody and hormone profiles after testicular Trucut biopsy. Fertility and Sterility 75(2):423–428

Templeton AA, Penney GC 1982 The incidence, characteristics and prognosis of patients whose infertility is unexplained. Fertility and Sterility 37:175–181

Thompson W 1995 Endometrial sampling. The Diplomate (Journal of the Diplomates of the Royal College of Obstetricians and Gynaecologists, London) 1(4):276–279

Tournaye H, Devroey P, Liu J, Nagy Z, Lissens W, van Steirteghem A 1994 Microsurgical epididymal sperm aspiration and intracytoplasmic sperm injection: a new effective approach to infertility as a result of congenital bilateral absence of the vas deferens. Fertility and Sterility 61:1045–1051

Tredway DR, Misschell DR Jr, Moyer D 1973 Correlation of endometrial dating with luteinizing hormone peak. American Journal of Obstetrics and Gynecology 117:1030–1033

van der Ven HH, Jeyendran RS, Al-Hasani S et al 1986 Correlation between human sperm swelling in hypoosmotic medium (hypoosmotic swelling test) and in vitro fertilization. Journal of Andrology 7:190–196

Wang CW, Lee CL, Lai YM, Tsai CC, Chang MY, Soong YK 1996 Comparison of hysterosalpingography and hysteroscopy in female infertility. Journal of the American Association of Gynecologic Laparoscopists 10:295–302

Wolff H, Politch JA, Martinez A, Haimovici F, Hill JA, Anderson DJ 1990 Leukocytospermia is associated with poor semen quality. Fertility and Sterility 53:528–536

World Health Organization 1992 WHO laboratory manual for the examination of human semen and sperm–cervical mucus interaction, 3rd edn. Cambridge University Press, Cambridge

World Health Organization 1999 WHO manual for the standardized investigation, diagnosis and management of the infertile male. Cambridge University Press, Cambridge

22
Disorders of male reproduction

Richard A. Anderson   Stewart Irvine

INTRODUCTION

There has been rapid progress during the past 20 years in our understanding of male reproductive physiology, with wide-ranging contributions from cell and molecular biologists, urologists and endocrinologists, whose efforts have contributed to establishing the discipline of andrology. Some of these advances are beginning to be translated into clinical practice, so that the management of male reproductive disorders can now be based on rational scientific principles and clinical evidence. Men with reproductive disorders often present to the gynaecologist and family practitioner through the intermediary of their female partners. It is therefore important for both the community doctors and hospital specialists to have a degree of awareness, in order to recognize potential problems, as well as an understanding of the newer diagnostic techniques and treatment options which are becoming increasingly available for male reproductive dysfunction.

This chapter aims to provide the practising gynaecologist with an overview of clinical andrology with an emphasis on male infertility. A description of normal physiology is given as the foundation for explaining pathophysiological mechanisms and as a basis for formulating rational treatment where possible.

Physiology

The testis can be thought of as having two major interconnected functions in the adult: the production of testosterone, which maintains a wide range of physiological processes, and the production of spermatozoa and thereby fertility.

Spermatogenesis
Spermatogenesis takes place in several hundred tightly coiled seminiferous tubules arranged in lobules (Fig. 22.1; Dym

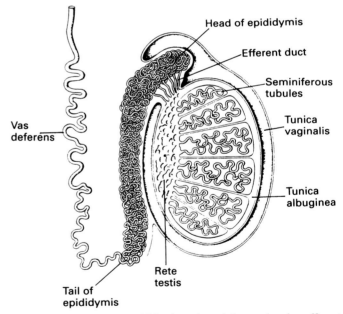

Fig. 22.1 Human testis, epididymis and vas deferens showing efferent ducts leading from the rete testis to the caput epididymis and the cauda epididymis, continuing to become the vas deferens. Reproduced with permission from Dym (1977).

1977) and which constitute some 80% of testicular volume in man. Each tubule resembles a loop draining at both ends into a network of tubules, the rete testis, and thence into the epididymis, a single but highly coiled tube which in turn drains into the unconvoluted and muscular-walled vas deferens.

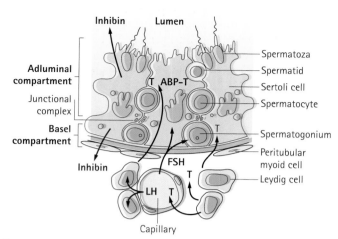

Fig. 22.2 Diagrammatic representation of the anatomical and functional relationship between germ cells, Sertoli cells and Leydig cells. Note the division of the seminiferous epithelium into adluminal and basal compartments by the tight junctions between adjacent Sertoli cells and the bidirectional secretion of Sertoli cell products (e.g. inhibin) into the lumen and interstitial space. ABP-T, androgen-binding protein testosterone; FSH, follicle-stimulating hormone; LH, luteinizing hormone.

The walls of the seminiferous tubules are composed of germ cells and Sertoli cells around a central lumen and surrounded by peritubular myoid cells and a basement membrane (Fig. 22.2). Spermatogenesis is a continuous sequence of closely regulated events, highly organized in space and time, whereby cohorts of undifferentiated diploid germ cells (spermatogonia) multiply and are then transformed into haploid spermatozoa. The following events, occurring within a precise sequence and duration, can be observed in the seminiferous epithelium during normal spermatogenesis.

1. Mitotic division (at least four) of stem cells to form cohorts of spermatogonia which, at intervals of 16 days, differentiate into primary preleptotene spermatocytes to initiate meiosis.
2. Meiotic reduction divisions of spermatocytes to form round spermatids.
3. Continuous remodelling of Sertoli cells in order to direct the migration of germ cells from basal to luminal positions.
4. Transformation (spermiogenesis) of large spherical spermatids into compact, virtually cytoplasm-free spermatozoa with condensed DNA in the head crowned by an apical acrosome cap, and a tail capable of propulsive beating movements.
5. Spermiation, whereby the spermatozoa are released from the Sertoli cell cytoplasm into the tubular lumen.

Cohorts of undifferentiated germ cells, joined to each other by cytoplasmic bridges, progress through these different steps in synchrony, so that several generations of developing germ cells are usually observed at any one part of the seminiferous epithelium at any one time. The total time taken for a cohort of spermatogonia to develop into spermatozoa is 74 days, during which time at least three further generations of spermatogonia have also successively, at intervals of 16 days, initiated their

development. In the human, spermatogenesis is arranged in a helical manner, so that cross-sections show more than one stage of spermatogenesis within individual seminiferous tubules. This organizational arrangement differs from that in many other species (e.g. rodents), in which spermatogenesis is arranged longitudinally and thus only one stage of spermatogenesis is seen in a cross-section of a tubule.

Sertoli cell function

Sertoli cells have extensive cytoplasm which spans the full height of the seminiferous epithelium from basement membrane to the lumen (Fig. 22.2). Where adjacent Sertoli cells come into contact with each other near the basement membrane, special occluding junctions are formed which divide the seminiferous epithelium into a basal (outer) compartment, which interacts with the systemic circulation, and an adluminal (inner) compartment enclosed by a functional permeability barrier, the blood–testis barrier (Fig. 22.2). Spermatogonia divide by mitosis in the basal compartment, while the two reduction divisions of the spermatocytes and spermiogenesis are confined to the unique avascular microenvironment of the adluminal compartment created by the blood–testis barrier. The developing germ cells are therefore completely dependent on Sertoli cells for metabolic support. In response to appropriate trophic stimuli (of which follicle-stimulating hormone (FSH) and testosterone are the best described), Sertoli cells secrete a wide range of substances including androgen-binding protein (ABP), inhibin, activin, plasminogen activator, transferrin, lactate, growth factors and a distinctive tubular fluid high in potassium and low in protein which bathes the mature spermatozoa.

Sertoli cells contribute directly to the feedback regulation of pituitary gonadotrophin secretion. The existence of an endocrine product of the testis termed 'inhibin' was postulated for many decades, but its nature has only recently been confirmed. This has allowed the demonstration that inhibin B, a dimeric glycoprotein, is secreted by the Sertoli cells and has a physiological role in the regulation of FSH secretion. Inhibin B concentrations reflect the functional activity of the seminiferous tubule and show a positive relationship to sperm production. Its production requires and reflects the interaction of the germ cell population with the Sertoli cells and is absent in men with Sertoli cell only syndrome. The measurement of inhibin B may be of clinical value as a marker of the activity of the seminiferous epithelium (Anderson & Sharpe 2000) but few data are so far available. Inhibin A, the product of the dominant follicle and corpus luteum in women, is not present in the circulation in men.

Unlike the actively dividing germ cells, Sertoli cells do not proliferate in the adult testis. However, the active cell division and morphogenesis are matched by the functional diversity and variation of Sertoli cells. Viewed from this perspective, spermatogenesis is a cyclical process, which is critically dependent on the periodic changes in Sertoli cell function associated with the constantly changing combination of germ cells in contact with its cytoplasm. Changes in the germ cell complement in contact with any one Sertoli cell occur at a fixed sequence and interval. Thus the synchronization of these repetitive cyclical changes in Sertoli cell function, associated with the variations in germ cell metabolic requirement as they divide and differentiate, has now become one of the central tenets of our conceptualization of normal spermatogenesis (Sharpe 1990). Although pituitary gonadotrophins provide obligatory trophic support for testicular function as a whole, the classic concept that luteinizing hormone (LH) stimulates Leydig cell steroidogenesis and FSH controls functions in the seminiferous tubules is far too simplistic in the light of our current understanding of spermatogenesis. There is now good evidence that the interstitial and tubular compartments are not functionally distinct but that there is a close and complex interrelationship between them (Skinner 1991). Thus testosterone from the interstitial Leydig cells stimulates Sertoli cell functions either directly or via the peritubular cells. Altered tubular/Sertoli cell function, on the other hand, can induce changes in Leydig cell steroidogenesis, although the identity of the intercompartmental regulator(s) is unknown.

Testosterone is the only and probably the most important paracrine hormone clearly identified and its presence in sufficient concentrations in the seminiferous tubules is an absolute requirement for spermatogenesis. How much testosterone is required and how it exerts its effects are just some of the fundamental questions that are still unanswered. Despite the large gaps in our existing knowledge, it is becoming increasingly accepted that local co-ordination of the multifarious functions in a variety of different cell types within the testis, orchestrated by the diverse functional capabilities of the Sertoli cells, holds the key to quantitatively normal spermatogenesis.

The Leydig cell

The adult human testis contains some 500 million Leydig cells clustered in the interstitial spaces adjacent to the seminiferous tubules. The biosynthesis of testosterone in Leydig cells is under the control of LH which binds to specific surface membrane receptors. Steroidogenesis is stimulated through a cyclic AMP–protein kinase C mechanism which mobilizes cholesterol substrate and promotes the conversion of cholesterol to pregnenolone by splitting the C21 side chain. The subsequent steps in the biosynthetic pathway involve the weakly androgenic intermediates dehydroepiandrosterone and androstenedione before testosterone, the principal secretory product, is obtained. Testosterone is secreted into the spermatic venous system, testicular lymphatics and tubular fluid.

Testosterone is the most important circulating androgen in the adult male, since most dihydrotestosterone is formed locally in androgen-responsive target tissues. When circulating in plasma, testosterone is bound to sex hormone-binding globulin (SHBG) and albumin. The latter binds to all steroids with low affinity, while SHBG, a glycoprotein synthesized in the liver, has a high affinity but a low capacity for testosterone. In man, 60% of circulating testosterone is bound to SHBG, 38% to albumin and 2% is free. Free and albumin-bound testosterone constitute the bioavailable fractions of circulating testosterone, but recent evidence suggests that SHBG-bound testosterone may also be extractable in some tissues, namely prostate and testis. The plasma concentration of SHBG is regulated by factors including steroid hormones, its synthesis being increased by oestrogens and reduced by testosterone. It is also related to body weight, being lower in the obese. These relationships are the same as in women.

Hormonal control of spermatogenesis

The hormonal control of spermatogenesis requires the actions of the pituitary gonadotrophins LH and FSH. There is general agreement that both LH and FSH are needed for the initiation of spermatogenesis during puberty. However, the specific roles and relative contributions of the two gonadotrophins in maintaining spermatogenesis are unclear (Sharpe 1987).

LH stimulates Leydig cell steroidogenesis, resulting in increased production of testosterone. Normal spermatogenesis is absolutely dependent on testosterone, but its mode of action and the amount required remain uncertain. Specific androgen receptors have not been demonstrated in germ cells but are present in Sertoli and peritubular cells. This implies that the actions of androgens in spermatogenesis must be mediated by somatic cells in the seminiferous tubules. The concentration of testosterone in the testis is 50 times higher than that in the peripheral circulation. There is thus an apparent gross overabundance of testosterone within the normal adult testis, the significance of which is uncertain. It is possible that some androgen-mediated functions in the testis are not mediated by classic androgen receptors. Steroids other than testosterone may also have important roles in the regulation of steroidogenesis. In particular, oestrogen receptors are widely distributed in the male reproductive tract, including the presence of the newly described oestrogen receptor β (ERβ) (Saunders 1998). However, testosterone on its own, in hypogonadotrophic conditions, can maintain qualitatively normal spermatogenesis but testicular weight and total sperm production remain subnormal (Matsumoto et al 1984).

FSH initiates function in immature Sertoli cells, prior to the onset of spermatogenesis, by stimulating the formation of the blood–testis barrier and the secretion of tubular fluid and other specific secretory products via FSH receptors which activate intracellular cyclic adenosine monophosphate (cAMP). Once spermatogenesis is established in the adult testis, Sertoli cells become less responsive to FSH. Evidence for the non-essential role of FSH is provided by individuals with inactivating mutations of the FSH receptor. Such men have been documented to have complete spermatogenesis but with low sperm concentrations (Tapanainen et al 1997). However, it can be shown, in animals immunized against FSH and in experimentally induced hypogonadotrophic men given gonadotrophin replacement, that both testosterone (depending on LH) and FSH are required for quantitatively normal spermatogenesis in the adult (testosterone-replete) testis by determining the number of spermatogonia available by meiosis. FSH therefore acts either by increasing spermatogonial mitosis or decreasing the number of cells that degenerate at each cell division. Testosterone is essential for the subsequent stages from meiosis to spermiogenesis.

Hypothalamic-pituitary-testicular axis

The secretion of gonadotrophins from the anterior pituitary gland is controlled by gonadotrophin-releasing hormone (GnRH) released into the pituitary portal circulation from axon terminals in the hypothalamic median eminence. These neurosecretory neurones in the medial basal hypothalamus are responsive to a wide variety of sensory inputs as well as to gonadal negative feedback. GnRH stimulates the secretion of both LH and FSH. In the adult male, GnRH is released

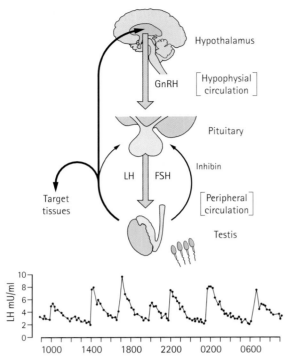

Fig. 22.3 **Top** Functional relationships in the hypothalamic-pituitary-testicular axis. Gonadotrophin-releasing hormone (GnRH) is secreted into the hypophysial circulation in an episodic manner, represented by a luteinizing hormone (LH) pulse in the peripheral circulation.
Bottom Peripheral blood LH concentration sampled in an adult male at 10-minute intervals for 24 hours from 0900 to 0900 hours.

episodically into the pituitary portal circulation at a frequency of about every 140 minutes; each volley of GnRH elicits an immediate release of LH, producing the typical pulsatile pattern of LH in the systemic circulation (Fig. 22.3; Wu et al 1989). Though also secreted episodically, FSH and testosterone pulses are not apparent in normal men, because of the slower secretion of newly synthesized rather than stored hormone and the longer circulating half-lives. The intermittent mode of GnRH stimulation, within a narrow physiological range of frequency, is obligatory for sustaining the normal pattern of gonadotrophin secretion. Continuous or high-frequency GnRH stimulation paradoxically desensitizes the pituitary gonado-trophin response in men as in women, because of depletion of receptors and refractoriness of postreceptor response mechanisms.

Testosterone exerts the major negative feedback action on gonadotrophin secretion. Its effect is predominantly to restrict the frequency of GnRH pulses from the hypothalamus to within the physiological range. Testosterone also acts on the pituitary to reduce the amplitude of LH reponse to GnRH. It is now recognized that these inhibitory effects on GnRH and gonadotrophin secretion are in part mediated following conversion of testosterone to oestradiol by the enzyme P450 aromatase. This is demonstrated both by administration of aromatase inhibitors to normal men and by the finding that men with either mutant, non-functional oestrogen receptors or absent aromatase activity have markedly elevated gonado-trophin concentrations despite high-normal testosterone con-

centrations (Morishima et al 1995, Smith et al 1994). Interestingly these men also showed marked osteoporosis, suggesting a distinct role for oestrogen in bone. These inhibitory actions are best seen in agonadal or castrated males where high-frequency and high-amplitude LH pulsatile secretion prevail. Feedback inhibition of pituitary FSH synthesis is also affected by testosterone, particularly at high concentrations, as well as by the recently purified glycoprotein Sertoli cell product, inhibin B. The regulation of FSH secretion by inhibin in addition to testosterone results in the selective rise in FSH but not LH concentrations in men with various disorders of spermatogenesis.

Progestogens are also potent inhibitors of gonadotrophin secretion. Progesterone receptors have been demonstrated in the hypothalamus of animal species and administration of progesterone reduces the amplitude of LH pulses in normal men. The physiological implications of this are uncertain, but this effect has been made use of in the development of progestogen-based hormonal male contraception (Merrigiola & Bremner 1997).

The spermatozoon

The primary function of the spermatozoon is the delivery of a male pronucleus to the fertilized egg. The spermatozoon must conserve its DNA and transport it to the site of fertilization, where it must recognize and fuse with a receptive egg. The ejaculated spermatozoon must first escape from the seminal plasma in which it is deposited beside the cervix and penetrate the barrier presented by cervical mucus. It must then travel through the uterus to the site of fertilization in the fallopian tube. During this journey it must complete the process of functional maturation known as capacitation, an ordered series of events involving reorganization of cell surface components and changes in cellular metabolism and motility patterns, which are a prerequisite for successful fertilization. Having reached the oviduct, the male gamete must recognize the oocyte, must penetrate the cumulus oophorus and bind to the zona pellucida. At this point, it must display a unique pattern of movement known as hyperactivated motility and must undergo the acrosome reaction. This process is initiated by a specific protein component of the zona pellucida (ZP3) and resuts in the release of the contents of the acrosomal matrix, which include the serine protease acrosin and other hydrolytic enzymes including hyaluronidase. In addition, the acrosome reaction results in the generation of a fusogenic equatorial segment, which is the zone of fusion with the oocyte plasma membrane. For a review of sperm structure and function, see Grudzinskas & Yovich (1995).

To enable it to undertake these complex functions, the human spermatozoon has developed a highly specialized morphology, with its various structural components tailored to specific functional attributes. The appearance of the spermatozoon was first described over 300 years ago, by Anthony van Leeuwenhoek. In outline, the spermatozoon has a dense oval head capped by an acrosome and is propelled by a motile tail (Fig. 22.4; Fawcett 1975). The head is made up largely of highly condensed nuclear chromatin constituting the haploid chromosome complement, complexed with highly basic proteins termed protamines. It is covered in its anterior half by the acrosome, a

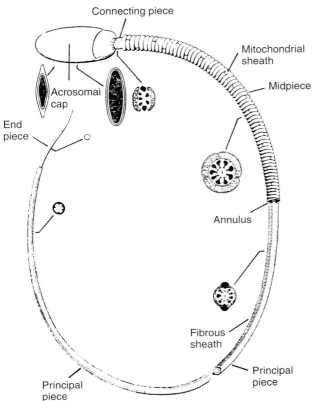

Fig. 22.4 The internal structure of a spermatozoon with the cell membrane removed. Reproduced with permission from Fawcett (1975).

membrane-enclosed sac of enzymes including acrosin and hyaluronidase. The area of the sperm head immediately behind the acrosome (the equatorial region) is important as it is this part which attaches to and fuses with the egg. The shape of the human sperm head is highly pleomorphic, making the morphological definition of a normal sperm head extremely challenging. Behind the head may be found a cytoplasmic droplet which consists of the remains of the residual cytoplasm left after the morphological remodelling of the cell during spermiogenesis.

The tail of flagellum is usually further divided into the midpiece, principal piece and terminal piece, joined to the head by the connecting piece. The motor apparatus of the tail is the axoneme which consists of a central pair (doublets) of microtubules of non-contractile tubulin protein enclosed in a sheath linked radially to nine outer pairs of microtubules. The axonemal complex is surrounded by columns of outer dense fibres, which are in turn covered by a helix of mitochondria in the midpiece and a fibrous sheath in the principal piece. The dense fibres and the fibrous sheath form the cytoskeleton of the flagellum. Through the hydrolysis of adenosine triphosphate, the dynein arms undergo a series of conformational changes resulting in adjacent doublets sliding over one another. Synchronized movement of groups of microtubules propagating waves of bending motions of the tail is the key to the various modes of co-ordinated sperm motility. Energy for sperm motility is provided by the sheath of mitochondria in the midpiece of the tail through a second messenger system, involving the calcium-mediated calmodulin-dependent conversion of adenosine triphosphate to cAMP and interaction with the adenosine triphosphatase of the dynein.

Sperm transport and maturation

Spermatozoa within the testis and male tract are quiescent and play little active role in their own transport along the tract. Moreover, they are functionally immature and a maturation process continues as they pass through the epididymis. Passage out of the seminiferous tubules and through the main testicular collecting duct, the rete testis, is due to the flow of secretions from Sertoli cells and rete epithelium and to the intrinsic smooth muscle contractions of the tubules. From the rete, the cells pass through the efferent ducts to the epididymis, a 3–4 m long single coiled tube whose function is under androgen and neural (adrenergic) control. It is typically subdivided into a caput or head region, a middle body or corpus and a distal tail or cauda region which leads into the proximal vas deferens. The epididymal epithelium actively reabsorbs testicular fluid but also secretes a hyperosmolar fluid rich in glycero-phosphorylocholine, inositol and carnitine. The specific transport of these compounds across the epithelium creates a favourable fluid environment where progressive motility and fertilizing capacity of the spermatozoa are normally acquired. Thus the cytoplasmic droplets decrease in size and move distally along the midpiece, the acrosome membrane swells and epididymal glycoproteins are incorporated into the plasma membrane. Some of these maturational changes are probably 'housekeeping' functions to ensure that the cell remains viable during its stay in the excurrent ducts, while others are associated with the development of fertilizing ability. In many animal species, spermatozoa retain fertility for several weeks in the cauda epididymis, which acts as a sperm reservoir prior to ejaculation. The human cauda epididymis, in contrast, has a relatively poor storage function, which diminishes further along the vas.

At ejaculation, spermatozoa pass along the vas and are mixed with the secretions of the accessory glands which form over 90% of the volume of the ejaculate. The seminal vesicles contribute the largest volume of alkaline fluid to the ejaculate and are also the souce of seminal fructose, prostaglandins and coagulating proteins. Prostatic secretion contains proteolytic enzymes (which normally liquefy the coagulated proteins in semen within 20–30 minutes) and are rich in citric acid and zinc. Seminal plasma provides a support medium for transporting male gametes out of the body and for buffering the acidic pH of the vagina so that a reservoir of functional sperm can be established after ejaculation. Just as testicular germ cells are subjected to constant attrition, ejaculated spermatozoa have to traverse the cervix, uterus and uterotubal junction before reaching the middle third of the oviduct, the site of fertilization, and at each barrier the sperm population is further reduced so that eventually only 200 or so of the most robust spermatozoa have the opportunity to fertilize the ovum. The number of these functionally competent sperm is more important than the total number ejaculated.

The cervical canal is the first selective filtering barrier to meet the ejaculated sperm (Fig 22.5). This barrier is virtually complete except during midcycle when oestrogenized cervical

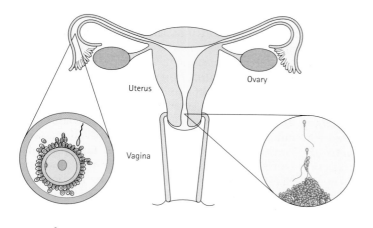

Oocyte

Fig. 22.5 Attributes of sperm function associated with fertility in vivo. The spermatozoon must escape from seminal plasma, penetrate and traverse the cervical mucus barrier, reach the site of fertilization, undergo capacitation, bind to and penetrate the zona pellucida, fuse with the plasma membrane of the egg and undergo nuclear decondensation within the cytoplasm of the oocyte.

mucus glycoprotein fibrils form parallel chains called micelles which permit spermatozoa with active progressive motility to swim through at a rate of 2–3 mm/min. Spermatozoa probably enter the uterine cavity from the internal os by virtue of their own motility and appear in the uterine cavity about 90 minutes after insemination. The uterotubal junction is the second of the major physical barriers for spermatozoa. The mechanism for selectivity is not clear, but may depend on factors other than sperm motility since inert particles can pass through. Once the uterotubal junction has been successfully negotiated, a minority of sperm immediately traverse the oviduct to the ampulla but the majority congregate in the isthmus until ovulation has occurred. At this time, capacitated sperm showing hyperactivated movements of the tail gradually progress towards the fimbriated end, helped on by the muscular contraction of the oviduct wall and the flow of fluid in the oviduct. A maximum number of spermatozoa is present in the cervix by 15–20 minutes following insemination and remains constant for 24 hours, although a rapid decline has commenced by 48 hours. Some spermatozoa may remain motile at the site of fertilization for up to 3 days (Mortimer 1995).

The physiology of male reproductive ageing

Reproductive ageing in the male is not accompanied by such an overt and abrupt fall in gonadal function as occurs in women, but by a more gradual decline. Indeed, fertility may be preserved until very old age. These differences reflect the consequence of a finite pool of gametes compared to one that continually replicates from a stock of stem cells, and in men there is a clearer distinction between the endocrine and gametogenic functions of the gonads.

The decline in function of the endocrine output of the hypothalamo-pituitary-testicular axis with age is well established and results in a fall of approximately 50% in plasma testosterone concentrations (Vermeulen 1991). This has both central and peripheral components; thus there is a relatively small increase

in LH. The 'andropause' is increasingly the subject of investigation, with large placebo-controlled studies of the effect of replacement under way (Snyder et al 1999). Changes in Sertoli cell function and spermatogenesis with ageing have received more limited investigation due to the lack of a biochemical marker and difficulties in the interpretation of minor changes in semen parameters. Inhibin B has been used to assess Sertoli cell function in a population of men aged up to 85 years (Mahmoud et al 2000). These data suggest that there is indeed an age-related fall in inhibin B concentrations, but need to be confirmed in a longitudinal study. This fall appears to occur at a relatively early age, inhibin B concentrations being fairly well maintained thereafter. This indirectly suggests that spermatogenesis is well maintained in elderly men, consistent with the limited direct data available from semen analysis, and contrasts with the decline in testosterone concentrations, which starts later in life and is progressive. The rise in FSH and thus fall in inhibin B/FSH ratio suggests that Sertoli cell functional activity is, however, significantly affected by ageing and complements detailed studies of hypothalamo-pituitary function (Veldhuis et al 1999).

MALE INFERTILITY

Definition and epidemiology

Infertility results in considerable distress for those couples affected. It is commonly defined as the failure of conception after at least 12 months of unprotected intercourse (Rowe et al 1993) but such a definition of 'infertility' serves to obscure the true complexity of the clinical situation. In reality, those couples who fail to achieve a pregnancy within 12–24 months include those who can be considered sterile (and who will never achieve a spontaneous pregnancy) and those who are more properly termed subfertile and who have reduced fecundability (probability of achieving a pregnancy within one menstrual cycle) and hence a prolonged time to pregnancy. Accurate assessment of the prevalence of infertility has always been difficult because of the scarcity of large-scale, population-based studies (Irvine 1998, Templeton et al 1990). Estimates suggest that some 14–17% of couples may be affected at some time in their reproductive lives (Hull et al 1985), with recent European data suggesting that as many as one in four couples who try may experience difficulties in conceiving (Schmidt et al 1995).

While infertility is relatively common, it is very difficult indeed to establish the relative contribution of the male partner, given the profound difficulties which exist in the accurate diagnosis of male infertility. Most studies which have attempted to evaluate the aetiology of infertility have used the conventional criteria of semen quality, promulgated by the World Health Organization (1999), to define the 'male factor'. Although of great importance, these criteria are of limited diagnostic value (Irvine & Aitken 1994) and a significant proportion of men with normal conventional criteria of semen quality will be infertile because of defects in sperm function (Aitken et al 1982a), while a significant number of men with abnormal semen quality will have normal sperm function (Aitken et al 1982b). Very few studies on the epidemiology of male infertility have used functional, as opposed to descriptive diagnostic criteria.

Nevertheless, one common theme to emerge is that, using the available diagnostic techniques, male factor infertility is, in many studies, the commonest single diagnostic category.

Pathophysiology

In the simplest terms, male infertility is a failure to fertilize the normal ovum arising from a deficiency of functionally competent sperm at the site of fertilization. Since less than 0.1% of ejaculated sperm actually reach the fallopian tube, it is defective sperm function rather than inadequate numbers of sperm ejaculated that constitutes the most important pathophysiological mechanism in male infertility. Specific lesions leading to defective sperm motility or transport and abnormal sperm–egg interaction are probably the key factors responsible for loss of fertilizing capacity in the gametes. In most instances, however, inadequate sperm function is usually but not invariably accompanied by reduced sperm production, suggesting that specific defects in spermatozoa commonly arise from disturbances in regulatory mechanisms which interfere with both germ cell multiplication and maturation in the seminiferous tubules. There is rarely any clinical evidence of systemic endocrine deficiency in men with male infertility; indeed, circulating gonadotrophins are frequently raised. By inference, therefore, disturbances in paracrine regulation within the testis could lead to low sperm output (oligozoospermia), from an increased rate of degeneration in the differentiating spermatogonia at successive mitotic divisions, as well as abnormal spermiogenesis giving rise to spermatozoa with poor motility (asthenozoospermia) and/or abnormal morphology (teratozoospermia). Abnormal epididymal function may lead to defective sperm maturation, impairment of sperm transport or even cell death. Interruption of the transport of normal sperm may be due to mechanical barriers between the epididymis and fallopian tube or abnormal coitus and/or ejaculation.

Aetiology

Notwithstanding the difficulties in diagnosis outlined above, the WHO has proposed a scheme for the diagnostic classification of the male partner of the infertile couple (Rowe et al 1993) (Box 22.1). This approach is of enormous value as a basis for standardization and for comparative multicentre studies. How-

ever, many of the male diagnostic categories are of a descriptive nature (e.g. idiopathic oligozoospermia) or of controversial clinical relevance (e.g. male accessory gland infection). Moreover, recent advances in our understanding of the causes of male infertility, particularly in the area of genetic problems (Hargreave 2000), mean that this classification is now in need of review. The relative frequency of the major diagnostic categories is shown in Figure 22.6, using data taken from a WHO study of over 8500 couples from 33 centres in 25 countries (Comhaire et al 1987). It can be seen that the largest single male 'diagnostic' category was men with seminal abnormalities of unknown cause. Beyond this, varicocoele was a relatively common pathology, as was male accessory gland infection; however, systemic, iatrogenic and endocrine causes were very infrequent.

Genetic causes

Perhaps the most striking advances in our understanding of the aetiology of male infertility in the past decade have been in the area of genetics. Many of the 'systemic' disorders commonly associated with male infertility (see below) are now understood to have a genetic basis and as our knowledge of the aetiology of disease expands, this will be increasingly the case. Traditionally, genetic causes of male infertility have been sought at the level of chromosomal abnormalities, with chromosomal abnormalities being detected in between 2.1% and 8.9% of men attending infertility clinics. Chandley, in a study of 2372 men attending

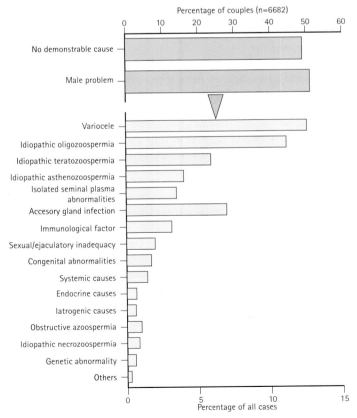

Fig. 22.6 Aetiology of male factor infertility. Reproduced with permission from Comhaire et al (1987).

Box 22.1 Diagnostic categories for the male partner of an infertile couple according to the WHO (data from Rowe et al 1993)

No demonstrable cause	Systemic causes
Idiopathic oligozoospermia	Endocrine causes
Idiopathic asthenozoospermia	Iatrogenic causes
Idiopathic teratozoospermia	Congenital abnormalities
Idiopathic azoospermia	Acquired testicular damage
Obstructive azoospermia	Varicocoele
Isolated seminal plasma abnormalities	Immunological infertility
Sexual or ejaculatory dysfunction	Male accessory gland infection

an infertility clinic in Edinburgh, found significant abnormalities in 21.5 per 1000 men, compared to a rate of 7 per 1000 newborn males in the same city (Chandley 1994). The frequency of chromosomal abnormalities increased as sperm concentration declined, with abnormal karyotypes being found in 15% of azoospermic patients, 90% of whom had Klinefelter's syndrome (47XXY), which accounted for half of the entire chromosomally abnormal group. In oligozoospermic patients, the incidence of chromosome abnormalities was 4%. However, it has been recognized for some time that structural anomalies of the Y chromosome, resulting in deletion of the distal fluorescent heterochromatin in the long arm, are associated with severe abnormalities of spermatogenesis. More recent studies have defined a family of genes on the Y chromosome involved in spermatogenesis and it has become clear that a little over 10% of cases of non-obstructive azoospermia may have deletions affecting these genes. A proprotion of cases of very severe oligozoospermia may have a similar aetiology. Microdeletions have been found in three non-overlapping regions of the Y chromosome, AZF a-b-c. Several genes have been described and these include RBM, DAZ, DFFRY, DBY and CDY. The abnormality most commonly reported in the literature is a microdeletion in the AZFc region and encompassing the DAZ gene. However, there is no exact correlation between DAZ deletion and the presence or absence of spermatogenesis, but this may be because of the DAZ gene there is also an autosomal copy. (For a review of the genetic basis of male fertility see Hargreave (2000).) The ability of microassisted fertilization to overcome severe deficits in spermatogenesis has reinforced the importance of understanding and investigating genetic causes of male subfertility.

Cryptorchidism

Undescended testis is a good example of a condition present at birth, and presumed to have its origins in intrauterine life, which is significantly associated with an increased risk of impaired spermatogenesis in later life and with an increased risk of testis cancer (Irvine 1997). The testis which is not in a low scrotal position by the age of 2 years is histologically abnormal; spontaneous descent rarely occurs after 1 year and there is little evidence that surgical orchidopexy for an undescended testis after 2 years of age improves fertility. For these reasons, treatment should ideally be undertaken between 1 and 2 years of age. Evidence suggests that fertility may also be impaired in boys with retractile testis who experience spontaneous descent during puberty. Apart from the association with infertility, cryptorchidism is a well-established risk factor for testicular cancer, the risk of which in a patient with a history of undescended testis, whether successfully treated or not, is 4–10 times higher than in the general population.

Orchitis

Symptomatic orchitis occurs as a complication in 27–30% of males over the age of 10–11 years who suffer from mumps. In 17% of cases, orchitis is bilateral and seminiferous tubular atrophy is a common sequela of mumps orchitis, although recovery of spermatogenesis even after persistent azoospermia for 1 year has been reported (Sandler 1954). The prevalence of infertility after mumps orchitis is unknown but fertility should only be significantly impaired if the orchitis is bilateral and occurs after puberty.

Varicocele

The subject of varicocoele has generated controversy amongst the andrological community since the Edinburgh urologist Selby Tulloch first reported the apparently beneficial effects of treatment (Tulloch 1952). The available evidence certainly suggests that varicocoele is a common pathology and that it is commoner in men with lower sperm counts. The diagnosis of visible (grade 3) and palpable (grade 2) varicocoeles is not difficult when the patient is examined in a standing position. The detection of subclinical (grade 1) varicocoeles, where spermatic vein reflux can only be detected during the Valsalva manoeuvre, requires more experience and has been aided by the use of Doppler or scrotal thermography. In a survey of over 10 000 military recruits, a population prevalence of just under 10% was observed (Damonte et al 1984), although prevalence figures from 5% to 25% have been reported in similar surveys of apparently healthy men (Hargreave 1994). In contrast, amongst men attending infertility clinics, varicocoele affects some 11% of men with normal semen and 25% of men with abnormal semen (WHO 1992). The difficulty has been in establishing with certainty whether or not varicocoele affects spermatogenesis and, most importantly, whether or not treatment of varicocoele improves fertility and if so, in which groups of men. It seems clear that varicocoele is associated with abnormal semen quality and while the mechanism of this relationship remains to be established with certainty, abnormal testicular temperature regulation is known to be associated with varicocoele and with impairment in semen quality.

Whatever the pathophysiology, there is a body of evidence suggesting that varicocoele causes progressive testicular damage, further complicating an assessment of its role in the aetiology of male infertility. Substantial controversy exists, however, over the question of whether or not the correction of varicocoele improves fertility. Most of the appropriately designed controlled studies suggest that treatment is clearly associated with an improvement in semen quality; however, when the achievement of pregnancy is used as the endpoint some studies find treatment to be effective while some suggest that it is of no benefit (Baker et al 1985, Laven et al 1992, Madgar et al 1995, Nieschlag et al 1995). Most recently a large multicentre randomized controlled trial conducted by the WHO suggested that treatment of varicocoele in men with oligozoospermia and a normal partner was beneficial in terms of both semen quality and pregnancy rates. In the context of contemporary assisted conception techniques, it is interesting that recent evidence suggests that the presence of varicocoele may even reduce the ability of the haploid male gamete to generate embryos when used for microassisted fertilization (Sofikitis et al 1996).

Occupational and environmental factors

The actively dividing male germ cells are one of the most sensitive cell types in the body with regard to the toxic effects of radiation, cytotoxic drugs and an increasing number of chemicals. Indeed, male gonadal function may be one of the most sensitive indices of overexposure to potential toxins (in the workplace, environment, foods, cosmetics and medicines)

(Sharpe 2000). Data on occupational hazards to male reproduction remain controversial. Exposure to heavy metals, such as cadmium, lead, arsenic and zinc, has been reported to impair spermatogenesis, although the data are conflicting. Certain pesticides and herbicides have more clearly been shown to be toxic to spermatogenesis, as have some organic chemicals. The best documented modern example is the pesticide dibromochloropropane (DBCP), which was responsible for azoospermic infertility in half of the male workers in a factory. There would seem to be clear evidence that occupational or environmental exposure to heat will have adverse consequences for spermatogenesis (Mieusset & Bujan 1995) and will prolong time to pregnancy (Thonneau et al 1996). Recreational drugs such as cigarettes, alcohol and cannabis have all been linked with lower semen quality and there is conflicting evidence on whether or not dress habit has a significant effect.

Recent data have demonstrated that male reproductive health is deteriorating, with evidence of a secular decline in semen quality (Auger et al 1995, Carlsen et al 1992, Irvine et al 1996), an increase in the incidence of congenital malformation of the male reproductive tract and an increase in the incidence of testicular cancer. It has been hypothesized that these changes may be due to perinatal exposure to environmental xeno-oestrogens (Sharpe & Skakkebaek 1993); however, there is (as yet) no evidence that these changes are having an influence on the prevalence of male infertility.

Iatrogenic infertility

Many general medical disorders are associated with male infertility, either directly (e.g. Kartagener's syndrome), indirectly as a consequence of systemic disturbance (e.g. diabetes) or as a consequence of medical or surgical intervention on account of the primary disease. A number of pharmaceuticals can impair sperm production, the most common example in clinical practice today being sulphasalazine for the treatment of inflammatory bowel diseases. A number of other drugs are also associated with detrimental effects on spermatogenesis, including nitrofurantoin, anabolic steroids, sex steroids and anticonvulsants. Cytotoxic treatment regimes for Hodgkin's disease, lymphoma, leukaemia and other malignancies damage the differentiating spermatogonia, so that most patients become azoospermic after 8 weeks. The degree of stem cell killing governs whether there is recovery of spermatogenesis or not after treatment. This is dependent on the cumulative dose of the drug combination used. Long-term follow-up has shown that following six or more courses of MOPP (mustine, vincristine, procarbazine and prednisolone), over 85% of patients remained azoospermic and recovery is unlikely after 4 years. Similarly, radiation exposure of over 6 Gy destroys germ cells with no chance of recovery. While 1–4 Gy produces complete cessation of spermatogenesis with only some stem spermatogonia surviving, there may be recovery after 12–36 months and spermatogenesis may continue to improve for several years but even then it may not be complete. Diagnostic procedures and therapeutic irradiation to other organs such as the thyroid usually expose the testis to 1 Gy.

Genital tract obstruction

The combination of azoospermia, normal testicular volume and normal FSH are the hallmarks of genital tract obstruction.

The incidence and relative importance of individual causes of obstruction differ according to geographic locality. Postcongenital and postvasectomy obstructions are the most common, but in some parts of the world infectious causes, particularly gonorrhoea and tuberculosis, are of greater importance.

Three specific congenital abnormalities are recognized. The commonest is agenesis or malformations of the wolffian duct-derived structures: the corpus/cauda epididymis, vas deferens and seminal vesicles. Diagnosis is usually quite easy: the scrotal vasa are not palpable and the ejaculate consists of low volumes (>1 ml) of acidic non-coagulating prostatic fluid devoid of fructose and sperm. Congenital bilateral absence of the vas deferens (CBAVD) is associated with CFTR mutations and is found in approximately 2% of men with obstructive azoospermia (Hargreave 2000). However, the incidence in men with obstructive azoospermia will vary in different countries depending on the prevalence of cystic fibrosis mutations in the population and the prevalence of other causes of obstruction; in those countries with a high prevalence of sexually transmitted infection, CBAVD as a cause of azoospermia will be relatively infrequent compared with azoospermia associated with postgonococcal epididymitis. In recent years, increasing numbers of mutations of the CFTR gene have been characterized and more than 400 have been described. In general, the more mutations tested for, the higher the percentage of men found to have mutations, so that in more recent publications detection rates have been almost 70–80%.

In Young's syndrome the obstruction is at the junction of the caput and body of the epididymis and there is marked inspissation of amorphous secretion in the lumen. In these patients, the high incidence of chronic sinopulmonary infection and bronchiectasis is presumably the consequence of the same abnormality in the respiratory tract and may be the result of mercury poisoning (Hendry et al 1990). Obstruction of the ejaculatory duct is an uncommon cause of obstructive azoospermis with semen abnormality as in CBAVD, but it may be distinguished by palpation of the scrotal vasa.

Male accessory gland infection

The second commonest diagnostic grouping in the WHO survey, is also an area of considerable aetiological controversy. Infection in the lower genital tract can be a treatable cause of male infertility and the incidence varies in different communities. Gram-negative enterococci, chlamydia and gonococcus are established pathogenic organisms which usually produce unequivocal clinical evidence of infection (adnexitis), such as painful ejaculation, pelvic or sacral pain, urethral discharge, haematospermia, dysuria, irregular tender epididymides and tender boggy prostate. This can be confirmed by semen culture, urethral swabs and the presence of more than 1 million peroxidase-positive polymorphonuclear neutrophils per millilitre of semen or in expressed prostatic fluid. Inflammation of the accessory glands and excurrent ducts may give rise to disturbed function, formation of sperm antibody and permanent structural damage with obstruction in the outflow tract.

Thus whilst there is little doubt that overt sexually transmitted disease may damage male fertility and should be appropriately managed, there is much more doubt about the relevance of subclinical infection. It is clear that gonorrhoea is implicated in the aetiology of obstructive azoospermia and that chlamydial infection in the male can lead to tubal infertility in his partner. It is much less clear whether subclinical infection in the male is causally associated with infertility and there is no clear consensus on diagnostic criteria. The entity of asymptomatic prostatitis is poorly defined and there is little evidence to support a genuine role for occult infections in male infertility. There is thus no place for microbiological screening investigations unless there is clinical suspicion of adnexitis. Furthermore, the isolation of non-pathogenic organisms such as staphylococcus, streptococcus, diptheroids, *Ureaplasma urealyticum* and *Mycoplasma hominis*, which are commensals in the normal urethra, does not warrant the indiscriminate use of antibiotics in the hope of correcting any abnormalities in the semen parameters.

One possible consequence of infection is seminal leucocytosis and one consequence of seminal leucocytosis is the excessive generation of reactive oxygen species (ROS) by these cells. There is good evidence linking the excessive generation of ROS with male infertility as an aetiological entity in its own right – prospective studies have shown that couples with elevated levels of ROS generation are less likely to conceive either spontaneously or in the context of in vitro fertilization.

Immunological causes

Suspected immunological infertility was found in some 3% of couples in a WHO survey on the basis of the finding of 10% or more of motile spermatozoa coated with antibody using assays such as the Immunobead test (IBT) or the mixed antiglobulin reaction (MAR). Whilst antisperm antibodies are found in perhaps one in six of the male partners of infertile couples, a prevalence which is higher than that for fertile controls, their effect on fertility is hard to determine. Some studies suggest that 'antibody-positive' couples conceive at a lower rate than those without immunological problems. Unfortunately, antibodies to sperm surface antigens are also found in fertile control populations and current techniques do not permit the meaningful separation of cases with autoimmunity to biologically relevant epitopes (Paradisi et al 1995). Given the consensus view that assisted conception is the treatment of choice, this may not now be a clinically relevant issue.

Gonadotrophin deficiency

The clinical features of gonadotrophin deficiency depend on the cause and time of onset, in particular whether the man is pre- or postpubertal. The spectrum includes patients with complete congenital deficiency in GnRH, which results in total failure of testicular and secondary sexual development. Other patients have less severe or partial GnRH deficiency, so that they have larger (4–10 ml) but still underdeveloped testes with more evidence of germ cell activity: this may be described as the so-called fertile eunuch syndrome. In three-quarters of these patients, anosmia or hyposmia and a variety of midline defects can be detected; this is the association known as Kallmann's syndrome.

In contrast to these congenital varieties of isolated hypogonadotrophic hypogonadism, postnatally or postpubertally acquired gonadotrophin deficiency may arise from tumours,

chronic inflammatory lesions, iron overload or injuries of the hypothalamus and pituitary, so that deficits in other pituitary hormones usually coexist. These patients have developed seminiferous tubules which have regressed through lack of trophic hormone support. Their testicular volumes are larger (10–15 ml) than in the former two groups.

Gonadotrophin treatment of these syndromes is discussed below. Androgen treatment is required by hypogonadal men for long-term replacement and is generally given by injection of testosterone esters every 3–4 weeks (Bagatell & Bremner 1996), aiming to maintain plasma testosterone concentrations in the physiological range. This is made more difficult by the high peaks and low troughs following administration of these preparations: monitoring of dosage should take place immediately before subsequent injection, i.e. at the trough. Other preparations include the orally active testosterone undecanoate, transdermal patches and subcutaneous testosterone pellets. The undecanoate avoids the extensive hepatic first-pass metabolism by being absorbed into the lymphatics after being incorporated into chylomicrons, but plasma concentrations are low and absorption erratic. It is therefore largely confined to paediatric practice, for pubertal induction. Testosterone patches frequently cause skin irritation, although this is not a problem with the scrotal patches as these do not contain the enhancers necessary to promote absorption across the skin. New injectable esters are becoming available with longer duration of action, with up to 3 months between administration. Testosterone will restore sexual interest and activity and penile erections during and on waking from sleep. Other symptoms of testosterone deficiency include tiredness and irritability and loss of body hair. Testosterone will not induce or improve fertility and there is no place for androgen treatment of men wishing to conceive.

Coital disorders

Inadequate coital technique (including the use of vaginal lubricants with spermicidal properties) and frequency and faulty timing of intercourse may contribute to continuing infertility, but are rarely the only aetiological factors in the infertile couple. Erectile and ejaculatory failure may be caused by psychosexual dysfunction, depression, spinal cord injuries, retroperitoneal and bladder neck surgery, diabetes mellitus, multiple sclerosis, vascular insufficiency, adrenergic blocking antihypertensive agents, psychotrophic drugs, alcohol abuse and chronic renal failure. Primary endocrine pathologies such as androgen deficiency, hyperprolactinaemia and hypothyroidism seldom present with infertility without diminished libido and clinical features specific to the hormonal disturbance, e.g. hypogonadism, loss of visual fields and myxoedema. Retrograde ejaculation must be differentiated from aspermia or anejaculation by examination of postejaculatory urine for the presence of spermatozoa.

Idiopathic impairment of semen quality

Regrettably, this descriptive label continues to be required for a very substantial proportion of men attending infertility clinics. Failure of seminiferous tubular function to the extent of producing azoospermia or severe oligozoospermia (>5 million) is usually associated with small (under 15 ml) and soft testes and elevated FSH. Histologically, the tubules may show completely absent or reduced numbers of germ cells, narrow tubular diameter and thickening and hyalinization of peritubular tissue. These changes are non-specific and are not always uniformly distributed throughout the testes. There is no evidence to support the contention that testosterone deficiency is the primary cause of defective spermatogenesis, nor that abnormalities in GnRH pulse frequency may be the underlying cause of idiopathic hypospermatogenesis. These patients usually remain infertile and there is no curative treatment available. Less severe degree of oligozoospermia are commonly associated with abnormal morphology and reduced motility.

Asthenozoospermia is the descriptive term applied to impaired sperm motility. Absent or extremely low sperm motility of only 1–2% may result from absence of dynein arms, radial spokes or nexin bridges and dysplasia of fibrous sheath. This is associated with similar defects in respiratory cilia and therefore frequently a history of chronic respiratory infection, bronchiectasis and sinusitis: the immotile cilia syndrome. In addition, some of these patients have situs inversus (Kartagener's syndrome). Based on this classic but extremely rare example, it is now becoming clear that more common but less severe degrees of asthenozoospermia may also be associated with more subtle structural malformations in the axonemal complex, recognizable only with ultrastructural examination and functionally evident as suboptimal sperm movements.

Teratozoospermia is the term used to describe altered morphology. Surface morphology directly reflects the maturity and functional integrity of the spermatozoa so that morphological analysis of ejaculated sperm is an important means of assessing spermatogenesis in the testis. Indeed, some workers believe that sperm morphology is the best predictor of spontaneous fertility or the outcome of in vitro fertilization (Kruger et al 1988, 1995). It has been reported that morphology in the individual spermatozoon is related to movement characteristics (swimming velocity, sperm head trajectories, flagellar beat frequency) and its ability to exhibit hyperactivation. Similarly, the ability to undergo the acrosome reaction has also been shown to be significantly higher in sperm with morphologically normal, compared with abnormal, sperm heads. Ultrastructural studies have also revealed a variety of structural malformations of the acrosome complex, the most extreme example being the round-headed sperm where the acrosome is completely missing, but lesser degrees of acrosomal defects are increasingly being identified. These attempts to relate specific functional defects to recognizable structural malformations in individual spermatozoa provide evidence that morphologically abnormal sperm are also functionally impaired.

CLINICAL MANAGEMENT

The essence of clinical management is to assess the prognosis (chances of conception per year or per cycle of assisted conception) and to advise the couple as to those treatment options that should improve the prognosis. This advice is based upon a sound knowledge of the causes of infertility and the treatment options available. In doing this, it is important to recognize that a number of general epidemiological factors will have a bearing on a couple's fertility. Examples of this include age, there being clear evidence that the age of the female partner is a major determinant of fertility (Templeton et al 1996) although the impact of male age is less certain. Similarly, a longer duration of infertility, even when allowing for age, results in a reduction in fertility. On the other hand, the occurrence of any previous pregnancy will enhance the outcome of treatment after IVF (Templeton 2000).

Recent advances in assisted conception technology have revolutionized the management of couples with male factor infertility and have advanced our understanding of the aetiology of male infertility by drawing attention to the major contribution of genetic factors. Paradoxically, they have also encouraged a minimalist clinical approach to the diagnosis of men with fertility problems, given the limited range of effective therapeutic options. The dangers of this approach have been highlighted in the light of existing concerns over the safety of microassisted fertilization (Cummins & Jequier 1994, 1995).

It is surprising how many clinicians endeavour to manage male infertility at one remove, a request for semen analysis preceding, even substituting for, taking a history from and performing a physical examination of the male partner. Those who take this attitude do their patients a disservice – they foster the idea that the male contribution to infertility is a limited one and while a semen analysis will only occasionally provide the clinician with a diagnosis, a careful history and examination may identify the cause of a couple's infertility. A number of significant features of the clinical history, together with their associated rates of azoospermia or abnormal semen quality, are shown in Table 22.1.

Table 22.1 Features in the clinical history with an influence on male fertility and their associated rates of azoospermia and abnormal semen quality (data from Comhaire et al 1987)

Feature	% of cases with azoospermia absent/present		% of cases with abnormal semen absent/present	
Diabetes mellitus	7.3	16.7	46.5	60.0
Bronchiectasis	7.2	32.0*	46.5	82.4*
Higher fever	7.3	5.2	46.4	64.4*
Long-term medication	7.2	12.3*	46.4	52.9
Urinary tract infection	7.2	8.9	45.3	60.1*
Sexually transmitted disease	7.2	7.6	45.7	50.4*
Epididymitis	7.1	17.3*	46.1	70.2*
Testicular injury	7.1	12.6*	46.2	56.9*
Testicular torsion	7.3	18.2*	46.5	88.9*
Unilateral maldescent	6.8	20.8*	46.1	65.7*
Testicular maldescent (bilateral)	6.8	40.8*	46.1	75.9*
Mumps orchitis (bilateral)	7.2	22.0*	46.2	84.4*
Excessive alcohol consumption	7.2	9.6	46.4	51.8*

* = differences significant at the 5% level

History

Infertility is, of course, the problem of a couple and must be managed as such, with the history being taken from both partners together. The duration of the present union and the duration of infertility complained of should be established at the outset, together with the history of any pregnancies for which the individual may have been responsible. In the patient's past medical history, areas which should receive special attention are a history of mumps virus infection, the age at which this occurred and whether or not there was an associated orchitis. As can be seen from Table 22.1, 84% of men with a history of bilateral mumps orchitis have abnormal semen and 22% are azoospermic. Diabetes mellitus and certain neurological diseases are known to be associated with ejaculatory disturbances and a history of these or of any other systemic illness should be sought, as should a history of recent pyrexial illness as this may compromise spermatogenesis for many weeks. A history of respiratory disease should be carefully sought, including recurrent respiratory tract infections, sinusitis, bronchiectasis or cystic fibrosis, as these conditions can be associated with ciliary dysfunction and therefore with impaired sperm motility, as in Kartagener's syndrome, or with obstructive azoospermia in Young's syndrome. As many as 82% of men with a history of bronchiectasis have abnormal semen and 32% are azoospermic. Parasitic diseases, such as schistosomiasis and filiariasis, are rare but must be borne in mind as potential causes of excurrent duct obstruction and prostatovesiculitis.

Any symptomatology related to the urinary tract, such as dysuria, urethral discharge, frequency or haematuria, is of self-evident importance. Likewise, aspects of the specific reproductive history which are of importance include any history of testicular maldescent, injury, torsion or epididymo-orchitis and any history of surgery which may have compromised the genital tract, such as herniorrhaphy, orchidopexy, drainage of hydrocoele, ligation of a varicocoele or bladder neck surgery. Other specific conditions may impair reproductive performance and a group of patients now requiring infertility investigations are those who have survived treatment for testicular or lymphatic malignancy and who may suffer the consequences of chemotherapy, radiotherapy or retroperitoneal lymph node dissection. A history of drug ingestion, including sulphasalazine, cimetidine or nitrofurantoin, or of exposure to other toxins, including alcohol and tobacco, known to impair spermatogenesis is important, as is the occupational history in terms of exposure to toxic chemicals and hyperthermia. The sexual history should endeavour to cover the adequacy of erectile function and if there is doubt, the presence of early morning and masturbatory erections should be enquired into in order to differentiate organic from psychogenic impotence. The occurrence of intravaginal ejaculation should be established and again, if there is doubt, the occurrence of nocturnal or masturbatory ejaculation sought, in addition to which the characteristics of ejaculation such as associated pain, prematurity or delay should be established. A number of couples attending infertility clinics will be infertile as a consequence of sexual dysfunction and a number of couples with sexual dysfunction will present to infertility clinics seeking primary help. Of course, any history of sexually transmitted disease and its

outcome is of note, as is a history of drug abuse or of other factors exposing the patient to high risk of infection with human immunodeficiency virus (HIV), due to the problems which this poses for the couple in terms of the risks of transmission and pregnancy and in terms of the problems presented to laboratory staff handling blood and semen samples.

Examination

The examination of the male partner should include a general medical examination covering height and weight, blood pressure and all of the major systems, including the respiratory system. The secondary sexual development of the patient must be assessed and signs of hypogonadism sought, including examination of the visual fields, to assess pituitary enlargement, and examination the sense of smell to exclude Kallman's syndrome if indicated. Gynaecomastia should be specifically examined for in this context. On examination of the abdomen, it is important to note the presence of scars or lymphadenopathy in the groins.

Turning to the urogenital examination, the penis is examined for evidence of phimosis, hypospadias or epispadias or the characteristic plaques of Peyronie's disease. The scrotum should be examined and the site of the testes determined, following which the testicular volume in millilitres should be determined with the aid of a Prader orchidometer (Fig. 22.7) and their consistency evaluated. It is known that a clear relationship exists between testicular volume and sperm production. Any tenderness of the gonads should be noted and the epididymides carefully palpated from caput to cauda, to exclude thickening, tenderness, cystic lesions, atrophy or absence of the epididymides. The vasa deferentia should next be palpated to establish that they are not congenitally absent and any thickening or induration noted. Scrotal swellings, such as hydrocoele or hernia, should be noted and the presence and grade of varicocoele established by asking the patient to perform Valsalva's manoeuvre. The inguinal regions should be inspected for hernia, scarring or the presence of lymphadenopathy. A rectal examination should be performed to assess the state of the prostate and seminal vesicles (although this seldom provides

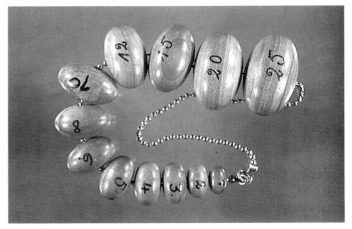

Fig. 22.7 Prader orchidometer for the assessment of testicular volume.

useful information and may be omitted unless ejaculatory duct obstruction or prostatovesciculitis is suspected).

The semen analysis

The conventional criteria of semen quality have changed little since van Leeuwenhoek first described spermatozoa in the human ejaculate in 1685. A standard semen analysis, performed according to clearly established guidelines promulgated by the WHO (1999) (Box 22.2), provides descriptive information concerning sperm number, motility and morphology, together with aspects of the physical characteristics of the ejaculate.

Sample collection and delivery

The sample should be collected after a minimum of 48 hours and not longer than 7 days sexual abstinence. Two semen samples should be collected for initial evaluation, not less than 7 days or more than 3 months apart. This is in order to take account of the effects of interejaculate variability and length of abstinence that are known to occur. The sample should be collected by masturbation into a clean wide-mouthed glass or plastic container and delivered to the laboratory within 1 hour of collection, if it is not possible for the patient to produce the sample at the laboratory. The sample should be evaluated by inspection and should normally be grey-opalescent and homogeneous, liquefying within 60 minutes. Abnormalities of appearance or failure of liquefaction are noted, following which the semen volume is measured. Abnormally low volumes are commonly due to incomplete sample collection, but may be due to ejaculatory dysfunction. A normal sample has a volume of 2.0 ml or more. The consistency or 'viscosity' of the liquefied sample should be evaluated and the pH of the sample should be in the range 7.2–7.8.

Microscopic evaluation

Motility. One hundred spermatozoa are examined at ×400–600, preferably using phase contrast optics, and their motility assessed and subjectively graded as rapid and linearly progressive motility (Grade 4), slower and sluggish linear or non-linear movement (Grade 3), non-progressive motility

Box 22.2   Normal values of semen analysis (WHO 1999)

Volume	2.0 ml or more
pH	7.2–7.8
Sperm concentration	20×10^6/ml more
Motility	50% or more with progressive motility (grade a + b) within 60 minutes of ejaculation
Morphology	Normal morphology below 15% is associated with reduced fertilization rates in the context of IVF
Viability	75% or more live
White blood cells	Fewer than 1×10^6/ml
MAR test	Fewer than 10% spermatozoa with adherent particles

(Grade 2) and immotile (Grade 1). The percentage of spermatozoa in each category is scored, WHO criteria requiring 50% or more cells with Grade 3 or 4 motility. Epithelial cells, spermatogenic cells and white blood cells may be seen, their concentration in a normal sample being less than 1×10^6/ml. If more are present, a specific stain should be performed for peroxidase-positive white blood cells. The adherence of spermatozoa to each other (agglutination) is noted and reported on an arbitrary scale. If the percentage of immotile spermatozoa exceeds 60%, the proportion of live spermatozoa may be determined.

Sperm concentration. This should be accurately determined by diluting a portion of the semen sample with a diluent to immobilize the spermatozoa and then loading this diluted preparation into a standard haemocytometer, the number of spermatozoa being counted by standard techniques and the result expressed as the concentration of spermatozoa (×10⁶/ml). This should be at least 20×10^6/ml.

Morphology. A smear slide of fresh semen is prepared, air dried and stained by the Giemsa, modified Papanicolau or Bryan–Leishman methods and examined by light microscopy for the various morphological abnormalities which are described. The result is expressed as the percentage of spermatozoa which are morphologically normal.

In addition to the above, a number of supplementary procedures may be undertaken in the evaluation of human semen, including semen culture, and biochemical evaluation for quantitation of acid phosphatases, citric acid and zinc (as markers of prostatic function), fructose and prostaglandins (as markers of seminal vesicular function) and free L-carnitine (as a marker of epididymal function). The WHO has issued a statement of the commonly accepted normal values for the parameters discussed above (Box 22.2), although making the point that it is preferable for each laboratory to establish its own normal ranges for each variable, by evaluating semen from individuals of proven fertility amongst its own local population.

Antisperm antibodies

The mixed agglutination reaction (MAR test) uses sheep red blood cells coated with rabbit antibodies to specific classes of human immunoglobulins, which will attach to motile sperm carrying immunoglobulins of the same class on their surface membrane (Bronsen et al 1984). This permits the detection of immunoglobulin gamma A, G or M on the surface of the sperm head or tail. The direct test uses washed sperm from the patient and the presence of surface-bound antibody, indicated by particulate binding in over 10% of spermatozoa, is considered to be a positive result. It depends on the availability of sufficient numbers of motile sperm in the patient's fresh semen sample and is currently the standard screening test in most laboratories. The indirect test uses decomplemented patient serum or seminal plasma which is incubated with motile donor sperm and is known as the tray agglutination test. Antisperm antibodies will bind to donor sperm and their presence is detected by attachment of particles to the sperm surface. The indirect test is therefore more convenient for screening larger numbers of patients. A positive screening test, however, must be substantiated by investigations to assess the biological significance of sperm antibody.

Additional diagnostic tests on semen

Although of central importance in the evaluation of the male partner of an infertile couple, the conventional criteria of semen quality are of a purely descriptive nature and there is widespread agreement that this information is of limited value in providing an assessment of the ability of a given individual to achieve a pregnancy. In an attempt to overcome this problem, numerous additional tests of sperm function have been evolved, including the study of human sperm movement characteristics, initially by time-exposure photomicrography and more recently by computer-assisted image analysis, the study of the penetration of human spermatozoa into cervical mucus and the zona-free hamster oocyte penetration test. This latter test examines a number of key aspects of human sperm function, including the ability of spermatozoa to capacitate, acrosome react and fuse with the vitelline membrane of the oocyte. More recently, biochemical tests, such as the measurement of reactive oxygen species production, have been developed. Although many of the advanced sperm function tests that have been described provide valuable diagnostic information in the hands of competent laboratories, they are typically difficult to perform and have poor predictive values when more widely applied. They are useful research tools and capable of identifying some of the specific causes for infertility. In clinical practice, in vitro fertilization remains the best test of sperm function and failed fertilization is probably best treated by intracytoplasmic sperm injection.

Hormone measurements

The measurement of plasma FSH is useful in distinguishing primary from secondary testicular failure and in identifying patients with obstructive azoospermia. In the presence of azoospermia or oligozoospermia, an elevated FSH, particularly with reduced testicular volume, is presumptive evidence of severe and usually irreversible seminiferous tubular damage. Low or undetectable FSH (usually associated with low LH and testosterone, with clinical evidence of androgen deficiency) is suggestive of hypogonadotrophism. Conversely, azoospermia with normal FSH and normal testicular volume usually indicates the presence of bilateral genital tract obstruction. Occasional exceptions to these general rules occur from time to time, as azoospermic men with the Sertoli cell only syndrome may be associated with normal FSH levels while some men with high FSH may have normal spermatogenesis.

Testosterone and LH measurements are indicated in the assessment of the infertile male when there is clinical suspicion of androgen deficiency, sex steroid abuse or steroid-secreting lesions such as functioning adrenal/testicular tumours. In men presenting with infertility, testosterone is usually within the normal range although some degree of Leydig cell dysfunction, as evidenced by statistically lower testosterone and higher LH compared to normal, is not uncommon. This may identify those who may be considered for androgen replacement, although this has no bearing on fertility. High LH and testosterone should raise the possibility of abnormalities in androgen receptors while low LH and testosterone suggest hypogonadotrophism.

Hyperprolactinaemia is not a frequent cause of male infertility, but prolactin measurement should be undertaken if there is clinical evidence of sexual dysfunction (particularly loss of interest in sex) or pituitary disease leading to secondary testicular failure. Oestradiol measurement is rarely indicated except in the presence of gynaecomastia, which is also a feature of Klinefelter's syndrome.

Dynamic tests of pituitary-testicular function such as GnRH, thyrotrophin-releasing hormone and human chorionic gonadotrophin stimulation generally do not add to the basal measurements already described. Bearing in mind the episodic nature of LH secretion, the diurnal variation in testosterone and the stress-related secretion of prolactin, it is usually sufficient to repeat their measurements in the morning under resting conditions if necessary.

Chromosome analysis

Chromosome karyotyping should be carried out in patients with azoospermia or severe oligospermia with reduced testicular volumes and elevated FSH. Cytogenetic abnormalities, by far the commonest being Klinefelter's syndrome, may be detected in about 10% of this group and are of importance if treatment by intracytoplasmic sperm injection is being contemplated.

Testicular biopsy

With the use of plasma FSH in recent years to differentiate between primary testicular failure and obstructive lesions, the need for testicular biopsy in the investigation of male infertility has largely been superseded, although it clearly has a place in the surgical retrieval of sperm for intracytoplasmic sperm injection. When genital tract obstruction is suspected, testicular biopsy is useful in confirming normal spermatogenesis and excluding spermatogenic arrest, but should only be undertaken under circumstances where sperm may be stored for subsequent use in assisted conception. When the clinical differentiation between spermatogenic failure and obstruction is uncertain (e.g. asymmetrical findings on examination between right and left testes or adnexae), scrotal exploration with testicular biopsy may be helpful, again with facilities for sperm storage to hand. Vasography during scrotal exploration is required to confirm the diagnosis of obstructed ejaculatory ducts. It is important to remember that even in primary testicular failure with small testes, elevated levels of FSH and a testicular biopsy showing Sertoli cell only syndrome, some areas of spermatogenesis may be present in the testis. There are many techniques for describing the appearances of a testicular biopsy but the combination of words and a qualitative assessment, using Johnsen scoring (Johnsen 1970), is useful. In the Johnsen score the histological features of spermatogenesis are scored from 1 to 10 (2, Sertoli cell only; 3, spermatogonia; 4, 5, spermatocytes; 6, 7, spermatids; 8, 9, 10, spermatozoa).

Treatment

The management of male infertility often remains a difficult and somewhat unsatisfactory experience for patients as well as doctors. Many patients present no recognizable or reversible aetiological factors for treatment and the doctor frequently fails to appreciate that normal semen values do not relate to fertility. In recent years there have been a number of advances which have made a significant impact on our therapeutic capabilities. It is important to improve semen quality and to treat those factors that impair fertility.

General measures

Although much has been written about the nature of general advice which should be given, objective evidence for its efficacy in improving fertility is sadly lacking. Commonly raised issues include avoidance of stress, a healthy diet and exercise. Recreational drugs such as cigarettes, excessive alcohol consumption and cannabis should certainly be withdrawn or reduced if possible. Occupational or social situations that may chronically elevate testicular temperature should be avoided. Medications that interfere with fertility, such as nitrofurantoin, anabolic steroids, sex steroids and anticonvulsants, should be avoided if possible. In patients with inflammatory bowel disease treated by sulphasalazine, changing treatment to 5-aminosalicylic acid removes the toxic agent, sulphapyridine, and leads to a rapid recovery of fertility without deterioration in disease activity. Although testicular function may improve in patients with chronic renal failure after successful transplantation, fertility impairment may be perpetuated by the continued use of immunosuppressive agents.

Medical treatment

Perhaps the most important point to stress is that empirical treatments for idiopathic oligozoospermia, such as anti-oestrogens, androgens, bromocriptine and kinin-enhancing drugs have not been shown to be effective in the treatment of men with abnormalities of semen quality and they should not be used. Although free radicals undoubtedly have a role to play in male infertility (Aitken et al 1989) few centres measure them as a routine and there is as yet no evidence that the antioxidant treatments which are used on an empirical basis are effective. Endocrine treatment is effective only in the presence of specific endocrine disturbances, which are rare.

Management of gonadotrophin deficiency. Patients with gonadotrophin deficiency due to acquired conditions and, to a lesser extent, those with partial GnRH deficiency usually respond to human chorionic gonadotrophin (1000–2500 iu once or twice weekly) alone for 6–12 months (Burger & Baker 1982). During this time the rise in testosterone will virilize the patient and the testes will usually increase in size. If there are no sperm in the ejaculate at the end of 12 months, FSH should be added, usually in the form of human menopausal gonadotrophin which contains both FSH and LH. This graded approach may take up to 2 years before one can ascertain if spermatogenesis is established or not. There is limited experience with recombinant FSH as yet, but developments such as longer-acting gonadotrophin preparations might be of clinical value in this context.

The treatment outcome of gonadotrophin induction of spermatogenesis is relatively successful, with up to 90% showing some degree of spermatogenesis and up to 70% can be expected to achieve pregnancies (Büchter et al 1998). Previous treatment with testosterone does not compromise the response to subsequent exogenous gonadotrophin, but there is a clear relationship between pretreatment testicular volume and duration of treatment required.

In patients with more profound degrees of GnRH deficiency, it might be anticipated that the most suitable form of replacement to induce maximal testicular growth and development is to emulate the physiological mode of pulsatile GnRH stimulation of the pituitary and, in turn, the testes. This has been made possible by the development of battery-driven portable infusion minipumps, which can automatically deliver a desired dose of GnRH subcutaneously at a set time interval, e.g. 5–20 µg every 120 minutes. While this form of treatment is effective (Büchter et al 1998), it is expensive and inconvenient to the patient.

Management of genital tract infection. Infection of the male genital tract should be treated if present, but there is no evidence that this will improve fertility. Symptomatic urethritis responds to treatment with the appropriate antibiotics. Chronic infection of the male genital tract is more difficult to diagnose and the presence of pus cells in the semen only indicates an infection in some patients. An alkaline pH (greater than 8.0) may occur in prostatitis due to decreased secretion of acid phosphatase by the prostate. Repeated growth on culture of the same organisms is probably of significance as is the finding of organisms during a modified Stamey test (Meares & Stamey 1972) where the semen culture replaces the culture of expressed prostatic secretions. If treatment is felt to be warranted, the antibiotics chosen to treat prostatoseminal vesiculitis (such as doxycycline, erythromycins, cephalosporins or oflaxacin) should be secreted by the male accessory glands and treatment should be continued for 4–12 weeks depending on the chronicity of the infection. In longer courses of treatment it is customary to rotate the antibiotics, but overall the current tendency is towards a shorter duration (6 weeks) of treatment consisting of two antibiotics each of which is taken for 3 weeks.

Management of antisperm antibodies. The presence of antisperm antibodies may be a cause of male factor infertility. The use of systemic corticosteroids for treatment of antisperm antibodies remains controversial and can only be recommended in the context of further research as the evidence of benefit is conflicting and there are potentially serious side-effects. Commonly, treatment by assisted conception is recommended.

Erectile failure. The inability of the man to obtain vaginal penetration may be overcome by various pharmacological approaches and this is particularly useful in men with neurological problems or with performance anxiety. If intracavernous agents are used, the physician should be familiar with the technique and avoid the tragedy of a priapism. Papaverine was for many years the drug of choice but this has been superseded by alprostadil, a prostaglandin E_1 preparation, and more recently by oral sildenafil. In those men with organic impotence, the implantation of a penile prosthesis may provide a solution to the problem.

Ejaculatory failure. Absent emission or retrograde ejaculation due to sympathetic denervation may respond to sympathomimetic drugs. The first choice is desipramine (50 mg on alternate days) for its noradrenaline reuptake blocking action. Ephedrine 30 mg twice daily, brompheniramine maleate 8 mg twice daily or imipramine 25 mg three times daily may also be tried. It is always worthwhile trying desipramine in those men with a diabetic autonomic neuropathy. Urine inhibits sperm motility and for this reason spermatozoa should be separated from the urine as soon as possible and used for artificial insemination or assisted conception. Surgical reconstruction of the bladder neck is rarely required.

Surgical treatments

Surgery on the male genital tract should be carried out only in centres where there are appropriate facilities and trained staff. Vasectomy reversal is an effective treatment for men who want to reverse their sterilization and surgical correction of epididymal blockage can be considered in cases of obstructive azoospermia. Testicular biopsy should be performed only in the context of a tertiary service where there are facilities for sperm recovery and cryostorage.

Relief of obstruction. Obstructive lesions of the seminal tract should be suspected in azoospermia or severe oligo-zoospermia with normally sized testes (greater than 4 cm in length or 15–20 ml in volume) and with normal plasma FSH levels. Where surgery is undertaken, it is convenient to explore and biopsy the testes, perform vasography and correct any obstruction that is identified, under the same general anaesthetic. A fuller account of the indications, techniques and outcomes of surgical treatments of male infertility may be found elsewhere (Hull et al 1985, Pryor et al 1997).

Epididymal obstruction. The results of reconstructive surgery on the epididymis are varied and depend upon the cause and duration of obstruction and the expertise of the surgeon. Congenital blockages and those that might be due to pink disease (Hendry et al 1990) have poor outcome, as do blockages resulting from tuberculous or chlamydial infections. The overall patency rate would appear to be about 10–15% of operations, as in many patients there is a great deal of scarring and the epididymis is filled with inspissated material. The best results are achieved when there is localized postgonococcal obstruction in the cauda epididymis and in these instances sperm may appear in 50% of ejaculates after surgery. A microsurgical technique would appear to give a 10% improvement in patency rates. Spermatozoa acquire motility as they pass through the epididymis and higher pregnancy rates occur when the blockage is in the distal part of the epididymis (Schoysman & Bedford 1986).

Vasal obstruction. Vasal obstruction is less common in infertility practice and is treated by vasovasostomy. Many techniques are described but an end-to-end one-layer anastomosis with 6–0 sutures is simple and effective. Vasal obstruction most commonly occurs following vasectomy and after vasovasostomy patency is to be expected in 80–90% of men with a conception rate of 40–50% in 1 year. Magnification is desirable and the use of an operating microscope for vasovasostomy is excellent training for the more difficult tubulovasostomy that is necessary in epididymal obstruction. The prognosis is worse for those men with a long interval between the vesectomy and reversal, but time does not prohibit any attempt to operate. The age of the female partner is of importance with regard to conception rates.

Ejaculatory duct obstruction. This is an uncommon cause of obstruction and is readily diagnosed by a low volume of semen, azoospermia or extreme oligozoospermia and an acid pH in a man with palpable vasa. Müllerian duct cysts are amenable to treatment (Pryor et al 1997) with sperm appearing in the ejaculate of 80% of men and conception in 33% of female partners. Other forms of ejaculatory duct obstruction do less well and are probably best treated by sperm retrieval.

Varicocoele treatment. As discussed above, this remains an area of considerable controversy. Varicocoele is a common finding amongst an infertility clinic population. In trying to interpret the available evidence and decide whether and when to treat, it is wise to remember the many other factors that have a considerable bearing on a couple's fertility. There is no evidence to suggest that treating varicocoele in the presence of normal semen quality is beneficial. Available evidence does suggest that treatment in men with oligozoospermia will improve semen quality, but evidence on whether this will result in pregnancy remains unclear, probably due to the heterogeneous populations studied. It is clear that any benefit is not substantial and in many cases, particularly where the age of the female partner is above 35, the duration of the couple's infertility prolonged or the deficit in semen quality severe, then assisted conception techniques have more to offer.

Assisted conception and male infertility

Early developments in *in vitro* fertilization (IVF) focused on couples with female factor infertility and particularly women suffering from bilateral tubal occlusion. Conventional IVF rapidly became established as an effective treatment option for couples with tubal disease and with unexplained infertility but it soon became apparent that it yielded generally poor pregnancy rates for couples with male factor infertility. Tournaye et al (1992), for example, compared IVF and embryo transfer (IVF-ET) in a group of couples with male infertility and a similar group with tubal infertility. In cases of male infertility, more oocytes were recovered but fewer oocytes were fertilized, fewer embryo transfers were performed, the average number of embryos per transfer was lower and the total pregnancy rate per cycle was also lower at 12.8 versus 22.9%. They concluded that male infertility could be treated by IVF-ET but that the results were disappointing when compared to a control group with normal spermatozoa. Although there was much discussion in the literature on the fine tuning of the IVF procedure for couples with problems in the male partner, management options for couples with poor semen quality remained very limited until the breakthrough of effective microassisted fertilization in 1992 (Palermo et al 1992). (For review, see Campbell & Irvine 2000.)

Micromanipulation techniques

Partial zona dissection (PZD) was the first micromanipulation technique studied in animal models with clinical intent and early reports in human practice of clinical pregnancies were encouraging, suggesting that monospermic fertilization and cleavage rates could be doubled by these appraoches. However, concerns existed over the risk of polyspermy, along with doubts about appropriate case selection. Subzonal insemination (SUZI) involves the injection of spermatozoa into the privitelline space and again, initial reports of its use were encouraging, although other groups found the technique to be less successful. The developments in human microassisted fertilization culminated in intracytoplasmic sperm injection (ICSI), with the first human pregnancies resulting from this technique being described by the Brussels group (Palermo et al 1992). This approach involves injection of a single spermatozoon directly into the cytoplasm of the oocyte through the intact zona pellucida and it very soon became apparent that this technique produced superior results to PZD or SUZI, with pregnancy rates of 22% per started cycle being reported (Abdalla et al 1995, van Steirteghem et al 1993). Indeed, such has been the success of ICSI that some commentators suggest that it might be considered the treatment of choice for all cases where in vitro conception is indicated.

A meta-analysis has concluded that for couples with normal semen there is no evidence of any benefit, either in fertilization rates per retrieved oocyte or in pregnancy rates, between ICSI and conventional IVF. In contrast, for couples with borderline semen, ICSI results in higher fertilization rates than IVF and couples with very poor semen will have better fertilization outcomes with ICSI than with SUZI or additional IVF (van Rumste et al 2000).

ICSI with epididymal spermatozoa.
Initially, clinical ICSI was used in the treatment of couples in whom the male partner had substantially abnormal semen quality, but it was not long before the technology was applied to the significant numbers of men who present with no sperm in their ejaculates. Amongst men with obstructive azoospermia, attention focused on spermatozoa derived from the epididymis. The first pregnancies achieved with epididymal sperm were described using conventional IVF. However, fertilization rates were low, so whilst it was established that sperm from the epididymis had a degree of functional competence, this was limited. Initially, the use of SUZI was described but this was rapidly replaced in clinical practice by ICSI (Liu et al 1994, Silber et al 1994), which achieved very statisfactory success rates.

As a consequence of the successful use of epididymal spermatozoa in ICSI, techniques have been described to facilitate the surgical retrieval of spermatozoa. The major approaches include microsurgical epididymal sperm aspiration (MESA) and percutaenous epididymal sperm aspiration (PESA). MESA involves a formal scrotal exploration, is commonly performed under general anaesthetic and hence is a significant surgical intervention. PESA is a widely used technique which is less invasive, can be performed under local anaesthesia and can be undertaken repeatedly. However, PESA provides less diagnostic information and the yield of spermatozoa may be lower, with one recent review suggesting that at least 20% of attempts at PESA are unsuccessful and require resort to MESA (Girardi & Schlegel 1999).

ICSI with testicular spermatozoa.
In contrast to the position in men with obstructive azoospermia, amongst men with non-obstructive azoospermia attention naturally focuses on the testis as a site for sperm recovery. With the availability of ICSI, it has become clear that non-obstructive azoospermia is a very heterogeneous condition and that testicular histology is similarly heterogeneous, with foci of apparently normal spermatogenesis adjacent to seminiferous tubules devoid of germ cells. Surgical sperm recovery from men with non-obstructive azoospermia has become a routine part of clinical infertility practice and as with the epididymis, cryopreservation of testis-derived spermatozoa has also become routine. A recent review concluded that surgical sperm recovery would be successful in some 48% of men with non-obstructive azoospermia. Undoubtedly one of the major problems confronting the process of surgical sperm recovery from men with non-obstructive azoospermia is the fact that there are currently no good predictors of which patients will have sperm recovered successfully and which will not. Against this background, a number of groups have argued that surgical recovery of sperm from the testis coupled with cryopreservation should precede ovarian stimulation in the female partner.

For those men in whom mature spermatozoa cannot be recovered, there is currently interest in the possibility of using less mature cells, commonly elongating or round spermatids, to achieve fertilization. Work in animal models has suggested that this may be a viable approach and there are a number of clinical case reports in the literature. At the present time, however, uncertainties over the safety and efficacy of this approach confine its use to properly designed clinical trials.

Success rates of ICSI.
ICSI has become well established as an effective form of treatment for couples with male factor infertility. In the last year for which data are available (1997–98) the United Kingdom's Human Fertilization and Embryology Authority reported 9295 cycles of ICSI alongside 24 889 cycles of IVF; in other words, some 27% of assisted conception treatment in the UK is for severe male factor infertility. In the same year, the reported live birth rate for ICSI was 20.7% per cycle compared to 14.9% for IVF. In keeping with the major issues in assisted conception in general, the multiple birth rate was high at over 25% and the age of the female partner was a major determinant of success, with a woman in her early 30s achieving a 20–25% per cycle success rate, dropping to 5% or less for a woman over the age of 40.

Outcomes of ICSI.
Given that ICSI is effective, is it also safe? The rapid development of microassisted conception techniques and the widespread use of ICSI in alleviating male infertility have raised concerns about the health of the offspring. ICSI, by directly injecting individual spermatozoa into a mature oocyte, bypasses the natural physiological processes of normal sperm selection, raising concerns over the potential risk of congenital malformations and genetic defects in children born after ICSI.

Without doubt, the most thorough and detailed follow-up studies of ICSI offspring have been those orchestrated by the Brussels group (Bonduelle et al 1999) who have undertaken a prospective follow-up study of 1987 children born after ICSI, aiming to compile data on karyotypes, congenital malformations, growth parameters and developmental milestones. They were able to collect data on 1699, 91 and 118 children born after ICSI with ejaculated, epididymal and testicular spermatozoa respectively, as well as on 79 children born from cryopreserved ICSI embryos. 1.66% of karyotypes determined by prenatal diagnosis were abnormal de novo (nine each of autosomal and sex chromosomal aberrations) and 0.92% were inherited structural aberrations. Most of these were transmitted from the father. Forty-six major malformations (2.3%) were observed at birth. Seven malformations, observed by prenatal ultrasound, were terminated. Twenty-one (1.1%) stillbirths, including four with major malformations, occurred later than 20 weeks of pregnancy.

Several other large cohort studies have been reported and as the database of ICSI offspring grows larger, the available evidence on the short-term health of these offspring is generally reassuring. It is important, however, to appreciate the important role that a genetic aetiology plays in the origins of much male subfertility and the ability of ICSI to promote the transgenerational transmission of genetic defects causing gametogenic failure. The significantly increased risk of chromosomal abnormalities in men with impaired semen quality is easily managed by the appropriate investigation and counselling which are required prior to treatment. It is less easy to be certain how to respond to the available evidence on microdeletions of the Y chromosome in men with severely impaired semen quality. The strength of the association between Y chromosome deletions and severely impaired semen quality is impressive and it is increasingly suggested that these lesions may result in progression from oligozoospermia to azoospermia over time. A recent study (Pryor et al 1997) found deletions in 7% of infertile men and in only 2% of normal men, but observed no clear relationships between the size and location of the deletions and the severity of the spermatogenic failure. Moreover, it is clear that these genetic deletions, if present, can be transmitted to offspring via ICSI. On the basis of this evidence, some authorities now advocate screening of men for Y chromosome microdeletions prior to ICSI and advocate testing of offspring and reproductive monitoring for those found to have inherited deletions.

CHANGES IN MALE REPRODUCTIVE HEALTH

During the past two decades, a number of reports have raised serious concerns about the development of reproductive problems in animals and man. There have been controversial reports of changes in human semen quality (Auger et al 1995, Carlsen et al 1992, Irvine 1996), alongside reports of an increasing incidence of congenital malformations of the male genital tract, such as cryptorchidism and hypospadias (Ansell et al 1992, Kallen et al 1986) and of an increasing incidence of testicular cancer (Adami et al 1994, Hoff Wanderas et al 1995). However, there is controversy over whether or not these reported changes in male reproductive health are genuine and if so, what the causes and implications are.

Testicular cancer

Although many of the changes seen in male reproductive health are controversial, there seems little argument that testis cancer is increasing in frequency, with unexplained increases in the age-standardized incidence being observed in Europe (Adami et al 1994, Bergstrom et al 1996, Hernes et al 1996) and the United States (Devesa et al 1995, Zheng et al 1996).

There would appear to be substantial geographical variation in both the incidence of testis cancer and in the observed rate of increase (Adami et al 1994). Of note, this geographical variation may be linked with that seen in semen quality: testis cancer is four times more common in Denmark where studies have revealed rather low sperm counts (Jensen et al 1996) than in Finland where semen quality appears to be better (Vierula et al 1996). Interestingly, the observed increases, both in Europe and the USA, would appear to be birth cohort related (Bergstorm et al 1996, Zheng et al 1996). Bergstrom and colleagues (1996) evaluated data from Denmark, Norway, Sweden, East Germany, Finland and Poland, including data on over 30 000 cases of testis cancer from 1945–89 in men aged 20–84. They found considerable regional variation in both the incidence of testis cancer and the observed rate of increase, ranging from a 2.3% increase annually in Sweden to 5.2% annually in East Germany. In all six countries, birth cohort was a stronger determinant of testis cancer risk than calendar time, such that men born in 1965 had a risk of testis cancer that was 3.9 times (95% CI 2.7–5.6; Sweden) to 11.4 times (95% CI 8.3–15.5; East Germany) higher than for men born in 1905.

A recent study has looked in detail at the risk of testicular cancer in subfertile men (Moller & Skakkebaek 1999), using a population-based case control design to study 514 men with cancer and 720 controls. They found that paternity was associated with a reduced risk of testis cancer (relative risk 0.63, 95% CI 0.47–0.85), that prior to the diagnosis of testis cancer, cases tended to have fewer children than expected for their age (RR 1.98, 95% CI 1.43–2.75) and suggested that these observations are consistent with the hypothesis that testicular cancer and male subfertility share important aetiological factors.

Cryptorchidism and congenital malformations of the male genital tract

The incidence of congenital malformation of the male genital tract may also be changing, with increases observed in the prevalence of cryptorchidism and hypospadias (Editorial 1985). Cryptorchidism, for example, has increased by as much as 65–77% over recent decades in the UK (Ansell et al 1992). In contrast, some data from the USA have tended to suggest that rates of cryptorchidism have not changed (Berkowitz et al 1993), although one recent large study from the USA reported that rates of hypospadias have doubled from the 1970s to the 1980s (Paulozzi et al 1997). Here too, though, regional differences have been observed, although the data are perhaps less robust than is the case with testicular cancer. In one multicentre study of 8122 boys from seven malformation surveillance systems around the world, Kallen et al concluded that, even when differences in ascertainment were taken into account, true geographical differences exist in the prevalence of hypospadias at birth (Kallen et al 1986).

Changing semen quality: historical data on normal men

In 1992, Carlsen et al reawakened concern over the possibility of secular trends in semen quality, publishing a meta-analysis of data on semen quality in normal men. The authors undertook a systematic review of available data on semen quality in normal men, published since 1930. Standard techniques applicable to meta-analysis were used to identify relevant papers and care was taken to exclude data on infertile couples, men selected on the basis of their semen quality and data generated using non-classical approaches to semen analysis. Data was obtained on 14 947 men, published in 61 papers between 1938 and 1990. Using weighted linear regression, the authors observed a decline in average ejaculate volume from 3.40 ml in 1940 to 2.75 ml in 1990. A similar analysis for sperm concentration suggested an apparent decline from 113×10^6/ml in 1940 to 66×10^6/ml in 1990, along with a decline in the proportion of men with a sperm concentration above 100×10^6/ml. Predictably, the central message of this meta-analysis, that sperm counts had declined by about 50% over the past 50 years, attracted enormous attention and generated much controversy.

Since the publication of the Carlsen meta-analysis, several papers have presented contemporary analyses of retrospective data. Unfortunately, the available data still fail to reach a conclusion on whether or not there is any secular trend in semen quality; at least as many studies have reported evidence of deteriorating semen quality as have reported evidence of no change. Most recently, a very careful reanalysis of the historical data (Carlsen et al 1992) on semen quality in normal men has been published (Swan et al 1997). These workers used multiple linear regression models, controlling for abstinence time, age, the proportion of the sample with proven fertility, specimen collection method, study goal and geographical location to examine regional differences and the interaction between region and year of publication. Using a linear model, they found that sperm concentrations and the rate of decline in sperm concentration differed significantly across regions. They concluded that there was evidence of a decline in sperm concentrations in the United States of -1.5×10^6/ml/year (95% CI -1.9 to -1.1), and in Europe of -3.13×10^6/ml/year (95% CI -4.96 to -1.30), but not in non-Western countries. Results were similar when other (non-linear) models were used and these workers concluded that their results were unlikely to be due to either confounding or selection bias (Swan et al 1997). More recently, the same group has reanalysed the data included in the Carlsen paper, together with 47 English language studies published in 1934–96 (Swan et al 2000). They concluded that the average decline in sperm count was virtually unchanged from that reported previously by Carlsen et al (slope = -0.94 vs -0.93). The slopes in the three geographic groupings were also similar to those we reported earlier. These results were consistent with those of Carlsen et al, suggesting that the reported trends are not dependent on the particular studies included by Carlsen et al and that the observed trends previously reported for 1938–90 are also seen in data from 1934 to 1996.

Whilst the available evidence is inconclusive and circumstantial, its weight is considerable and at the very least, it should raise concerns that deserve to be addressed by properly designed, co-ordinated and funded research. Delay may compromise the fertility and reproductive health of future generations (de Kretser 1996, Irvine et al 1996).

KEY POINTS

1. The male partner should normally have two semen analyses performed during the initial investigation (B). Further investigations of the male partner should be preceded by a clinical examination including an assessment of secondary sexual characteristics and testicular size (B).
2. In considering the results of semen analysis for the individual couple, it is important to take into account the duration of infertility, the woman's age and the previous pregnancy history (B).
3. Sperm function tests are specialized tests and should not be used in the routine investigation of the infertile couple (C).
4. Men with poor-quality sperm should be advised to wear loose-fitting underwear and trousers and avoid occupational or social situations that might cause testicular hyperthermia (B).
5. Antioestrogens, androgens, bromocriptine and kinin-enhancing drugs have not been shown to be effective in the treatment of men with abnormalities of semen quality (A). The use of systemic corticosteroids for treatment of antisperm antibodies can only be recommended in the context of further research as the evidence of benefit is conflicting and there are potentially serious side-effects (C).
6. Where a diagnosis of hypogonadotrophic hypogonadism is made in the male partner the use of gonadotrophin drugs is an effective fertility treatment (B).
7. There is evidence that semen quality and pregnancy rates may improve in oligozoospermic men after treatment of a clinically apparent varicocoele (A).
8. Intrauterine insemination with or without ovarian stimulation is an effective treatment where the man has abnormalities of semen quality, but it has to be remembered that the pregnancy rates even after treatment remain very low (A).
9. Prior to treatment by ICSI, couples should undergo appropriate investigations including the male partner's karyotype, both to establish a diagnosis and to enable informed discussion about the implications of treatment (C)
10. Testing for Y chromosome microdeletions should not be regarded as a routine investigation prior to ICSI. However, it is likely that a significant proportion of male infertility results from abnormalities of genes on the Y choromosome (C).

Adapted from the Royal College of Obstetricians and Gynaecologists *Evidence-based infertility guidelines* (1999). The letter in parentheses indicates the level of evidence: (A) based on randomized controlled trials; (B) based on other robust experimental or observational trials; (C) based on more limited evidence.

REFERENCES

Abdalla, H, Leonard T, Pryor J, Everett D 1995 Comparison of SUZI and ICSI for severe male factor. Human Reproduction 10:2941–2944
Adami HO, Bergstrom R, Mohner M et al 1994 Testicular cancer in nine Northern European countries. International Journal of Cancer 59:33–38

Aitken RJ, Clarkson JS, Hargreave TB, Irvine DS, Wu FCW 1989 Analysis of the relationship between defective sperm function and the generation of reactive oxygen species in cases of oligozoospermia. Journal of Andrology 10(3):214–220

Aitken RJ, Best FSM, Richardson DW et al 1982a An analysis of sperm function in cases of unexplained infertility: conventional criteria, movement characteristics, and fertilizing capacity. Fertility and Sterility 38:212–221

Aitken RJ, Best FSM, Richardson DW, Djahanbakhch O, Templeton A, Lee MM 1982b An analysis of semen quality and sperm function in cases of oligozoospermia. Fertility and Sterility 38:705–711

Anderson RA, Sharpe RM 2000 Regulation of inhibin production in the human male and its clinical applications. International Journal of Andrology 23(3):136–144

Ansell PE, Bennet V, Bull D et al 1992 Cryptorchidism: a prospective study of 7500 consecutive male births, 1984–8. Archives of Disease in Childhood 67:892–899

Auger J, Kunstmann JM, Czyglik F, Jouannet P 1995 Decline in semen quality among fertile men in Paris during the past 20 years. New England Journal of Medicine 332:281–285

Bagatell CJ, Bremner WJ 1996 Androgens in men—uses and abuses. New England Journal of Medicine 334(11):707–714

Baker HW, Burger HG, de Kretser DM, Hudson B, Rennie GC, Straffon WG 1985 Testicular vein ligation and fertility in men with varicoceles. British Medical Journal 291:1678–1680

Bergstrom R, Adami HO, Mohner M et al 1996 Increase in testicular cancer incidence in six European countries: a birth cohort phenomenon. Journal of the National Cancer Institute 88:727–733

Berkowitz GS, Lapinski RH, Dolgin SE, Gazella JG, Bodian CA, Holzman IR 1993 Prevalence and natural history of cryptorchidism. Pediatrics 92:44–49

Bonduelle M, Camus M, de Vos A et al 1999 Seven years of intracytoplasmic sperm injection and follow-up of 1987 subsequent children. Human Reproduction 14 (suppl):243–264

Bronsen RA, Cooper GW, Rosenfeld D 1984 Sperm antibodies: their role in infertility. Fertility and Sterility 42:171–183

Büchter D, Behre HM, Kleisch S, Nieschlag E 1998 Pulsatile GnRH or human chorionic gonadotrophin/human menopausal gonadotrophin as effective treatment for men with hypogonadotrophic hypogonadism: a review of 42 cases. Clincial Endocrinology 139:298–303

Burger HG, Baker HWG 1982 Therapeutic considerations and results of gonadotrophic treatment in male hypogonadotrophic hypogonadism. Annals of the New York Academy of Science 438:447–453

Campbell AJ, Irvine DS 2000 Male infertility and intracytoplasmic sperm injection (ICSI). British Medical Bulletin 56(3):616–629

Carlsen E, Giwercman A, Keiding N, Skakkebæk NE 1992 Evidence for decreasing quality of semen during past 50 years. British Medical Journal 305:609–613

Chandley A 1994 Chromosomes. In: Hargreave T (Ed) Male infertility. Springer-Verlag, London

Comhaire FH, de Kretser D, Farley TMM et al 1987 Towards more objectivity in diagnosis and management of male infertility. Results of a World Health Organization Multicentre Study. International Journal of Andrology 10(S7):1–53

Cummins JM, Jequier Am 1994 Treating male infertility needs more clinical andrology, not less. Human Reproduction 9:1214–1219

Cummins JM, Jequier AM 1995 Concerns and recommendations for intracytoplasmic sperm injection (ICSI) treatment. Human Reproduction 10(suppl 1):138–143

Damonte P, Ciprandi G, Giberti C, Martorana G 1984 Incidence of idiopathic varicocele in young men of military age. IRCS Medical Science 12:176

de Kretser DM 1996 Declining sperm counts. Environmental chemicals may be to blame. British Medical Journal 312:457–458

Devesa SS, Blot WJ, Stone BJ, Miller BA, Tarone RE, Fraumeni Jf Jr 1995 Recent cancer trends in the United States. Journal of the National Cancer Institute 87:175–182

Dym M 1977 In: Weiss L, Greep RO (eds) Histology. McGraw Hill, New York

Editorial 1985 An increasing incidence of cryptorchidism and hypospadias. Lancet i:1311

Fawcett DW 1975 The mammalian spermatozoa: a review. Developmental Biology 44:394–436

Girardi SK, Schlegel PN 1999 Techniques for sperm recovery in assisted reproduction. Reproductive Medicine Review 7:131–139

Grudzinskas JG, Yovich LJ (eds) 1995 Gametes – the spermatozoon. Cambridge Reviews in Human Reproduction. Cambridge University Press, Cambridge

Hargreave TB 1994 Varicocele. In: Hargreave TB (ed) Male Infertility. Springer-Verlag, London

Hargreave TB 2000 Genetic basis of male fertility. British Medical Bulletin 56:650–671

Hendry W, Levison DA, Parkinson MC, Parslow JM, Royle MG 1990 Testicular obstruction: clinicopathological studies. Annals of the Royal College of Surgeons England 72:396–407

Hernes EH, Harstad K, Fossa SD 1996 Changing incidence and delay of testicular cancer in southern Norway (1981–1992). European Urology 30:349–357

Hoff Wanderas, E, Tretli S, Fossa SD 1995 Trends in incidence of testicular cancer in Norway 1955–1992. European Journal of Cancer Part A 31:2044–2048

Hull MGR, Glazener CMA, Kelly NJ et al 1985 Population study of causes, treatment and outcome of infertility. British Medical Journal 291:1693–1697

Irvine DS 1996 Is the human testis still an organ at risk? British Medical Journal 312:1557–1558

Irvine DS 1997 Declining sperm quality, a review of facts and hypotheses. In: Van Steirteghem A, Devroey P, Tournaye H (eds) male infertility. Baillière Tindall, London

Irvine DS 1998 Epidemiology and aetiology of male infertility. Human Reproduction 13 (suppl 1):33–44

Irvine DS, Aitken RJ 1994 Seminal fluid analysis and sperm function testing. Endocrinology and Metabolism Clinics of North America 23:725–748

Irvine DS, Cawood EHH, Richardson DW, MacDonald E, Aitken RJ 1996 Evidence of deteriorating semen quality in the UK: birth cohort study in 577 men in Scotland over 11 years. British Medical Journal 312:471–476

Jensen TK, Giwercman A, Carlsen E, Scheike T, Skakkebaek NE 1996 Semen quality among members of organic food associations in Zealand, Denmark. Lancet 347:1844

Johnsen SG 1970 Testicular biopsy score count – a method for registration of spermatogenesis in human testes: normal values and results in 335 hypogonadal males. Hormones 1:2–25

Kallen B, Bertollini R, Castilla E et al 1986 A joint international study on the epidemiology of hypospadias. Acta Paediatrica Scandinavica 324(suppl):1–52

Kruger TF, Acosta AA, Simmons KF, Swanson RJ, Matta JF, Oehninger S 1988 Predictive value of abnormal sperm morphology in vitro fertilization. Fertility and Sterility 49:112–117

Kruger TF, du Toit TC, Franken DR, Menkveld R, Lombard CJ 1995 Sperm morphology: assessing the agreement between the manual method (strict criteria) and the sperm morphology analyser IVOS. Fertility and Sterility 63:134–141

Laven JS, Haans LC, Mali WP, te Velde ER, Wensing CJ, Eimers JM 1992 Effects of varicocele treatment in adolescents: a randomized study. Fertility and Sterility 58:756–762

Liu J, Lissens W, Silber SJ, Devroey P, Liebaers I, van Steirteghem A 1994 Birth after preimplantation diagnosis of the cystic fibrosis delta F508 mutation by polymerase chain reaction in human embryos resulting from intracytoplasmic sperm injection with epididymal sperm. Journal of the American Medical Association 272:1858–1860

Madgar I, Weissenberg R, Lunenfeld B, Karasik A, Goldwasser B 1995 Controlled trial of high spermatic vein ligation for varicocele in infertile men. Fertility and Sterility 63:120–124

Mahmoud AM, Goemaere S, de Bacquer D, Comhaire FH, Kaufman JM 2000 Serum inhibin B levels in community-dwelling elderly men. Clinical Endocrinology 53:141–147

Matsumoto AM, Paulsen CA, Bremner WJ 1984 Stimulation of sperm production by human luteinizing hormone in gonadotrophin-suppressed normal men. Journal of Clinical Endocrinology and Metabolism 59:882–887

Meares EM Jr, Stamey TA 1972 The diagnosis and management of bacterial prostatitis. British Journal of Urology 44(2):185–179

Meriggiola MC, Bremner WJ 1997 Progestin-androgen combination regimens for male contraception. Journal of Andrology 18:240–244

Mieusset R, Bujan L 1995 Testicular heating and its possible contributions to male infertility: a review. International Journal of Andrology 18:169–184

Moller H, Skakkebaek NE 1999 Risk of testicular cancer in subfertile men: case-control study. British Medical Journal 318:559–562

Morishima A, Grumbach MM, Simpson ER, Fisher C, Qin K 1995 Aromatase deficiency in male and female siblings caused by a novel mutation and the physiological role of estrogens. Journal of Clinical Endocrinology and Metabolism 80:3689–3698

Mortimer D 1995 Sperm transport in the female genital tract. In: Grudzinskas JG, Yovich LJ (eds) Gametes – the spermatozoon. Cambridge Reviews in Human Reproduction. Cambridge University Press, Cambridge

Nieschlag E, Hertle L, Fischedick A, Behre HM 1995 Treatment of varicocele: counselling as effective as occlusion of the vena spermatica. Human Reproduction 10:347–353

Palermo G, Joris H, Devroey P, van Steirteghem AC 1992 Pregnancies after intracytoplasmic injection of single spermatozoon into an oöcyte. Lancet 340:17–18

Paradisi R, Pession A, Bellavia, E, Focacci M, Flamingni C 1995 Characterization of human sperm antigens reacting with antisperm antibodies from autologous sera and seminal plasma in a fertile population. Journal of Reproductive Immunology 28:61–73

Paulozzi LJ, Erikson JD, Jackson RJ 1997 Hypospadias trends in two US surveillance systems. Pediatrics 100:831–834

Pryor JL, Kent-First M, Muallem A et al 1997 Microdeletions in the Y choromsome of infertile men. New England Journal of Medicine 336(8):534–539

Rowe PJ, Comhaire FH, Hargreave TB, Mellows HJ 1993 WHO manual for the standardized investigation and diagnosis of the infertile couple. Cambridge University Press, Cambridge

Sandler B 1954 Recovery from sterility after mumps orchitis. British Medical Journal 2:795

Saunders PTK 1998 Oestrogen receptor beta (ERb). Reviews of Reproduction 3:164–171

Schmidt L, Münster K, Helm P 1995 Infertility and the seeking of infertility treatment in a representative population. British Journal of Obstetrics and Gynaecology 102:978–984

Schoysman RJ, Bedford JM 1986 The role of the human epididymis in sperm maturation and sperm storage as reflected in the consequences of epididymovasostomy. Fertility and Sterility 46(2):293–299

Sharpe RM 1987 Testosterone and spermatogenesis. Journal of Endocrinology 113:1–2

Sharpe RM 1990 Intratesticular control of steroidogenesis. Clinical Endocrinology 33:787–807

Sharpe RM 2000 Lifestyle and environmental contribution to male infertility. British Medical Bulletin 56:630–642

Sharpe RM, Skakkebaek NE 1993 Are oestrogens involved in falling sperm counts and disorders of the male reproductive tract? Lancet: 341:1392–1395

Silber SJ, Nagy ZP, Liu J, Godoy H, Devroey P, van Steirteghem AC 1994 Conventional in-vitro fertilization versus intracytoplasmic sperm injection for patients requiring microsurgical sperm aspiration. Human Reproduction 9(9):1705–1709

Skinner MK 1991 Cell-cell interaction in the testis. Endocrinology Reviews 12:45–77

Smith EP, Boyd J, Frank JR et al 1994 Estrogen resistance caused by a mutation in the estrogen-receptor gene in a man. New England Journal of Medicine 331:1056–1061

Snyder PJ, Peachey H, Hannoush P et al 1999 Effect of testosterone treatment on body composition and muscle strength in men over 65 years of age. Journal of Clinical Endocrinology and Metabolism 84:2647–2653

Sofiktis NV, Miyagawa I, Incze P, Andrighetti S 1996 Detrimental effect of left varicocele on the reproductive capacity of the early haploid male gamete. Journal of Urology 156:267–270

Swan SH, Elkin EP, Fenster L 1997 Have sperm densities declined? A reanalysis of global trend data. Environmental Health Perspectives 105:1228–1232

Swan SH, Elkin EP, Fenster L 2000 The question of declining sperm density revisited: an analysis of 101 studies published 1934–1996. Environmental Health Perspectives 108(10):961–966

Tapanainen TS, Aittomaki K, Min J, Vasivko T, Huhtaniemi IT 1997 Men homozygous for an inactivating mutation of the follicle-stimulating hormone (FSH) receptor gene present variable suppression of spermatogenesis and fertility. Nature Genetics 15:205–206

Templeton A 2000 Infertility and the establishment of pregnancy – overview. British Medical Bulletin 56:577–587

Templeton A, Fraser C, Thompson B 1990 The epidemiology of infertility in Aberdeen. British Medical Journal 301:148–152

Templeton A, Morris JK, Parslow W 1996 Factors that affect outcome of in vitro fertilisation treatment. Lancet 348:1402–1406

Thonneau P, Ducot B, Bujan L, Mieusset R, Spira A 1996 Heat exposure as a hazard to male fertility. Lancet 347:204–205

Tournaye H, Devroey P, Camus M et al 1992 Comparison of in-vitro fertilization in male and tubal infertility: a 3 year survey. Human Reproduction 7:218–222

Tulloch WS 1952 A consideration of sterility factors in the light of subsequent pregnancies: subfertility in the male. Transaction of the Edinburgh Obstetrical Society 52:29–34

van Rumste MM, Evers JL, Farquhar CM, Blake DA 2000 Intra-cytoplasmic sperm injection versus partial zona dissection, subzonal insemination and conventional techniques for oocyte insemination during in vitro fertilisation. Cochrane Database of Systematic Reviews(2):CD001301

van Steitreghem AC, Liu J, Joris H et al 1993 Higher success rate by intracytoplasmic sperm injection than by subzonal insemination. Report of a second series of 300 consecutive treatment cycles. Human Reproduction 8:1055–1060

Veldhuis JD, Iranmanesh A, Damers M, Mulligan T 1999 Joint basal and pulsatile hypersecretory mechanisms drive the monotropic follicle-stimulating hormone (FSH) elevation in healthy older men: concurrent preservation of the orderliness of the FSH release process: a general clinical research centre study. Journal of Clinical Endocrinology and Metabolism 84:3506–3514

Vermeulen A 1991 Androgens in the aging male. Journal of Clinical Endocrinology and Metabolism 73:221–224

Vierula M, Niemi M, Keiski A, Saaranen M, Saarikoski S, Suominen J 1996 High and unchanged sperm counts of Finnish men. International Journal of Andrology 19:11–17

World Health Organization 1992 The influence of varicocele on parameters of fertility in a large group of men presenting to infertility clinics. Fertility and Sterility 57:1289–1293

World Health Organization 1999 WHO laboratory manual for the examination of human semen and semen–cervical mucus interaction. Cambridge University Press, Cambridge

Wu FCW, Taylor PL, Sellar RE 1989 LHRH pulse frequency in normal and infertile men. Journal of Endocrinology 123:149–158

Zheng T, Holford TR, Ma Z, Ward BA, Flannery J, Boyle P 1996 Continuing increase in incidence of germ-cell testis cancer in young adults: experience from Connecticut, USA, 1935–1992. International Journal of Cancer 65:723–729

23

Assisted reproduction treatments

Nazar N. Amso   Robert W. Shaw

INTRODUCTION

There have been considerable advances in the field of assisted reproduction treatments (ART) in the past two decades, which resulted in about 200 000 babies born worldwide. ART are now widely available and in one year (1998), more than 200 000 treatment cycles were carried out in Europe. In the UK, a total of 35 363 in vitro fertilization (IVF)/micromanipulation and frozen embryo replacement (FER) cycles were reported in the year 2000, resulting in 6450 live-birth events (HFEA 2000). The number of conventional IVF cycles dropped slightly in 1998 and 1999 while the number of intracytoplasmic sperm injection (ICSI) treatment cycles has been steadily increasing since their introduction (Fig. 23.1). Conversely, the number of donor insemination (DI) cycles has dropped by 57% since the 1992–1993 reporting period (HFEA 2000).

The Human Fertilization and Embryology Authority (HFEA) was established in 1991 by the Human Fertilization and Embryology Act 1990 (HFE Act) and was the first statutory body of its kind in the world. Over the past decade assisted reproduction technology has encountered many clinical challenges and difficult social, ethical and regulatory issues. New drugs have become available, treatments were introduced and became established over an incredibly short period of time, creating more ethical dilemmas and encouraging continuing debate. Widespread provision of these treatments remains a hotly debated topic socially, medically and politically.

The introduction of clinical guidelines into clinical practice in general and in assisted reproduction in particular has led to an ever-increasing role for an evidence-based approach to the provision of these services. Clinical guidelines for the management of infertility in primary and secondary care centres were published by the Royal College of Obstetricians and Gynaecologists (RCOG 1998a,b) to streamline services and avoid unnecessary waste of resources. More recently, evidence-based clinical guidelines for the management of infertility in tertiary care centres were published (RCOG 1999). The demand to introduce new technology into clinical practice, often before adequate scientific evidence has accumulated,

317

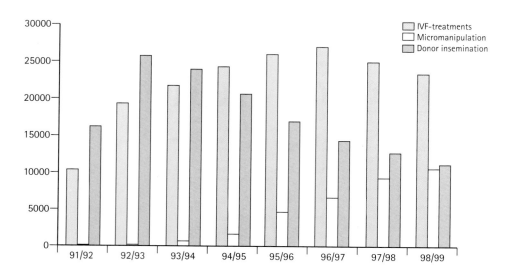

IVF-treatments
Micromanipulation
Donor insemination

Fig. 23.1 Number of treatment cycles 1991–99 (HFEA 2000).

may have serious consequences. Hence, it is essential that clinical practice evolves appropriately in order to protect both the public and the profession. Additionally, there may be adverse consequences for related specialties such as the high multiple pregnancy rate and its implications for the cost of neonatal services. These issues are also regularly discussed between the HFEA and the relevant professional and ethical bodies.

In this chapter we will review the current status of conventional IVF, ICSI and other treatments, new developments in ART and current ethical dilemmas as well as the clinical risks associated with these techniques. The obstetric and neonatal consequences of these treatments and in particular the impact of the number of embryos transferred on the outcome will be discussed.

SELECTION AND PREPARATION OF PATIENTS

Although IVF was initially introduced to bypass tubal blockage, the currently available techniques enable the treatment of various causes of infertility. The current indications are:

- tubal disease
- unexplained infertility
- treated endometriosis
- male factor infertility
- failed artificial insemination by donor (AID)
- cervical hostility
- failed ovulation induction
- absent or inappropriate ovaries
- IVF in association with preimplantation genetic diagnosis (PGD)
- therapy for female cancer.

Over the past decade great emphasis has been placed on the pretreatment evaluation of the couple. Assessment of the welfare of the child that may result from this treatment, including its need for a father, has become central to the provision of treatment. With that in mind there should be careful consideration of the duration and stability of the couple's relationship, their medical and social backgrounds and other relevant issues which may be known to their general practitioners.

In addition, information-giving and decision-making aspects of counselling should be made available by a specially trained counsellor as a matter of routine, to all couples. These couples have frequently undergone extensive investigations, are under considerable stress, and their relationship is often strained. ART should not be used as a panacea for marital or psychosexual disorders, but to fulfil the wishes of a well-adjusted couple to have a baby.

The male and female partner should be interviewed together and appropriate history and clinical examination are undertaken for both. For the female partner, baseline hormone profile, midluteal phase progesterone assay and rubella status must be determined. Additional tests such as thyroid function, high vaginal or endocervical swabs and cytomegalovirus (CMV) status are carried out where necessary. Hepatitis B and C and human immunodeficiency virus (HIV) screening are now commonly carried out before ART for both partners to ensure safety of the staff, to prevent spread of infection should the woman's serum be used for culture media or when oocytes or embryos are being donated. Laparoscopy should be carried out to confirm a normal pelvis if gamete intrafallopian transfer (GIFT) is the treatment of choice. Genetic tests before, during or after ART should be done to give adequate counselling to couples and their families in cases such as women with Turner's syndrome, men with 47XXY, men or women with structural chromosomal aberrations and men with either Yq11 deletion or congenital bilateral absence of vas deferens (ESHRE Capri Workshop Group 2000).

The male partner should be evaluated carefully. Clinical examination, semen analysis including sperm function tests and biochemical tests show that the aetiology of male subfertility can be divided into four main groups as follows.

1. Primary spermatogenic failure, which is a testicular disorder, resulting in the reduction of sperm count and abnormal sperm function. A number of different factors can induce this condition including testicular maldescent, trauma, karyotype abnormalities, severe infection and antimitotic therapy, but in many patients a cause cannot be ascertained.

2. Congenital or acquired obstructive lesions. Men with failed reversal of vasectomy are increasingly seen in infertility clinics and at present constitute up to 10% of all male problems.
3. Disturbances of erection or ejaculatory disorders including those following spinal injuries.
4. Endocrine disorders such as Cushing's disease, thyroid disorders and androgen receptor abnormalities.

Many causes of male infertility may have considerable congenital implications for the children of such patients. The majority of men with congenital bilateral absence of the vas deferens were shown to have one or more of the cystic fibrosis genes (Rigot 1991). The use of ICSI in these circumstances should be carefully considered and men must be screened with the appropriate tests before their treatment.

The couple must be well informed about the treatment options that are suitable for them, the indications for the tests they have to undergo, details of the proposed treatment and its success rate, risks and complications.

Assisted reproduction involves four principal steps:

1. the induction and timing of ovulation
2. egg collection/sperm production
3. fertilization (IVF)
4. the replacement of gametes/embroyos.

CLINICAL MANAGEMENT OF THE TREATMENT CYCLE

The first successful birth from IVF-embryo transfer (ET) in 1978 resulted from a single oocyte obtained from the dominant follicle in a natural ovarian cycle. Success rates were found to be improved when multiple embryos were transferred; thus at present, the majority of assisted reproduction programmes undertake ovarian stimulation to induce multiple follicular development.

Normal folliculogenesis

This involves several important and interrelated steps.

1. *Follicular recruitment* – this occupies the first few days of the ovarian cycle and allows the follicle to continue to mature in the correct gonadotrophic environment and to progress towards ovulation.
2. *Selection* – the mechanism whereby a single follicle is chosen and ultimately achieves ovulation.
3. *Dominance* – the selected follicle maintains its pre-eminence over all other follicles and occupies days 8–12 of the primate ovarian cycle.

Follicular development beyond the antral stage depends on the concentration of follicle-stimulating hormone (FSH) in the circulation. Once a threshold level has been attained, follicular growth beyond 4 mm occurs. The interval during which FSH remains elevated above threshold level can be regarded as a gate through which a follicle must pass to avoid atresia. The width of the gate will therefore determine the number of follicles that can be selected for ovulation (Fig. 23.2). The preovulatory luteinizing hormone (LH) surge is triggered by the positive feedback of estradiol (E_2) from the dominant follicle as well as other follicular contributory factors. Ovulation occurs between 24 and 36 hours after the onset of the LH surge.

Stimulation protocols

Pregnancy rate with unstimulated IVF remains much lower than in stimulated cycles, achieving a live birth rate of 2.3% per initiated cycle and 4.7% per ET (HFEA 2000). These results have remained low over the past decade. Although an unstimulated cycle is simpler, faster, less painful or expensive and with no risk of ovarian hyperstimulation, it requires relatively extensive monitoring which increases the cost and results in inconvenience in the timing of the oocyte retrieval. Additionally, women with irregular cycles and/or hormonal imbalance or couples with male factor infertility, where fertilization may be a problem, are not suitable for natural-cycle IVF. The aims of superovulation regimens in assisted reproduction are to maximize the number of follicles which mature to minimize the degree of asynchrony amongst developing follicles and to minimize the deleterious effects of the abnormal follicular environment on luteal function and endometrial receptivity. Multiple follicular development and ovulation can be achieved by widening the FSH gate. Several drug combinations have been used to achieve this.

Oocyte retrieval may be programmed to coincide with a working day by manipulating the onset of the menstrual cycle using norethisterone tablets, the combined oral contraceptive pill, or utilizing the hypogonadotrophic effect of gonadotrophin-releasing hormone (GnRH) agonists prior to commencing gonadotrophins on a predetermined day of the week. The GnRH agonist is either commenced in the midluteal phase and continued until complete down regulation is achieved (long protocol) or started on the first day of the menstrual cycle (short protocol). The downregulatory phase may be prolonged to allow a fixed number of patients to be treated each week. Follicular response is monitored by ultrasound scans and serum hormone assays for oestrogen and LH commencing on the 8th day of the treatment cycle. The gonadotrophin dosage is adjusted according to ovarian response. When three or more follicles are greater than 18 mm in diameter, 5000–10 000 U of human chorionic gonadotrophin (hCG) are given intra-muscularly 34–36 hours prior to oocyte collection. Oocyte retrieval takes place on a weekday, 13 days or more after commencing gonadotrophin stimulation.

Typically, follicles are noted to grow at a rate of 2–3 mm/day accompanied by a steady increase in serum E_2 levels. Unfortunately, not all stimulation cycles progress in this typical pattern and many may have to be abandoned before oocyte collection, primarily due to poor ovarian response. The impact of superovulation protocols on outcome of assisted reproduction treatment will be discussed later.

Abnormal ovarian response

Ovarian response is poor when no or less than three follicles develop after 14 days of gonadotrophin treatment and generally results in cancellation of the stimulation cycle. This

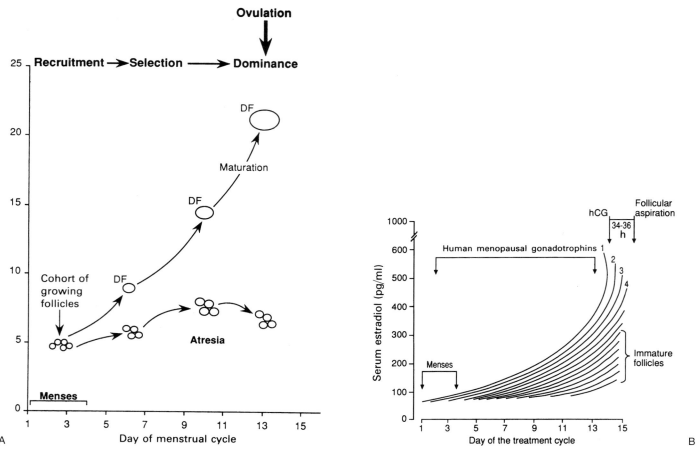

Fig. 23.2   A Selection and maturation of the dominant follicle (DF) during a natural cycle. B Induced follicular maturation with gonadotrophin therapy overriding selection of a single dominant follicle, as in the natural cycle.

problem is frequently encountered in women over the age of 37 years and those with severe ovarian endometriosis, where few oocytes of low quality are obtained and pregnancy rates are usually poor. Increasing the starting dose of gonadotrophins may sometimes improve the response and enable recruitment of a larger number of follicles. Conversely, excessive ovarian response may result in ovarian hyperstimulation syndrome (OHSS), which will be discussed later. Other problems such as premature LH surge or preoperative ovulation have been largely eliminated by the introduction of GnRH analogues in superovulation protocols.

OOCYTE COLLECTION

Methods of egg collection have improved considerably since the introduction of ART. The main motivation for these technical advances was to limit the high cost of IVF treatment, which was largely due to time spent in hospital, the type of anaesthesia and the degree of invasiveness of the procedure and its morbidity. At first, all egg collections were laparoscopic while presently this is reserved for patients being treated with GIFT or when the ovaries are inaccessible through the transvaginal route. The need for general anaesthesia and the frequently encountered limited access to adherent or covered ovaries meant that simpler ultrasound-guided techniques

such as the transvesical and transurethral methods replaced laparoscopy as the principal methods for egg collection. They were easy to learn, quick and did not require prolonged hospitalization. However, discomfort was often experienced when filling the bladder and haematuria was a frequent complication of the transurethral approach.

With the introduction of endovaginal transducers, the transvaginal route became the predominant method for egg collection. In this, the specially designed transducer is used to visualize the follicles and the aspirating needle is passed alongside it. This method is generally well tolerated when carried out under light intravenous sedation, can be learnt very quickly and is associated with minimal morbidity. It has almost completely replaced all previously described ultrasound methods. Ideally, both laparoscopy and ultrasound-guided techniques should be available to accommodate the anatomical needs of all patients.

Equipment and preparation

Several ultrasound machines are now equipped with slim-line vaginal probes with frequencies between 6 and 7.5 MHz. The probes may have a diametaer of 1.5 cm and, together with the needle guide, occupy minimum space in the vagina, causing least discomfort.

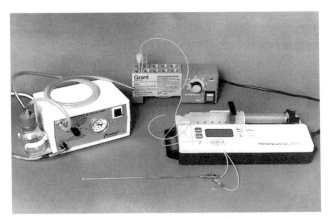

Fig. 23.3 An assembled follicle aspiration needle connected to a test tube and a flushing syringe pump. The test tube is in turn connected to a suction pump.

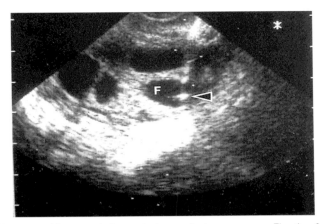

Fig. 23.5 Ultrasound picture during vaginal egg recovery. The tip of the needle (arrow) is seen within the follicle (F). The two parallel dotted lines demarcate the path of the needle. The dots are 1 cm apart.

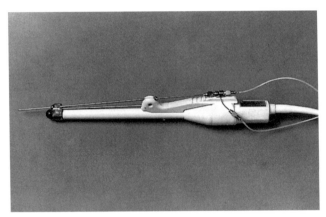

Fig. 23.4 Vaginal ultrasound transducer with needle bracket and guide. The needle tip is protruding from the proximal end of the probe.

Several designs of aspiration needles are available. They may have a single or double lumen to enable aspiration and flushing through different routes. The needle must have a very sharp tip to enable easy puncture of mobile ovaries and its distal 2 cm should be roughened to enhance ultrasound visualization. The needle is connected to a test tube by tubing and suction is applied from a foot-operated pump (Fig. 23.3).

The ultrasound transducer (Fig. 23.4) is enclosed in a special sterile condom and plastic sleeve prior to insertion into the vagina and should be thoroughly cleaned with a damp cloth after each procedure.

Anaesthesia

Vaginal egg collections may be performed under general anaesthesia or conscious sedation. The latter involves intravenous or intramuscular medication to induce sedation (e.g. diazepam or midazolam) and provide effective pain relief (e.g. pethidine or fentanyl citrate) during the operation. The dose given varies according to the patient's tolerance, level of pain relief and the time taken to complete the operation.

Technique

The patient is placed in the lithotomy position and the vagina is cleaned carefully. Prior to puncture of the lateral vaginal vault, the ovaries should be carefully scanned to determine the plane that enables the best access to the largest follicles. The needle is pushed through the vaginal wall and into the first follicle by a single, firm thrusting movement. Suction is applied as soon as the needle tip is seen to be within the follicle which will be seen to collapse as the follicular fluid is aspirated (Fig. 23.5). During aspiration, the needle is rotated and moved gently in all directions within the follicle to increase the chance of oocyte retrieval. If the oocyte is not recovered in the first aspirate, the follicle may be flushed either manually or using a foot-controlled pump to facilitate delivery of flushing media at a steady rate. Once the egg is obtained, the needle is lined against a neighbouring follicle without removing it from the ovarian surface. Unanaesthetized patients will experience pain or discomfort when the external follicular surface is entered. However, the procedure is well tolerated and usually completed in about 30 minutes. At the end, the vaginal vault should be inspected to exclude bleeding from puncture sites. The patient recovers quickly and will be able to leave the hospital after a few hours.

Generally, very few technical difficulties are encountered during vaginal egg collections. Mobile ovaries may be stabilized with gentle suprapubic or iliac fossa pressure and the use of sharp needles usually overcomes this difficulty. If the uterus lies between the vaginal vault and the ovary, manual suprapubic pressure or redirection of the transducer will often bring the ovary in direct line with the needle. Occasionally, the ovary will need to be accessed by passing the needle through the uterus. This is rather painful for the unanaesthetized patient but appears to have minimal risk of damage or bleeding. Complications of the procedure are discussed later.

LABORATORY TECHNIQUES

Sperm utilized for conventional IVF is obtained by masturbation. However, when there is obstructive azoospermia, it is aspirated from the epididymis and/or testis (percutaneous epididymal

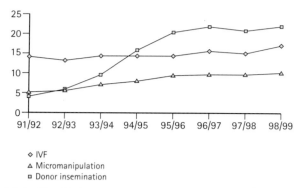

◇ IVF
△ Micromanipulation
□ Donor insemination

Fig. 23.6 Live-birth rates per treatment cycle 1991–99 (HFEA 2000).

sperm aspiration – PESA, testicular sperm aspiration – TESA) or extracted from the testes (testicular sperm extraction – TESE). Sperm preparation, oocyte insemination and other related laboratory techniques are varied and the reader is advised to consult specialist books for further information.

OUTCOME MEASURES AND FACTORS AFFECTING SUCCESS RATE

Pregnancy and live-birth rates per treatment cycle for IVF, ICSI and DI have steadily improved worldwide over the past decade. Figure 23.6 shows the improvement in the live-birth rate per treatment cycle in the UK between 1991 and 1999 (HFEA annual reports). It is now widely accepted that when attempting to ascertain whether or not a treatment is required, it is essential that the time-specific or cycle-specific conception rate is used. Crude pregnancy rate per couple is almost meaningless. Pregnancy rate per cycle can also be misleading if limited to the first cycle or two because the rate may fall in subsequent cycles. Thus, cumulative conception or cumulative live-birth rates have been increasingly used in reporting conventional and ART outcomes. Cumulative conception rates for some of the most common causes of infertility in the untreated population were compared to those in couples following treatment with conventional methods (Hull 1992). The results showed that in some conditions such as amenorrhoea and oligomenorrhoea, or in those being treated with donor insemination, the cumulative conception rate following conventional therapy is almost the same as in normal women. However, in other circumstances, such as salpingostomy for distal tubal occlusion, or the use of high-dose glucocorticosteroids for seminal antisperm antibodies, the prognosis is worse and the cumulative conception rates are lower than that which can now be expected in a single cycle of IVF treatment.

The effectiveness of infertility treatments (IVF, ICSI, egg and sperm donation, embryo donation) is dependent on a reasonable likelihood that embryos can be created in vitro and then placed in the uterus with a reasonable expectation that implantation will occur. Many factors determine the outcome of treatment, such as patient selection, age, cause and duration of infertility and the number of attempts that couples undergo. A recent randomized trial reported that even non-medical factors, such as intercessory prayer, resulted in a significantly

higher clinical pregnancy rate (Cha et al 2001)! However, the decision to recommend ART should be based on the likelihood that a pregnancy will occur without treatment, the possibility that a less invasive form of treatment might be effective and the likely outcome of IVF treatment (RCOG 1999). The likelihood of treatment-independent pregnancy depends on the woman's age, cause and duration of infertility and history of previous pregnancy (Collins et al 1995, Eimers et al 1995, Vardon et al 1995). In a retrospective study (Vardon et al 1995), the incidence of spontaneous treatment-independent pregnancy in couples enlisted on an IVF programme was reported to be 11% of couples with low fertility. The main difference from those in whom pregnancy did not occur was a shorter duration of infertility.

Success of ART is also dependent on where the provision of service takes place. It is clear from the HFEA annual reports that the outcome of treatment varies between small and large centres. When discussing the likelihood of birth following IVF treatment with any couple, it is essential to consider the factors that can significantly affect the outcome. These include female age, cause and duration of infertility, previous pregnancy history, number of embryos replaced, availability of surplus embryos for cryopreservation and the number of any previous treatment cycles. Such advice is particularly relevant and important in women over the age of 40 in whom success rates are considerably reduced and the risk of miscarriage is increased.

Female age

The woman's age at the time of treatment is an important prognostic factor when the success of IVF is discussed with any couple. The number of oocytes and consequently the number of embryos decline with age. However, the cleavage rate does not seem to alter in the same manner. The number of embryos replaced compounds the effect of age and embryo implantation rates on pregnancy rate. The total number of embryos available for replacement further influences this. When a larger number of embryos is available for replacement, the selection of the most appropriate embryos for transfer would improve the implantation and pregnancy rates respectively.

Indeed, when women over the age of 40 had four or more embryos transferred, their pregnancy rate was not significantly different from younger women, whether following IVF (Widra et al 1996) or ICSI (Alrayyes et al 1997). Hence, it may be concluded that older women with good ovarian response, producing three or more embryos suitable for transfer, have similar prospects to establishing a pregnancy to younger patients. It should be noted, however, that early reports (Piette et al 1990) were contradictory to more recent findings. This may reflect improvements in ovarian stimulation protocols and laboratory practices.

Fertilization rates decrease with age. Women attempting pregnancy over the age of 40 have approximately 50% less fertility rate in comparison with younger women (Toner & Flood 1993). Numerous reports have found significantly lower fertilization rates in older women undergoing IVF or ICSI (Ashkenazi et al 1996, Cordiero et al 1995, Tucker et al 1995a), while others (Sharif et al 1998) reported that age had no significant association with fertilization rates. Similarly, cumulative conception rates (Prietl et al 1998) and implantation rates appeared to decline significantly with age. However, maternal age alone was not found to be a useful predictor of embryo implantation or endometrial receptivity in IVF treatment cycles (Arthur et al 1994, van Kooij et al 1996).

Age and pregnancy, live-birth and miscarriage rates

Although live-birth rates per treatment cycle following IVF, ICSI, and DI have increased consistently over the past decade, they decline with advancing age of women when using their own eggs (Fig. 23.7). A number of investigators have examined different age cut-offs such as 40 years (Sharif et al 1998, Widra et al 1996) or 35 years (Preutthipan et al 1996). Mardesic et al (1994) reported that the cut-off point of effectiveness for an IVF programme was 36–37 years, with marked decline in pregnancy rate per ET in women over the age of 38.

Similarly, Tan et al (1992a) found that both conception and live-birth rates per cycle declined with age. The cumulative conception and live-birth rates after five treatment cycles were about 54% and 45% respectively at 20–34 years, 39% and 29% at 35–39 years and 20% and 14.4% at 40 years and older. It is likely that pregnancy rates are related to the quality of the embryos. When adjustment is made for equal embryonic quality, maternal age did not interfere significantly with pregnancy rates (Parneix et al 1995). Thus, women over the age of 40 with good response to controlled ovarian hyperstimulation have better prognosis and success rates than those who have poor response.

In an attempt to identify factors that affect the outcome of treatment, Templeton and colleagues (1996) analysed the HFEA database between 1991 and 1994. The authors reported that the overall live-birth rate per cycle of treatment was 13.9%. The highest live-birth rates were in the 25–30 years age group, with younger women (under 25 years) having lower rates, while a sharp decline was noted in older women. At all ages over 30 years, the use of donor eggs was associated with significantly higher live-birth rates compared with the use of women's own eggs, though there was equally a downward trend in success rates with age. After adjustment for age, increasing duration of infertility was associated with a

significant decrease in live-birth rates. The indications for treatment had no significant effect on the outcome, while previous pregnancy and live birth significantly increased treatment success.

Miscarriage rates have been reported to be higher in all the women following IVF and there is a 2–3-fold increase in the rate of spontaneous abortion in women aged 40 or more (Toner & Flood 1993). However, others (Al-Shawaf et al 1992, Mardesic et al 1994) have not detected higher pregnancy loss in older women. It is more likely that embryo quality is the main factor influencing the poor reproductive performance of women with advancing age rather than defective response of uterine vasculature to steroids or uterine ageing. Increasing maternal age correlates with a higher risk of fetal chromosomal anomalies, which results in an increased abortion rate.

Cause of infertility

Reports have differed in their analysis of the impact of infertility factors on the cumulative conception and live-birth rates. While some have found significant differences, with the lowest rates being reported in patients with male infertility or multiple infertility factors (Tan et al 1992a), others found no significant effect on the outcome (Dor et al 1996, Templeton et al 1996). However, history of previous pregnancy and live birth significantly increased treatment success (Prietl et al 1998, Templeton et al 1996). The IVF clinical pregnancy and live-birth rates in the HFEA report of 2000 show similar results for tubal disease, endometriosis and unexplained infertility (Fig. 23.8). Reports of higher fertilization rates after ICSI suggested that this technique may be better than the conventional method for all couples seeking IVF. A multicentre randomized controlled trial comparing clinical outcome after ICSI or conventional IVF in couples with non-male factor infertility showed higher implantation and pregnancy rates per cycle after IVF, hence supporting the practice of reserving ICSI for severe male factor infertility (Bhattacharya et al 2001).

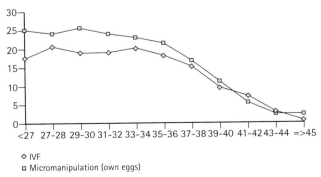

Fig. 23.7   Live-birth rates by age of women (using own eggs and including frozen embryo replacements) (HFEA 2000).

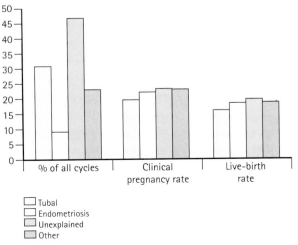

Fig. 23.8   IVF clinical pregnancy and live-birth rates for female causes of infertility (HFEA 2000).

All stages of endometriosis are viewed as suitable indications for ART. The timing of treatment is dependent on the severity of the disease, previous therapy and other factors, such as female age and duration of infertility. In women with severe endometriosis with mechanical tubal blockage and where surgery is inappropriate, IVF should be expedited. IVF should also be recommended 1–2 years after previous unsuccessful medical or surgical therapy, while in minimal or mild endometriosis, the balance of choice seems to be in favour of IVF or GIFT after more than 2 years of expectant management.

Initially, poor results were reported in women with severe disease (Matson & Yovich 1986). The introduction of ultrasound-guided techniques for oocyte collection resulted in retrieving larger number of oocytes and hence achieving higher pregnancy and implantation rates in advanced-stage disease (Geber et al 1995, Olivennes et al 1995). The use of GnRH agonists in stimulation protocols or as a pretreatment of women with endometriosis has also resulted in a higher number of preovulatory oocytes retrieved and transferred, lower cancellation of treatment cycles and a higher pregnancy rate, especially in women with advanced-stage disease. The effect that assisted reproduction treatment may have on the progression of endometriosis has been insufficiently studied and evidence suggests that one or repeated superovulations for IVF has minimal deleterious effect on the disease or chances of subsequent spontaneous pregnancy (Amso 1995a).

For male factor infertility, ICSI was successfully introduced in 1992 (Palermo et al 1992) and since then, the annual number of treatment cycles has increased steadily (see Fig. 23.1). Previous techniques such as partial zona dissection (PZD) and subzonal insemination (SUZI) were very disappointing (Cohen et al 1991) and comparative studies indicated that ICSI was a much more efficient technique than either of the others (Tarin 1995). It gave men who had previously been diagnosed with severe male factor infertility the chance to have their own genetic children. The sperm may be obtained either by ejaculation, percutaneous aspiration from the epididymis (PESE) or testis (TESA) or testicular extraction (TESE), resulting in equally high fertilization, pregnancy and implantation rates, especially in men with borderline or very poor sperm quality (Tucker et al 1995b). Recognized indications for ICSI include:

- very poor sperm quality
- obstructive azoospermia
- non-obstructive azoospermia.
- previously failed or very poor fertilization.

Live-birth rates following ICSI, overall and by age of women, are shown in Figures 23.6 and 23.7. A remarkable change in fertilization rate with a significant increase in the percentage of two pronuclei oocytes occurred when the technique was slightly modified by breaking the sperm tail before injection (Fishel et al 1995, Gerris et al 1995). The technique requires a high-quality inverted microscope and special equipment with holding and injection pipettes being used to stabilize and inject the oocyte respectively. The injecting pipette is pushed almost entirely through the ooplasm before the spermatozoon is deposited inside the oocyte (Fig. 23.9).

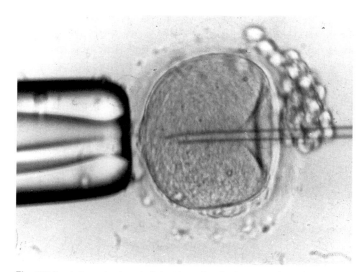

Fig. 23.9 Intracytoplasmic injection of a single sperm into the egg (courtesy of Dr Simon Fishel, Scientific Director, Park Fertility Services Nottingham).

The duration of infertility

The duration of infertility remains one of the most important variables that influence the outcome of assisted reproduction, with lower pregnancy and live-birth rates associated with a longer period of infertility. Analysis of the HFEA database between 1991 and 1994 showed that, even with adjustment for age, there was a significant decrease in live-birth rate with increasing duration of infertility from 1 to 12 years (Templeton et al 1996).

Superovulation protocols

In the early years, clomiphene citrate alone or in conjunction with human menopausal gonadotrophins were the main drugs used in superovulation protocols. The use of GnRH agonists (GnRH-a) in stimulation protocols has increased steadily since their introduction into clinical practice and has resulted in a reduction in the cancellation rates and an increase in the number of oocytes retrieved. A meta-analysis comparing the efficacy of GnRH-a in superovulation cycles for IVF (Hughes et al 1992) reported significantly improved clinical pregnancy rate and decreased cancellation rate in GnRH-a cycles in comparison with non-downregulated cycles. More recently, the long downregulation protocol was found to be superior to the short or ultrashort regimens (Daya 1998) and the type of GnRH-a (short acting or depot preparation) did not appear to affect pregnancy or miscarriage rates (Dada et al 1999, Daya 1997).

The use of GnRH-a often prolongs the stimulation phase and may be associated with poor response in some patients as well as introducing a higher risk of ovarian hyperstimulation syndrome (OHSS). Some of the disadvantages can be obviated with the use of GnRH antagonists. However, some prospective studies had showed lesser pregnancy rates in antagonist cycles and the question remains whether this is inherent to the medication, any adverse effects on the luteal phase, the type of patient population or is due to the limited experience with follicle stimulation in antagonist cycles (Devroey 2000). Others (van Os & Jansen 2000) have compared the antagonist Cetrorelix (ASTA Medica AG) in two groups of patients: previous poor responders (less than three oocytes retrieved in previous IVF/ICSI treatment) or normal responders. Cetrorelix was started when the mean follicular diameter of the leading follicle was 14–15 mm which corresponded to day 5 or 6 of gonadotrophin stimulation. The pregnancy rate, ongoing/delivery rate in the previously poor responders was poor and clearly showed that this group did not benefit from this new treatment strategy. In the normal responders group, the results were more encouraging and an overall pregnancy rate and implantation rates per ET were 45% and 22% respectively. These data should be interpreted with caution and further randomized controlled studies in predefined patient subgroups should be carried out to further establish any benefit from this new treatment.

Commercially available gonadotrophin preparations used in superovulation protocols were originally extracted from the urine of menopausal women. They had been shown to be of low purity with the major protein components not being gonadotrophins! The repeated injection of non-gonadotrophin proteins may be the cause of unwanted effects, such as pain and allergic reactions. The desirability of having high-purity preparations led to the development of an immunopurified FSH product of >95% purity. The introduction of high-purity gonadotrophins (high-purity FSH) was associated with a small but significant increase in pregnancy rate in comparison with conventional hMG preparations (Daya et al 1995).

However, variations in bio-activity and continued dependence on human menopausal urine collection remained as major obstacles in the production of these compounds. Recent progress in purification technology, as well as genetic and molecular engineering, led to the production of recombinant human FSH (rFSH) with high purity (>99%), high specific bio-activity (>10 000 IU/mg protein), and absent intrinsic LH activity which is suitable for intramuscular or subcutaneous administration (Mannaerts et al 1991). Its use produces similar results to high-purity FSH when fresh embryo replacement only is considered (Bergh et al 1997). It also results in the production of significantly more oocytes and if pregnancies from FER cycles are included, significantly more pregnancies are produced (Out et al 1995).

Timing of embryo transfer

The convention has been to replace embryos on the second day post insemination. It can be argued that there are advantages from delaying embryo transfer to allow selection of those embryos with greater potential for implantation and to replace them at a more physiological time into the uterine cavity. Some retrospective studies have failed to demonstrate any increase in the ongoing pregnancy rates whether embryos were replaced 2, 3 or 4 days post insemination (Dawson et al 1995, Huisman et al 1994). However, others have demonstrated significantly higher pregnancy rates after day 3 transfers and even more so if the embryos replaced had eight or more blastomeres (Carrillo et al 1998). Significantly higher implan-

tation rates (Carrillo et al 1998, Dawson et al 1995) and lower miscarriage rates (Dawson et al 1995) were also reported following day 3 transfers.

Transfer of embryos at blastocyst stage has potential advantages. It is a more physiological approach, allowing synchronization of the embryo with the endometrium and the selection of viable embryos for transfer will be more efficient. Furthermore, the reduction of the number of embryos transferred, even if only one is transferred, leads to acceptable pregnancy rates while eliminating the risk of high-order multiple pregnancy rates (Gardner et al 1998). Assessment of blastocyst viability is mainly based on morphological appearance but this is a notoriously poor method. Early reports indicated that transfer of two or three blastocysts resulted in high viable pregnancy rates of 62% and 58% respectively. However, the advantage of two-blastocyst transfer is a lower multiple pregnancy rate of 39% compared with 79% for three blastocysts and the absence of triplet pregnancies (Milki et al 1999). Culture of human blastocyst in sequential media and the use of a systematic scoring and grading system can achieve much higher pregnancy and implantation rates when top-quality blastocyst(s) are transferred. This will be an important area of future research.

Endometrial thickness

Endometrial thickness on its own is a poor predictor for pregnancy. However, no conception was recorded when endometrial thickness was below 5 mm on the day of transfer and hence it is recommended that consideration should be given to cryopreserving all embryos and preparing the endometrium with exogenous hormones at a subsequent cycle (Friedler et al 1996).

Uterine or tubal embryo transfer/gamete intrafallopian transfer (GIFT)

Uterine embryo replacement is a relatively simple procedure, which must be carried out meticulously to ensure appropriate placement of the embryos (Fig. 23.10). Variations among clinicians in the technique of embryo transfer may influence the pregnancy rate. Avoidance of blood, mucus, bacterial contamination, excessive uterine contractions and trauma to the endometrium is associated with optimal pregnancy and implantation rates after transcervical embryo transfer. A trial transfer, ultrasonographic guidance, usually transabdominal to determine the precise depth of embryo placement within the

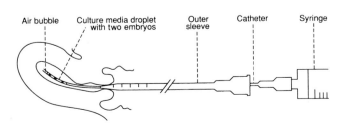

Fig. 23.10 Loaded ET catheter. Two embryos are ready to be deposited within 1 cm of the uterine fundus.

uterus, and the use of 'soft' catheters appear to facilitate successful embryo transfer (Schoolcraft et al 2001).

Tubal embryo transfer was the subject of considerable interest in the late 1980s following reports of high pregnancy rates with GIFT. Randomized controlled trials have failed to demonstrate any significant difference in the overall results between fresh tubal embryo transfer and uterine transfer (Amso 1996, Fluker et al 1993), though significantly higher pregnancy rates were reported after frozen tubal embryo transfers (van Voorhis et al 1995). Interestingly, a randomized trial comparing transcervical tubal cannulation and embryo transfer with uterine embryo transfer reported higher pregnancy and implantation rates following uterine transfer.

Initial reports of high pregnancy rates with GIFT generated considerable excitement with this technique. However, controlled trials comparing GIFT with IVF failed to demonstrate any significant benefit. Many factors may have contributed to the early reports, including patients' profile and differences in the number of gametes or embryos transferred per patient. The effect of restriction of the number of gametes transferred to a maximum of four was reflected in the subsequent dramatic decline in pregnancy and live-birth rates reported by a number of studies as well as the UK annual reports.

Luteal phase support

Pregnancy rates are higher when the luteal phase is supported in GnRH agonist cycles. Human chorionic gonadotrophin is superior to progestogerone but is associated with a higher incidence of ovarian hyperstimulation syndrome (OHSS) (Soliman et al 1994). There is no evidence that any method of progesterone administration (oral, parenteral, vaginal) is superior to the other. Similarly, luteal phase support in non-downregulated GnRH-a cycles does not increase pregnancy rates.

Number of embryos transferred

Assisted reproduction treatment involving ovarian stimulation is associated with increased multiple pregnancy rate. In England and Wales, multiple birth rate increased from 9.9 per thousand pregnancies in 1975 to 13.6 in 1994. During the same period, an increase in the prescription for fertility drugs was reported which led to the conclusion that fertility treatments were responsible for this increase in multiple pregnancies, especially triplet births. Unmonitored or poorly supervised ovulation induction treatment results in multiple pregnancy due to surplus of oocytes. However, with IVF treatment the multiple pregnancy rate is very much dependant on the number of embryos replaced.

Retrospective studies, as early as 1985, had argued that multiple pregnancies and births increased with the increase in the number of embryos replaced (Tucker et al 1991, Waterstone et al 1991, Wood et al 1985). Randomized studies comparing two- with three-embryo transfers (Staessen et al 1993) or four-embryo transfers (Vauthier-Brouzes et al 1994) reported similar pregnancy rates as long as there were sufficient morphologically regular embryos available for transfer. However, there were no higher order multiple births when two

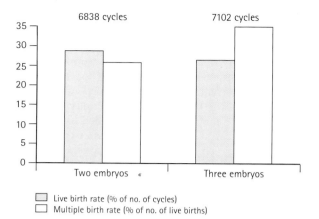

Fig. 23.11 IVF live and multiple births for two or three fresh embryos transferred where four or more embryos created (HFEA 2000).

embryos only were transferred. Analysis of the HFEA database of more than 44 000 cycles (Templeton & Morris 1998) and the HFEA reports (1999, 2000) showed that when four or more fertilized eggs were available, the transfer of three embryos did not result in improved pregnancy rates compared to the elective transfer of two embryos only. However, the incidence of triplets or higher order multiple births decreased considerably when two embryos were replaced (Fig. 23.11).

When two embryos only are available for transfer in women at or above the age of 40, the pregnancy rate is markedly reduced. Interestingly, the multiple pregnancy rate is only marginally reduced in these women when only two embryos are electively replaced (Templeton & Morris 1998). Further, the HFEA report (2000) indicated that the IVF live-birth rate per treatment cycle was slightly higher when two embryos were electively replaced. Another study involving women aged >40 years and undergoing ICSI between 1991 and 1995 demonstrated a significant difference in the clinical pregnancy rate when four or more embryos were replaced in comparison with 1–3 only. However, there were no differences in the delivery, multiple pregnancy or spontaneous abortion rates between the two groups (Adonakis et al 1997).

The British Fertility Society (1997) advocates the transfer of a maximum of two embryos only in each treatment cycle as a measure of good practice. Additionally, reduction in the number of embryos transferred from three to two has economic implications. A clinical audit in Scotland (Liao et al 1997) demonstrated that the cost of neonatal intensive care was reduced ninefold when a two-embryo policy was adopted for the majority of women. Martikainen and colleagues (2001) have even argued for the transfer of one embryo only when there are at least four good-quality embryos available for transfer after IVF or ICSI. Their study showed similarly high pregnancy rates for one- or two-embryo transfers while dizygotic twins were avoided. Elective single-embryo transfer combined with embryo cryopreservation resulted in very high pregnancy rates of 39% per fresh ET and a cumulative delivery rate per oocyte retrieval of 53% with low risk (8%) of twins (Tiitinen et al 2001). In 2001 the HFEA circulated guidance to all UK centres requiring them to transfer two embryos only unless there are exceptional circumstances.

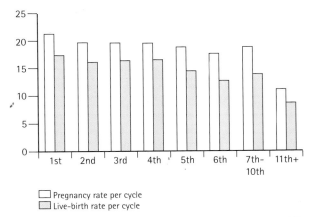

Fig. 23.12 Live-birth rates by number of attempts following IVF (HFEA 1998).

Number of ART attempts

The literature appears to be somewhat divided when the pregnancy and live-birth rates in relation to the number of ART attempts are examined. In one study (Padilla & Garcia 1989), the pregnancy rate per ET was similar for at least seven attempts, while other studies (FIVNAT 1994, Tan et al 1992a, Templeton et al 1996) reported decline in the chances of pregnancy and live-birth rates with successive treatment cycles. The data from the HFEA 1998 annual report showed a steady decline after the fifth attempt with pregnancy and live-birth rates per cycle, being 11.1% and 8.6% respectively at the 11th attempt (Fig. 23.12).

When IVF cumulative pregnancy rates were estimated for a cohort of women, the rates showed a constant rise during the six initial IVF treatments and plateaued subsequently (Dor et al 1996). Similarly, the rates were reported to be as high as 80% after seven cycles and a history of previous pregnancy significantly improved a couple's probability of conception (Croucher et al 1998).

Embryo cryopreservation

The ability to cryopreserve embryos enables any supernumerary embryos to be stored for some time before subsequent replacement when fresh ET has failed or if further children are desired. Additionally, cryopreservation has the added benefit of increasing the number of potential embryo replacement cycles without the need to undergo superovulation and oocyte retrieval, hence reducing the risk of ovarian hyperstimulation syndrome. Embryo quality has the most significant impact on post-thaw survival and ultimately pregnancy and implantation rates. As with fresh embryos, factors such as patient's age, the number of embryos transferred and whether a pregnancy resulted from the original stimulation cycle will affect the outcome of the FER cycle.

In 2000, the HFEA annual register reported a clinical pregnancy rate of 15% and a live-birth rate of 12.2% per FER cycle in women using their own gametes. Over the past decade considerable improvement has taken place. The French register (FIVNAT 1996) reported an increase in the pregnancy rates per transfer from 11.5% to 16% between 1987 and 1995. It has been estimated that one FER cycle increases the take home baby rate by 5% (Kahn et al 1993) while treatment involving one fresh and two FER cycles achieves a cumulative viable pregnancy rate of 41% (Home et al 1997). Frozen thawed embryos can be replaced in natural or hormonally adjusted cycles utilizing GnRH agonist and oestrogen/progestogen preparations with comparable results. The use of GnRH agonist is useful in anovulatory or irregular cycles and the use of different progestogens for luteal phase support is equally effective. The cost per delivery for an FER cycle has been estimated to be between 25% and 45% of a fresh cycle. In view of these advantages, cryopreservation should be accessible and discussed with all couples where surplus good-quality embryos are available.

Sperm and oocyte donation

Donor insemination (DI) is an effective treatment for male factor infertility (azoospermia, severe oligoasthenospermia), though treatment-independent pregnancy may occur in some non-azoospermic couples while awaiting treatment. The success of DI depends on the availability of a suitable semen donor with high fertilizing potential and the adequate investigation of women for factors that influence the probability of conception. Factors that may affect the success of DI include the woman's age, ovulatory status, fallopian tube patency and the quality of frozen-thawed semen. The use of fresh semen in previous years resulted in cycle fecundity rates that approached natural conceptions (Mackenna et al 1992, Peek et al 1984). Pregnancy and live-birth rates per cycle are slightly lower in natural (10.9% and 9%) than stimulated cycles (13.6% and 11%) respectively (HFEA 2000). The multiple pregnancy rate is, however, higher with stimulated than natural cycles, 2.8% and 1.3% respectively, while 13% of all births in stimulated cycles were multiple compared with 1.4% in unstimulated cycles. This resulted in a three- and ninefold increase in the stillbirth and neonatal deaths per thousand births for twins and triplets compared to singleton births (HFEA 2000).

Interestingly, stillbirth and neonatal death rates for singleton pregnancies are slightly higher in unstimulated DI cycles. It is recommended that at first, a minimum of six cycles of insemination without ovarian stimulation should be carried out in regularly ovulating women (RCOG 1999). The use of donated sperm in IVF resulted in clinical pregnancy and live-birth rates of 30.2% and 24.9% per treatment cycle for fresh replacements and 16.9% and 11.5% respectively for FER (HFEA 2000).

Egg donation is an effective treatment for women with premature ovarian failure, gonadal dysgenesis such as Turner's syndrome, following oophorectomy, chemo- or radiotherapy-related ovarian failure and where repeated failure of fertilization is attributed to poor oocyte quality. High pregnancy rates have been reported following oocyte donation for Turner's syndrome patients (Khastgir et al 1997). However, Turner's patients were reported to have significantly higher biochemical pregnancy rates and early miscarriages, lower clinical pregnancy and delivery rates when compared to other women with premature ovarian failure (Yaron et al 1996). An important factor in the establishment of pregnancy is an endometrial thickness of greater than 6.5 mm. Other factors include the number of previous natural conceptions and live births and the fertilization rate, while increasing female age does not affect the outcome (Burton et al 1992).

Oocyte donation has considerable emotional and social effects on both the donor and recipient, more so if the donor is undergoing IVF treatment herself. Pregnancy and live-birth rates per treatment cycle following oocyte donation in comparison with other treatments are depicted in Figure 23.13, where fresh embryos are replaced, and Figure 23.14 where frozen-thawed embryos are replaced (HFEA 2000).

POTENTIAL HEALTH RISKS ASSOCIATED WITH ASSISTED REPRODUCTIVE TECHNOLOGY

Potential health risks arising from ART have been the subject of important debate. Seamark & Robinson (1995) voiced concerns regarding the effect of such treatments on fetal development antenatally and the long-term postnatal outcome. They also drew our attention to 'disconcerting' results from

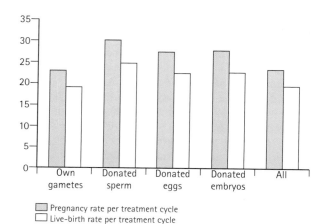

Fig. 23.13   IVF clinical pregnancy and live-birth rates with fresh embryo transfer – stimulated cycles (HFEA 2000).

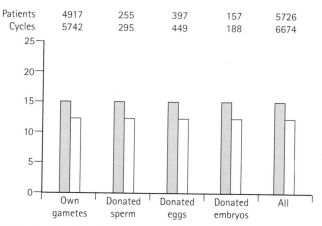

Fig. 23.14   IVF clinical pregnancy and live-birth rates – frozen embryo replacements (HFEA 2000).

animal research and sounded a caution on the potential harmful effect on human reproduction. It is likely that more studies and several years of observation will be needed before we establish the full impact and potential health problems arising in the resultant babies. Equally pressing is the need to address the risks to couples and in particular women undergoing such treatments (Amso 1995b).

In most centres, women undergoing assisted reproduction treatments such as IVF or GIFT receive medication to induce multiple follicular development. Problems may arise due to inadvertent exposure of the developing embryo to these medications or side-effects resulting from their pharmacological effects. More serious complications such as ovarian hyper-stimulation syndrome (OHSS), the potential risk of genital cancer and physical/psychological health problems related to ART will be addressed in this section.

Ovarian hyperstimulation syndrome (OHSS)

The pathophysiology of OHSS is poorly understood. It remains the most serious and potentially lethal complication of ovulation induction, correlates positively with conceptual cycles and is almost exclusively related to either exogenous or endogenous hCG stimulation. The risk increases with the total number of follicles in the preovulatory period, including immature and intermediate follicles and it may present 3–7 days (early presentation) or 12–17 days (late presentation) after the hCG injection. The overall prevalence of moderate to severe OHSS varies from 1% to 10% of IVF/ICSI cycles (Brinsden et al 1995). The key to prevention is proper identification of the population at risk before treatment and close monitoring of hormone levels as well as follicular response on ultrasound (Fig. 23.15). When a high-risk situation is recognized, withholding the ovulatory dose of hCG injection and can-cellation of the treatment cycle will almost certainly prevent OHSS. The couple should be advised to avoid intercourse as spontaneous ovulation may occur up to 11 days after discontinuing gonadotrophin treatment, resulting in conception and development of severe OHSS.

Alternative strategies have been attempted and when effective, they usually ameliorate the severity of OHSS rather than prevent it absolutely. They include:

- reduction of the ovulatory hCG dose and avoiding its use in the luteal phase
- triggering ovulation with GnRH agonist (intranasal or subcutaneous administration) instead of hCG in suitable subjects
- reduction of the gonadotrophin dose in subsequent treatment cycles has been attempted with varying degrees of success
- the use of intravenous albumin infusion or hydroxyethyl starch solution. Albumin infusion after hCG injection or at the time of oocyte recovery has been reported to increase the carrier-protein capacity and prevent the development of severe OHSS or to markedly reduce its incidence and severity (Asch et al 1993, Shoham et al 1994). However, it is expensive and, being a human derivative, carries a potential risk of viral transmission

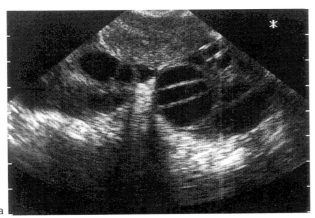 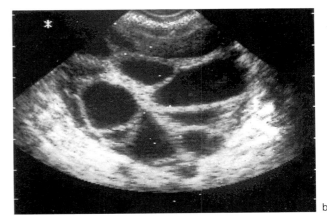

Fig. 23.15 **a** Vaginal ultrasound appearance of the hyperstimulated ovaries. The enlarged ovaries almost completely occupy the pelvis and contain excessive number of large, intermediate and small follicles. **b** Vaginal ultrasound appearance of the mature follicles in a normal ovary prior to vaginal egg collection.

- laparoscopic ovarian electrocautery in women with polcystic ovarian disease or previous OHSS
- use of GnRH antagonist
- early follicular aspiration of one ovary 10–12 hours after hCG injection
- a delay in the administration of hCG (controlled drift period or prolonged coasting) results in rapid decline of serum oestradiol levels but an increase in the size of the lead follicles. Clinical pregnancy rates between 25% and 35% have been reported (Urman et al 1992), but with unacceptably high multiple pregnancy rate (50%) and severe OHSS in 2.5% of all cases
- conversion of a superovulation ± intrauterine insemination cycle to IVF
- elimination of the endogenous pregnancy-derived hCG by aspiration of all follicles, fertilization of oocytes and elective cryopreservation of all embryos (Amso et al 1990). Subsequent frozen/thawed embryo replacement cycles result in pregnancies and live births, though believed to be at lower rates than in fresh ET
- the use of steroids in high-risk patients has been found to be ineffective in reducing the rate of OHSS after superovulation for IVF.

A systematic Cochrane Review of interventions for the treatment of OHSS showed significantly lower incidence of severe OHSS when intravenous albumin was given and no difference in the incidence of clinical pregnancy per woman when cryopreservation of all embryos was compared to fresh ET. However, a slightly lower clinical pregnancy rate was reported in albumin and fresh ET women than when all embryos were cryopreserved (D'Angelo & Amso 2002). A Cochrane Review of 'Coasting' for the treatment of OHSS is still under way. Clearly there is a need for well-designed randomized studies to determine the most appropriate treatment for women at risk of OHSS.

Treatment of established OHSS depends on its severity, the stage at which the diagnosis is made and whether the patient is pregnant or not. In mild/moderate OHSS (haematocrit <45%), bed rest, increased fluid intake and close monitoring of electrolyte balance may be sufficient. The patient's progress

can be supervised daily as an outpatient procedure. Patients with severe OHSS (haematocrit ≥45%, massive ascites) should be hospitalized and if critically ill, should be cared for in intensive care units. Paracentesis, for symptomatic relief or failing renal function, was reported to result in dramatic improvement in clinical symptoms with almost instantaneous diuresis, decrease in haematocrit, improved creatinine clearance and prevention of respiratory distress (Aboulghar et al 1992). In an extreme situation, therapeutic interruption of an early pregnancy may be the only life-saving action when other measures have failed.

Risk of genital cancer

The potential risk of genital cancer from follicular stimulation has initiated considerable debate (Cohen et al 1993, Fishel & Jackson 1989, Rossing et al 1994, Whittemore 1994). Excessive oestrogen secretion has been implicated in ovarian, endometrial and breast carcinoma, and excessive gonadotrophin secretion may have a direct carcinogenic effect as well. Although a number of case reports of ovarian tumours (benign, borderline malignancy, carcinoma) in women undergoing infertility treatment have raised questions about the potential neoplastic effects of ovulation induction medication, none proves a causal relationship. Results of case control and case cohort studies are conflicting. Whittemore et al (1992) pooled data from case control studies of ovarian cancer between 1956 and 1986 and reported that in nulligravid women there was positive association between the use of fertility medications and the risk of invasive and borderline epithelial tumours. There was a possible association between the use of such medications and the risk of non-epithelial cancers. However, the study had many limitations and a causal link between fertility medications and ovarian cancer cannot be confirmed (Whittemore 1994). In a case control study, Franceschi et al (1994) analysed the relationship between fertility drugs and ovarian cancer in four areas of Italy and the authors were able to exclude any association between the use of fertility drugs and the risk of epithelial ovarian cancer. Rossing et al (1994) examined the risk of ovarian tumours in a cohort of infertile women and reported a higher risk of malignant ovarian tumours in gravid and nulligravid women treated for infertility and in particular those who used clomiphene citrate for 12 or more treatment cycles.

All of the above studies had their limitations and included a relatively small number of tumours during the follow-up period. Other studies (Mosgaard et al 1997, Parrazzini et al 1997, Shushan et al, 1996) also failed to show strong or any association between fertility drugs and a subsequent risk of ovarian cancer. However, the previously documented increased risk of ovarian cancer in nulliparous women or those with infertility but not undergoing treatment was confirmed (Mosgaard et al 1997). All authors agreed on the need for further studies with appropriate control groups to determine whether the link is causal and, if so, the magnitude of the risks, the treatments that are more risky and the women who are most susceptible. In an attempt to characterize ovarian and uterine tumours in a cohort of in vitro fertilization patients, Venn and colleagues (2001) examined pathology reports in a large cohort of IVF patients, who later developed ovarian or uterine cancer. The authors reported a broad range of patient and tumour characteristics and an increased incidence of uterine sarcoma.

Concerns relating to the effect of high oestrogen and progesterone levels on the potential risk for the development of breast cancer have also been expressed. A case control study (Braga et al 1996) failed to show any relation between fertility treatment and breast cancer risk. In another report (Venn et al 1995) the incidence of breast cancer in women who had had IVF treatment with ovarian stimulation in a single IVF clinic was not different from the incidence of the general population or in women referred for IVF but not treated. An interesting finding in the study was the significant association between unexplained infertility and both invasive ovarian and uterine body cancers independent of IVF exposure. The same group later reported their findings on a larger cohort of women (n = 29 700) attending 10 Australian IVF clinics (Venn et al 1999). Their previous findings were confirmed and further-more, they found a transient but significantly higher than expected incidence of breast and uterine cancer within 12 months of exposure to fertility drugs, though the incidence overall was no greater than expected. They also found no association between the number of IVF treatment cycles with ovarian stimulation and the incidence of breast, ovarian or uterine cancers. Further large studies are required to allow for variations between different populations in the expected incidence of these cancers and the effect of fertility drugs on the later development of cancer.

Procedure-related health problems

Whilst ultrasound-guided transvaginal oocyte recovery is at present the most commonly used method, the laparoscopic approach is still used in certain circumstances and is associated with risks related to anaesthesia, pneumoperitoneum, visceral and vascular injuries and infections. In women undergoing transvaginal oocyte retrievals, intestinal, vascular, uterine and tubal injury with the aspiration needle have been reported. Bleeding and infections may be serious, sometimes even fatal,

complications. Previous history of pelvic inflammatory disease may imply a higher risk of pelvic reinfection. Appropriate preoperative vaginal preparation and minimizing the number of repeated vaginal penetrations may serve to lower the risk of infection.

The long-term effect of repeated oocyte collections on the pelvic structures has not been fully evaluated. In one study of 15 women with endometriosis undergoing tubal embryo transfer, only one patient was noted to have a change in that one fallopian tube had become tethered to the corresponding ovary. Similarly, the culture of micro-organisms in peritoneal samples obtained at the time of laparoscopic tubal embryo transfer (coagulase-negative staphylococcus, β-haemolytic streptococcus and *Chlamydia trachomatis*) was not associated with the development of symptoms or signs of pelvic infection. Neither did it prevent three conceptions and subsequent normal deliveries without any sequelae to the newborn. Furthermore, spontaneous pregnancies were also reported up to 18 months after an unsuccessful attempt (Amso 1996). The results in this small group of women are very assuring, but larger studies are required to determine the full impact of these techniques on the pelvic organs.

Psychological and emotional effects

The intensive monitoring that is commonly required during ovulation induction may cause undue stress and anxiety. In the immediate aftermath of a failed treatment cycle or following early pregnancy loss, the couple may experience shock, frustration and depression. Long-term effects of failed treatment(s) may result in profound consequences on physical and mental health and may lead to marital discord and breakdown of the relationship. There is very little evidence to determine whether psychological distress is a consequence or cause of infertility (Brkovich & Fisher 1998). The precise effects of stress and anxiety on the outcome of treatment are not clear. Infertile women are more depressed and anxious than fertile ones (van Balen & Trimbos-Kemper 1993) and the stress of IVF treatment may have important psychoendocrinological responses. Indeed, reduction of stress associated with IVF may even improve conception rates (Eugster & Vingerhoets 1999).

In addition to the increased antenatal medical risks associated with multiple pregnancy, mothers encounter considerable psychological difficulties after birth. The increased perinatal mortality and morbidity are well known and further increase the couple's anxiety and emotional strain. The majority of these mothers report considerable fatigue and stress, social isolation, strain on marital relationship, emotional detachment and difficulties in their relationship with their children (Garel & Blondel 1992). Emotional distress and high depression scores with regrets about having triplets persisted for up to 4 years (Garel et al 1997).

Risk of congenital anomalies and malignancy in the newborn

Tan et al (1992b) reported comparable malformation rates in children born following conventional IVF with matched normally conceived pregnancies. ICSI enabled men with severe oligospermia or azoospermia to pass their genes on to their own progeny, an event that may not have been possible just a few years ago. This raised certain questions about the genetic constitution of any resulting pregnancies after ICSI (Liebaers et al 1995). The quality of the sperm used for ICSI treatment may adversely affect the chromosome constitution of the resulting embryo (Obasaju et al 1999). This case report utilized fluorescent in situ hybridization (FISH) to determine any chromosomal abnormalities in embryos prior to implantation. An infertile couple with severe male infertility and endometriosis underwent two ICSI cycles with the husband's sperm and one IVF cycle with donor sperm. Preimplantation genetic diagnosis with FISH showed that all the embryos derived from the cycle in which donor sperm was used were chromosomally normal, whereas 82% of the embryos derived from cycles in which the husband's sperm was used were chromosomally abnormal. It was concluded that paternal factors, thought to be derived from the paternal centrosome, could have contributed to the numerical chromosomal abnormalities and may in turn predispose to implantation failure. It is possible that they would be manifested as congenital abnormalities that present to the paediatrician. The cycle in which donor sperm was used resulted in an ongoing pregnancy.

Short- and long-term follow-up data on children born by ICSI have thus far been encouraging. Bider et al (1999) did not note any major malformations or difference between ICSI and conventional IVF. Similarly, a retrospective study comparing 132 children born after IVF and 120 after ICSI reported no differences between the two groups for early embryonic development and obstetric outcome (van Golde et al 1999). The congenital malformation rate was 3% after IVF and 1.7% after ICSI, though in both groups only 30% of women underwent prenatal chromosomal diagnosis. A long prospective follow-up study (Bonduelle et al 1999) of 1987 children born after ICSI, with subgroups depending on whether ejaculated, epididymal or testicular spermatozoa were used, reported no increase in the incidence of congenital malformations or abnormal karyotypes. Physical examination of these children was carried out at 2 months, 1 year and 2 years after birth and noted similar growth parameters and developmental milestones in all subgroups. A more recent case control population study (Sutcliffe et al 2001) did not show any significant difference between children conceived after ICSI and their naturally conceived peers in term of physical health and their neurodevelopment.

One condition that does appear to be directly associated with ICSI is hypospadias, a malformation of the penis. In one study (Wennerholm et al 2000) of over 1000 babies born after ICSI seven cases of hypospadias were identified, with an expectation in the general population of around two. Hypospadias appears to be associated with paternal subfertility so a link with ICSI is possible. The same study showed an increased risk of abnormalities in babies born after ICSI compared to babies born without the use of fertility treatments; however, this was mainly due to conditions associated with multiple or premature births rather than the ICSI treatment itself.

Couples requiring ICSI appear to have an increased incidence of chromosomal disorders and this appears to manifest itself in a low implantation rate (Scholtes et al 1998). This may increase the risk of transmitting chromosomal aberrations, though it can be minimized by karyotyping potential parents, preimplantion genetic diagnosis and prenatal fetal karyotyping. There is also the risk of transmitting fertility problems to the offspring. Overall, about 20 000 babies have been born worldwide through ICSI in the last decade and the vast majority of these are healthy normal children. However, since ICSI is still a relatively new procedure, the fertility potential of these children cannot be determined at present and further follow-up studies are required. Potential parents, however, may be reassured that generally there appears to be no increased incidence of major congenital malformations.

Retrospective comparison of births resulting from cryopreserved embryos with those after fresh replacement reported significantly lower incidence of major congenital malformation (Wada et al 1994). However, more recently children born following FER were compared and matched for maternal age, parity, single or twin pregnancy and gestational age at birth with those born after fresh IVF and those conceived spontaneously (Wennerholm et al 1998). The authors reported similar growth rates, incidence of major malformations and prevalence of chronic disease at 18 months.

Risk of malignancy

It is important for potential parents undergoing assisted reproduction treatments to be counselled on the likely outcome of their unborn children having any life-threatening illnesses such as cancer. There have been case reports (Toren et al 1995) suggesting a possible association between IVF and paediatric malignancies such as hepatoblastoma and clear cell carcinoma of the kidney. Two recent studies (Bruinsma et al 2000, Lerner-Geva et al 2000) did not detect any significant increase in the incidence of cancer among cohorts of children born after IVF in comparison with the expected age-adjusted rates of the general population. Larger prospective studies are needed to provide the necessary power to reach definite conclusions.

In view of the above risks and potential health problems, it is imperative that clinicians should define the risks as those not only associated with the medication itself but also the short and long-term effects which are either physical, emotional or pregnancy related. As many of the long-term effects are still undetermined, clinicians must offer couples appropriate counselling and exercise extreme care and caution before and during treatment.

Obstetric and perinatal outcome of ART

The obstetric risks and outcome of assisted reproduction treatments have always been the subject of considerable debate. Indeed, the first pregnancy following in vitro fertilization was an ectopic pregnancy. In the context of pregnancy outcomes, the aim of assisted reproduction treatments should be a healthy singleton delivery at term. However, infertile couples may not share this target (Goldfarb et al 1996, Murdoch 1997). They do not appreciate the risks associated with multiple pregnancy and indeed, between 67% and 90% of couples may desire a twin birth (Gleicher et al 1995), while less than a third regard a single child as an ideal outcome. Increasing age or duration of infertility has been associated with greater desire for multiple births (Murdoch 1997).

The risk of multiple pregnancy is greater with super-ovulation with or without IUI than IVF/ICSI treatments due to the overabundance of oocytes released from multiple follicles. The latter treatments allow greater control on the incidence of multiple pregnancy as the number of embryos replaced determines it. Indeed, when there are more than four developing follicles with intrauterine insemination (IUI) treatments, follicle reduction using the transvaginal ultrasound guidance prior to insemination reduced the multiple pregnancies without compromising pregnancy rates.

Antenatal and intrapartum complications following IVF/oocyte donation

Many studies have examined the obstetric outcome after fertility treatments. In early reports of IVF pregnancies, the miscarriage rate appeared to be higher in general (Australian In Vitro Fertilization Collaborative Group 1985) and more so when one or two embryos were transferred compared with three or four (Balen et al 1993). However, no increase in the spontaneous miscarriage rate was identified in a large series involving over 5000 cycles in more than 2391 women (Alsalili et al 1995). Comparison of the obstetric outcome of IVF pregnancies with matched normally conceived pregnancies (Tan et al 1992b) showed a higher multiple pregnancy rate of 25%, significantly increased incidence of vaginal bleeding and hypertension requiring hospitalization and caesarean births. Among IVF singleton pregnancies, there was a significantly increased incidence of intrauterine growth restriction, placenta praevia and preterm delivery. The increased obstetric risks may reflect the women's history of infertility, a relatively high incidence of poor obstetric history and the lower threshold for intervention in these patients. A more recent retrospective cohort study in Sweden (Bergh et al 1999) compared the obstetric outcome of IVF babies born between 1982 and 1995 with all babies born in the general population during the same period. It reported an approximately fivefold increase in preterm birth and low birthweight rates in IVF babies compared to controls. The study concluded that a high frequency of multiple births and maternal characteristics were the main factors leading to adverse outcome and not the IVF technique itself.

Others have also reported that IVF mothers may have higher incidences of pregnancy-induced hypertension, premature labour, labour induction and preterm delivery (Tallo et al 1995). Multiple pregnancies have a higher prevalence of pre-eclampsia and more so with triplets than in twins. A case control study (Skupski et al 1996) concluded that fetal number, placental mass or other factors unrelated to the success of implantation are more important to the development of pre-eclampsia than is the successful implantation alone. Comparison of singleton IVF pregnancies with matched controls showed longer first stage of labour, greater intrapartum blood loss and a trend towards a higher caesarean delivery rate than controls (Howe et al 1990). The authors concluded that

these differences probably do not arise from the physiology of IVF and are of minimal clinical significance; hence, these pregnancies should not be regarded as high risk in the absence of other predisposing factors.

The obstetric outcome of natural and IVF twin pregnancies was compared in a multicentre study. The mean gestational age was equal in the two groups at 36 weeks but the elective caesarean section rate was higher in the assisted conception group. Induction of labour rates did not differ and once labour commenced there was no difference in the mode of delivery or neonatal short-term morbidity between the two groups. Similarly, birth weight, gestational length and perinatal mortality rates by conventional and extended classification were not different (Agustsson et al 1997). Others have also reported comparable outcome between the two groups in terms of mean duration of gestation, birth weight and incidence of congenital malformations (Dhont et al 1999) despite earlier suggestion of a higher incidence of preterm deliveries (Dhont et al 1997). There was also no difference in preterm labour, preterm premature rupture of membranes, pregnancy-induced hypertension and incidence of gestational diabetes (Fitzsimmons et al 1998).

Interestingly, for both singleton and twin IVF pregnancies the incidence of caesarean section is increased (Dhont et al 1999). In Agustssen's study (1997), it was noted that only the elective caesarean section rate was significantly higher. This may in part be a reflection of the generally held medical perception of ART pregnancies being 'precious' but may also indicate a higher complication rate necessitating operative delivery.

Women who conceive following oocyte donation, especially with a history of ovarian failure, should be considered as 'high risk'. Analysis of 232 ovum donation pregnancies reported a higher risk of pregnancy-induced hypertension and postpartum haemorrhage as well as an increased incidence of small-for-gestational-age infants. Of the 151 babies born, the overall operative delivery rate was 85% and the caesarean section rate was 69% (Abdalla et al 1998).

Antenatal and intrapartum complications following ICSI

Pregnancy following ICSI treatment has generated interest due to the additional tests involved with these pregnancies, namely the microinjection technique and the prenatal diagnostic tests often performed on the resulting pregnancies. The incidence of pregnancy loss in early observational reports ranged from 22% to 38% depending on the use of ejaculated, epididymal or testicular spermatozoa respectively (Wisanto et al 1996) and was not different from conventional IVF outcome in historical controls. Similarly other complications such as prematurity and low birth weight were related to the multiplicity of pregnancy. A national cohort study of all ICSI pregnancies in Denmark between 1994 and 1997 confirmed that ICSI pregnancy outcome was comparable with other studies, except that no sex chromosome abnormalities were found (Loft et al 1999). In ICSI pregnancies where prenatal diagnosis (amniocentesis, chorion villus sampling) was carried out, the preterm delivery, low or very low birthweight rates were not increased when compared with cycles where no such tests were carried out. Furthermore, the fetal loss rates were comparable (Aytoz et al 1998).

Retrospective comparison of ICSI pregnancies with matched IVF controls (Govaerts et al 1998) showed no difference in the early pregnancy loss, congenital malformation or multiple pregnancy rates nor the singleton mean birth weight and gestational ages at birth. However, these last two parameters were significantly higher in ICSI twins than in IVF. Couples undergoing ICSI for severe male infertility (oligoasthenoteratozoospermia) have slightly reduced fertilization rates but have similar pregnancy loss and delivery rates to other couples undergoing ICSI and IVF for non-male factor infertility (Mercan et al 1998).

Embryo cryopreservation and obstetric outcome

Comparative retrospective studies of births resulting from cryopreserved embryos and conventional IVF reported similar incidence of twins and triplet births, mean gestation age and birth weight for singleton, twins and triplets in the two groups (Wada et al 1994). More recently, pregnancies resulting from the transfer of fresh or frozen conventional IVF or ICSI embryos were compared (Aytoz et al 1999). The frozen ICSI group showed a significantly higher miscarriage rate than the frozen conventional IVF patients. The incidence of preterm deliveries, very low birth weights, major malformations and intrauterine deaths was similar in all groups. However, the low birthweight rates in frozen IVF and ICSI were significantly lower than in the fresh embryo transfer groups.

Perinatal outcome of assisted reproduction pregnancies

Multiple pregnancy and prematurity

An increase in twinning and triplet rates in developed countries such as England and Wales, Germany, the Netherlands, Switzerland and others had been attributed to the higher proportion of mothers treated with ovulation-inducing hormones and partially attributed to IVF (Imaizumi 1998). The vast majority of multiple pregnancies are dizygotic. The rate of monozygotic twinning after ART, irrespective of treatment modality or micromanipulation, increased more than twofold over the background rate in the general population (Schachter et al 2001).

It is widely accepted that multiple pregnancies account for a disproportionately large share of adverse pregnancy outcomes (Powers & Kiely 1994) including increased incidence of very low birth weight, low birth weight, perinatal and neonatal mortality, as well as infant death. The increased incidence of death and morbidity in twin as compared to singleton pregnancy has been attributed mainly to prematurity (Ho & Wu 1975) and to adverse outcomes associated with premature delivery such as hyaline membrane disease, hypocalcaemia, hypoglycaemia, hyperbilirubinaemia, small for dates and low Apgar scores. In one recent study (Tough et al 2000), the contribution of IVF to changes in the incidence of low birth weight, preterm delivery and multiple birth over a 3-year period was substantial. The increased incidence of preterm

delivery and low birth weight is partially related to multiple births, though an increase in preterm deliveries has also been seen in IVF singleton pregnancies (Dhont et al 1999). The high multiple pregnancy rate is related to the number of embryos transferred. The evidence supports the view that transferring two embryos instead of three does not compromise the chance of pregnancy but reduces the risk of triplets (Matson et al 1999, Preutthipan et al 1996). It results in an overall multiple pregnancy rate of 14.3% for double embryo transfers and 32.4% for triple embryo transfers, with no significant difference in the pregnancy rate if at least one good-quality embryo was available for transfer (Tasdemir et al 1995).

In one report (Slotnick & Ortega 1996), it was suggested that monoamniotic multiple gestations may be increased in zona-manipulated cycles (ICSI, zona drilling, assisted hatching) and although all resulting monoamniotic pregnancies ended in live births, there was high incidence of intrauterine discordance in fetal growth. Some early evidence suggested that ART twin pregnancies have a higher incidence of preterm deliveries and need more neonatal intensive care when compared to matched control twin pregnancies (Dhont et al 1997).

Perinatal mortality/morbidity

Early reports (Tan et al 1992b) suggested that stillbirths and perinatal mortality rates following IVF were comparable with national maternal age-standardized rates. Twins conceived with IVF have comparable perinatal mortality and morbidity rates to spontaneously conceived controls (Dhont et al 1999). However, a retrospective cohort study (Fitzsimmons et al 1998) reported a significantly increased perinatal mortality in spontaneous twin gestations but not in triplets when compared with those resulting from ART. Singleton IVF pregnancies were reported to have significantly worse perinatal outcome in comparison to spontaneously conceived pregnancies, mainly due to the increased rate of preterm birth (Dhont et al 1999). Others (Ishii et al 1994) reported a doubling of the premature birth rate in singleton post-infertility pregnancy when compared to normal controls, with an increased mortality rate. IVF infants may have a lower mean birth weight and shorter gestations. Additionally, these infants may require more days of oxygen therapy and continuous positive airway pressure and longer hospitalization as well as having an increased prevalence of respiratory distress syndrome, patent ductus arteriosus and sepsis (Tallo et al 1995). The same authors concluded that couples who underwent IVF appear to be at increased risk of having low birthweight and preterm infants, but that multiple gestations accounted for most of the neonatal morbidity. ICSI treatment does not appear to differ from conventional IVF when the incidences of multiple pregnancies and perinatal outcome are compared (Bider et al 1999).

Retrospective comparison of births resulting from cryopreserved embryos with those after conventional IVF and fresh embryo transfer showed no difference in the perinatal mortality between the two groups (Wada et al 1994).

It is logical to assume that women with infertility problems are likely to have an increased incidence of pelvic or systemic pathology to account for their infertile status. It therefore follows that such women, having achieved a pregnancy, would be susceptible to an increase in the complication rate. Indeed, women with a past medical history of infertility, whether treated or untreated, have a significantly increased risk of perinatal death (Draper et al 1999). In this study, women with untreated infertility were at increased risk of perinatal death and any association with multiple births did not explain this finding. The same was true for women with treated infertility where the risks of associated multiple births explained some but not all of this excess. The authors advocated that at antenatal booking a history of infertility, irrespective of treatment, should be sought as these women have a significantly increased risk of perinatal death.

PREIMPLANTATION GENETIC DIAGNOSIS: BREAKING THE BARRIERS

Preimplantation genetic diagnosis (PGD) is a new procedure that has been developed in the past decade as an alternative to prenatal diagnosis for carriers of chromosomal or sex-linked disorders (Handyside et al 1990). As with other forms of prenatal diagnosis, its primary aim is to avoid severe genetic disease in the offspring of a couple who have a high probability of passing on mutant genes, but with an added advantage that it avoids termination of pregnancy. The procedure involves biopsy of a single cell from the human cleavage stage embryo at around the eight-cell stage followed by the application of a sensitive diagnostic technique to that cell. At present, biopsied polar body and/or blastomeres have been used and pregnancies as well as healthy babies have resulted from such biopsied and diagnosed embryos. The diagnostic technique, specific for the disorder being tested, may be analysis of enzymes, chromosomes or specific mutation in the DNA. If the cell shows no abnormality in the course of this analysis, the embryo is judged to be normal and transferred to the mother to initiate pregnancy.

The enzyme approach has been disregarded, for the few genes studied, as it has been difficult to differentiate between maternal gene expression (mRNA inherited in the egg cytoplasm) and embryonic gene expression in the early embryo (Braude et al 1989). However, the analysis of sex chromosomes using FISH and the analysis of specific gene sequences using sensitive polymerase chain reaction (PCR) for sexing or detection of a specific gene mutation such as cystic fibrosis have been used successfully.

Preimplantation diagnosis of single gene defects and chromosomal abnormalities by analysis of the first and second polar bodies had been proposed as an alternative to embryonic biopsy. The limitations of this approach lie in the fact that the genotype of polar bodies is not identical to that of the oocyte and that the validity of predicting chromosome abnormalities in the pre-embryo from observations of the chromosome complement of either polar bodies has been subject to uncertainty. The variety of combinations that may arise through random segregation of each single chromatid either to the second polar body or oocyte indicate that it would not be possible to predict the chromosome normality or otherwise of the female gamete (Angell 1994) and more data are needed. It has also been reported that polar bodies are more difficult to manipulate than blastomeres due to their size and that for some reason, embryos obtained after polar body biopsy show a reduced implantation rate (Egozcue 1994). Hence, subject to the success of polar body analysis techniques, the possible application in clinical practice would be limited to those couples who, on moral grounds, reject embryo selection after preimplantation diagnosis.

Since the introduction of PGD, attempts have been made to maximize the results through simultaneous detection of more than one mutation, increase efficiencies and further be able to analyse these biopsied cells for chromosomal abnormalities. Avner et al (1994) reported the successful development of a PCR-based method for the simultaneous detection of the two most common mutations of the cystic fibrosis gene in a single blastomere. The diagnostic system allowed the identification of affected embryos as well as phenotypically normal carriers. The completion of the multiple loci analysis with this method required about 17 hours and embryo transfer was possible on the same day or within 24 hours of biopsy.

Thornhill et al (1994) introduced the concept of recycling the single cell to detect specific chromosomes and investigate unique gene sequences. The two techniques, PCR and FISH, were carried out on the same single cell. In this system a fixed cell is used as a DNA template for PCR prior to the FISH analysis. The combination of the two techniques provided an even greater potential for the efficiency and accuracy of preimplantation diagnosis. It was also proposed that the potential of cell recycling could be extended using multiplex PCR with different sets of primers to examine between five and 10 specific gene sequences simultaneously. The FISH analysis can also be extended to employ up to seven specific chromosomal DNA probes using combinatorial labelling.

Muggleton-Harris et al (1995) demonstrated that dual-stage biopsies are possible where blastomeres are taken from the 8–10 cell embryos and the biopsied cleavage stage embryo was cultured to the blastocyst stage, where the serial biopsy of 3–5 mural trophectoderm cells provided two further cell samples. Repeat or additional preimplantation diagnostic analyses were undertaken again. This approach answers to a certain extent the uncertainty as to how representative is the chromosome constitution of the single blastomere of the whole embryo. Equally there would be a significant advantage for genetic diagnosis studies if retrospective PCR analysis could be undertaken on stored cell samples used previously for preimplantation genetic diagnosis. Pregnancy rates have continued to improve following replacement of cleavage stage embryos and cultured blastocysts. So far, the techniques have been used to diagnose cystic fibrosis, sickle cell disease, haemophilia, Marfan's syndrome, retinitis pigmentosa and Duchenne muscular dystrophy as well as the identification (using FISH technique) of human chromosomes X, Y, 13, 18 and 21. Preimplantation diagnosis may also be achieved after natural conceptions by obtaining blastocysts through a uterine lavage procedure.

Data collected by the European Society for Human Reproduction and Embryology (ESHRE) special interest group on reproductive genetics showed that over a period of seven years, 886 couples were referred for 1318 PGD cycles resulting in 163 pregnancies and 162 babies. It confirmed that the technique is becoming more established for increasing applications and that such data have become invaluable for patients, clinicians and governmental bodies alike (ESHRE PGD Consortium Steering Committee 2000).

The psychological implications and acceptability of pre-implantation diagnosis is an area that requires further evaluation. Palomba et al (1994) examined the degree of acceptability of preimplantation diagnosis with blastocyst stage biopsy in women at risk of β-thalassaemia who were awaiting chorionic villous sampling. The authors reported that all women who had had previous therapeutic termination of pregnancy found blastocyst biopsy acceptable, while only 30% of women who had not had a previous therapeutic abortion favoured the technique, and 25% of primigravid women also favoured blastocyst biopsy over chorionic villous sampling. In this group of women, blastocysts were anticipated to have been obtained through uterine lavage, hence the diagnosis would have been made on the 5th day after fertilization, offering psychological advantages, both by reducing the waiting time of 11 weeks and by avoiding therapeutic abortion in the first trimester of pregnancy when there was an affected fetus. In women undergoing in vitro fertilization, PGD also offers the option of replacing only healthy embryos and possibly increasing the chances of implantation and pregnancy.

ETHICAL DILEMMAS IN ASSISTED REPRODUCTION

Edwards & Sharpe (1971) first raised the problems related to social values and research on the human embryo. The Human Fertilization and Embryology Act (1990) resulted in the establishment of a statutory body, the Human Fertilization and Embryology Authority, within the UK to regulate and monitor, by means of an inspection and licensing system, the provision of treatment and research using human gametes and embryos.

The authority has also issued consultation documents on a number of ethical and social dimensions of the new aspects of assisted human reproduction. The use of oocytes from donated ovarian tissue for infertility treatment and embryo research has generated considerable debate and views were obtained from a wider public before determining the authority's position. The current opinion is that it would be acceptable to use ovarian tissue for treatment purposes only from live donors. In the case of a deceased woman over the age of 18 there appears to be no objection in principle to the use of donated ovarian tissue for the treatment of other women but informed consent should be provided before death. Not unexpectedly, there was widespread and fundamental objection to the use of fetal tissue for treatment in view of the difficult psychological consequences for the resulting offspring.

The debate in the UK has contributed to the establishment in many countries of similar public mechanisms to review clinical and ethical questions relating to ART and provide counsel. Self-regulation, supported by national and/or local codes of practice, appears to be the most popular means but countries like Germany and the UK impose strict codes underlined by the power of the law. In the USA, the National Advisory Board on Ethics and Reproduction was set up in 1992 to fill the vacuum created by the lack of systematic reflection on the ethical questions raised by reproductive research and medicine. However, in parts of the United States, legislation relating to assisted reproduction has been implemented, such as the State of Florida Assisted Reproduction Technology Act of 1993.

Pregnancies in postmenopausal women have been controversial. The introduction of oocyte donation, with its high clinical pregnancy, implantation and live-birth rates, has meant that pregnancy is now possible in virtually any woman with a uterus and no definitive physiological limitation appears to exist based solely on the age of the patient. There are arguments and counter-arguments on either side of the debate with respect to this treatment. At present, the consensus of opinion in the UK is that no category of women should automatically be denied treatment, that it is not necessary nor advisable to fix an upper age limit for the treatment of infertility and that each case should be considered individually. It is also required by law to consider the welfare of the prospective child and the implications for the couple concerned. A survey of community attitudes to maternal age and pregnancy after assisted reproduction technology reported support for the use of a woman's own eggs or embryos after the menopause, but only minority support for oocyte or embryo donation to postmenopausal women (Bowman & Saunders 1994). The psychosocial effects of such treatment are largely unknown and the nature of obstetric complications will not be known without greater numbers being reported. Epidemiological statistics from the USA suggest that one in five mothers and one in three fathers having a child at the age of 50 years will not survive to see the child at college; if the age of delivery is 55 years, then one in three mothers and one in two fathers will not survive the same length of time (Meldrum 1993).

Equally controversial has been treatment by IVF with surrogacy. Appropriate and genuine indications exist and more than 300 births are known to have occurred in the United Kingdom following this treatment. HFEA guidance and governmental legislation are in place to regulate its provision, but ethical dilemmas are often encountered with surrogacy. The host's wish to keep the child, an abnormal child rejected by parents, payment or no payment for the host and the long-term psychological effects on all parties are just a few of these dilemmas (Brinsden et al 2000). Public opinion may alter over time, especially if the attitudes of the younger portion of the community, as reflected in the above survey, are maintained and furthermore, opinion expressed in one community may or may not reflect that of other communities.

Other ethical controversies have attracted worldwide debate such as the control of human sex ratios and 'sex selection', posthumous reproduction, and artificial insemination of single and lesbian women with donor sperm. Posthumous reproduction can result in complex and expensive legal proceedings and generate undue anxieties for the parties involved. It has also been argued that it lacks the very values that most people find in the reproductive experience, such as interests in rearing one's child or giving birth. Several countries (Canada, France, Germany and Sweden) have legislation that forbids posthumous reproduction on the basis of moral commitment to fairness and respect for children and an obligation to treat them as ends in themselves (Aziza-Shuster 1994).

Even more controversy has been generated lately by the success of cloning techniques, stem cell research and the ethics of using PGD to select stem cell donors for an existing person. The aims of PGD are to select embryos that do not have the genetic mutation that affects the family (e.g. Fanconi's anaemia or thalassaemia). However, to select an HLA-compatible stem cell donor from these embryos not because of a familial genetic disease but to treat a sick sibling raises ethical concerns. Many argue that the unborn child becomes a commodity and its best interest may not be best addressed while others point to the benefits for treating an existing person (Boyle & Savulescu 2001).

The HFEA has recently approved the use of genetic tests in conjunction with IVF by a couple to have a child where stem cells harvested from umbilical cord blood could be used for bone transplant to treat their 3-year-old-child (Dyer 2002a). In a further development, a Parliamentary committee set up to review the rules governing stem cell reserch concluded that researchers should continue to have access to human embryos and that further review is warranted towards the end of the decade to consider the continuing need for stem cell research. Furthermore, the committee argued that there was no ethical difference between the use of embryos obtained from IVF and those created by cell nuclear replacement (CNR) or cloning, with the proviso that 14 days should remain the limit for research on early embryos (Dyer 2002b).

Whilst all these issues are brought about through advances in technology it is clear that, irrespective of the current guidelines, clinicians need a better understanding of the background and needs of such women and their views towards the resulting child and its future development. Similarly, clinicians must have the right of non-participation should their conscience forbid it.

LOOKING INTO THE FUTURE

As we enter a new century and indeed a new millennium, rapid developments are taking place in ART and will certainly lead to new challenges. It is tempting to speculate on the areas that are most likely to witness such developments over the next few years.

Recombinant FSH compounds are now well established in superovulation protocols. Early results from efficacy and safety studies comparing recombinant human hCG with urinary hCG for induction of final follicular maturation in IVF indicate that these compounds are well tolerated and as effective as the urinary products. Equally exciting are results of efficacy and safety studies of recombinant human LH to induce final follicular maturation in IVF or when used in association with FSH in ovarian stimulation protocols. Such developments will enable clinicians to fine-tune follicular development by choosing the precise LH and FSH dose independently of each other to suit individual patient needs. It also appears that when used for final follicular maturation, there is less risk of severe OHSS.

Improving pregnancy and live-birth rates will remain a challenge for the future. Reports of high pregnancy rates following elective transfer of one or two embryos stressed the need for accurate selection of the highest quality embryo(s). However, this is notoriously difficult and often subjective.

Numerous embryo-scoring protocols, based on embryo morphology, have been proposed over the years. A recent report (Fisch et al 2001) showed correlation between a high 'graduated embryo score', based on morphological assessment of the embryo at the first cell division stage and on day 3, and blastocyst formation and consequently high pregnancy rate. More accurate assessment methods, possibly including biochemical markers, are desperately needed. Vascular changes in the ovaries and endometrium have been proposed to influence the outcome of ART. Highly vascular follicles or endometrial layers are believed to result in high-quality oocytes or better embryo receptivity respectively (Bhal et al 1999). Colour Doppler indices have not reflected outcome in a consistent manner while power Doppler energy images were evaluated subjectively. Development of computer software programs to analyse and quantify these colour or power Doppler images may provide more consistent and reproducible indices for follicular development or endometrial receptivity (Amso et al 2001).

The unravelling of the human genome and the increase in our knowledge of the genetic basis for many more diseases than we had ever imagined previously will lead to a greater understanding of the factors involved in male infertility and how to increase fecundity. This, coupled with advances in preimplantation genetic diagnosis, will enable accurate screening of parents for specific genes before treatment, biopsied embryos before replacement and the resulting child afterwards. Additionally, these advances will permit rapid progress in gene therapy for single or multiple gene disorders where a normal cloned gene(s) is used to replace the faulty genome.

Another challenging area for research is that of preserving fertility in children or young adults treated for cancer. As survival rates continue to improve more young people want to know if they will be fertile, if their children will have a greater risk of developing cancer and what alternatives exist should pelvic irradiation or chemotherapy adversely affect their fertility permanently. Sperm banking is a well-recognized preservation technique for pubertal males and adults. In women, several approaches are being explored but none is yet clinically established. Oocyte cryopreservation requires superovulation treatment to induce multifollicular development followed by oocyte retrieval and its availability is limited. Endocrine function and oocyte retrieval after autologous transplantation of ovarian cortical strips to the forearm has been reported (Oktay et al 2001). This approach may be useful for women undergoing pelvic irradiation only, but its efficacy is questionable for women undergoing chemotherapy where ovarian tissue damage is very likely. Other interventions requiring surgical harvesting of gonadal tissue or germ cells remain experimental. There are many ethical concerns with these interventions, particularly their experimental nature in emotionally vulnerable patients, who often present to ART units with unrealistic expectations, the possibility of harvesting malignant cells with the germ cells and the potential for continued transmission of germ-line mutations in cancer predisposition genes. All these highlight the need for further research and well-designed controlled clinical trials.

As anticipated in the previous edition, the 'Internet' has become an important facet of medicine. It offers several opportunities such as information resources, communication tools and new consulting modes for patients and has resulted in a major change in the patient–doctor relationship. Thousands of pages on infertility and ART are found on the Worldwide Web, providing medical information and self-help solutions for patients. Ironically, the Internet creates more challenges, such as the threat of misleading information, unlicensed drug usage, inequity between the digital 'haves' and 'have nots', and legal and security problems. It even has its own disease, the Internet print-out (IPO) syndrome, in which patients present their clinicians with pages of information, sometimes useless, at their consultation! It is the duty of ART units to be proactive in this revolution and disseminate general information, specific instructions and up-to-date success rates of the different techniques in their units to any couple requiring such therapy.

Such ethical issues will continue to be the focus of ethics committees and legislators worldwide. Developments in one country have often led to 'global' ethical and societal debates with establishment of voluntary or statutory bodies to consult and develop guidelines and implement laws, where necessary. It is our duty to ensure the continued trust and support of society for the scientists and clinicians working in this field. In the UK, it is reassuring to see that such measures are in place and are fulfilling their role.

KEY POINTS

1. In vitro fertilization should not be used as a panacea for marital or psychosexual disorders, but to fulfil the wishes of a well-adjusted couple to have a baby.
2. The aims of superovulation regimens in assisted reproduction are to maximize the number of follicles which mature, minimize the degree of asynchrony amongst developing follicles and minimize the deleterious effects of the abnormal follicular environment on luteal function and endometrial receptivity.
3. The use of GnRH agonists in stimulation protocols has increased steadily since their introduction into clinical practice and appears to result in a reduction in the cancellation rates, an increase in the number of oocytes retrieved and a significantly higher clinical pregnancy rate.
4. Past history of infertility significantly increases the risk of perinatal death.
5. A history of unexplained infertility is significantly associated with invasive ovarian and uterine body cancers independent of IVF exposure. There is also a transient but significantly higher than expected incidence of breast and uterine cancer within 12 months of exposure to fertility drugs, though the incidence overall is no greater than expected.
6. Pregnancy and live-birth rates in national registers in the US, France and Britain have improved by about 50% since the first annual reports were published in these countries.

KEY POINTS (CONTINUED)

7. Crude pregnancy rates per couple are almost meaningless and cumulative conception or live-birth rates should be increasingly used in reporting conventional and assisted reproduction treatment outcomes.
8. The outcome of assisted reproduction treatment depends on the age of the female partner, the duration of infertility, the multiplicity of factors responsible for the couple's subfertility, the number of embryos transferred and the number of treatment cycles that a couple undergo.
9. When four or more embryos are available for transfer, the transfer of only two embryos results in equally high pregnancy and live-birth rates. However, the rate of multiple pregnancy with all its pregnancy and perinatal complications is dramatically reduced.
10. One FER cycle increases the take home baby rate by 5% while one fresh and two FER cycles achieve a cumulative viable pregnancy rate of 41%. The cost per delivery for FER cycle has been estimated to be between 25% and 45% of a fresh cycle.
11. In view of the potential health risks arising from assisted reproduction techniques, it is imperative that clinicians should define the risks as those associated with the medication itself as well as the short- and long-term physical, emotional and pregnancy-related effects.
12. Male infertility is a very common cause of childlessness.
13. Rate of pregnancy complications following ICSI treatment is comparable with matched IVF controls. So far, hypospadias appears to be the only congenital anomaly directly associated with ICSI treatment.
14. Preimplantation genetic diagnosis is now an established technique and is only one facet of the genetic revolution.
15. Ethical dilemmas in assisted reproduction continue to provoke considerable global debate and some treatments have been controversial.
16. Clinicians must have the right of non-participation should their conscience forbid it.

REFERENCES

Abdalla HI, Billet A, Kan AK et al 1998 Obstetric outcome in 232 ovum donation pregnancies. British Journal of Obstetrics and Gynaecology 105(3):332–337
Aboulghar MA, Mansour RT, Serour GI, Riad R, Ramzi AM 1992 Autotransfusion of the ascitic fluid in the treatment of severe ovarian hyperstimulation syndrome. Fertility and Sterility 58:1056–1059
Adonakis G, Camus M, Joris H, Vandervorst M, van Streitegham A, Devroey P 1997 The role of the number of replaced embryos on intracytoplasmic sperm injection outcome in women over the age of 40. Human Reproduction 12(11):2542–2545
Agustsson T, Geirsson RT, Mires G 1997 Obstetric outcome of natural and assisted conception twin pregnancies is similar. Acta Obstetricia et Gynecologica Scandinavica 76(1):45–49
Alrayyes S, Fakih H, Khan I 1997 Effect of age and cycle responsiveness in patients undergoing intracytoplasmic sperm injection. Fertility and Sterility 68(1):123–127
Alsalili, Yuzpe A, Tummon I et al 1995 Cumulative pregnancy rates and pregnancy outcome after in-vitro fertilization. Human Reproduction 10:470–474
Al-Shawaf T, Nolan A, Guirgis R, Harper J, Santis M, Craft I 1992 The

influence of ovarian response on gamete intra-Fallopian transfer outcome in older women. Human Reproduction 7(8):1106–1110

Amso NN 1995a Role of assisted reproduction in endometriosis. In: Shaw RW (ed) Endometriosis: current understanding and management. Blackwell Science, Oxford, pp 282–295

Amso NN 1995b Potential health hazards of assisted reproduction: problems facing the clinician. Human Reproduction 10:1628–1630

Amso NN 1996 Studies of the Fallopian tube environment and an assessment of its role in assisted reproduction. PhD thesis, Faculty of Medicine, University of London

Amso NN, Ahuja KK, Morris N, Shaw RW 1990 The management of predicted ovarian hyperstimulation involving gonadotropin-releasing hormone analog with elective cryopreservation of all pre-embryos. Fertility and Sterility 53:1087–1090

Amso NN, Watermeyer SR, Pugh N, O'Brien S, d'Angelo A 2001 Quantification of power Doppler energy and its future potential. Fertility and Sterility 76(3):583–587

Angell RR 1994 Polar body analysis: possible pitfalls in preimplantation diagnosis of chromosomal disorders based on polar body analysis. Human Reproduction 9:181–182

Arthur ID, Anthony FW, Masson GM, Thomas EJ 1994 The selection criteria on an IVF program can remove the association between maternal age and implantation. Acta Obstetrica et Gynecologica Scandinavica 73(3):562–566

Asch RH, Ivery G, Goldsman M, Frederick JL, Stone SC, Balmaceda JP 1993 The use of intravenous albumin in patients at high risk for severe ovarian hyperstimulation syndrome. Human Reproduction 8:1015–1020

Ashkenazi J, Orvieto R, Gold-Deutch R et al 1996 The impact of woman's age and sperm parameters on fertilization rates in IVF cycles. European Journal of Obstetrics, Gynecology and Reproductive Biology 66(2):155–159

Australian In Vitro Fertilisation Collaborative Group 1985 High incidence of preterm births and early losses in pregnancy after in vitro fertilisation. British Medical Journal 291(6503):1160–1163

Avner R, Laufer N, Safran A, Karem B-S, Friedmann A, Mitrani-Rosenbaum S 1994 Preimplantation diagnosis of cystic fibrosis by simultaneous detection of the W1282X and delta F508 mutations. Human Reproduction 9:1676–1680

Aytoz A, de Catte L, Camus M et al 1998 Obstetric outcome after prenatal diagnosis in pregnancies. Human Reproduction 13:2958–2961

Aytoz A, van den Abbeel E, Bonduelle M et al 1999 Obstetric outcome of pregnancies after transfer of cryopreserved and fresh embryos obtained. Human Reproduction 14:2619–2624

Aziza-Shuster E 1994 A child at all costs: posthumous reproduction and the meaning of parenthood. Human Reproduction 9:2182–2185

Balen AH, MacDougall J, Tan SL 1993 The influence of the number of embryos transferred in 1060 in-vitro fertilization pregnancies on miscarriage rates and pregnancy outcome. Human Reproduction 8(8):1324–1328

Bergh C, Howels CM, Borg K et al 1997 Recombinant human follicle stimulating hormone (r-hFSH; Gonal-F) versus highly purified urinary FSH (Metrodin HP) results of a randomized comparative study in women undergoing assisted reproductive techniques. Human Reproduction 12:2133–2139

Bergh T, Ericson A, Hillensjo T, Nygren KG, Wennerholm UB 1999 Deliveries and children born after in-vitro fertilisation in Sweden 1982–95: a retrospective cohort study. Lancet 354(9190):1579–1585

Bhal PS, Pugh ND, Chui DK, Gregory L, Walker SM, Shaw RW 1999 The use of transvaginal power Doppler ultrasonography to evaluate the relationship between perifollicular vascularity and outcome in in-vitro fertilization treatment cycles. Human Reproduction 14(4):939–945

Bhattacharya S, Hamilton MPR, Shaaban M et al 2001 Conventional in-vitro fertilisation versus intracytoplasmic sperm injection for the treatment of non-male factor infertility: a randomised controlled trial. Lancet 357:2075–2079

Bider D, Livshitz A, Tur Kaspa I, Shulman A, Levron J, Dor J 1999 Incidence and perinatal outcome of multiple pregnancies after intracytoplasmic sperm injection compared to standard in vitro fertilization. Journal of Assisted Reproduction and Genetics 16(5):221–226

Bonduelle M, Camus M, de Vos A et al 1999 Seven years of intracytoplasmic sperm injection and follow up of 1987 subsequent children. Human Reproduction 14 (suppl 1):243–264

Bowman MC, Saunders DM 1994 Community attitudes to maternal age and pregnancy after assisted reproductive technology: too old at 50 years? Human Reproduction 9:167–171

Boyle RJ, Savulescu J 2001 Ethics of using preimplantation genetic diagnosis to select a stem cell donor for an existing person. British Medical Journal 323:1240–1243

Braga C, Negri E, La Vecchia et al 1996 Fertility treatment and risk of breast cancer. Human Reproduction 11:300–303

Braude PR, Monk M, Pickering SJ, Cant A, Johnson MH 1989 Measurement of HPRT activity in the human unfertilised oocyte and pre-embryo. Prenatal Diagnosis 9:839–850

Brinsden PR, Wada I, Tan SL, Balen A, Jacobs HS 1995 Diagnosis, prevention, and management of ovarian hyperstimulation syndrome. British Journal of Obstetrics and Gynaecology 102:767–772

Brinsden PR, Appleton TC, Murray E, Hussein M, Akagbosu F, Marcus SF 2000 Treatment by in vitro fertilisation with surrogacy: experience of one British centre. British Medical Journal 320:924–929

British Fertility Society 1997 Human reproduction 12 Natl Suppl. Journal of the British Fertility Society 2(2):88–92

Brkovich AM, Fisher WA 1998 Psychological distress and infertility: forty years of research. Journal of Psychosomatic Obstetrics and Gynaecology 19:218–228

Bruinsma F, Venn A, Lancaster P, Speirs A, Healy D 2000 Incidence of cancer in children born after in-vitro fertilization. Human Reproduction 15(3):604–607

Burton G, Abdalla HI, Kirkland A, Studd JWW 1992 The role of oocyte donation in women who are unsuccessful with in-vitro fertilization treatment. Human Reproduction 7(8):1103–1105

Carrillo AJ, Lane B, Pridman DD et al 1998 Improved clinical outcomes for in-vitro fertilisation with delay of embryo transfer from 48 to 72 hours after oocyte retrieval: use of glucose and phosphate-free media. Fertility and Sterility 69:329–334

Cha KY, Wirth DP, Lobo RA 2001 Does prayer influence the success of in vitro fertilization-embryo transfer? Report of a masked randomised trial. Journal of Reproductive Medicine 46:781–787

Cohen J, Alikani M, Malter HE, Adler A, Talansky BE, Rosenwaks Z 1991 Partial zona dissection or subzonal sperm insertion: microsurgical fertilization alternatives based on evaluation of sperm and embryo morphology. Fertility and Sterility 56:696–706

Cohen J, Forman R, Harlap S et al 1993 IFFS Expert Group Report on the Whittemore study related to the risk of ovarian cancer associated with the use of fertility agents. Human Reproduction 8:996–999

Collins JA, Burrows EA, Willan AR 1995 The prognosis for live birth among untreated infertile couples. Fertility and Sterility 64(1):22–28

Cordiero I, Calhaz-Jorge C, Barata M, Leal F, Proenca H, Coelho AM 1995 Repercussao da idade da mulher na taxa de clivagem e da qualidade embrionaria, na obtencao de gravidez por fertilizacao in vitro. Acta Medica Portuguesa 8(3):145–150

Croucher CA, Lass A, Margara R, Winston RM 1998 Predictive value of the results of a first in-vitro fertilization cycle on the outcome of subsequent cycles. Human Reproduction 13(2):403–408

Dada T, Salha O, Baillie HS, Sharma V 1999 A comparison of three gonadotrophin-releasing hormone analogues in an in-vitro fertilisation programme: a prospective randomised study. Human Reproduction 14(2):288–293

D'Angelo A, Amso NN 2002 Interventions for the treatment of ovarian hyperstimulation syndrome (OHSS): a Cochrane review. (in press)

Dawson KJ, Conaghan J, Ostera RM, Winston RM, Hardy Y 1995 Delaying transfer to the third day post-insemination, to select non-arrested embryos, increases development to the fetal heart stage. Human Reproduction 10:177–182

Daya S 1997 Optimal agonist protocol for GnRH agonists. Journal of Assisted Reproduction and Genetics 14:39S

Daya S 1998 Comparison of gonadotrophin releasing hormone agonist (GnRHa) protocols for pituitary desensitization in in vitro fertilization (IVF) and gamete intrafallopian transfer (GIFT) cycles (Cochrane Review). The Cochrane Library, issue 4. Update Software, Oxford

Daya S, Gunby J, Hughes EG, Collins JA, Sagle MA 1995 Follicle-stimulating hormone versus human menopausal gonadotrophin for in vitro fertilization cycles: a meta-analysis. Fertility and Sterility 64(2):347–354

Devroey P 2000 GnRH antagonists. Fertility and Sterility 73:15–17

Dhont M, de Neubourg F, van der Elst J, de Sutter P 1997 Perinatal outcome of pregnancies after assisted reproduction: a case-control study. Journal of Assisted Reproduction and Genetics 10:575–580

Dhont M, de Sutter P, Ruyssinck G, Martens G, Bekaert A 1999 Perinatal outcome of pregnancies after assisted reproduction: a case-control study. American Journal of Obstetrics and Gynecology 3:688–695

Dor J, Seidman DS, Ben-Shlomo I, Levran D, Ben-Rafael Z, Maschiach S 1996 Cumulative pregnancy rate following in-vitro fertilization: the significance of age and infertility aetiology. Human Reproduction 11(2):425–428

Draper ES, Kurinczuk JJ, Abrams KR, Clarke M 1999 Assessment of separate contributions to perinatal mortality of infertility history and treatment: a case-control analysis. Lancet 353(9166):1746–1749

Dyer C 2002a Watchdog approves embryo selection to treat three year old child. British Medical Journal 324:503

Dyer C 2002b Embryo cell research should continue, committee says. British Medical Journal, 324:502

Edwards RG, Sharpe DJ 1971 Social values and research in human embryology. Nature 231:87–91

Egozcue J 1994 Polar body analysis: possible pitfalls in preconception diagnosis of single gene and chromosome disorders. Human Reproduction 9:1208

Eimers JM, te-Velde ER, Gerritse R, Vogelzang ET, Looman CWN, Habbema JDF 1995 The prediction of the chance to conceive in subfertile couples. Fertility and Sterility 61(1):44–52

ESHRE Capri Workshop Group 2000 Optimal use of infertility diagnostic tests and treatments. Human Reproduction 15(3):723–732

ESHRE PGD Consortium Steering Committee 2000 ESHRE preimplantation genetic diagnosis (PGD) consortium: data collection II (May 2000). Human Reproduction 15(12):2673–2683

Eugster A, Vingerhoets AJJM 1999 Psychological aspects of in vitro fertilization: a review. Social Science and Medicine 48:575–589

Fisch JD, Rodriguez H, Ross R, Overby G, Sher G 2001 The Graduated Embryo Score (GES) predicts blastocyst formation and pregnancy rate from cleavage-stage embryos. Human Reproduction 16(9):1970–1975

Fishel S, Jackson P 1989 Follicular stimulation for high tech pregnancies: are we playing it safe? British Medical Journal 299:309–311

Fishel S, Lisi F, Rinaldi L et al 1995 Systematic examination of immobilizing spermatozoa before intracytoplasmic sperm injection in the human. Human Reproduction 10:497–500

Fitzsimmons BP, Bebbington MW, Fluker MR 1998 Perinatal and neonatal outcomes in multiple gestations: assisted reproduction. American Journal of Obstetrics and Gynecology 179:1162–1167

FIVNAT 1994 Evolutions des criteres pronostiques de fecondation in vitro selon le rang de la tentative. Contraception Fertilite Sexualite 22(5):282–286

FIVNAT 1996 Evaluation of frozen embryo transfers from 1987 to 1994. Contraception Fertilite Sexualite 24:700–705

Fluker MR, Zouves CG, Bebbington MW 1993 A prospective randomised comparison of zygote intrafallopian transfer and in vitro fertilisation-embryo transfer for non-tubal factor infertility. Fertility and Sterility 60:515–519

Franceschi S, La Vecchia C, Negri E et al 1994 Fertility drugs and risk of epithelial ovarian cancer in Italy. Human Reproduction 9:1673–1675

Friedler S, Schenker JG, Herman A, Lewin A 1996 The role of ultrasonography in the evaluation of endometrial receptivity following assisted reproductive treatments: a critical review. Human Reproduction Update 2:323–335

Gardner DK, Vella P, Lane M, Wagley L, Schlenker T, Schoolcraft 1998 Culture and transfer of human blastocysts increases implantation rates and reduces the need for multiple embryo transfers. Fertility and Sterility 69(1):84–88

Garel M, Blondel B 1992 Assessment at 1 year of the psychological consequences of having triplets. Human Reproduction 7:729–732

Garel M, Salobir C, Blondel B 1997 Psychological consequences of having triplets: a 4-year follow-up study. Fertility and Sterility 67:1162–1165

Geber S, Paraschos T, Atkinson G, Margara R, Winston RML 1995 Results of IVF in patients with endometriosis: the severity of the disease does

not affect the outcome, or the incidence of miscarriage. Human Reproduction 10:1507–1511

Gerris J, Mangelshcots K, van Royen E, Joostens M, Eestermans W, Ryckaert G 1995 ICSI and severe malefactor infertility: breaking the sperm tail prior to injection. Human Reproduction 10:484–486

Gleicher N, Campbell DP, Chan CL et al 1995 The desire for multiple births in couples with infertility problems contradicts present practice patterns. Human Reproduction 10:1079–1084

Goldfarb J, Kinzer DJ, Boyle M, Kurit D 1996 Attitudes of in vitro fertilization and intrauterine insemination couples toward multiple gestation pregnancy and multifetal pregnancy reduction. Fertility and Sterility 65:815–820

Govaerts I, Devreker F, Koenig I, Place I, van den Bergh M, Englert Y 1998 Comparison of pregnancy outcome after intracyoplasmic sperm injection and in vitro fertilization. Human Reproduction 13:1514–1518

Handyside AH, Kontogianni EH, Hardy K, Winston RML 1990 Pregnancies from biopsied human pre-implantation embryos sexed by Y-specific DNA amplification. Nature 344:768–770

Ho SK, Wu PY 1975 Perinatal factors and neonatal morbidity in twin pregnancy. American Journal of Obstetrics and Gynecology 122(8):979–987

Home G, Critchlow JD, Newman MC, Edozien L, Matson PL, Lieberman BA 1997 A prospective evaluation of cryopreservation strategies in a two-embryo transfer programme. Human Reproduction 12:542–547

Howe RS, Sayegh RA, Durinzi KL, Tureck RW 1990 Perinatal outcome of singleton pregnancies conceived by in vitro fertilization: a controlled study. Journal of Perinatology 10(3):261–266

Hughes EG, Fedorkow DM, Daya S, Sagle MA, van de Koppel P, Collins JA 1992 The routine use of gonadotrophin-releasing agonists prior to in vitro fertilisation and gamete intrafallopian transfer: a meta-analysis of randomised controlled trials. Fertility and Sterility 58(5):888–896

Huisman GJ, Alberda AT, Leerenveld RA, Verhoeff A, Zellmaker GH 1994 A comparison of in vitro fertilisation results after embryo transfer after 2, 3 and 4 days of embryo culture. Fertility and Sterility 61:970–971

Hull MGR 1992 Infertility treatment: relative effectiveness of conventional and assisted conception methods. Human Reproduction 7:785–796

Human Fertilization and Embryology Authority 1998 Seventh annual report and accounts. The Stationery Office, London

Human Fertilization and Embryology Authority 1999 Eighth annual report and accounts. The Stationery Office, London

Human Fertilization and Embryology Authority 2000 Ninth annual report and accounts. The Stationery Office, London

Imaizumi Y 1998 A comparative study of twinning and triplet rates in 17 countries, 1972–1996. Acta Genetica Medica Gemellol (Roma) 47(2):101–114

Ishii S, Tanaka K, Okai T et al 1994 Perinatal outcome of pregnancies following therapy of infertility. Nippon Sanka Fujinka Gakkai Zasshi. Acta Obstetricia et Gynecologica Japonica 46(12):1305–1310

Kahn JA, von During V, Sunde A, Sordal T, Molne K 1993 The efficacy and efficiency of an in-vitro fertilization programme including embryo cryopreservation: a cohort study. Human Reproduction 8:247–252

Khastgir G, Abdalla H, Thomas A, Korea L, Latarche L, Studd J 1997 Oocyte donation in Turner's syndrome: an analysis of the factors in recipients with or without premature ovarian failure. Human Reproduction 12(2):279–285

Lerner-Geva L, Toren A, Chetrit A et al 2000 The risk of cancer among children of women who underwent in vitro fertilization. Cancer 88(12):2845–2847

Liao X H, de Crestecker L, Gemnell J, Lees A, Mcllwaine G, Yates R 1997 The neonatal consequences and neonatal cost of reducing the number of embryos transferred following IVF. Scottish Medical Journal 42:76–78

Liebaers I, Bonduelle M, van Assche E, Devroey P, van Steirteghem 1995 Sex chromosome abnormalities after intracytoplasmic sperm injection. Lancet 346:1095–1097

Loft A, Petersen K, Erb K et al 1999 A Danish national cohort of 730 infants born after intracytoplasmic sperm injection (ICSI) 1994–1997. Human Reproduction 14:2143–2148

Mackenna A, Zegers-Hochild F, Fernandez EO, Fabres CV, Huidobro CA,

Guadarrama AR 1992 Intrauterine insemination: critical analysis of a therapeutic procedure. Human Reproduction 7:351–354

Mannaerts B, de Leeuw R, Geelen J et al 1991 Comparative in vitro and in vivo studies on the biological characteristics of recombinant human follicle stimulating hormone. Endocrinology 129:2623–2630

Mardesic T, Muller P, Zetova L, Mikova M 1994 Faktory ovlivnujici vysledky in vitro fertilizace-1. Vliv veku. Ceska Gynekologie 59(5):259–261

Martikainen H, Tiitinen A, Tomas C et al 2001 One versus two embryo transfer after IVF and ICSI: a randomized study. Human Reproduction 16:1912–1921

Matson PL, Yovich JL 1986 The treatment of infertility associated with endometriosis by in vitro fertilization. Fertility and Sterility 46:432–434

Matson PL, Browne J, Deakin R, Bellinge B 1999 The transfer of two embryos instead of three to reduce the risk of multiple pregnancy: a retrospective analysis. Journal of Assisted Reproduction and Genetics 16(1):1–5

Meldrum DR 1993 Female reproductive aging – ovarian and uterine factors. Fertility and Sterility 59:1–5

Mercan R, Lanzendorf SE, Mayer JJr, Nassar A, Muasher SJ, Oehninger S 1998 The outcome of clinical pregnancies following intracytoplasmic sperm injection is not affected by semen quality. Andrologia 30(2):91–95

Milki AA, Fisch JD, Behr B 1999 Two-blastocyst transfer has similar pregnancy rates and a decreased multiple gestation rate compared with three-blastocyst transfer. Fertility and Sterility 72(2):225–228

Mosgaard BJ, Lidegaard O, Kjaer SK et al 1997 Infertility, fertility drugs, and invasive ovarian cancer: a case-control study. Fertility and Sterility 67:1005–1012

Muggleton-Harris AL, Glazier AM, Pickering S, Wall M 1995 Genetic diagnosis using polymerase chain reaction and fluorescent in-situ hybridization analysis of biopsied cells from both the cleavage and blastocyst stages of individual cultured human preimplantation embryos. Human Reproduction 10:183–192

Murdoch A 1997 Triplets and embryo transfer policy. Human Reproduction 12 88–92

Obasaju M, Kadam A, Sultan K, Fateh M, Munne S 1999 Sperm quality may adversely affect the chromosome constitution of embryos that result from intracytoplasmic sperm injection. Fertility and Sterility 72(6):1113–1115

Oktay K, Economos K, Kan M, Rucinski J, Veeck L, Rosenwaks Z 2001 Endocrine function and oocyte retrieval after autologous transplantation of ovarian cortical strips to the forearm. Journal of the American Medical Association 286:1490–1493

Olivennes F, Feldberg D, Liu H-C, Cohen J, Moy F, Rosenwaks Z 1995 Endometriosis: a stage by stage analysis – the role of in vitro fertilization. Fertility and Sterility 64:392–398

Out HJ, Mannaerts BM, Driessen SG, Bennink HJ 1995 A prospective, randomised, assessor-blind multicentre study comparing recombinant and urinary follicle stimulating hormone (Puregon versus Metrodin) in in-vitro fertilization. Human Reproduction 10:2534–2540

Padilla SL, Garcia JE 1989 Effect of maternal age and number of in vitro fertilization procedures on pregnancy outcome. Fertility and Sterility 52(2):270–273

Palermo G, Joris H, Devroey P, van Steirteghem A 1992 Pregnancies after intracytoplasmic injection of single spermatozoon into an oocyte. Lancet 340:17–18

Palomba ML, Monni G, Lai R, Cau G, Olla G, Cao A 1994 Psychological implications and acceptability of preimplantation diagnosis. Human Reproduction 9:360–362

Parneix I, Jayot S, Verdaguer S, Discamps G, Audebert A, Emperaire JC 1995 Age et fertilite: apport des coc ultures sur cellules endometriales. Contraception Fertilite Sexualite 23(11):667–669

Parrazzini F, Negri E, La Vecchia C et al 1997 Treatment for infertility and risk of invasive ovarian cancer. Human Reproduction 12:2159–2161

Peek JC, Godfrey B, Matthews CD 1984 Estimation of fertility and fecundity in women receiving artificial insemination by donor semen and in normal fertile women. British Journal of Obstetrics and Gynaecology 91:1019–1024

Piette C, de-Mouzon J, Bachelot A, Spira A 1990 In-vitro fertilization: influence of women's age on pregnancy rates. Human Reproduction 5(1):56–59

Powers WF, Kiely JL 1994 The risks confronting twins: a national perspective. American Journal of Obstetrics and Gynecology 170(2):456–461

Preutthipan S, Amso N, Curtis P, Shaw RW 1996 The influence of number of embryos transferred on pregnancy outcome in women undergoing in vitro fertilization and embryo transfer (IVF-ET). Journal of the Medical Association of Thailand 79(10):613–617

Prietl G, Engleberts U, Maslanka M, van-der-Ven HH, Krebs D 1998 Kumulative Schwangerschaftsraten Der Konventionellen In Vitro Fertilisation In Abhangigkeit Der Diagnose Und Des Alters Der Patientinnen: Ergebnisse Des Bonner Ivf-Programms. Geburtshilfe-und-Frauenheilkunde 58(8):433–439

Rigot JM 1991 Cystic fibrosis and congenital absence of the vas deferens. New England Journal of Medicine 325:64–65

Rossing MA, Daling JR, Weiss NS, Moore DE, Self SG 1994 Ovarian tumors in a cohort of infertile women. New England Journal of Medicine 331:771–776

Royal College of Obstetricians and Gynaecologists 1998a The initial management of the infertile couple. Evidence-based guideline no. 2. RCOG Press, London

Royal College of Obstetricians and Gynaecologists 1998b The management of infertility in secondary care. Evidence-based guideline no. 3. RCOG Press, London

Royal College of Obstetricians and Gynaecologists 1999 Guidelines for the management of infertility in tertiary care. Evidence-based guideline no. 6. RCOG Press, London

Schachter M, Raziel A, Friedler S, Strassburger D, Bern O, Ron-E1R 2001 Monozygotic twinning after assisted reproductive techniques: a phenomenon independent of micromanipulation. Human Reproduction 16(6):1264–1269

Scholtes MC, Behrend C, Dietzel-Dahmen J et al 1998 Chromosome aberrations in couples undergoing intracytoplasmic sperm injection: influence on the implantation and ongoing pregnancy rates. Fertility and Sterility 70(5):933–937

Schoolcraft WB, Surrey ES, Gardner DK 2001 Embryo transfer: techniques and variables affecting success. Fertility and Sterility 76(5):863–870

Seamark RF, Robinson JS 1995 Potential health hazards of assisted reproduction: potential health problems stemming from assisted reproduction programmes. Human Reproduction 10:1321–1322

Sharif K, Elgendy M, Lashen H, Afnan M 1998 Age and basal follicle stimulating hormone as predictors of in vitro fertilisation outcome. British Journal of Obstetrics and Gynaecology 105(1):107–112

Shoham Z, Weissman A, Barash A, Borenstein R, Schachter M, Insler V 1994 Intravenous albumin for the prevention of severe ovarian hyperstimulation syndrome in an in vitro fertilization programme: a prospective, randomized, placebo-controlled study. Fertility and Sterility 62:137–142

Shushan A, Paltiel O, Iscovich J et al 1996 Human menopausal gonadotropin and the risk of epithelial ovarian cancer. Fertility and Sterility 65:13–18

Skupski DW, Nelson S, Kowalik A et al 1996 Multiple gestations from in vitro fertilization: successful implantation alone is not associated with subsequent pre-eclampsia. American Journal of Obstetrics and Gynecology 175:1029–1032

Slotnick RN, Ortega JE 1996 Monoamniotic twinning and zona manipulation: a survey of U.S. IVF centers correlating zona manipulation and high risk twinning frequency. Journal of Assisted Reproduction and Genetics 13(5):381–385

Soliman S, Daya S, Collins J, Hughes EG 1994 The role of luteal phase support in infertility treatment: a meta-analysis of randomized trials. Fertility and Sterility 61:1068–1076

Staessen C, Janssenswillen C, van den Abbeel E, Devroey P, van Streitegham AC 1993 Avoidance of triplet pregnancies by elective transfer of two good quality embryos. Human Reproduction 8(10):1650–1653

Sutcliffe AG, Taylor B, Saunders K, Thornton S, Lieberman BA, Grudzinskas JG 2001 Outcome in the second year of life after in-vitro fertilisation by intracytoplasmic sperm injection: a UK case-control study. Lancet 357:2080–2084

Tallo CP, Vohr B, Oh W, Rubin LP, Seifer DB, Haning RV Jr 1995 Maternal and neonatal morbidity associated with in vitro fertilization. Journal of Pediatrics 127(5):794–800

Tan SL, Royston P, Campbell S et al 1992a Cumulative conception and livebirth rates after in-vitro fertilisation [see comments]. Lancet 339(8806):1390–1394. Comment in Lancet 340(8811):116

Tan SL, Doyle P, Campbell S et al 1992b Obstetric outcome of in vitro fertilization pregnancies compared with normally conceived pregnancies. American Journal of Obstetrics and Gynecology 167(3):778–784

Tarin JJ 1995 Subzonal insemination, partial zona dissection or intracytoplasmic sperm injection? An easy decision? Human Reproduction 10:165–170

Tasdemir M, Tasdemir I, Kodama H, Fukuda J, Tanaka T 1995 Two instead of three embryo transfer in in vitro fertilisation. Human Reproduction 10(8):2155–2158

Tekay A, Martikainen H, Jouppila P 1995 Blood flow changes in uterine and ovarian vasculature, and predictive value of transvaginal pulsed colour Doppler ultrasonography in an in-vitro fertilization programme. Human Reproduction 10:688–693

Templeton AA, Morris JK 1998 Reducing the risk of multiple births by transfer of two embryos after in-vitro fertilization. New England Journal of Medicine 339:573–577

Templeton AA, Morris JK, Parslow W 1996 Factors that affect outcome of in-vitro fertilisation treatment. Lancet 348(9039):1402–1406

Thornhill A, Holding C, Monk M 1994 Recycling the single cell to detect specific chromosomes and to investigate specific gene sequences. Human Reproduction 9:2150–2155

Tiitinen A, Halttunen M, Harkki P, Vuorist P, Hyden-Granskog C 2001 Elective single embryo transfer: the value of cryopreservation. Human Reproduction 16(6):1140–1144

Toner JP, Flood JT 1993 Fertility after the age of 40. Obstetric and Gynecologic Clinics of North America 20(2):261–272

Toren A, Sharon N, Mandel M et al 1995 Two embryonal cancers after in vitro fertilisation. Cancer 76(11):2372–2374

Tough SC, Greene CA, Svenson LW, Belik J 2000 Effects of in vitro fertilisation on low birth weight, preterm delivery, and multiple birth. Journal of Pediatrics 136(5):618–622

Tucker M, Kost HI, Massey JB 1991 How many IVF embryos to transfer. Lancet 337:1482

Tucker MJ, Morton PC, Witt MA, Wright G 1995b Intracytoplasmic injection of testicular and epididymal spermatozoa for treatment of obstructive azoospermia. Human Reproduction 10:486–489

Tucker MJ, Morton PC, Wright G, Ingargiola PE, Jones AE, Sweitzer CL 1995a Factors affecting success with intracytoplasmic sperm injection. Reproduction, Fertility and Development 7(2):229–236

Urman B, Pride SM, Yuen BH 1992 Management of overstimulated gonadotrophin cycles with a controlled drift period. Human Reproduction 7:213–217

Van Balen F, Trimbos-Kemper TCM 1993 Long-term infertile couples: a study of their well-being. Journal of Psychosomatic Obstetrics and Gynaecology (Special Issue):53–60

Van Golde R, Boada M, Veiga A, Evers J, Geraedts J, Barri P 1999 A retrospective follow-up study on intracytoplasmic sperm injection. Journal of Assisted Reproduction and Genetics 16(5):227–232

Van Kooij RJ, Looman CW, Habbema JD, Dorland M, te-Velde ER 1996 Age-dependent decrease in embryo implantation rate after in vitro fertilization. Fertility and Sterility 66(5):769–775

Van Os HC, Jansen CAM 2000 The use of GnRH antagonist for COH as a second line strategy in IVF or ICSI. In: Proceedings of the 16th Annual Meeting of the European Society of Human Reproduction and Embryology. Human Reproduction 15 (Abstracts Book 1):134(P-089)

Van Voorhis BJ, Syrop CH, Vincent RD Jr, Chestnut DH, Sparks AE, Chapler FK 1995 Tubal versus uterine transfer of cryopreserved embryos: a prospective randomised trial. Fertility and Sterility 63:578–583

Vardon D, Burban C, Collomb J, Stolla V, Emy R 1995 Spontaneous pregnancies in couples after failed or successful in vitro fertilization. Journal de Gynecologie Obstetrique et Biologie de la Reproduction Paris 24(8):811–815

Vauthier-Brouzes D, Lefebvre G, Lesourd S, Gonzales J, Darbois Y 1994 How many embryos should be transferred in in vitro fertilization? A prospective randomised study. Fertility and Sterility 62(2):339–342

Venn A, Watson L, Lumley J, Giles G, King C, Healy D 1995 Breast and ovarian cancer incidence after infertility and in vitro fertilisation. Lancet 346:995–1000

Venn A, Watson L, Bruinsma F, Giles G, Healy D 1999 Risk of cancer after the use of fertility drugs with in-vitro fertilisation. Lancet 354:1586–1590

Venn A, Jones P, Quinn M, Healy D 2001 Characteristics of ovarian and uterine cancers in a cohort of in vitro fertilization patients. Gynecological Oncology 82(1):64–68

Wada I, Macnamee MC, Wick K, Bradfield JM, Brinsden PR 1994 Birth characteristics and perinatal outcome of babies conceived from cryopreserved embryos. Human Reproduction 9:543–546

Waterstone J, Parsons J, Bolton V 1991 Embryo transfer of two embryos. Lancet 337:975–976

Wennerholm UB, Albertsson Wikland K, Bergh C et al 1998 Postnatal growth and health in children born after cryopreservation as embryos. Lancet 351:1085–1090

Wennerholm UB, Bergh C, Hamberger L et al 2000 Incidence of congenital malformations in children born after ICSI. Human Reproduction 15(4):944–948

Whittemore AS 1994 The risk of ovarian cancer after treatment for infertility. New England Journal of Medicine 331:805–806

Whittemore AS, Harris R, Intyre J 1992 The collaborative ovarian cancer group. Characteristics relating to ovarian cancer risk: collaborative analysis of 12 U.S. case control studies. II. Invasive epithelial ovarian cancers in white women. American Journal of Epidemiology 136:1184–1203

Widra EA, Gindoff PR, Smotrich DB, Stillman RJ 1996 Achieving multiple-order embryo transfer identifies women over 40 years of age with improved in vitro fertilization outcome. Fertility and Sterility 65(1):103–108

Wisanto A, Bonduelle M, Camus M et al 1996 Obstetric outcome of 904 pregnancies after intracytoplasmic sperm injection. Human Reproduction 11 (suppl 4):121–129

Wood C, McMaster R, Rennie G 1985 Factors influencing pregnancy rates following in vitro fertilization and embryo transfer. Fertility and Sterility 43:245–250

Yaron Y, Ochshorn Y, Amit A, Yovel I, Kogosowski A, Lessing JB 1996 Patients with Turner's syndrome may have an inherent endometrial abnormality affecting receptivity in oocyte donation. Fertility and Sterility 65(6):1249–1252

341

24

Sporadic and recurrent miscarriage

William Buckett   Lesley Regan

INTRODUCTION

Miscarriage is the most common complication of pregnancy and accounts for a high proportion of gynaecology consultations and hospital admissions. It can be a traumatic and highly emotional event for a woman and her partner and the impact may be greatly underestimated by all who are involved in their care.

Current recommendations are that in early pregnancy loss, the term 'abortion' should be avoided and more sensitive terminology substituted.

- *Spontaneous abortion* should be replaced by *miscarriage*.
- *Blighted ovum, missed abortion or anembryonic pregnancy* should be replaced by *early embryonic* or *fetal demise*.
- *Incomplete abortion* should be replaced by *incomplete miscarriage*.
- *Recurrent* or *habitual abortion* should be replaced by *recurrent miscarriage*.

At the present time in the United Kingdom, miscarriage is defined as the loss of an intrauterine pregnancy before 24 completed weeks of gestation. The World Health Organization definition of miscarriage is the expulsion of a fetus or embryo weighing 500 g or less and also a gestational limit of less than 22 completed weeks of pregnancy.

Threatened miscarriage is defined as uterine bleeding prior to 24 weeks of pregnancy. Inevitable miscarriage can be subdivided into complete or incomplete depending on whether all or not all fetal and placental tissues have been expelled from the uterus. *Early embryonic or fetal demise* is where failure of the pregnancy is identified before expulsion of the fetal and placental tissues (usually by repeated ultrasound examination). *Recurrent miscarriage* is defined as three or more consecutive miscarriages (Stirrat 1990). This can be further subdivided into primary recurrent miscarriage, where there have been no previous live births, and secondary recurrent miscarriage where at least one previous successful pregnancy has occurred.

In terms of investigation and further medical and surgical management, there should be a clear distinction between sporadic miscarriage and recurrent miscarriage.

SPORADIC MISCARRIAGE

Epidemiology

Problems of definition and ascertainment

Problems of definition arise very early in pregnancy, where reliable detection of pregnancy is possible only with biochemical testing using urinary or serum β-human chorionic gonadotrophin (β-HCG), and also in late pregnancy, where the distinction between a late mid-trimester miscarriage and a stillbirth can be difficult (Chard 1991). The ideal research model for determining rates of miscarriage is a prospective longitudinal study of a representative cross-section of the population which is capable of recognizing all conceptions immediately, takes account of termination of pregnancy and follows women through the first 20 weeks of pregnancy (Regan et al 1989, Alberman 1992).

Early histological work from the 1950s (Hertig et al 1959), in which fertilized ova were directly observed in 107

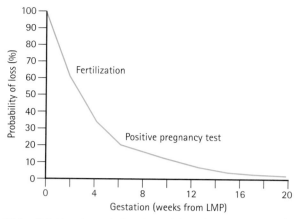

Fig. 24.1 Fetal loss by gestational age. Adapted from Kline et al (1989).

Table 24.1 Preclinical and clinical miscarriage rates

Authors	Preclinical loss rate (%)	Clinical loss rate (%)
French & Bierman (1962)	–	22
Miller et al (1980)	33	14
Edmonds et al (1982)	58	12
Wilcox et al (1988)	22	12
Regan et al (1989)	–	12
Brambati (1990)	–	14
Nybo Andersen et al (2000)	–	13

Table 24.2 Frequency of chromosomal abnormalities

Authors	Number of conceptions	Chromosomally abnormal	% abnormal
Dhalial et al (1970)	547	128	23
Boué et al (1975)	1498	921	61
Creasy et al (1976)	986	290	29
Takahara et al (1997)	505	237	47
Therkelsen et al (1997)	254	139	54
Hassold et al (1980)	1000	463	46
Kajii et al (1980)	402	215	54
Warburton et al (1980)	967	312	32
Takakuwa et al (1997)	148	89	60
	6307	3093	49

hysterectomy specimens from women who had intercourse around the time of expected ovulation prior to their operation, suggests a postimplantation pregnancy rate of 58% (21 of 36 possible conceptions). In a mathematical model, total pregnancy loss rates have been estimated at 78% (Roberts & Lowe 1975).

Rate of miscarriage

Following critical review of the literature, a reasonably coherent picture is emerging (Fig. 24.1). Estimates of early reproductive loss rates in the peri-implantation period of about 50–70% still rest largely on the early work of Hertig, although data derived from IVF studies support losses of this order of magnitude (Chard 1991).

Postimplantation and biochemical pregnancy loss rates appear to be in the order of 30%, whereas recognized pregnancy losses after clinical recognition of pregnancy remain consistent in most studies as 10–15% (Table 24.1).

Aetiology

Chromosomal abnormalities

Miscarriage is a heterogeneous condition but the single largest cause of sporadic miscarriages is fetal chromosomal abnormalities, accounting for about 50% of all cases (Table 24.2)

It is difficult to establish the precise contribution made by fetal chromosomal abnormalities. The figures in Table 24.2 are probably an underestimate since miscarriages occurring as a result of fetal chromosomal anomalies are maximal at the earliest and least well-documented stages of pregnancy. Evidence from preimplantation genetic diagnosis studies of embryos created as a result of in vitro fertilization (IVF) suggests that at least 65% of all embryos are chromosomally abnormal (Gianaroli et al 2000). However, extrapolation of these results to miscarriage in the general population must be cautious, given the high degree of selectivity of these patients and a different microenvironment at fertilization.

Trisomies are the major fetal chromosomal abnormality in sporadic cases of miscarriage, being found in 30% of all miscarriages and 60% of chromosomally abnormal miscarriages. Trisomies, together with monosomy X (15–25%) and triploidy (12–20%), account for over 90% of all chromosomal abnormalities found in sporadic cases of miscarriage.

Trisomies for all chromosomes have been described, with the exception of chromosomes 1 and Y, although the relative frequencies are vastly different. Chromosome 16, and to a lesser extent chromosomes 2, 13, 15, 18, 21 and 22, account for the majority of trisomic abnormalities (Fig. 24.2). Most trisomies are believed to be a consequence of non-disjunction during maternal meiosis. Trisomy 16 gives rise to only the most rudimentary embryonic growth with an empty sac (Edmonds 1992) and other trisomies often result in early embryonic demise.

Monosomy X (45XO) is thought to result from paternal sex chromosome loss (which can be either X or Y). It is usually associated with the presence of a fetus although focal abnormalities, such as encephalocoele or hygromata, may occur (Edmonds 1992).

Polyploidy results from the addition of complete haploid sets of chromosomes. Most common are triploid micarriages, usually 69XXY or 69XXX, which are thought to result from dispermic fertilization. These pregnancies are also characterized by multiple fetal and placental changes, such as neural tube defects, omphalocoele, hydropic villi and intrachorial haemorrhage. Tetraploid pregnancies are rare

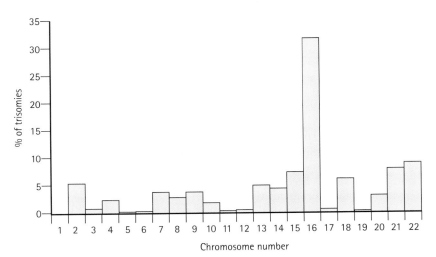

Fig. 24.2 Distribution of differing trisomies in sporadic cases of miscarriage.

and usually do not progress beyond the third week of embryonic life.

Structural chromosome abnormalities have been reported although minor abnormalities are no less frequent in live births compared with miscarriages. Major structural defects may arise de novo or be inherited. They are rarely a cause of sporadic miscarriage but are associated with recurrent miscarriage.

There appears to be a difference in the gestational age of pregnancy loss between different types of chromosomal abnormality, with trisomic and monosomic pregnancies miscarrying at a modal peak of 9 weeks and triploid pregnancy losses spanning 5–16 weeks of gestation (Alberman 1992).

Fetal malformations other than those caused by chromosomal anomaly

There is little doubt that the risk of miscarriage is increased with fetal malformation (Alberman 1992). However, since there has been no systematic search for malformations in fetal loss and since, in some cases, the malformation is secondary to a chromosomal anomaly, it is very difficult to assess the size of the increased risk. A single published study after 20 years (Shephard et al 1989) demonstrated an increased neural tube defect rate (3.6%) and an increased facial cleft rate (2.7%) amongst spontaneous miscarriages. Overall, the proportion of miscarriages as a result of fetal abnormalities without any associated chromosomal anomaly is small.

Placental abnormalities

Histological analysis of placental tissue from sporadic miscarriages has revealed several different patterns (Rushton 1995). These either point towards early fetal or embryonic demise, with essentially normal placentation, or they have shown abnormal placental villous development, either with marked villous hypoplasia, reduced vascularization, enlarged intravillous spaces, often with clots and lacking significant extravillous trophoblastic infiltration, or with acute necrotic changes in the villi and associated clots which can either be patchy or global. Other reported placental changes have included inflammatory changes or a mixture of the above changes.

Box 24.1 Infective causes associated with sporadic miscarriage

Bacteria	Parasites
Listeria monocytogenes	*Toxoplasma gondii*
Group B streptococcus	*Trichomonas vaginalis*
Gonococcus	*Plasmodium falciparum*
Chlamydia trachomatis	
Spirochaetes	Viruses
Treponema pallidum	Herpes simplex
	Varicella zoster
	Rubella
	Cytomegalovirus
	Parvovirus B19
	Hepatitis B
	Human immunodeficiency virus

Amongst sporadic miscarriages, abnormalities of villous development have been reported fairly consistently at 30–40% (Hustin & Jauniaux 1997). However, the causes leading to the majority of these cases of abnormal placentation and therefore subsequent miscarriage remain unknown. Although autoimmune and infective causes can be associated with abnormal villous development, most inherently abnormal embryos probably also have an abnormal placentation.

At present, although routine histological analysis of all products of conception is indicated in order to exclude molar and ectopic pregnancies, it is of little benefit in determining the cause of sporadic miscarriage.

Infection

Infection has been cited as a cause of late pregnancy loss and also early pregnancy loss for the past century. However, the precise role of infection as a cause of sporadic miscarriage is poorly and inconsistently reported (Simpson et al 1996). In many cases, whether infection has actually preceded any fetal demise or merely arose afterwards remains satisfactorily unanswered.

Several organisms have been associated with miscarriage (Box 24.1). Listeria, toxoplasmosis, herpes varicella zoster and malaria (*Plasmodium falciparum*) appear to be the most clinically important pathogens in women with early miscarriage.

Rubella infection, although a cause of first-trimester miscarriage, is now rare. The role of cytomegalo virus is unclear, although primary infection may cause miscarriage. The role of chlamydia infection, whether via an acute primary infection or a resultant chronic endometritis, also remains unclear. An association between herpes simplex virus infection and early pregnancy loss was first reported in the 1970s (Nahmias et al 1971), although later prospective studies have failed to show any association with sporadic or recurrent miscarriage even when primary infection occurred in the first trimester (Stray-Pedersen 1993). Whether human inmunodeficiency virus (HIV) is an important cause of early pregnancy loss remains unknown. Some studies demonstrate an increased rate of early pregnancy loss with HIV (d'Ubaldo et al 1998) while others do not (Bakas et al 1996). Whether any increased risk of miscarriage is the result of the virus, the mother's general health or her immunocompromised status remains unclear.

Syphilis (*Treponema pallidum*) and parvovirus B19 are more commonly a cause of late second-trimester miscarriage and stillbirth whilst group B streptococcus has been implicated in late miscarriage and preterm labour. Bacterial vaginosis (*Trichomonas vaginalis*) is also associated with late second-trimester miscarriage and preterm labour but the use of metronidazole or other antibiotics in women with demonstrable BV infection does not reduce late miscarriage or preterm delivery rates (Carey et al 2000).

Fetal sex, multiple pregnancy, maternal age and parity

Most studies have reported an excess of males in miscarriage and pregnancies complicated by varying degrees of placental dysfunction (Edwards et al 2000, Kellokumpu-Lethtinen & Pelliniemi 1984). However, the sex ratio of most early conceptions still remains unknown.

Multiple pregnancy is associated with an increased risk of fetal loss, via either early resorption, postimplantation loss or second-trimester miscarriage. In early pregnancy, the risk of miscarriage is twice that of singleton pregnancies (Sebire et al 1997a). The rate of late pregnancy loss is also increased, particularly in monochorionic twin pregnancy where late miscarriage rates can approach 12% (Sebire et al 1997b).

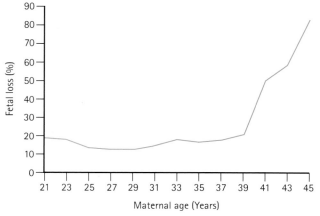

Fig. 24.3 The risk of miscarriage in first pregnancies with maternal age. Adapted from Alberman (1987).

The risk of miscarriage rises with parity; however, the rise is a result of reproductive compensation (Alberman 1987). The risk of miscarriage in first pregnancies is low in young women (Regan et al 1989), but rises significantly after the age of 39 years (Fig. 24.3). This rise is not only found in association with trisomic pregnancies (which rise with maternal age) but also in chromosomally normal pregnancies.

Maternal health

Virtually every maternal medical disorder has been associated with sporadic miscarriage. Women with severe medical disease rarely become pregnant but if they do, their disease may deteriorate during pregnancy. Various mechanisms, including endocrinological, immunological or infective, have been suggested. Poorly controlled diabetes is associated with an increased risk of miscarriage (Mills et al 1988), whereas well-controlled and subclinical diabetes can rarely be considered a cause. Overall, only a small fraction of all early pregnancy losses can be considered attributable to severe maternal disease.

Cigarette smoking has been positively correlated with miscarriage and a review of the effects of nicotine on ovarian, uterine and placental function suggests that cigarette smoking has an adverse effect on trophoblast invasion (Schiverick & Salafia 1999). Cocaine use has also been reported as increasing the risk of miscarriage (Ness et al 1999). Alcohol consumption has been shown to be higher in women whose pregnancies ended in miscarriage compared with pregnancies which proceeded beyond 28 weeks of gestation (Harlap & Shapiro 1980, Kline et al 1980), although other studies have not confirmed this observation (Halmesmäki et al 1989, Parazzini et al 1990). There is some evidence to suggest that even moderate maternal alcohol consumption is associated with an increased risk of miscarriage (Windham et al 1997). Many studies have shown a relationship between coffee/caffeine intake and spontaneous miscarriage, although these have not controlled for other confounding variables. Only high levels of caffeine metabolites in maternal serum are associated with miscarriage so it would appear that moderate consumption of caffeine is unlikely to increase the risk of miscarriage (Klebanoff et al 1999).

Some chemical agents including lead, ethylene oxide, solvents, pesticides, vinyl chloride and anaesthetic gases have been shown to have some association with fetal loss (Cohen et al 1971, McDonald et al 1998, Mur et al 1992, Rowland et al 1996). Although many environmental toxicologists accept these agents as proven, the evidence for low levels of exposure remains far from convincing.

Radiotherapy and chemotherapeutic agents are accepted causes of miscarriage (Zemlickis et al 1992), although they are only administered during pregnancy in seriously ill women. Although significant ionizing radiation for diagnostic purposes can lead to fetal malformation and miscarriage, a dose of >25 rads is associated with a 0.1% risk of abnormality (1 rad is the equivalent of 8–10 abdominal/pelvic X-ray films).

There is a small increase in the risk of spontaneous miscarriage with general anaesthesia and incidental surgery during the first and second trimesters, although this is higher with gynaecological surgery (Duncan et al 1986).

It has been claimed that impaired psychological well-being predisposes to fetal loss (Stray-Pedersen & Stray-Pedersen 1984), although it has been difficult to exclude other confounding variables. Despite problems with recall bias, there are an increased number of negative life events in women with chromosomally normal as compared with chromosomally abnormal miscarriages (Neugebauer et al 1996) but no differences in hormonal markers of stress have been determined.

Pathophysiology

The exact pathophysiology resulting in the uterine expulsion of early pregnancy remains unknown. Abnormal placentation (either primary or itself secondary to early fetal demise) can either lead to reduced or shallow uterine invasion by the trophoblast or can itself be caused by reduced invasion. In this situation, the usual reduction in maternal vascular tone cannot occur. It is presumed that this blood flow enters the intervillous space and dislodges the conceptus, thereby leading to embryonic demise if this has not already occurred (Rushton 1995). Nevertheless, even quite large intrauterine haematomata visualized by ultrasound have not prevented live births at term (Pedersen & Mantoni 1990) and the presence of haematomata per se does not increase the risk of miscarriage (Tower & Regan 2001).

Once the conceptus is dislodged, there is further intrauterine bleeding. Local prostaglandin release will lead to pain and ultimately expulsion of the conceptus and any associated blood.

Presentation

Threatened miscarriage

This can be defined as uterine bleeding before 24 weeks of pregnancy (the time of presumed fetal viability) with no evidence of any fetal or embryonic demise. It is usually painless. Characteristically, the bleeding is initially bright red, followed by a reducing brown loss. This can affect up to 25% of all pregnancies and is one of the commonest indications for emergency early pregnancy referral. Clinical examination reveals a soft, non-tender uterus, usually of the appropriate gestational size, and a closed cervix. Transvaginal or transabdominal ultrasound scan confirms an ongoing pregnancy (Fig. 24.4).

The non-specific nature of abdominal pain, vaginal bleeding and pelvic tenderness precludes their use as predictors of ultimate outcome in women with threatened miscarriage. However, continued vomiting (rather than nausea alone) in early pregnancy is associated with an increased chance of live birth (Weigel & Weigel 1989), presumably because it indicates continued placental hormone production.

Inevitable miscarriage

Miscarriage is a process rather than a single event. Of all women presenting with bleeding in early pregnancy, about 50% will ultimately miscarry (Stabile et al 1987). Whilst the cervix remains closed, any pain and bleeding may subside and the pregnancy may continue otherwise normally to term. However, once the cervix opens, miscarriage is inevitable.

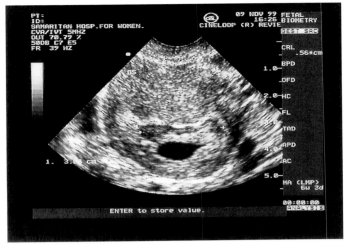

Fig. 24.4 Ultrasound picture of an ongoing pregnancy with an intrauterine haematoma in a woman who presented with a threatened miscarriage.

Usually women present with crampy abdominal pains and fresh bleeding. Symptoms alone are unreliable and the diagnosis is determined by the confirmation of cervical dilatation at vaginal examination. Examination often reveals a tender, firm uterus, which may be smaller than the expected gestational size, and the cervical os is open. Products of conception may also be felt through the os.

Occasionally, the woman may present with severe shock. This can either be secondary to massive haemorrhage, which will require appropriate emergency resuscitation, blood transfusion and uterine evacuation, or the degree of shock may be out of proportion to the blood loss and is due to the distension of the cervix by products of conception and the resultant sympathetic stimulation. This is termed cervical shock syndrome and is often severe. Quick removal of the products from the os, at the bedside, results in relief of the shock. In rare cases, endotoxic shock secondary to sepsis may occur.

Complete and incomplete miscarriage

Inevitable miscarriage is either complete or incomplete depending on whether all fetal and placental tissues have been expelled from the uterus. The typical features of incomplete miscarriage are heavy bleeding (which may be intermittent) and abdominal cramps. The finding of a dilated cervix on examination in the presence of continued pain and bleeding is usually diagnostic. Ultrasound scan will confirm the presence of retained products of conception (Fig. 24.5).

If the symptoms of incomplete miscarriage resolve spontaneously, then complete miscarriage may have occurred. Nevertheless, following abdominal and pelvic examination, ultrasound may need to be performed to confirm that the uterus is indeed empty. Occasionally the cervix may close despite the presence of retained products. The number of complete miscarriages is unknown. Many such early miscarriages may go unreported. Early studies of women with threatened miscarriage showed complete miscarriage rates of less than 1% (Stabile et al 1987), although more recent evidence suggests

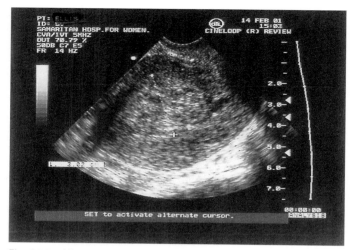

Fig. 24.5 Ultrasound picture of incomplete miscarriage demonstrating retained products of conception within the endometrial cavity.

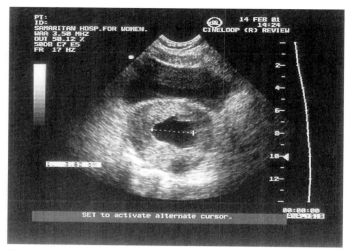

Fig. 24.6 Ultrasound picture of early fetal demise, showing a collapsing gestation sac.

around 20–30% of miscarriages are complete (Chung et al 1994, Mansur 1992). Similarly, expectant management of early fetal demise has demonstrated that, with time, up to 25% women go on to have complete miscarriage (Jurkovic et al 1998).

Early fetal demise (missed abortion/miscarriage)

Early embryonic or fetal demise rather than missed abortion or missed miscarriage is now the preferred term both in the UK and the United States. Previously this has also been termed an anembryonic pregnancy (all pregnancies develop from an embryo) or blighted ovum (the pregnancy cannot result from an ovum alone). These terms should also be abandoned.

Early fetal demise is where failure of pregnancy is identified before any expulsion of the products of conception occurs. The woman may report a disappearance of the symptoms and signs of early pregnancy such as nausea and vomiting or breast tenderness. A brown vaginal loss may also be reported. The diagnosis may also be made in otherwise asymptomatic women at routine obstetric/dating ultrasound examination. The diagnosis is made by the lack of fetal heart activity in a pregnancy with a crown–rump length of over 5 mm (Pennell et al 1991) or when two ultrasound examinations 1 or 2 weeks apart have shown no growth and no fetal heart activity. In cases of doubt, a repeat ultrasound is always indicated. Occasionally, a collapsing gestational sac or a failed pregnancy surrounded by clot in utero may be seen (Fig. 24.6). Abdominal and pelvic examination often reveals a uterus smaller than expected for the gestational age and a closed cervical os.

Sepsis

This occurs when infection complicates miscarriage or termination of pregnancy. Intrauterine sepsis rarely follows incomplete miscarriage, although the incidence is considerably higher at around 3.6% following termination of pregnancy (Frank 1985). The most common infecting organisms are *E. coli*, Bacteroides, streptococci (both anaerobic and occasionally aerobic) and *Clostridium welchii*. Occasionally, a history of intrauterine instrumentation may be withheld. The woman usually presents with suprapubic pain, malaise, fever and occasionally vaginal bleeding. Findings on examination include abdominal rigidity, uterine and adnexal tenderness and a closed cervical os. Rarely, a septicaemia may ensue leading to bacteraemic endotoxic shock and possibly maternal death.

Trophoblastic tumours

Trophoblastic tumours include complete and partial hydatidiform moles, choriocarcinoma and placental site tumours. These occasionally present as threatened miscarriage and suggestive features are noted at ultrasound examination. They are discussed elsewhere in this volume.

Investigations

Ultrasound, usually transvaginal, is essential in the diagnosis of miscarriage. It will determine the presence of an ongoing pregnancy in cases of threatened miscarriage and distinguish between early fetal demise, incomplete miscarriage and complete miscarriage in failing pregnancies. Ultrasound is also important in the diagnoses of ectopic pregnancy and trophoblastic disease.

Reliable pregnancy testing, whether by urinary or serum β-HCG, is also essential in order to distinguish an early complete miscarriage or an ongoing ectopic pregnancy.

All women with uterine bleeding in early pregnancy should have their blood group determined and all women who are rhesus (D) negative should receive anti-D immunoglobulins regardless of the gestational age of the pregnancy.

The measurement of other fetoplacental hormones and proteins, such as α-fetoprotein (AFP), schwangerschaftprotein 1 (SP1), human placental lactogen (HPL), pregnancy-associated plasma protein (PAPP-A), oestrogen and progesterone have all been reported as diagnostic tests in early pregnancy. In rare cases they may improve the prediction of both early fetal demise and ectopic pregnancy (Grudzinskas & Chard 1992), but their routine use is not indicated.

Treatment

Threatened miscarriage

Early studies demonstrated that the presence of fetal heart activity at ultrasound examination in women who present with a history of bleeding in early pregnancy was associated with a high chance (97–98%) ultimately of a live birth (Stabile et al 1987). More recent evidence confirms live birth rates of 90–95% for younger women, but for women over 40 years miscarriage rates of 15–30% are reported even after the identification of fetal heart activity (Deaton et al 1997, Schmidt-Sarosi et al 1998). Nevertheless, for most women, reassurance and continued medical and emotional support are all that is required.

Bedrest and avoiding penetrative intercourse have historically been advised. If the vascular hypothesis for the pathophysiology of miscarriage is accepted (Hustin & Jauniaux 1997), bedrest may improve pressure variation and flow changes and therefore improve the outcome. However, there is a paucity of clinical evidence to support this hypothesis. Initial presentation is usually in primary care and, currently, over 96% of general practitioners still advise bedrest and the avoidance of intercourse, although many believe that it does not improve the eventual outcome.

Progesterone supplementation in early pregnancy has been prescribed for over 30 years for women presenting with threatened (and also recurrent) miscarriage. The historical rationale was that a progesterone deficiency would lead to miscarriage. Obviously, the converse may also be true – that a failed pregnancy may lead to a progesterone deficiency. There is a wealth of published data, mostly from uncontrolled treatment trials. However, several meta-analyses (Daya 1989, Goldstein et al 1989) have been unable to demonstrate a beneficial effect for progesterone treatment. The routine use of progesterone in threatened miscarriage cannot be justified.

Incomplete miscarriage

Surgical evacuation of the uterus after cervical dilatation, if necessary, has remained the cornerstone of the management of incomplete miscarriage in the industrialized world since the 1940s (Hertig & Livingstone 1944). Evacuation and curettage have been regarded as essential to ensure that the uterine cavity is empty, otherwise haemorrhage, infection and later complications such as Ashermann's syndrome may result. Early studies showed a maternal mortality of 1.6% in women who did not undergo surgical treatment (Russell 1947). In cases of haemodynamic compromise of cervical shock appropriate resuscitation and urgent surgical evacuation are indicated. Most cases are performed under general anaesthesia, although effective outpatient curettage has been reported (Fawcus et al 1997). Suction evacuation is generally regarded as a safer technique than sharp curettage, with lower rates of perforation, blood loss and subsequent intrauterine adhesion formation (Edmonds 1992, Verkuyl & Crowther 1993).

The routine use of syntocinon or ergometrine has shown no benefit in reducing blood loss during the surgical treatment of first-trimester incomplete miscarriage (Beeby et al 1984). Because of the risk of ascending infection and its sequelae, whenever uterine instrumentation is performed, screening for chlamydia infection is recommended, although the use of prophylactic doxycycline is likely to be of benefit only in areas of relatively high prevalence (Prieto et al 1995).

Although a minor procedure, surgical evacuation is associated with rare but serious morbidity. Complications include tearing or lacerations to the cervix, perforation of the uterus, which may also lead to bowel perforation, bladder perforation, damage to the broad ligament, infection, Ashermann's syndrome (intrauterine adhesions) and haemorrhage (Ratnam & Prasad 1990). The incidence of serious morbidity has been estimated at 2.1% (Lawson et al 1994, RCGP/RCOG 1985), of which the most common problem is infection. This can lead to later sequelae including secondary infertility, ectopic pregnancy and Ashermann's syndrome. The incidence of mortality associated with surgical evacuation of the uterus has been estimated at 0.5 per 100 000 (Lawson et al 1994).

Recent studies demonstrate the efficacy of expectant management or 'observation alone' in women with incomplete miscarriage (Hurd et al 1997, Nielsen & Hahlin 1995). In cases where there was no haemodynamic compromise or maternal anaemia, spontaneous resolution occurred within 3 days in up to 80% of cases with minimal retained products (15–50 ml). Therefore, in women with minimal intrauterine tissue (after ectopic pregnancy has been excluded), expectant management is safe. However, large volumes of retained products are associated with an increase in complications, primarily infection and prolonged bleeding (Hurd et al 1997). There is no evidence that future fertility is impaired following expectant management (Kaplan et al 1996).

Herbal remedies have been used in the past to encourage the uterus to expel its contents but an effective non-surgical alternative to termination of pregnancy and miscarriage had to await the development of the anti-progesterone mifepristone and the prostaglandin analogues gemeprost and misoprostol. Their efficacy has been demonstrated in the treatment of incomplete miscarriage (Ashok et al 1998, Henshaw et al 1993), leading to complete miscarriage rates of around 95%.

The use of medical treatment or the adoption of an expectant approach in appropriately selected cases may have many medical and economic benefits. However, many women continue to express a preference for surgical treatment (Hamilton-Fairley & Donaghy 1997), citing fears regarding pain, bleeding and the length of time to resolution in the non-surgical group.

Early fetal demise

The treatment options for early fetal demise are essentially the same as for incomplete miscarriage. Surgical treatment should be preceded by cervical ripening agents (mifepristone or prostaglandins) in order to reduce the risks of cervical trauma or uterine perforation associated with forced cervical dilatation. Gemeprost, mifepristone and oral or vaginal misoprostol seem to be equally effective (Ayres de Campos et al 2000, Gupta & Johnson 1992, Platz-Christiansen et al 1995). Expectant management is feasible although less effective than in cases of incomplete miscarriage, with only 25% proceeding to complete miscarriage (Jurkovic et al 1998). The efficacy of medical treatment is also less when compared with incomplete miscarriage, although complete miscarriage rates of up to 90%

have been reported with higher doses of mifepristone and misoprostol and a longer surveillance period (El-Refaey et al 1992).

Psychological aspects

Psychological consequences of early pregnancy loss differ widely among different women, different families and even different pregnancies in the same woman. Nevertheless, most women, irrespective of their attitude towards the pregnancy at the time, experience feelings of depression and anxiety following miscarriage (Seibel & Graves 1980) and up to 36% of women are 'highly symptomatic' in terms of clinical depression 4 weeks after miscarriage (Neugebauer et al 1992).

All workers caring for women with miscarriage and their families need to understand the increased psychiatric morbidity associated with pregnancy loss and be able to offer appropriate support both at the time of diagnosis and also after treatment. Good communication with providers of primary care for the whole family and access to counselling are important, since 'miscarriages do not occur in a uterus but in a woman, and miscarriages do not occur solely in a woman but in a family' (Cain et al 1964). For some couples, the use of ritual can help them through the bereavement process (Hopper 1997).

In subsequent pregnancies, many women will need considerable reassurance and support (Hamilton 1989) and early access to ultrasound and hospital services may be required.

RECURRENT MISCARRIAGE

In contrast to sporadic miscarriage, recurrent miscarriage is relatively uncommon. A history of three or more consecutive miscarriages occurs in 0.5–2% women (Daya 1993, Katz & Kuller 1994, Stirrat 1990). Recurrent miscarriage is obviously distressing and frustrating for both the couple concerned and those treating them. In many cases, the cause may not be apparent despite intensive and expensive clinical and laboratory testing and there remains only a limited understanding of the causes of recurrent miscarriage.

The aetiologies are outlined below and summarized in Box 24.2. The management of recurrent miscarriage, including unexplained recurrent miscarriage, will be discussed below under specific headings. Unexplained miscarriage occurs in around 50% of women attending specialist recurrent miscarriage clinics (Clifford et al 1994, Li 1998, Stephenson 1996).

Genetic factors

Parental chromosomal abnormalities
Parental chromosomal abnormalities are the most important genetic anomalies currently detectable amongst couples with recurrent miscarriage. Most studies report an incidence of 3–5% (Clifford et al 1994, Li 1998, Stephenson 1996, Stray-Pedersen & Stray-Pedersen 1984) compared to an incidence of 0.5% in the general population.

Balanced or reciprocal translocations are the most frequently detected parental chromosomal anomaly in couples with

Box 24.2 Summary of the potential causes of recurrent miscarriage

Genetic	Parental chromosomal abnormalities Recurrent aneuploidy Other genetic causes
Anatomical	Uterine anomalies Cervical imcompetence
Infective	Predisposition to infection Possible pathogens
Endocrine	Luteal phase deficiency Thyroid disease Hypersecretion of LH/polycystic ovary syndrome
Immunological	Antiphospholipid syndrome Other thrombophilic defects Alloimmune

recurrent miscarriage. The male-to-female ratio is about 1:2. A portion of one chromosome is exchanged with a portion of another, resulting in two abnormal chromosomes but overall a normal chromosomal complement. Translocations have been reported for all chromosomes in many different combinations. At gametogenesis, there is a 50% chance of a chromosomally abnormal gamete being produced. However, there appears to be a lower fertilization or implantation rate with abnormal gametes, since chorionic villus sampling and amniocentesis have demonstrated a 40% and 11% risk respectively of a chromosomally unbalanced fetus (Mikkelson 1985).

Robertsonian translocations are less frequent, occurring in about 1% of couples with recurrent miscarriage. Here, two chromosomes adhere to each other at either the centromere or the short arms of the chromosome short arms. This leads to a total chromosome count of 45 but a normal chromosome complement overall. The risks of recurrence and miscarriage vary in different Robertsonian translocations. The most common translocation (involving chromosomes 14 and 21) result in 10–15% of pregnancies with trisomy 21 (Boué & Gallano 1984). If homologous chromosomes are involved the risk of a chromosomally abnormal conceptus is 100%.

Pericentric chromosomal inversions occur in about 1% of the general population and are not considered of clinical significance for recurrent miscarriage.

Peripheral blood karyotyping should be performed in both partners of all couples with recurrent miscarriage to determine any parental chromosome abnormality. Specialized genetic counselling is essential and offers the couple a prognosis for future pregnancies which may in some cases not be as bleak as anticipated. There should also be the opportunity to discuss preimplantation genetic diagnosis and antenatal fetal karyotyping, including chorionic villus sampling and amniocentesis. In cases of homologus Robertsonian translocations gamete donation and/or effective contraception should be discussed.

It is important to note that over 35% of couples with a significant parental chromosomal abnormality have already achieved a successful pregnancy in addition to their miscarriages (Clifford et al 1994).

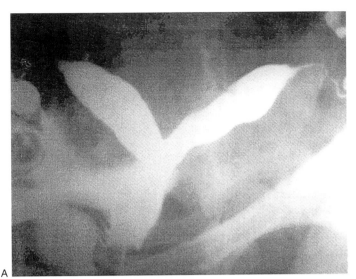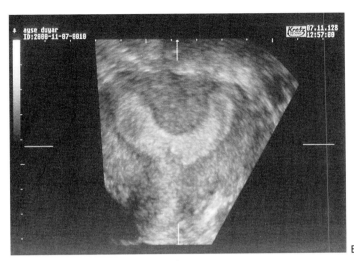

Fig. 24.7 A Hysterosalpingogram demonstrating a septate uterus. B Three-dimensional ultrasound demonstrating a septate uterus.

Recurrent aneuploidy

Some couples have an increased risk of miscarriage because they produce recurrent aneuploid fetuses. This may be the result of an increased tendency to non-disjunction, either inherited or induced environmentally. Chromosomal abnormalities are seen with a higher frequency amongst preimplantation embryos created during in vitro fertilization from couples with a history of recurrent miscarriage (Vidal et al 2000). Presumably these are the results of errors in gametogenesis and much current research is focused on the role of sperm chromosome abnormalities in recurrent miscarriage.

Other genetic factors

The karyotype of many recurrent miscarriage conceptions may be euploid (46XX or 46XY) and in the absence of any other identifiable cause or association, these unexplained recurrent early pregnancy losses may be the result of molecular mutations or single gene defects. Chromosome analysis itself is a very crude tool to determine genetic abnormalities. So far there has only been one report of a specific single gene locus abnormality associated with recurrent miscarriage (Pegoraro et al 1997), but much work remains to be done. The impact of other genetic factors on recurrent miscarriage is confirmed by the increased incidence amongst consanguinous couples (Hendrick 1988).

Anatomical factors

Uterine anomalies

The reported incidence of uterine anomalies in women with recurrent miscarriage varies widely from as low as 1% up to 27% (Regan 1997). Described anomalies vary from uterus didelphis to subseptate uteri and some studies even include submucosal fibroids. The incidence of such anomalies in the fertile population has been reported as 1.8–3.6% (Ashton et al 1988).

The significance of such anomalies, particularly intrauterine septae, arcuate uterus and submucosal fibroids, in women

with recurrent miscarriage is unclear. Historically, uterine anomalies were associated with second-trimester miscarriages but later reports have also shown an increase in early miscarriages. The exact aetiology is unknown although implantation over a septum or similar defect may result in decreased vascularity of the placenta.

Hysterosalpingography (HSG), laparoscopy and hysteroscopy, magnetic resonance imaging, computed tomography and three-dimensional ultrasound have all been used in the diagnosis and evaluation of uterine anomalies. Although HSG has traditionally been used as the primary screening test, three-dimensional ultrasound shows promise as a less invasive screening tool (Jurkovic et al 1995). In most cases, further evaluation at laparoscopy and hysteroscopy is indicated (Fig. 24.7).

Treatment of uterine anomalies in women with recurrent miscarriage remains controversial. Many reports demonstrate a benefit of hysteroscopic or conventional metroplasty in women with septate, subseptate or bicornuate uterus who have suffered mid-trimester miscarriage compared with matched controls (Ayhan et al 1992, Candiani et al 1990, Heinonen 1997, Pabuccu et al 1995). However the likelihood of a live birth in untreated women is as high as 66% (Heinonen 1997) and a similar percentage of women presenting with recurrent miscarriage have already achieved a live birth (Clifford et al 1994). Open pelvic surgery, in particular, has been associated with subsequent infertility (Bennett 1987). The value of corrective uterine surgery in women with these anomalies and a history of early pregnancy loss is uncertain (Ben-Rafael et al 1991). Similarly, the value of transcervical myomectomy in women with submucous fibroids remains unknown, although there have been initial successful reports (Egwuatu 1989).

Cervical incompetence

Cervical incompetence is usually associated with miscarriage occurring after 12–14 weeks or premature labour. It usually presents as silent dilatation of the cervix without painful contractions. The membranes bulge through the cervical canal and eventually rupture spontaneously.

The diagnosis of cervical incompetence poses a difficult problem (MRC/RCOG 1993). It is usually based on a previous history of mid-trimester miscarriages in the absence of painful uterine contractions. Vaginal ultrasound may be useful to detect early features of cervical incompetence (Shortening or funnelling) (Althuisius et al 2000) but neither ultrasound nor HSG has been found to be useful in the diagnosis of cervical incompetence before pregnancy.

Treatment of cervical incompetence is cervical cerclage in pregnancy, usually after 12–14 weeks when the toll of first-trimester miscarriages has occurred and after screening for chromosomal abnormalities has been performed. It has traditionally involved the insertion of a MacDonald suture, where a tape is inserted round the exposed vaginal cervix (MacDonald 1957), or a Shirodkar suture, where the vaginal mucosa is incised and the bladder reflected, allowing insertion of the suture at a higher level of the cervical canal (Shirodkar 1960). Modifications of this procedure have included burying the suture under the vaginal mucosa at the end of the procedure. In our experience, this is rarely accompanied by significant vaginal discharge. The MacDonald suture is more widely used and less traumatic to the cervix than the Shirodkar suture, although the exposed tape remains a possible focus for later infection. More recently, the emergency cervical cerclage in women who present acutely in the mid-trimester with silent cervical dilatation and/or herniation of the membranes through the cervix has been reported with live-birth rates of 50–60% (Aarts et al 1995, Wong et al 1993). Nevertheless, there are high rates of premature delivery and infection, including chorioamnionitis, in over 30% of cases.

In some women, particularly where the diagnosis is unsure or in those who have other risk factors, regular ultrasound monitoring of the cervix can be performed and if there is funnelling or shortening of the cervix, emergency cerclage can be performed (Althuisius et al 2000). Ultrasound may also be useful in women who have already had cervical cerclage in order to warn of problems (Dijkstra et al 2000). Transabdominal cervical cerclage may be useful in a highly selected group of women with anatomical defects in the cervix and previous mid-trimester miscarriages or preterm labours following failed vaginal cervical cerclage (Gibb & Salaria 1995). Laparoscopic transabdominal cervical cerclage has also been reported (Scibetta et al 1998), but neither of these procedures has been assessed in appropriate trials.

Infective factors

Although any severe infection may lead to sporadic miscarriage, for infection to be a cause of repeated pregnancy failure, it must persist in the genital tract and usually be asymptomatic.

Syphilis (*Treponema pallidum*) is a cause of recurrent late second-trimester miscarriage and stillbirth. This is routinely screened for and treatment with penicillins is effective. It is a rare cause of recurrent miscarriage in developed countries. Malaria infection in non-immune women is also associated with recurrent miscarriage in endemic areas (RCOG 2001).

Baterial vaginosis (*Trichomonas vaginalis*) is associated with recurrent late second-trimester miscarriage and preterm labour (Hay et al 1994), although there is no association with early pregnancy loss (Llahi-Camp et al 1996). Treatment with metronidazole has not been shown to be effective (Carey et al 2000).

The identification of individual organisms has proven to be disappointing in the search for causes of early or late recurrent miscarriage, which suggests that pregnancy outcome may be determined by maternal or fetal response to infection rather than the infective organism itself. Gene mutations, such as those associated with mannose-binding protein (MBP) deficiency, are an important cause of inherited immunodeficiency and increased susceptibility to infection. Early studies demonstrate a trend in association between late miscarriage and MBP genes (Baxter et al 2001). Future research regarding the role of infection in recurrent miscarriage needs to explore genetic susceptibility.

In women with a history of recurrent mid-trimester miscarriage regular gentle sterile speculum examination to assess any cervical change and regular high and low vaginal swabs to screen for any infection can be performed. This approach is empirical but it is difficult not to treat women with demonstrable infection. Similarly, low-dose maintenance antibiotic therapy may be used in women with repeated positive results although this is also empirical.

Endocrine factors

Systemic endocrine disease

As discussed previously, diabetic women with good metabolic control are no more likely to miscarry than non-diabetic women. However, diabetic women with high glycosylated haemoglobin A_{1c} levels in the first-trimester are at significantly higher risk of both miscarriage and fetal malformation (Hanson et al 1990). As the risk of miscarriage is only increased in women with poorly controlled diabetes mellitus, there is no value in screening for occult disease in asymptomatic women.

Although thyroid autoantibodies are associated with an increased risk of miscarriage, this is secondary to a generalized autoimmune abnormality rather than a specific thyroid dysfunction (Singh et al 1995). Screening asymptomatic women with thyroid function test is unhelpful as they are usually normal (Clifford et al 1994, Rushworth et al 2000).

Luteal phase deficiency

A functional corpus luteum is essential for the implantation and maintenance of early pregnancy, primarily through the production of progesterone, which is responsible for the conversion of a proliferative endometrium into a secretory endometrium available for embryo implantation. Disorders or removal of the corpus luteum can result in infertility and early pregnancy loss (Csapo et al 1973, Miller et al 1969). Although much controversy exists about luteal function, the success of oocyte donation with oestradiol and progesterone support in the absence of any ovarian activity would suggest that its effects are primarily progesterone determined.

The prevalence of luteal phase defect is reported to occur in 23–60% of women with recurrent miscarriage (Li & Cooke 1991), although it is difficult to determine the exact proportion of women with luteal-phase problems because of difficulties in diagnosis. The diagnosis is usually determined by low luteal-phase progesterone level and/or a non-secretory endometrium, by biopsy, in non-fertile, non-pregnant cycles (Jordan et al 1994, Serle et al 1994). Between 30% and 50% of cases of luteal-phase defect as determined by endometrial histology are found in the presence of normal circulating progesterone levels, suggesting that a primary endometrial defect is as common as deficient progesterone production (Li et al 1991). There is no reliable way of demonstrating luteal-phase defect in conception cycles or early pregnancy as low levels of progesterone in early pregnancy are a reflection that the pregnancy has already failed because the trophoblast cannot produce sufficient progesterone. The use of colour-flow pulsed Doppler ultrasound may offer a non-invasive tool for diagnosis and has been used in the diagnosis of luteal-phase defect, although only at a preliminary stage (Glock & Brumsted 1995).

There have been many reports of successful pregnancies following treatment with progesterone following the diagnosis of luteal-phase defect. These studies have for the most part been uncontrolled. The only meta-analysis of controlled trials of progesterone treatment in women with recurrent miscarriage has not demonstrated any benefit (Daya 1989).

Treatment with HCG should stimulate progesterone production from the corpus luteum and has been used in the treatment of luteal-phase defect. Although one small study demonstrates a beneficial effect of HCG treatment in women with oligomenorrhoea (Quenby & Farquharson 1994), meta-analysis has concluded that there is insufficient evidence at present concerning the effectiveness of HCG to recommend its use for women with unexplained recurrent miscarriage (Prendiville 1995).

Polycystic ovary syndrome and hypersecretion of luteinizing hormone

The prevalence of polycystic ovarian morphology in women with recurrent miscarriage is 40% (Rai et al 2000) and there have been numerous reports of an increased risk of miscarriage in women with hypersecretion of luteinizing hormone (LH), hyperandrogenaemia and more recently hyperprolactinaemia, all the classic endocrinopathies of polycystic ovary syndrome (PCOS) (Bussen et al 1999, Homburg et al 1988, Howles et al 1987, Regan et al 1990, Stanger & Yovich 1985). Nevertheless, a degree of controversy exists.

Several reports have not confirmed the relationship between hypersecretion of LH and an increased risk of miscarriage in women with recurrent miscarriage (Liddell et al 1997, Tulppala et al 1993). Whether this is due to the radioimmunoassays or a genetic variant of LH is unclear. Also, suppression of high endogenous LH secretion with GnRH analogues in a prospective randomized placebo-controlled trial did not improve the live-birth rate (Clifford et al 1996).

The association between raised androgens and recurrent miscarriage has similarly not been confirmed with later studies (Liddell et al 1997, Rai et al 2000), although these are not universal findings and some reports demonstrate retarded endometrial development and increased risk of miscarriage in association with raised testosterone levels (Okon et al 1998, Tulppala et al 1993).

Hyperprolactinaemia is a common finding in women with PCOS and has been also associated with recurrent miscarriage (Bussen et al 1999, Hirahara et al 1998). Although one study has demonstrated a beneficial effect of bromocriptine treatment this has not been corroborated elsewhere (Hirahara et al 1998).

In summary, PCOS is over-represented in women with recurrent miscarriage but the exact mechanism or individual endocrinopathy by which miscarriage is mediated remains unclear. Until this is determined, any corrective treatment is unlikely to be effective.

Autoimmune and thrombophilic factors

Autoimmune disease

Sporadic and recurrent miscarriage are recognized complications of systemic lupus erythematosus (SLE), the most common autoimmune disorder in women of reproductive age. Since the 1980s it has been recognized that recurrent miscarriage is associated with an increase in the detection of many autoantibodies, even in asymptomatic women. The two most common groups of autoantibodies detected have been the antiphospholipid antibodies, which in conjunction with a history of recurrent miscarriage is now known as the antiphospholipid syndrome (APS) (Harris 1987), and thyroid autoantibodies (Bussen & Steck 1995). However, with the exception of APS, the mechanisms by which a generalized increase in the autoantibody pool leads to miscarriage remain unclear. Although intravenous immunoglobulins (IVIG) therapy has been used in women with recurrent miscarriage associated with non-specific autoimmunity, at present, the collective evidence indicates that IVIG does not have a therapeutic effect that is clinically meaningful (Daya et al 1999).

Antiphospholipid syndrome

The antiphospholipid syndrome (APS) refers to the relationship between antiphospholipid antibodies (aPL), namely lupus anticoagulant (LA) and anticardiolipin antibodies (aCL), and recurrent miscarriage, thrombosis or thrombocytopenia (Harris 1987). Since this original description it has become apparent that the three defining clinical features are too limiting and aPL are implicated in a wide range of clinical conditions (Box 24.3).

In women with recurrent miscarriage, a previous personal or family history of thrombosis, cardiovascular disease, epilepsy and migraine is strongly predictive of a positive aPL status (Regan 1997). The overall prevalence of aPL in women with recurrent miscarriage is around 15% (Li 1998).

Women with APS without treatment have a miscarriage risk of 85–90%, the majority of which occur in the first trimester after establishment of a fetal heart (Rai et al 1995a, b). Pregnancy loss associated with APS is attributed initially to defective embryonic implantation and later to thrombosis of the uteroplacental vasculature and placental infarction (Rai & Regan 1998).

Diagnosis of APS and detection of aPL are subject to widespread interlaboratory variation and the fluctuating nature of the antibodies themselves. Testing for LA should follow internationally agreed guidelines (Lupus Anticoagulant

Box 24.3 Clinical features associated with antiphospholipid antibodies

Obstetrics and gynaecology	Recurrent miscarriage Pre-eclampsia Placental abruption Intrauterine growth retardation Chorea gravidarum
Dermatological	Livido reticularis Cutaneous necrosis
Vascular	Venous thrombosis Arterial thrombosis Mitral valve disease Thrombotic endocarditis
Neurological	Transient ischaemic attacks Cerebrovascular accidents Migraine Epilepsy Multiple sclerosis

Working Party 1991) and the test of choice is the dilute Russell's viper venom time (dRVVT) which is more sensitive than the activated partial thromboplastin time (aPTT) and the kaolin clotting time (KCT). Testing for aCL is by standardized enzyme-linked immunosorbent assay (ELISA). Testing must be repeated on at least two occasions 8 weeks apart in order to make a diagnosis of APS. Testing for aPL other than LA and aCL is of no clinical use in women with recurrent miscarriage.

Although a variety of treatments have been described for APS, including corticosteroids (Lubbe et al 1983), low-dose aspirin (Silver et al 1993), heparin alone (Rosove et al 1990) and IVIG therapy (Carreras et al 1998), treatment with subcutaneous heparin and low-dose aspirin until 34 weeks gestation has been shown to be currently the most effective treatment for women with APS and recurrent miscarriage (Rai et al 1997). In cases where there are additional medical complications, such as thrombocytopenia, IVIG may be appropriate (Cowchock 1998, Piette et al 2000).

Other thrombophilic abnormalities

While APS is an acquired autoimmune thrombophilic state, recurrent miscarriage is also associated with other inherited and acquired causes of thrombophilia (Blumenfeld & Brenner 1999). Most studies are retrospective and interpretation must be cautious, because of problems with acquisition and ascertainment.

Activated protein C resistance, usually but not always inherited via factor V Leiden mutation, is an important cause of acquired venous thrombosis and thrombophilia (Bertina et al 1994). It is also associated with recurrent fetal loss (Brenner et al 1997). Successful treatment with low-dose aspirin and also heparin has been reported, although there are no prospective controlled studies to date.

Hyperhomocystainaemia, as a result of congenital enzyme deficiencies or vitamin B6, B9 and B12 deficiencies, is associated with thrombosis and premature vascular disease (Boers et al 1985). It has also been reported in association with recurrent pregnancy loss (Wouters et al 1993). Thromboprophylaxis and

vitamin supplementation have been reported (Aubard et al 2000), but currently there are no prospective data.

Other inherited thrombophilias, including protein S and protein C deficiency and anti-thrombin III deficiency, are associated with recurrent miscarriage as well as late pregnancy complications (Girling & de Swiet 1998). These need to be managed with appropriate haematological experience because of the increased risk of thromboembolism during pregnancy.

Screening women who have a history of recurrent miscarriage has shown increased incidence of thrombin generation, a global marker of a pro-thrombotic state, even when not pregnant (Vincent et al 1998). Further research is needed to determine whether thromboprophylaxis is appropriate for these women.

Alloimmune factors

The possibility that maternal alloimmune abnormalities lead to recurrent miscarriage has been proposed but remains contentious and there is no reliable test. Treatments involving immunization with trophoblast or paternal leucocytes or third-party leucocytes have been successfully used in women with recurrent miscarriage. However, results of prospective randomized trials and meta-analyses have shown only minimal benefit or no benefit with treatment (Daya & Gunby 1994, Ober et al 1999, Recurrent Miscarriage Immunotherapy Trialists Group 1994). Any potential benefit must be balanced against the risk of the treatment and at the present time allogenic immunization should only be offered in the context of a clinical trial. Current recommendations, both in the UK and the US, are against treatment.

Investigations

The known causes and management of recurrent miscarriage have been detailed above. Necessary investigations to identify such causes are indicated in women with recurrent miscarriage (Box 24.4). Testing thyroid function, random glucose, auto-antibody screen and TORCH screen are no longer appropriate (Li 1998).

Women with recurrent miscarriage are best cared for by a careful history (ideally with a structured history sheet or questionnaire), thorough investigation, sympathetic explanation and counselling. This is best managed in the context of a dedicated recurrent miscarriage clinic. Women who conceive

Box 24.4 Investigation for recurrent miscarriage

Male and female chromosome analysis
Anticardiolipin antibody
Lupus anticoagulant
Clotting studies
Activated and modified protein C resistance
Factor V Leiden mutation
Early follicular phase LH and FSH
Pelvic ultrasound scan
Hysterosalpingogram
Hysteroscopy
Laparoscopy

should then be offered early pregnancy clinic follow-up with ultrasonography and supportive care.

Treatment of unexplained recurrent miscarriage

Treatment of recurrent miscarriage where a potential cause has been identified has been discussed above. In about 50% of recurrent miscarriages, no cause is determined. The prognosis for this group is usually good. The value of continued reassurance and psychological support has been demonstrated (Stray-Pedersen & Stray-Pedersen 1984), with a 75% chance of a live birth in unexplained recurrent miscarriage. This support should include care in a specialist clinic, psychological support, easy access to a named contact, close monitoring including ultrasonography, appropriate reassurance and helpful and caring staff.

Treatment of unproven value should not be offered. Any empirical treatment or treatment in clinical trials needs to have a sound scientific and statistical basis and should include careful counselling and informed consent (Clifford et al 1994, Liddel et al 1997).

Counselling

Counselling should be offered to all patients attending a recurrent miscarriage clinic. It should include an explanation of the possible underlying causes and prognoses. After three consecutive early pregnancy losses there remains a 60–70% chance that the next pregnancy will be successful (Edmonds 1992, Li 1998). This chance decreases with each subsequent miscarriage, although even after six miscarriages the chance of a successful pregnancy is still over 45%.

CONCLUSION

Recurrent miscarriage needs to be differentiated from sporadic miscarriage and thoroughly investigated as outlined above. Careful evaluation and treatment of this aetiologically diverse condition are necessary as detailed above. Continued research into the causes and effective treatments is appropriate and best managed through a dedicated recurrent miscarriage clinic.

Sporadic miscarriage is common and increasing in incidence because of increasing maternal age. The majority of these are unlikely to recur. Management may involve expectant and medical treatment as well as surgical evacuation.

KEY POINTS

1. Miscarriage is the most common complication of pregnancy and accounts for the majority of emergency gynaecology consultations and admissions.
2. The term 'abortion' should be avoided and more sensitive terminology substituted.
3. Miscarriage is defined as the loss of a intrauterine pregnancy before 24 completed weeks of gestation.
4. Sporadic miscarriage occurs in about 15% of all clinically recognized pregnancies, but rises with maternal age.

KEY POINTS (*CONTINUED*)

5. Most early miscarriages are the result of chromosomal abnormalities. The most common is trisomy.
6. Treatment of miscarriage is usually with surgical uterine evacuation, although medical and expectant management should be discussed. There is a small mortality rate with miscarriage, usually due to haemorrhage or sepsis.
7. Recurrent miscarriage is defined as three consecutive miscarriages. Recurrent miscarriage should be distinguished from sporadic miscarriage.
8. Recurrent miscarriage should be investigated and managed in a specialist clinic. Empirical treatments should be avoided.
9. All treatments for recurrent miscarriage need to be evaluated in controlled randomized prospective trials because of the high likelihood of live birth in any placebo group.

REFERENCES

Aarts JM, Brons JT, Bruinse HW 1995 Emergency cerclage: a review. Obstetrical and Gynecological Survey 50:459–469

Alberman E 1987 Maternal age and spontaneous abortion. In: Bennett MJ (ed) Spontaneous and recurrent abortion. Blackwell Science, Oxford

Alberman E 1992 Spontaneous abortions: epidemiology. In: Stabile I, Grudzinskas G, Chard T (eds) Spontaneous abortion – diagnosis and treatment. Springer-Verlag, London

Althuisius SM, Dekker GA, van Geijin HP et al 2000 Cervical incompetence prevention randomized cerclage trial: study design and preliminary results. American Journal of Obstetrics and Gynecology 183:823–829

Ashok PW, Penney GC, Flett GM et al 1998 An effective regimen for early medical abortion: a report of 2000 consecutive cases. Human Reproduction 13:2962–2965

Ashton D, Amin HK, Richart RM et al 1998 The incidence of asymptomatic uterine anomalies in women undergoing transcervical tubal sterilization. Obstetrics and Gynecology 72:28–30

Aubard Y, Darodes N, Cantaloube M et al 2000 Hyperhomocysteinemia and pregnancy: a dangerous association. Journal of Obstetrics, Gynecology and Reproduction (Paris) 29:363–372

Ayhan A, Yucel I, Tuncer ZS et al 1992 Reproductive performance after conventional metroplasty: an evaluation of 102 cases. Fertility and Sterility 57:1194–1196

Ayres de Campos D, Teixeira da Silva J, Campos I et al 2000 Vaginal misoprostol in the management of first trimester missed abortions. International Journal of Gynecology and Obstetrics 71:53–57

Bakas C, Zarou DM, de Caprariis PJ 1996 First-trimester spontaneous abortions and the incidence of human immunodeficiency virus seropositivity. Journal of Reproductive Medicine 41:15–18

Baxter N, Sumiya M, Cheng S et al 2001 Recurrent miscarriage and variant alleles of mannose binding lectin and tumour necrosis factor genes. Clinical and Experimental Immunology 126:529–534

Beeby D, Morgan Hughes JO 1984 Oxytocic drugs and anaesthesia. A controlled clinical trial of ergometrine, syntocinon and normal saline during evacuation of the uterus after spontaneous abortion. Anaesthesia 39:764–767

Bennett MJ 1987 Congenital abnormalities of the fundus. In: Bennett MJ, Edmonds DK (eds) Spontaneous and recurrent abortion. Blackwell Science, Oxford

Ben-Rafael Z, Seidman DS, Recabi K et al 1991 Uterine anomalies: a retrospective matched-control study. Journal of Reproductive Medicine 36:223–227

Bertina RM, Koeleman BP, Koster T et al 1994 Mutation in blood coagulation factor V associated with resistance to activated protein C. Nature 369:64–67

Blumenfeld Z, Brenner B 1999 Thrombophilic-associated pregnancy wastage. Fertility and Sterility 72:765–774

Boers GH, Smals AG, Trijbels FJ et al 1985 Heterozygosity for homocystinuria in premature peripheral and cerebral occlusive arterial disease. New England Journal of Medicine 313:709

Boué A, Gallano P 1984 A collaborative study of the segregation of inherited structural arrangements in 1356 prenatal diagnoses. Prenatal Diagnosis 4:45–67

Boué J, Boué A, Lazar P 1975 Retrospective and prospective epidemiological studies of 1500 karyotyped spontaneous human abortions. Teratology 12:11–26

Brambati B 1990 Fate of human pregnancies. In: Edwards RG (ed) Serono Symposia: establishing a successful human pregnancy, vol. 66 Raven Press, New York

Brenner B, Mandel H, Lanir N et al 1997 Activated protein C resistance can be associated with recurrent fetal loss. British Journal of Haematology 97:551–554

Bussen S, Steck T 1995 Thyroid autoantibodies in euthyroid non-pregnant women with recurrent spontaneous abortions. Human Reproduction 10:2938–2940

Bussen S, Sutterlin M, Steck T 1999 Endocrine abnormalities during the follicular phase in women with recurrent spontaneous abortion. Human Reproduction 14:18–20

Cain AC, Erikson ME, Fast I et al 1964 Children's disturbed reaction to their mothers' miscarriage. Psychosomatic Medicine 26:58–66

Candiani GB, Fedele L, Parazzini F et al 1990 Reproductive prognosis after abdominal metroplasty in bicornuate or septate uterus: a life-table analysis. British Journal of Obstetrics and Gynaecology 97:613–617

Carey JC, Klebanoff MA, Hauth JC et al 2000 Metronidazole to prevent preterm delivery in pregnant women with asymptomatic bacterial vaginosis. National Institute of Child Health and Human Development of Maternal-Fetal Medicine Units. New England Journal of Medicine 342:534–540

Carreras LO, Perez GN, Vega HR et al 1988 Lupus anticoagulant and recurrent fetal loss: successful treatment with gammaglobulin. Fertility and Sterility 54:991–994

Chard T 1991 Frequency of implantation and early pregnancy loss in natural cycles. Baillière's Clinical Obstetrics and Gynaecology 5:179–189

Chung TK, Cheung LP, Lau WC et al 1994 Spontaneous abortion: a medical approach to management. Australia and New Zealand Journal of Obstetrics and Gynaecology 34:432–436

Clifford K, Rai R, Watson H et al 1994 An informative protocol for the investigation of recurrent miscarriage: preliminary experience of 500 cases. Human Reproduction 9:1328–1332

Clifford K, Rai R, Watson H et al 1996 Does suppressing luteinising hormone secretion reduce the miscarriage rate? Results of aa randomised controlled trial. British Medical Journal 312:1508–1511

Cohen EN, Belville JW, Brown BW 1971 Anesthesia, pregnancy and miscarriage: a study of operating room nurses and anesthetists. Anesthesiology 35:343–347

Cowchock S 1998 Treatment of antiphospholipid syndrome in pregnancy. Lupus 7(suppl 2):S95–S97

Creasy MR, Crolla JA, Alberman ED 1976 A cytogenetic study of human spontaneous abortions using banding techniques. Human Genetics 31:177–196

Csapo AI, Pulkinnen MO, Wiest WG 1973 Effects of lutectomy and progesterone replacement therapy in early pregnant patients. American Journal of Obstetrics and Gynecology 115:759–765

Daya S 1989 Efficacy of progesterone support for pregnancy in women with recurrent miscarriage. A meta-analysis of controlled trials. British Journal of Obstetrics and Gynaecology 96:275–280

Daya S 1993 Evaluation and management of recurrent spontaneous abortion. Current Opinion in Obstetrics and Gynecology 8:188–192

Daya S, Gunby J 1994 The effectiveness of allogeneic leukocyte immunization in unexplained primary recurrent spontaneous abortion. Recurrent Miscarriage Immunotherapy Trialists Group. American Journal of Reproductive Immunology 32:294–302

Daya S, Gunby J, Porter F et al 1999 Critical analysis of intravenous immunoglobulins therapy for recurrent miscarriage. Human Reproduction 5:475–482

Deaton JL, Honore GM, Huffman CS et al 1997 Early transvaginal ultrasound following an accurately dated pregnancy: the importance of finding a yolk sac or fetal heart motion. Human Reproduction 12:2820–2823

Dhalial RK, Machin AM, Tait SM 1970 Chromosomal anomalies in spontaneously aborted human fetuses. Lancet 2:20–21

Dijkstra K, Funai EF, O'Neill L et al 2000 Change in cervical length as a predictor of preterm delivery. Obstetrics and Gynecology 96:346–350

D'Ubaldo C, Pezzotti P, Rezza G et al 1998 Association between HIV-1 infection and miscarriage: a group retrospective study. DIANAIDS Collaborative Study Group. AIDS 12:1087–1093

Duncan PG, Pope WD, Cohen MM et al 1986 Fetal risk of anesthesia and surgery during pregnancy. Anesthesiology 64:790–794

Edmonds DK 1992 Spontaneous and recurrent abortion. In: Shaw R, Soutter P, Stanton S (eds) Gynaecology, 2nd edn. Churchill Livingstone, Edinburgh

Edmonds DK, Lindsay KS, Miller JF et al 1982 Early embryonic mortality in women. Fertility and Sterility 38:447–453

Edwards A, Megens A, Peek M et al 2000 Sexual origins of placental dysfunction. Lancet 355:203–204

Egwuatu VE 1989 Fertility and fetal salvage among women with uterine leiomyomas in a Nigerian teaching hospital. International Journal of Fertility 34:341–346

El-Refaey H, Hinshaw K, Henshaw R et al 1992 Medical management of missed abortion and anembryonic pregnancy. British Medical Journal 305:1399

Fawcus S, McIntyre J, Jewkes RJ et al 1997 Management of incomplete abortions at South African public hospitals. National Incomplete Abortion Study Reference Group. South African Medical Journal 87:438–442

Frank P 1985 Sequelae of induced abortion. In: Abortion: medical and social implications. Pitman, London

French FE, Bierman JM 1962 Probabilities of fetal mortality. Public Health Report 77:835–847

Gianaroli L, Magli MC, Ferraretti AP et al 2000 Gonadal activity and chromosomal constitution of in vitro generated embryos. Molecular and Cellular Endocrinology 161:111–116

Gibb DM, Salaria DA 1995 Transabdominal cervicoisthmic cerclage in the management of recurrent second trimester miscarriage and preterm delivery. British Journal of Obstetrics and Gynaecology 102:802–806

Girling J, de Swiet M 1998 Inherited thrombophilic and pregnancy. Current Opinion in Obstetrics and Gynecology 10:135–144

Glock JL, Brumsted JR 1995 Color-flow pulsed Doppler ultrasound in diagnosing luteal phase defect. Fertility and Sterility 64: 500–504

Goldstein P, Berrier J, Rosen S et al 1989 Hormone administration for the maintenance of pregnancy. In: Chalmers I, Enkin M, Kierse MJNC (eds) Effective care in pregnancy and childbirth. Oxford University Press, Oxford

Grudzinskas JG, Chard T 1992 Assessment of early pregnancy: measurement of fetoplacental hormones and proteins. In: Stabile I, Grudzinskas G, Chard T (eds) Spontaneous abortion. Springer-Verlag, Berlin

Gupta JK, Johnson N 1992 Should we use prostaglandins, tents, or progesterone antagonists for cervical ripening before first trimester abortion? Contraception 46:489–497

Halmesmäki E, Valimaki M, Roine R et al 1989 Maternal and paternal alcohol consumption and miscarriage. British Journal of Obstetrics and Gynaecology 96:188–191

Hamilton SM 1989 Should follow-up be provided after miscarriage? British Journal of Obstetrics and Gynaecology 96:743–745

Hamilton-Fairley D, Donaghy J 1997 Surgical versus expectant management of first trimester miscarriage: a prospective observational study. In: Grudzinskas JG, O'Brien PMS (eds) Problems in early pregnancy. RCOG Press, London

Hanson U, Persson B, Thunell S 1990 Relationship between haemoglobin A1C in early type (insulin dependent) diabetic pregnancy and the occurrence of spontaneous abortion and fetal malformation in Sweden. Diabetologia 33:100–104

Harlap S, Shapiro PH 1980 Alcohol, smoking and incidence of spontaneous abortions in the first and second trimester. Lancet 2:2

Harris EN 1987 Syndrome of the black swan. British Journal of Rheumatology 26:324–326

Hassold T, Chen N, Funkhouser J et al 1980 A cytogenetic study of 1000 spontaneous abortions. Annals of Human Genetics 44:151–178

Hay PE, Lamont RF, Taylor-Robinson D 1994 Abnormal bacterial colonisation of the genital tract and subsequent pre-term delivery and late miscarriage. British Medical Journal 308:295–299

Heinonen PK 1997 Reproductive performance of women with uterine anomalies after abdominal or hysteroscopic metroplasty or no surgical treatment. Journal of the American Association of Gynecological Laparoscopy 4:311–317

Hendrick PW 1988 HLA-sharing, recurrent spontaneous abortion, and the genetic hypothesis. Genetics 119:199–204

Henshaw RC, Cooper K, El-Refaey H et al 1993 Medical management of miscarriage: non-surgical uterine evacuation of incomplete and inevitable spontaneous abortion. British Medical Journal 306:894–895

Hertig AC, Rock J, Adams E et al 1959 Thirty-four fertilised human ova, good, bad and indifferent, recovered from 210 women of known fertility. A study of biologic wastage in early human pregnancy. Pediatrics 23:202–211

Hertig AT, Livingstone RG 1944 Spontaneous, threatened and habitual abortion: their pathogenesis and treatment. New England Journal of Medicine 230:797–806

Hirahara F, Andoh N, Sawia K et al 1998 Hyperprolactinaemic recurrent miscarriage and results of randomised bromocriptine treatment trials. Fertility and Sterility 70:246–252

Homburg R, Armar NA, Eshel A et al 1998 Influence of serum luteinising hormone concentrations on ovulation, conception, and early pregnancy loss in polycystic ovary syndrome. British Medical Journal 297:1024–1026

Hopper E 1997 Psychological consequences of early pregnancy loss. In: Grudzinskas JG, O'Brien PMS (eds) Problems in early pregnancy. RCOG Press, London

Howles CM, Macnamee MC, Edwards RG 1987 Follicular development and early luteal function of conception and non-conception cycles after in-vitro fertilization: endocrine correlates. Human Reproduction 2:17–21

Hurd WW, Whitfield RR, Randolph JF Jr et al 1997 Expectant management versus elective curettage for the treatment of spontaneous abortion. Fertility and Sterility 68: 601–606

Hustin J, Jauniaux E 1997 Mechanisms and pathology of miscarriage. In: Grudzinskas JG, O'Brien PMS (eds) Problems in early pregnancy. RCOG Press, London

Jordan J, Craig K, Clifton DK et al 1994 Luteal phase defect: the sensitivity and specificity of diagnostic methods in common clinical use. Fertility and Sterility 62:54–62

Jurkovic D, Geipel A, Gruboeck K et al 1995 Three-dimensional ultrasound for the assessment of uterine anatomy and detection of congenital anomalies: a comparison with hysterosalpingography and two-dimensional ultrasound in Obstetrics and Gynecology 5:233–237

Jurkovic D, Ross JA, Nicolaides KH 1998 Expectant management of missed miscarriage. British Journal of Obstetrics and Gynaecology 105:670–671

Kajii T, Ferrier A, Nikawa N et al 1980 Anatomic and chromosomal anomalies in 639 spontaneous abortuses. Human Genetic 55:87–98

Kaplan B, Pardo J, Rabinerson D et al 1996 Future fertility following conservative management of abortion. Human Reproduction 11:92–94

Katz VL, Kuller JA 1994 Recurrent miscarriage. American Journal of Perinatology 11:386–397

Kellokumpu-Lethtinen P, Pelliniemei LJ 1984 Sex ratio of human conceptuses. Obstetrics and Gynecology 64:220–222

Klebanoff MA, Levine RJ, Der Simonian R et al 1999 Maternal serum paraxanthine, a caffeine metabolite, and the risk of spontaneous abortion. New England Journal of Medicine 341:1639–1644

Kline J, Shrout P, Stein ZA et al 1980 Drinking during pregnancy and spontaneous abortion. Lancet 2:176–180

Kline J, Stein Z, Susser M 1989 Conception to birth – epidemiology of prenatal development. Monographs in epidemiology and biostatistics vol.14. Oxford University Press, Oxford

Lawson HW, Frye A, Atrash HK et al 1994 Abortion mortality, United States, 1972 through 1987. American Journal of Obstetrics and Gynecology 171:1365–1372

Li TC 1998 Recurrent miscarriage: principles of management. Human Reproduction 13:478–482

Li TC, Cooke ID 1991 Evaluation of the luteal phase: a review. Human Reproduction 6:484–499

Li TC, Dockery P, Cooke ID 1991 Endometrial development in the luteal phase of women with various types of infertility: comparison of women with normal fertility. Human Reproduction 6:325–330

Liddell HS, Sowden K, Farquhar CM 1997 Recurrent miscarriage: screening for polycystic ovaries and subsequent pregnancy outcome. Australia and New Zealand Journal of Obstetrics and Gynaecology 37:402–406

Llahi-Camp JM, Rai R, Ison C et al 1999 Association of bacterial vaginosis and a history of second trimester miscarriage. Human Reproduction 11:1575–1578

Lubbe WF, Butler WS, Palmer SJ et al 1983 Fetal survival after prednisone suppression of maternal lupus anticoagulant. Lancet 1:1361–1363

Lupus Anticoagulant Working Party on behalf of the BSCH Homeostasis and Thrombosis Task Force 1991 Guidelines on testing for the lupus anticoagulant. Journal of Clinical Pathology 44:885–889

MacDonald IA 1957 Suture of the cervix for inevitable miscarriage. Journal of Obstetrics and Gynecology of the British Empire 64:731–735

MacDonald AD, McDonald JC, Armstrong B et al 1988 Fetal death and work in pregnancy. British Journal of Industrial Medicine 45:148–157

Mansur MM 1992 Ultrasound diagnosis of complete abortion can reduce need for curettage. European Journal of Obstetrics, Gynecology and Reproductive Biology 44:65–69

Mikkelson M 1985 Cytogenetic findings in first trimester chorionic villus sampling. In: Fraccaro G, Simoni G, Brambati B (eds) First trimester fetal diagnosis. Springer-Verlag, Berlin

Miller H, Durant JA, Ross DM et al 1969 Corpus luteum deficiency as a cause of early recurrent abortion: a case history. Fertility and Sterility 20:433–438

Miller JF, Williamson E, Glue J et al 1980 Fetal loss after implantation: a prospective study. Lancet 2:554–556

Mills JL, Simpson JL, Driscoll SG et al 1988 Incidence of spontaneous abortion amongst normal women and insulin dependent diabetic women whose pregnancies were identified within 21 days of conception. New England Journal of Medicine 319: 1617–1623

MRC/RCOG Working Party on Cervical Cerclage 1993 Final report of the Medical Research Council/Royal College of Obstetricians and Gynaecologists multicentre randomised trial of cervical cerclage. British Journal of Obstetrics and Gynaecology 100:516–523

Mur JM, Mandereau L, Deplan F et al 1992 Spontaneous abortion and exposure to vinyl chloride. Lancet 339:127–128

Nahmias AJ, Josey WE, Naib WM et al 1971 Perinatal risk associated with maternal genital herpes simplex virus infection. American Journal of Obstetrics and Gynecology 110:825–837

Ness RB, Grisso JA, Hirschinger N et al 1999 Cocaine and tobacco use and the risk of spontaneous abortion. New England Journal of Medicine 340:333–339

Neugebauer R, Kline J, O'Connor P et al 1992 Depressive symptoms in women in the six months following miscarriage. American Journal of Obstetrics and Gynecology 166:104–109

Neugebauer R, Kline J, Stein Z et al 1996 Association of stressful life events with chromosomally normal spontaneous abortion. American Journal of Epidemiology 143:588–596

Nielsen S, Hahlin M 1995 Expectant management of spontaneous first trimester abortion. Lancet 345:84–86

Nybo Andersen AM, Wohlfahrt J, Christens P et al 2000 Maternal age and fetal loss: population based register linkage. British Medical Journal 320:1708–1712

Ober C, Karrison T, Odem RR et al 1999 Mononuclear-cell immunisation in prevention of recurrent miscarriages: a randomised trial. Lancet 354:365–369

Okon MA, Laird SM, Tuckerman EM et al 1998 Serum androgen levels in women who have recurrent miscarriages and their correlation with markers of endometrial function. Fertility and Sterility 69:682–690

Pabuccu R, Atay V, Urman B et al 1995 Hysteroscopic treatment of septate uterus. Gynaecological Endoscopy 4:213–215

Parazzini F, Boccialone L, La Vecchia C et al 1990 Maternal and paternal moderate alcohol consumption and unexplained miscarriages. British Journal of Obstetrics and Gynaecology 97:618–622

Pedersen JF, Mantoni M 1990 Large intrauterine haematomata in threatened miscarriage. Frequency and clinical consequences. British Journal of Obstetrics and Gynaecology 97:75–77

Pegoraro E, Whitaker J, Mowery-Rushton P et al 1997 Familial skewed X inactivation: a molecular trait associated with high spontaneous abortion rate maps to Xq28. American Journal of Human Genetics 61:160–170

Piette JC, Le Thi Huong D, Wechsler B 2000 Therapeutic use of intravenous immunoglobulins in the antiphospholipid syndrome. Annales de Médicine Interne (Paris) 151(suppl 1):S51–S54

Platz-Christiansen JJ, Nielsen S, Hamberger L 1995 Is misoprostol the drug of choice for induced cervical ripening in early pregnancy termination? Acta Obstetrica et Gynaecologica Scandinavica 74: 809–812

Pennell RG, Needleman L, Pajak T et al 1991 Prospective comparison of vaginal and abdominal sonography in normal early pregnancy. Journal of Ultrasound in Medicine 10:63–67

Prendiville WG 1995 HCG for recurrent miscarriage. In: Enkin MW, Keirse MJNC, Renfrew MJ et al (eds) Pregnancy and childbirth module (CD-Rom). Cochrane Database. Update Software, Oxford

Prieto JA, Eriksen NL, Blanco JD 1995 A randomised trial of prophylactic doxycycline for curettage in incomplete abortion. Obstetrics and Gynecology 85:692–696

Quenby SM, Farquharson RG 1994 Human chorionic gonadotrophin supplementation in recurring pregnancy loss: a controlled trial. Fertility and Sterility 62:708–710

Rai R, Regan L 1998 Antiphospholipid syndrome and pregnancy loss. Hospital Medicine 59:637–639

Rai RS, Clifford K, Cohen H et al 1995 High prospective fetal loss rate in untreated pregnancies of women with recurrent miscarriage and antiphospholipid antibodies. Human Reproduction 10:3301–3304

Rai RS, Regan L, Clifford K et al 1995 Antiphospholipid antibodies and beta2-glycoprotein-I in 500 women with recurrent miscarriage: results of a comprehensive screening approach. Human Reproduction 10:2001–2005

Rai R, Cohen H, Dave M et al 1997 Randomised controlled trial of aspirin and aspirin plus heparin in pregnant women with recurrent miscarriage associated with phospholipid antibodies (or antiphospholipid antibodies). British Medical Journal 314:253–257

Rai R, Backos M, Rushworth F et al 2000 Polycystic ovaries and recurrent miscarriage – a reappraisal. Human Reproduction 15:612–615

Ratnam SS, Prasad RNV 1990 Medical management of abnormal pregnancy. Baillière's Clinical Obstetrics and Gynaecology 4:361–374

RCGP/RCOG Joint Study Group 1985 Induced abortion operations and their early sequelae. Journal of the Royal College of General Practitioners 35:175–180

RCOG 40th Study Group 2001 Infection and pregnancy. RCOG Press, London

Recurrent Miscarriage Immunotherapy Trialists Group 1994 Worldwide collaborative observational study and meta-analysis on allogenic leukocyte immunotherapy for recurrent spontaneous abortion. American Journal of Reproductive Immunology 32:55–72

Regan L 1997 Sporadic and recurrent miscarriage. In: Grudizinskas JG, O'Brien PMS (eds) Problems in early pregnancy – advances in diagnosis and management. RCOG Press, London

Regan L, Braude P, Trembath PL 1989 Influence of past reproductive performance on risk of spontaneous abortion. British Medical Journal 299:541–545

Regan L, Owen EJ, Jacobs HS 1990 Hypersecretion of luteinising hormone, infertility, and miscarriage. Lancet 336:1141–1144

Roberts CJ, Lowe DB 1975 Where have all the conceptions gone? Lancet 1:498

Rosove MH, Tabsh K, Wasserstrum N et al 1990 Heparin therapy for pregnant women with lupus anticoagulant or anticardiolipin antibodies. Obstetrics and Gynecology 75:630–634

Rowland AS, Baird DD, Shore DL et al 1996 Ethylene oxide exposure may increase the risk of spontaneous abortion, preterm birth and postterm birth. Epidemiology 7:363–368

Rushton DI 1995 Pathology of abortion. In: Fox H (ed) Haines and Taylor obstetrical and gynecological pathology. Churchill Livingstone, Edinburgh

Rushworth FH, Backos M, Rai R et al 2000 Prospective pregnancy outcome in untreated recurrent miscarriers with thyroid autoantibodies. Human Reproduction 15:1637–1639

Russell PB 1947 Abortions treated conservatively: a twelve year study covering 3739 cases. Southern Medical Journal 40:314–324

Schiverick KT, Salafia C 1999 Cigarette smoking and pregnancy I: ovarian, uterine and placental effects. Placenta 20:265–272

Schmidt-Sarosi C, Schwartz LB, Lublin J et al 1998 Chromosomal analysis of early fetal losses in relation to transvaginal ultrasonographic detection of fetal heart motion after infertility. Fertility and Sterility 69:274–277

Scibetta JJ, Sanko SR, Phipps WR 1998 Laparoscopic transabdominal cervicoisthmic cerclage. Fertility and Sterility 69:161–163

Sebire NJ, Thornton S, Hughes K et al 1997a The prevalence and consequences of missed abortion in twin pregnancies at 10 and 14 weeks of gestation. British Journal of Obstetrics and Gynaecology 104:847–848

Sebire NJ, Snijders RJ, Hughes K et al 1997b The hidden mortality of monochorionic twin pregnancies. British Journal of Obstetrics and Gynaecology 104:1203–1207

Seibel M, Graves WL 1980 The psychological implication of spontenous abortion. Journal of Reproductive Medicine 25:161–172

Serle E, Aplin JD, Li TC et al 1994 Endometrial differentiation in the preimplantation phase of women with recurrent miscarriage: a morphological and immunohistochemical study. Fertility and Sterility 62:989–996

Shephard TH, Fantel AG, Fitzsimmons J 1989 Congenital defect rates among spontaneous abortuses: twenty years of monitoring. Teratology 39:325–331

Shirodkar VM 1960 Contributions to obstetrics and gynaecology. Churchill Livingstone, Edinburgh

Silver RK, MacGregor SN, Sholl JS et al 1993 Comparative trial of prednisone plus aspirin versus aspirin alone in the treatment of anticardiolipin antibody-positive obstetric patients. American Journal of Obstetrics and Gynecology 169:1411–1417

Simpson JL, Gray RH, Queenan JT et al 1996 Further evidence that infection is an infrequent cause of first trimester spontaneous abortion. Human Reproduction 11:2058–2060

Singh A, Dantas ZN, Stone SC, Asch RH 1995 Presence of thyroid antibodies in early reproductive failure: biochemical versus clinical pregnancies. Fertility and Sterility 63:277–281

Stabile I, Campbell S, Grudzinskas JG 1987 Ultrasound assessment in complications of first trimester pregnancy. Lancet 2:1237–1242

Stanger JD, Yovich JL 1985 Reduced in vitro fertilisation of human oocytes from patients with raised basal luteinising hormone levels during the follicular phase. British Journal of Obstetrics and Gynaecology 92:385–393

Stephenson MD 1996 Frequency of factors associated with habitual abortion in 197 couples. Fertility and Sterility 66:27–29

Stirrat GM 1990 Recurrent miscarriage: I. Definitions and epidemiology. Lancet 336:673–675

Stray-Pedersen B 1993 New aspects of perinatal infections. Annals of Medicine 25:295

Stray-Pedersen B, Stray-Pedersen S 1984 Etiological factors and subsequent reproductive performance in 195 couples with a prior history of habitual abortion. American Journal of Obstetrics and Gynecology 148:140–146

Takahara H, Ohama K, Fukiwara A 1977 Cytogenetic study in early spontaneous abortion. Hiroshima Journal of Medical Science 26:291–296

Takakuwa K, Asano K, Arakawa M et al 1997 Chromosome analysis of aborted conceptuses of recurrent aborters positive for anticardiolipin antibody. Fertility and Sterility 68:54–58

Therkelsen AJ, Grunnet N, Hjort T et al 1977 Studies in spontaneous abortion. In: Boué A, Thibault C (eds) Chromosomal errors in relation to reproductive failure INSERM, Paris

Tower CL, Regan L 2001 Intrauterine haematomas in a recurrent miscarriage population. Human Reproduction 16:2005–2007

Tulppala M, Stenman UH, Cacciatore B et al 1993 Polycystic ovaries and levels of gonadotrophins and androgens in recurrent miscarriage: a prospective study of 50 women. British Journal of Obstetrics and Gynaecology 100:438–352

Tulppala M, Huhtaniemi I, Ylikorkala O 1998 Genetic variant of luteinizing hormone in women with a history of recurrent miscarriage. Human Reproduction 13:2699–2702

Verkuyl DA, Crowther CA 1993 Suction v. conventional curettage in incomplete abortion. A randomised controlled trial. South African Medical Journal 83:13–15

Vidal F, Rubio C, Simon C et al 2000 Is there a place for preimplantation genetic diagnosis screening in recurrent miscarriage patients? Journal of Reproduction and Fertility 55:143–146

Vincent T, Rai R, Regan L et al 1998 Increased thrombin generation in women with recurrent miscarriage. Lancet 352:116

Warbuton D, Stein Z, Kline J et al 1980 Chromosome abnormalities in spontaneous abortions. In: Porter IH, Hook EB (eds) Human embryonic and fetal deaths. Academic Press, New York

Weigel MM, Weigel RM 1989 Nausea and vomiting of early pregnancy and pregnancy outcome. An epidemiological study. British Journal of Obstetrics and Gynaecology 96:1304–1311

Wilcox AJ, Weinberg CR, O'Connor JF et al 1988 Incidence of early loss in pregnancy. New England Journal of Medicine 319:189–194

Windham GC, von Behren J, Fenster I et al 1997 Moderate maternal alcohol consumption and the risk of spontaneous abortion. Epidemiology 8:509–514

Wong GP, Farquharson DF, Dansereau J 1993 Emergency cervical cerclage: a retrospective review of 51 cases. American Journal of Perinatology 10:341–347

Wouters MG, Boers GH, Blom HJ et al 1993 Hyperhomocysteinemia: a risk factor in women with unexplained recurrent early pregnancy loss. Fertility and Sterility 60:820

Zemlickis D, Lishner M, Degendorfer P et al 1992 Fetal outcome after in utero exposure to cancer chemotherapy. Archives of Internal Medicine 152:573–576

25
Tubal disease

Ovrang Djahanbakhch   Ertan Saridogan

INTRODUCTION

The fallopian tube has many active roles in the process of reproduction. As the fallopian tube provides the environment in which fertilization and early development take place, these events may have a significant effect on all the subsequent events of the pregnancy. The role of the fallopian tube in the process of natural conception begins when the oocyte is released by the ruptured ovarian follicle and is picked up by the fimbrial end of the fallopian tube. It also facilitates the final maturation of sperm, which have passed through the uterus. Both the sperm and oocytes are transported within the fallopian tube to the site of fertilization and meet within well-defined, species-dependent time limits. Fertilization takes place at the ampullary-isthmic junction, then the pre-embryo is transported to the uterine cavity at the optimum time for nidation. Significantly, the sperm and pre-embryo, which differ antigenically from the mother, are not attacked by the immune system. The mechanisms by which all these complex processes are controlled are not well understood.

ANATOMY

The fallopian tubes are situated in the upper margin of the broad ligament, on each side, extending from the uterine cornua to the sides of the pelvis. Since they are contractile organs, their length is determined by muscle tone. The average length of the fallopian tube is 11 cm, ranging from 6 to 15 cm. The fallopian tube consists of three layers: serosa, muscle layer and mucosa. The external layer or serosa is peritoneal. It surrounds the fallopian tube by a double fold peritoneum and fuses inferiorly to form the mesosalpinx, the primary supporting mesentery of the tube. The muscle layer or myosalpinx consists of longitudinal and circular muscular fibres continuous with those of the uterus. Their thickness depends on the segment of the tube. The internal layer of the tube consists of an intricately folded mucosa or endosalpinx which surrounds a lumen whose space is determined by the amount of secretion and the segment of the tube.

Four distinct segments of the fallopian tubes can be identified depending on the anatomical position, thickness of the smooth muscle, complexity of mucosal folding and cellular composition of the mucosa. Starting from the uterine end of the fallopian tube, these regions are termed the intramural or interstitial segment, the isthmus, the ampulla and the infundibulum. The zone between the ampulla and the isthmus is known as the ampullary-isthmic junction, while that between the isthmus and the uterus is the utero-tubal junction.

The intramural (interstitial) segment of the tube passes through the uterine wall and is surrounded by myometrium. It is about 1 cm in length and varies from 0.2 mm to 0.4 mm in diameter. The endosalpinx is composed of four or five folds.

The isthmus, which is 2–3 cm in length, is the most densely muscular segment of the tube. The diameter of the lumen of the isthmus varies between 0.2 mm and 2 mm. The proximal endosalpinx with its cruciform, narrow lumen becomes progressively wider and more complex toward the ampulla.

The ampulla constitutes about half the length of the tube and it usually follows a straight course devoid of abrupt angulations and convolutions. The myosalpinx is thin, surrounding a large lumen measuring 1–2 mm at the ampullary-isthmic junction and 1 cm at its lateral end. The endosalpinx is extensively folded; there are 6–8 primary folds which comprise numerous complex secondary and tertiary folds.

The infundibulum is the funnel-shaped distal portion of the fallopian tube and the abdominal opening of the tubal ostium is about 3 mm in diameter. The internal surface of the infundibulum is occupied by complex folds of mucosa and these evert to form numerous irregular slender processes called fimbriae. One such fimbria, the fimbria ovarica, is longer, reaching to the tubal pole of the ovary, to which it is closely applied.

HISTOLOGY

The mucosa is arranged into longitudinal folds. Each fold is lined with a single layer of columnar epithelium underlined by a layer of connective tissue, the lamina propria. Four types of epithelial cells have been identified: ciliated cells, secretory cells, intercalary or peg cells and basal or indifferent cells (Fig. 25.1). Ciliated cells are most frequently found on the apices of mucosal folds. Secretory cells have secretory granules and their apical surface contains protrusions or domes and numerous microvilli. The apical protrusions are released into the lumen with the granules in them, as a form of apocrine or decapitation secretion. This release of cytoplasmic fragments is also accompanied by

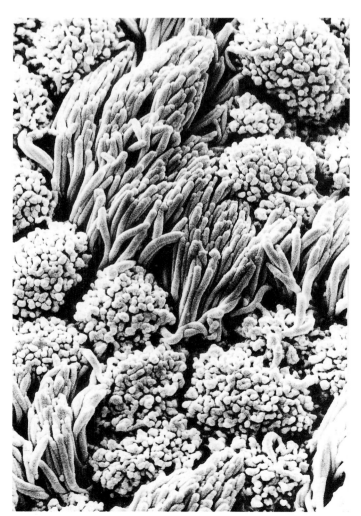

Fig. 25.1 Scanning electron micrograph showing ciliated and non-ciliated cells of the fallopian tube mucosa.

extrusion of larger cell fragments, sometimes including nuclei and greater numbers of whole cells (Crow et al 1994). Intercalary cells probably represent the degenerative or end phase of the secretory cell. While some authors believe that basal cells are T-lymphocytes of predominantly cytotoxic/suppressor type, others postulate that they may represent 'stem cells' from which mature epithelial cells, and possibly stroma, regenerate.

The myosalpinx is made up of the outer longitudinal and inner circular layers of smooth muscle, thickest in the proximal isthmus and intramural regions where there is also an inner longitudinal layer (Lindblom & Norstrom 1986).

The general morphology of the fallopian tube mucosa varies during the ovarian cycle, although the variations are much less pronounced than those observed in the endometrium (reviewed by Jansen 1984).

FUNCTIONAL ASPECTS

Ovum and embryo transport is probably the result of an interaction between the egg/embryo and the muscle contractions, ciliary activity and flow of tubal secretions. The relative importance of these factors is debatable, although it is generally accepted that there are regional differences in the contribution made by each of these factors (Croxatto & Ortiz 1975). Both myosalpingeal and ciliary activity are affected by a diverse range of chemical, biological and hormonal agents including ovarian steroids, sympathomimetic agents, prostaglandins and angiotensin II (Jansen 1984, Mahmood et al 1998, Saridogan et al 1996).

Tubal secretions contain proteins that derive from the plasma and also some specific substances synthesized within the oviduct itself (reviewed by Maguiness et al 1992b). Both tubal proteins and the physical contact between the gametes and tubal epithelium may play a role in gamete function (i.e. capacitation), fertilization and early embryo development (Djahanbakhch et al 1994, Kervancioglu et al 2000).

AETIOLOGY OF TUBAL DISEASE

Tubal disease is usually defined as tubal damage caused by pelvic infection such as pelvic inflammatory disease, tuberculosis, salpingitis isthmica nodosa or iatrogenic disease with varying degrees of tubal damage or obstruction, sometimes involving the surrounding ovary or pelvic peritoneum, and adhesion formation. As a result, patients with tubal damage suffer from infertility and/or pelvic pain. However, this definition does not include functional aspects of the fallopian tube as currently our ability to describe the tubal disease is limited to demonstrating its patency and macroscopic normality. Tubal disease is accountable for 30–40% of cases of female infertility.

Salpingitis

Most salpingitis is the result of an ascending infection from the lower genital tract (Fig. 25.2). The mechanisms whereby the infection ascends through the cervical canal and reaches the tubes are still unknown. It is possible that cervical resistance diminishes, allowing the bacteria to pass through, and is at its lowest during ovulation and menstruation. This theory fits with observations that in cases of cervical gonorrhoea the

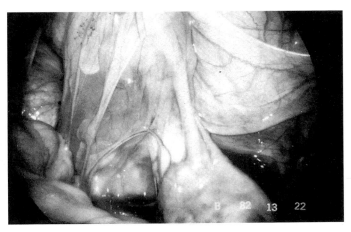

Fig. 25.2 Laparoscopic view of a pelvis after pelvic inflammatory disease. There is a 'curtain' of adhesions covering the pelvic organs.

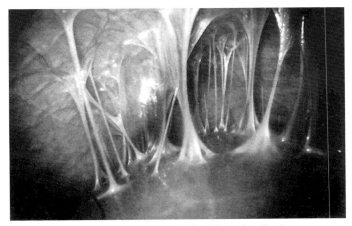

Fig. 25.3 Laparoscopic photograph of perihepatic adhesions: Fitz-Hugh–Curtis syndrome.

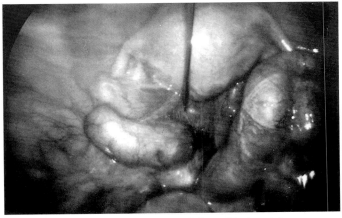

Fig. 25.4 Laparoscopic appearance of bilateral hydrosalpinges as a result of previous inflammatory disease.

symptoms of salpingitis appear after menstruation and patients on oral contraception appear to be 'protected' due to anovulation.

Salpingitis is not generally seen in women who are not sexually active and it is possible that coitus produces uterine contractions, facilitating the spread of infection into the uterus and tubes. In other cases, iatrogenic manoeuvres such as insertion of an intrauterine device, termination of pregnancy, hysterosalpingography or curettage can spread a cervical infection into the uterus and tubes.

Iatrogenic tubal disease is tubal damage caused by surgical procedures which damage the peritoneum and tubes, rendering young women infertile.

Pelvic inflammatory disease has by tradition been associated with gonorrhoea. Improvement of microbiological techniques has allowed the identification of numerous other organisms capable of producing salpingitis, including *Chlamydia trachomatis*, *Mycoplasma hominis* and anaerobic bacteria. In developed countries there has been a shift observed in microbial aetiology of PID and chlamydia has emerged as the most prevalent sexually transmitted disease (Washington 1996) (Figs 25.3 and 25.4) (see also Chapters 61 and 62). Mycobacterium tuberculosis is still seen in developed countries, although rarely.

Other causes

Endometriosis, fibroids, previous pelvic/tubal surgery, salpingitis isthmica nodosa, endosalpingiosis and cornual polyps can be the cause of cornual obstruction or tubal damage. Endometriosis is reviewed in Chapter 34. In some patients tubal damage is secondary to previous tubal or pelvic surgery such as salpingotomy for ectopic pregnancy, ovarian cystectomy, myomectomy, ovarian wedge resection and shortening of round ligaments. Salpingitis isthmica nodosa was described by Chiari (1887) as nodular thickening of the proximal part of the fallopian tube. The aetiology of this entity is unknown but it is probably due to a non-inflammatory process.

DIAGNOSIS

Assessment of the fallopian tube should normally determine patency, a normal external and internal appearance, the

ability to transport gametes and the embryo, and provision of an environment for the early steps of reproduction to occur. It is possible that, apart from the obvious need for tubal patency to allow passage of gametes, factors that affect the gametes and embryo, the effectors of tubal transport, the cilia, flow of tubal fluid and tubal contractions appear to constitute a higher-order system in which intact function of each may not be needed to achieve pregnancy (Verdugo 1986). However, dysfunction of this higher-order system may be the reason for unsuccessful tubal surgery even when tubal patency has been achieved. Similarly a functional disorder of this system may be accountable for subfertility in some cases of unexplained infertility. Currently, tubal function is determined by demonstrating patency and normal appearance at endoscopy.

The methods commonly used to determine tubal patency are hysterosalpingography (HSG), laparoscopy and hysterosalpingo contrast sonography (HyCoSy). The first two have been used for many years, whereas HyCoSy is a relatively new technique. All these methods have some degree of false-negative and false-positive results in determining tubal patency. A comparison of HSG and laparoscopy showed that a complete agreement of tubal patency was found in 80.2% of cases (Maguiness et al 1992a). Laparoscopy has the ability to identify

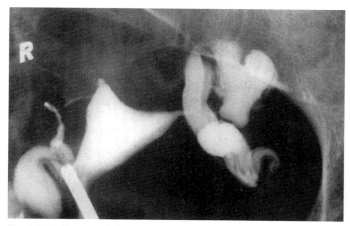

Fig. 25.5 Hysterosalpingogram of a patient with bilateral hydrosalpinges.

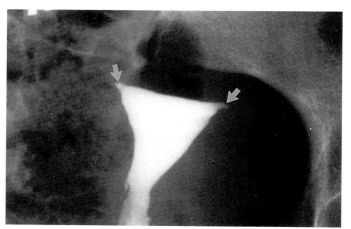

Fig. 25.7 Hysterosalpingogram of a patient with bilateral tubal block (arrows).

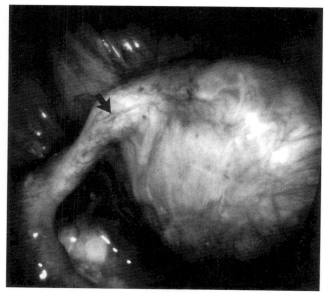

Fig. 25.6 Tubal cornual block: there are irregular vessels on the peritoneum surface as a result of previous inflammation (arrow).

peritubal adhesions, endometriosis, polycystic ovaries and other pelvic and intra-abdominal pathology. However, it is usually performed under general anaesthesia and does not give information about the uterine cavity.

In general, these methods are considered complementary investigations, offering very important information (Figs 25.5, 25.6 and 25.7). Laparoscopy should be performed by the surgeon or a member of the team who will eventually operate on the patient, if surgery is the treatment of choice, because of the variation between units in experience and approaches to varying tubal diseases.

Internal appearance of the fallopian tubes can be assessed by falloposcopy or salpingoscopy. Falloposcopy is the transcervical assessment of the tubal lumen using a fibreoptic endoscope. It can be performed as an outpatient procedure and allows assessment of the isthmic lumen. However, due to its narrow diameter and lack of fluid distension, it does not give as good a view of the tubal folds in the rest of the tube.

Salpingoscopy is the transabdominal examination of the tubal lumen by introducing an endoscope through the fimbrial end. Rigid endoscopes with a 2.8 mm diameter allow excellent visualization of the infundibulum and ampulla as far as the ampullary-isthmic junction. The presence of minor intratubal lesions is not necessarily incompatible with fertility (Maguiness & Djahanbakhch 1992); however, loss of mucosal folds and intratubal fibrosis are significant. Nowadays, salpingoscopic assessment of the tubal lumen is recommended by some groups before tubal surgery for hydrosalpinges (Puttemans et al 1998). De Bruyne et al (1989) proposed a classification of ampullary findings in hydrosalpinges: grades 1 and 2 refer to normal salpingoscopic findings, whereas grade 3 (intermediate group) has focal adhesions and grades 4 and 5 have severe adhesions and loss of mucosal folds.

Selective transcervical salpingography and tubal catheterization can be done in cases where it is doubtful that there is cornual obstruction (Ataya & Thomas 1991). Mucus plugs and debris can be mobilized and a tube that was apparently obstructed can be 'opened'.

TREATMENT

The treatment of tubal disease in the infertile patient is surgical. Selective transcervical salpingography and tubal catheterization can be used for the treatment of proximal tubal obstruction in selected cases. The use of magnification and microsurgical techniques has been the traditional method. With the development of laparoscopic instruments the laparoscopic approach is very much favoured by many gynaecologists for patients with minor tubal disease and/or adhesions.

The criteria for patient selection for treatment depend very much on the surgeon's experience and on the possibility of being able to offer alternative treatment. Other points to be considered when making the decision regarding treatment are the patient's wishes about the type of treatment that she prefers and the problem of pain. Large numbers of patients with tubal disease have pelvic pain due to adhesions. In some of them the surgical freeing of the ovaries and tubes from adhesions can give symptomatic relief.

Microsurgical treatment

The microscope was first used for tubal surgery by Walz (1959). Whilst others used delicate electrosurgery and magnification (loupes) in the treatment of hydrosalpinges, Paterson & Wood (1974) in Australia and Winston & McClure-Browne (1974) in England adapted their experience from animal experiments to humans and operated on infertile women, under high magnification, using an operating microscope.

Microsurgery is not only the use of a microscope; it is based on gentle tissue handling, reperitonealization of raw areas, the use of non-resorbable suture materials and irrigation of the tissues using Ringer's lactate solution as this tends to prevent adhesion formation.

The use of the microscope was originally much debated but now microsurgery is well established and is a routine procedure for tubal infertility.

Coadjuvants

The use of coadjuvants can sometimes help to avoid adhesion formation, but it is important to keep in mind that no coadjuvant will replace good surgical technique. Recent reviews of methods for preventing adhesions suggest that none of the methods is clearly shown to improve pregnancy rates; however, some methods such as steroids, oxidized regenerated cellulose (Interceed) and polytetrafluoroethylene (Gore-Tex) reduce adhesion formation (Farquhar et al 2000, Watson et al 2000).

Cornual occlusion

Cornual occlusion due to inflammatory causes was treated by uterotubal implantation with very poor results. Ehrler (1963) described his technique and suggested that in most patients the intramural portion of the tube could be spared. Since Winston (1977) and Gomel (1977) described their methods based on the use of the microscope it has become the surgical technique of choice. Cornual implantation is now rarely used, except in cases of severe damage of the intramural portion of the tubes, and is reserved for cases where there is a severe degree of adenomyosis or tubal damage. Tubocornual implantation is avoided whenever possible. Destroying a possible sphincter at the uterotubal junction is associated with excessive bleeding and damage to the tubal blood supply; it shortens the tube and may increase the risk of rupture of the uterus in the event of subsequent pregnancy, which means that patients must be delivered by caesarean section.

The use of magnification allows the surgeon better identification of the intramural portion of the tube by careful shaving of the cornua until healthy tissue is found, permitting a more accurate tissue apposition with a watertight anastomosis between healthy tubal tissues. Once the ends are well defined the anastomosis is done in two layers, using 8/0 nylon as a suture. The suture material should not penetrate the mucosa, only the muscularis (Seki et al 1977). In some cases the use of a temporary splint gives considerable help, especially in deep cornual tubal anastomosis (Fig. 25.8), but it should be removed at the end of the surgical procedure and if left in situ, should not remain more than 48 hours. Longer periods of time cause mucosal damage. Tension between the anastomosed ends must be avoided.

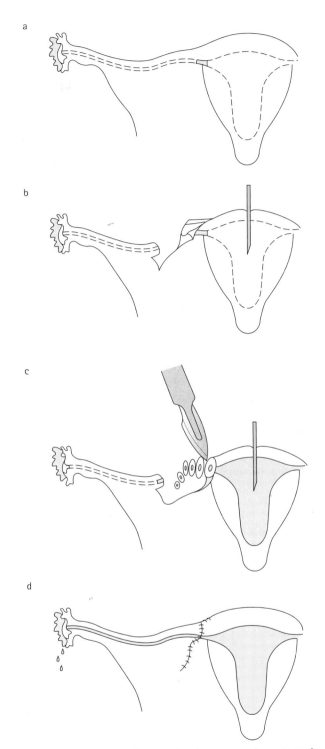

Fig. 25.8 Cornual block diagram showing a cornual anastomosis. **a** Superficial cornual block. **b** Opening of the cornua to expose the intramural part of the tube. **c** Shaving of the tube to find healthy mucosa for anastomosis. **d** Cornual anastomosis completed.

A stitch of 6/0 Prolene between both ends of the mesosalpinx should be applied as a stay suture. More details about the technique have been given elsewhere (Margara 1982, Winston 1977).

Cornual polyps

Removal of cornual polyps is still a matter of controversy. Glazener et al (1987) stated that the removal of cornual polyps does not improve fertility and they are not a cause of infertility. However, consideration should be given to removal of large polyps present in the intramural or isthmic portion of the tube. This can involve salpingotomy and resection of the polyp without tubal resection or the opening of the cornu, and removal of the affected portion of the tube followed by cornual-isthmic anastomosis in two layers. In some cases when a large polyp is implanted deep in the intramural portion of the tube, the anastomosis can be difficult due to disparity of the lumen of the tubal ends. The portion where the polyp was present is wider than the isthmic portion of the tube and it is not always easy to achieve a watertight anastomosis. For this reason some surgeons prefer salpingotomy whenever possible.

Tubal anastomosis

Tubal anastomosis for reversal of sterilization is the most successful technique in microsurgery for the following reasons: healthy tissues are anastomosed, the localized damage is removed completely (Fig. 25.9) and these patients are in general fertile.

Success depends on the length of the remaining tube. The minimum length of tube necessary to maintain fertility in women is not known. In animal experiments, fertility diminished in a linear fashion depending on the length of the ampulla resected; when more than 70% was missing, none of the animals became pregnant. Resection of the ampullary-isthmic junction did not appear to alter fertility (Winston et al 1977). The rabbit is far from an ideal model for human tubal physiology, but these results emphasize the fact that the ampulla seems to be important in maintaining fertility.

The length of time between sterilization and reversal is important and has a prognostic value. Vasquez et al (1980) demonstrated that after 5 years of sterilization the proximal

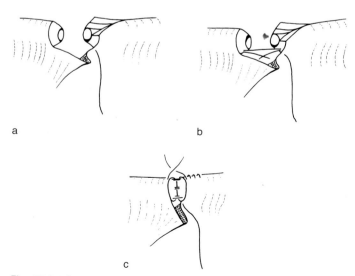

a   b

c

Fig. 25.9 Anastomotic procedure. **a** Both tubal lumens are exposed (healthy mucosa); **b** the first stitch is at 6 o'clock and must be extra-mucosal; **c** the anastomosis is completed in two layers. The suture material used is 8/0 nylon.

portion of the tube had a severely damaged mucosa with flattening of the epithelium and polyp formation. The surgical technique of reversal of sterilization has been described by Winston (1977) and Margara (1982).

Hydrosalpinges

As well as being a cause of infertility, hydrosalpinges also have a detrimental effect on the outcome of in vitro fertilization-embryo transfer treatment with reduced pregnancy and implantation rates and increased miscarriage rates. The hydrosalpinx fluid is known to be embryotoxic and may also reduce the endometrial receptivity. Removal of hydrosalpinges prior to IVF-ET seems to lead to better results (Nackley & Muasher 1998, Zeyneloglu et al 1998). However, some groups believe that salpingectomy should be performed only when there is severe tubal pathology and the other patients should be given the chance of tubal surgery (Puttemans & Brosens 1996).

The value of microsurgery varies in the treatment of hydrosalpinges. In some cases, where the tube is completely free of adhesions, the use of loupes suffices. Where complex adhesions are present, the use of the microscope is mandatory. When performing a salpingostomy, the following points should be borne in mind. Before starting the salpingostomy, mobilization of the tube must be completed. Division of adhesions between tube and ovary or other pelvic organs is very important in order to leave the tube fully mobile, with the possibility of the new ostium being able to cover the whole ovarian surface and make egg pick-up more likely.

While dividing adhesions, special care must be taken to avoid damage to the fimbrial blood supply. These vessels are in the area of the connecting ligament between the ovary and the tube at the outer margin of the mesosalpinx. The hydrosalpinx must be opened at the most terminal part, the 'pucker point'. This is where the fimbrial end has closed; it is clearly seen under the microscope as a thin fibrous line, often with an H-shaped configuration, and is not always the thinnest part of the tube. Linear salpingostomy has a high chance of healing over. Using fine diathermy, the tube is then opened and a glass probe introduced, following the fibrous tracts parallel to the blood vessels and ensuring that the mucosal folds are not cut. Using small incisions the new tubal ostium is completed and then the mucosa can be everted (Fig. 25.10).

Two or three stitches of 8/0 nylon are used to secure the mucosal eversion. If the ovarian surface is damaged during the division of adhesions, the raw area should be repaired using fine non-absorbable suture material to avoid recurrence of adhesions.

Adhesions

Omental adhesions are not infrequent and when they are more than minimal, a partial omentectomy is performed. It is best done at the beginning of the operation. Fine 2/0 linen is used to secure the pedicles. It is not used as a routine procedure, but is seems to be a very effective way of avoiding recurrent adhesion in the pelvis (Fig. 25.11).

The most frequent adhesions are between the ampulla, the ovary and the mesosalpinx. It is easy to work from the isthmus towards the fimbrial end. Using a glass probe, the adhesions are hooked and incised with monopolar diathermy. Care

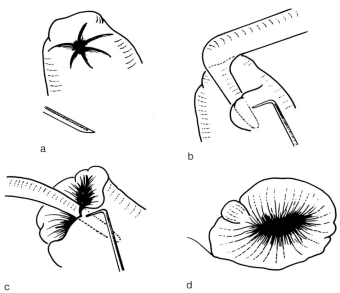

c   d

Fig. 25.10   Salpingostomy. **a** Identification of the terminal part of the hydrosalpinx where the incision must be made. **b** An incision is made using diathermy and the tip of the glass probe is inserted into the hole in the tube. **c** The salpingostomy is enlarged using the diathermy needle and glass rods. **d** The salpingostomy is completed.

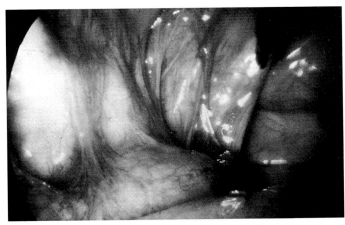

Fig. 25.11   Laparoscopic appearance in a patient with severe periovarian adhesions after pelvic inflammatory disease.

should be taken not to damage the tubal peritoneum. The use of the microscope simplifies the process because the peritoneal edges can be easily seen. If the tubal peritoneum is incised it must be repaired using 8/0 nylon as a suture material.

Ovarian adhesions should be removed from the ovarian capsule using diathermy or scissors, leaving the ovarian capsule as free as possible. Ovulation and egg release seem to improve after careful ovariolysis and may depend on the amount of the ovarian surface left free.

Special attention must be paid to raw areas. The uterine surface and the surrounding peritoneum must be carefully inspected. Peritonealization is very important and all raw areas must be covered. If the ovarian fossa has been damaged in order to free or liberate a firmly adherent ovary, the raw area should be closed using a linear suture of 4/0 Prolene. If the

raw area cannot be peritonealized using the surrounding peritoneum, a peritoneal graft can be applied. The peritoneum should be thin and without fatty tissue. It is attached to the raw area using 8/0 nylon or 6/0 Prolene. The donor areas can be the peritoneum layer of the anterior abdominal wall, the peritoneal space between the round ligament and the bladder and, in some cases, the peritoneum of the mesentery of the small or large bowel. This technique has proved very effective in experimental animals and the results with humans are very encouraging. Synthetic materials are available to replace peritoneum (Haney & Dotty 1992, Hunter et al 1988). They can be applied during open surgery as well as laparoscopic procedures and can remain in situ, apparently without side-effects, but if removal is necessary, this can be done through a laparoscope.

It must be emphasized that the treatment of tubal damage due to tuberculosis is always medical and the tubal damage cannot be repaired by surgery. In this group of patients, if the uterine cavity remains unaffected or without damage, in vitro fertilization is the only option.

Laparoscopic surgery

With the development of endoscopic techniques in the last two decades, gynaecologists, using the laparoscope, have been able to perform numerous operations in the field of infertility as well as in general gynaecology.

Since the first diagnostic use of the endoscope in the 1800s, developments in optics and related technology have revolutionized the use of the laparoscope. In the 1940s Palmer in France promoted the laparoscope as a diagnostic instrument. In the 1970s Gomel published the first results of laparoscopic surgery. He performed salpingo-ovariolysis and fimbrioplasties using this approach, with results comparable to those he achieved using magnification in open procedures. At the same time Semm in Germany also developed the technique and a large number of new instruments were available for laparoscopic surgery.

The development of laser beams for medical use had an impact in laparoscopic surgery too. The use of video-laparoscopy has become a standard part of laparoscopic surgery. It is less tiring, the assistant has a more active role during surgical procedures and so it facilitates training and teaching. Different methods of dissection using laser diathermy (Donnez & Nisolle 1989) or cold cutting (Serour et al 1989) have been discussed. There is no evidence that one is better than the other.

After the initial experiences, procedures that can now be performed safely using operative laparoscopy include salpingo-ovariolysis, fimbrioplasty, salpingostomies, tubal reanastomosis and management of ectopic pregnancy and endometriosis.

One of the most important attributes of this method is that it apparently has a low rate of adhesion formation. There is no doubt that laparoscopic adhesiolysis is very effective for pain and open surgery may cause more adhesion formation (Lundford et al 1991). The question still remains whether patients with severe tubal damage, not suitable for open procedures, should be operated upon using the laparoscopic approach when the prognosis is very poor anyway and there are alternative methods available to them.

Great financial advantages are offered by this method. This procedure can be done as a day case or overnight stay and the

Table 25.1 Cornual anastomosis after inflammatory damage

	Patients	Pregnancies	Miscarriages	Ectopic pregnancies
Isolated cornual block	29	14	5	1
Salpingitis isthmica nodosa	15	4	1	0
Total	44	18	6	1

Data from Hammersmith Hospital, London

patient resumes her normal activities in a very short period of time. Laparoscopic surgery, as with any other surgical procedure, has its risks and therefore intensive training is fundamental in order to diminish complications and achieve good results.

RESULTS

Cornual anastomosis

Cornual anastomosis offers very good results in selected groups of patients (Table 25.1).

Postoperative laparoscopies show a high patency rate amongst those patients who have not conceived. The major limiting factors seem to be the recrudescence of the disease or extension of the original inflammation into the anastomotic site, rather than lack of patency. Gomel (1980) has reported similar results: 53% of his patients conceived and had at least one term pregnancy.

Following tubocornual anastomosis by microsurgery, the reported term pregnancy rates in the literature varied between 22% and 57% and ectopic pregnancy rates were 2–12%. These results are similar to cumulative delivery rates following five cycles of IVF-ET (reviewed by Posaci et al 1999). In contrast, the outcome of tubouterine anastomosis is much poorer and this procedure has mostly been replaced by tubocornual anastomosis.

Salpingitis isthmica nodosa

The surgical treatment of salpingitis isthmica nodosa in the infertile patient is similar to that of cornual block. In nearly half of the patients the tubes are open and the diagnosis is made on the basis of the typical images of diverticular on the hysterosalpingogram and at laparoscopy. The anastomotic procedure is in general much easier but the length of isthmic portion that must be removed can be difficult to assess. The prognosis depends on the length of tube removed, but if we do not remove enough tissue the surgical procedure will probably fail.

The use of the microscope and the experience of the surgeon are very important in the evaluation of the amount or length of tissue that must be resected. In general, this condition involves most of the isthmic portion of the tube, so the anastomosis is between the cornu and the ampullary-isthmic junction.

Where the intramural portion of the tube is extensively involved in the process, the patient probably should not be treated surgically. The surgical procedure itself does not vary from that of tubocornual anastomosis. When the whole of the isthmus is removed, the problem of tension at the anastomotic level can be solved using stay sutures of 6/0 Prolene between the uterus and the mesosalpinx in order to approximate the tubal ends.

Reversal of sterilization

Reversal of tubal sterilization is the most successful procedure in tubal microsurgery. At Hammersmith Hospital, in a series of 126 patients, 58% conceived; the pregnancy rates varied according to the site of the anastomosis (Table 25.2). Results with reversal of sterilization are very much influenced by the length of tube remaining (Table 25.3).

The pregnancy rates in the literature following reversal of sterilization with microsurgery vary between 33% and 86% with ectopic pregnancy rates of 1–14%. The success rates are lower after sterilization with cautery or Pomeroy's technique compared with clip or ring sterilization (Posaci et al 1999).

Salpingostomy

In general, it is difficult to assess the results of salpingostomy because a very heterogeneous group of patients is involved. Patient selection varies widely between units and there is no agreement regarding classification, especially where salpingostomy and fimbrioplasty are concerned.

Many gynaecologists think that salpingostomy is obsolete, because in vitro fertilization techniques offer comparable or

Table 25.2 Reversal of sterilization according to the site of the anastomosis

Site of anastomosis	Number of patients	Number of pregnant patients	Number of ectopic pregnancies	Percentage of pregnancies
Cornu-isthmus	17	12	0	71
Cornu-ampulla	26	14	1	54
Isthmus-isthmus	16	12	0	75
Isthmus-ampulla	27	17	2	63
Ampulla-ampulla	19	8	0	42
Other	21	10	0	48
Total	126	73	3	58

Data from Hammersmith Hospital, London

Table 25.3 Reversal of sterilization in 95 patients: pregnancy rates according to the length of the longer tube

Length of tube, cm	Patients	Number of pregnancies	Percentage
<2.5	7	2	28
2.5–4	15	4	30
4.1–6	30	14	46
6.1–8	25	16	64
>8	20	18	90

Data from Hammersmith Hospital, London

better results in some cases. As in any other surgical procedure, if we select the patients well, good results will be achieved.

Boer-Meisel et al (1986), in a prospective study, classified hydrosalpinges as grades I, II and III, based on the nature and extent of the adhesions, the microscopic aspect of the endo-salpinx, the thickness of the tubal wall and the diameter of the hydrosalpinx. In their series, 77% of patients with grade I hydro-salpinx had the possibility of conception, 21% with grade II and only 3% with grade III. Thus surgery is the obvious treatment for patients with grade I hydrosalpinges. Patients with grade III hydrosalpinges should avoid salpingostomy and be treated using in vitro fertilization techniques after salping-ectomy. The difficult group is that of grade II hydrosalpinx, where treatments with in vitro fertilization or tubal surgery have the same prognosis. Age, social and religious background, the possibility of alternative treatment and the patient's wishes must be considered very carefully.

In a series of 323 patients from Hammersmith Hospital, 81 (25%) of the patients conceived, most of them during the first 8 months following surgery or after the second year. After the second year the ectopic pregnancy rate seemed to be higher. Of these patients, 20 have more than one child (Tables 25.4 and 25.5).

The success of tubal microsurgery for distal tubal lesions depends on several factors. Patients with extensive pelvic adhesions, thick tubal wall and abnormal tubal mucosa at salpingoscopy have poor results. Type of surgery also affects the outcome. Pregnancy rates as high as 59–60% can be achieved with fimbrioplasty but the results after salpingostomy may not be as good (Posaci et al 1999). Patients with poor prognostic factor will have a higher chance of achieving pregnancy with IVF, whereas in the absence of poor prognostic factors tubal microsurgery should be the first choice.

Laparoscopic surgery

Laparoscopic adhesiolysis for pelvic adhesions results in very good results with term pregnancy rates of 47–62% and ectopic pregnancy rates of 4–8%. These results are similar to those achieved after microsurgery so laparoscopic surgery should be the first option for suitable patients (Posaci et al 1999).

Table 25.4   Results of salpingostomies (1971–1985)

Patients	Pregnancies	Miscarriages	Ectopic pregnancies
323	81 (25%)	54 (16.7%)	32 (10%)

Data from Hammersmith Hospital, London

Table 25.5   Results of laparoscopic salpingostomy

		Pregnancies		
	Patients	Term	Intrauterine	Ectopic
Primary	33	4	6 (18%)	2
Repeat	45	2	4 (8%)	4
Total	78	6	10 (13%)	6

Data from Hammersmith Hospital, London

Success rates of laparoscopic surgery for distal tubal lesions again depend on several prognostic factors, including the presence of extensive pelvic adhesions, thick tubal wall and severe endo-tubal damage. The reported intrauterine pregnancy rates following laparoscopic surgery for distal tubal lesions vary between 13% and 51% with ectopic pregnancy rates of 3–23% (Posaci et al 1999).

CONCLUSION

Currently, in the absence of detailed information about early reproductive events which take place within the fallopian tube, the assessment of tubal function mainly depends on checking its patency and appearance at endoscopy. A better understanding of the tubal physiology may enable us to test its function more effectively and may also improve our understanding of so-called unexplained infertility. There is no doubt that we can treat a large group of patients with tubal disease using in vitro fertilization techniques. In a well-selected group of infertile patients with tubal damage, surgical procedures, performed using laparoscopy or open surgery (microsurgery), offer a very good prognosis and many patients can conceive more than once after only one treatment. In a highly specialized reproductive unit these methods should be available and the choice of procedure adapted to each individual case.

KEY POINTS

1. Tubal disease is tubal damage caused by pelvic infection, endometriosis or iatrogenic disease with varying degrees of damage, and sometimes involving surrounding structures.
2. Tubal disease is accountable for 30–40% of cases of female infertility.
3. Salpingitis most commonly results from ascending infection from the lower genital tract.
4. Cervical resistance diminishes during ovulation and menstruation, possibly allowing bacteria to ascend.
5. Salpingitis is not generally seen in women who are not sexually active.
6. *Chlamydia trachomatis* is responsible for a significant amount of salpingitis, postpartum endometritis and perihepatic adhesions.
7. Many organisms are capable of producing salpingitis. Gonococcal infection seems to pave the way for other micro-organisms to cross the cervical mucus and affect the uterus or tubes.
8. Tubal damage of tuberculous origin is rare in developed countries.
9. A significant proportion of patients with tubal disease are best treated by in vitro fertilization techniques.
10. In a well-selected group of infertile patients with tubal damage, surgical procedures, performed using laparoscopy or open surgery (microsurgery), offer a very good prognosis and many patients can conceive more than once after only one treatment.

REFERENCES

Ataya K, Thomas M 1991 New techniques for selective transcervical osteal salpingography and catheterisation in the diagnosis and treatment of proximal tubal obstruction. Fertility and Sterility 56:980–983

Boer-Meisel ME, te Velde ER, Habbema JD, Kardaun JW 1986 Predicting the pregnancy outcome in patients treated for hydrosalpinx: a prospective study. Fertility and Sterility 45:23–29

Chiari H 1887 Zur pathologischen Anatomic des Eileiter-Catrrhs. Zeitschrift fur Heilkunde 8:457–473

Crow J, Amso NN, Lewin J, Shaw RW 1994 Morphology and ultrastructure of fallopian tube epithelium at different stages of the menstrual cycle and menopause. Human Reproduction 9:2224–2233

Croxatto HB, Ortiz ME 1975 Egg transport in the fallopian tube. Gynecological Investigation 6:215–225

De Bruyne F, Puttemans P, Boeckx W, Brosens IA 1989 The clinical value of salpingoscopy in tubal infertility. Fertility and Sterility 51:339–340

Djahanbakhch O, Kervancioglu E, Maguiness SD, Martin JE 1994 Fallopian tube epithelial cell culture. In: Grudzinskas JG, Chapman MG, Chard T, Djahanbakhch O (eds) The fallopian tube. Clinical and surgical aspects. Springer-Verlag, London, pp 37–51

Donnez J, Nisolle M 1989 CO_2 laser laparoscopy surgery. Adhesiolysis, salpingostomy, laser uterine nerve ablation and tubal pregnancy. Baillière's Clinics in Obstetrics and Gynaecology 3:525–543

Ehrler P 1963 Die intramurale tubenanastomoze (ein Beitrag zur Uberwindung der Tubaren Steritat). Zentralblatt für Gynaekologie 85:393–400

Farquhar C, Vandekerckhove P, Watson A, Vail A, Wiseman D 2000 Barrier agents for preventing adhesions after surgery for subfertility. In: The Cochrane Library, Issue 4. Update Software, Oxford

Glazener CMA, Loveden LM, Richardson SJ, Jeans WD, Hull MGR 1987 Tubocornual polyps: their relevance in subfertility. Human Reproduction 2:59–65

Gomel V 1977 Tubal reanastomosis by microsurgery. Fertility and Sterility 28:59

Gomel V 1980 Clinical results of infertility microsurgery. In: Crosignani PG, Rubin BL (eds) Microsurgery in female infertility. Academic Press, New York, pp 77–94

Haney AF, Dotty E 1992 Murine peritoneal injury and de novo adhesion formation caused by oxidized-regenerated cellulose (Interceed TC7) but not expanded polytetrafluoroethylene (Gore-Tex surgical membrane). Fertility and Sterility 57:202–208

Hunter SK, Scott JR, Hull D, Urry RL 1988 The gamete and embryo compatibility of various synthetic polymers. Fertility and Sterility 50:110–116

Jansen RP 1984 Endocrine response in the fallopian tube. Endocrine Reviews 5:525–551

Kervancioglu ME, Saridogan E, Aitken RJ, Djahanbakhch O 2000 Importance of sperm to epithelial cell contact for the capacitation of human spermatozoa in human Fallopian tube-epithelial cell coculture. Fertility and Sterility 74:780–784

Lindblom B, Norstrom A 1986 The smooth-muscle architecture of the human fallopian tube. In: Siegler AM (ed) The fallopian tube. Basic studies and clinical contributions. Futura Publishing, Mount Kisco, pp 13–20

Lundford P, Hahlin M, Kallfelt B, Thourburn J, Lindblom B 1991 Adhesion formation after laparoscopic surgery in tubal pregnancy: a randomised trial versus laparotomy. Fertility and Sterility 55:911–915

Maguiness SD, Djahanbakhch O 1992 Salpingoscopic findings in women undergoing sterilization. Human Reproduction 7:269–273

Maguiness SD, Djahanbakhch O, Grudzinskas JG 1992a Assessment of the Fallopian tube. Obstetrical and Gynecological Survey 47:587–603

Maguiness SD, Shrimanker K, Djahanbakhch O, Grudzinskas JG 1992b Oviduct proteins. Contemporary Reviews in Obstetrics and Gynaecology 4:42–50

Mahmood T, Saridogan E, Smutna S, Habib AM, Djahanbakhch O 1998 The effect of ovarian steroids on epithelial ciliary beat frequency in the human Fallopian tube. Human Reproduction 13:2991–2994

Margara RA 1982 Tubal reanastomosis. In: Chamberlain G, Winston RML (eds) Tubal infertility. Blackwell Science, Oxford, pp 106–119

Nackley AC, Muasher SJ 1998 The significance of hydrosalpinx in in vitro fertilization. Fertility and Sterility 69:373–384

Paterson P, Wood C 1974 The use of microsurgery in the reanastomosis of the rabbit fallopian tube. Fertility and Sterility 25:757–761

Posaci C, Camus M, Osmanagaoglu K, Devroey P 1999 Tubal surgery in the era of assisted reproductive technology: clinical options. Human Reproduction 14(suppl 1):120–136

Puttemans PJ, Brosens IA 1996 Preventive salpingectomy of hydrosalpinx prior to IVF. Salpingectomy improves in-vitro fertilization outcome in patients with hydrosalpinx: blind victimization of the fallopian tube. Human Reproduction 11:2079–2084

Puttemans PJ, de Bruyne F, Heylen SM 1998 A decade of salpingoscopy. European Journal of Obstetrics, Gynecology and Reproductive Biology 81:197–206

Saridogan E, Djahanbakhch O, Puddefoot JR et al 1996 Angiotensia II receptors and angiotensin II stimulation of ciliary activity in human fallopian tube. Journal of Clinical Endocrinology and Metabolism 81:2719–2725

Seki K, Eddy CA, Smith Nk, Pauerstein CJ 1977 Comparison of two techniques of suturing in microsurgical anastomosis of the rabbit oviduct. Fertility and Sterility 28:1215–1219

Serour GI, Bandroui MH, Agizi HM, Hamed AF, Abdel-Aziz F 1989 Laparoscopic adhesiolysis for infertile patients with pelvic adhesive disease. International Journal of Gynaecology and Obstetrics 30:249–252

Vasquez G, Winston RML, Boeckx W, Brosens I 1980 Tubal lesions subsequent to sterilisation and their relation to fertility after attempts at reversal. American Journal of Obstetrics and Gynecology 138:86–92

Verdugo P 1986 Functional anatomy of the fallopian tube. In: Insler V, Lunenfeld B (eds) Infertility: male and female. Churchill Livingstone, London, pp 26–55

Walz W 1959 Fertilitäts Operationen mit Hilfe eines Operationemkroscopes. Geburtshilfe und Gynaekologe 153:49–53

Washington AE 1996 Pelvic inflammatory disease: linking epidemiological trends, determinants and prevention. In: Templeton A (ed) The prevention of pelvic infection. RCOG Press, London, pp 3–13

Watson A, Vandekerckhove P, Lilford R 2000 Liquid and fluid agents for preventing adhesions after surgery for subfertility. In: The Cochrane Library, Issue 4. Update Software, Oxford

Winston RML 1977 Microsurgical tubocornual anastomosis for reversal of sterilisation. Lancet i:284–285

Winston RML, McClure-Browne JC 1974 Pregnancy following autograft transplantation of the fallopian tube and ovary in the rabbit. Lancet i:494–497

Winston RML, Frantzen C, Oberti C 1977 Oviduct function following resection of the ampullary-isthmic junction. Fertility and Sterility 28:284–289

Zeyneloglu H, Arici A, Olive DL 1998 Adverse effects of hydrosalpinx on pregnancy rates after in vitro fertilization-embryo transfer. Fertility and Sterility 70:492–499

26

Ectopic pregnancy

Lukas D. Klentzeris

INTRODUCTION

Ectopic pregnancy is a pregnancy that is implanted outside the uterine cavity, i.e. at a site that by nature is not designed anatomically or physiologically to accept the conceptus or to permit its growth and development. The fallopian tube is the most common site of ectopic pregnancy.

Over 100 years ago, Tait, in one of his classic articles, indicated how deaths from ectopic pregnancy can be avoided: 'If an operation is to be done, it must be done without delay' (Tait 1884). Prior to his paper most women with ectopic pregnancy died of either haemorrhage or infection. Ectopic pregnancy has been described as 'the great masquerader' because it can present with a wide spectrum of symptoms and signs. The possibility of ectopic pregnancy must be excluded in all women of reproductive age who present with lower abdominal pain.

INCIDENCE

The incidence of ectopic pregnancy ranges between 0.25% and 1.5% of all pregnancies, including live births, induced abortions and ectopic gestations. There are, however, two factors that need to be considered. First, comparison of the incidence of ectopic pregnancy in different countries becomes difficult because various authors use different denominators to express the results. The most commonly used denominators are: per 1000 live births; per 1000 reported pregnancies; per 10 000 women aged 15–44 years. Second, the exact incidence of ectopic pregnancy remains largely unknown because the diagnosis is missed when the ectopic pregnancy resolves spontaneously at an early stage. Recently the problem has been magnified with the introduction of techniques of assisted procreation. Sensitive serum assays for β-hCG detect a rise and later a fall of the concentration of the hormone but the exact location of the pregnancy cannot be detected.

In England and Wales between 1966 and 1996 the incidence of ectopic pregnancy increased by 3.1-fold from 30.2 to 94.8 per 100 000 women aged 15–44 and 3.8-fold from 3.25 to 12.4 per 1000 pregnancies (Rajkhowa et al 2000). A recently published article from Sweden (Kamwendo et al 2000) indicates a 33% decrease of the incidence of ectopic pregnancy between 1990 and 1997. The declining trend was a consequence of a reduced incidence of pelvic inflammatory disease (PID), particularly in women less than 24 years of age.

In the USA the Center for Disease Control and Prevention (CDCP) has the most comprehensive data available on ectopic pregnancy. Between 1970 and 1989, there was a fivefold increase in the incidence of ectopic pregnancy; from 3.2 to 16 ectopic pregnancies per 1000 reported pregnancies (Goldner et al 1993). Women between 35 and 44 years of age have the highest risk of developing an ectopic pregnancy (27 per 1000 reported pregnancies). Data from the same centre indicate that the risk of ectopic pregnancy in African women (21 per 1000) is 1.6 times greater than the risk amongst whites (13 per 1000). Women from Saigon and Jamaica have unusually high rates. A more critical interpretation of these risks, however, reveals that the problem is not the origin of the individuals but the high incidence of PID and low socioeconomic status occurring in certain populations.

MORTALITY AND MORBIDITY

Ectopic pregnancy still causes significant mortality and morbidity. In 1988 in the USA, according to data from the CDCP, 44 deaths were attributed to complications of ectopic pregnancy, which represent 15% of all maternal deaths. The risk of death is higher for African women. Teenagers have the highest mortality rates.

In the United Kingdom the number of deaths from ectopic pregnancies increased from nine (1991–93) to 12 (1994–96). The death rate per 1000 estimated ectopic pregnancies was 0.3% and 0.4% in the first and second trimester respectively.

AETIOLOGY AND RISK FACTORS

The aetiology of ectopic pregnancy remains enigmatic. In contrast to intrauterine implantation there is no suitable animal model for the study of ectopic implantation and extrapolation of data. Ectopic pregnancy is unknown in lower animals and is very rare in subhuman primates. Only three tubal pregnancies have been reported in 3000 pregnancies observed in monkeys in captivity.

The common denominator in most aetiological theories of ectopic pregnancy is delay in ovum transport. A likely consequence of the delay is that the ovum becomes too large to pass through certain areas of fallopian tube, particularly the isthmic segment and uterotubal junction. Also in ectopic gestations the growth and proliferation of the trophoblast may

be so advanced that implantation of the fertilized ovum begins prior to departure of the ovum from the fallopian tube. Myoelectrical activity of the wall of the fallopian tube allows approximation and fertilization of gametes as well as propulsion of the zygote and cleaving embryo from the ampulla to the uterine cavity. Oestrogens increase smooth muscle activity and progesterone decreases muscular tone. Increased incidence of tubal pregnancy in perimenopausal women may be related to progressive loss of myoelectrical activity along the fallopian tube which is observed with ageing (Pulkkinen & Talo 1987).

The cilia of the ciliated tubal epithelium are also involved in transportation of oocytes towards the uterine cavity. At the ampulla, the cilia beat towards the isthmus. Salpingitis results in loss of ciliated epithelium and subsequently delayed propulsion of zygote towards the uterine cavity.

Steroid hormones, oestrogens and progesterone influence cilia formation and movements. Oestrogens stimulate epithelial cell hyperplasia and ciliogenesis. High levels of serum progesterone are associated with deciliation and atrophy of the epithelium. These changes of the ciliated epithelium of the fallopian tube may explain the increased incidence of tubal pregnancy observed in women who take the progesterone-only pill or have a progesterone-containing IUCD in situ.

Theoretically, all sexually active women are at risk of experiencing an ectopic pregnancy. However, women of reproductive age who are associated with one (or more) of the risk factors shown in Box 26.1 have a much higher risk.

Independent risk factors consistently shown to increase the risk of tubal pregnancy include the following.

Previous tubal pregnancy

History of a prior ectopic pregnancy is a significant risk factor (Ankum et al 1996). A woman who has experienced one ectopic pregnancy has a 10–20% chance of presenting with an ectopic gestation in her subsequent pregnancy. However, her chance of an intrauterine pregnancy is still 60–80%. Accurate assessment of the risk for recurrent ectopic pregnancy is difficult because it depends on the size, location of the previous ectopic pregnancy, status of the contralateral adnexa, treatment method and history of infertility.

Previous tubal surgery

Sterilization
Following sterilization the absolute risk of ectopic pregnancy is reduced. However, the ratio of ectopic to intrauterine

---

Box 26.1 Risk factors for ectopic pregnancy

- Previous tubal pregnancy
- Previous tubal surgery
- Previous laparoscopically proven PID
- Current IUCD users
- Abortion
- Endocrine disorders: luteal phase defects; ovulatory dysfunction
- Assisted conception
- Salpingitis isthmica nodosa (SIN)
- Smoking
- Diethylstilboestrol (DES)

pregnancy is higher. The greatest risk for pregnancy, including ectopic, occurs in the first 2 years after sterilization. The risk of ectopic pregnancy depends on the sterilization technique. Approximately 15% of pregnancies following tubal ligation are ectopic. Fistula formation and recanalization of the proximal and distal stumps of the fallopian tube are implicated for the ectopic gestation. Approximately 50% of postlaparoscopic electrocautery failures are ectopic pregnancies (McCausland 1980). Tubal coagulation has a lower risk of pregnancy compared with mechanical devices (spring-loaded clips or fallope rings) but the risk of ectopic pregnancy is 10 times higher when a pregnancy does occur (DeStefano et al 1982).

Reversal of sterilization
The risk depends on the method of sterilization. Following reconstruction of a cauterized tube, approximately 15% of women who conceive have an ectopic pregnancy. The risk of ectopic pregnancy is reduced to 5% when the reversal is performed following Pomeroy's method or clip sterilization.

Tubal reconstruction and repair
Reconstructive tubal surgery is a predisposing factor for ectopic pregnancy. However, it remains unclear whether the increased risk results from the surgical procedure or from the underlying pathology of the ciliated tubal epithelium and pelvis. In a consecutive series of 232 tubal microsurgical operations, including salpingostomies, proximal anastomoses and adhesiolyses, 12 patients (5%) presented with an ectopic pregnancy whereas 80 patients (35%) achieved an intrauterine pregnancy (Singhal et al 1991). Other studies reported a sixfold increase in ectopic pregnancy following salpingostomy. The risk of recurrent ectopic pregnancy following conservative surgery (salpingostomy) is not significantly different to that observed following radical surgery (salpingectomy): 14% versus 10%.

Previous laparoscopically proven pelvic inflammatory disease

The relationship between PID, tubal obstruction and ectopic pregnancy is well documented. Infection of tubal endothelium results in damage of ciliated epithelium and formation of intraluminal adhesions and pockets. A consequence of these anatomical changes is entrapment of the zygote and ectopic implantation of the blastocyst. Westrom et al (1981) studied 450 women with laparoscopically proven PID (case control study). The authors reported that the incidence of tubal obstruction increased with successive episodes of PID; 13% after one episode, 35% after two episodes and 79% after three. Following one episode of laparoscopically verified acute salpingitis the ratio of ectopic to intrauterine pregnancy was 1:24, a sixfold increase over the incidence for control women with laparoscopically negative results.

Chlamydia trachomatis-induced tubal damage is associated with tubal pregnancy. Many cases of Chlamydia infections are subclinical. The relationship of Chlamydia trachomatis endosalpingitis and tubal pregnancy originates from the following observations:

- Chlamydia has been cultured from 7–30% of patients with tubal pregnancy (Berenson et al 1991, Diquelou et al 1988).

- Patients with ectopic pregnancy have higher Chlamydia trachomatis-specific titre than controls (Svensson et al 1985).
- Patients with anti-Chlamydia trachomatis titre of ≥1:64 are three times more likely to have an ectopic pregnancy compared with negative controls (Chow et al 1990).

Although PID is a high risk factor for ectopic pregnancy, it should be remembered that only 50% of the fallopian tubes removed for an ectopic pregnancy have histological evidence of salpingitis.

Current IUCD users
Unmedicated, medicated and copper-coated IUCDs prevent both intrauterine and extrauterine pregnancies. However, a woman who conceives with an IUCD in situ is seven times more likely to have a tubal pregnancy compared with a woman who conceives without contraception (Vessy et al 1974). IUCDs are more effective in preventing intrauterine than extrauterine implantation. With copper IUCDs, 4% of all accidental pregnancies are tubal whereas with progesterone-coated IUCDs 17% of all contraceptive failures are tubal pregnancies. The different mechanism of action of the two devices could partially explain the different in failure rates. Although both devices prevent implantation, copper IUCDs also interfere with fertilization by inducing cytotoxic and phagocytotic effects on the sperm and oocytes. Progesterone-containing IUCDs are probably less effective in preventing fertilization. Although the incidence of pregnancy diminishes with long-term use of the IUCD, among the women who become pregnant the likelihood of ectopic pregnancy increases. Ory (1981) reported that the risk for ectopic pregnancy was the same in current and never-users of IUCDs. However, women who had used the IUCD for more than 24 months were 2.6 times more likely to have an ectopic pregnancy compared to short-term users (<24 months). The 'lasting effect' of the IUCD may be related to the loss of the cilia from the tubal epithelium, especially if the IUCD has been in situ for 3 years or more (Wollen et al 1984.)

Abortion
Data from two French case control studies suggest that induced abortion may be a risk factor for ectopic pregnancy for women with no history of ectopic pregnancy. There is an association between number of previous induced abortions and ectopic pregnancy (odds ratio 1.4 for one previous induced abortion and 1.9 for two or more) (Tharaux-Deneux et al 1998).

Endocrine disorders
Luteal phase defects
Luteal phase defects (LPD) and inadequate corpus luteum have been associated with ectopic pregnancy. Although the exact link remains unkown, a possible explanation is that the oestradiol-to-progesterone ratio observed in LPD affects myoelectrical activity of the fallopian tubes and motility of ciliated epithelium.

Ovulatory dysfunction
Induction of ovulation with either clomiphene citrate or HMG is a predisposing factor for tubal implantation. A number of

studies (Gemzell et al 1982, Marchbanks et al 1985, McBain et al 1980) indicate that 1–4% of pregnancies achieved following induction of ovulation are ectopic pregnancies. The majority of these patients had a normal pelvis and patent tubes.

Assisted conception

The incidence of tubal pregnancy following oocyte retrieval and embryo transfer is approximately 4.5%. It must be noted, however, that some women who undergo an IVF cycle have in their history high risk factors for an ectopic pregnancy, i.e. previous ectopic, tubal pathology or surgery. However, even after GIFT procedures, 4% of all pregnancies achieved will be tubal (Assisted Reproductive Technology in the United States and Canada 1995).

Salpingitis isthmica nodosa (SIN)

A typical histological feature of SIN is the invasion of tubal epithelium into the myosalpinx and the formation of a true diverticulum. This condition occurs more often in the tubes of women with an ectopic pregnancy than in non-pregnant women. Persaud (1970) reported that 49% of fallopian tubes excised for tubal pregnancy had diverticula and evidence of SIN. The reason for the high incidence of ectopic gestation in women with SIN remains largely unknown. Defective myoelectrical activity has been demonstrated over the diverticula. Entrapment of embryo into the diverticula is a possible mechanical complication.

Smoking

A French study found that the risk of ectopic pregnancy was significantly higher in women who smoke. The risk increases according to the number of cigarettes per day (Bouyer et al 1998). The relative risk for ectopic pregnancy is 1.3 for women who smoke 1–9 cigarettes per day, 2 for 10–12 cigarettes per day and 2.5 for more than 20 cigarettes per day. Inhibition of oocyte cumulus complex pick-up by the fimbrial end of the fallopian tube and reduction of ciliary beat frequency are associated with nicotine intake (Knoll & Talbot 1998).

Diethylstilboestrol (DES)

Results of a collaborative study indicate that the risk of ectopic pregnancy in DES-exposed women was 13% compared with 4% for women who had a normal uterus (Barnes et al 1980). A meta-analysis on risk factors for ectopic pregnancy confirms that exposure to DES in utero increases significantly the risk of ectopic pregnancy (Ankum et al 1996).

PATHOLOGY

Sites of ectopic pregnancy

A 21-year survey of 654 ectopic pregnancies (Breen 1970) revealed that the most common sites of ectopic pregnancy are as shown in Box 26.2.

Box 26.2 Most common sites of ectopic pregnancy

- Fallopian tube:

Ampullary segment	80%
Isthmic segment	12%
Fibrial end	5%
Interstitial and cornual	2%

• Abdominal	1.4%
• Ovarian	0.2%
• Cervical	0.2%

Natural progression of a tubal pregnancy

Unruptured tubal pregnancy

Occasionally in the very early stages of a tubal pregnancy there are no obvious macroscopic features and an ectopic pregnancy could be overlooked even after a laparoscopy. As pregnancy progresses, however, local enlargement of the tube occurs at the point of implantation. At a later stage a large segment of the tube is distended and the tubal wall appears discoloured, dark red or purple.

Tubal rupture

One of the fundamental aspects of ectopic pregnancy is the inability of the tissues into which the blastocyst implants to project resistance or respond to the invading trophoblast. Uncontrolled invasion of the trophoblast results in destruction of vessels, local haemorrhage and thinning of the tubal wall. Rupture of the tubal wall results in the escape of large amounts of blood, with or without the products of conception, into the peritoneal cavity. The embryo rarely survives. In rare cases pregnancy continues if an adequate portion of the placenta is retained or if secondary implantation occurs in other organs of the pelvic or peritoneal cavity. Rupture occurs more often at the antimesenteric part of the tubal wall. Rupture of the inferior, mesenteric, part of the tubal wall results in haemorrhage between the two layers of the broad ligament. Intraligamentous haemorrhage could cause rupture of anterior or posterior layers of the broad ligament.

Spontaneous involution

Usually the conceptus dies at an early stage without production of any notable symptoms.

Complete tubal abortion

At an early stage the conceptus is excluded via the fimbriated end of the fallopian tube into the peritoneal cavity and subsequently absorbed by the surrounding tissues (abortion and absorption).

Incomplete tubal abortion

The conceptus is partially excluded via the fimbriated ostium. Intervention is usually required.

Tubal blood mole or carneous mole

In some cases recurrent choriodecidual haemorrhage around the dead conceptus contributes to the formation of a tubal blood mole or carneous mole. The presence and development of cellular and biochemical elements of connective tissue around the mole give rise to a semi-solid structure which could remain unresolved for years.

Time of rupture at various sites in the tube

Isthmic implantation
The isthmic segment of the fallopian tube is narrow and less distensible than the ampullary or interstitial segments. Isthmic rupture often occurs at 6–8 weeks and is usually dramatic.

Ampullary implantation
Rupture of an ampullary pregnancy usually occurs at 8–12 weeks gestation. The ampulla is the wider segment of the fallopian tube and the site of 80% of all ectopic pregnancies.

Interstitial implantation
The interstitial segment of the fallopian tube is surrounded by myometrium which can hypertrophy to accommodate the enlarging conceptus. Rupture therefore occurs at a relatively later stage (12–14 weeks). Rupture of an interstitial pregnancy results in damage of the highly vascularized cornual end of the uterus and very severe intra-abdominal haemorrhage.

Histological changes

In the early stages of pregnancy, under the influence of hormones, the myometrium responds with an identical pattern regardless of the location of gestation, ectopic or utopic. The uterus becomes softened and slightly enlarged as a consequence of hypertrophy and hyperplasia of the myometrial cells.

The endometrial glands demonstrate an atypical histological pattern (Arias-Stella phenomenon). The characteristic histological features of the Arias-Stella reaction are: hyperplasia of glandular cells; closely packed glands with evidence of hypersecretion; large irregular hyperchromatic nuclei; cytoplasmic vacuolation and loss of cellular polarity. It must be emphasized that the Arias-Stella reaction is a non-specific finding and it can be observed in patients with an intrauterine pregnancy. However, the presence of the Arias-Stella reaction and the absence of chorionic villi from endometiral curettings are both signs highly suspicious for an extrauterine pregnancy. The presence of chorionic villi is the most reliable histological finding for the definite diagnosis of an ectopic (or utopic) gestation.

The endometrial stroma is converted into decidual tissue containing large polyhydral cells with hyperchromatic nuclei. Declining pregnancy and lower levels of hormones result in gradual disintegration of the decidua, giving rise to the intermittent, occasionally heavy, vaginal bleeding that occurs in ectopic pregnancy. The vaginal bleeding in tubal pregnancy is of uterine origin. In some cases the decidua may be detached abruptly and be passed as a flat, triangular, reddish-brown piece of tissue called a decidual cast.

DIAGNOSIS

Symptoms and signs

Ectopic pregnancy remains a diagnostic challenge. The doctor

Table 26.1 Symptoms and signs in 300 consecutive cases of ectopic pregnancy at admission

Symptoms and signs	Cases (%)
Abdominal pain	99
Generalized	44
Unilateral	33
Radiating to the shoulder	22
Abnormal uterine bleeding	74
Amenorrhoea $\leq$ 2 weeks	68
Syncopal symptoms	37
Adnexal tenderness	96
Unilateral adnexal mass	54
Uterus	
Normal size	71
6–8 week size	26
9–12 week size	3
Uterine cast passed vaginally	7
Admission temperature >37°C	2

should 'think ectopic first' for any woman of reproductive age who presents with the triad of abdominal pain, irregular vaginal bleeding and amenorrhoea. This philosophy is particularly useful if the patient has high risk factor(s) for ectopic pregnancy such as a history of sterilization or reversal, history of tubal surgery or PID or an IUCD in situ. The admission symptoms and signs in 300 consecutive cases of ectopic pregnancy are shown on Table 26.1 (Droegemueller 1982).

Abdominal pain
In cases of ectopic pregnancy the abdominal pain has three different forms:

- generalized
- localized in the pelvis, unilateral or bilateral
- radiating to the shoulder.

The generalized abdominal pain is usually due to rupture of ectopic pregnancy and intraperitoneal haemorrhage. The pain is often severe. Shoulder pain is also an indirect indication of intraperitoneal haemorrhage. Accumulation of blood in the subdiaphragmatic region stimulates the phrenic nerve and creates shoulder tip pain. Localized pain may be due to distension of the fallopian tube.

It should be emphasized, however, that there is no pathognomonic pain that is diagnostic of ectopic pregnancy. The pain may be sudden or progressive and continuous or intermittent.

Amenorrhoea and abnormal uterine bleeding
Most patients present with amenorrhoea of at least 2 weeks duration. One-third of the women will not recall the date of the last menstrual period (LMP) or have irregular menstruation. This problem contributes to the diagnostic challenge. Abnormal uterine bleeding occurs in 75% of women with ectopic pregnancy. The bleeding is light, recurrent and results from detachment of the uterine decidua. According to Stabile (1996a,b): 'If a patient who is a few weeks pregnant complains of a little pain and heavy vaginal bleeding, the pregnancy is probably intrauterine, whereas if

she has much pain and little bleeding, she is more likely to have an ectopic pregnancy'.

Physical examination

The physical examination should include assessment of the vital signs and examination of the abdomen and pelvis.

Depending on the rate and amount of blood loss the general condition of the patient may vary from slight pallor to haemodynamic shock. Palpation of the abdomen may reveal generalized or localized mild tenderness. Occasionally guarding and rebound tenderness are also seen.

An unusual feature is the Cullen's sign. This is bluish discoloration of the skin around the umbilicus caused by a considerable quantity of free blood in the peritoneal cavity. However, the sign is rare and even if it is absent massive intraperitoneal haemorrhage cannot be excluded.

On pelvic examination the findings vary from completely negative to the presence of a large, fixed, soft and tender mass. An adnexal mass may be palpable in up to 55% of cases. In many cases the mass is ill defined; it may consist not only of tubal pregnancy but also of adherent omentum, small and large bowel. The mass could also be an enlarged corpus luteum. The uterus may be slightly enlarged but its size does not normally correspond to the gestational age. Cervical excitation may or may not be present. A tender boggy mass in the pouch of Douglas, when present, represents either a collection of blood in the area or a dilated tube adherent to the posterior uterine wall.

Clinical presentation of an ectopic pregnancy

The presentation of symptomatic patients with a tubal ectopic pregnancy may be acute or subacute.

Acute presentation

Acute presentation is usually a consequence of rupture of the ectopic gestation, intraperitoneal haemorrhage and haemodynamic shock. On physical examination the patient is pale, hypotensive and tachycardic. She may complain of shoulder tip pain or the urge to defaecate. These symptoms are due to intra-abdominal haemorrhage and collection of blood into specific areas – subdiaphragmatic and pouch of Douglas. Abdominal examination reveals generalized severe tenderness and rebound tenderness. Vaginal examination will reveal tenderness in both iliac fossae and cervical excitation. However, vaginal examination in patients who present with acute abdomen due to a ruptured ectopic pregnancy is unnecessary and potentially dangerous for the following reasons: due to generalized haemoperitoneum and pain, specific information cannot be elicited; the patient is very uncomfortable and the assessment is often difficult and inadequate; it could result in total rupture of the ectopic pregnancy and delay management of the patient.

Acute presentation of an ectopic pregnancy is becoming less common because not only are patients more aware of the disease and seek medical advice earlier but more doctors 'think ectopic first' and refer women to hospital at an earlier stage. Finally the availability of more sensitive and rapid biochemical tests for β-hCG and the wider availability of other diagnostic tests such as transvaginal ultrasonography and laparoscopy have significantly reduced the interval between presentation and treatment.

Subacute presentation

When the process of tubal rupture or abortion is very gradual the presentation of ectopic pregnancy is subacute. According to Stabile (1996a,b), this is the group of women who are symptomatic but clinically stable. A history of a missed period and recurrent episodes of light vaginal bleeding may exist. The circulatory system adjusts the blood pressure and haemodynamically the patient is stable. Progressively deteriorating lower abdominal pain and occasionally shoulder pain are reported. On bimanual examination there may be localized tenderness in one of the fornices and cervical excitation.

Subacute presentation occurs in 80–90% of ectopic pregnancies. The establishment of an accurate diagnosis becomes more difficult and hence further investigations are necessary.

FURTHER INVESTIGATIONS

Quantitation of β-hCG subunit

Using highly sensitive assays (detection limit 0.1–0.3 iu/l), β-hCG can be detected in the maternal circulation around the time of blastocyst implantation, i.e. 6–7 days after conception. The hCG will appear in the urine approximately 2 days after it appears in the blood. The hCG level changes with the gestational age and during the first 6 weeks of pregnancy the serum hCG concentration increases exponentially. After the 6th week of gestation when the hCG concentration is >6000–10 000 iu/l, the hCG rise is slower and not constant. The sensitivity of modern assays is 99–100%.

Single hCG measurement

A single assessment of β-hCG has limited clinical value because there is a considerable overlap of values between normal and abnormal pregnancies. When using radioimmunometric assays with a detection limit of 5 iu/l a single measurement of β-hCG may be useful because, if negative, it can exclude the diagnosis of ectopic pregnancy.

Serial hCG measurements

Serial quantitative assessments of β-hCG may distinguish normal from abnormal pregnancies. Kadar et al (1981) reported a method for screening for ectopic pregnancy based on the hCG doubling time: if hCG increases by <66% over 48 hours an ectopic pregnancy should be considered (85% confidence limits). Approximately 15% of patients with an ectopic pregnancy will have a >66% rise in hCG within 48 hours. However, the hCG pattern that is highly suggestive of an ectopic pregnancy is a 'plateau' in hCG levels. Plateau is defined as an hCG doubling time of 7 days or more (Kadar & Romero 1988). Falling levels of hCG can distinguish ectopic pregnancy from spontaneous miscarriage. If serial measurements of hCG every 48 hours reveal a half-life of <1.4 days then spontaneous abortion is the most likely diagnosis.

Other protein and steroid markers

In an effort to detect an ectopic pregnancy at an early stage, various steroid and protein markers have been studied including Schwangerschafts protein-1 (SP1), human placental lactogen (HPL), pregnancy-associated plasma protein A (PAPP-A) and others.

However, none of these markers has made a significant impact in clinical practice. For more details see excellent reviews by Stabile (1996a,b).

Ultrasonography

In cases of suspected ectopic pregnancy the role of ultra-sonography is to locate the pregnancy. The presence of an intrauterine pregnancy does not absolutely exclude the possibility of an ectopic but the simultaneous coexistence of a heterotopic pregnancy is very rare (1:30 000). Transvaginal ultrasonography is superior to abdominal ultrasonography. The proximity of the vaginal probe to the pelvic structures allows use of high-frequency transducers (5–7 MHz) which improve resolution.

The earliest normal intrauterine gestational sac (approximately 2 mm) is seen at 4 weeks of gestation with transvaginal ultrasound and at 5 weeks with abdominal ultrasound. In 20% of patients with an ectopic pregnancy collection of fluid within the uterine cavity results in formation of a pseudo-gestational sac which mimics a true intrauterine sac.

An ultrasonographic sign used to differentiate between a true gestational sac and a pseudo-sac is the double ring or double decidual sac sign (DDSS). The double sac is likely to be created by the decidual capsularis and parietalis. The DDSS, however, may also be seen in one-third of ectopic pregnancies and therefore its usefulness in clinical practice is limited.

The most reliable sign to differentiate between a pseudo-sac and a true sac is the appearance of the yolk sac within the true gestational sac. The presence of a yolk sac confirms an intrauterine pregnancy before a living embryo is detected. A yolk sac is identified by ultrasound when the mean gestational sac diameter is greater than 8 mm.

A review of the world literature by Brown & Doubilet (1994) indicates that in cases of ectopic pregnancy the following images may be seen if transvaginal sonography is applied.

- An empty uterus (28%).
- An empty uterus and an adnexal mass (35%).
- An intrauterine sac or pseudo-gestational sac (25%).
- An empty uterus and an ectopic gestational sac (12%) with or without a yolk sac; anembryonic cardiac activity (Fig. 26.1).
- Images in the pouch of Douglas (25%); various amounts of fluid: these are features of a tubal pregnancy that is aborting or is ruptured.

Quantitative assessment of β-hCG levels is essential for the accurate interpretation of ultrasonographic findings. All viable intrauterine pregnancies should be visualized by transvaginal ultrasound if serum β-hCG levels are ≥1500 iu/l and by abdominal ultrasound if serum β-hCG levels are ≥6500 iu/l.

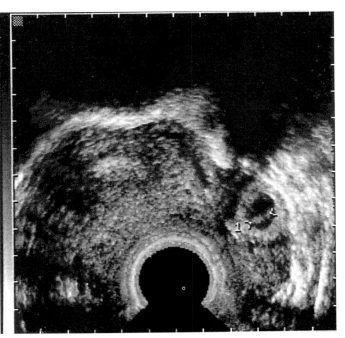

Fig. 26.1 Vaginal scan of pelvis. Transverse view of the pelvis. Arrow shows an empty uterine cavity. Dots show an ectopic pregnancy of the left tube lying on the ovary.

Failure to visualize an intrauterine gestational sac by transvaginal ultrasound if β-hCG is >1500 iu/l indicates either an abnormal intrauterine gestational sac or a recent abortion or an ectopic pregnancy. It must be emphasized that although the discriminatory zone for intrauterine pregnancy is well established there is no discriminatory zone for ectopic pregnancy.

Doppler ultrasonography

Doppler ultrasound is a non-invasive biophysical method of investigating patterns of blood flow and its changes in the human cardiovascular system. Ectopic pregnancy is one of the conditions changing the normal high-resistance blood flow from the uterine or ovarian artery branches.

Jurkovic et al (1992), in a prospective study, used colour Doppler to detect and compare changes of blood flow in the uterine and spiral arteries and the corpus luteum in ectopic and intrauterine pregnancies. In both uterine arteries the impedance to flow (resistance index) decreases with the gestational age in intrauterine pregnancies but remains constant in ectopic pregnancies. Peak blood velocity in the uterine arteries increases with the gestational age in intrauterine pregnancies and the values are significantly higher than those seen in ectopic pregnancies. However, uterine blood flow velocity is lower in the ectopic group, indicating an overall reduction in uterine blood supply. Local vascular changes associated with a true gestational sac differentiate an intrauterine pregnancy from the pseudo-sac of an ectopic pregnancy. Doppler flow imaging can suggest that the adnexal mass is an ectopic pregnancy by detecting high vascularity at the periphery of the adnexal mass, lower resistance to flow and a relatively cool uterine vasculature.

Colour and pulsed Doppler increase the sensitivity of vaginal ultrasonography and allow earlier detection of ectopic pregnancy, a consequence of which is application of medical treatment or conservative surgery for the management of this disease.

Three-dimensional ultrasound

Three-dimensional ultrasound is emerging as a possible additional diagnostic tool for ectopic pregnancy. Rempen (1998) conducted a prospective follow-up study in order to evaluate the potential ability of 3D ultrasound to differentiate intrauterine from extrauterine gestations. Fifty-four pregnancies with a gestational age of <10 weeks and with an intrauterine gestational sac <5 mm in diameter were included in the study. The configuration of the endometrium in the frontal plane of the uterus was correlated with pregnancy outcome: it was found to be asymmetrical in 84% of intrauterine pregnancies whereas the endometrium showed asymmetry in the frontal plane in 90% of extrauterine pregnancies ($p = 0.0000001$). The conclusion was that evaluation of the endometrial shape in the frontal plane is a useful additional mean of distinguishing intrauterine from extrauterine pregnancies.

Harika et al (1995) conducted a study to assess the role of 3D imaging in the early diagnosis of ectopic pregnancy. Twelve asymptomatic patients were included in the study; the gestational age was <6 weeks in all patients. Laparoscopy showed ectopic pregnancy in nine cases. Three-dimensional transvaginal ultrasonography showed a small ectopic gestational sac in four cases. These preliminary results suggest that 3D ultrasonography is likely to be an effective procedure for the diagnosis of ectopic pregnancy in asymptomatic patients prior to sixth gestational week.

Laparoscopy

Laparoscopy represents the gold standard for the diagnosis of ectopic pregnancy with distension of the tubal wall seen in the majority of cases. In the very early stages a small ectopic pregnancy may not be visualized and in 3–4% of cases the diagnosis will be missed. Free blood in the peritoneal cavity is another pointer suggesting careful examination of the fallopian tubes.

Culdocentesis

The introduction of transvaginal ultrasonography, laparoscopy and highly sensitive hCG assays has made culdocentesis redundant.

DIFFERENTIAL DIAGNOSIS

The differential diagnosis of ectopic pregnancy should include: ruptured corpus luteum cyst; threatened or incomplete abortion; pelvic inflammatory disease; degeneration of fibroid. Quantitative assessment of β-hCG, transvaginal ultrasonography and occasionally laparoscopy are powerful tools to solve the diagnostic problem.

SURGICAL TREATMENT

Salpingectomy

Removal of the fallopian tube is still the most common method for the treatment of ectopic pregnancy. It can be performed via laparotomy or laparoscopy. When laparotomy is performed the easiest way to remove the fallopian tube is by progressive division and ligation of the mesosalpinx. Laparoscopic salpingectomy can be performed with one of the following methods: pretied loop ligatures, bipolar diathermy or disposable stapling devices. However, the cost associated with use of the stapling devices has limited their popularity.

Several methods have been proposed for the removal of the fallopian tube from the peritoneal cavity following laparoscopic salpingectomy:

- placement of the fallopian tube into a specially designed plastic bag introduced via a 10 mm port, the bag being sealed at its neck and then removed intact through the port
- morcellation of the fallopian tube and removal by a 10 mm grasping forceps
- posterior colpotomy and removal of the tube intact via the pouch of Douglas.

When to consider salpingectomy

Salpingectomy is indicated in the following groups of patients.

- Ruptured tubal pregnancy
- Recurrent ectopic pregnancy in a tube already treated conservatively
- Previous sterilization and reversal of sterilization
- Previous tubal surgery for infertility
- Pre-existing tubal damage as a consequence of frozen pelvis.

Finally, the debate over salpingectomy or salpingo-oophorectomy does not exist any more. Removal of a healthy ovary is now considered both unnecessary and unjustified.

Linear salpingotomy

An incision is made on the antimesenteric border of the fallopian tube with the needle-point monopolar cutting diathermy, scalpel, scissors or laser and the tubal lumen is exposed. The products of conception are removed with grasping forceps. Sometimes the laparoscopic suction/irrigation probe is very useful for aqua dissection and removal, by suction, of the products of conception. Irrigation of the tubal lumen after removal of products of conception is essential. Haemostasis is achieved with electrocoagulation. The incision can either be closed with a fine non-absorbable suture material, such as 6/0 Prolene, or left open (salpingotomy) to complete second-intention healing. Either approach results in satisfactory healing of the tubal wall. A study by Tulandi & Guralnilk (1991) showed that there was no signficant difference in the number of subsequent intrauterine pregnancies, number of ectopic pregnancies or incidence of adhesion formation with either method.

Linear salpingotomy can be performed via an open or laparoscopic approach. However, regardless of the route used

Fig. 26.2 Conservative surgical management of an ampullary ectopic pregnancy. **a** Linear salpingotomy. **b** Removal of the gestational sac. **c** Salpingotomy left open to heal without closure.

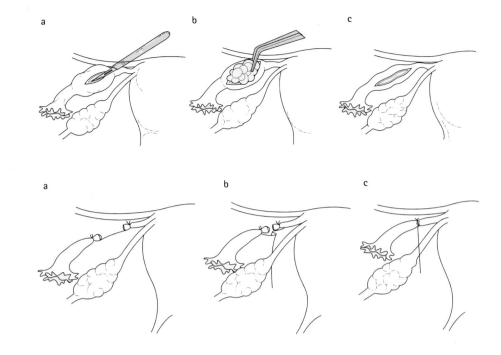

Fig. 26.3 Conservative surgical management of an isthmic ectopic pregnancy. **a** Resection of the gestational sac. **b** Blind ends left tied in order to perform a reanastomosis as a second procedure. **c** Reanastomosis done during the same procedure.

to access the ectopic pregnancy, the surgeon should remember that the fallopian tubes are delicate and sensitive structures. The basic microsurgical principles should always be applied: gentle handling of tissues; avoidance of peritoneal damage; thorough irrigation and suction of the peritoneal cavity to remove all the blood clots and minimize post-operative adhesion formation. Laparoscopic linear salpingotomy is currently the procedure of choice when the patient has an unruptured ectopic pregnancy and wishes to retain her potential for future fertility (Fig. 26.2).

Segmental resection

When the ectopic pregnancy is located in the isthmic segment of the fallopian tube, segmental resection and end-to-end anastomosis constitute one of the conservative surgical therapeutic options (Fig. 26.3). The anastomosis is usually isthmo-ampullary and can be performed either at the time of the resection (primary) or at a later stage (secondary). However, for isthmic tubal pregnancy linear salpingotomy is technically less difficult and has a shorter operative time.

Fimbrial evacuation

Fimbrial evacuation is indicated when the pregnancy lies in the fimbrial segment of the fallopian tube. It involves gentle and progressive compression of the tube starting just proximal to the side of the pregnancy and moving systematically to the fimbrial end of the tube. When the pregnancy is located at the ampullary part, fimbrial evacuation or 'milking of the tube' is not recommended because the external pressure required to propel the ectopic pregnancy and achieve a tubal abortion is likely to cause severe damage to the endosalpinx, fail to stop the bleeding from the implantation site and came a risk of

persistent trophoblast (Brosens et al 1984). Also when milking is compared with linear salpingotomy for ampullary ectopic pregnancy, milking is associated with a twofold increase in the recurrent ectopic pregnancy rate (Smith et al 1987).

Laparoscopy or laparotomy?

All the surgical procedures for treatment of ectopic pregnancy can be accomplished via laparoscopy or laparotomy. The main factors which will determine the preferred approach are:

- the haemodynamic condition of the patient
- the size and the location of the ectopic mass
- the laparoscopic experience of the surgeon
- availability of the appropriate equipment for laparoscopic surgery.

Laparotomy should be considered in the following cases: the patient is haemodynamically unstable; extensive abdominal and pelvic adhesions making laparoscopy difficult; cornual or ovarian pregnancy. A ruptured ectopic pregnancy does not necessarily require laparotomy. In the hands of an experienced laparoscopist all the indications for laparotomy are relative rather than absolute if the patient is haemodynamically stable.

A meta-analysis of three studies involving 228 haemodynamically stable women with a small unruptured tubal pregnancy was undertaken. In the laparoscopy and laparotomy groups the rates of subsequent intrauterine pregnancy were 61% and 53% and the rates of recurrent ectopic pregnancy were 7% and 14% respectively. The figures show that there is no statistically significant difference in the reproductive outcome after salphingotomy by laparoscopy and by laparotomy. However, laparoscopic conservative surgery was associated with a higher persistent trophoblast rate (RR 3.6, 95% CI 0.63,21). It is likely that the failure represent problems occurring during the learning curve of the laparoscopists (Hajenius et al 2000).

The laparoscopic approach provides a shorter duration of hospitalization and canvalescence.

An additional benefit of the laparoscopic approach is that patients who undergo laparoscopic treatment of ectopic pregnancy have significantly fewer adhesions at the surgical site compared with those treated by laparotomy (Lundorff et al 1991).

Reproductive outcome

The evaluation of reproductive outcome following surgical treatment for ectopic pregnancy is based on three main parameters.

- Tubal patency as assessed by hysterosalpingography or second-look laparoscopy
- The subsequent intrauterine pregnancy rate
- The recurrent ectopic pregnancy rate

In patients who underwent radical surgery (salpingectomy) the subsequent intrauterine pregnancy rate was 49.3% (36.6–71.4%) and the recurrent ectopic pregnancy rate was 10% (5.8–12%). In those patients, however, who underwent conservative surgery the subsequent intrauterine pregnancy rate was 53% (38–83%) and the recurrent ectopic pregnancy rate was 14% (6.4–21.2%). These results are based on a retrospective analysis of nine studies in a total of 2635 patients (Yao & Tulandi 1997) and indicate that conservative surgery is associated with higher subsequent intrauterine pregnancy and higher recurrent ectopic rates compared with radical surgery. However, the variations in the design of each study make strict comparison of the results very difficult.

MEDICAL TREATMENT WITH METHOTREXATE

Early detection of ectopic pregnancy, desire to improve fertility, minimizing cost and surgical morbidity are the main reasons for incorporating medical treatment in the spectrum of therapeutic options for ectopic pregnancy. Currently the most frequently used drug is methotrexate and therefore its application will be discussed in detail although other agents have been used.

Gynaecologists are familiar with methotrexate (MTX) because the drug has been used very effectively for the treament of gestational trophoblastic disease since 1955 (Li et al 1956). Hreschchyshyn et al (1965) were the first to report use of MTX in the management of ectopic pregnancy. It was successfully adminsitered to a patient who had a mid-trimester missed abortion. In 1982 Tanaka et al reported the treatment of an unruptured interstitial pregnancy with a course of intramuscular methotrexate.

Mode of action and pharmacokinetics

Methotrexate, formerly known as amethopterin, is a potent folic acid antagonist. It inhibits the action of the enzyme dehydrofolate reductase and the coenzyme methyl tetrahydro-folate. These enzymes are essential for the conversion of dehydrofolic acid into tetrahydrofolic acid and the conversion of deoxyuridylic acid into thymidylic acid which is critical for the synthesis of DNA during the S phase of the cell cycle. Prevention of incorporation of thymidylic acid into DNA results in lack of DNA synthesis and subsequently arrest of cellular division and multiplication.

Methotrexate is ideal for inhibition of rapidly growing cells such as trophoblasts. It is almost completely absorbed if administered intramuscularly, with peak serum concentrations reached within 30–60 minutes. Only 10% of methotrexate undergoes hepatic and intracellular metabolism to poly-glutamated products which also act as active antimetabolites. Up to 90% of the drug is secreted unchanged in the urine within 48 hours and therefore impaired renal function can result in prolonged exposure of tissues to high levels of methotrexate or its metabolic products.

Side-effects of methotrexate

The two most significant factors that determine the intensity of methotrexate toxicity are the serum concentration of drug and the duration of exposure to methotrexate. The drug affects all rapidly proliferating cells and therefore the main side-effects originate from suppression of bone marrow cells and epithelial cells of the gastrointestinal tract. The spectrum of possible side-effects of methotrexate is shown below.

- Myelosuppression
- Stomatitis
- Gastritis
- Diarrhoea
- Alopecia (reversible)
- Liver toxicity
- Abdominal pain
- Photosensitivity (skin reaction)
- Pneumonitis
- Renal toxicity
- Anaphylaxis

The incidence of side-effects among patients treated with high-dose or multidose methotrexate is reported at 20–30%. Single-dose regimes, however, currently used for non-surgical treatment of ectopic pregnancy are associated with minor or no side-effects. Resolution of the adverse effects usually occurs within 72 hours after termination of therapy.

Guidelines for the prescription of methotrexate

In order to achieve early identification and prevention of serious side-effects, the Committee on the Safety of Medicines has issued the following guidelines for the prescription of methotrexate.

Myelosuppression
Pretreatment full blood count needs to be documented as a baseline blood count. If an acute decrease in the white cell or platelet count occurs, treatment should be discontinued immediately.

Liver toxicity
Pre-existing abnormal liver function or concurrent abnormal liver function tests should alert medical staff to potential liver toxicity. Again, pretreatment baseline liver function tests are essential.

Renal function

Assessment of renal function is essential prior to treatment because the primary route of excretion of methotrexate is the kidney. Caution should be applied in concurrent medication with non-steroidal anti-inflammatory drugs as they may adversely affect renal function and hence increase even further the serum concentration of methorexate.

Folinic acid rescue

Methorexate morbidity can be minimized by concurrent administration of the 'antidote' folinic acid in the form of calcium folinate which is converted to 5-methyltetrahydrofolate. The enzymatic cell deficiency is corrected via bypassing the methotrexate block.

Who will benefit from methotrexate?

The key for successful and safe medical treatment of ectopic pregnancy is proper selection of patients. Methotrexate should be reserved for patients who have an unruptured tubal pregnancy who are clinically asymptomatic and haemodynamically stable. The indications and contraindications for methotrexate therapy are presented below.

Indications
- Initial pretreatment plasma β-hCG level should be <10 000 iu/l.
- The tubal diameter should be <2 cm as defined by direct visualization or by ultrasound.
- Fetal heartbeat must be absent on ultrasound scan.

Contraindications
- Symptomatic patients
- Haemodynamically unstable patients
- Presence of haemoperitoneum
- Initial pretreatment β-hCG concentration >10 000 iu/l
- Tubal diameter >2 cm
- Presence of fetal heart on ultrasound scan
- Evidence of liver disease, renal insufficiency or myelo-suppression
- Inability of the patient to return for follow-up care

A review of 24 studies indicated that the incidence of tubal ruptured is 10 times higher in women who have initial β-hCG serum concentration >10 000 iu/l than in those with β-hCG <10 000 iu/l (32% versus 3%). Shalev et al (1995) reported that following intratubal administration of methotrexate the failure rate was 24% when the tubal diameter was <2 cm and 48% when the diameter was >2 cm. The authors recommend that methotrexate should be used only when the size of the ectopic pregnancy is <2 cm. Stovall & Ling (1993) found that administration of methotrexate to patients who had evidence of fetal heartbeat on ultrasound scan was associated with 14.3% failure rate. In the group of patients without evidence of fetal cardiac activity the failure rate was 4.7%.

Routes of administration and dose

Methotrexate can be administered systemically (intravenously or intramuscularly) or locally using a laparoscopic or trans-vaginal or ultrasound-guided approach. The published literature includes a wide spectrum of protocols for the systemic administration of methotrexate, including:

- standard single dose (60–200 mg IM)
- multiple individualized doses (1 mg/kg per day × 3–5 days IM)
- single individualized dose (1 mg/kg or 50 mg/m^2 of body surface)

The success rate of all three regimes is comparable. Three trials have shown that administration of methotrexate in a single IM dose of 50 mg per m^2 of body surface area is associated with a complete resumption rate of 92%, a subsequent intrauterine pregnancy rate of 58% and a recurrent ectopic rate of 9%. Resumption rate is defined as the time interval between initiation of therapy and undetectable serum hCG concentration. The mean resumption time is 30 days, ranging from 5 to 100 days. Tubal patency is reported to be 50–100%, with a mean of 71%, after systemic administration of methotrexate.

Two randomized controlled trials (Cohen et al 1996, Fernandez et al 1994) suggested that local injection of methotrexate was equivalent in effect to systemic methotrexate. The major advantages of direct injection of methotrexate into the tube include smaller dose of the drug, higher tissue concentration and fewer systemic side-effects.

Laparoscopic surgery versus methotrexate

O'Shea et al (1994) published the results of a prospective randomized trial comparing intra-amniotic methotrexate versus CO_2 laser laparoscopic salpingotomy. The salpingotomy group and the local methotrexate group have comparable success rates, 87.5% and 89.7% respectively. However, another study by Shalev et al (1995) revealed a success rate of 93% in 55 patients treated by laparoscopic salpingotomy and a significantly lower rate of 61% in 44 patients treated by laparoscopic injection of methotrexate.

Methotrexate appears to be effective in a selective group of patients with ectopic pregnancy. Intramuscular administration eliminates anaesthetic and surgical risks arising from laparoscopic injection of the drug. However, the long-term effect of locally injected pharmacological substances upon the endosalpinx remains largely unknown.

A suggested algorithmic approach for the medical managment of tubal ectopic gestation is shown in Figure 26.4. It is important to recognize that abdominal pain occurs in 30–50% of patients 6–7 days after administration of methotrexate. The gynaecologist has to decide if the pain is due to imminent tubal rupture, already existing tubal rupture or simply represents post-methotrexate administration pain. Post-methotrexate pain is localized in the lower abdomen and its precise aetiology remains largely unknown but it is likely to be due to a combination of factors, including destruction of the trophoblastic tissue, a small amount of transtubal haemorrhage and irritation of the gastrointestinal mucosa. Close monitoring of the patient is essential in order to avoid unnecessary surgical intervention in the form of laparoscopy or laparotomy. According to Stovall (1995), regular assessment of haemo-

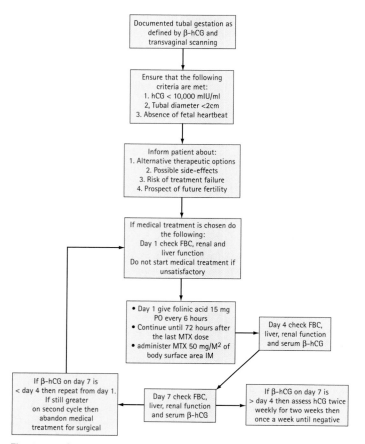

Fig. 26.4 Suggested protocol for the medical management of tubal ectopic gestation.

globin is the most useful parameter. The pain usually subsides within 24–48 hours and occasionally precedes or follows an episode of vaginal bleeding.

The concentration of serum β-hCG is likely to increase between days 1 and 4 after treatment. It has been suggested that although methotrexate is arresting mitosis in the cytotrophoblast, the syncytiotrophoblast may still be able to produce hCG. Also, destruction of the cells releases more hCG into the systemic circulation.

Brown et al (1991) assessed the clinical value of serial transvaginal ultrasonography in ectopic pregnancies treated with methotrexate and concluded that routine ultrasonography is not necessary after methotrexate treatment. There was no correlation between the pattern of resolution of β-hCG and sonographic findings.

Mifepristone and methotrexate

Mifepristone (RU486) has been used in combination with methotrexate for the medical treatment of ectopic pregnancy (Gazvani & Emery 1999). A non-randomized study from France (Perdu et al 1998) reported only one failure in the 30 patients treated with IM methotrexate and oral mifepristone and 11 failures in 42 patients treated with methotrexate alone. The authors concluded that the combination of mifepristone and methotrexate decreased the risk of failure in medical

treatment of ectopic pregnancy. However, further prospective randomized studies are needed to evaluate the role of mifepristone in the medical management of ectopic pregnancy.

CONTROLLED EXPECTANT MANAGEMENT

When only expectant management was available, it was associated with a very high degree of morbidity and mortality because the patients who failed expectant management had significant clinical symptoms indicating rupture of the ectopic pregnancy. Since then, due to the advancement in ultrasound scanning and rapid access to quantitative β-hCG assays, the natural history of the expectant management of ectopic gestation has changed in that it is now controlled and monitored.

Ten prospective studies with a total of 347 patients managed expectantly demonstrated that 69% of the ectopic gestations resolved spontaneously. All patients were haemodynamically stable and had decreasing serum β-hCG levels. However, other variables such as size and location of ectopic prenancy or presence of fetal cardiac activity were not always specified (Yao & Tulandi 1997).

The essential prerequisite for successful expectant management of ectopic gestation is appropriate selecion of patients. The Royal College of Obstetricians & Gynaecologists (1999) issued guidelines for the management of tubal pregnancy. The conclusion was that expectant management is more likely to be successful in the following circumstances:

- baseline serum β-hCG concentration <1000–2000 iu/l
- haemoperitoneum of <50 ml
- a tubal mass of <2 cm
- absence of recognizable fetal parts on ultrasound
- absence of clinical symptoms.

It must be emphasized, however, that tubal rupture has been reported in cases of very low and decreasing serum β-hCG levels and expectant management often involves long periods of hospitalization and follow-up.

NON-TUBAL ECTOPIC PREGNANCY

Cervical pregnancy

Cervical pregnancy is one that implants entirely within the cervical canal. The reported incidence ranges from 1:2500 to 1:18 000 deliveries (0.2% of ectopic pregnancies). A variety of conditions are thought to predispose to the development of cervical pregnancy, including previous therapeutic abortion, previous caesarean delivery, Asherman's syndrome and exposure to DES. Sporadic cases of cervical pregnancy have been reported after controlled ovarian stimulation with human menopausal gonadotrophins and intrauterine insemination as well as IVF (Weyerman et al 1989).

Cervical pregnancy produces profuse vaginal bleeding without associated cramping pain. The clinical and ultrasound criteria for the diagnosis of cervical pregnancy are summarized below (Hofmann et al 1987).

- *Clinical criteria* – the uterus surrounding the distended cervix feels smaller on vaginal examination. Curettage of the endometrial cavity reveals no evidence of trophoblastic tissue. The products of conception are confined within the cervix. The internal cervical os is closed.

- *Ultrasound criteria* – balloon cervical canal; gestational sac in the endocervix; closed internal os; no evidence of an intrauterine gestational sac.

The differential diagnosis should include cervical carcinoma, cervical or prolapsed submucosal myoma, placenta praevia, trophoblastic tumour or an ongoing spontaneous intrauterine abortion.

Early forms of cervical pregnancy are managed conservatively. Removal of the products of conception from the cervical canal by suction curettage is likely to stop the haemorrhage. Other measures which have been used to control bleeding include packing of the uterus and cervix, insertion of an intracervical 30 ml Foley catheter to arrest the bleeding, insertion of sutures to ligate the lateral placement of cervical vessels and placement of a cervical cerclage. In some cases, because of the depth of trophoblastic invasion, major blood vessels are involved and more radical measures are necessary to control the bleeding. Bilateral internal iliac artery ligation has been recommended. When all the conservative measures have failed to arrest the bleeding, hysterectomy is required. Preoperatively the patient must be informed about the possibility of hysterectomy and sign the appropriate consent.

Ovarian pregnancy

Ovarian pregnancy represents the most common type of non-tubal ectopic pregnancy and it occurs in 0.2–1% of all ectopic pregnancies. The incidence range from 1:40 000 to 1:7000 deliveries. Ovarian pregnancy has been reported after IVF treatment (Marcus & Brinsden 1993) and clomiphene ovulation induction (De Muylder et al 1994). The only risk factor associated with the development of an ovarian pregnancy is the current use of an IUCD.

The symptoms and signs of an ovarian pregnancy are similar to those of tubal pregnancy. Usually the diagnosis is made during a laparoscopy or laparotomy. The classic criteria of Spiegelberg (1878) for the diagnosis of an ovarian pregnancy are as follows.

- The gestational sac must occupy a portion of the ovary.
- The gestational sac must be connected to the uterus by the ovarian ligament.
- Ovarian tissue must be identified in the wall of the sac.
- The fallopian tube on the affected side of the pelvis must be intact.

Conditions to be considered for the differential diagnosis include tubal pregnancy or complications of an ovarian cyst. Treatment consists of resection of the trophoblast from the ovary, preserving as much ovarian tissue as possible. Salpingo-oophorectomy is rarely necessary.

Abdominal pregnancy

There are two types of abdominal pregnancy:

- primary peritoneal implantation of blastocyst

- secondary peritoneal implantation of conceptus following tubal abortion or rupture or, less often, after uterine rupture with subsequent implantation within the abdomen.

Secondary abdominal pregnancies are by far the most common. Abdominal pregnancy represents approximately 1.4% of all ectopic pregnancies and its incidence varies from 1:3000 to 1:10 000 deliveries. Abdominal pregnancies are associated with high maternal (0.5–1.8%) and perinatal mortality (40–95%) (Atrash et al 1987). The incidence of congenital fetal abnormality ranges from 35% to 75%. Most of the abnormalities are caused by growth restriction and external pressure of the fetus; common problems include fetal pulmonary hypoplasia, facial asymmetry and talipes.

The classic criteria for the diagnosis of primary abdominal pregnancy are:

- no evidence of uteroplacental fistula
- presence of normal tubes and ovaries with no evidence of recent or past pregnancy
- pregnancy attached only to peritoneal surface.

Diagnosis of abdominal pregnancy must be made early enough to eliminate the possibility of secondary implantation after primary tubal nidation. In the first and early second trimesters, the symptoms may be the same as with tubal ectopic gestation. As the pregnancy advances, however, unexplained abdominal pain, occasional vomiting, diarrhoea or constipation may occur. Fetal movements are very marked or painful and felt high in the abdomen. Braxton-Hicks contractions are absent. Abdominal palpation may disclose persistently abnormal fetal lie, abdominal tenderness and easy palpation of the fetal parts. The fetus gives the impression that it lies just under the skin of the abdomen. On bimanual examination the uterus is usually normal in size and the cervix is long, firm and displaced. Abdominal ultrasound provides an unequivocal diagnosis although computerized tomography and magnetic resonance imaging have also been used to confirm the diagnosis.

The treatment is laparotomy as soon as the diagnosis is made. This is not to be undertaken lightly. The objectives are to remove the fetus and to ligate the umbilical cord close to the placenta without disturbing it. The placenta is allowed to be absorbed; if left alone it rarely presents problems of bleeding or infection. The placenta should only be removed when the surgeon is absolutely certain that total haemostasis can be achieved. Removal of placenta is possible if it is attached to the ovary, broad ligament and posterior surface of the uterus. Attempts to remove the placenta from other intra-abdominal organs are likely to cause massive haemorrhage due to the invasive properties of the trophoblast and the lack of cleavage planes. Placental involution can be monitored using serial ultrasonography and hCG levels. Potential complications of leaving the placenta in place include bowel obstruction, fistula formation, haemorrhage and peritonitis.

Interstitial pregnancy

In interstitial pregnancy the zygote/blastocyst implants in the portion of the uterine fallopian tube that traverses the uterine wall. It occurs in 1:2 500–5000 live births and comprises 2% of all ectopic pregnancies. Predisposing factors are similar to those of other tubal pregnancies.

The implantation site may be in the utero interstitial (inner segment), the true interstitial (middle segment) or the tubo interstitial (outer segment) region. The duration of pregnancy depends on its location. Implantation in either the inner or outer segments results in early rupture. Implantation in the middle segment involves greater mass of myometrium and permits the pregnancy to advance to a somewhat later date. Rupture of the uterine wall is the most frequent outcome and the haemorrhage is usually severe. The signs and symptoms are similar to those of tubal ectopic pregnancy. Intermittent recurrent, sharp abdominal pain occurs at 4–6 weeks. Sudden severe abdominal pain is followed by collapse.

An asymmetric pregnant uterus with a tender mass in the cornual area may be the first sign alerting the physician to the possibility of an interstitial pregnancy. Laparoscopy will reveal an asymmetrical enlargement of the uterus, displacement of the uterine fundus to the opposite side, elevation of the involved cornu and rotation of the uterus on its long axis. The round ligament may be lateral to the gestational sac.

Interstitial pregnancy must be differentiated from cornual myoma, pregnancy in one horn of a bicornuate uterus and large endometrioma at the uterotubal junction.

Treatment involves management of the haemorrhagic shock, as in any other case, followed by surgical intervention. Immediate laparotomy is required. Simple wedge resection, reconstruction of the uterine wall and salpingectomy will be neccessary. The extent of surgery will depend on the degree of damage to the uterus. In some cases, if the uterine wall is severely damaged the only way to control the haemorrhage is to perform a total abdominal hysterectomy and unilateral salpingo-oophorectomy. Cornual resection and uterine reconstruction has been associated with uterine rupture later in pregnancy or during labour in subsequent gestations.

Intraligamentous pregnancy

Intraligamentous pregnancy is another rare form of non-tubal pregnancy and occurs in approximately 1:300 ectopic pregnancies. This kind of pregnancy is secondary as a result of penetration of the tubal wall by the trophoblastic tissue and advancement of the trophoblast between the two layers of the broad ligament. Clinical findings are similar to those of abdominal pregnancy. The uterus is felt separately and is usually displaced to the opposite side. If the pregnancy persists the mass may become palpable abdominally. The diagnosis is usually made at the time of surgery. The surgical principles are similar to those applied for abdominal pregnancy. Problems with extensive placental invasion of nearby structures are less likely. If possible, the placenta should be removed; when this is not possible it can be left in situ and allowed to resolve.

Heterotopic pregnancy

Heterotopic pregnancy is the combination of an intrauterine and an extrauterine pregnancy. In spontaneous conception the incidence of this phenomenon varies from 1:4000 to 1:30 000 pregnancies. Patients who have undergone infertility treatment, particularly in vitro fertilization and embryo transfer, have a much higher incidence of heterotopic pregnancy compared to those who have a spontaneous conception. After IVF/ET 1–3% of all clinical pregnancies are heterotopic. Delay in diagnosis is common because even after a transvaginal ultrasound scan attention is concentrated on the viable intrauterine pregnancy. It is, however, essential for the gynaecologist to remember the relatively high incidence of heterotopic pregnancy following infertility treatment and aim to visualize the adnexae at 6–7 weeks gestation when usually the first transvaginal scan is performed after assisted conception.

Unusual abdominal pain in the presence of spontaneous abortion or profuse uterine bleeding with signs of peritoneal irritation should suggest a combined pregnancy. Serial assessments of serum β-hCG concentration are often not helpful and therefore unnecessary. The diagnosis depends on maintaining a high index of suspicion, particularly for patients who are in the high-risk group. The diagnosis is usually made either via transvaginal ultrasound scan or laparoscopy. If the diagnosis of heterotopic pregnancy is established at an early stage the prognosis of the intrauterine pregnancy is more favourable.

The treatment of the ectopic pregnancy is operative. Once the ectopic pregnancy has been removed the intrauterine pregnancy continues in approximately 75% of patients.

Cornual pregnancy

The term cornual pregnancy indicates that the pregnancy has occurred in one side of a double uterus or in one horn of a bicornuate uterus. It is very rare (1:100 000 pregnancies) but it carries a 5% maternal mortality. Asymmetrical enlargement of the early pregnant uterus should suggest a uterine anomaly. Unusual discomfort and tenderness may be described. Abdominal or transvaginal ultrasound scan should be able to detect the problem and locate the pregnancy. If the fetus is mature, caesarean section is indicated. If the condition is diagnosed in the early stages of pregnancy the treatment is excision of the rudimentary horn and tube of the affected side. Congenital abnormalities of the müllerian duct are associated with renal anomalies and therefore studies of the renal tract should be ordered postoperatively to visualize the anatomy.

KEY POINTS

1. Ectopic pregnancy is a pregnancy that is implanted outside the uterine cavity. The ampullary segment of the fallopian tube is the most common site of ectopic pregnancy.
2. Independent risk factors consistently shown to increase the risk of tubal pregnancy include previous tubal pregnancy, previous laparoscopically proven pelvic inflammatory disease, previous tubal surgery and current intrauterine contraceptive device users.

KEY POINTS (*CONTINUED*)

3. The doctor should 'think ectopic first' for any woman of reproductive age who presents with the triad of abdominal pain, irregular vaginal bleeding and amenorrhoea. The presentation of symptomatic patients with a tubal ectopic pregnancy may be acute or subacute.

4. The introduction of highly sensitive biochemical assays for the measurement of β-hCG and transvaginal sonography have made possible the diagnosis of ectopic pregnancy at an early stage.

5. Laparoscopic surgery is the treatment of choice for most tubal pregnancies, particularly if laparoscopy is needed for diagnosis.

6. Laparoscopic surgery is superior to laparotomy. Following salpingectomy the subsequent intrauterine pregnancy rate is 50% and the recurrent ectopic pregnancy rate is 10%. Following salpingotomy or salpingostomy the subsequent intratuerine pregnancy rate is 53% and the recurrent ectopic pregnancy rate is 14%.

7. Systemic administration of methotrexate in combination with non-surgical diagnosis allows non-invasive outpatient management of tubal pregnancy.

8. Methotrexate should be considered when the initial pretreatment β-hCG concentration is <10 000 iu/l, the tubal diameter is <2 cm, there is no evidence of fetal heartbeat on ultrasound scan and the patient is haemodynamically stable and asymptomatic.

9. Expectant management of tubal ectopic pregnancy is more likely to be successful if the initial serum β-hCG concentration is <1000 iu/l, the diameter of the tubal mass is <2 cm, there is absence of recognizable fetal parts on ultrasound and absence of clinical symptoms.

10. Non-tubal ectopic pregnancies are rare but recently the incidence of heterotopic pregnancy has increased significantly following the introduction of techniques of assisted conception.

REFERENCES

Ankum WM, Mol BW, van der Veen F et al 1996 Risk factors for ectopic pregnancy: a meta-analysis. Fertility and Sterility 65(6):1093–1099

Assisted Reproductive Technology in the United States and Canada 1995 1993 results generated from the American Society for Reproductive Medicine/Society for Assisted Reproductive Registry. Fertility and Sterility 64:13–21

Atrash HK, Frieda A, Hogue CJ 1987 Abdominal pregnancy in the United States: frequency and maternal mortality. Obstetrics and Gynecology 69:333–337

Barnes AB, Colton T, Gundersen J et al 1980 Fertility and outcome of pregnancy in women exposed in utero to diethylstibestrol. New England Journal of Medicine 302(11):609–613

Berenson A, Hammill H, Martens M et al 1991 Bacteriologic findings with ectopic pregnancy. Journal of Reproductive Medicine 36(2):118–120

Bouyer J, Coste J, Fernandez H et al 1998 Tobacco and ectopic pregnancy. Arguments in favour of a causal relation. Revue de Epidemologie et de Sante Publique 46(2):93–99

Breen JL (1970) A 21 year survey of 654 ectopic pregnancies. American Journal of Obstetrics and Gynecology 106:1004–1019

Brosens I, Gordts S, Vasquez G et al 1984 Function-retaining surgical management of ectopic pregnancy. European Journal of Obstetrics Gynecology and Reproductive Biology 18(5–6):395–402

Brown DL, Felker RE, Stovall TG et al 1991 Serial endovaginal sonography of ectopic pregnancies treated with methotrexate. Obstetric and Gynecology 77(3):406–409

Brown DL, Doubilet PM 1994 Transvaginal sonography for diagnosing ectopic pregnancy: positive criteria and performance characteristics. Journal of Ultrasound in Medicine 13(4):259–166

Chow JM, Yonekura ML, Richwald GA et al 1990 The association between Chlamydia trachomatis and ectopic pregnancy. A control study. JAMA 263(23):3164–3167

Cohen DR, Falcone T, Khalife S 1996 Methotrexate: local versus intramuscular. Fertility and Sterility 65(1):206–207

De Muylder X, De Loecker P, Campo R 1994 Heterotopic ovarian pregnancy after clomiphene ovulation induction. European Journal of Obstetrics, Gynecology and Reproductive Biology 53(1):65–66

DeStefano F, Peterson HB, Layde PM 1982 Risk of ectopic pregnancy following tubal sterilization. Obstetrics and Gynecology 60(3):326–330

Diquelou JY, Pia P, Tesquier L et al 1988 The role of Chlamydia trachomatis in the infectious etiology of extra-uterine pregnancy. Journal de Gynecologie, Obstetrics et Biologie de la Reproduction (Paris) 17(3):325–332

Droegemueller W 1982 Ectopic pregnancy. In: Danforth D (ed) Obstetrics and Gynaecology, 4th edn. Harper and Row, Philadelphia

Fernandez H, Bourget P, Ville Y et al 1994 Treatment of unruptured tubal pregnancy with methotrexate: pharmacokinetic analysis of local versus intramuscular administration. Fertility and Sterility 62:943–947

Gazvani MR, Emery SJ 1999 Mifepristone and methotrexate: the combination for medical treatment of ectopic pregnancy. American Journal of Obstetrics and Gynecology 180(6 Pt 1):1599–1600

Gemzell C, Guillome J, Wang EF 1982 Ectopic pregnancy following treatment with human gonadotropins. American Journal of Obstetrics and Gynecology 143(7):761–765

Goldner TE, Lawson HW, Xia Z et al 1993 Surveillance for ectopic pregnancy – United States 1970–1989. Morbidity and Mortality Weekly Report 42(6):73–85

Hajenius PJ, Mol BW, Bossuyt PM et al 2000 Interventions for tubal ectopic pregnancy. Cochrane Database of Systematic Reviews. Issue 2

Harika G, Gabriel R, Carre-Pigeon F et al 1995 Primary application of three-dimensional ultrasonography to early diagnosis of ectopic pregnancy. European Journal of Obstetrics Gynecology and Reproduction Biology 60(2):117–120

Hofmann HM, Urdl W, Holfer H et al 1987 Cervical pregnancy: case reports and current concepts in diagnosis and treatment. Archives of Gynecology and Obstetrics 241(1):63–69

Hreschchyshyn MM, Naples JD, Randall CL 1965 Amethopterin in abdominal pregnancy. American Journal of Obstetrics and Gynecology 93:286–287

Jurkovic D, Bourne TH, Jauniaux E et al 1992 Transvaginal color Doppler study of blood flow in ectopic pregnancies. Fertility and Sterility 57(1):68–73

Kadar N, Romero R 1988 Serial human chorionic gonadotrophin measurements in ectopic pregnancy. American Journal of Obstetrics and Gynecology 158(5):1239–1240

Kadar N, Caldwell BV, Romero R 1981 A method of screening for ectopic pregnancy and its indications. Obstetric and Gynecology 58(2):162–166

Kamwendo F, Forslin L, Bodin L et al 2000 Epidemiology of ectopic pregnancy during a 28 year period and the role of pelvic inflammatory disease. Sexually Transmitted Infections 76(1):28–32

Knoll M, Talbot P 1998 Cigarette smoke inhibits oocyte cumulus complex pick-up by the oviduct ciliary beat frequency. Reproductive Toxicology 12(2):57–68

Li MC, Nerts R, Spence DB 1956 Effect of methotrexate therapy on choriocarcinoma and chorioadenoma. Proceedings of the Society for Experimental Biology and Medicine 93:361–366

Marchbanks PA, Coulman CB, Annegers JF 1985 An association between clomiphene citrate and ectopic pregnancy: a preliminary report. Fertility and Sterility 44(2):268–270

Marcus SF, Brinsden PR 1993 Primary ovarian pregnancy after in vitro fertilisation and embryo transfer: report of seven cases. Fertility and Sterility 60(1):167–169

McBain JC, Evans JH, Pepperell RJ et al 1980 An unexpectedly high rate of ectopic pregnancy following the induction of ovulation with human pituitary and chorionic gonadotrophin. British Journal of Obstetrics and Gynaecology 87(1):5–9

McCausland A 1980 High rate of ectopic pregnancy following laparoscopic tubal coagulation failure: incidence and etiology. American Journal of Obstetrics and Gynecology 136(1):97–101

Ory HW 1981 Ectopic pregnancy and intrauterine contraceptive devices: new perspectives. The Women's Health Study. Obstetrics and Gynecology 57(2):137–144

O'Shea RT, Thompson GR, Harding A 1994 Intra-amniotic methotrexate versus CO_2 laser laparoscopic salpingotomy in the management of tubal ectopic pregnancy – a prospective randomized trial. Fertility and Sterility 62(4):876–878

Perdu M, Camus E, Rozenberg P et al 1988 Treating ectopic pregnancy with the combination of mifeperistone and methotrexate: a phase II nonrandomized study. American Journal of Obstetrics and Gynecology 179(pt 3):640–643

Persaud V 1970 Etiology of tubal ectopic pregnancy. Radiologic and pathologic studies. Obstetrics and Gynecology 36(2):257–263

Pulkkinen MO, Talo A 1987 Tubal physiologic consideration in ectopic pregnancy. Clinical Obstetrics and Gynecology 30(1):164–172

Rajkhowa M, Glass MR, Rutherford AJ et al 2000 Trends in the incidence of ectopic pregnancy in England and Wales from 1966–1996. British Journal of Obstetrics and Gynaecology 107(3):369–374

Rempen A 1998 The shape of the endometrium evaluated with three-dimensional ultrasound: an additional predictor of extrauterine pregnancy. Human Reproduction 13(2):450–454

Royal College of Obstetricians and Gynaecologists 1999 The management of tubal pregnancies. Guideline no. 21. RCOG, London

Shalev E, Peleg D, Bustan M et al 1995 Limited role for intratubal methotrexate treatment of ectopic pregnancy. Fertility and Sterility 63:20–24

Singhal V, Li TC, Cooke ID 1991 An analysis of factors influencing the outcome of 232 consecutive tubal micro surgery cases. British Journal of Obstetrics and Gynaecology 98(7):628–636

Smith HO, Toledo AA, Thompson JD 1987 Conservative surgical management of isthmic ectopic pregnancies. American Journal of Obstetrics and Gynecology 157(3):604–610

Spiegelberg O 1878 Zur casuistik der ovarialschwangerschaft. Archives of Gynecology 13:73–77

Stabile I 1996a Clinical presentation of ectopic pregnancy. In: Stabile I (ed) Ectopic pregnancy: diagnosis and management. Cambridge University Press, Cambridge

Stabile I 1996b Biochemical diagnosis of ectopic pregnancy. In: Stabile I (ed) Ectopic pregnancy: diagnosis and management. Cambridge University Press, Cambridge

Stovall TG 1995 Medical management should be routinely used as primary therapy for ectopic pregnancy. Clinical Obstetrics and Gynecology 38(2):346–352

Stovall TG, Ling FW 1993 Ectopic pregnancy. Diagnostic and therapeutic algorithms minimizing surgical intervention. Journal of Reproduction Medicine 38(10):807–812

Svensson I, Mardh PA, Ahigren M et al 1985 Ectopic pregnancy and antibodies to chlamydia trachomatis. Fertility and Sterility 44:313–317

Tait T 1884 Five cases of extrauterine pregnancy operated upon at the time of rupture. British Medical Journal 1:1250–1251

Tanaka T, Hayashi H, Kutsuzawa T et al 1982 Treatment of interstitial ectopic pregnancy with methotrexate: report of a successful case. Fertility and Sterility 37(6):851–852

Tharaux-Deneux C, Bouyer J, Job-Spira N et al 1998 Risk of ectopic pregnancy and previous induced aborton. American Journal of Public Health 88(3):401–405

Tulandi T, Guralnick M 1991 Treatment of tubal ectopic pregnancy by salpingotomy with or without tubal suturing and salpingectom. Fertility and Sterility 55(1):53–55

Vessey MP, Johnson B, Doll R et al 1974 Outcome of pregnancy in women using an intrauterine device. Lancet 1(7856):495–498

Westrom L, Bengtsson LP, Mardh PA 1981 Incidence, trends and risks of ectopic pregnancy in a population of women. British Medicine Journal 282:(6257):15–18

Weyerman PC, Verhoeven AT, Alberda AT 1989 Cervical pregnancy after in vitro fertilisation and embryo transfer. American Journal of Obstetrics and Gynecology 161(5):1145–1146

Wollen AL, Flood PR, Sandvei R et al 1984 Morphological changes in tubal mucosa associated with the use of intrauterine contraceptive devices. British Journal of Obstetrics and Gynaecology 91(11):1123–1128

Yao M, Tulandi T 1997 Current status of surgical and nonsurgical managment of ectopic pregnancy. Fertility and Sterility 67(3):421–433

27

Hirsutism and virilization

Carole Gilling-Smith   Stephen Franks

INTRODUCTION

Hirsutism is defined as the excessive growth of terminal hair in a typical male pattern distribution. Virilization refers to more severe effects of hyperandrogenism in a female, including male hair pattern and body habitus, clitoromegaly, increased libido, deepening of the voice and increased muscle mass. Since androgens are the principal endocrine regulators of terminal hair growth, hirsutism may be caused by increased androgen production by the ovaries and/or adrenal glands, increased target tissue sensitivity to androgens or an increase in the level of biologically active free circulating androgens. Virilization usually results from a rapidly growing, androgen-producing tumour or use of certain androgenic drugs.

The key to successful diagnosis and treatment of any problem depends on understanding the pathogenesis of the condition. This chapter reviews the biology of hair growth and androgen metabolism in the female before presenting a systematic approach to diagnosis and therapeutic management.

BIOLOGY OF HAIR GROWTH

Hair follicles start to develop from the epidermis between 8 and 10 weeks of intrauterine life and the total complement of hair follicles is reached by 22 weeks. Hair cells are formed from the dermal papilla at the base of the hair follicle. The column of dead, keratinized cells so formed elongates to form a hair shaft consisting of a central medulla of loosely connected cells surrounded by a cortex of compressed cells and a hard external cuticle. Sebaceous glands are connected to the hair follicle. Hair colour is provided by the pigment melanin, produced in the medulla. If the dermal papilla is damaged or degenerates, there will be no further hair growth from that follicle.

The hair cycle

Hair grows in cyclical fashion with alternate growing and resting phases, as shown in Figure 27.1. In telogen, the resting phase, the hair is short and the follicle inactive. Anagen, the active growing phase, involves rapid division of the basal matrix cells and upward extension of the hair shaft. During catagen, the bulb shrivels and the hair is shed. Final hair length on different parts of the body is determined by the relative duration of each phase. Scalp hair has a relatively long anagen of 3 years and only a short telogen. Conversely, on other parts of the body, the hair has a long telogen and short anagen phase, resulting in much shorter hair.

Normally, hair growth is asynchronous. Pregnancy and certain drugs can increase the synchrony of hair growth, resulting in periodic growth and shedding.

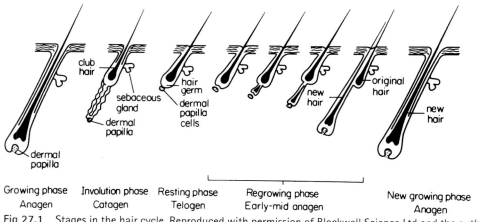

Fig 27.1   Stages in the hair cycle. Reproduced with permission of Blackwell Science Ltd and the author from Randall (1994).

Types of hair

1. Lanugo hair is lightly pigmented, short, fine hair which covers the fetal body until about 7 months of intrauterine life.
2. Vellus hair is fine downy hair which covers most of the body during the prepubertal period.
3. Terminal hair is coarse, pigmented hair which grows on certain parts of the body, primarily during adult years.
4. Sexual hair is terminal hair which responds specifically to sex steroids and characteristically grows on the face, chest, axillae, pubic area, lower abdomen and anterior thighs.

Hirsutism in characterized by the conversion of vellus to sexual hair, primarily under the influence of androgens, in a male-pattern distribution. This is in contrast to hypertrichosis in which there is excessive growth of fine lanugo hair in a non-androgenic pattern, a condition often resulting from the use of certain drugs, starvation (anorexia) or malignancy.

Genetic and ethnic influences on hair growth

The number of hair follicles per unit area of skin is genetically predetermined. Significant differences exist between races, e.g. Caucasian women have significantly more hair follicles than their oriental counterparts. More importantly, with respect to management, body hair which may be socially acceptable to a Mediterranean woman may be a source of great distress to a woman of Nordic descent.

Hormonal influences on hair growth

1. Androgens are the principal hormonal regulators of hair growth. They initiate growth and increase the diameter and pigmentation of the hair column of facial, axillary and pubic hair. Conversely, on the scalp, they cause regression of terminal hair to vellus hair to produce androgenic alopecia or male-pattern balding in genetically susceptible individuals (Randall 1994). These two opposing actions of androgens are illustrated in Figure 27.2.
2. Oestrogens reduce the rate of hair growth, resulting in finer, less pigmented hair.

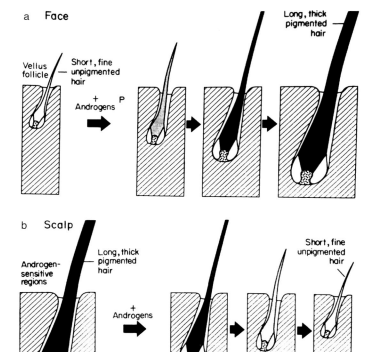

Fig 27.2   Effect of androgens on hair follicles. a In areas stimulated by androgens, e.g. face. b On scalp of genetically predisposed individuals. Reproduced with permission of Blackwell Science Ltd and the author from Randall (1994).

3. Progestogens have a variable effect on hair growth depending on their androgenic potency.

During pregnancy the combined effect of high oestrogen and progesterone can increase the synchrony of hair growth such that some women experience increased hair growth whilst others notice loss of hair.

Generalized endocrine disturbances can affect hair growth

through an indirect effect on either adrenal or ovarian hormone secretion. In hypopituitarism, hair growth may slow down; conversely hirsutism develops in 15% of acromegalics and is also associated with Cushing's disease and hyper-prolactinaemia.

Non-hormonal influences on hair growth

Hair growth is affected by skin temperature and blood flow and therefore is faster during the summer months. Central nervous system lesions such as cranial trauma or encephalitis may enhance growth. Certain non-hormonal drugs, e.g. phenytoin, may produce hirsutism.

ANDROGEN BIOSYNTHESIS AND METABOLISM IN THE FEMALE

The principal circulating androgens are testoterone and its metabolite dihydrotestosterone (DHT), androstenedione, dehydroepiandrosterone (DHA) and dehydroepiandrosterone sulphate (DHAS). All are C19 steroids derived from the conversion of cholesterol in either the ovaries or adrenals. DHT is the most biologically potent, followed by testosterone. Androstenedione, DHA and DHAS are comparatively weak androgens, with minimal effect on skin and hair growth under normal circumstances.

In the normal female, 25% of the circulating testosterone is produced by the ovary and 25% by the adrenal cortex. The remainder is derived from peripheral conversion of androstenedione. Of the circulating androstenedione, 50% is produced by the ovary and 50% by the adrenal. In contrast the adrenal secretes 90% of the DHA and virtually all the DHAS (Fig. 27.3). DHT is derived exclusively from the peripheral conversion of circulating testosterone and androstenedione in target tissues, principally in the liver and skin, in a reaction catalysed by the enzyme 5α-reductase.

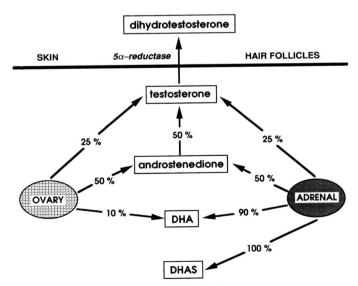

Fig 27.3   Ovarian and adrenal contributions to circulating androgens. (DHA, dehydroepiandrosterone; DHAS, dehydroepiandrosterone sulphate.)

Factors affecting the concentration of circulating androgens

Both testosterone and DHT circulate partly in a free state and partly bound to either albumin or to a β-globulin called sex hormone-binding globulin (SHBG) (Anderson 1974). DHA, DHAS and androstenedione are not significantly protein bound. In the case of testosterone, 80% is bound to SHBG, 19% is weakly bound to albumin and 1% is unbound. Since the biological effect of circulating androgens depends primarily on the unbound fraction, care needs to be taken when interpreting the results of serum testosterone concentration tests as these will measure both protein-bound and free hormone. It is not unusual therefore to find a normal total testosterone concentration in a hirsute woman. Nevertheless, it is not helpful, clinically, to measure non-SHBG testosterone or free testosterone, both of which may also be normal in hirsute subjects.

Liver SHBG production is decreased by both androgens and insulin. In hyperandrogenic, hirsute women, SHBG levels are depressed and the percentage of free testosterone is increased to about 2% (in men the level of free testosterone is about 3%). Hyperinsulinaemia enhances this effect and can exacerbate the degree of hirsutism. Conversely, oestrogens increase SHBG production so that binding is increased in women on oral contraceptives and during pregnancy, often resulting in a reduction of hirsutism.

Androgen action in target tissues

Androgen action in target tissues depends on the interaction of the steroid with intracellular cytoplasmic receptors. The androgen–receptor complex is then transported into the nucleus where it interacts with specific receptor sites on the DNA, thereby influencing protein synthesis. The binding affinity of DHT to the androgen receptor is about 10 times that of testosterone. Hence the conversion of testosterone to DHT by the enzyme 5α-reductase is a key step in androgen action.

These is poor correlation between the presence or severity of hirsutism and serum levels of either testosterone or DHT (Franks 1989). This has prompted considerable interest in the measurement of DHT metabolites such as 3α-androstenediol-glucuronide (adiol-G) and other androgen conjugates. These reflect 5α-reductase activity and in theory should be more sensitive biochemical markers for cutaneous androgen (Greep et al 1986, Horton et al 1982). Although early studies showed an excellent correlation between serum levels of adiol-G and hirsutism (Horton et al 1982, Serafini et al 1985), more recent studies have shown marked overlap in levels between normal and hirsute women (Matteri et al 1989, Thompson et al 1990). Furthermore, studies performed during medical therapy are controversial, some showing no change in adiol-G levels in response to treatment (Lobo et al 1985, Marcondes et al 1992) and others showing good correlation with clinical response (Kirschner et al 1987). These discrepancies are thought, in part, to be related to the fact that circulating adiol-G is not derived exclusively from peripheral DHT metabolism but also reflects both hepatic and adrenal metabolism.

Thus, in practice, androgen conjugates are of little additional benefit over serum testosterone or DHT levels in the clinical

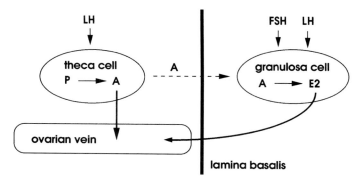

Fig 27.4 Two-cell two-gonadotrophin theory of steroidogenesis. (P, progesterone; A, androstenedione; E2, oestradiol.)

evaluation or management of hyperandrogenism (Rittmaster 1993).

Ovarian androgen production

The specialized steroid-secreting cells of the ovary are the theca and granulose cells. Theca cells convert cholesterol to androstenedione under the stimulation of pituitary luteinizing hormone (LH). Androstenedione crosses the basement membrane to the avascular granulosa layer where follicle-stimulating hormone (FSH) and, in the preovulatory follicle, both FSH and LH stimulate aromatization of androgens. This is referred to as the two-cell two-gonadotrophin theory of steroidogenesis (Fig. 27.4). Theca cell androgen production varies during the ovarian cycle in parallel with development of the dominant follicle and corpus luteum, but cyclical changes of androstenedione and testosterone in the peripheral circulation are not very great, showing a small midcycle increment only.

Adrenal androgen production

Adrenal androgens are secreted by the zona fasciculata and zona reticularis under ACTH stimulation. During prepubertal life, adrenal androgen secretion remains low until adrenarche, during which there is a selective increase in secretion of androgenic steroids leading to pubic and axillary hair development. This heralds the onset of puberty which is associated with the growth spurt, breast development and finally menarche. Adrenal androgen secretion continues to rise for a short while after puberty but then plateaus until the menopause, when it declines slowly. In contrast to ovarian androgen production, which is minimal, the adrenal gland becomes the main source of both androgen and oestrogen production in the postmenopausal woman.

The biosynthetic pathways of ovarian and adrenal androgen metabolism are summarized in Figure 27.5. In summary, hirsutism may result from any one or a combination of these factors:

1. increased circulating androgens derived from the ovaries or adrenals
2. increased percentage of unbound testosterone reflecting decreased levels of SHBG
3. increased peripheral conversion of testosterone to DHT reflecting increased 5α-reductase activity
4. genetic or racial predisposition for an increased number of hair follicles per unit of skin area.

OTHER CUTANEOUS SIGNS OF HYPERANDROGENAEMIA

Although hirsutism is the commonest cutaneous manifestation of hyperandrogenaemia, increased circulating androgens affect the entire pilosebaceous unit and acne and increased oiliness of the skin are commonly reported. Up to 60% of women with acne have increased peripheral 5α-reductase activity (Carmina & Lobo 1993).

As previously discussed, in some women the principal effect of androgenization is to decrease scalp hair, resulting in temporal recession and, in severe cases, frontal balding. This is referred to as male-pattern or androgen-dependent alopecia. Although alopecia may be due to a period of synchronous hair growth and shedding or even drugs, its persistence beyond 6 months to a year warrants investigation for underlying hyperandrogenaemia.

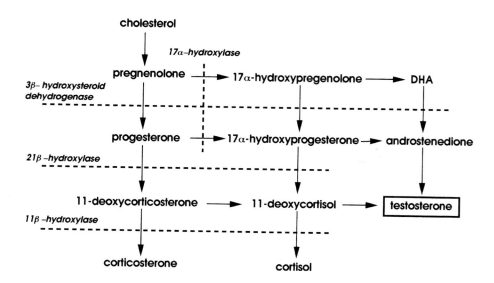

Fig 27.5 Ovarian and adrenal androgen biosynthesis.

Table 27.1 Principal causes of hirsutism

1. *Ovarian*	Polycystic ovary syndrome (PCOS)
	Tumour
	— Sex-cord stromal cell
	— Adrenal-like
2. *Adrenal*	Congenital adrenal hyperplasia
	Tumour
	— Adenoma
	— Adenocarcinoma
3. *Pituitary*	Tumour
	— ACTH secreting → Cushing's disease
	— Growth hormone-secreting → acromegaly
4. *Ectopic ACTH*	Tumour
	— Bronchus
	— Pancreas
	— Thyroid
	— Thymus
5. *Iatrogenic*	Androgenic drugs
	— Testosterone
	— Danazol
	— Glucocorticoids
6. *Idiopathic*	

Acanthosis nigricans is a grey-brown velvety discoloration of the skin usually found in the axillae, neck and groin. It is a characteristis cutaneous manifestation of hyperinsulinaemia often found in association with obesity (Dunaif et al 1991).

CAUSES OF HIRSUTISM

The principal causes of hirsutism are listed in Table 27.1.

Polycystic ovary syndrome (PCOS)

This syndrome, first described by Stein & Leventhal (1935), is a heterogeneous disorder, both clinically and biochemically (Conway et al 1989, Franks 1989). Classic features of anovulation, hirsutism and obesity are variably expressed and serum levels of LH and testosterone are elevated in only 50% of cases. Recent advances in ultrasound imaging have made it a reliable means of identifying polycystic ovaries (PCO) (Adams et al 1986) and this is now used in preference to endocrine indices alone in making the diagnosis of PCOS (Gilling-Smith & Franks 1993). Using pelvic ultrasound, the prevalence of PCO in different populations of women has been extensively studied. Although PCO are found in up to 20% of normal women (Polson et al 1988), they have a much higher prevalence in women with androgen-related disorders such as acne, hirsutism and alopecia (Adams et al 1986, Conway et al 1989, O'Driscoll et al 1994) as well as being the commonest cause of anovulation (Adams et al 1986). However, many women presenting with hirsutism have regular menstrual cycles, while those with cycle disturbance often show no clinical signs of hyperandrogenaemia.

The relative importance of PCOS in the differential diagnosis of hirsutism has, until recently, remained controversial. In the largest prospective study to date, of 350 women presenting with hirsutism and/or androgenic alopecia, 60% (170/350) had PCO on ultrasound. By comparison only eight women had other clearcut causes (mainly adrenal) for their hyperandrogenaemia, of whom three coincidentally had PCO. The remainder had normal ovaries and were therefore classified as having idiopathic hirsutism (O'Driscoll et al 1994). Jahanfar & Eden (1993) reported an even higher incidence of ultrasound PCO in their series of 173 women presenting with hirsutism, ranging from 86% in the ovulatory group to 97% in the non-ovulatory group, casting doubt on the existence of the condition 'idiopathic hirsutism'. In a similar study, 83% of women presenting with acne vulgaris were found to have ultrasound polycystic ovaries (Bunker et al 1989). These data clearly identify PCOS as the single most common cause of hirsutism, acne or alopecia, in contrast to adrenal, pituitary or other ovarian causes, which are relatively rare.

Source of androgen excess in PCOS

The relative role of ovarian and adrenal androgens in the pathogenesis of PCOS remains a subject of considerable debate. Selective venous catheterization of ovarian and adrenal veins has produced controversial results, primarily due to methodological difficulties (Azziz 1993). Adrenal androgen secretion is episodic and sampling should ideally be serial. Furthermore, the stress induced by such invasive techniques necessarily tends to increase adrenal secretion. Similarly, selective adrenal suppression by glucocorticoids has not yielded useful information (Azziz 1993). Conversely, studies measuring serum androgens, following either ovarian wedge resection (Katz et al 1978) or laparoscopic ovarian diathermy (Aakvaag & Gjonnaess 1985, Greenblatt & Casper 1987) in hyperandrogenic women with PCOS have provided more direct evidence for an ovarian role. Both treatments produce a significant fall in both androstenedione and testosterone within 3–4 days of ovarian tissue reduction. More recently, Barnes has demonstrated an exaggerated ovarian androgen response to the acute administration of a long-action gonadotrophin hormone-releasing hormone analogue (GnRH-A) in women with PCO compared to normal controls. On the basis of these data, this group has proposed that PCOS results from dysregulation of the key enzyme involved in theca cell androgen biosynthesis, P450c17α (Barnes et al 1989).

In some series, up to 50% of women with hirsutism in association with PCOS have been shown to have elevated DHAS levels, suggesting an adrenal component to their hyperandrogenaemia. However, obesity may be an independent effect on elevating serum levels of DHAS and thus the prevalence of raised DHAS concentration is likely to reflect the proportion of obese subjects in these series. In our own series of subjects with PCOS, 35% of whom were overweight, fewer than 10% had higher than normal serum levels of DHAS. Furthermore, ACTH levels are within the normal range in PCOS (Horrocks et al 1983) and, in the absence of coexisting adrenal pathology such as CAH or Cushing's syndrome, the adrenal response to ACTH stimulation is not significantly different from that in control populations (Hudson et al 1990).

If, as is suggested by the above data, the underlying cause of PCOS is an abnormality of ovarian androgen production, the obvious question must be, is this a primary event or one which is secondary to the increased pituitary LH secretion? Several investigators have addressed this issue by studying the effect of

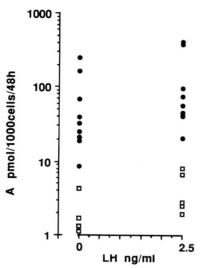

Fig 27.6 Comparison of androstenedione (A) accumulation from five normal (□) and nine polycystic (●) ovaries under basal and LH-stimulated conditions during the first 48h of culture. Each data point is the average of duplicate or triplicate experiments. The plating density range was 10–15 × 10⁴ cells/well. Reproduced with permission from Gilling-Smith et al (1994).

stimulating the ovary with human chorionic gonadotrophin (hCG), the bioequivalent of LH. Most studies show no significant increase in androgenic responsiveness to hCG in PCO women (Abraham et al 1975, Rosenfield et al 1972, Gilling-Smith et al 1997). More importantly, if hCG is administered after endogenous LH levels have first been suppressed by GnRH-A, androstenedione and testosterone levels remain significantly higher in the PCO women, while DHAS levels, unaltered by the effect of the GnRH-A, remain similar in both groups (Gilling-Smith et al 1997), suggesting a primary ovarian disturbance in androgen secretion.

In view of the ovarian morphology, hyperandrogenaemia in PCOS could be due simply to increased follicle number or theca cell hyperplasia. However, in vitro studies have found that human theca cells isolated from polycystic ovaries produce significantly more androstenedione per cell than theca from normal ovaries, although the magnitude of response to LH is similar, as shown in Figure 27.6 (Gilling-Smith et al 1994). These data are consistent with the hypothesis that PCOS results from a primary abnormality of androgen biosynthesis and hence, effective therapy should be directed primarily against ovarian, not adrenal, androgen production.

The role of insulin and insulin-like growth factors (IGFs)
Both insulin and the IGFs have been shown to potentiate the actions of LH on theca cell androgen production in vitro (Bergh et al 1993). However, there appears to be no difference between PCO and normal ovaries in the response to these factors, either in vitro or in vivo (Franks et al 1994, Gilling-Smith et al 1993). Hyperinsulinaemia and insulin resistance are features of anovulatory women with PCOS and both are exacerbated in the presence of obesity (Sharp et al 1991). Body mass index (BMI) is positively correlated to serum insulin and testosterone levels and inversely correlated to SHBG levels.

Weight loss results in a fall in circulating insulin and testosterone levels and a significant improvement in symptoms (Kiddy et al 1990, 1992).

Idiopathic hirsutism

This is defined as hirsutism in women with regular cycles, normal ovaries on ultrasound and no identifiable pathology to account for the symptoms. A recent report would suggest the true incidence of this condition to be far lower than previously described (Jahanfar & Eden 1993). Both free and total serum testosterone levels are often elevated and SHBG levels suppressed.

As with PCOS, there is controversy over whether the source of excess circulating androgens is adrenal or ovarian. In contrast to PCOS, LH levels are within the normal range and the response to GnRH-A is normal.

The most likely explanation for excessive hair growth in these women is increased end-organ sensitivity to normal androgen levels, possibly secondary to increased 5α-reductase activity. This argument is supported by the observation that there is an inverse correlation between adiol-G levels and clinical response to medical therapy (Kirschner et al 1987).

Late-onset congenital adrenal hyperplasia

Congenital adrenal hyperplasia (CAH) is caused by an enzyme deficiency resulting in an inability or reduced capacity to synthesize glucocorticoids. In response to the low cortisol levels, ACTH levels rise, increasing secretion of both androgens and glucocorticoid precursors and producing hyperplasia of the adrenal cortex. In the majority of cases, the condition is inherited in an autosomal recessive mode and presents, in its most severe form, at birth with virilization of the female external genitalia. Late-onset CAH represents a milder form, which often does not present until childhood or early adult life and is thought to affect up to 5% of women with hirsutism (Kuttenn et al 1985). The majority of cases are characterized by partial 21-hydroxylase deficiency, although other enzyme defects can occur. Features suggestive of late-onset CAH worth noting are onset of hirsutism at or shortly after puberty, a strong family history of hirsutism and serum testosterone levels greater than 5 nmol/l. Diagnosis is based on the short Synacthen test in which 17α-hydroxyprogesterone and cortisol levels are measured before, and 1 hour after, the administration of a single dose (250 µg IM or IV) of synthetic ACTH.

The coexistence of PCO on ultrasound has been reported to be as high as 83% in adult females with CAH (Hague et al 1990). As in Cushing's syndrome, it is likely that the ovarian changes occur secondarily to the elevation in adrenal androgens, but these figure emphasize the importance of ACTH testing in women with PCOS with markedly elevated testosterone levels.

Cushing's syndrome

This is due to overproduction of cortisol by the adrenal and may result from the following conditions:

1. overproduction of ACTH by the pituitary (Cushing's disease)
2. ectopic ACTH secretion by a non-pituitary tumour

3. autonomous secretion of cortisol by an adrenal or ovarian tumour
4. ectopic corticotrophin-secreting hormone production (very rare).

Hyperstimulation of the adrenal by ACTH invariably results in varying degrees of hirsutism or alopecia, acne and occasionally virilization. The most useful screening tests for suspected Cushing's syndrome are 24-hour urine free cortisol or an overnight, low-dose (1 mg) dexamethasone suppression test. If these tests prove positive, further investigations should be undertaken, including diurnal serum cortisol and ACTH measurements and a high-dose dexamethasone suppression test (2 mg at night for 5 days). Pituitary-dependent Cushing's disease is characterized by normal or elevated serum levels of ACTH in the face of an elevated diurnal serum level of cortisol, although cortisol is typically suppressed by high-dose dexamethasone. If ACTH levels are undetectable and cortisol not suppressed, this strongly suggests an autonomous adrenal or ovarian tumour, whilst high ACTH levels with failure of cortisol to suppress are consistent with an ectopic source of ACTH.

Further evaluation of the ACTH-producing tumour involves computed tomography (CT) or magnetic resonance imaging (MRI) of the adrenals, chest or pituitary, which is by far the most accurate means of detecting the site of ACTH production. An ectopic ACTH-producing tumour is found in up 15% of cases, typically located in the thorax or abdomen and associated with bilateral adrenal enlargement. In the absence of an adrenal or etopic tumour on imaging, inferior petrosal sinus sampling of the blood draining the pituitary is recommended. In contrast to patients with an ectopic tumour, those with Cushing's disease show a significant rise in ACTH levels after CRH stimulation (Findling et al 1991).

Androgen-producing tumour of the ovary or adrenal

These are extremely rare but should always be excluded in a woman who develops hirsutism or virilization over a short time course, particularly if there are coexisting features of Cushing's syndrome.

Adrenal tumours are divided into the benign adenoma and malignant adenocarcinoma. Typically these are small and impalpable and, in half the reported cases, occur in pre-menopausal women.

Androgen-secreting ovarian tumours comprise less than 1% of all ovarian tumours. Previously these tumours were classified according to their supposed cell of origin. The currently accepted classification has been simplified and divides the tumours into two groups: sex cord stromal cell tumours, formerly knows as androblastomas, arrhenoblastomas or gynandroblastomas, and adrenal-like tumours of the ovary which include luteomas, virilizing lipoid cell tumours, hypernephromas and adrenal rest tumours. The latter are associated with Cushingoid features in 50% of cases. Most androgen-secreting ovarian tumours are benign and they present in young women, typically under the age of 30 (Young & Scully 1985).

Unlike PCOS, in which the hirsutism develops over a period of years and is associated with relatively low testosterone levels (<5 nmol/l), androgen-secreting tumours grow rapidly, resulting in relatively fast onset and progression of both hirsutism and menstrual cycle disturbance. Serum testosterone is usually >5 nmol/l, which is more than twice the upper limit of the normal range (0.5–2.6 nmol/l). Virilization together with serum testosterone concentrations in the male range (>10 nmol/l) are particularly ominous signs. Although androgen production is increased overall, different steroid pathways can be involved, which limits the value of endocrine studies as a method of delineating whether the source of excess androgen production is ovarian or adrenal. The most useful screening tests are serum DHAS and 17α-hydroxyprogesterone levels. Adrenal or adrenal-like ovarian tumours are often associated with elevated DHAS levels (>20 nmol/l), while 17α-hydroxyprogesterone production is specifically increased in CAH, particularly in response to ACTH stimulation. In the presence of elevated DHAS levels, dexamethasone suppression tests are advisable, as described for the investigation of Cushing's syndrome, to exclude ACTH-dependent tumours.

Further evaluation of androgen-producing tumours relies on imaging. Although functional ovarian tumours are often palpable on pelvic examination, ultrasound imaging is always indicated and when an ovarian mass is not present on clinical examination or ultrasound, CT or MRI imaging of both adrenals and ovaries must be carried out (see above). Selective adrenal or ovarian vein sampling is technically demanding and should be restricted to those few cases in which the source of excess androgen secretion remains equivocal after imaging.

Virilization presenting during pregnancy may be associated with a luteoma in which the ovarian stroma shows an exaggerated response to the high levels of hCG. These regress spontaneously postpartum and pose little threat to the pregnancy (Garcia-Bunuel et al 1975). The risk of masculinization of a female fetus is very small since the fetus is protected from excess androgen secretion by the high SHBG levels in the maternal circulation and by the ability of the placenta to metabolize androgens. True androgen-secreting tumours are extremely rare in pregnancy (McClamrock & Adashi et al 1992).

Acromegaly

This condition arises from the excessive secretion of growth hormone by a pituitary adenoma and may occasionally present with hirsutism. Clinical suspicion should be raised if associated symptoms include headaches, arthropathy and carpal tunnel syndrome. Classic signs are an increase in the size of the skull, supraobital ridges and jaw, vertebral enlargement often with kyphosis and spade-shaped hands and feet. Hypertension and diabetes mellitus are present in 10–15% of cases. Investigations, which should be carried out in conjunction with an endocrinologist, include growth hormone (GH) measurements during a standard glucose tolerance test (which, normally, is associated with complete suppression of serum GH), skull X-ray and, where indicated, a CT or MRI scan of the pituitary.

Table 27.2 The Ferriman–Gallwey scoring system

Site	Grade	Definition
Upper lip	1	A few hairs at outer margin
	2	Small moustache at outer margin
	3	Moustache extending halfway from outer margin
	4	Moustache extending to midline
Chin	1	A few scattered hairs
	2	Small concentrations of scattered hairs
	3	Light complete cover
	4	Heavy complete cover
Chest	1	Circumareolar hairs
	2	Additional midline hairs
	3	Fusion of these areas with three-quater cover
	4	Complete cover
Upper back	1	A few scattered hairs
	2	Rather more, still scattered
	3	Light complete cover
	4	Heavy complete cover
Lower back	1	A sacral tuft of hair
	2	With some lateral extension
	3	Three-quarter cover
	4	Complete cover
Upper abdomen	1	A few midline hairs
	2	Rather more, still midline
	3	Half-cover
	4	Full cover
Lower abdomen	1	A few midline hairs
	2	A midline streak of hair
	3	A midline band of hair
	4	An inverted V-shaped growth
Upper arm	1	Sparse growth affecting not more than a quarter of the limb surfaces
	2	More than this, cover still incomplete
	3	Light complete cover
	4	Heavy complete cover
Forearm	1–4	Complete cover of dorsal surface: very light (1) to very heavy (4) growth
Thigh	1–4	As for arm
Leg	1–4	As for arm

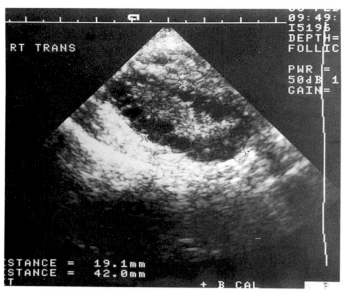

Fig 27.7 Transabdominal ultrasound image of a polycystic ovary (courtesy of Miss D. Kiddy). To make the diagnosis of PCO at least three of the following four features should be present: (i) peripheral distribution of follicles; (ii) 10 or more follicles, typically 2–8 mm in diameter; (iii) increased stroma; (iv) increased ovarian volume (Adams et al 1986).

Iatrogenic hirsutism

A number of drugs may produce hirsutism in susceptible individuals. It is a commonly reported side-effect of danazol, testosterone and glucocorticoids. Drugs which interfere with the hair cycle, such as chemotherapy agents or interferons, will result in hair loss. In either case, there should be a prompt return to normal hair growth once the drug is withdrawn (Tosi et al 1994).

CLINICAL ASSESSMENT

Attention to the patient's general body habitus (height, weight and muscle distribution) is important. This will identify obesity and signs of virilism and, in some cases, classic features of general endocrine disorders such as Cushing's syndrome or acromegaly. If there is coexisting cycle disturbance, careful examination of the breasts (for galactorrhoea) and thyroid should be performed. Care should be taken to exclude any abdominal or pelvic masses and, on pelvic examination, note taken of clitoromegaly. Acanthosis nigricans, typically found in the neck and axillae, is also commonly seen in the vulval region (Grasinger et al 1993).

In the case of patients presenting with hirsutism, a semiquantitative assessment of the degree of hirsutism using the Ferriman–Gallwey chart (Ferriman & Gallwey 1961) is helpful both as a baseline and in subsequent assessment of response to treatment, particularly if follow-up is to be carried out by different clinicians (Table 27.2). Measurements of hair thickness or growth rate require complex equipment and are limited to research trials. Another useful index of growth rate is to ask the patient how frequently various cosmetic measures, such as shaving or waxing, are being carried out and look for a fall once treatment has been initiated.

INVESTIGATIONS

The two most useful initial investigations are a pelvic ultrasound scan, best performed in the early follicular phase in an ovulatory patient, and a serum testosterone, taken at any time in the cycle.

The purpose of ultrasound is to define ovarian morphology and, at the same time, exclude rare androgen-secreting ovarian tumours. The typical features of the polycystic ovary on ultrasound are shown in Figure 27.7.

Total serum testosterone is elevated in only 40% of women with hirsutism and there is considerable variation in levels between individuals. The levels do not correlate well with severity of hirsutism or acne (Conway et al 1989, Franks 1989). Indeed, as previously discussed, serum testosterone

Fig 27.8   Investigation of women presenting with hirsutism or virilization (USS, ultrasound scan; DHAS, dehydroepiandrosterone sulphate; 17OHP, 17α-hydroxyprogesterone; CAH, congenital adrenal hyperplasia.)

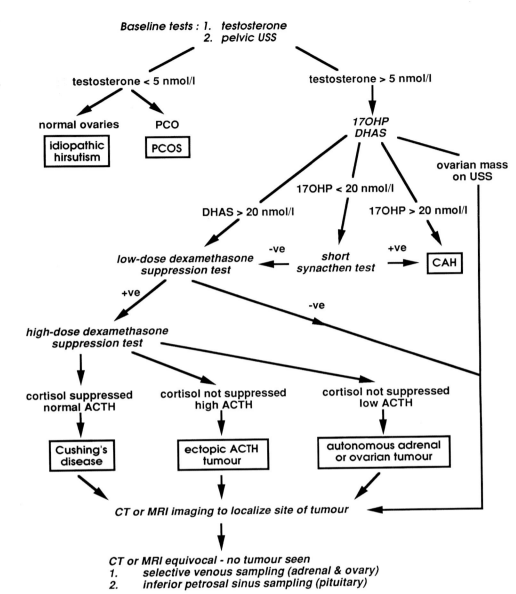

Baseline tests : 1. **testosterone**
                        2. **pelvic USS**

testosterone < 5 nmol/l   **testosterone > 5 nmol/l**

normal ovaries   **PCO**   *17OHP*
                                               DHAS
| idiopathic hirsutism | | PCOS | **ovarian mass on USS**

                                    17OHP < 20 nmol/l
         DHAS > 20 nmol/l   **17OHP > 20 nmol/l**

                              -ve   +ve
low-dose dexamethasone ← *short* → | CAH |
suppression test   *synacthen test*

+ve
                                              -ve
high-dose dexamethasone
suppression test

cortisol suppressed normal ACTH   **cortisol not suppressed high ACTH**   **cortisol not suppressed low ACTH**

| Cushing's disease | | ectopic ACTH tumour | | autonomous adrenal or ovarian tumour |

CT or MRI imaging to localize site of tumour

CT or MRI equivocal - no tumour seen
1.   selective venous sampling (adrenal & ovary)
2.   inferior petrosal sinus sampling (pituitary)

Table 27.3   Steps in the management of hirsutism due to benign causes, i.e. polysyctic ovary syndrome (PCOS) or idiopathic

1. Cosmetic measures
2. Weight reduction (BMI >25 kg/m²)
3. Antiandrogens   ● Cyproterone acetate or Dianette
                          ● Spironolactone
                          ● Flutamide
4. Ovarian suppression   ● Combined oral contraceptives
                          ● GnRH analogues
5. Bilateral oophorectomy

may be within the normal range in markedly hirsute women due to the suppressive effect of androgens and insulin on SHBG levels. However, in such cases, androgen production rate is always increased along with the percentage of unbound, free testosterone. There is no additional benefit to be gained by measuring free testosterone, as women with cutaneous signs of hyperandrogenaemia of sufficient severity to seek medical advice warrant treatment, irrespective of their serum testosterone levels.

The main reason for measuring serum testosterone levels at initial assessment is to exclude more serious disorders of androgen secretion such as CAH, Cushing's or adrenal or ovarian tumours. In women with normal ovaries and idiopathic hirsutism, testosterone levels are usually less than 3 nmol/l while in those with polycystic ovaries, levels greater than 5 nmol/l are rare. If a testosterone level of greater than 5 nmol/l is found, further tests of adrenal function should be performed, along with ultrasound, CT or MRI imaging as summarized in Figure 27.8. If a benign cause for the hirsutism is found and medical treatment initiated, testosterone levels need only be checked in those patients in whom the clinical response is poor. The initial diagnosis should be reviewed and, if appropriate, an alternative treatment offered.

TREATMENT

When possible, this should be directed at treatment of the underlying pathology, e.g adrenal or ovarian tumours should be surgically removed and congenital adrenal hyperplasia treated with corticosteroids. If the cause is iatrogenic, the drug should be stopped.

For the remainder of patients, who will have either PCOS or idiopathic hirsutism, the treatment plan outlined in Table 27.3 should be adopted. First and foremost, it is important to reassure the patient that the underlying cause is benign and self-limiting. In cases of mild hirsutism, cosmestic measures alone are often sufficient but if these fail or the degree of hirsutism is more severe, medical and, in certain cases, surgical treatment should be offered.

Obesity significantly exacerbates the severity of hirsutism and weight loss should therefore be encouraged in subjects who are overweight, preferably prior to therapy but certainly in addition to medical treatment.

Cosmestic treatment

The value of waxing, shaving, electrolysis, the use of depilatory creams and bleaching is often underestimated. With either medical or surgical therapy, androgen levels usually decline rapidly, but the effect on hair growth typically takes 3–6 months to become apparent and often an acceptable improvement is not achieved until after a year of therapy. It is important to forewarn patients of this so that cosmestic measures are continued during this time.

Women concerned that shaving increases the rate of hair growth should be reassured that this is not the case. Electrolysis is the only permanent way of removing hair and gives the best cosmetic result, but it is costly and needs to be performed by an experienced operator to minimize the risk of scarring or infection (Schriock & Schriock 1991).

Antiandrogens

These drugs inhibit androgen action primarily by competing with the androgen receptor in target tissues. They are usually prescribed in combination with oestradiol which has the additional effects of suppressing gonadotrophin production and consequently ovarian androgen production, inhibiting 5α-reductase and stimulating SHBG levels.

Cryproterone acetate (CPA)

This is the most widely prescribed antiandrogen in the UK. It is also a potent progestogen and when prescribed in a reverse sequential regimen for the first 10 days of a 21-day treatment cycle, combined with either a low-dose birth control pill or 30 µg ethinyl oestradiol taken daily, it suppresses ovulation and, in the majority of women, produces regular withdrawal bleeds. The dosage of CPA in the preparation can be varied according to the severity of hirsutism.

In mild to moderate hirsutism Dianette (35 µg ethinyl oestradiol plus 2 mg CPA daily for 21 days) should be prescribed. It is effective in improving symptoms in up to 50% of cases (Prelevic et al 1989) and is a useful 'maintenance' preparation once a response has been achieved with higher doses. If there is no response to Dianette or the hirsutism is more severe (Ferriman–Gallwey score >10), CPA (25–100 mg) should be given for 10 days in each Dianette cycle in a reverse sequential regimen. Over 70% of women treated in this way report a significant improvement in symptoms within 1 year (McKenna 1991). Side-effects of CPA include depression, weight gain and breast tenderness and limit the time for which the higher dose regimens can be tolerated. A review of the literature would suggest that there is no overall benefit to be gained from using higher doses of CPA in preference to Dianette, although the rate of response appears to be faster at higher doses (Jeffcoate 1993). These data are, however, not necessarily consistent with the clinical experience in many centres and most practitioners advocate using higher doses of CPA in more severe cases.

CPA should always be prescribed with either a combined oral contraceptive or an anti-oestrogen in order to suppress ovulation since feminization of a male fetus could occur if a woman conceived when on antiandrogen therapy. If for any reason this is not feasible, alternative contraceptive measures should be taken.

Spironolactone

This is an aldosterone antagonist which also has androgen-receptor blocking activity. Like CPA, it is usually administered with oestrogen or a combined oral contraceptive. It is widely used in the United States, as CPA is not available there, and has been shown to be effective in reducing hair growth and androgen levels (Barth et al 1989, Chapman et al 1985). In the UK the Committee on the Safety of Medicines has not approved its use in the treatment of hirsutism. In the only trial to date comparing spironolactone with CPA, there was no significant difference in response between the two groups (O'Brien et al 1991).

Flutamide

This is a non-steroidal antiandrogen acting on peripheral target tissues which has been used successfully in the treatment of prostatic cancer. There have been few trials evaluating its use in hirsutism but those to date would suggest that, at a daily dose of 500 mg in combination with an oral contraceptive, results are comparable to those with spironolactone (Cusan et al 1994, Erenus et al 1994).

Although, in theory, it may be effective in cases where CPA or spironolactone treatment has proved unsuccessful, our own clinical experience suggests that it is no more efficacious than these more commonly used antiandrogens.

Ketoconazole

This is a synthetic imidazole derivative which blocks gonadal and adrenal steroidogenesis by inhibiting key enzymatic steps in androgen biosynthesis. Data on its role in the management of hirsutism remain controversial. Most trials express concern over marked side-effects (nausea, asthenia and alopecia) which necessitate close monitoring and produce a high drop-out rate (Martikainen et al 1988, Venturoli et al 1990). In addition, clinical response is relatively poor and, in the light of the available data, few would advocate its routine clinical use.

Ovarian suppression

Combined oral contraceptives

The combined low-dose pill provides the simplest means of suppressing pituitary FSH and LH and hence ovarian androgen production. In addition oestrogen stimulates SHBG production by the liver and inhibits 5α-reductase. The choice of progestogen in the preparation is critical. Most progestogens have some androgenic activity and suppress the synthesis of SHBG. For this reason desogestrel- (Porcile & Gallardo 1991) and gestodone-based pills are favoured and should still be considered, despite recent data suggesting a higher risk of thromboembolism with these progestogens. Nevertheless, only 30% of patients will notice an improvement with such formulations, which is why we would only recommend these preparations as second line in cases where Dianette is not tolerated.

GnRH analogues

These have been used to suppress ovarian steroid production in moderate to severe hirsutism and results are comparable to those achieved with CPA. Side-effects of vasomotor symptoms and bone loss limit the duration for which these drugs can be prescribed. However, more recent trials would suggest that low-dose oestrogen replacement therapy may enhance the antiandrogenic effect of the GnRH-A, as well as minimizing the side-effects (Carmina et al 1994).

Adrenal suppression

Glucocorticoids only have a place in the treatment of hirsutism when there is an underlying adrenal component such as late-onset CAH. Dexamethasone (0.25–5.0 mg) taken at night suppresses the morning ACTH surge and hence adrenal androgen production. The dose of glucocorticoid given needs to be monitored carefully and particular care should be taken with obese subjects due to the appetite-stimulating effect of the glucocorticoid.

Interestingly, a randomized trial comparing the use of CPA with hydrocortisone in women with late-onset CAH found that CPA produced a significantly better clinical response: 54% responded in the CPA arm vs 26% in the hydrocortisone arm (Spritzer et al 1990).

5α-Reductase inhibitor

Finasteride is a non-steroidal specific competitive inhibitor of 5α-reductase which has been used with success in the treatment of prostatic hyperplasia. The incidence of side-effects is low and therefore it has potential therapeutic application in the treatment of cutaneous hyperandrogenaemia, particularly in those cases where the predominant feature appears to be end-organ sensitivity to androgens (Sudduth & Koronkowski 1993). Trials to evaluate this compound are awaited, but it should be noted that finasteride is predominantly an inhibitor of type 2 5α-reductase, whereas the enzyme thought to be active in hair follicles is type 1 5α-reductase.

Surgical methods

Surgery has a limited place in the management of hyper-androgenaemia. It should be reserved for those women who have completed their families and in whom long-term steroid therapy is either unacceptable or contraindicated (due to age or cardiovascular risk).

Traditionally, ovarian wedge resection was the only treatment available for PCOS and was found to effectively lower LH and testosterone levels, restore ovarian cyclicity and produce an improvement in hirsutism (Katz et al 1978). Newer, less invasive laparoscopic technique have to a large extent replaced wedge resection since they achieve the same end result but theoretically pose less risk of producing pelvic adhesions. Although they have been shown to be effective in the management of anovulatory subfertility (Armar et al 1990, Gadir et al 1990) the effect on serum androgens appears to be short-lived which limits their application to the management of hirsutism. Bilateral oophorectomy (usually combined with hysterectomy) may, in some cases, be a more appropriate option. The numbers of patients treated in this way, and hence follow-up data, are limited. In our centre, we have performed bilateral oophorectomy in only three cases of severe hirsutism in over 15 years and obtained a satisfactory clinical response in two. A short trial of GnRH analogues may be useful in predicting those cases likely to benefit from surgery.

HIRSUTISM IN THE MENOPAUSAL WOMAN

Hirsutism arising de novo in the menopause should be fully investigated as described earlier and particular care taken to exclude a tumour. CPA remains the therapy of choice for postmenopausal women with PCOS or idiopathic hirsutism and is best prescribed in a reverse sequential regimen with physiological doses of oestrogen (i.e. hormone replacement therapy). A small proportion of women will be found to have ovarian hyperthecosis and their response to antiandrogen treatment is usually poor. The high LH levels associated with ovarian failure may play a role and some benefit may be gained by a course of GnRH-A. Oophorectomy is often the only real long-term solution if the hirsutism is severe.

PSYCHOLOGICAL CONSIDERATIONS

Hirsutism can be an extremely distressing condition, both cosmetically and psychosexually. For this reason, women requesting medical help should always be investigated, counselled as to the underlying cause and offered medical treatment if response to cosmetic measures alone has been inadequate. In more severe cases additional psychotherapy sessions may be beneficial (Sonino et al 1993).

ACNE AND ALOPECIA

The treatment principles outlined above are equally applicable to women with other cutaneous sign of hyperandrogenaemia. Alopecia is best treated with CPA, as described above. In contrast to the significant improvement reported in women with hirsutism, results with alopecia are often poor. GnRH analogues have been used in difficult cases, but again response is poor. Hair loss is usually limited although some women may get full restoration of hair growth.

Acne responds well to Dianette. Higher doses of CPA are often used when there is coexisting hirsutism or alopecia.

Antibiotics (tetracycline derivatives) or retinol derivatives can be used when Dianette is not tolerated, contraception is not required and there is no associated hirsutism or alopecia.

KEY POINTS

1. Hirsutism is the excessive growth of facial and body hair in a male-pattern distribution.
2. It may result from increased androgen production by the ovaries and/or adrenal glands, increased target tissue sensitivity to androgens or an increase in biologically active circulating androgens.
3. Virilization involves more severe features of hyperandrogenism including male body habitus, clitoromegaly, voice deepening and increased libido, and is characteristically associated with androgen-stimulating or- producing tumours or use of androgenic drugs.
4. The commonest cause of hirsutism is PCOS. Diagnosis is based on ultrasound appearance. Serum testosterone is usually elevated (>2.5 nmol/l but <5 nmol/l).
5. All women with a serum testosterone >5 nmol/l should be further investigated to exclude CAH or an androgen-secreting tumour. Investigations should include pelvic ultrasound scan, measurement of serum DHAS and 17α-hydroxyprogesterone levels and, where indicated, CT or MRI imaging of the abdomen and pelvis.
6. The diagnosis of idiopathic hirsutism should be limited to those cases in which there is no identifiable pathology to account for the symptoms; the menstrual cycle is regular, the ovaries normal on ultrasound scan and serum testosterone <5 nmol/l.
7. Medical treatment should be offered to all women with hirsutism due to benign causes in whom cosmetic measures alone have failed.
8. Weight reduction should be encouraged in women with a BMI >25 kg/m^2 prior to starting medical treatment.
9. Cyproterone acetate is the antiandrogen of choice in the management of benign hirsutism, given either in low-dose form as Dianette or at higher doses (25–100 mg) in more severe cases.
10. Ovarian suppression with GnRH analogues should be considered in all cases resistant to cyproterone acetate therapy.

REFERENCES

Aakvaag A, Gjonnaess H 1985 Hormonal response to electrocautery of the ovary in patients with polycystic ovarian disease. British Journal of Obstetrics and Gynaecology 92:1258–1264

Abraham GE, Chakmakjian ZH, Buster JE, Marshall JR 1975 Ovarian and adrenal contributions to peripheral androgens in hirsute women. Obstetrics and Gynecology 46:169–173

Adams J, Polson DW, Franks S 1986 Prevalence of polycystic ovaries in women with anovulation and idiopathic hirsutism. British Medical Journal 293:355–359

Anderson DC 1974 Sex hormone binding globulin. Clinical Endocrinology 3:69–73

Armar NA, McGarrigle HH, Honour J, Holownia P, Jacobs HS, Lachelin GC 1990 Laparoscopic ovarian diathermy in the management of anovulatory infertility in women with polycystic ovaries: endocrine changes and clinical outcome. Fertility and Sterility 53:45–49

Azziz R 1993 The role of the ovary in the genesis of hyperandrogenism. In: Adashi EY, Leung PCK (eds) The ovary. Raven Press, New York, pp 581–605

Barnes RB, Rosenfield RL, Burstein S, Ehrmann DA 1989 Pituitary–ovarian responses to nafarelin testing in the polycystic ovary syndrome. New England Journal of Medicine 320:559–565

Barth JH, Cherry CA, Wojnarowski F, Drawber RPR 1989 Spironolactone is an effective and well tolerated systemic anti-androgen therapy for hirsute women. Journal of Clinical Endocrinology and Metabolism 68:966–970

Bergh C, Carlsson B, Olsson J-H, Selleskog U, Hillensjo T 1993 Regulation of androgen production in cultured human thecal cells by insulin-like growth factor 1 and insulin. Fertility and Sterility 59:323–331

Bunker CB, Newton JA, Kilborn et al 1989 Most women with acne have polycystic ovaries. British Journal of Dermatology 121:675–680

Carmina E, Lobo RA 1993 Evidence for increased androsterone metabolism in some normoandrogenic women with acne. Journal of Clinical Endocrinology and Metabolism 76:1111–1114

Carmina E, Janni A, Lobo RA 1994 Physiological estrogen replacement may enhance the effectiveness of the gonadotrophin-releasing hormone agonist in the treatment of hirsutism. Journal of Clinical Endocrinology and Metabolism 78:126–130

Chapman MG, Dowsett M, Dewhurst CG, Jeffcoate SL 1985 Spironolactone in combination with an oral contraceptive: an alternative treatment for hirsutism. British Journal of Obstetrics and Gynaecology 92:983–985

Conway GS, Honour JW, Jacobs HS 1989 Heterogeneity of the polycystic ovary syndrome: clinical, endocrine and ultrasound features in 556 patients. Clinical Endocrinology 30:459–470

Cusan L, Dupont A, Gomez JL, Tremblay RR, Labrie F 1994 Comparison of flutamide and spironolactone in the treatment of hirsutism: a randomized controlled trial. Fertility and Sterility 61:281–287

Dunaif A, Green G, Phelps RG, Lebwohl M, Futterweit W, Lewy L 1991 Acanthosis nigricans, insulin action, and hyperandrogenism: clinical, histological, and biochemical findings. Journal of Clinical Endocrinology and Metabolism 73:590–595

Erenus M, Gurbuz O, Durmusoglu F, Demircay Z, Pekin S 1994 Comparison of the efficacy of spironolactone versus flutamide in the treatment of hirsutism. Fertility and Sterility 61:613–616

Ferriman D, Gallwey JD 1961 Clinical measurement of body hair growth in women. Journal of Clinical Endocrinology and Metabolism 21:1440–1447

Findling JW, Kehoe ME, Shaker JL, Raff H 1991 Routine inferior petrosal sinus sampling in the differential diagnosis of adrenocorticotropin (ACTH) dependent Cushing's syndrome: early recognition of the occult ectopic ACTH syndrome. Journal of Clinical Endocrinology and Metabolism 73:408–413

Franks S 1989 Polycystic ovary syndrome: a changing perspective. Clinical Endocrinology 31:87–120

Franks S, Willis D, Hamilton-Fairley D, White DM, Mason HD 1994 The evidence against a role for the growth hormone/insulin-like growth factor system in the polycystic ovary syndrome. In: Adashi EY, Thorner MO (eds) The somatotrophic axis of the reproductive process in health and disease. Springer-Verlag, New York, pp 220–228

Gadir AA, Mowafi RS, Alnaser HMI, Alrashid AH, Alonezi OM, Shaw RW 1990 Ovarian electrocautery versus human menopausal gonadotrophins and pure follicle stimulating hormone therapy in the treatment of patients with polycystic ovarian disease. Clinical Endocrinology 33:585–592

Garcia-Bunuel R, Berek JS, Woodruff JD 1975 Luteomas of pregnancy. Obstetrics and Gynecology 45:407

Gilling-Smith C, Franks S 1993 Polycystic ovary syndrome. In: Smith S (ed) Reproductive medicine review. Edward Arnold, London, pp 15–32

Gilling-Smith C, Willis D, Mason HD, Franks S 1993 Comparison of androgen production by theca cells from normal and polycystic ovaries. Human Reproduction 8:Abstract 207

Gilling-Smith C, Willis DS, Beard RW, Franks S 1994 Hypersecretion of androstenedione by isolated thecal cells from polycystic ovaries. Journal of Clinical Endocrinology and Metabolism 79:1158–1165

Gilling-Smith C, Story H, Rogers V, Franks S 1997 Evidence for a primary abnormality of thecal cell steroidogenesis in the polycystic ovary syndrome. Clinical Endocrinology 47:93–99

Grasinger CC, Wild RA, Parker IJ 1993 Vulvar acanthosis nigricans: a marker for insulin resistance in hirsute women. Fertility and Sterility 59:583–586

Greenblatt E, Casper RF 1987 Endocrine changes after laparoscopic ovarian cautery in polycystic ovarian syndrome. American Journal of Obstetrics and Gynecology 156:279–285

Greep N, Hoopes M, Horton R 1986 Androstenediol glucuronide plasma clearance and production rates in normal and hirsute women. Journal of Clinical Endocrinology and Metabolism 62:22–27

Hague WM, Adams J, Rodda C et al 1990 The prevalence of polycystic ovaries in patients with congenital adrenal hyperplasia and their close relatives. Clinical Endocrinology 33:501–510

Horrocks PM, Kandeel FR, London DR et al 1983 ACTH function in women with the polycystic ovary syndrome. Clinical Endocrinology 19:143–150

Horton R, Lobo RA, Hawks D 1982 Androstenediol glucuronide in plasma: a marker of androgen action. Journal of Clinical Investigation 69:1203–1206

Hudson RW, Lochnan HA, Danby FW, Margesson LJ, Strang BK, Kimmett SM 1990 11 beta-hydroxyandrostenedione: a marker of adrenal function in hirsutism. Fertility and Sterility 54:1065–1071

Jahanfar S, Eden JA 1993 Idiopathic hirsutism or polycystic ovary syndrome? Australian and New Zealand Journal of Obstetrics and Gynaecology 33:414–416

Jeffcoate W 1993 The treatment of women with hirsutism. Clinical Endocrinology 39:143–150

Katz M, Carr PJ, Cohen BM, Millar RP 1978 Hormonal effects of wedge resection of polycystic ovaries. Obsterics and Gynecology 52:437–443

Kiddy DS, Sharp PS, White DM et al 1990 Differences in Clinical and endrocrine features between obese and non-obese subjects with polycystic ovary syndrome: an analysis of 263 consecutive cases. Clinical Endocrinology 32:213–220

Kiddy DS, Hamilton-Fairley D, Bush A et al 1992 Improvement in endocrine and ovarian function during dietary treatment of obese women with polycystic ovary syndrome. Clinical Endocrinology 36:105–111

Kirschner MA, Samojlik E, Szmal E 1987 Clinical usefulness of plasma androstenediol glucuronide measurements in women with idiopathic hirsutism. Journal of Clinical Endocrinology and Metabolism 65:597–601

Kuttenn F, Couillin P, Girard F et al 1985 Late-onset adrenal hyperplasia in hirsutism. New England Journal of Medicine 313:224–231

Lobo RA, Shoupe D, Serafini P, Brinton D, Horton R 1985 The effects of two doses of spironolactone on serum androgens and anagen hair in hirsute women. Fertility and Sterility 43:200–205

Marcondes JAM, Minnani SL, Luthold WW, Wajchenberg BL, Samojlik E, Kirschner MA 1992 Treatment of hirsutism in women with flutamide. Fertility and Sterility 57:543–547

Martikainen H, Heikkinen J, Ruokonen A, Kauppila A 1988 Hormonal and clinical effects of ketoconazole in hirsute women. Journal of Clinical Endocrinology and Metabolism 66:987–991

Matteri RK, Stanczyk FZ, Gentzschein EE, Delgado C, Lobo RA 1989 Androgen sulfate and glucuronide conjugates in nonhirsute and hirsute women with polycystic ovary syndrome. American Journal of Obstetrics and Gynecology 161:1704–1709

McClamrock HD, Adashi EY 1992 Gestational hyperandrogenism. Fertility and Sterility 57:257

McKenna TJ 1991 Cyproterone acetate in the treatment of hirsutism. Clinical Endocrinology 35:5–10

O'Brien RC, Cooper ME, Murray RM, Seeman E, Thomas AK, Jerums G 1991 Comparison of sequential cyproterone acetate/estrogen versus spironolactone/oral contraceptive in the treatment of hirsutism. Journal of Clinical Endocrinology and Metabolism 72:1008–1013

O'Driscoll JB, Mamtora H, Higginson J, Pollock A, Kane J, Anderson DC 1994 A prospective study of the prevalence of clear-cut endocrine disorders and polycystic ovaries in 350 patients presenting with hirsutism or androgenic alopecia. Clinical Endocrinology 41:231–236

Polson DW, Adams J, Wadsworth J, Franks S 1988 Polycystic ovaries – a common finding in normal women. Lancet 1:870-872

Porcile A, Gallardo E 1991 Oral contraceptives containing desogestrel in the maintenance of the remission hirsutism: monthly versus bimonthly treatment. Contraception 44:533–539

Prelevic GM, Wurzburger MI, Balint PL, Puzigaca Z 1989 Effects of a low-dose estrogen antiandrogen combination (Diane-35) on clinical signs of androgenization, hormone profile and ovarian size in patients with polycystic ovary syndrome. Gynecological Endocrinology 3:269–280

Randall VA 1994 Androgens and human hair growth. Clinical Endocrinology 40:439–457

Rittmaster RS 1993 Androgen conjugates: physiology and clinical significance. Endocrine Reviews 14:121–132

Rosenfield RL, Ehrlich EN, Clearly RE 1972 Adrenal and ovarian contributions to the elevated free plasma androgen levels in hirsute women. Journal of Clinical Endocrinology 34:92–98

Schriock EA, Schriock ED 1991 Treatment of hirsutism. Clinical Obstetrics and Gynecology 34:852–863

Serafini P, Ablan F, Lobo RA 1985 5α-reductase activity in the genital skin of hirsute women. Journal of Clinical Endocrinology and Metabolism 60:349–355

Sharp PS, Kiddy DS, Reed MJ, Anyaoku V, Johnston DG, Franks S 1991 Correlation of plasma insulin and insulin-like growth factor-I with indices of androgen transport and metabolism in women with polycystic ovary syndrome. Clinical Endocrinology 35:253–257

Sonino N, Fava GA, Mani E, Belluardo P, Boscaro M 1993 Quality of life of hirsute women. Postgraduate Medical Journal 69: 186–189

Spritzer P, Billaud L, Thalabard J-C et al 1990 Cyproterone acetate versus hydrocortisone treatment in late-onset adrenal hyperlasia. Journal of Clinical Endocrinology and Metabolism 70:642–646

Stein IF, Leventhal ML 1935 Amenorrhea associated with bilateral polycystic ovaries. American Journal of Obstetrics and Gynecology 29:181–191

Sudduth SL, Koronkowski MJ 1993 Finasteride: the first 5 alpha-reductase inhibitor. Pharmacotherapy 13:309–325

Thompson DL, Horton N, Rittmaster RS 1990 Androsterone glucuronide is a marker of adrenal hyperandrogenism in hirsute women. Clinical Endocrinology 32:283–292

Tosi A, Misciali C, Piraccini BM, Peluso AM, Bardazzi F 1994 Drug-induced hair loss and hair growth. Incidine, management and avoidance. Drug Safety 10:310–317

Venturoli S, Fabbri R, Dal PL et al 1990 Ketoconazole therapy for women with acne and/or hirsutism. Journal of Clinical Endocrinology and Metabolism 71:335–339

Young RH, Scully RE 1985 Ovarian Sertoli-Leydig cell tumours. A clinicopathological analysis of 207 cases. American Journal of Surgical Pathology 9:543–569

28

Premenstrual syndrome

P.M. Shaughn O'Brien   Khaled M.K. Ismail
Paul Dimmock

INTRODUCTION

Premenstrual syndrome (PMS) is a psychological and somatic disorder of unknown aetiology. However, hormonal and other, possibly neuroendocrine, factors probably contribute (O'Brien 1993, Rapkin et al 1997). Most menstruating women exhibit some premenstrual symptomatology but hormonal differences do not appear to account for the severity of the symptoms seen in some women. There has been a reluctance, until relatively recently, to accept PMS as a serious condition. This has arisen because of a failure to distinguish true PMS from the milder physiological premenstrual symptoms occurring in the normal menstrual cycle of the majority of women.

THE SYNDROME

Premenstrual syndrome was traditionally thought to affect multiparous middle-class articulate women in their late 30s and 40s, the symptoms beginning after childbirth and often following postnatal depression. It is probable, however, that this group of women report their symptoms, whilst younger and less educated women experience equally severe problems but do not recognize them as such.

There is now a trend, especially with psychiatrically trained clinicians, to define PMS in terms of the American Psychiatric Association Diagnostic and Statistical Manual of Mental Disorders (DSM-IV) (American Psychiatric Association 1994). This was late luteal phase dysphoric disorder (LLPDD) in DSM-III and is now premenstrual dysphoric disorder (PMDD) under DSM-IV. Box 28.1 shows the criteria for a DSM-IV PMDD diagnosis. It is important to be clear what is meant by the terms PMDD and PMS as current literature often uses them interchangeably. PMDD is the extreme, predominantly psychological end of the PMS spectrum.

Some patients may additionally have an underlying psychological disorder that coexists with PMS; others self-diagnose PMS but actually have depression unrelated to their cycle. These patients are characterized by the fact that their symptoms fail to resolve after menstruation.

Box 28.1   DSM-IV PMDD diagnostic symptoms

1*	markedly depressed mood, feelings of hopelessness or self-deprecating thoughts
2*	marked anxiety, tension, feelings of being 'keyed up' or 'on edge'
3*	marked affective lability
4*	persistent and marked anger, irritability or increased interpersonal conflicts
5	decreased interest in usual activities
6	subjective sense of difficulty in concentrating
7	lethargy, easy fatigability or lack of energy
8	marked change in appetite
9	hypersomnia or insomnia
10	subjective sense of being overwhelmed or out of control
11	other physical symptoms

*=PMS defining symptoms

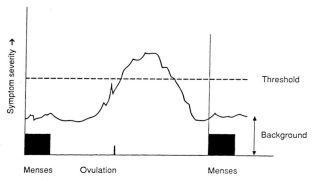

Fig. 28.1 Hypothetical representation of the components of PMS.

Definition

A woman has PMS if she complains of recurrent psychological or somatic symptoms (often both), occurring specifically during the luteal phase of the menstrual cycle and resolving by the end of menstruation. These symptoms are so severe that they disrupt the patient's normal functioning, quality of life and interpersonal relationships. Symptoms must have occurred in at least four of the previous six cycles (Fig. 28.1).

PMDD is defined in the DSM-IV as five or more of the diagnostic symptoms listed in Box 28.1 being present for most of the last week of the luteal phase and remitting within a few days after the onset of the follicular phase. At least one of the symptoms must be from the cluster of PMDD-defining symptoms. The disturbance caused by the symptoms must interfere markedly with work, school or usual social activities and relationships with others. The disturbance must not be an exacerbation of another psychiatric disorder such as major depression disorder, panic disorder, dysthymic disorder or personality disorder.

Prevalence

Only 5% of women are completely free from symptoms premenstrually. At least one premenstrual symptom occurs in 95% of all women of reproductive age; severe, debilitating symptoms (PMS) occur in about 5% of those women (O'Brien 1987) (Fig. 28.2).

SYMPTOMS

An enormous range of symptoms has been described (Box 28.2). The character of the symptoms is less important than their timing and severity.

The classic symptoms of irritability, aggression, depression, tension, bloatedness and mastalgia are well known; there are many others (Box 28.2).

Behavioural changes are also recognized and include suicide, child abuse, examination failures, absence from and poor performance at work, alcohol abuse and criminal acts. Indeed, there have been several legal cases where PMS has been cited in defence of serious crime such as murder. It is also clear that medical disorders such as epilepsy, cardiac disease and asthma worsen premenstrually. Not all of these assertions have been borne out by adequate scientific studies.

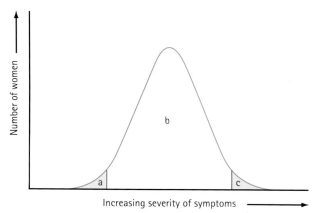

Fig. 28.2 Diagrammatic representation of PMS in the population of women of reproductive age. **a** Represents totally symptom-free women. **b** Represents symptom severity ranges from physiological to moderate PMS. **c** Represents most severe PMS and PMDD.

Box 28.2 Commonly reported symptom groups in women with PMS

Psychological symptoms	Irritability, depression, crying/tearfulness, anxiety, tension, mood swings, lack of concentration, confusion, forgetfulness, unsociableness, restlessness, temper outbursts/anger, sadness/blues, loneliness
Pain symptoms	Headache/migraine, breast tenderness/soreness/breast pain/breast swelling (collectively known as premenstrual mastalgia), back pain, abdominal cramps, general pain
Bloatedness	Weight gain, abdominal bloating, oedema of extremities (arms and legs), abdominal swelling, water retention
Appetite symptoms	Increased appetite, food cravings, nausea
Behavioural symptoms	Fatigue, dizziness, sleep/insomnia, decreased efficiency, accident prone, sexual interest changes, increased energy, tiredness

AETIOLOGY

The definitive aetiology of PMS is not known though it appears to be directly related to the ovarian cycle trigger. The concept of hormonal imbalance has been popular, but there is no supportive evidence. The hormone status of PMS patients does not appear to differ from that of asymptomatic women.

The range of proposed theories is enormous (Fig. 28.3).

Sodium and water retention

There can be few articles on PMS which do not refer to premenstrual sodium and water retention. It is surprising, then, to find few scientific data which demonstrate the phenomenon. Women experience an extremely severe subjective sensation of premenstrual bloatedness in the absence of weight increase, changes in abdominal dimensions or any true water or sodium

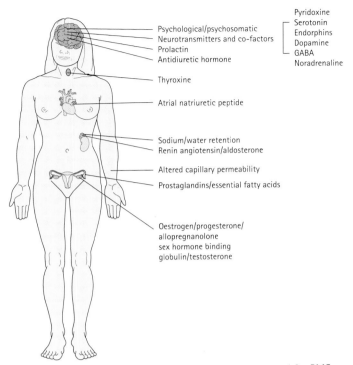

Pyridoxine
Serotonin
Endorphins
Dopamine
GABA
Noradrenaline

Psychological/psychosomatic
Neurotransmitters and co-factors
Prolactin
Antidiuretic hormone

Thyroxine

Atrial natriuretic peptide

Sodium/water retention
Renin angiotensin/aldosterone

Altered capillary permeability

Prostaglandins/essential fatty acids

Oestrogen/progesterone/
allopregnanolone
sex hormone binding
globulin/testosterone

Fig. 28.3 Aetiological theories which have been suggested for PMS.

retention (Faratian et al 1984, Hussain 1994). It seems that bloatedness is either perceived or due to gut distension as a result of progesterone-induced relaxation of the gut muscle. Evidence for this is limited though one study has demonstrated delay in intestinal transit during the luteal phase of the cycle (Wald et al 1981).

Endocrine effects on fluid and electrolytes

Lack of a premenstrual water and electrolyte shift is paralleled by a similar lack of difference in those hormones which control sodium and water transport. The factors which could promote water retention include oestrogen, prolactin, antidiuretic hormone, oxytocin, renin, angiotensin, aldosterone and corticosteroids. Deficiencies of progesterone, atrial natriuretic peptide or renal prostaglandins could also permit water retention by the lack of a natriuretic effect. No clear differences have been demonstrated in any of these, with the exception of atrial natriuretic peptide, which appears to be low in the luteal phase in PMS patients (Hussain et al 1990).

Prostaglandins and essential fatty acids

The ubiquitous nature of the prostaglandins makes them candidates for an aetiological role in PMS. Inhibition of synthesis and enhancement using precursors (essential fatty acids) have been claimed to relieve PMS. The underlying theory on which essential fatty acid supplementation is based is unconvincing. In the absence of a demonstrable endocrine abnormality in PMS a differential sensitivity to the endocrine changes of the ovarian cycle has been suggested. In in vitro studies, interactions at a cellular and receptor level have been demonstrated between polyunsaturated essential fatty acids and the activity of oestrogen and progesterone. Defective essential fatty acid/prostaglandin metabolism may give rise to a breakdown in the normal balance or a change in steroid receptor status, allowing an exaggerated response to normal circulating levels of these different hormone systems (Kosikawa et al 1982).

Investigation of essential fatty acid levels in PMS has produced interesting but as yet inconclusive information. Brush and colleagues (1984) have demonstrated abnormalities in essential fatty acid levels in one study. These findings have not been replicated by others (Menden-Vrtovec & Vujic 1992, O'Brien & Massil 1990).

Prolactin

Prolactin promotes retention of sodium, potassium and water, stimulates the breast and is a so-called stress hormone. Consequently many researchers have investigated its role in PMS. However, prolactin does not undergo change during the cycle; PMS patients have normal levels of prolactin and women with hyperprolactinaemia do not report PMS. Therapeutic studies of bromocriptine show no effect on PMS symptoms, but found limited evidence for treatment of cyclical mastalgia.

Ovarian hormones

It has long been suggested that fluctuation in mood may be related to ovarian hormone imbalance (Dalton 1977). Research has produced data which could support theories of oestrogen excess, progesterone deficiency, oestrogen/progesterone imbalance and progesterone excess. None of these has been confirmed and thus, factors other than differences in the levels of individual hormones must be important. Interactions with other endocrine or biochemical systems may operate or differences in receptor status may be relevant.

A link with ovarian hormone changes, particularly progesterone, seems likely, however, since the temporal relationship between progesterone secretion and symptoms is so close. Ablation of the ovarian endocrine cycle by oophorectomy or more conveniently by the administration of analogues of GnRH is associated with the parallel elimination of PMS symptoms (Hussain et al 1992) (Fig. 28.4). Furthermore, in women whose ovarian cycles have ceased (due to the menopause or bilateral oophorectomy) and who subsequently receive HRT, a significant percentage re-develop PMS symptoms during the progesterone phase of therapy (Hammarback et al 1985).

In a pilot study, women with severe PMS who had undergone hysterectomy and bilateral salpingo-oophorectomy were recruited to assess the effects of hormone replacement on their PMS symptoms (Henshaw et al 1993). During oestrogen-only replacement therapy they remained asymptomatic; when progesterone was administered PMS symptoms recurred (Fig. 28.5), demonstrating fairly clearly that patients remained sensitive to the effects of progesterone.

Investigations of the metabolites of progesterone have shown that women with PMS had lower levels of the

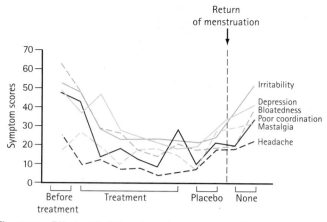

Fig. 28.4 Effect of GnRH analogue on premenstrual symptoms, showing elimination of symptoms whilst ovarian function is suppressed with return of symptoms prior to the return of menstruation during placebo. Adapted from Hussain et al (1992).

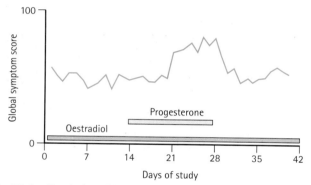

Fig. 28.5 Simulation of PMS symptoms on PMS patients after bilateral oophorectomy and hysterectomy. PMS symptoms recur during progesterone treatment but not during unopposed oestrogen. Adapted from Henshaw et al (1993).

progesterone metabolite allopregnanolone in the luteal phase (Rapkin et al 1997) (Table 28.1). This provides a plausible theory because allopregnanolone has γ-aminobutyric acid (GABA)-ergic activity; deficiency may lose this, giving rise to PMS.

Opioids

Diminished levels of luteal phase β-endorphin have been shown (Chuong et al 1985, Rapkin et al 1996). Symptoms such as anxiety, food craving and physical discomfort have been associated with a significant premenstrual decline in β-endorphin levels (Giannini et al 1994).

Serotonin

The role of serotonin in depression has been extended into PMS research. Low serotonin levels in red cells and platelets (Rapkin 1992) have been demonstrated in PMS patients. This serotonin deficiency has been proposed to enhance sensitivity to progesterone (Rapkin et al 1997). Selective serotonin reuptake

Table 28.1 Progesterone and allopregnanolone (progesterone metabolite) levels through the menstrual cycle. Adapted from Rapkin et al (1997).

Hormone	Day	PMS	Control
Allopregnanolone	19	6.32 ± 1.35	7.70 ± 1.01
	26	3.60 ± 0.75*	7.51 ± 1.25
Progesterone	19	10.66 ± 0.64	8.88 ± 0.79
	26	7.64 ± 0.91	6.39 ± 0.84
Ratio A:P	19	0.68 ± 0.15	1.17 ± 0.25
	26	0.91 ± 0.26*	3.24 ± 1.25

*=statistical significance

inhibitors (SSRIs), such as fluoxetine and sertraline, have been shown to be an extremely efficacious treatment for severe PMS/PMDD (Dimmock et al 2000). This gives further support to the involvement of serotonin in PMS aetiology. Vitamin B6 (pyridoxine) is a co-factor in the final step in the synthesis of serotonin and dopamine from tryptophan. However, no data have yet demonstrated consistent abnormalities either of brain amine synthesis or deficiency of co-factors such as vitamin B6.

Other neurotransmitters may have relevance to PMS, for example GABA, dopamine and acetylcholine, although research data are less convincing for these in comparison to β-endorphin and serotonin.

If these theories are true, it would seem that PMS is not caused by an endocrine imbalance. However, it appears that there is increased sensitivity to normal circulating level of ovarian hormones, particularly progesterone following ovulation, secondary to a neuroendocrine disturbance, probably serotonin deficiency. Accordingly, as we will see later, approaches to treatment fall into two broad strategies: (a) correction of the neuroendocrine anomaly and (b) suppression of ovulation.

MANAGEMENT

Diagnosis

PMS is unusual in that women usually present themselves with the presumed diagnosis of PMS and it is the clinician's role to determine the validity of this. It may be confused with many other disorders and the diagnosis of PMS itself may be difficult. For practical clinical purposes reliance is placed on the history, prospective quantification of symptoms and the exclusion of certain specific disorders.

Symptoms quantification

Quantification of PMS is difficult. Ideally we would wish to measure:

- the degree of underlying psychological dysfunction
- the severity of cyclical symptoms
- the degree of disruption of that patient's normal functioning.

It is possible to quantify underlying psychopathology using established psychiatric questionnaires such as the General Health Questionnaire (GHQ) (Goldberg & Hillier 1979). These must be completed only in the follicular phase. Many methods are available to measure the cyclical symptoms (Budeiri et al

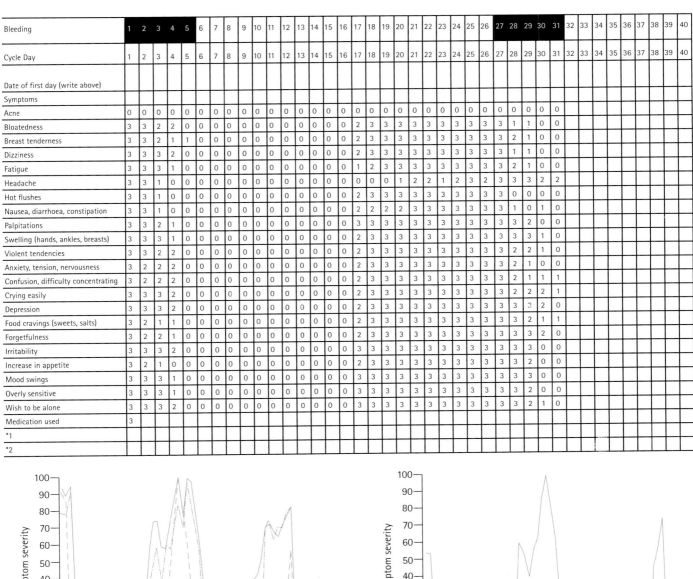

	1	2	3	4	5	6	7	8	9	10	11	12	13	14	15	16	17	18	19	20	21	22	23	24	25	26	27	28	29	30	31	32	33	34	35	36	37	38	39	40
Bleeding						6	7	8	9	10	11	12	13	14	15	16	17	18	19	20	21	22	23	24	25	26						32	33	34	35	36	37	38	39	40
Cycle Day	1	2	3	4	5	6	7	8	9	10	11	12	13	14	15	16	17	18	19	20	21	22	23	24	25	26	27	28	29	30	31	32	33	34	35	36	37	38	39	40
Date of first day (write above)																																								
Symptoms																																								
Acne	0	0	0	0	0	0	0	0	0	0	0	0	0	0	0	0	0	0	0	0	0	0	0	0	0	0	0	0	0	0	0									
Bloatedness	3	3	2	2	0	0	0	0	0	0	0	0	0	0	0	0	2	3	3	3	3	3	3	3	3	3	3	1	1	0	0									
Breast tenderness	3	3	2	1	1	0	0	0	0	0	0	0	0	0	0	0	2	3	3	3	3	3	3	3	3	3	3	2	1	0	0									
Dizziness	3	3	3	2	0	0	0	0	0	0	0	0	0	0	0	0	2	3	3	3	3	3	3	3	3	3	3	1	1	0	0									
Fatigue	3	3	3	1	0	0	0	0	0	0	0	0	0	0	0	0	1	2	3	3	3	3	3	3	3	3	3	2	1	0	0									
Headache	3	3	1	0	0	0	0	0	0	0	0	0	0	0	0	0	0	0	1	2	2	1	2	3	2	3	3	3	2	2										
Hot flushes	3	3	1	0	0	0	0	0	0	0	0	0	0	0	0	0	2	3	3	3	3	3	3	3	3	3	3	0	0	0	0									
Nausea, diarrhoea, constipation	3	3	1	0	0	0	0	0	0	0	0	0	0	0	0	0	2	2	2	2	3	3	3	3	3	3	3	1	0	1	0									
Palpitations	3	3	2	1	0	0	0	0	0	0	0	0	0	0	0	0	0	3	3	3	3	3	3	3	3	3	3	2	0	0										
Swelling (hands, ankles, breasts)	3	3	3	1	0	0	0	0	0	0	0	0	0	0	0	0	2	3	3	3	3	3	3	3	3	3	3	1	0											
Violent tendencies	3	3	2	2	0	0	0	0	0	0	0	0	0	0	0	0	2	3	3	3	3	3	3	3	3	3	3	2	2	1	0									
Anxiety, tension, nervousness	3	2	2	2	0	0	0	0	0	0	0	0	0	0	0	0	0	3	3	3	3	3	3	3	3	3	3	2	1	0	0									
Confusion, difficulty concentrating	3	2	2	2	0	0	0	0	0	0	0	0	0	0	0	0	0	3	3	3	3	3	3	3	3	3	3	2	1	1	1									
Crying easily	3	3	3	2	0	0	0	0	0	0	0	0	0	0	0	0	2	3	3	3	3	3	3	3	3	3	3	2	2	2	1									
Depression	3	3	3	2	0	0	0	0	0	0	0	0	0	0	0	0	2	3	3	3	3	3	3	3	3	3	3	3	2	0										
Food cravings (sweets, salts)	3	2	1	1	0	0	0	0	0	0	0	0	0	0	0	0	2	3	3	3	3	3	3	3	3	3	3	2	1	1										
Forgetfulness	3	2	2	1	0	0	0	0	0	0	0	0	0	0	0	0	2	3	3	3	3	3	3	3	3	3	3	3	2	0										
Irritability	3	3	3	2	0	0	0	0	0	0	0	0	0	0	0	0	3	3	3	3	3	3	3	3	3	3	3	3	0	0										
Increase in appetite	3	2	1	0	0	0	0	0	0	0	0	0	0	0	0	0	2	3	3	3	3	3	3	3	3	3	3	2	0	0										
Mood swings	3	3	3	1	0	0	0	0	0	0	0	0	0	0	0	0	3	3	3	3	3	3	3	3	3	3	3	3	0	0										
Overly sensitive	3	3	3	1	0	0	0	0	0	0	0	0	0	0	0	0	3	3	3	3	3	3	3	3	3	3	3	2	0	0										
Wish to be alone	3	3	3	2	0	0	0	0	0	0	0	0	0	0	0	0	3	3	3	3	3	3	3	3	3	3	3	2	1	0										
Medication used	3																																							
*1																																								
*2																																								

a

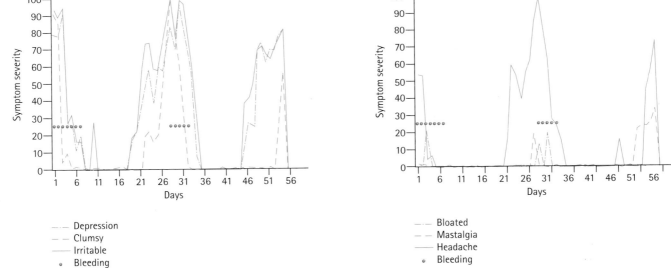

Depression
Clumsy
Irritable
• Bleeding

Bloated
Mastalgia
Headache
• Bleeding

b

Fig. 28.6 **a** A typical calendar of premenstrual experience (COPE) for a PMS sufferer. This shows the range of symptoms, the severity of symptoms and resolution of symptoms with menses. **b** A plot of daily visual analogue scores of typical PMS sufferer symptoms. With permission from the RCOG.

1994). The Moos' Menstrual Distress Questionnaire is most commonly used despite its limitations (Moos 1985). Visual analogue scales (Faratian et al 1984) are patient friendly and precise. The calendar of premenstrual experience (COPE) (Fig. 28.6) provides a good tool for measuring PMS symptoms in a routine clinic.

Measuring the degree to which the patient's life is disrupted is less simple. Quality of life health surveys, for example the SF-36 questionnaire (Ware & Sherbourne 1992), have been applied to quantify the degree of life disruption in PMS patients (Wyatt et al 2001a).

A user-friendly hand-held PMS Symptometrics computer

device has recently been developed at Keele and Nottingham universities in the UK. The instrument incorporates validated visual analogue scales, the GHQ and SF-36 and is capable of measuring, recording, calculating and transferring to a computer database all these measures of PMS and producing 'clinician-friendly' graphic displays (Crowe et al 2000). The program also includes measures of dysmenorrhoea and menstrual blood loss in millilitres.

Physical examination

Though the physical examination of the PMS patient will make little contribution to her diagnosis, the importance of opportunistic screening and the exclusion of disorders which may mimic somatic symptoms (i.e. pelvic pain and abdominal bloatedness), may be considered. Reassurance that there is no breast, cervical or pelvic cancer is of particular value and, of course, patients should not receive hormonal therapy without such an examination.

Blood tests

There is no objective measure, such as a biochemical test, available to diagnose the condition and its severity. However, blood tests may be useful to exclude other disorders such as menopause, polycystic ovary syndrome, hyper- and hypo-thyroidism and anaemia (Table 28.2).

Differential diagnosis

Many disorders have been wrongly attributed to PMS (Box 28.3). We have already suggested that physiological premenstrual changes often cause patients to seek advice although such symptoms are not particularly severe. Women with psychiatric disorders unrelated to the menstrual cycle often find it more acceptable to label their problem as PMS than to have the stigma of depression.

The essence of diagnosis is the cyclicity of the symptoms. If they are not relieved by the end of menstruation, then an alternative explanation must be sought. This is equally true for somatic problems. Non-cyclical breast pain may well be due to non-cyclical underlying breast pathology. Cyclical mastalgia is a part of PMS and may respond to similar therapeutic measures.

Premenstrual pelvic pain must be distinguished from that due to endometriosis, by laparoscopy if necessary.

Cyclical or idiopathic oedema is a separate problem from PMS though its cyclical nature and frequent association with psychological symptoms may cause confusion. There is nearly always a history of diuretic abuse. The original reason for the diuretic use may have been for the treatment of premenstrual bloatedness or as an adjunct to diet for weight reduction; both are relatively inappropriate indications for diuretics.

Lethargy due to hypothyroidism or anaemia may rarely be confused with PMS. Anxiety and irritability may result from hyperthyroidism. The presence of other characteristic symptoms will usually distinguish these and the diagnosis can be excluded by the appropriate blood tests.

Two gynaecological problems which are confused with PMS are dysmenorrhoea and the menopause; these are distinctly different problems. The latter is frequently confused in older menstruating women but this may be identified by measuring gonadotrophin levels.

Is there a definitive test for PMS?

In difficult cases it may be of value to use a GnRH depot for 3 months to distinguish to what degree the ovarian cycle contributes to symptoms, i.e. to carry out the goserelin test. Those symptoms persisting after suppression of the cycle must be the consequence of the underlying psychological disorder

Table 28.2 Blood tests

Test	Findings	Value of diagnosis
Progesterone, day 21	No consistent differences	No value
Oestrogen	No consistent differences	No value
Sex hormone-binding globulin	Marked differences between symptomatic patients shown in one study, not confirmed by others	No value
Prolactin	No consistent differences	No value
Follicle-stimulating hormone (FSH)	No differences in PMS	Excludes menopause
Leuteinizing hormone (LH)	No differences in PMS	May assist in diagnosis of polycystic ovary syndrome (ovarian scan more appropriate)
Thyroid function test (TFTs)	No differences in PMS	Exclusion of hypo- and hyperthyroidism
Electrolytes	No differences in PMS	No diagnostic value
Haemoglobin	No differences in PMS	Excludes anaemia as a cause of lethargy
Serotonin	Low luteal phase serotonin	No proven diagnostic value; not readily available
Allopregnanolone	Low luteal phase allopregnanolone: progesterone ratio	No proven diagnostic value; not readily available

Box 28.3   Differential diagnosis of PMS

Psychiatric disorders
- May be confused because of the similarity in symptoms and because of the bipolar and periodic nature of some psychiatric disorders.
- Many women prefer to 'label' their psychological inadequacies as gynaecological rather than psychiatric.
- There are no objective tests but there are many questionnaires. The General Health Questionnaire may help (Goldberg & Hillier 1979).

Intrafamilial and psychosexual problems
- Distinguish between cause and effect.

Other causes of breast symptoms
- Cyclical breast pain may be considered part of PMS. Can be distinguished from noncyclical breast disease by history
- Noncyclical disease includes severe disorders requiring breast examination and possibly mammography, ultrasonography, aspiration and biopsy.
- Breast cancer must, of course, be excluded.

Other causes of abdominal bloatedness and water retention
- Only a few women exhibit significant water retention in PMS.
- More women have idiopathic oedema which is also cyclical but only occasionally coincides by chance with the menstrual cycle.
- Some women call progressive obesity 'PMS bloatedness'.
- These can all be distinguished by twice daily weighing.

Endometriosis, pelvic and dysmenorrhoea
- Primary dysmenorrhoea occurs with period.
- Secondary dysmenorrhoea is related to pelvic pathology.
- Laparoscopy will exclude endometriosis or pelvic infection.

Medical causes of lethargy/tiredness and anxiety/irritability
- Occasionally anaemia; haemoglobin estimation.
- Rarely hypothyroidism or hyperthyroidism; thyroid function tests.

Menopause
- May be confused with PMS in patients over 40.
- Flushes may occur in PMS.
- Usually distinguished from history.
- Raised follicle-stimulating hormone level.

Box 28.4   Range of treatment approaches for PMS for which success has been claimed

Non-pharmacological	Non-hormonal	Hormonal
Rest	Pyridoxine	Progestogens
Isolation	Essential fatty acids	Progesterone
Psychotherapy	Vitamins	Oral contraception
Education	Diuretics	Testosterone
Yoga	Aldosterone	Danazol
Self-help groups	antagonists	Bromocriptine
Counselling	Clonidine	Hormone implants
Intravaginal electrical	Non-steroidal anti-	GnRH analogues
stimulation	inflammatories	Mifepristone
Diet	β-blockers	Drospirenone
Music therapy		
Hypnosis	Zinc	
Homeopathy	Tranquillizers	
Agnus castus		
Acupuncture	Antidepressants	
Stress management	Phenobarbital	
Nutritional manipulation	Lithium	
Salt restriction	Immune complexes	
Irradiation of ovaries	Antifungals	
Bilateral oophorectomy	Naltrexone	
Endometrial ablation	Selective serotonin	
Hysterectomy	reuptake inhibitors	
	(SSRIs)	

- show the existence of PMS before treatment by prospectively administered, validated scales
- include a prerandomization placebo cycle to exclude women who have a non-specific response
- contain sufficient cycles to allow for symptom variability between cycles.

The wide range of diagnostic scales, outcome criteria and dosing regimens makes comparison between trials difficult.

Drug treatments

Progesterone
Progesterone as pessaries, injections and the oral micronized form has been advocated as replacement for the so-called progesterone deficiency. It is licensed in the UK for treating PMS, even though there is insufficient evidence to support its effectiveness. A recent systematic review of progesterone versus placebo found no improvement in overall premenstrual symptoms (Wyatt et al 2001b) (Fig. 28.7). The very small positive effect shown is unlikely to arise from the correction of progesterone deficiency, but more likely from the relatively large amounts of exogenous progesterone acting as a 'minor tranquillizer'. Despite the limitation of the quality of evidence, progesterone and progestogens continue to be the most commonly prescribed therapies for PMS in the UK, US and Australia.

Progestogens (synthetic progesterone-like drugs)
Dydrogesterone and many other progestogens have been advocated on the basis of the unproven progesterone deficiency theory for PMS. These are also licensed in the UK for

and not related to ovarian acivity. Many clinicians have now utilized this approach even though it has never been scientifically validated. Additionally, a clearer answer may be obtained by giving 'add-back' tibolone to eliminate 'menopausal' physical and mood symptoms.

TREATMENT

There is a wide range of proposed therapeutic regimens for the treatment of PMS (Box 28.4). This may result partly from the high but short-lived placebo effect, the lack of long-term benefit leading to the quest for new methods. When considering claims for drug efficacy it must be remembered that placebo responses in excess of 90% have been reported in some studies (Magos et al 1986).

Although many therapeutic modalities have been assessed by randomized controlled trials (RCTs), only some of these trials have been well controlled. A well-controlled trial should:

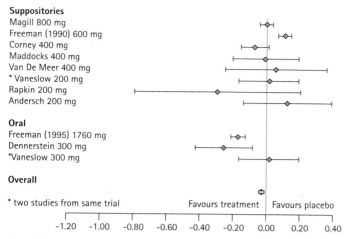

Suppositories
Magill 800 mg
Freeman (1990) 600 mg
Corney 400 mg
Maddocks 400 mg
Van De Meer 400 mg
* Vaneslow 200 mg
Rapkin 200 mg
Andersch 200 mg

Oral
Freeman (1995) 1760 mg
Dennerstein 300 mg
*Vaneslow 300 mg

Overall

* two studies from same trial

Favours treatment | Favours placebo

-1.20   -1.00   -0.80   -0.60   -0.40   -0.20   0.00   0.20   0.40

Fig. 28.7 A meta-analysis of trials of progesterone in the management of PMS. Adapted from Wyatt et al (2001b).

the treatment of PMS. The evidence available from a systematic review and meta-analysis of 10 RCTs showed progestogens to be clinically ineffective in the treatment of PMS (Wyatt et al 2001b). Moreover, as we have seen above, progestogens may actually cause PMS when given as part of hormone replacement therapy (see Fig. 28.5).

Oestrogen

There is limited evidence to suggest benefit from oestradiol in the treatment of PMS patients. However, there are studies to suggest that oestrogenic ovarian suppression may eliminate PMS (de Lignieres et al 1986, Watson et al 1989). Oestradiol has been used in the form of patches (100–200 µg), subcutaneous implants (50–100 mg) or gel. The latter was shown in one study to reduce premenstrual migraine (de Lignieres 1986). Progestogens, used to protect the endometrium from the untoward effects of unopposed oestrogen, may reintroduce PMS-like symptoms. To avoid this systemic effect, progestogen may be used locally (i.e. levonorgestrel intrauterine system (LNG-IUS), when systemic levels remain low and restimulation is not seen, or progesterone gel). Research on the use of oestrogen plus the LNG-IUS has not yet been published, although there is RCT evidence to demonstrate that suppression of ovulation by oestrogen treats PMS symptoms. There is also evidence to demonstrate that the LNG-IUS successfully protects the endometrium from or even reverses hyperplasia. This combination has the potential to eliminate PMS, treat flushes, reduce heavy periods, give endometrial protection and provide contraception.

Most gynaecologists would reserve oestradiol implants for severe cases and in those for whom the menopause is imminent. Testosterone implants have also been given empirically when diminished libido is a significant symptom.

Tibolone

There is limited evidence of benefit from two small RCTs (Taskin et al 1998). The use of tibolone as an 'add-back' therapy with GnRH analogues looks encouraging (Di Carlo et al 2001).

Danazol

Danazol suppresses the ovarian cycle in most women and has been shown to be an effective treatment for PMS in several RCTs (Wyatt et al 2000). It has, however, important side-effects and there may be significant risks associated with long-term use. Masculinizing effects, such as hirsutism, weight gain and voice changes, are notable, but osteoporosis appears not to be a problem. There are also possible long-term cardiovascular risks via effects on plasma lipids. Because of concerns of potential side-effects, it is no longer licensed for the treatment of PMS.

Luteal-phase danazol seems to be effective for premenstrual breast pain (but not other PMS symptoms) and without significant short-term adverse effects (O'Brien & Abukhalil 1999, Sarno et al 1987).

GnRH analogues

Agonist analogues of GnRH have been used in several clinical disorders where it is necessary to suppress the gonadal production of steroids. These include prostate and breast cancer, endometriosis and fibroids and recently the value of GnRH analogues in PMS has been assessed. In the first trials an unclear picture emerged which was probably related to incomplete suppression of ovarian function. A recent review of the literature (Wyatt et al 2000) revealed 10 RCTs assessing the use of GnRH analogues, including buserelin and goserelin, in PMS. Nine of these demonstrated an improvement with the drug over placebo (Brown et al 1994, Freeman et al 1997, Hammarback & Backstrom 1988, Leather et al 1999, Mezrow et al 1994, Mortola et al 1991, Muse et al 1984, Sundstrom et al 1999, West & Hillier 1994). 'Add-back' treatments with oestrogen/progestogen or tibolone have proved beneficial (Mezrow et al 1994, Mortola et al 1991) and low-dose GnRH may avoid the need for add-back therapy (Sundstrom et al 1999).

GnRH analogues do not provide a permanent 'cure' for PMS and this is not surprising. To provide effective therapy the analogue treatment would need to be given indefinitely. Such treatment, used alone, will be precluded by the genesis of menopausal side-effects, the most worrying of which is probably osteopenia. It has been well documented that significant trabecular (albeit reversible) bone loss occurs after only 6 months of analogue treatment.

The use of GnRH analogues in PMS serves the following purposes.

- It allows us to determine what proportion of symptoms are of ovarian endocrine origin.
- It pinpoints which patients with severe PMS would benefit from bilateral oophorectomy (relevant particularly where a patient is to undergo hysterectomy for another gynaecological indication)
- It offers short-term therapy of 6 months in particular circumstances.
- It may be useful (combined with add-back) in women in whom higher dose oestrogens are contraindicated and who are shortly to reach the menopause.

Bromocriptine

Although prolactin had originally been considered a potential candidate as the pathogenic agent in PMS, no studies have demonstrated differences in PMS nor have cyclical changes been clearly shown. Several workers have assessed the efficacy of bromocriptine in PMS treatment, which have been reviewed by Andersch (1983). There is no evidence to support its use in the treatment of PMS, but there is limited evidence of its effectiveness for the treatment of premenstrual mastalgia.

Bromocriptine has a high incidence of side-effects which have been well documented in these trials. They include nausea, dizziness, headache, weight increase and swelling.

Oral contraceptives

There is limited and conflicting evidence from RCTs on the effects of oral contraceptives in PMS. Some women develop PMS-like symptoms for the first time when taking the oral contraceptive pill. Because many women who present with PMS will also request contraception, it seems worthwhile trying this empirically to achieve both aims. Continuous combined regimens (those without a week break) should, in theory, suppress ovulation and provide symptom relief, but this has not yet been researched.

The response in an individual patient cannot be predicted but any of the following results could be expected:

- complete relief of symptoms
- continuation of symptoms but limited to 1 or 2 days premenstrually
- intolerance of the pill
- no change.

Diuretics

The majority of women who experience bloatedness and a feeling of weight increase have no objectively demonstrable premenstrual weight increase, sodium or water retention (Hussain 1994) but there is a small group of women who experience true premenstrual water retention. Those with clearly demonstrable oedema or measured weight increase (and not simply bloatedness) may benefit from treatment with an aldoesterone antagonist. Most published evidence is on spironolactone (Burnet et al 1991, Hellberg et al 1991, O'Brien et al 1979, Smith 1975, Vellacott et al 1987, Wang et al 1995). Most of these trials showed beneficial effects, particularly on breast tenderness and bloating (Wyatt et al 2000c). The positive effects of diuretics must be carefully weighed against the side-effects, which can be significant.

Prostaglandin inhibitors

Mefenamic acid and naproxen sodium have been assessed in good studies (Budoff 1980, 1987, Facchinetti et al 1989, Gunston 1986, Jakubowicz et al 1984, Mira et al 1986, Wood & Jakubowicz 1980). These have found benefit for a range of premenstrual symptoms but not for premenstrual breast pain. Despite this evidence, they seem to be prescribed relatively infrequently for PMS.

Selective serotonin reuptake inhibitors (SSRI)

Significant improvement of premenstrual symptoms has been shown in patients treated with this group of drugs. Altered serotonergic function has been reported in patients with

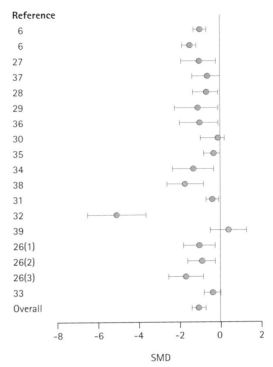

Fig. 28.8 A meta-analysis of trials for SSRIs in the management of PMS. Reproduced with permission from Dimmock et al (2000).

premenstrual syndrome (Rapkin 1992). Serotonin deficiency possibly makes women with severe PMS more sensitive to their endogenous ovarian steroid cycle than women with physiological premenstrual symptoms. SSRIs have been shown to be very efficacious in the treatment of both behavioural and physical symptoms of PMS. A recent meta-analysis of 15 trials showed an overall odds ratio of 6.91 in favour of SSRIs (Dimmock et al 2000) (Fig. 28.8). SSRIs used in the trials were fluoxetine, sertraline, citalopram, fluovoxamine and paroxetine. Common adverse effects were headache, nervousness, insomnia, drowsiness/fatigue, sexual dysfunction and gastrointestinal disturbances. Unlike anxiolytics and non-SSRI antidepressants, they do not cause dependence. Fluoxetine (Prozac) is now licensed for PMDD. Most of these trials used continuous dosing regimes, but targeted luteal-phase regimens may offer minimal side-effects whilst maintaining efficacy.

Anxiolytics and other (non-SSRI) antidepressants

Antidepressants (bupropion, clomipramine, nortriptyline and desipramine), β-blockers (atenolol and propranolol) and anxiolytics (alprazolam and buspirone) have been assessed in adequately controlled trials (Wyatt et al 2000). These found benefit for one or more symptoms of PMS, but a significant proportion of women stop treatment because of adverse effects. Side-effects such as drowsiness, nausea, anxiety and headache led to problems with adherence to treatment in many of the trials.

There are also published preliminary data on newer drugs such as venlafaxine, which is a combined serotonin and noradrenaline reuptake inhibitor.

Trials

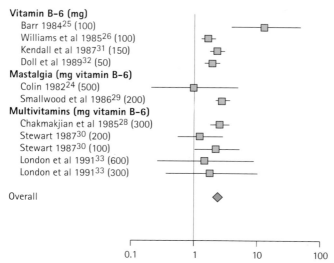

Vitamin B-6 (mg)
Barr 1984[25] (100)
Williams et al 1985[26] (100)
Kendall et al 1987[31] (150)
Doll et al 1989[32] (50)
Mastalgia (mg vitamin B-6)
Colin 1982[24] (500)
Smallwood et al 1986[29] (200)
Multivitamins (mg vitamin B-6)
Chakmakjian et al 1985[28] (300)
Stewart 1987[30] (200)
Stewart 1987[30] (100)
London et al 1991[33] (600)
London et al 1991[33] (300)

Overall

0.1   1   10   100

Fig. 28.9 A meta-analysis of trials for vitamin B6 in the management of PMS. Reproduced with permission from Wyatt et al (1999).

Nutritional supplements

Dietary manipulations

There may be limited evidence to support the use of calcium and magnesium supplements. There is also no supportive evidence for regular carbohydrate intake (Wyatt et al 2000).

Vitamin B6

Vitamin B6 is a co-factor in the final stages of neurotransmitter synthesis, particularly of serotonin and dopamine, from tryptophan. No abnormalities directly related to vitamin B6 have been identified. A recent definitive systematic review of all extant vitamin B6 trials in the treatment of PMS found a beneficial effect (Wyatt et al 1999) (Fig. 28.9). However, the trials were of low methodological quality, so conclusive recommendations on its use are not possible. There has been concern about side-effects (reversible peripheral neuropathy) at higher doses of vitamin B6 (>200 mg/d). Concerns regarding the toxicity of vitamin B6 causing peripheral neuropathy are unfounded at the 100 mg/d level recommended to show efficacy. In practice, many patients will have self-prescribed vitamin B6 before consulting their doctor.

Evening primrose oil

Oil of evening primrose contains the polyunsaturated essential fatty acids linoleic and gammalinolenic acids. These are dietary precursors of several prostaglandins, mainly E_2 and E_1. It has been postulated that deficiency of E series prostaglandins and polyunsaturated fatty acids allows an enhanced response to physiological levels of ovarian hormones.

Evening primrose oil is one of the most popular 'self-help' remedies for PMS, although in the UK it is only licensed for the treatment of premenstrual mastalgia. There are rare reports of evening primrose oil causing seizures in people with epilepsy.

Evidence from one systematic review of eight small RCTs

suggests that evening primrose oil may have a small beneficial effect (Budeiri et al 1996).

Non-drug treatment

Cognitive behavioural treatment

There is conflicting evidence from five RCTs (Blake et al 1998, Christensen & Oei 1995, Corney et al 1990, Kirkby 1994, Morse et al 1991). Two of these trials found cognitive behavioural therapy to be better than a control group, who were those remaining on a waiting list and not receiving therapy (Blake et al 1998, Kirkby 1994).

Exercise and physical therapy

Although the evidence is limited, RCTs have found that both exercise and physical therapy improve symptoms of PMS (Bibi 1995, Lemos 1991, Prior et al 1986).

Relaxation treatment

There is insufficient evidence on the effects of relaxation treatment in PMS. Most studies of relaxation techniques have used them as an adjunct to other treatment.

Surgical treatment

Hysterectomy with or without oophorectomy

Hysterectomy with bilateral oophorectomy is curative (Casson et al 1990) but rarely justified; it may be indicated if there are co-existing gynaecological problems of sufficient severity to justify pelvic surgery. Additionally it appears more justifiable if symptoms have been demonstrated to be eliminated by the GnRH test. Patients must first be identified as being treatable in this fashion following a positive goserelin test. Surgery must be followed by oestrogen replacement, which should be unopposed. Hysterectomy alone may reduce the symptoms in the short term. Evidence for both is limited by the difficulty in providing controls.

Side-effects include the potential risks of major surgery and of course the fact that infertility and surgical menopause are irreversible effects.

Endometrial ablation

There is no reason why endometrial ablation should be effective as no 'menotoxin' has ever been identified. Studies claiming that endometrial ablation may relieve symptoms of PMS have been undertaken within the context of menorrhagia and thus subjects were not randomized on the basis of PMS.

These are two important points to make in relation to surgery for severe unresponsive PMS. First, it would seem wise to perform a goserelin test before embarking on surgery. Second, it is appropriate for all women undergoing hysterectomy to be assessed with respect to PMS prior to any discussions of ovarian conservation or removal. Consent to removal of the ovaries in relatively young women must be very informed, detailed and documented.

The current clinical evidence for the different treatment modalities is provided in Box 28.5.

Box 28.5   Evidence of different interventions

Beneficial	Selective serotonin reuptake inhibitors (SSRIs)
	Oestrogen suppressing ovulation
	Bromocriptine (breast symptoms only)
	Diuretics (bloatedness and swelling only)
	Prostaglandin inhibitors
Likely to be beneficial	Vitamin B6 (poor quality of trials)
	Evening primrose oil (limited quality of trials)
	Exercise
Trade-offs between benefits and harms	Danazol (androgenic side-effects)
	GnRH analogues (risk of oesteoporosis)
	Antidepressants
	Hysterectomy ± bilateral oopherectomy (curative but rarely appropriate)
Unknown effectiveness	Cognitive-behavioural therapy (conflicting results)
	Relaxation therapy
	Oral contraceptives (conflicting evidence)
	Endometrial ablation (information only available for menorrhagia trials)
	Mineral supplements (limited evidence)
Likely to be ineffective	Progesterone
	Progestagens

CONCLUSIONS

In the absence of a clearly identifiable endocrine abnormality it is possible that PMS should not be considered a gynaecological disorder, as it is likely that it represents a psychological or biochemical predisposition to the normal physiological endocrine events of the ovarian cycle. However, women may prefer to label their problem as gynaecological rather than psychiatric or psychological. Gynaecologists, who are often accused of being unsympathetic to women's needs, should not be coerced into dealing with a problem which is not necessarily gynaecological and frequently has a large psychological component. As we have seen, many patients presenting at the gynaecology clinic have other disorders, which do not fall within the sphere of training of gynaecologists.

If we were to treat PMS symptoms only with regimens which have conclusively been shown to be superior to placebo we would be limited to a narrow range of pharmacological treatments. There is no justification that all PMS women should receive long-term treatment with danazol, oestrogen implants, GnRH analogues or bilateral oophorectomy and it would be inappropriate to suggest so. Only patients with a severity of PMS which warrants such major intervention should be referred for gynaecological evaluation.

It is probably justified to suggest the use of SSRIs as an early drug intervention in moderate-to-severe PMS. It is likely that formulations specifically for PMS (given in the luteal phase only) will become available over the next 5 years.

The future of the management of severe PMS/PMDD lies in the acceptance by departments of health and medical bodies that this is a serious disorder that must be distinguished from the mild physiological premenstrual symptoms that are experienced by the majority of normal women.

KEY POINTS

1. Premenstrual syndrome (PMS) is a psychological and somatic disorder of unknown aetiology. It appears to be directly related to the ovarian cycle trigger.
2. At least one premenstrual symptom occurs in 95% of women of reproductive age, but severe, debilitating symptoms (PMS) occur in about 5% of those women.
3. Premenstrual dysphoric disorder (PMDD) is the extreme, predominantly psychological end of the PMS spectrum.
4. An enormous range of symptoms have been described. For a diagnosis of PMS the timing and severity of the symptoms are more important than their character.
5. The main value of physical examination and investigations is the exclusion of other disorders which might be confused with PMS.
6. In difficult cases it may be of value to use a GnRH depot for 3 months to distinguish to what degree the ovarian cycle contributes to symptoms. (This GnRH test has not been scientifically validated.)
7. Progesterone and progestogens continue to be the most commonly prescribed therapies for PMS in the UK, US and Australia. However, there is no evidence that they are better than placebo and no evidence exists to support the hypothesis of progesterone deficiency.
8. PMS appears to be due to an increased sensitivity to *normal* circulating levels of ovarian hormones, particularly progesterone. This enhanced sensitivity is thought to be secondary to a neuroendocrine disturbance, probably serotonin deficiency.
9. Approaches to treatment fall into two broad strategies: (a) suppression of ovulation and (b) correction of the neuroendocrine anomaly.
10. Significant improvement of premenstrual symptoms has been shown following ovulation suppression, using oestrogen, danazol, GnRH agonists and hysterectomy with bilateral oophorectomy, and in patients treated with SSRIs. Fluoxetine is now licensed in the UK for the treatment of PMDD.

REFERENCES

American Psychiatric Association 1994 DSM-IV. APA, Washington

Andersch B 1983 Bromocriptine and premenstrual symptoms: a survey of double blind trials. Obstetrical and Gynecological Survey 38:643–646

Bibi KW 1995 The effects of aerobic exercise on premenstrual syndrome symptoms. Dissertation Abstracts International 56:6678

Blake F, Salkovskis P, Gath D, Day A, Garrod A 1998 Cognitive therapy for premenstrual syndrome: a controlled trial. Journal of Psychosomatic Research 45:307–318

Brown CS, Ling FW, Andersen RN, Farmer RG, Arheart KL 1994 Efficacy of depot leuprolide in premenstrual syndrome: effect of symptoms severity and type in a controlled trial. Obstetrics and Gynecology 84:779–786

Brush MG, Watson SJ, Horrobin DF, Manku MS 1984 Abnormal essential fatty acid levels in plasma of women with premenstrual syndrome. American Journal of Obstetrics and Gynecology 50:262–266

Budeiri DJ, Li Wan Po A, Dornan JC 1994 Clinical trials of treatments of premenstrual syndrome: entry criteria and scales for measuring treatment outcomes. British Journal of Obstetrics and Gynaecology 101:689–695

Budeiri D, Li WP, Dornan JC 1996 Is evening primrose oil of value in the treatment of premenstrual syndrome? Controlled Clinical Trials 17:60–68

Budoff PW 1980 No more menstrual cramps and other good news. GP Putman's Sons, New York

Budoff PW 1987 Use of prostaglandin inhibitors in the treatment of PMS. Clinical Obstetrics and Gynecology 30(2):453–464

Burnet RB, Radden HS, Easterbrook EG, McKinnon RA 1991 Premenstrual syndrome and spironolactone. Australia and New Zealand Journal of Obstetrics and Gynaecology 31:366–368

Casson P, Hahn PM, van Vugt DA, Reid RL 1990 Lasting response to ovariectomy in severe intractable premenstrual syndrome. American Journal of Obstetrics and Gynecology 162:99–105

Christensen AP, Oei TPS 1995 The efficacy of cognitive behaviour therapy in treating premenstrual dysphoric changes. Journal of Affective Disorders 33:57–63

Chuong CJ, Coulam CB, Kao PC, Bergstrahl EJ, Go VLW 1985 Neuropeptide levels in premenstrual syndrome. Fertility and Sterility 44:760–765

Corney RH, Stanton R, Newell R 1990 Comparison of progesterone, placebo and behavioural psychotherapy in the treatment of premenstrual syndrome. Journal of Psychosomatic Obstetrics and Gynaecology 11:211–220

Crowe J, Hayes-Gill B, Francon B et al 2000 Customisation of personal digital assistant (PDA) for logging premenstrual syndrome (PMS) symptoms. British Journal of Healthcare Computing and information Management 17:33–35

Dalton K 1977 The premenstrual syndrome and progesterone therapy. Heinemann, London

de Lignieres B, Vincens M, Mauvais-Jarvis P et al 1986 Prevention of menstrual migraine by percutaneous oestradiol. British Medical Journal 293:1540

Di Carlo C, Palomba S, Tommaselli GA, Guida M, Di Spiezio Sardo A, Nappi C 2001 Use of leuprolide acetate plus tibolone in the treatment of severe premenstrual syndrome. Fertility and Sterility 75:380–384

Dimmock PW, Wyatt KM, Jones PW, O'Brien PMS 2000 Efficacy of selective serotonin-reuptake inhibitors in premenstrual syndrome. A systematic review. Lancet 356:1131–1136

Facchinetti F, Fioroni L, Sances G, Romano G, Nappi G, Genazzani AR 1989 Naproxen sodium in the treatment of premenstrual symptoms. A placebo-controlled study. Gynecological and Obstetrics Investigation 28:205–208

Faratian B, Gaspar A, O'Brien PMS, Filshie GM, Johnson IR, Prescott P 1984 Premenstrual syndrome: weight, abdominal size and perceived body image. American Journal of Obstetrics and Gynecology 50:200–204

Freeman EW, Sondheimer SJ, Rickels K 1997 Gonadotrophin-releasing hormone agonist in the treatment of premenstrual symptoms with and without ongoing dysphoria: a controlled study. Psychopharmacology Bulletin 33:303–309

Giannini AJ, Melemis SM, Martin DM, Folts DJ 1994 Symptoms of premenstrual syndrome as a function of beta-endorphin: two subtypes. Progress in Neuro-Psychopharmacology and Biological Psychiatry 18(2):321–327

Goldberg DP, Hillier B 1979 A scaled version of the general health questionnaire. Psychological Medicine 9:139–145

Gunston KD 1986 Premenstrual syndrome in Cape Town. Part II. A double-blind placebo-controlled study of the efficacy of mefenamic acid. South African Medical Journal 70:159–160

Hammarback S, Backstrom T 1988 Induced anovulation as treatment of premenstrual tension syndrome. A double-blind cross-over study with GnRH-agonist versus placebo. Acta Obstetrica and Gynaecologica Scandinavica 67:159–166

Hammarback S, Backstrom T, Hoist J, von Schoultz B, Lyrenas S 1985 Cyclical mood changes as in the premenstrual tension syndrome using sequential oestrogen-progestagen postmenopausal replacement therapy. Acta Obstetrica et Gynaecologica Scandinavica 64:393–397

Hellberg D, Claessan B, Nilssan S 1991 Premenstrual tension: a placebo-controlled efficacy study with spironolactone and medroxyprogesterone acetate. International Journal of Gynecology and Obstetrics 34:243–248

Henshaw C, O'Brien PMS, Foreman D, Belcher J, Cox J 1993 An experimental model for PMS. Neuropsychopharmacology (25):713

Hussain SY 1994 The compartmental distribution of fluid and electrolytes in relation to the symptomatology of the ovarian cycle and premenstrual cycle. PhD thesis, University of London

Hussain SY, Massil JH, Matta WH, Shaw RW, O'Brien PMS 1992 Buserelin in premenstrual syndrome. Gynaecological Endocrinology 6:57–64

Hussain SY, O'Brien PMS, de Souza VF, Okonofua F, Dandona P 1990 Reduced atrial natriuretic peptide concentrations in premenstrual syndrome. British Journal of Obstetrics and Gynaecology 97:397–401

Jakubowicz DL, Godard E, Dewhurst J 1984 The treatment of premenstrual tension with mefenamic acid: analysis of prostaglandin concentrations. British Journal of Obstetrics and Gynaecology 91:78–84

Kirkby RJ 1994 Changes in premenstrual symptoms and irrational thinking following cognitive–behavioural coping skills training. Journal of Consulting and Clinical Psychology 62:1026–1032

Kosikawa N, Tatsunuma T, Furuya K, Seki K 1992 Prostaglandins and premenstrual syndrome. Prostaglandins, Leukotrienes and Essential Fatty Acids 45(1):33–36

Leather AT, Studd JWW, Watson NR, Holland EFN 1999 The treatment of severe premenstrual syndrome with goserelin with and without 'add-back' estrogen therapy: a placebo-controlled study. Gynecology Endocrinology 13:48–55

Lemos D 1991 The effects of aerobic training on women who suffer from premenstrual syndrome. Dissert Abstracts International 52:563

Magos AL, Brincat M, Studd JW 1986 Treatment of premenstrual syndrome by subcutaneous oestradiol implants and cyclical oral norethisterone: placebo controlled study. British Medical Journal 292:1629–1633

Menden-Vrtovec H, Vujic D 1992 Bromocriptine (Bromergon, Lek) in the management of premenstrual syndrome. Clinical and Experimental Obstetrics and Gynecology 19(4):242–249

Mezrow G, Shoupe D, Spicer D, Lobo R, Leung B, Pike M 1994 Depot leuprolide acetate with estrogen and progestin add-back for long-term treatment of premenstrual syndrome. Fertility and Sterility 62:932–937

Mira M, McNeil D, Fraser IS, Vizzard J, Abraham S 1986 Mefenamic acid in the treatment of premenstrual syndrome. Obstetrics and Gynecology 68:395–398

Moos R 1985 Premenstrual symptoms: a manual and overview of research with the menstrual distress questionnaire. Department of Psychiatry and Behavioural Sciences, Stanford University School of Medicine, Palo Alto, CA, USA

Morse C, Dennerstein L, Farrell E 1991 A comparison of hormone therapy, coping skills training and relaxation for the relief of premenstrual syndrome. Journal of Behavioural Medicine 14:469–489

Mortola JF, Girton L, Fischer U 1991 Successful treatment of severe premenstrual syndrome by combined use of gonadotrophin-releasing hormone agonist and estrogen/progestin. Journal of Clinical Endocrinology and Metabolism 72:252A–252F

Muse KN, Cetel NS, Futterman LA, Yen SC 1984 The premenstrual syndrome. Effects of 'medical ovariectomy'. New England Journal of Medicine 311:1345–1349

O'Brien PMS 1987 Premenstrual syndrome. Blackwell Science, London

O'Brien PMS 1993 Helping women with premenstrual syndrome. British Medical Journal 307:1471–1475

O'Brien PMS, Abukhalil IEH 1999 Randomised controlled trial of the management of premenstrual syndrome and premenstrual mastalgia using luteal phase only danazol. American Journal of Obstetrics and Gynecology 180:18–23

O'Brien PMS, Massil H 1990 Premenstrual syndrome: clinical studies on essential fatty acids. In: Horrobin DF (ed) Omega-6-essential fatty acids: pathology and role in clinical medicine. Wiley/Liss, New York

O'Brien PM, Craven D, Selby C, Symonds EM 1979 Treatment of premenstrual syndrome by spironolactone. British Journal of Obstetrics and Gynaecology 86:142–147

Prior JC, Vigna Y, Alojada N 1986 Conditioning exercise decreases premenstrual symptoms. A prospective controlled three month trial. European Journal of Applied Physiology 55:349–355

Rapkin AJ 1992 The role of serotonin in premenstrual syndrome. Clinical Obstetrics and Gynecology 35:658–666

Rapkin AJ, Shoupe D, Reading A et al 1996 Decreased central opioid activity in premenstrual syndrome: Lutenizing hormone response to naloxone. Journal of the Society of Gynecological Investigation 3:93–98

Rapkin AJ, Morgan M, Goldman L, Brann DW, Simone D, Mahesh VB 1997 Progesterone metabolite allopregnanolone in women with premenstrual syndrome. Obstetrics and Gynecology 90:709–714

Sarno APJ, Miller EJJ, Lundblad EG 1987 Premenstrual syndrome: beneficial effects of periodic, low-dose danazol. Obstetrics and Gynecology 70:33–36

Smith SL 1975 Mood and the menstrual cycle. In: Sachar EJ (ed) Topics in psychoendocrinology. Grune and Stratton, New York

Sundstrom I, Nyberg S, Bixo M, Hammarback S, Backstrom T 1999 Treatment of premenstrual syndrome with gonadotrophin-releasing hormone agonists in a low dose regimen. Acta Obstetrica et Gynecologica Scandinavica 78:891–899

Taskin O, Gokdeniz R, Yalcinoglu A et al 1998 Placebo-controlled crossover study of effects of tibolone on premenstrual symptoms and peripheral beta-endorphin concentrations in premenstrual syndrome. Human Reproduction 13:2402–2405

Vellacott ID, Shroff NE, Pearce MY, Statford ME, Akbar FA 1987 A double-blind, placebo-controlled evaluation of spironolactone in the premenstrual syndrome. Current Medical Research and Opinion 10:450–456

Wald A, van Thiel DH, Hoechsletter I et al 1981 Gastrointestinal transit: the effect of the menstrual cycle. Gastroenterology 80:1497–1500

Wang M, Hammarback S, Lindhe BA, Backstrom T 1995 Treatment of premenstrual syndrome by spironolactone: a double-blind, placebo-controlled study. Acta Obstetrica et Gynecologica Scandinavica 74:803–808

Ware JE, Sherbourne CD 1992 The MOS 36-item short-form health survey (SF-36): I Conceptual framework and item selection. Medical Care 30:473–483

Watson NR, Studd JW, Savvas M, Garnett T, Baber RJ 1989 Treatment of severe premenstrual syndrome with oestradiol patches and cyclical oral norethisterone. Lancet 2: 730–732

West CP, Hillier H 1994 Ovarian suppression with the gonadotrophin-releasing hormone agonist gosereline (Zoladex) in management of the premenstrual tension syndrome. Human Reproduction 9:1058–1063

Wood C, Jakubowicz D 1980 The treatment of premenstrual symptoms with mefenamic acid. British Journal of Obstetrics and Gynaecology 87:627–630

Wyatt KM, Dimmock PW, O'Brien PMS 1999 Vitamin B6 therapy: a systematic review of its efficacy in premenstrual syndrome. British Medical Journal 318:1375–1381

Wyatt KM, Dimmock PW, Walker TW, O'Brien PMS 2001a Fertility and Sterility 76:125–131

Wyatt KM, Dimmock PW, O'Brien PMS 2000 Premenstrual syndrome. Clinical Evidence 4:1121–1133

Wyatt KM, Dimmock PW, Jones PW, Obhrai M, O'Brien PMS 2001b Efficacy of progesterone and progestagens in management of premenstrual syndrome: systematic review. British Medical Journal 323:776–780

29

The Menopause

Margaret Rees

INTRODUCTION

Overall the median age of reproductive cessation in humans is 51 years and, when compared with other species such as non-human primates, rodents, whales, dogs, rabbits, elephants and domestic livestock, happens unusually early in the lifespan (Morabia & Costanza 1999, Packer et al 1998). The human menopause has been considered to be an evolutionary adaptation and several theories have been proposed. One theory is that menopause follows from the extreme dependence of human babies, coupled with the difficulty in giving birth due to the large neonatal brain size and the growing risk of child bearing at older ages. There may be little advantage for an older mother in running the increased risk of a further pregnancy when existing offspring depend critically on her survival. An alternative theory is that within kin groups menopause enhances fitness by producing post-reproductive grandmothers who can assist their adult daughters. It appears that a combined model incorporating both hypotheses can explain why menopause may have evolved (Shanley & Kirkwood 2001).

Worldwide increasing life expectancy and falling fertility rates mean that by 2025:

- life expectancy, currently 68 years, will reach 73 years – a 50% improvement on the 1955 average of only 48 years
- the global population, about 5.8 billion now, will increase to about 8 billion
- there will never have been so many older people, with women forming the majority of the oldest old and so relatively few young ones (see Table 29.1 for UK population)
- the number of people aged over 65 will have risen from 390 million in 1997 to 800 million – from 6.6% of the total population to 10%
- the proportion of young people under 20 years will have fallen from 40% in 1997 to 32% of the total population, despite reaching 2.6 billion – an actual increase of 252 million.

Table 29.1   United Kingdom population aged 45–85+(000s)

Age band	2000 Male	2000 Female	2025 Male	2025 Female
45–49	1888	1883	1854	1767
50–54	2026	2043	2047	1965
55–59	1610	1644	2272	2238
60–64	1412	1473	2214	2238
65–69	1233	1352	1772	1877
70–74	1060	1287	1406	1599
75–79	832	1186	1235	1549
80–84	447	796	721	1032
85+	292	838	604	1248

Adapted from IDB summary demograpic data for the United Kingdom (US Census Bureau, international database 5.10.2000)

These demographic trends, which have profound implications for human health, follow on the many positive changes that have occurred in the past 50 years. For example, the number of hip fractures worldwide due to osteoporosis is expected to rise threefold by the middle of this century, from 1.7 million in 1990 to 6.3 million by 2050. At the present time, the majority of hip fractures occur in Europe and North America. Demographic changes over the next 50 years will lead to unprecedented increases in the number of the elderly in Asia, Africa and South American. As a result, up to 75% of all hip fractures will be occurring in the developing countries 50 years from now (WHO 1998).

DEFINITIONS

Various definitions are used which are detailed below (Utian 1999, WHO 1994).

- *Menopause* – is the permanent cessation of menstruation resulting from loss of ovarian follicular activity. Natural menopause is recognized to have occurred after 12 consecutive months of amenorrhoea, for which there is no other obvious pathological or physiological cause. Menopause occurs with the final menstrual period which is known with certainty only in retrospect a year or more after the event. No adequate biological marker exists.

- *Perimenopause* – includes the period beginning with the first clinical, biological and endocrinological features of the approaching menopause (e.g. vasomotor symptoms, menstrual irregularity) and ending 12 months after the last menstrual period.
- *Menopausal transition* – is that period of time before the final menstrual period when variability in the menstrual cycle is usually increased.
- *Climacteric* – is the phase in the ageing of women marking the transition from the reproductive to the non-reproductive state. This phase incorporates the perimenopause by extending for a longer variable period before and after the perimenopause.
- *Climacteric syndrome* – the climacteric is sometimes but not always associated with symptomatology. When this occurs, the term 'climacteric syndrome' may be used.
- *Premenopause* – this term is often used ambiguously to refer to 1 or 2 years immediately before the menopause or to the whole of the reproductive period prior to the menopause. Currently it is recommended that this term be used in the latter sense to encompass the entire reproductive period up to the final menstrual period.
- *Postmenopause* – should be defined as dating from the final menstrual period, regardless of whether the menopause was induced or spontaneous. However, it cannot be determined until after a period of 12 months of spontaneous amenorrhoea has been observed.
- *Premature menopause* – ideally premature menopause should be defined as menopause that occurs at an age less than two standard deviations below the mean estimated for the reference population. In practice, in the absence of reliable estimates of the distribution of age of natural menopause in developing countries, the age of 40 years is frequently used as an arbitrary cut-off point, below which the menopause is said to be premature.
- *Induced menopause* – is defined as the cessation of menstruation which follows either surgical removal of both ovaries or iatrogenic ablation of ovarian function (e.g. by chemotherapy or radiotherapy).

OVARIAN FUNCTION

The menopause is caused by ovarian failure. It occurs earlier in smokers than in non-smokers (Adena & Gallagher 1982). The age of menopause may be determined in utero with growth restriction in late gestation and low weight gain in infancy leading to an earlier menopause (Cresswell et al 1997). It also occurs earlier in women with Down's syndrome (Seltzer et al 2001).

The ovary has a finite endowment of germ cells with a maximum number of 7 million ovarian follicles at 20 weeks of fetal life. From mid-gestation onwards there is a logarithmic reduction in germ cells until the oocyte store becomes exhausted,

on average at the age of 51. Fewer than 0.5% are ovulated and follicles are lost through atresia or apoptosis. This results in a fall in production of estradiol and inhibin and an increase in gonadotrophin levels. The ovary gradually becomes less responsive to gonadotrophins several years before the final menstrual period (Burger 1999, Ebbiary et al 1994). Thus there is gradual increase in circulating levels of FSH and later LH, and a decrease in estradiol and inhibin levels. FSH levels fluctuate markedly from premenopausal to postmenopausal values virtually on a daily basis during the menopausal transition. These changes in circulating hormone levels frequently occur in the face of ovulatory menstrual cycles. Complete failure of follicular development eventually occurs and estradiol production is no longer sufficient to stimulate the endometrium, amenorrhoea follows and FSH and LH levels become persistently elevated. FSH levels greater than 30 iu/l are generally considered to be in the postmenopausal range.

Sequelae of ovarian failure

Short term

The short-term sequelae are vasomotor symptoms, mood disorder, urogenital and sexual changes. There are cultural differences in attitudes to the menopause; for example, menopausal complaints are fewer in Japanese and Chinese than in North American women (Lock 1998, Tang 1994). Furthermore, a recent Swedish study showed that women with a higher education and those who exercised regularly were more often symptom free (Stadberg et al 2000).

Vasomotor symptoms. Hot flushes and night sweats are episodes of inappropriate heat loss. Sympathetic nervous control of skin blood flow is impaired in women with menopausal flushes in that reflex constriction to an ice stimulus cannot be elicited (Rees & Barlow 1988). Serotonin and its receptors have now been implicated (Berendsen 2000). Hot flushes can occur at any time and at night disturb sleep. Chronically disturbed sleep can in turn lead to insomnia, irritability and difficulties with short-term memory and concentration.

Mood disorders. The mood disorders that have been associated with the menopause include depression, anxiety, irritability, mood swings, lethargy and lack of energy. However, general population studies suggest that the majority of women do not experience major mood changes during the menopause transition (Avis et al 1994, Bebbington et al 1998, Pearlstein et al 1977). Studies of depressive symptoms in menopausal women indicate that menopause is not associated with increased rates of depression. Previous mood changes and affective disorders may be a risk factor for depression at menopause (Dennerstein et al 2001, Morse et al 1998).

Urogenital atrophy. Embryologically the female genital tract and urinary systems develop in close proximity, both arising from the primitive urogenital sinus. Steroid receptors have been identified in the human female urethra, urinary bladder, the vagina and the pelvic floor muscles. Urogenital complaints such as vaginal discomfort, dysuria, dyspareunia, recurrent lower urinary tract infections and urinary incontinence are more common in women after the menopause and more than 50% of postmenopausal women suffer from at least one of these symptoms (Milsom & Molander 1998, Schaffer

& Fantl 1996). The vaginal microenvironment changes with increasing age, mostly in response to the fall in ovarian steroid concentrations. The vaginal mucosa often becomes quite thin and heavily infiltrated with neutrophils. Changes in the bacterial colonization of the vagina occur. After the menopause the vagina is colonized with a predominantly faecal flora in contrast to the dominance with lactobacilli premenopausally. The presence of lactobacilli provides protection against vaginal and periurethral colonization by Gram-negative bacteria, which have been implicated in the pathogenesis of cystitis and urethritis.

Sexual dysfunction. Interest in sexual activities declines in both men and women with increasing age and this change appears to be more pronounced in women. The US National Health and Social Life survey of 1749 women aged 18–59 years reported a prevalence of sexual dysfunction of 43% (Laumann et al 1999). Female sexual dysfunction (FSD) consists of four recognized components: decreased sexual desire, decreased sexual arousal, dyspareunia and inability to achieve orgasm. The underlying reasons for FSD are obviously multifactorial.

Changes in sex hormones may be involved but other factors such as a general well-being, psychosocial factors and presence of diseases are probably even more important (McCoy 1998).

Long term

The long-term complications of greatest interest are osteoporosis, cardiovascular disease and connective tissue atrophy and are likely to have a greater impact than the acute short-term symptoms.

Osteoporosis. Osteoporosis has been defined by the WHO as 'a disease characterized by low bone mass and microarchitectural deterioration of bone tissue, leading to enhanced bone fragility and a consequent increase in fracture risk' (Consensus Development Conference 1993). It is estimated to affect 75 million people in the US, Europe and Japan combined. One in three postmenopausal women has osteoporosis.

Osteoporosis affects both sexes, but in general men have fewer fractures than women. There is an ethnic variation in the susceptibility to osteoporosis with, for example, Caucasian women having a higher rate of fracture than those of Afro-Caribbean origin. It is unlikely that there is a single gene defect for osteoporosis, but several possible ones have been examined which include those for the vitamin D receptor, oestrogen receptor and collagen.

Bone density increases during childhood and adolescence, reaching a peak during the third decade. Following the menopause there is an accelerated period of bone loss, which lasts for 6–10 years and which does not occur in men. Thereafter bone loss continues but at a much slower rate. The development of osteoporosis depends on the peak bone density attained and subsequent bone loss.

The main clinical manifestations of osteoporosis are fractures of the wrist (Colles), hip and vertebrae. Furthermore, hip fractures are associated with considerable excess mortality (Sernbo & Johnell 1993) (Fig. 29.1). As an order of magnitude, annual NHS expenditure on the acute and aftercare of osteoporosis-related fracture is close to £1 billion.

Risk factors for the development of osteoporosis These are shown in Box 29.1 (Cummings et al 1995, Royal College of

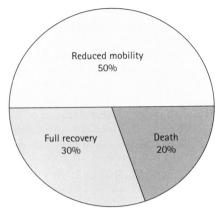

Fig. 29.1 Consequences of hip fracture after 1 year. Data taken from Sernbo & Johnell (1993).

Box 29.1 Risk factors for the development of osteoporosis

Genetic	Positive family history, especially first-degree relative
Constitutional	Low body mass index/anorexia nervosa Early menopause (<45 years of age)
Endocrine disease	Cushing's syndrome Hyperparathyroidism Hyperthyroidism Hypogonadism Type I diabetes
Drugs	Corticosteroids, >75 mg prednisolone or equivalent daily GnRH analogues
Environmental	Cigarette smoking Alcohol abuse Low calcium intake Sedentary lifestyle/immobilization Excessive exercise leading to amenorrhoea
Diseases	Rheumatoid arthritis Neuromuscular disease Chronic liver disease Malabsorption syndromes Post-transplantation bone loss

Physicians 1999). In clinical practice the most important risk factors are early ovarian deficiency and corticosteroid use.

Cardiovascular disease. The primary endpoints of cardiovascular disease are myocardial infarction and stroke. Although cardiovascular disease is rarely the cause of death in women before the sixth decade it is the most common cause after the age of 60. The incidence of coronary heart disease (CHD) increases after the menopause but the exponential rise with age when age-specific rates are examined is remarkably constant in both sexes (Newton 1998). Even in the oldest groups, CHD mortality never 'catches up' with that of men. The 'gender gap' for CHD arises because the exponential rise in mortality rates starts earlier in men.

The incidence of stroke increases with age and is again a

leading cause of death in women. Many survivors are left with significant physical and mental impairment and have serious long-term disability.

Connective tissue atrophy. Skin ageing in women is due to a combination of factors including intrinsic biological ageing, extrinsic damage, particularly ultraviolet radiation and oestrogen deficiency. The most obvious signs of ageing are atrophy, laxity, wrinkling, dryness, mottled pigmentation and sparse grey hair; most of these are attributable to chronic ultraviolet exposure rather than intrinsic ageing itself.

Premature ovarian failure

Women with premature ovarian failure are at increased risk of developing osteoporosis and cardiovascular disease. In the absence of oophorectomy premature ovarian failure could be more appropriately called premature ovarian dysfunction since spontaneous return of ovarian acitivity may occur, leading to pregnancy (Kalantaridou & Nelson 2000).

Primary premature ovarian failure

Primary premature ovarian failure can present as either primary or secondary amenorrhoea. It can occur at any age, even in teenagers. In the vast majority of cases no cause can be found.

- *Chromosome abnormalities* – particularly of the X chromosome, have been implicated. X chromosome mosaicisms are the most common abnormality in women with premature ovarian failure. In Turner's syndrome (45XO) accelerated follicular loss causes ovarian failure. Familial premature ovarian failure has been linked with fragile X permutations. Women with Down's syndrome also have an early menopause.
- *Autoimmune disease* – autoimmune endocrine disease such as primary hypothyroidism, Addison's and diabetes may be associated with premature ovarian failure.
- *FSH receptor abnormalities* – mutations of gonadotrophin receptors have been reported.
- *Disruption of oestrogen synthesis* – specific enzyme deficiencies (e.g. 17-α hydroxylase) can prevent oestradiol synthesis, leading to primary amenorrhoea and elevated gonadotrophin levels even though developing follicles are present.
- *Metabolic* – galactosaemia is associated with premature ovarian failure. It is thought that galactose and its metabolites may be toxic to the ovarian parenchyma.

Secondary premature ovarian failure

This is becoming more important as survival following the treatment of malignancy continues to improve. However, the development of techniques to conserve ovarian tissue/oocytes before therapy is instigated should help at least with maintaining fertility.

Radiotherapy and chemotherapy. Chemotherapy can cause either temporary or permanent ovarian damage, which depends on the cumulative dose received and duration of treatment, so that long-term treatment with small doses is more toxic than short-term acute therapy. These changes occur at all ages but especially so in women aged more than 30 years. With regard to radiotherapy, ovarian damage is dose and age dependent.

Bilateral oophorectomy or surgical menopause. This results in immediate menopausal symptoms such as hot flushes and night sweats. The implications of this procedure require detailed discussion with the patient in view of the increased morbidity and mortality in those who do not take oestrogen replacement.

Hysterectomy without oophorectomy. This can cause ovarian failure either in the immediate postoperative period, where in some cases it may be temporary, or at a later stage where it occurs sooner than the time of the natural menopause. This is an area of controversy and may depend on ovarian function preceding hysterectomy (Raven et al 1995, Siddle et al 1987, Watson et al 1995). The diagnosis may be difficult since not all women suffer acute symptoms and in the absence of a uterus the pointer of amenorrhoea is absent. A case could be made for annual FSH estimation in women who have had a hysterectomy before the age of 40 to allow early detection.

Infection may rarely affect the ovaries. Tuberculosis and mumps are infections which have been implicated. In most cases normal ovarian function continues after mumps infection.

THERAPEUTIC OPTIONS

The three main options available are oestrogen-based hormone replacement therapy, bisphosphonates or selective oestrogen receptor modulators. The approach used depends on the endpoints of treatment for each individual woman. Some may not wish to consider any of the above and want to take alternative therapies.

Worldwide there has been a dramatic increase in the number of licensed HRT preparations available, with over 50 in the UK. The essential component is oestrogen, which is combined with a progestogen to reduce the risk of endometrial neoplasia in women whose uterus is intact. HRT can be delivered by a variety of routes: oral, transdermal, subcutaneous, vaginal and intranasal.

Oestrogens and progestogens

Oestrogens are classed into two types: natural and synthetic. Natural oestrogens include estradiol, estrone and estriol of which most are chemically synthesized from soya beans or yams. Conjugated equine estrogens, also classed as natural, contain about 50–65% estrone sulphate and the remainder consists of equine oestrogens, mainly equilin sulphate. Synthetic oestrogens such as ethinyl oestradiol and mestranol are less suitable for HRT because of their greater metabolic impact.

The progestogens used in HRT are nearly all synthetic, are structurally different to progesterone and are also derived from plant sources. Progestogens are added to reduce the risk of endometrial hyperplasia and malignancy.

The two classes of progestogens most commonly used in HRT are 17-hydroxyprogesterone derivatives (dydrogesterone, medroxyprogesterone acetate) and 19-nortestosterone derivatives (norethisterone, norgestrel). Other progestogens such as trimegestone, gestodene, desogestrel, norgestimate, drospirenone and nomegestrol acetate are becoming available (Ross et al 1997, Rozenberg et al 2001). Currently progestogens are mainly given orally, though norethisterone and levonorgestrel are available in transdermal patches combined with estradiol, and levonogestrel can be delivered directly to the uterus (Antoniou et al 1997, Archer et al 1999a, Jenkins et al 1997). Trimegestone is also becoming available in a matrix patch (Maillard-Salin et al 2000). Progesterone itself is formulated as a 4% vaginal gel and is licensed for use in HRT (Fanchin et al 1997).

In general hysterectomized women need to be given oestrogen alone and there is no requirement for a progestogen. Non-hysterectomized women require combined therapy of progestogen and oestrogen to reduce the increased risk of endometrial hyperplasia and carcinoma which occurs with oestrogen alone (Grady et al 1995, Weiderpass et al 1999a,b). Progestogen must be given to women who have undergone endometrial ablative techniques since it cannot be assumed that all the endometrium has been removed, even if they have been amenorrhoeic.

Progestogen can either be given for 10–14 days every 4 weeks, for 14 days every 13 weeks or every day continuously. The first leads to monthly bleeds, the second to 3-monthly bleeds and the last aims to achieve amenorrhoea. Monthly sequential HRT is suitable for perimenopausal women and continuous combined therapy for postmenopausal women.

Delivery systems

In routine clinical practice the oral route is the usual first line of treatment unless there is a pre-existing medical condition.

Estradiol and progestogens can penetrate through skin. Two transdermal systems are now available: patch and gel. There are two patch technologies: alcohol-based reservoir patches with an adhesive outer ring and matrix patches where the hormone is evenly distributed throughout the adhesive. Skin reactions are less common with matrix than reservoir patches. At present only estradiol is delivered in a gel. Estradiol implants are crystalline pellets of estradiol which are inserted subcutaneously under local anaesthetic, releasing estradiol over many months.

Implants have the advantage that once inserted the patient does not have to remember to take medication. A significant concern is tachyphylaxis defined as recurrence of menopausal symptoms while the implant is still releasing adequate levels of estradiol. A check on plasma estradiol should be considered prior to reimplantation to ensure that the level is in the normal range (<1000 pmol/l).

Estradiol and progestogen can also be absorbed from the vagina and nasal mucosa, leading to the development of vaginal rings and nasal sprays (Mattsson et al 2000, Nash et al 1999).

The levonorgestrel intrauterine system delivers intrauterine progestogen and can provide the progestogen component of HRT (Suvanto-Luukkonen et al 1998). The oestrogen can then be given by any route. It also provides a solution to the problem of contraception in the perimenopause. It is also the only way in which a 'no bleed' regimen can be achieved in perimenopausal women.

The advantages of oral versus transdermal therapy are highly debated mainly for oestrogen. The transdermal route avoids the gut and first-pass effect on the liver. After oral administration the dominant circulating oestrogen is estrone, but after parenteral administration it is estradiol. However, all oestrogens regardless of the route of administration eventually pass through the liver and are recycled by the enterohepatic circulation.

Substances produced by the liver may be differentially affected by the two routes. For example, oral oestrogens lower plasma levels of low-density lipoproteins (LDL) and lipoprotein (a) (Lp(a)), protect these lipoproteins from oxidation and increase levels of high-density lipoproteins (HDL). These changes would be considered desirable, but may be accompanied by an increase in fasting triglyceride levels. Non-oral oestrogens have less effect on plasma levels of LDL and Lp(a), but protect them from oxidation and either have no effect on or in some cases reduce levels of HDL and fasting triglyceride (Spencer et al 1999). Currently there appears to be no clear advantage of the transdermal over the oral route.

Tibolone

Tibolone is a synthetic compound which has mixed oestrogenic, progestogenic and androgenic actions due to its three different metabolites and is used in postmenopausal women who wish to have amenorrhoea. The Δ4 metabolite, as opposed to the other two, has no oestrogenic activity and binds only to androgen and progesterone receptors. This metabolite is produced in the endometrium and accounts for the amenorrhoea found in the majority (80%) of women (Hammar et al 1998). It is used to treat vasomotor, psychological and libido problems. It can be used for osteoporosis prevention and the bone-sparing dose is 2.5 mg daily.

Vaginal oestrogens

Some women only wish to have treatment of urogenital symptoms and not take systemic HRT. Synthetic oestrogens should be avoided since they are well absorbed from the vagina. The options available are low-dose natural oestrogens such as vaginal oestriol (cream or pessary) or estradiol (tablet or ring). Long-term treatment is required since symptoms return on cessation of therapy. With the recommended dose regimens no adverse endometrial effects should be incurred and progestogen need not be added for endometrial protection with such low-dose preparations.

Urogenital symptoms can occur even with systemic HRT in doses sufficient to deal with hot flushes. In these women vaginal oestrogens need to be added.

Benefits of HRT

Vasomotor symptoms Hot flushes and night sweats can usually improve within 4 weeks of starting therapy. Maximum therapeutic response to any particular formulation is usually achieved within 3 months. It is now becoming apparent that low doses of estrogen are useful in treating hot flushes. Oral estradiol 1 mg is as effective as 2 mg in reducing hot flushes (Heikkinen et al 2000a, Notelovitz et al 2000). Treatment should be continued for at least 1 year, as otherwise vasomotor symptoms will often recur. Patterns of HRT prescribing would suggest that most women take it for symptom control rather than prophylaxis of long-term disease such as osteoporosis (Hope et al 1998).

Osteoporosis   The efficacy of HRT to conserve bone mass is well established (Komulainen et al 1999, Lufkin et al 1992). Some bone gain may be anticipated in the initial 18–24 months but thereafter bone mineral density values tend to plateau. The bone protection of HRT lasts as long as the regimen is taken and stops on cessation of treatment. Therefore for HRT to be effective in preventing hip fracture it needs to be taken lifelong and continuously.

The 'standard' bone-protective doses of oestrogen are said to be estradiol 2 mg, conjugated equine oestrogens 0.625 mg and transdermal 50 μg patch. However, it is now evident that lower doses are protective (Delmas et al 2000, Heikkinen et al 2000b, Naessen et al 1997a, Prestwood et al 2000). HRT has been given an A grade of recommendation for antifracture efficacy at the spine and a B at the hip (Royal College of Physicians 2000). With regard to progestogens, there is some evidence that 19-nortestosterone derivatives may enhance oestrogenic bone gain. Tibolone is also bone protective. Women with a pre-existing vertebral fracture are a particularly good group to target any antifracture treatment as they have a 1.5–4-fold increased risk of appendicular fractures compared with women without vertebral fractures.

Some women have no bone response to HRT, despite good compliance with therapy. Current smokers and women with low body weight appear to be at increased risk of poor bone response to HRT (Komulainen et al 2000).

Cardiovascular disease   Until recently it was accepted that HRT reduced the incidence of cardiovascular disease. Observational epidemiological studies strongly suggested a protective effect. The protective effect was supported by experimental in vitro and in vivo animal and human studies of arterial function and biochemical markers such as plasma lipoproteins. The beneficial effects of HRT on the cardiovascular system may be mediated by several mechanisms which include alterations in lipids, coagulation, insulin sensitivity and endothelial function. Opinions have varied on the strength of the evidence that HRT reduces the risk of CHD since observational studies could have significant bias related to the inclusion of healthy women who were HRT users.

Primary and secondary prevention randomized placebo-controlled trials are probably necessary to quantify benefits and risks reliably. It is important to distinguish between primary and secondary prevention since it is likely that an endothelium with an established atherosclerotic plaque will respond differently from one that has not.

Coronary heart disease   Observational studies of primary prevention of coronary heart disease showed a reduction in risk of on average 50% (Barrett-Connor & Grady 1998, Grodstein et al 1997, 2000). Two randomized placebo-controlled primary prevention trials are in progress. The Women's Health Initiative (WHI), which started in 1993 and will run to 2007, tests the effect of HRT and that of calcium and vitamin D supplementation and dietary modification, using a factorial design (Women's Health Initiative Study Group 1998). In the HRT arms of the trial, the WHI has enrolled 27 300 women aged 50–79 from 45 centres in the USA. The other similar study is the Women's International Study of Long Duration Oestrogen after the Menopause (WISDOM) which will randomize 34 000 women aged 50–64 years, about half of whom will be from the UK

(MacLennan et al 2000). This started in 1998 and will treat women for 10 years and follow them for a further 10 years. Both WHI and WISDOM will compare combined HRT with oestrogen-only HRT in women who have had a hysterectomy.

The most positive results of secondary prevention with HRT come from angiographic studies. These showed very marked survival benefits which were greatest in women with the most severe coronary stenosis. The Nurses Health Study reported a relative risk for all-cause mortality in current HRT users with at least one major CHD risk factor of 0.51 (0.45–0.57) compared with only 0.89 (0.62–1.28) for current users with no risk factors (Grodstein et al 1997).

A number of randomized trials have been set up, which may be confounded by the fact that the women involved may have other coronary risk factors (diabetes, smoking, obesity) and multiple drugs may be taken as a secondary intervention (statins, antihypertensives, aspirin). The Heart and Estrogen/ Progestin Replacement Study (HERS), which enrolled 2763 women with established CHD with an average follow-up of 4 years, reported its essentially negative findings at least in the first year of treatment (Hulley et al 1998). The treatment group was given continuous combined conjugated equine oestrogens and medroxyprogesterone acetate. There were significant trends for a reduction with time in primary CHD events and non-fatal myocardial infarction. However, on a year-to-year basis there was no statistically significant difference between the HRT and placebo groups. However, women with high initial Lp(a) levels may have a more favourable response than women with low ones (Shlipak et al 2000).

The Estrogen Replacement and Atherosclerosis (ERA) trial was a three-arm, randomized, placebo-controlled, double-blind trial to evaluate the effects of oestrogen replacement therapy (0.625 mg/day oral conjugated oestrogen) with or without continuous progestogen (2.5 mg oral medroxyprogesterone acetate/day) versus placebo on progression of atherosclerosis in 309 women over 3 years. The primary outcome of interest was the change in minimum diameter of the major epicardial segments, as assessed by quantitative coronary angiography. The study has shown that neither oestrogen alone nor oestrogen plus medroxyprogesterone affected the progression of coronary atherosclerosis in women with established disease (Herrington et al 2000).

Other secondary prevention trials are under way.

Stroke   The data for stroke are unclear and few randomized trials are available at present. A substantial body of observational data on the use of HRT exists (see, for example, Grodstein et al 2000). However, interpretation is complicated by the differences in study design, failure to differentiate between ischaemic and haemorrhagic stroke and status of HRT use (current versus ever-users). There is no evidence which either supports or refutes the use of HRT in women with a previous stroke.

Alzheimer's disease   Several epidemiological studies have suggested that oestrogen use may delay or prevent the onset of Alzheimer's disease with the risk decreasing with both increasing dose and duration of use (Baldereschi et al 1998, Paganini-Hill & Henderson 1996). Furthermore, the age of onset of Alzheimer's disease was later in women who had taken oestrogen. However, HRT does not slow disease progression or improve global, cognitive or functional outcomes in women with established mild to moderate AD (Henderson et al 2000, Mulnard et al 2000, Shaywitz et al 1999, Wang et al 2000). Oestrogen stimulates neuronal function, increases the number of developed gliacytes, increases cerebral blood flow, suppresses amyloid deposition, improves cholinergic transmission and protects from the oxidative stress induced by amyloid deposition (Green & Simpkins 2000).

Urogenital ageing The symptoms resulting from urogenital ageing such as vaginal dryness and urinary problems may take as long as a year to respond to oestrogen therapy. Recurrent urinary tract infections may be prevented by oestrogen replacement but the appropriate dose and duration of therapy have yet to be established (Cardozo et al 1998).

Psychological benefits Many women report an improvement of psychological well-being after starting HRT. There has been much controversy about what this actually means. It has been suggested that oestrogen is a treatment for depressive illness, will restore flagging vigour and confidence and will dispel a host of troublesome psychological difficulties including sleep disturbance, loss of sexual interest, fatigue, anxiety, oversensitivity, tearfulness, guilt and aggression. However, it must be remembered that there is a large placebo effect. Relief of vasomotor symptoms, especially night sweats, may also contribute (von Holst & Salbach 2000).

Other benefits There is now evidence that women taking HRT have a lower risk of colon cancer, but the mechanisms involved have not been elucidated. Meta-analysis has shown a 20% reduction in the risk of colon cancer among current users (Grodstein et al 1999). It may also be involved in wound healing (Ashcroft et al 1997). It can also improve balance and reduce tooth loss (Grodstein et al 1996, Naessen et al 1997b). A reduction in falls has the potential to have a significant effect on fracture. Age-related macular degeneration and cataract are leading causes of blindness and several studies now show a reduction in its incidence of these conditions in HRT users (Smith et al 1997). Cataract and dry eye are also improved. Recently long-term HRT use has been reported as having a non-significant protective effect against the development of osteoarthritis (Wluka et al 2001).

Risks of HRT
The risks of HRT are one of the major reasons for stopping therapy. The three main areas of concern are breast and endometrial cancer and venous thromboembolic disease.

Breast cancer Breast cancer is the most common reason given by women for not wanting to take long-term HRT, with a 50-year-old having about a 10% chance of developing it during her remaining lifetime (Hope et al 1998). In North America and Europe the cumulative incidence of breast cancer between the ages of 50 and 70 in never-users of HRT is about 45 per 1000 women. A reanalysis undertaken in 1997 of 51 epidemiological studies including 52 705 women with and 108 411 without breast cancer found that HRT increases the risk by 2.3% per year of use, when it is started in the 50+ age group (Collaborative Group on Hormonal Factors in Breast Cancer 1997). This magnitude of increase is roughly equivalent to the rise in relative risk of breast cancer associated with each year the menopause is delayed after the age of 50. Such an effect is not seen in women who start HRT early for a premature

Table 29.2 HRT and breast cancer risk

Years of HRT use	Extra cases per 1000 HRT users
5	2
10	6
15	12

Data derived from Collaborative Group on Hormonal Factors in Breast Cancer (1997).

menopause, indicating that it is the duration of lifetime oestrogen exposure which is relevant (Table 29.2). After cessation of HRT use, the effect on breast cancer falls and has disappeared within 5 years.

Breast cancers occurring in women taking HRT appear to have a better prognosis than non-users with a 16% reduction in mortality (Willis et al 1996). While this may be due to increased surveillance, it might be due to differences in the biology of these tumours. The tumours are more localized and less aggressive than in never-users. There is little evidence that use of HRT in patients with a family history of breast cancer will further increase their risk. Similarly there is no convincing evidence that breast cancer risk is increased in patients with benign disease.

Studies of combined oestrogen/progestin HRT versus oestrogen alone so far have not been randomized and data have been presented in slightly different ways. It would appear that breast cancer risk is greater in combined HRT users and this may be more pronounced in lean women (Ross et al 2000, Schairer et al 2000). The studies refute the notion that progestogens protect against breast cancer development and their use in hysterectomized women for this indication. It must also be remembered that the increased risk of breast cancer found in nulliparous women, those who delay their first birth or who have a family history of breast cancer may be higher than that conferred by HRT.

Breast cancer survivors who request HRT pose a management problem since there is no evidence from randomized controlled trials (Cobleigh 1998, Creasman 1999). Standard advice is to stop medication at the time of diagnosis and avoid future use of exogenous oestrogens. Various clinical studies of breast cancer patients have not shown that HRT has an adverse effect on survival. However, these involved small numbers with short-term follow-up. Low-dose vaginal oestrogens such as estradiol and estriol are not absorbed systemically to any significant degree and are not contraindicated in women with a previous breast cancer.

Endometrial cancer The link between unopposed postmenopausal oestrogen replacement therapy and endometrial cancer was first reported in the 1970s. The effect of unopposed oestrogen therapy increasing the risk of developing endometrial hyperplasia and carcinoma has been reviewed in a meta-analysis of 30 studies (Grady et al 1985). The summary relative risk (RR) was 2.3 for oestrogen users compared to non-users with a 95% confidence interval (CI) of 2.1–2.5. The risk of endometrial cancer death is also raised. The relative risk increased with prolonged duration of use (RR 9.5 for 10 or more years). The risk of endometrial cancer remained elevated for 5 or more years after discontinuation of unopposed oestrogen therapy (RR 2.3). Interrupting oestrogen for 5–7 days per month does not reduce risk. Recent case-control studies have shown similar findings. Relative risk increase by 17% per year of use (Weiderpass et al 1999a). With regard to low-potency oestrogen, oral but not vaginal estriol increases the risk of endometrial cancer and atypical hyperplasia (Weiderpass et al 1999b).

Progestogen addition has been advocated for many years with the intention of preventing hyperplasia and carcinoma. Meta-analysis shows that the overall summary RR for endometrial cancer was 0.8 (CI 0.6–1.2) (Grady et al 1985). In contrast with unopposed oestrogen, no substantial elevation of relative risk remains 5 years or more after stopping therapy. Ten days or more of progestogen are recommended for monthly sequential regimens, but there has been some debate (Beresford et al 1997, Pike et al 1997, Weiderpass et al 1999a). No increased risk of endometrial cancer has been found with continuous combined regimes (Hill et al 2000a, Pike et al 1997, Weiderpass et al 1999a). There is debate about the relative merits of different progestogens but studies have not examined equivalent doses.

The increased risk of endometrial cancer in HRT users has to be compared to that found in obese and diabetic women, where it is higher (Weiderpass et al 2000).

Management in women with a previous endometrial cancer depends on the extent of myometrial invasion, histology and whether or not there is cervical involvement (Creasman 1999). Patients with stage I endometrial cancer can be considered for oestrogen therapy. There is debate about whether opposed or unopposed HRT should be used.

Venous thromboembolic disease Case-control studies and one randomized controlled trial provide clear evidence linking HRT and venous thromboembolic disease (VTE), with a relative risk of between 2 and 4 and an absolute risk of around 3 per 10 000 users per year (Hulley et al 1998, Keeling 1999). The baseline risk of VTE in menopausal women is low, being of the order of 1 in 10 000 per year. This means that for 10 000 women-years of use, HRT would be responsible for two extra cases of VTE that would otherwise not have occurred. The mortality of VTE is 1–2%. The mechanisms as to why HRT provokes an increased risk of VTE are unclear. The study suggesting that the increased risk is restricted to the first year of use raises the possibility that HRT interacts with and unmasks previously undiagnosed thrombophilic abnormalities.

The haemostatic system is altered with HRT, but does not appear to be the sole mechanism by which the risk of VTE is increased (van Baal et al 2000). The evidence base relating VTE risk factors and HRT is scanty and advice and management strategies have to depend on clinical 'logic' and opinion (RCOG 1999). Women commencing HRT should be evaluated for VTE risk factors on an individual basis and advised not only of the potential benefits but also of the small risk of venous thrombosis. When taking the history it is essential to assess the family history, the severity of personal events and whether or not any were objectively confirmed. A personal history of VTE is the single biggest risk of a future episode. After a single episode of VTE when anticoagulation is discontinued there is a constant risk of recurrence of 5% per annum.

Data regarding the combination of HRT use and thrombophilias are limited (Lowe et al 2000). It would appear that it increases the relative risk of VTE substantially, especially if the thrombophilic defects are multiple. The evidence as to whether the transdermal route is superior to the oral one is poor, though many experts tend to favour the former. Until recently it was thought that progestogens in high dose did not increase the risk of VTE and were a useful option for vasomotor symptom control in women at increased risk of VTE. However, recent studies show that progestogens in non-contraceptive doses also increase the risk of VTE (Vasilakis et al 1999). Raloxifene also increases the risk of venous thromboembolism (Ettinger et al 1999).

Specific pre-existing medical conditions and HRT
Women wishing to take HRT may have a pre-existing medical condition, which data sheets may list as a contraindication to therapy. Some conditions commonly seen in clinical practice are evaluated below.

Hypertension. There is no evidence that HRT elevates blood pressure or has an adverse effect in women with hypertension. Rarely conjugated equine oestrogens cause severe hypertension but this returns to normal when treatment is stopped.

Hyperlipidaemia. In women the most significant lipid risk factors for cardiovascular disease are HDL, triglyceride and Lp(a). The increased risk associated with raised triglyceride and LDL can be offset by elevated HDL (Seed 1999). In terms of lipids, the ideal HRT would increase HDL without increasing triglyceride, decrease LDL cholesterol and Lp(a). The effects depend on the type of steroid and the route of administration. Oral oestrogen reduces Lp(a) and LDL and increases HDL and triglycerides. The transdermal route is less effective at reducing Lp(a) and LDL but does not increase triglyceride or HDL. The type of progestogen is also important. Oral HRT with a non-androgenic progestogen will increase HDL, decrease LDL, Lp(a) and increase triglyceride. Oral HRT with a 19-nortestosterone derivative will decrease LDL, Lp(a) but will not increase HDL and be neutral for triglyceride. Thus HRT in these women needs to be tailored to their lipid profile for example, in women with hypertriglyceridaemia the transdermal is preferred to the oral route. HRT can be combined with statins.

Rolaxifene and tamoxifen reduce total cholesterol and LDL while remaining neutral towards triglyceride and HDL. Although much discussed, as yet there is no randomized controlled trial evidence available for SERMS for cardiovascular events. A large randomized controlled trial of the effects of raloxifene on cardiovascular endpoints is currently under way.

Migraine. This condition usually occurs in the reproductive years, starting during the teens and 20s. It is unusual for migraines to start after the age of 50. Menstruation is often a significant trigger. Migraine often improves after a natural menopause, but may be worsened after bilateral oophorectomy if HRT is not given. There is no good evidence to support the idea that HRT aggravates migraine (MacGregor 1997). Since migraine can be triggered by fluctuating oestrogen concentrations the transdermal route is favoured over the oral one since it produces more stable levels. Too high an oestrogen dose can trigger migraine aura which usually resolves as the dose is reduced. Unlike the contraceptive pill, there are no data to suggest that the risk of ischaemic stroke is increased in women with migraine with aura taking HRT. Sequential progestogen therapy may be a trigger for migraine. The strategies that can be employed are changing the type of progestogen (19-nortestosterone to 17-hydroxyprogesterone derivatives), changing to continuous combined therapy, delivering the progestogen transdermally or into the uterus using the levonorgestrel device.

Epilepsy. The data regarding HRT and the menopause and epilepsy are limited (Abbasi et al 1999, Harden et al 1999). Of concern is that some antiepileptics are liver enzyme inducers; however, there are no data as yet as to whether the transdermal is preferable to the oral route. It is also not known whether these women taking oral therapy should take an increased dose extrapolating from combined oral contraceptives. Furthermore, there are data that anticonvulsant therapy causes changes in calcium and bone metabolism and may lead to decreased bone mass with the risk of osteoporotic fractures. The two widely used antiepileptic drugs phenytoin and carbamazepine are recognized to have direct effects on bone cells, leading to impaired bone formation (Feldkamp et al 2000).

Gallbladder disease. The data on the effect of HRT on cholelithiasis are limited. A recent randomized placebo-controlled trial of oral HRT in elderly women for the secondary prevention of cardiovascular disease has shown an increased incidence of gallbladder disease (Hulley et al 1998). As a confounder, women receiving HRT may have pre-existing silent disease. It is usually recommended that in women with pre-existing disease the non-oral route should be used, but there is little evidence to support this.

Liver disease. It is advisable to use a non-oral route of oestrogen therapy. Treating such women should be undertaken in collaboration with the gastroenterologists and liver function monitored.

Crohn's disease. A major consideration in such women is the increased risk of osteoporosis which may result either from the disease itself or long-term use of corticosteroids (Schoon et al 2000). The transdermal route of HRT is usually preferred to ensure adequate absorption.

Diabetes mellitus. The prevalence of type 2 diabetes mellitus is increasing in postmenopausal women. The condition raises the risk of developing coronary heart disease. There is now emerging evidence that oestrogen improves insulin sensitivity, dysplidaemia, fibrinolysis and may improve endothelial dysfunction with no apparent adverse effect on blood pressure or body weight. The North American Menopause Society (2000) has recently provided a consensus statement on the management of diabetic women. It is currently believed that the greatest benefits may be obtained from the use of transdermal oestrogen preparations or low doses of oral 17β-estradiol rather than conjugated equine oestrogens, especially with regard to improvement in dyslipidaemia and the threat of oestrogen-induced hypertriglyceridaemia. The choice of progestogen is less clear but micronized progesterone or dydrogesterone would appear to have the least adverse effect on insulin sensitivity and HDL cholesterol concentration. Glucose levels should be monitored closely and insulin dose adjusted, if necessary.

Thyroid disease. A past history of hyperthyroidism of any aetiology is associated with an increased risk of osteoporosis and hip fracture. This effect is found mainly in the short rather than long term (Affinito et al 1996, Cummings et al 1995, Hallengren et al 1999, Jodar et al 1997). This may result from either endogenous overproduction of thyroxine or over-replacement in hypothyroidism. Patients presenting with hyperthyroidism should be screened for osteoporosis. Thyroxine replacement should be adjusted so the TSH is not suppressed. Thyroxine replacement therapy in patients with suppressed thyroid-stimulating hormone levels increases postmenopausal bone loss. Thyroid replacement is not a contraindication for HRT.

Malignant melanoma. This is a controversial area. It is generally accepted that there is no association between the risk of melanoma and use of HRT (Persson et al 1996, Smith et al 1998).

Bisphosphonates

Several bisphosphonates such as etidronate, alendronate, risedronate, clodronate and pamidronate have been use (Fig. 29.2), mainly in the field of Paget's disease and the hypercalcaemia of malignancy. The first three are used in the prevention and treatment of osteoporosis and also corticosteroid-induced osteoporosis. All bisphosphonates are poorly absorbed from the gastrointestinal tract and must be given on an empty stomach. Food or calcium-containing drinks (except water) inhibit the absorption which at best is only 5–10% of the administered dose. Thus they must be administered in the fasting state. A side-effect of all bisphosphonates is irritation of the upper gastrointestinal tract. Symptoms resolve quickly after drug withdrawal.

Historically bisphophonates are linked to inorganic pyrophosphates. Inorganic pyrophosphate is a polyphosphate,

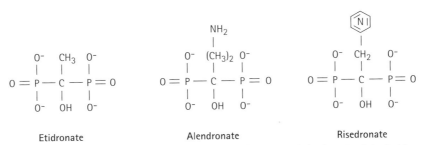

Fig. 29.2 Chemical structure of etidronate, alendronate and risedronate. Adapted from Francis (1995).

a member of a family of compounds characterized by the presence of at least one phosphorus-oxygen-phosphorus (POP) bridge. Replacement of the P-O-P bond with a phosphorus-carbon-phosphorus (PCP) bond results in a stable compound resistance to degradation by pyrophosphatases which occur in vivo. Bisphosphonates become incorporated into bone at sites of mineralization and in resorption cavities. They also diffuse into osteoclasts and promote apoptosis, thus inhibiting bone resorption. High doses of bisphosphonates can also inhibit bone formation and mineralization, but for most bisphosphonates there is a wide window of safety between a dose which blocks resorption and one which inhibits formation.

Etidronate

Etidronate has been widely investigated in postmenopausal osteoporosis (Storm et al 1990, van Staa et al 1998). The concentration at which etidronate inhibits bone resorption is a little lower than that which inhibits bone formation. The use of high-dose etidronate results in impaired mineralization and focal osteomalacia. Thus etidronate is given intermittently (14 out of every 90 days) and 1.250 mg of calcium salts is given during the remaining 76. This preparation can be given indefinitely. It has been given an A and a B grade rating for antifracture efficacy at the spine and hip respectively (Royal College of Physicians 2000). Furthermore cyclical etidronate therapy also prevents bone loss in the spine and proximal femur in early postmenopausal women (Health et al 2000). When etidronate is combined with HRT bone gain may be superior to that observed with either agent alone (Wimalawansa 1998).

Alendronate

Alendronate is an aminobisphosphonate which has an anti-resorptive potency 1000 times greater than etidronate. Approximately 1% of an administered dose enters the circulation and half of this is excreted unchanged in the urine. Unlike etidronate, the antiresorptive dose is far less than the dose required to inhibit mineralization and so it may be administered daily. A recent study has shown that intermittent dosing is also effective at maintaining BMD at spine and hip.

Long-term double-blind multicentre studies have shown that continuous daily doses of 10 or 20 mg increased bone mineral density at both the lumbar spine and hip (Black et al 1996, Bone et al 2000, Liberman et al 1995). The changes are most marked in the first year with a plateau occurring after 2–3 years. Bone mass is preserved for at least 1 year after treatment is stopped. Intermittent dosing is also effective (Rossini et al 2000). It has been given an A grade rating for antifracture efficacy at both the spine and hip (Royal College of Physicians 2000). Combined use of alendronate and oestrogen produces somewhat larger increases in BMD than either agent alone.

Risedronate

Risedronate is a pyridinyl bisphosphonate which has recently become available for the management of osteoporosis (Harris et al 1999b, Reginster et al 2000, Reid et al 2000). In women with established osteoporosis 5 mg daily over 3 years reduces the incidence of new vertebral fractures by about 45% and non-vertebral fracture by about 36%. It has been given an A grade rating for antifracture efficacy at both the spine and hip

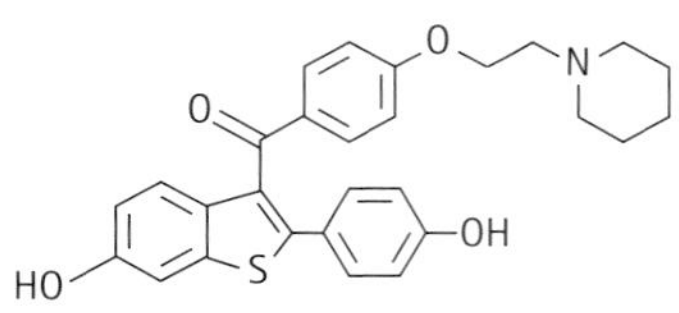

Raloxifene

Fig. 29.3 Chemical structure of raloxifene.

(Royal College of Physicians 2000). It is also effective in the prevention of corticosteroid-induced osteoporosis.

Selective oestrogen receptor modulators (SERMS)

The term selective oestrogen receptor modulators or SERMs is used for compounds that possess tissue-specific oestrogen agonist and antagonist effects.

Tamoxifen was the first SERM. It is used as an adjuvant and preventive treatment for breast cancer, since it behaves as an oestrogen antagonist in that tissue. It also displays oestrogen agonist-like effects on bone and lipids. Raloxifene (Fig. 29.3) is the first SERM to be licensed for the prevention and treatment of oesteoporosis-related vertebral fracture. Studies have shown that at 24 months, the mean ($\pm$SE) difference in the change in bone mineral density between the women receiving 60 mg of raloxifene per day and those receiving placebo was 2.4$\pm$0.4% for the lumbar spine, 2.4$\pm$0.4% for the total hip and 2.0$\pm$0.4% for the total body ($p < 0.001$ for all comparisons). Raloxifene reduces vertebral fracture by 30–50%, depending on dose in women with established osteoporosis. However, it does not significantly reduce the risk of non-vertebral fracture (Drug and Therapeutics Bulletin 1999, Ettinger et al 1999). No comparative studies of raloxifene and other treatments of osteoporosis such as HRT and bisphosphonates are currently available.

The dose is 60 mg daily and it is suitable for post-menopausal but not perimenopausal women. It is a 'no bleed' therapy since it does not stimulate the endometrium (Delmas et al 1997). It also does not stimulate breast tissue. It may reduce the risk of breast cancer but this is currently being evaluated. Its beneficial effects on lipids are also being examined in studies with cardiovascular endpoints (de-Valk-de-Roo et al 1999). Side-effects include vasomotor flushes and calf cramps. Therefore it is not suitable for women with vasomotor symptoms. It increases the risk of venous thrombo-embolism to the same extent as oestrogen-based HRT.

Other therapies for osteoporosis

Calcium salts

Calcium is the most important nutritional factor in osteoporosis. Some 99% of total body calcium is located in the skeleton and a form of calcium phosphate makes up about 65% of bone by weight (Nordin 2000). Balance studies in premenopausal women have shown that mean calcium intake at which absorbed and urinary calcium are equal is 520 mg. However, there is good evidence of an additional insensible loss of calcium through the skin which increases the requirement to 700 mg and implies an allowance of about 900 mg. The evidence that oestrogen deficiency increases requirement has been demonstrated in calcium balance studies across the menopause. These studies show a decrease in absorption and an increase in urinary calcium excretion at the menopause. An appropriate allowance would perhaps be 1100–1200 mg.

The most rigorous situation to test the effect of calcium salts is after oophorectomy where placebo-controlled studies show that high doses of calcium reduce bone loss. The effect of calcium appears to be due to a reduction in bone turnover. Epidemiological studies have conflicting results with some showing that a high dietary intake reduces risk of osteoporotic fracture and others showing an increased risk. However, women who have a high dietary intake of calcium differ from those who do not in terms of general health, education and other possibly confounding factors. Such studies have to be distinguished from those that examine the pharmacological use of calcium. Here vertebral fracture risk is reduced by about 30–40%. The data for hip fracture are more limited, but benefits have also been observed (Cumming & Nevitt 1997, Tilyard et al 1992). Calcium supplementation has been given an A and a B grade rating for antifracture efficacy at the spine and hip respectively (Royal College of Physicians 2000).

Most studies show that about 1.5 g of elemental calcium is necessary to preserve bone health in postmenopausal women and the elderly (NIH Consensus Conference 1994). It must be noted, however, that while this benefit has been found in elderly women there is no evidence that calcium on its own is capable of reversing bone loss in the perimenopause.

Calcium and vitamin D

This combination may be particularly relevant to populations in northern latitudes such as the UK, where there is much evidence of vitamin D insufficiency especially in the elderly. In northern latitudes the cutaneous synthesis of vitamin D only occurs in summer months and in the UK the national diet lacks sufficient amounts of this vitamin for adequate intake in the absence of solar exposure. Other more southerly countries, e.g. the United States, fortify foods by adding vitamin D to dairy products.

In the United States a significant reduction in long bone fractures was found in adults aged 65 years and over taking an additional 500 mg of elemental calcium and 700 iu of vitamin D daily. This study, which was double blinded and placebo controlled, recorded the incidence of falls which was no different between the two groups. An earlier French study had shown a 30% lower risk of hip fracture in elderly women given 1.2 g of elemental calcium and 800 iu of vitamin D. There was also a significant reduction in all long bone fractures in women treated for 18 months (Chapuy et al 1992). The benefits of vitamin D alone are less clear and the evidence is conflicting.

Calcitriol, alfacalcidol and related analogues

The vitamin D derivatives most widely used are calcitriol and alfacalcidol. Alfacalcidol is the synthetic analogue of calcitriol and is metabolized to the active hormone in the liver. Studies on vertebral fracture have produced conflicting results and no protective effect has been shown for hip fracture (Tilyard et al 1992).

Calcitonin

Calcitonin may be given either parenterally or by nasal spray. Much of the evidence for the efficacy of calcitonin is derived from experience with the nasal spray. Calcitonin has been used for over 20 years and has not been associated with serious adverse effects. Parenteral calcitonin can cause nausea, diarrhoea and flushing and results in the production of neutralizing antibodies in some patients. Nasal calcitonin has also been shown to reduce vertebral fractures (Chesnut et al 2000). There is also evidence for its efficacy as an analgesic in acute vertebral fracture.

Fluorides

Fluoride is one of the few agents that has a marked anabolic effect on the skeleton. The efficacy of fluoride regimens continues to be controversial. While vertebral bone mineral density is increased, this has not consistently been translated as a reduction in fracture risk. No protective effect has been shown on hip fracture risk.

Exercise

Animal studies have shown that bone responds to strain. Furthermore, many epidemiological studies have shown an association between the level of physical exercise and bone mass and risk of fracture. However, studies have shown a rather limited role for weight-bearing exercise in the prevention of osteoporosis at the menopause. In contrast, exercise regimes can be very helpful in the management of established osteoporosis. The benefits are mainly related to increased well-being, muscle strength, postural stability and a reduction of chronic pain rather than skeletal mass. Exercise has to be carefully structured because of concerns of further fractures.

Prevention and treatment of falls

Except for vertebral fractures, the majority of fragility fractures result from falls. The risk of falling increases with age and is greater in women than in men. The importance of falls relative to the decline of bone mineral density in promoting fracture is controversial. Home exercise programmes may prevent falls (Robertson et al 2001).

Hip protectors

These are used to reduce the impact of falling directly on the hip. A randomized controlled study of padded polypropylene hip protectors has shown a reduction of hip fracture in the treatment wing. However, hip protectors are not particularly attractive and are uncomfortable in hot weather.

Complementary and alternative therapies

The evidence from randomized trials that alternative therapies improve menopausal symptoms or have the same benefits as hormone replacement therapy is poor. However, many women use them, believing them to be safer and 'more natural'. The choice of therapies is confusing (Zollman & Vickers 1999).

Progesterone transdermal creams

Progesterone creams are being advocated for the treatment of menopausal symptoms and skeletal protection. They have been recently examined in a randomized controlled trial. Although no protective effect on bone density was found after 1 year, a significant improvement in vasomotor symptoms was seen in the treated group (Leonetti et al 1999). There are concerns that women may use progesterone creams for endometrial protection. However, the available evidence shows no effect and thus women using such a combination are increasing their risk of endometrial cancer (Drug and Therapeutics Bulletin 2001, Wren et al 1999).

Herbalism

Herbalism needs to be used with caution in women with a contraindication to oestrogen since some herbs, e.g. ginseng, have oestrogenic properties. Furthermore, there is little control over the quality of the products and thus it is difficult to know what is actually in herbal preparations and dietary supplements (Ernst 1999). Severe adverse reactions, including renal failure and cancer, have recently been reported due to a manufacturing error where a nephrotoxic and carcinogenic herb was included in a Chinese herbal preparation given for weight loss (Nortier et al 2000). The safety of some herbs such as aloe vera, kava and milk thistle is being tested. Dong quai contains coumarins and can interact with anticoagulants.

Black cohosh has been certified by the German Commission E to have a favourable risk:benefit ratio for use in 'climacteric neurovegetative complaints'. The precise mechanism of action is unclear, but some of the constituents bind to oestrogen receptors.

St John's wort can be used successfully to treat depression and has been examined in randomized controlled trials (Grube et al 1999). There are concerns that it is a liver enzyme inducer and could potentially interact with HRT.

Ginseng is another popular therapy for postmenopausal women, but there are concerns regarding its potential oestrogenic properties (Wiklund et al 1999).

Phytoestrogens

Phytoestrogens are plant substances that are structurally or functionally similar to oestradiol (Fig. 29.4) and which are found in many foods. The preparations used vary from enriched foods such as bread and drinks (soy milk) to tablets. They consist of a number of classes of which the lignans and isoflavones are the most important in humans. Oilseeds such as flaxseed contain the highest concentrations of lignans and they are also found in cereal bran, whole cereals, vegetables, legumes and fruits. Isoflavones occur in high concentrations in soybeans, chick peas and possibly other legumes as well as clovers. The major lignans are enterolactone and enterodiol. The major isoflavones are genistein and daidzein.

The role of phyto-oestrogens has stimulated considerable interest since populations consuming a diet high in isoflavones, such as the Japanese, have a lower incidence of menopausal vasomotor symptoms, cardiovascular disease, osteoporosis, breast, colon, endometrial and ovarian cancers. Furthermore, women with breast cancer in Japan have a better prognosis than those with breast cancer in the United States or Great Britain. Phyto-oestrogens have a variety of activities: oestrogenic, antioestrogenic, antiviral, anticarcinogenic, bactericidal, antifungal, antioxidant, antimutagenic, antihypertensive, anti-inflammatory and antiproliferative effects. Genistein, the most extensively studied isoflavone, is an inhibitor of tyrosine kinase, DNA topoisomerases I and II and ribosomal S6 kinase. Other properties include inhibition of angiogenesis and differentiation of cancer cell lines.

Data regarding the ability of genistein and the synthetic isoflavone ipriflavone to maintain bone mass are conflicting (Alexandersen et al 2001, Gennari et al 1997). In the USA the Food and Drug Administration has approved food or food substances containing specific amounts of soya protein to reduce the risk of heart disease. Randomized placebo-controlled trials, however, are required. With regard to menopausal symptoms the evidence is conflicting and soy seems to be no more effective than placebo (Quella et al 2000). Similarly there are also debates about the effects on lipoproteins, endothelial function and blood pressure (Clarkson et al 2001, Simons et al 2000, Washburn et al 1999).

Thus it would appear that phyto-oestrogens represent a group of compounds worthy of further investigations for the treatment of menopausal syndrome.

Dehydroepiandrosterone (DHEA)

DHEA is a steroid secreted by the adrenal cortex. The secretion and the blood levels of DHEA and its sulphate ester (DHEAS) decrease profoundly with age, leading to the suggestion that old age represents a DHEA deficiency syndrome and that the effects of ageing can be counteracted by DHEA 'replacement therapy'. DHEA is increasingly being used in the USA, where it is classed as a food supplement, outside medical supervision, for its supposed antiageing effects (Baulieu et al 2000, Hinson & Raven 1999). Some studies have shown benefits on the skeleton, cognition, well-being and the vagina. The short-term effects of DHEA administration are, however, still controversial and possible adverse effects in long-term use are, as yet, unrecorded.

Other

Other complementary therapies include acupressure, acupuncture, Alexander technique, Ayurveda, osteopathy and

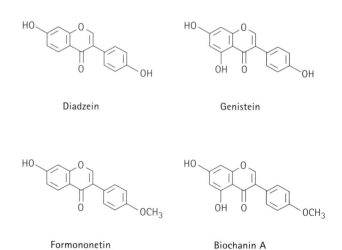

Diadzein   Genistein

Formononetin   Biochanin A

Fig. 29.4 Chemical structure of genistein, diadzein, biochanin A and formononetin.

Reiki. These have been covered in recent reviews and need further examination in relation to the menopause (Zollman & Vickers 1999).

Assessment and monitoring the menopausal woman taking HRT

Long-term therapy is advised to obtain the long-term benefits of HRT. However, there is controversy about the frequency of follow-up and what examinations should be undertaken (Page & Glasier 2000). There are no randomized controlled trials. It would be prudent to undertake an initial patient assessment with discussion of the endpoints of treatment and assessment of risks (e.g. personal or family history of venous thrombo-embolism or breast cancer) before starting therapy. The next review could be at 3 months to determine whether the HRT preparation is suitable and controlling menopausal symptoms. Thereafter, women could be seen 6 monthly or annually. Some experts recommend measuring blood pressure at each visit and undertaking pelvic and breast examination every 12–18 months, but this is not evidence based. There is no evidence that HRT increases blood pressure even in hypertensive women.

Irregular bleeding or heavier withdrawal bleeds should always be taken seriously and are an indication for pelvic examination and investigation such as vaginal ultrasound, endometrial biopsy or hysteroscopy (Archer et al 1999b, Gull et al 2001, Korhonen et al 1997, Lindgren et al 1999).

Contraception is an important issue for perimenopausal women and pregnancies and births have been documented in women in their 50s. High maternal age is a significant risk factor for spontaneous abortion, ectopic pregnancy and stillbirth (Nybo et al 2000). There is an increasing risk of fetal malformation, with a rise in chromosomal disorders. The normal recommendation is to continue contraception after the final menstrual period for at least 2 years if the woman is under 50 and at least 1 year if she is over 50 years old (Wordsworth 1999). However, the final menstrual period may be difficult to identify in women using a contraceptive method that renders them amenorrhoeic, those taking a combined oral contraceptive or monthly sequential HRT.

Endocrine investigations are undertaken to diagnose ovarian failure where appropriate and other causes of vasomotor symptoms such as abnormalities of thyroid function, phaeochromocytoma, carcinoid syndrome and, very rarely, mastocytosis. FSH levels are only helpful in the diagnosis of ovarian failure (Burger 1999). The menopausal range is greater than 30 iu/l. FSH need only be measured if the diagnosis of the menopause is in doubt and need not be measured in women of normal menopausal age. However, this needs to be measured in women with suspected premature ovarian failure, i.e. aged less than 40 years. In the perimenopause the daily variation in FSH levels renders this parameter of limited value. FSH levels are of little value in monitoring hormone replacement therapy since in normal physiology it is controlled by inhibin as well as oestradiol.

Breast examination and mammography
The role of breast self-examination and breast awareness is controversial and there are no specific data for women taking HRT. Similarly conflicting advice has been given by UK government authorities regarding the frequency of breast examination in primary care in HRT users.

Policies regarding mammography vary from country to country. The use of HRT can lead to various changes, including mammographic density, and may reduce the sensitivity of screening (Boyd et al 1998, Litherland et al 1999). Most increases in density occur in the first year of treatment (Sterns & Zee 2000). The effect of different regimes (oestrogen alone, oestrogen with monthly sequential progestogen, continuous combined therapy) varies in individual studies (Lundstrom et al 1999). The effect of different doses and types of oestrogen and progestogen needs to be examined. Further study of the magnitude and meaning of increased mammographic density due to use of HRT is required.

Assessment of the skeleton
Various methods are available with measurement of bone mineral density using dual-energy X-ray absorptiometry (DXA) currently being considered the 'gold standard' (Purdie & Steele 2001). It is generally agreed that population screening for osteoporosis is not advised. However, it is important to identify women at increased risk of osteoporosis, and therefore fracture, and monitor response to treatment.

DXA uses an X-ray beam with two different energy peaks which are differentially absorbed by bone and soft tissue. The bone mineral content in the area of interest can then be calculated. Measurements using this technique are conventionally made at the spine and proximal femur but can be made at other sites such as forearm. DXA results are reported as T scores (comparison with young adult mean) and Z scores (comparison with reference values of the same age). The T score relates to absolute fracture risk whereas the Z score relates to the individual's relative risk for their age. A normal T score is greater than −1, osteopenia <−1 to >−2.5 and osteoporosis <−2.5 (Department of Health 1998).

Biochemical markers of bone turnover are classified as markers of resorption or formation (Seibel & Woitge 1999). A potential use of these markers is to monitor antiosteoporotic therapy since they will show changes within 3–6 months while DXA will take more than 1 year. However, these markers have not yet been fully evaluated for routine clinical practice. The principal markers of bone formation are the procollagen peptides of type I collagen, osteocalcin and the bone isoenzyme of alkaline phosphatase. The most widely used markers of bone resorption are hydroxyproline, hydroxylysine glycosides, pyridinium crosslinks and tartrate-resistant acid phosphatase.

Quantitative ultrasound (QUS) involves the transmission of a low-amplitude ultrasound beam, usually through the calcaneus, and measures bone strength. It has the attraction of being portable and not using ionizing radiation. It remains to be fully evaluated before it can be used in routine clinical practice (Frost et al 2001). In terms of diagnostic capability the majority of data involve fracture prediction in elderly women where it appears to be a competent measure of hip fracture risk. However, it remains to be determined whether it can predict fracture at other sites or in younger menopausal women.

Concordance with therapy

One of the reasons for monitoring HRT is to aid concordance with therapy (Bastian et al 1998, Bradley 1999). There are many reasons why women elect to take HRT or not (Hope & Rees 1995). The frequency of HRT use in different populations varies greatly. In Western Europe rates vary between 3% and 44%. In most the percentage is below 20% (Hope et al 1998). Concordance is greater in female gynaecologists or general practitioners or the spouses of their male counterparts, suggesting that good information and a positive attitude to therapy are important (Isaacs et al 1997). Furthermore, a number of studies have reported that a major reason for taking HRT was a positive attitude of and recommendation by the physician (Andersson et al 1998). The gender of the doctor is also an important factor, with non-compliance being greater with male than with female practitioners. Concordance is greater in women following hysterectomy and bilateral oophorectomy: this could be because these women often have severe vasomotor symptoms on stopping therapy, have no vaginal bleeding and no progestogenic side-effects.

Ethnic differences in HRT use have been noted with, for example, a lower rate of use in non-Caucasian women in the UK: uptake of other preventive health measures is also lower in these groups (Harris et al 1999a). Over 50% of women will have stopped therapy after 1 year (Hill et al 2000b). This is even found in women with low bone mineral density who are advised to take HRT.

Various strategies can be employed to improve concordance (North American Menopause Society 1998, Ettinger et al 1998).

- Involvement of the women in the decision-making process.
- Clear and personalized explanation of the benefits, risks and duration of therapy.
- Discussion of the woman's preferences and which regime she wishes to use.
- Provide written information.
- Arrange follow-up.

Poor concordance is not limited to HRT and has been found with patients taking antihypertensives or antituberculous drugs. Studies which have examined the reasons why women stop therapy emphasize the dislike of continued menstruation, side-effects, lack of efficacy and concerns about long-term risks. Some women consider HRT to be unnatural and in those with no symptoms or at low risk of osteoporosis, the benefits of therapy are limited.

CONCLUSION

Increased longevity, particularly in women, means that the menopause can now be considered to be a mid-life stage. There are major concerns about the implications, especially with regard to osteoporosis. The development of various continuous combined therapies should in theory improve long-term use. However, in those where this is still problematic bisphosphonates provide an alternative strategy. Maintaining an adequate intake of calcium and vitamin D is also of help. Some women do not wish to take standard medication and wish to use alternative or complementary therapies. The evidence regarding their benefits and safety needs to be fully evaluated and discussed.

KEY POINTS

1. The menopause is the permanent cessation of menstruation resulting from loss of ovarian follicular activity. In Western societies women will spend over one-third of their lives in the postmenopausal state.
2. Worldwide the elderly population is increasing, with women forming the majority.
3. The major issues in menopausal women are vasomotor symptoms, mood disorders, urogenital atrophy, sexual dysfunction, osteoporosis and cardiovascular disease. Osteoporosis affects 1 in 3 women and 1 in 12 men.
4. Hormone replacement therapy relieves menopausal symptoms and conserves bone mass. The role of oestrogen in coronary heart disease is currently unclear with secondary prevention studies showing no clear benefit. The results of primary prevention studies are awaited. In women where the sole endpoint of treatment is prevention of fracture, bisphosphonates are useful.
5. With regard to risks of HRT, the areas of concern are breast and endometrial cancer and venous thromboembolism. The increase in risk of breast cancer is roughly equivalent to the rise in relative risk in breast cancer associated with each year the menopause is delayed after the age of 50. In non-hysterectomized women progestogen is added to oestrogen to reduce the risk of endometrial cancer. HRT is responsible for one extra case of venous thromboembolism per 5000 women-years of use.
6. The evidence that complementary therapies are effective is poor and there are concerns about the quality control of herbal preparations.

REFERENCES

Abbasi F, Krumholz A, Kittner SJ, Langenberg P 1999 Effects of menopause on seizures in women with epilepsy. Epilepsia 40:205–210

Adena MA, Gallagher HG 1982 Cigarette smoking and the age at menopause. Annals of Human Biology 9:121–130

Affinito P, Sorrentino C, Farace MJ et al 1996 Effects of thyroxine therapy on bone metabolism in postmenopausal women with hypothyroidism. Acta Obstetrica et Gynecologica Scandinavica 75:843–848

Alexandersen P, Toussaint A, Christiansen C et al 2001 Ipriflavone in the treatment of postmenopausal osteoporosis: a randomized controlled trial. JAMA 285:1482–1488

Andersson K, Pedersen AT, Mattsson LA, Milsom I 1998 Swedish gynecologists' and general practitioners' views on the climacteric period: knowledge, attitudes and management strategies. Acta Obstetrica Gynecologica et Scandinavica 77:909–916

Antoniou G, Kalogirou D, Karakitsos P, Antoniou D, Kalogirou O, Giannikos L 1997 Transdermal estrogen with a levonorgestrel-releasing intrauterine device for climacteric complaints versus estradiol-releasing vaginal ring with a vaginal progesterone suppository. Clinical and endometrial responses. Maturitas 26:103–111

Archer DF, Furst K, Tipping D, Dain MP, Vandepol C 1999a A randomised comparison of continuous combined transdermal delivery of estradiol-norethindrone acetate and estradiol alone for menopause. Obstetrics and Gynecology 94:498–503

Archer DF, Lobo RA, Land HF, Picker JH 1999b A comparative study of transvaginal uterine ultrasound and endometrial biopsy for evaluating the endometrium of postmenopausal women taking hormone replacement therapy. Menopause 6:201–208

Ashcroft GS, Dodsworth J, Boxley EV et al 1997 Estrogen accelerates

30
Fertility control
Anna F. Glasier

INTRODUCTION

Over the last 40 years there has been a significant rise in the use of contraception worldwide. In 1998 it was estimated that up to 58% of all married women of reproductive age or their partners were using contraception. The prevalence of contraceptive use remains low, however, in many less developed countries: only 14% of couples use contraception in some African countries. It has been estimated (Division of Reproductive Health 1998) that some 120 million women in developing countries who do not wish to become pregnant are unable, for a variety of reasons, to use contraception.

In Great Britain (Oddens et al 1994) over 95% of sexually active women who wish to avoid pregnancy use a method of contraception. The highest percentages of women not using contraception, despite being sexually active and not wanting to get pregnant, are among adolescents (9%), women over 40 (9%), women with lower educational standards and those with occasional sexual partners (13%).

Worldwide between 8 and 30 million unplanned pregnancies are the result of contraceptive failure. Despite the apparently high prevalence of contraceptive use in the UK, it has been estimated that 30% of babies delivered are the result of unplanned or unintended pregnancies. Moreover, large numbers of unplanned pregnancies are terminated. Scotland has an abortion rate which is one of the lowest in countries in which abortion is legal, yet for every six babies born, one pregnancy is terminated. Although abortion is a safe procedure in Western countries, it has been estimated that of the annual figure of 46 million abortions performed around the world, 20 million are unsafe and some 78 000 women die as a result (Division of Reproductive Health 1998).

Different methods of contraception are prevalent in different countries. The intrauterine device (IUD) is the commonest method in China, while the vast majority of couples in Japan, where the combined oral contraceptive pill has only very recently been licensed, use the condom. In some of the less developed parts of the world breastfeeding is still the most important method of birth spacing. The prevalence of method use in the UK is shown in Table 30.1.

CONTRACEPTION

Combined oral contraceptives

The combined oral contraceptive pill (COC) was developed during the 1950s and approved for use in Britain in 1961. The first preparations were thought to contain only progestogen but when purified preparations were tried, cycle control

Table 30.1   Use of contraceptive methods in the UK. From Oddens et al (1994)

Method	%
Oral contraceptives (OC)	36
Barrier methods	20.8
Vasectomy	16
Female sterilization	10.1
Intrauterine devices (IUD)	7.3
OC with barrier	3.3
Natural family planning (NFP)	1.5
Coitus interruptus	1.1
No method	3.6

deteriorated. The impurity had been oestrogen and when it was reinstated the combined pill as we know it today was created.

The COC contains oestrogen, usually ethinyl estradiol, and a synthetic progesterone (progestogen). Most modern pills contain 20–35 µg ethinyl estradiol with either a second-generation progestogen (norethisterone, levonorgestrel or ethynodiol diacetate) or a so-called third-generation progestogen (gestodene, desogestrel or norgestimate). The 20 µg-containing pills are as effective as 30 µg pills but, not surprisingly, are associated with poorer cycle control (Akerlund et al 1993).

Third-generation progestogens have a lower affinity for androgen receptors and are therefore less androgenic than the older progestogens. For this reason they are associated with a less adverse effect on serum lipids (Rebar & Zeserson 1991). Women taking pills containing modern progestogens have higher circulating concentrations of high-density lipoproteins (HDL) and lower concentrations of low-density lipoproteins (LDL). Since this profile of lipoproteins, at least in men, appears to be associated with a lower risk of cardiovascular disease, it was thought that the risk of myocardial infarction (MI) and perhaps stroke would be lower among women using third- as compared with second-generation progestogen-containing pills and the shift from second- to third-generation pills seen in the early 1990s was largely based on claims of superior cardiac safety. Since myocardial infarction is a very rare event among young women it is hard to demonstrate a significant difference in risk with different types of COC. However, in the recent MICA study from the UK no difference in risk of MI was identified between second- and third-generation pills (Dunn et al 1999).

In October 1995, however, the UK Committee on Safety of Medicines (CSM) considered evidence from four well-designed studies (Bloemenkamp et al 1995, Jick et al 1995, Spitzer et al 1996, WHO 1995) which suggested that the risk of venous thromboembolic (VTE) disease was roughly double among women taking pills containing either gestodene or desogestrel compared with women taking pills containing levonorgestrel. The CSM subsequently advised that women with an increased risk of thrombosis (risk factors identified were obesity, varicose veins, a family history of thrombosis and a personal history of pregnancy-induced hypertension) should change to a second-generation pill and that other women taking third-generation pills should seriously consider their position. Second-generation pills were to be regarded as the pill of first choice with third-generation pills reserved for women who experienced unwanted side-effects on second-generation pills *and* who were prepared to accept an increased risk of thrombosis.

Many people believed that the CSM acted hastily in issuing this advice (Weiss 1995) and a confusing and often acrimonious debate is still ongoing, fuelled by new studies showing no difference and by endless reanalysis of the original studies. While it has been argued that the original data were flawed or incorrectly analysed, the authors of three of the original studies stand by their conclusions and two well-reasoned editorials (O'Brien 1999, Skegg 2000) have concluded that caution is still justified. In 1999, accepting that the absolute risk of VTE is very small indeed, the CSM removed the restriction on prescribing, suggesting that the choice of pill was a matter for the clinician and the user but that the latter should be made aware of the evidence relating to a higher risk of VTE of third-generation pills (Medicines Commission 1999). It is not clear through what mechanism third-generation pills may act to increase the risk of thromboembolism but it has been demonstrated that acquired resistance to activated protein C (which downregulates in vitro thrombin formation) is more pronounced during use of a pill containing desogestrel compared with one containing levonorgestrel (Rosing et al 1999).

Combined pills are available in monophasic, biphasic and triphasic preparations. Phasic pills were developed in order to reduce the total dose of progestogen and, by mimicking the fluctuating pattern of steroid concentrations in the normal ovarian cycle, in an attempt to produce better cycle control. There is no good evidence that cycle control is superior compared with that achieved by monophasic pills. Moreover, while the older triphasic pills do expose the user to a lower total dose of progestogen than their monophasic equivalent, the newer third-generation brands do not.

Mode of action

The COC works primarily by inhibiting ovulation. Exogenous oestrogen inhibits FSH secretion, while progestogens inhibit the development of the LH surge. The COC also alters cervical mucus, rendering it hostile to the passage of sperm, and causes endometrial atrophy.

The COC is a highly effective method of contraception (Table 30.2). The failure rates associated with all forms of contraception depend on the inherent efficacy of the method but also on the potential for incorrect or inappropriate use. Since ovulation is inhibited in most women who use the combined pill, failure rates of the method itself are low. However, as inhibition of ovulation depends on reliable pill taking, the overall failure rate of the COC, which includes user failures, is higher.

Contraindications

In an analysis of 25 years of follow-up of 46 000 women who took part in the Royal College of General Practitioners' (RCGP) Oral Contraceptive Study comparing 517 519 years of pill use with 335 998 years of never-use, the risk of death from all causes was similar in ever-users and never-users of oral contraception (Beral et al 1999). Among current and recent users (within 10 years) the relative risk of death from ovarian cancer was significantly decreased (RR 0.2) while the risks of dying from cervical cancer (RR 2.5) and from cerebrovascular disease (RR 1.9) were increased.

Absolute contraindications to COC use are listed in Box 30.1. They include either a past history of, or existing cardiovascular disease, including migraine, and most liver diseases. Women often describe headaches as migraine. The COC is contraindicated in migraine which is or may be associated with transient cerebral ischaemia; this includes crescendo migraine and focal migraine with asymmetric symptoms. Symmetrical blurring of vision, generalized flashing lights or photophobia associated with unilateral headache are not features which are regarded as absolute contraindications. A recent study designed to investigate the risk between migraine and stroke in young women demonstrated a significant increase in the risk of ischaemic

Table 30.2 Pregnancy rates for birth control methods (for 1 year of use). Data adapted from Trussel (1998).

Method	Typical use rate of pregnancy (%)	Lowest expected rate of pregnancy (%)
Sterilization		
Male sterilization	0.15	0.1
Female sterilization	0.5	0.5
Hormonal methods		
Implant (Norplant®)	0.05	0.05
Hormone injection (Depo-provera™)	0.3	0.3
Combined pill (oestrogen/ progestogen)	5	0.1
Minipill (progestogen only)	5	0.5
Intrauterine methods (IUDs)		
Copper T	0.8	0.6
LNG-IUS	0.2	0.2
Barrier methods		
Male condom[1]	14	3
Diaphragm[2]	20	6
Female condom	21	5
Spermicide (gel, pessary,)	26	6
Emergency contraception		
Levonelle-2 (within 24h)	5	
Schering PC4 (within 24h)	23	
Copper IUD	<5	
Natural methods		
Withdrawal	19	4
'Natural family planning' (calendar, temperature, mucus)	25	1–9
No method	85	85

[1]Used without spermicide, [2]used with spermicide
This table provides estimates of the per cent of women likely to become pregnant while using a particular contraceptive method for 1 year. These estimates are based on a variety of studies.
'Typical use' rate means that the method either was not always used correctly or was not used with every act of sexual intercourse or was used correctly but failed.
'Lowest expected' rates mean that despite being used correctly with every act of sexual intercourse, the method failed.

but not haemorrhagic stroke in women with a personal history of migraine both with and without aura (classic and simple). Coexistent use of the COC further increased this risk (Chang et al 1999). It is important therefore to take a clear and detailed history before refusing to prescribe the COC because the woman has an occasional migraine.

Relative contraindications to COC use include the following.

- Factors which increase the risk of cardiovascular disease or venous thrombosis such as obesity, smoking, hypertension and family history.
- Sex steroid-dependent conditions, including cancer, e.g. breast cancer.

Box 30.1 Absolute contraindications to the combined oral contraceptive pill

Arterial or venous thrombosis
Ischaemic heart disease including myopathy
Most valvular heart disease
Past cerebral haemorrhage
Hypercholesterolaemia
Conditions predisposing to thrombosis, e.g. polycythaemia
Migraine
Pulmonary hypertension
Active liver disease
Porphyria
History of a serious condition affected by sex steroids, e.g. trophoblastic disease

- Factors which adversely affect liver function.
- Factors which predispose to arterial wall disease.

Comprehensive discussions and lists of contraindications are available in most textbooks of contraception.

Side-effects of combined oral contraception

Oestrogen and progestogens are both metabolized by the liver and as such alter the metabolism of most substances, including carbohydrates and lipids. Oestrogens also alter coagulation factors. A reduction in antithrombin III and alteration in platelet function increase the risk of venous thromboembolism by up to sevenfold. A clear history of thromboembolism is a contraindication to the COC. A possible history or a very strong family history are indications for investigating haemostasis, particularly circulating concentrations of antithrombin III and the factor V Leiden thrombogenic mutation. Population screening for inherited thrombophilias is not currently considered to be cost effective.

Arterial disease, including myocardial infarction and cerebrovascular accident, results from the (mainly) progestogen-related alteration to lipid profiles together with the oestrogen-associated changes in blood coagulation. A WHO expert group recently reviewed the data on myocardial infarction, stroke and hormonal contraception; the conclusions are a useful summary of current knowledge and are as follows (WHO Scientific Group 1998).

Acute myocardial infarction

- Acute myocardial infarction (MI) is uncommon in women of reproductive age.
- The risk of MI, regardless of age, is not increased among pill users who do not smoke and do not have either hypertension or diabetes.
- Women who have hypertension and who take the COC have an increased relative risk of MI of at least three times that of women who take the COC and are normotensive.
- Smoking increases the risk of MI by 10 times when compared with COC users who do not smoke.
- There is insufficient evidence to allow any conclusion on whether the risk of MI is influenced by the type or dose of progestogen.

Thus women who have no other risk factors can be reassured that they have no increased risk of myocardial infarction. There was no increased risk of mortality due to ischaemic heart disease either during or after COC use in the report of the RCGP study (Beral et al 1999).

Stroke

- Ischaemic and haemorrhagic stroke are both uncommon among women of reproductive age.
- The risk of ischaemic stroke is increased by about 1.5-fold in pill-users who do not smoke and are not hypertensive. In contrast, the risk of haemorrhagic stroke is not increased in these women until they reach the age of 35, after which the increasing natural risk of haemorrhagic stroke is magnified by COC use.
- Hypertension increases the risk of both ischaemic (by three times) and haemorrhagic (10-fold) stroke when compared with never-users.
- Smoking increases the risk of ischaemic and haemorrhagic stroke ($\times 2$–3) compared with pill users who do not smoke.
- There is insufficient evidence to determine whether the risk of either type of stroke is influenced by the type or dose of progestogen.

Thus the data are reassuring for haemorrhagic stroke, but the risk of ischaemic stroke is increased by COC use and once again, this is supported by the findings of the RCGP study (Beral et al 1999) in which the relative risk of death from stroke was significantly increased to 1.9 (confidence intervals 1.2–3.1, $p = 0.009$). After 10 years of stopping the pill the risk of death from stroke is no longer elevated.

Breast cancer.   Overviews of the risks and benefits of the COC are dominated by breast cancer. Published data are difficult to interpret because pill formulations and patterns of reproduction (particularly age at first pregnancy) have changed with time. In 1996 the Collaborative Group on Hormonal Factors in Breast Cancer reported a meta-analysis of 54 studies involving over 53 000 women with breast cancer and 100 000 control subjects. The groups concluded that use of the COC was associated with a small increase in breast cancer and that the increased risk persisted for 10 years after stopping the pill. The relative risk for current users was 1.24; for 1–4 years after stopping 1.16 and for 5–9 years after stopping 1.07. Since the absolute risks of breast cancer increase with age, the effect of this is more significant in population terms among older women who are taking or have recently taken the COC. After 10 years the relative risk of breast cancer was no longer increased. Although the relative risk was higher for women who started the pill at a young age (because breast cancer is rare in this age group) there was little added effect from the duration of use, dose or type of hormone. Somewhat reassuringly, ever-users were significantly less likely (RR 0.88) to have cancer which had spread beyond the breast even if they had stopped the pill more than 10 years earlier. The RCGP study (Beral 1999) is also reassuring in this respect since the risk of dying from breast cancer is not significantly increased among current or recent (within 10 years) COC users.

The relationship between the pill and breast cancer is difficult to explain because the risk appears to increase soon after exposure, does not increase with duration of exposure and returns to normal 10 years after stopping. It has been suggested that starting to use the pill may accelerate the appearance of breast cancer in susceptible women, i.e. late-stage promotion of existing dysplasia. It is also possible that women using the pill have their tumours diagnosed earlier although it is difficult to explain why a tendency to earlier diagnosis would persist for years after stopping. In the large meta-analysis, the risk of breast cancer was also increased among current users of both the progestogen-only pill (RR 1.17) and Depo-provera (RR 1.07) although the numbers of women using progestin-only methods was small. These findings strengthen the argument for increased detection rather than late-stage promotion of breast cancer. None the less, a biological effect of hormonal contraception has still not been ruled out.

Other side-effects.   Around 2% of women become clinically hypertensive after starting the pill. The incidence increases with age and duration of use, obesity and family history. It does not, however, appear to be increased in women with a history of pregnancy-induced hypertension.

A modest increase in the risk of squamous carcinoma of the cervix (RR 1.3–1.8) has been recognized for some time (WHO 1992) and is borne out by the increased risk of death from the disease among current and recent users demonstrated in the 25-year follow-up study (Beral et al 1999). The relationship is complicated by a number of confounding factors such as patterns of sexual behaviour and the likelihood of having cervical smears. An increase in the risk of the much less common cervical adenocarcinoma (RR 2.1, and increasing to 4.4 after 12 years of use) has also been demonstrated (Ursin et al 1994).

An increased risk of gallstones is significant only during the early years of pill use.

A few women develop chloasma on the COC and it appears that both oestrogen and progestogens contribute to this. The chloasma may be slow to fade after the pill is stopped.

Minor side-effects are commonest during the first 3 months of use and often lead to discontinuation of the method. More common problems include breakthrough bleeding or spotting, nausea, breast tenderness, acne and loss of libido. Many of these resolve with time. If side-effects persist after 4 months it is often worth changing the brand of pill, opting for a lower dose of oestrogen or a different type of progestogen. Pills containing antiandrogens (Dianette) are particularly useful for acne.

While the combined pill, in general, improves menstrual bleeding patterns, one common reason for presentation to a gynaecologist is breakthrough bleeding (BTB). BTB is common during the first three cycles of use. Persistence beyond 3 months may be a result of poor compliance or a coexisting gynaecological disorder such as cervical ectropion (probably more common among COC users), cervical or uterine polyp. If pelvic examination is normal, it is worth trying a formulation containing a higher dose of oestrogen or different type of progestogen. After 3 months use of a pill containing 50 µg ethinyl estradiol the bleeding will often settle and the woman can then resume a lower-dose pill. If bleeding persists, try stopping hormonal contraception altogether and if it does not resolve it should be investigated as intermenstrual bleeding, i.e. by endometrial biopsy and hysteroscopy.

Benefits of combined oral contraception

In addition to being an effective and acceptable method of contraception, the pill confers a number of health benefits.

Withdrawal bleeds are usually more regular, lighter and less painful and the COC is often the treatment of choice for women with irregular heavy periods (resulting from anovulatory dysfunctional uterine bleeding) and for dysmenorrhoea. COC use is associated with a decreased incidence of benign breast disease and functional ovarian cysts and is often used as the first line in the management of premenstrual syndrome. Inhibition of ovarian activity for the treatment of endometriosis can be achieved without the need for additional contraception (in contrast to danazol).

COC use is associated with a reduction in the risk of endometrial cancer which is related to the duration of use and reaches 50% after 4 years. The protective effect may be maintained for up to 15 years after discontinuation (WHO 1992). There is a similar duration-dependent reduction in the risk of ovarian cancer (Beral et al 1999, WHO 1992), which probably acts through the inhibition of ovulation. Protection is apparent after as little as 6 months of use and lasts at least 10 years after discontinuation. After 10 years non-users are five times more likely to develop ovarian cancer than women who have used the COC. It is interesting to note that the incidence of ovarian cancer is declining in all developed countries except Japan where the COC was only approved for contraception in 2000.

Significant numbers of unplanned pregnancies are a result of women stopping the pill for 'a break'. There is no evidence that breaks in pill taking reduce the long-term risks. There is also no evidence that it is necessary to stop the COC before planning a pregnancy. There is no evidence of any adverse effect on the fetus of COC use prior to conception, neither is exposure during pregnancy associated with increased risk of fetal malformation.

Fertility is restored after a delay of 1–3 months although some women take longer to resume normal cycles. So-called post-pill amenorrhoea is almost always associated with cycle irregularity before starting the pill or with coincidental factors associated with secondary amenorrhoea such as weight loss or stress.

Progestogen–only contraception

Progestogen-only contraception is much less commonly used than combined hormonal contraception. It is, however, available in a wider variety of systems including pills, implants, long-acting injectables and hormone-releasing IUDs. New delivery systems include vaginal rings, patches and a gel preparation.

The mechanism of action of progestogen-only contraceptives depends on the dose of steroid administered. High doses, e.g. DMPA, inhibit ovulation. Low doses inhibit ovulation only inconsistently, depending on the individual response. By all routes of administration, progestogens affect both the quantity and physical characteristics of cervical mucus, reducing sperm penetrability and transport. All methods have an effect on the endometrium which probably compromises implantation.

The absence of oestrogen in this group of hormonal methods has long been thought to be associated with an absence of cardiovascular risks including VTE. In a recent case control study undertaken by the WHO (1998), there was no significant increase in the risk of MI, stroke or VTE associated with use of oral or injectable progestogen-only methods.

The progestogen-only pill (POP or mini-pill) is a useful alternative for women who like the convenience of the COC but for whom oestrogen is contraindicated. It should be emphasized that not only does the POP not contain oestrogen, but the dose of progestogen is significantly lower than in equivalent combined preparations. The POP is still a good alternative for women with medical contraindications to the COC such as migraine and hypertension. It is often advocated for women with diabetes who are at increased risk of cardiovascular disease and who may find that insulin requirements fluctuate with COC cycles. It should be said, however, that the COC is not absolutely contraindicated for diabetic women without long-term complications, whose diabetes is well controlled and for whom pregnancy would be a disaster. The commonest indication for POP use in the UK is probably for women who are breast-feeding since the POP (unlike the COC) does not interfere with either the quantity or constituents of breast milk. It is no longer considered necessary to advise women routinely to change from the COC to the POP when they reach the age of 35 since the combined pill, in the absence of risk factors for cardio-vascular disease, is so very safe.

Mode of action

Around 50% of POP users continue to ovulate and menstruate regularly. In these women the POP works by altering cervical mucus and probably by interfering with implantation. In some 10–20% of women, follicular development is completely inhibited with resultant amenorrhoea. The remainder will experience irregular bleeding associated with follicular growth without ovulation or with inadequate luteal phase cycles.

Side-effects

The mode of action of the POP explains its side-effects. Erratic bleeding is the commonest cause for discontinuation of the pill; around 20% of women will stop using it for this reason.

Follicular growth without ovulation is associated with an increased incidence of functional ovarian cysts. Up to 20% of women using the POP will have a cyst identifiable by ultrasound. Most are symptomless and nearly all resolve spontaneously. A woman found to have a symptomless ovarian cyst should be reviewed after her next menstrual period.

POP use is associated with a slightly increased risk of ectopic pregnancy. Some 2% of pregnancies among POP failures will be ectopic, perhaps as a result of an effect of the progestogen on tubal motility.

Because of its mechanism of action (50% of women continue to ovulate) and its relatively short half-life (around 19 hours) the POP has a higher failure rate than the COC (see Table 30.2). This failure rate is dependent on age and is almost as low as the COC in women over 35 years. Women weighing more than 70 kg have higher failure rates and should be advised to take two pills each day.

Injectable progestogens

Long-acting injectable progestogens are available in two forms: depot medroxyprogesterone acetate (DMPA or Depo-provera,

150 mg IM every 12 weeks) and norethisterone oenanthate (NET-EN, 200 mg IM every 8 weeks). NET-EN is seldom used in the UK.

Worldwide, DMPA is a popular method of contraception used by some 9 million women in over 90 countries. Early reports of mammary tumours in beagle dogs and endometrial cancer in rhesus monkeys led to reluctance on the part of some governments, notably the USA, to approve its use and data on the risk of cancer and DMPA in women were scarce until the 1990s. A WHO expert group was convened in 1993 to review a number of recently published large epidemiological studies. DMPA appears to exert a powerful protective effect against endometrial cancer with a relative risk of 0.2. No association has been described between DMPA use and the risk of ovarian cancer which is surprising if the protective effect of the COC is due to the inhibition of ovulation. Nor is there any association with cervical cancer, which is reassuring. The slight increase in the risk of breast cancer among users of both the POP and DMPA identified in the large meta-analysis (Collaborative Group on Hormonal Factors in Breast Cancer 1996) may be due to detection bias; however, there are some concerns that progestins alone may be associated with a real increase in risk. Depo-provera was licensed for use in the UK in 1984 as a short-term method of contraception – one injection covered the period of infertility required after rubella vaccination, for example – or as a long-term method for women who were unable to use any existing methods. These conditions were removed in 1994.

Depo-provera is a highly effective (Table 30.2) long-acting method which only requires the user to attend for injection four times a year. It inhibits ovulation and after 1 year of use 80% of women are either amenorrhoeic (40%) or have very scanty, infrequent periods (40%). The remaining 20% will have prolonged regular or more usually irregular bleeding episodes and around 2% of women will present, often to a gynaecologist, with troublesome menorrhagia. After excluding any pathology the most effective treatment of menorrhagia is oestrogen (Fraser 1983) and it is most easily given as one packet of the COC. If bleeding problems persist, an alternative method of contraception should be considered.

Other significant long-term side-effects include the following.

- Weight gain; many women will gain up to 6 pounds during the first year of use.
- A delay in the resumption of fertility of up to 1 year or more after cessation of use.
- A possible reduction in bone mineral density (BMD). Studies from New Zealand (Cundy et al 1991, 1994) have demonstrated a small but reversible loss of BMD in women using Depo-provera for 5 years or more. Although MPA has been shown in some circumstances to protect bone after the menopause, most women using Depo-provera become relatively hypo-oestrogenic. The loss in bone density is almost certainly not sufficient to cause an increased risk of fracture in premenopausal women and a cross-sectional study from the UK (Gbolade et al 1998) of 185 women using Depo-provera for more than 5 years or amenorrhoeic after 1 year of use showed only a minimal change in BMD which was thought unlikely to be of clinical significance.

Similarly no significant difference in BMD is demonstrable when past users are compared with controls (Orr-Walker et al 1998). Concerns remain, however, about the use of DMPA in adolescents who have yet to achieve their peak bone mass.

It has been suggested that long-term users of Depo-provera should be managed by measuring serum estradiol and, if it is low, by treating with oestrogen patches in addition to the DMPA. This seems to make it a complicated and relatively expensive method of contraception and there is no evidence to support the practice. A more pragmatic approach may be to suggest that women stop using Depo-provera at the age 45 to allow for recovery of bone mineral density before postmenopausal bone loss ensues. Depo-provera was licensed in the USA in 1992 on condition that the effect on bone mineral density of long-term use was investigated; the results of a longitudinal study should be available in 2003.

Progestogen-only implants

The progestogen-only implant Norplant® was licensed for use in the UK in 1993. Comprising six Silastic rods containing a total of 216 mg of crystallized levonorgestrel (LNG), Norplant® is inserted subdermally on the inner aspect of the upper arm. Circulating levels of levonorgestrel are around 80 μg/day during the first 8 weeks and decline slowly to around 50 μg at the end of the first year and 25–30 μg at 60 months (see Fraser et al 1998 for review). The implants must be inserted and removed using local anaesthetic and the contraceptive effect lasts for 5 years. Although the implants are not difficult to insert, removal can be troublesome, particularly if the rods are inserted subcutaneously rather than subdermally. Failure rates are extremely low (Table 30.2) and obviously comprise only method failures as implants do not depend on compliance. Ovulation is inhibited in many cycles, particularly in the first year of use, and when it does occur it is associated with an inadequate luteal phase. Cervical mucus is scanty and allows poor sperm penetration.

The dose of progestogen is similar to that of the POP and the mode of action is therefore similar. Erratic bleeding occurs in around 70% of users and some 10% of women become amenorrhoeic. Fertility resumes as soon as the implants are removed. Bleeding irregularity is the commonest side-effect and reason for removal, but others include acne, hirsutism, headache, mood change and weight gain or bloating (i.e. the metabolic side-effects of progestogens).

In 1999 Norplant® ceased to be marketed in the UK because of adverse publicity; extensive threatened litigation (which failed); relatively poor sales and the imminent arrival of a single implant Implanon®. The two-rod version of Norplant® (Norplant 2 or Jadelle), although now marketed in many countries, is unlikely to become available in the UK. Implanon® contains 68 mg of 3-keto-desogestrel, a metabolite of the third-generation progestogen desogestrel. The implant provides contraception for 3 years. The initial release rate is around 60–70 μg/day, falling gradually to around 25–30 μg/day at the end of 3 years. Implanon® comes as a single rod preloaded into a sterile disposable inserter. The rod is inserted subdermally under local anaesthetic into the upper arm. Insertion and removal are immeasurably easier than with Norplant®. The dose of progestogen is sufficient to inhibit ovulation in every cycle throughout the 3 years and there have as yet been no pregnancies reported as a result of failure of the method. Bleeding patterns are disrupted in a manner very similar to Norplant® although slightly more women (up to 20%) will experience amenorrhoea. For a useful review of Implanon see Archer et al (1998).

Intrauterine devices

The intrauterine device (IUD) is an effective long-acting method of contraception which is perhaps under-rated in the developed world. It exerts a local inflammatory reaction within the cavity of the uterus which probably, acting through tubal and uterine fluid, interferes with the viability of both sperm and eggs. It also inhibits implantation. Inert devices are no longer recommended nor marketed but some older women do still have them in utero. Modern copper-containing devices are licensed for use over 5 (Nova T 380) to 10 (Copper T 380) years. After a woman reaches 40 the device need not be changed and can be removed 1 year after the last menstrual period. Copper IUDs consist of a plastic frame with copper wire round the stem and, in some cases, copper caps on the arms. The surface area of the copper determines the lifespan and efficacy of the device. IUDs with a surface area of copper of less than 200 mm^2 are associated with higher pregnancy rates and are no longer recommended for long-term use. A frameless IUD (Gynefix®; Wildemeersch et al 1999) comprises six copper beads threaded on to a nylon line. The beads at the top and bottom are crimped to hold them all in place and the string has a knot at the proximal end which is embedded, using a special inserter, into the myometrium, anchoring it in place. Anchored in this way, the device is 'free' to move within the uterine cavity and as such may be associated with lower rates of dysmenorrhoea.

The levonorgestrel-releasing device (known as a system – IUS – to distinguish it from copper IUDs) has been licensed in the UK since 1995 under the trade name Mirena®. It consists of a column of LNG within a rate-limiting membrane wrapped around the stem of a Nova-T frame. A total dose of 52 mg of LNG is released at a rate of 20 mg/day. It is licensed for 5 years for contraception. A small amount of levonorgestrel is absorbed systemically and can give rise to androgenic side-effects such as acne. Menstrual bleeding is significantly reduced, with periods being replaced by light spotting and eventually, in many women, amenorrhoea. In the classic study of the effects of the LNG-IUS on menstrual blood loss (Andersson & Rybo 1990), women complaining of menorrhagia experienced a reduction in blood loss of 86% at 3 and 97% at 12 months after LNG-IUS insertion. Mirena® is now widely used in the UK, and indeed recommended, for the management of menorrhagia (RCOG 1999a) and can also provide the progestogen component of HRT. It is not yet licensed for either of these indications but is likely to be within the near future.

Perforation is a rare event (1 in 1000 insertions); if it is recognized early it may be possible to remove the IUD via the laparoscope before adhesions form. For this reason it is probably wise to see women for follow-up to check the tails of the device within 4–6 weeks of insertion.

Expulsion occurs in 3–10% of women in the first year of use and is related to parity, age, type of IUD and timing of insertion. The incidence of both expulsion and perforation is influenced by the skill of the person inserting the device. Both are increased with postpartum insertions which should be delayed until 6 weeks among bottlefeeding women and 8 weeks among breastfeeders.

The risk of pelvic infection among IUD users has been greatly exaggerated. In countries where IUDs are inserted under appropriate sterile conditions the risk of pelvic infection is only increased for 20 days after insertion. Women infected with gonorrhoea or chlamydia have an increased risk of infection if an IUD is inserted compared with uninfected women but the risk of salpingitis is not increased when compared with infected women who are not undergoing IUD insertion. Even women who are HIV positive do not appear to have an increased risk of complications, including infection, associated with IUD insertion and there is no evidence that IUD use increases viral shedding (Grimes 2000). There is no evidence for an increased risk of infertility among past or current IUD users. However, if an IUD user becomes pregnant the probability of that pregnancy being ectopic is greater than for women using no contraception or another method because the IUD does not prevent tubal implantation. In women at risk of pre-existing infection IUD insertion can be covered with a broad-spectrum antibiotic. Routine screening for infection may be more cost effective in services where the background rate of infection, especially with chlamydia, is high (SIGN 2000).

The commonest reason for discontinuation of the copper IUD is menorrhagia. The local inflammatory response, together with an increased production of prostaglandins, causes both menorrhagia and dysmenorrhoea. All IUDs are removed by steady traction on the tail of the device. Occasionally, the string snaps off during removal. It is sometimes possible to remove the device with a pair of artery forceps or a specially designed IUD remover but some IUDs, particularly the old inert devices, appear to become deeply embedded in the endometrium and may only be removed under a general anaesthetic. Whether an IUD without its tails can be left in the cavity of the uterus for a woman's lifetime without causing any problems is not known. There is a small risk of actinomycosis but the inconvenience of admission to hospital for a general anaesthetic may outweigh this. It is probably best discussed with the individual concerned.

Natural family planning

Although few couples in the UK use so-called natural methods of family planning (NFP), nevertheless in some parts of the world these methods are common. All involve 'periodic abstinence', that is, avoidance of intercourse during the fertile period of the cycle. Methods differ in the way in which they recognize the fertile period. The simplest is the calendar or rhythm method in which the woman calculates the fertile period according to the length of her normal menstrual cycle. Others use symptoms which reflect fluctuating concentrations of circulating oestrogen and progesterone, themselves reflecting follicular development, impending ovulation and completed ovulation. The mucus or Billings method relies on identifying changes in the quantity and quality of cervical and vaginal mucus as a reflection of the steroid environment. As circulating oestrogens increase with follicle growth the mucus becomes clear and stretchy, allowing the passage of sperm. With ovulation, and in the presence of progesterone, mucus becomes opaque, sticky and much less stretchy or disappears altogether. Intercourse must stop when fertile-type mucus is identified and can start again when infertile-type mucus is recognized. Progesterone secretion is also associated with a rise in basal body temperature (BBT) of about 0.5°C. The BBT method is thus able to identify the end of the fertile period. Other signs and symptoms such as ovulation pain, position of cervix and degree of dilatation of the cervical os can be used additionally to help define the fertile period. A personal fertility monitor called Persona, which measures urinary oestrogen and LH using a dipstick, can help to identify the fertile period but does not significantly reduce the number of days of abstinence required and is expensive (Bonnar et al 1999).

Whatever method is used, all rely on a period of abstinence and many couples find this difficult. Failure rates are high (Table 30.2) and most of the failures are due to conscious rule breaking. Perfect use of the mucus method is in fact associated with a failure rate of only 3.4%. There is no evidence that accidental pregnancies occurring among NFP users, which are conceived with ageing gametes, are associated with a higher risk of congenital malformations.

Lactational amenorrhoea method (LAM)

Breastfeeding delays the resumption of fertility and in developing countries it still has a major impact on fertility rates. It has been calculated that breastfeeding provides more than 98% protection from pregnancy during the first 6 months postpartum, if the mother is fully or nearly fully breastfeeding and has not yet experienced vaginal bleeding after the 56th day postpartum. On the basis of this statement, guidelines (Labbok et al 1990) have been developed for women who wish to use lactational amenorrhoea as a means of fertility regulation. The guidelines advise that as long as the baby is less than 6 months old a woman can rely on breastfeeding alone until she menstruates or until she starts to give her baby significant amounts of food other than breast milk. Prospective studies of the LAM confirm its effectiveness (Perez et al 1992). In societies where women breastfeed for prolonged periods the guidelines can probably be extended beyond 6 months.

Barrier methods

The male condom remains one of the most popular methods of contraception in the UK. It is cheap, widely available over the counter and, with the exception of the occasional allergic reaction, is free from side-effects. Use of the condom has increased significantly during the last decade as a result of concern over the spread of HIV and AIDS as it is, of course, the only method of contraception which also prevents sexually transmitted infections (STI).

In addition to protection against STI, use of the condom – and diaphragm – is associated with a significant reduction in cervical disease (Celentano et al 1987). Female barrier methods are less popular. The diaphragm and cervical cap must be fitted by a professional and do not confer the same degree of protection from STI/HIV. The female condom, by virtue of covering the mucus membranes of the vagina and vulva, is more effective in preventing sexually transmitted diseases but has a high failure rate and low acceptability (Bounds et al 1992).

Spermicides alone are not a very effective method of contraception and are only recommended for use with a condom (most of which are already lubricated with spermicide) or diaphragm. There have been concerns that nonoxynol-9 (N9, the active ingredient of all spermicides available in the UK) may increase the risk of HIV/AIDS transmission by causing local irritation and breaching of the vaginal epithelium. A recent double-blind placebo-controlled multicentre study of sex workers demonstrated a higher rate of seroconversion in the women using N9 than in the controls (van Damme et al 2000). Studies of this type are extremely difficult to perform and there may be bias or confounding variables which explain the effect. Moreover, the studies were undertaken in regions where the prevalence of HIV/AIDS is high and among women with very frequent intercourse with a large number of partners. For these reasons the results are being interpreted with caution and there has been no change in the recommendations regarding the routine use of N9 with condoms and diaphragms. An immense research effort is ongoing to develop microbicides/virucides, with and without contraceptive properties, which are effective against HIV as well as chlamydia and other organisms responsible for STI.

Emergency contraception

Hormonal preparations and the IUD can be used to prevent pregnancy after intercourse has taken place. In the UK one hormonal preparation is available: Levonelle-2 (levonorgestrel 0.75 mg, Schering). Both compounds are given as two doses separated by 12 hours with the first dose given within 72 hours of intercourse (see Glasier 2000 for review). Recent data suggest that both are much more effective given within 24 hours (Table 30.2) and women should be encouraged to present as soon as possible for treatment. Levonelle-2 is thought to be the more effective method although this assertion is based on the results of only one RCT in which the failure rate of the Yuzpe regimen was unusually high (Task Force on Postovulatory Methods of Fertility Regulation 1998). It is in any case very difficult to estimate the efficacy of any emergency contraceptive (EC) since the true risk of pregnancy for any one individual cannot be calculated with any degree of certainty and many of the 'failures' are pregnancies which are in fact conceived with an act of intercourse which occurred earlier in the cycle or some time after the act for which EC was sought. Levonelle-2 is now available off prescription from pharmacists although it is expensive to buy (all contraception is, of course, free of charge in the UK if prescribed by a doctor). Levonelle-2 is certainly better tolerated with significantly less nausea and vomiting.

IUD insertion is probably even more effective (Table 30.2) and can be used up to 5 days after the estimated day of ovulation which may be significantly longer than 5 days after the act of intercourse.

The mechanism of action of the hormonal methods of EC remains unclear. Both methods have been shown to delay or impair ovulation in some 50% of users but there is no good evidence that either method will inhibit implantation. Neither of them will have any contraceptive/contragestive effect once implantation is complete. Although there has been a tendency to confuse the risks of the Yuzpe regimen with those of long-term use of the combined pill (particularly the risk of VTE) there is no evidence for any serious risks with either method.

Recent efforts to find a more effective, orally active emergency contraceptive with fewer side-effects have resulted in trials of the antiprogesterone mifepristone (Task Force on Postovulatory Methods of Fertility Regulation 1999). Since mifepristone is known to inhibit both ovulation and implantation it is likely to be more effective than either the Yuzpe regimen or levonorgestrel alone but its properties as an abortifacient limit its further development at present.

Future prospects

Steroidal contraception

Steroid hormones remain the most successful approach to modern methods of contraception, and in addition to adjusting pill formulations, the research efforts of both pharmaceutical companies and international organizations have centred round new delivery systems for steroids.

Combined oestrogen-progestogen once-a-month injectables (Cyclofem and Mesigyna) have been developed by the WHO. With failure rates of less than 0.5%, they are associated with a significant reduction in menstrual irregularities compared with DMPA. These preparations are particularly useful in societies where injectables are popular and easy to deliver but where amenorrhoea is unacceptable.

Soft Silastic or vinyl vaginal rings have also been developed, releasing progestogen either alone or in combination with oestrogen. Steroids are readily absorbed vaginally, avoiding the first pass through the liver, and thus the dose can be reduced. In most studies, around 8% of women are unable to use rings because of expulsion or local side-effects such as vaginal discharge. The levonorgestrel ring has a daily release rate of 20 µg and is designed to be worn continuously. Efficacy, ectopic pregnancy rates and the incidence of bleeding irregularities are equivalent to those of the mini-pill (WHO 1990a). Combination rings have been developed by the Population Council in the USA and by Organon. The Organon ring releases etonorgestrel and only 15 µg of ethinyl oestradiol per day, thus significantly reducing the dose of oestrogen. Use will be for 3 weeks in and 1 week out. The vaginal ring has been licensed in the US, and it is also available in every European country except France and the UK.

Transdermal delivery of contraceptive steroids lags strangely far behind the development of this route of administration of ovarian steroids for postmenopausal hormone replacement therapy. Research in this area continues and a phase 3 study of a combination patch was recently completed successfully. The patch has now been licensed for use in the US. (Audet et al 2001).

Vaccines

The development of contraceptive vaccines has been disappointingly slow. A vaccine against part of the β-subunit of hCG is being tested by the WHO. It appears to be capable of inducing a level of antibodies sufficient to prevent pregnancy for 6–12 months but is associated with troublesome local allergic reactions. In India a vaccine against the whole β-subunit is effective and, despite cross-reacting with LH, appears to be associated with little menstrual disturbance. Individual variability in response and long-term safety, however, still needs to be addressed.

Vaccines directed towards the zona pellucida have been developed and produce reversible contraception in monkeys. Disappointingly, anti-zona vaccines appear to lead ultimately to irreversible interference with ovarian function, permanent sterility and premature menopause. Anti-sperm vaccines are proving difficult to develop despite the existence of apparently non-toxic anti-sperm antibodies in vivo.

Hormone agonists and antagonists

Hormone agonists and antagonists offer perhaps the most promising lead for reversible non-steroidal contraception.

Ovulation is inhibited during chronic intranasal administration of the gonadotrophin-releasing hormone (GnRH) agonist buserelin. If ovarian activity is completely suppressed, however, the deleterious effects of a prolonged hypo-oestrogenic state on bone and the cardiovascular system would probably necessitate some form of replacement therapy. In contrast, incomplete suppression, with residual ovarian activity, might lead to an increased risk of endometrial hyperplasia and cancer, due to the effects of unopposed oestrogen. GnRH agonists may nevertheless have a place where there is a need for short-term contraception and indeed, have been shown to be effective during breastfeeding when minimal quantities of agonist pass into the milk (Fraser 1993).

Antagonists of progesterone offer considerable potential for the regulation of fertility. Progesterone is essential for the establishment and maintenance of pregnancy. Antagonists such as mifepristone block the action of progesterone on the endometrium and hence produce an environment hostile to pregnancy. Mifepristone is licensed as an emergency contraceptive in China. Administration of daily doses as low as 2 mg and weekly doses of 100 mg are effective in inhibiting ovulation and daily, weekly and once-per-month preparations are all being investigated as regular contraceptives. Given in combination with prostaglandins, these compounds would probably also be effective as a late luteal-phase contraceptive and a single dose of 200 mg administered at the time of the LH surge has promise as a once-a-month pill (see Baird 1993 for review). Unfortunately the politics surrounding the use of mifepristone and other anti-progesterones has seriously hindered their further development.

Male methods

The development of reliable methods of hormonal contraception has proved much more difficult for men than for women. The regulation of spermatogenesis is poorly understood and the link between sexual activity and hormones is much more direct in men than in women. Any method that compromises the endocrine activity of the testes must also involve testosterone replacement if sexual function is to be maintained. Testosterone must be given systemically because orally active synthetic androgens may cause liver damage. The WHO undertook a trial

441

of testosterone enanthate 200 mg once per week (WHO 1990b). Complete azoospermia occurred in only 58% of 271 men, although it was more likely to occur in Asian men than in caucasians. In men who achieved azoospermia the method had a failure rate of <1%. Oligozoospermia (counts of <3.0 million/ml) induced in this way is associated with a failure rate of 1.5/100 person-years.

The combination of a potent antagonist of GnRH and testosterone causes azoospermia more reliably, but the need for daily injections of antagonist, the cost and the high incidence of local allergic reactions make this regimen impractical.

A hormonal contraceptive method for men may become available within the next 10 years. For a review of future developments in contraception, see Baird & Glasier 2000.

STERILIZATION

Over 42 million couples worldwide, the majority of whom live in developing countries (particularly China and India), rely on vasectomy. More than three times that number rely on female sterilization. In Britain almost 50% of couples aged 35–44 are using either female or male sterilization as their method of contraception.

Female sterilization

Female sterilization usually involves the blocking of both fallopian tubes either by laparotomy or minilaparotomy or, more commonly, by laparoscopy. It may also be achieved by bilateral salpingectomy (or by hysterectomy when there is coexistent gynaecological pathology such as hydrosalpinx or fibroids).

Minilaparotomy and laparoscopic female sterilization are probably equally safe and effective; however, the latter allows sterilization to be done as a day-case procedure and is recommended by the Royal College of Obstetricians and Gynaecologists (RCOG) as the method of choice in the UK (RCOG 1999b). Minilaparotomy is most commonly used when sterilization is performed immediately postpartum as at that time the uterus is large, the pelvis very vascular and the risks of laparoscopy are increased. An incision in the posterior fornix allows an alternative approach to the tube (culdotomy) but has largely been abandoned because of higher complication rates.

A variety of techniques exist for occluding the tube.

Ligation. This is used when laparotomy or minilaparotomy are performed. The tubes can be tied with absorbable or non-absorbable sutures and the ends left free or buried in the broad ligament or uterine cornu. Postpartum sterilization is associated with a higher failure rate.

Electrocautery. With this technique one or more areas of the tube are cauterized by diathermy. Bipolar diathermy allows only the tissues held between the jaws of the forceps to be cauterized. The temperature of the cauterized tube may reach 300–400°C and if allowed to touch adjacent structures, can cause local burns. Failure to cauterize all the layers of the tube results in a relatively high failure rate (2–5/1000) and cautery close to the cornual portion of the tube is thought to increase the risk of ectopic pregnancy. The RCOG guidelines (RCOG 1999b)

recommend the use of diathermy only if tubal occlusion proves to be difficult and mechanical methods have failed.

Falope ring. A ring of silicone rubber is placed over a loop of tube with a specially designed applicator. The ring destroys 2–3 cm of tube and may be difficult to apply if the tube is fat or rigid. Ischaemia of the loop causes significant postoperative pain.

Clips. A variety of clips is available. They destroy a much smaller length of tube, allowing easier reversal, but special care must be taken to ensure that the whole width of the tube is occluded; some surgeons routinely apply two clips to each tube. The Hulka–Clemens clip (stainless steel and a polycarbonate) and the smaller Filshie clip (titanium lined with silicone rubber) are probably the most commonly used in the UK.

Laser. Laser vaporization can be used to divide the tubes; however, the carbon dioxide laser divides them very cleanly and may allow a high incidence of recanalization. The Nd:YAG laser, although probably more effective, is extremely expensive.

Efficacy

A report from the US Collaborative Review of Sterilization (Peterson et al 1996) evaluated prospectively over 10 000 women who underwent sterilization in nine US cities. The women were followed up for between 8 and 14 years. The failure rate varied with age and the method of tubal occlusion. The 10-year life table cumulative probability of pregnancy for all ages combined (18–44) ranged from 7.5 pregnancies per 1000 procedures (for unipolar coagulation and postpartum partial salpingectomy) to 36.5 pregnancies per 1000 procedures (for clips). Failure rates were highest for women under the age of 28, with 52 pregnancies per 1000 procedures for spring clips.

New developments

A number of chemical agents have been tested for their ability to occlude the fallopian tube when instilled into the tube either directly or transcervically into the uterus. The quinacrine pellet is the only one ready for large-scale use. The method involves insertion of a 252 mg quinacrine pellet into the uterine cavity through a modified IUD inserter passed through the cervical canal. Two insertions, 1 month apart, are made during the follicular phase of the cycle. Occlusion is caused by inflammation and fibrosis of the intramural segment of the tube. Efficacy can be increased by adding adjuvants such as antiprostaglandins or by increasing the number of quinacrine insertions. A failure rate of 2.6% after 1 year of follow-up has been reported (Hieu et al 1993).

The method is cheaper than surgical sterilization, avoids the use of any anaesthesia and can be performed by non-medical personnel. Large numbers of women in Asia and Pakistan have been sterilized using this method. However, although quinacrine is widely used for malaria prophylaxis, the safety of quinacrine sterilization has not yet been determined and some question the ethics of using a technique which has not been approved in developed countries. Toxicology studies are presently under way.

Counselling for sterilization

Most couples seeking sterilization have been thinking about the operation for some considerable time. The initial consultation should include a discussion of:

- the procedure involved
- the failure rate
- the risks and side-effects
- the possibility of wanting more children
- which partner should be sterilized
- the issue of reversibility. Despite careful counselling, a few couples will inevitably request reversal of sterilization. This is most likely to happen with remarriage. Immediate postpartum or postabortion sterilization is more likely to be regretted and should be avoided if possible. Although as many as 10% of couples regret being sterilized, only 1% of these will request reversal
- alternative long-acting methods of contraception which are reversible and equally effective, such as contraceptive implants.

The RCOG guidelines (1999b) recommend that verbal counselling advice be backed up by accurate impartial printed information which the couple may take away.

Reversal of female sterilization is more likely to be successful after occlusion with clips which have been applied to the isthmic portion of the tube since only a small section of tube will have been damaged. Patients should realize that reversal involves laparotomy, does not always work (microsurgical techniques are associated with around 70% success) and carries a significant risk of ectopic pregnancy (up to 5%). Ovulation should be confirmed and a normal semen analysis obtained from the partner before reversal is undertaken. Reversal is unlikely to be available on the NHS in most parts of the UK.

The history should include the following.

- The reason for the request: some women seek sterilization as a cure for menstrual dysfunction, sexual problems or abdominal pain.
- Gynaecological and obstetric history and relevant medical histories of both partners.
- Ages, occupations and social circumstances of both partners.
- Numbers, ages and health of their children.
- Previous and current contraception and any problems experienced. Some women request sterilization because they are unable to find any other acceptable method of contraception; this is not a good reason for sterilization.
- The stability of the marriage and the possibility of its breakdown.
- The quality of the couple's sex life.

It is seldom possible to arrange sterilization for a particular time of the cycle and women should be told to continue using their current method of contraception until their operation. It is not necessary to stop the combined pill before sterilization as the risk of thromboembolic complications is negligible.

If an IUD is in situ it should be removed at the time of sterilization, unless the operation is being done at mid-cycle and intercourse has taken place within the previous few days, in which case it can be removed after the next menstrual period.

Complications
Immediate complications

1. The operation carries a small operative mortality of <8 per 100 000 operations. In a large series from the USA (Peterson et al 1983) the commonest cause of death was anaesthesia. In the UK laparoscopic sterilization is commonly performed under general anaesthesia but local anaesthesia is an acceptable alternative.
2. Vascular damage or damage to bowel or other internal organs may occur during the procedure and is usually recognized at the time of operation. Nevertheless, patients should be aware that the rare possibility of a laparotomy and longer stay in hospital does exist.
3. Gas embolism.
4. Thromboembolic disease is rare, but more likely if the procedure is done immediately postpartum.
5. Wound infection.
6. Postoperative pain is common because of local tissue ischaemia and necrosis at the site of occlusion of the tube. It can be reduced by the use of local tubal anaesthesia.

Long-term complications

1. Menstrual disorders: women who stop using the combined pill will almost certainly notice that their periods become heavier, perhaps more painful and less predictable, and they should be warned of this. In contrast, women whose previous method of contraception was an IUD will notice an improvement in their bleeding patterns. Kasonde & Bonnar (1976) were unable to demonstrate a measurable change in menstrual blood loss following sterilization in women who had been using barrier methods of contraception and a recent review of the evidence concluded that female sterilization does not alter ovarian activity or menstruation (Gentile et al 1998). Despite this there have been a number of studies which have demonstrated an increased incidence of gynaecological consultation and an increased incidence of hysterectomy among women who have been sterilized (Hillis et al 1998, Templeton & Cole 1982). Bearing in mind the inevitable changes in menstrual bleeding patterns associated with advancing age and with stopping the combined pill (the most commonly used method of reversible contraception) it may be that women who have been sterilized are more likely to seek hysterectomy, or more willing to accept it, if they are already incapable of further child bearing.
2. The term *post-tubal sterilization syndrome* was coined to describe a variety of symptoms that have been reported after sterilization and which women may attribute to the procedure. These symptoms include abdominal pain, dyspareunia, exacerbation of PMS or dysmenorrhoea and emotional and psychosexual problems. Laparoscopy fails to demonstrate any pathology. A recent review of the literature (Gentile et al 1998) concluded that sterilization is not associated with an increased risk of these problems except among young women sterilized before the age of 30 in whom the symptoms may sometimes be a manifestation of regret.
3. Psychological and psychosexual problems are rare and when they do arise, tend to do so in those who have had problems before sterilization. Many studies in fact report a better mental state after sterilization.
4. Bowel obstruction from adhesions is a very rare complication.
5. Ectopic pregnancy is a well-recognized complication of

sterilization. In the US Collaborative Review (Peterson et al 1997) the risk was influenced by age and the method of occlusion. The 10-year cumulative probability of ectopic pregnancy for all ages combined ranged from 1.5 (for post-partum partial salpingectomy) to 17 (for bipolar coagulation) pregnancies per 1000 procedures, while for women aged <30 the figures were 1 and 33 respectively. Women should be advised that if they miss a period and have symptoms of pregnancy they should seek medical advice urgently.

Vasectomy

Vasectomy involves the division or occlusion of the vas deferens to prevent the passage of sperm. The vas is exposed through a small skin incision and ligated or occluded with small silver clips or by unipolar diathermy with a specially designed probe which can be passed into the cut end of the vas.

Excising a small portion of vas makes reversal more difficult and probably does not increase the effectiveness unless at least 4 cm is removed. It does allow histological confirmation of a correct procedure which may help in any subsequent litigation but adds to the expense. Interposing the fascial sheath between the cut ends or looping the cut ends of the vas back on itself may increase effectiveness. The RCOG guidelines (1999b) recommend that fascial interposition or diathermy should accompany division of the vas which, on its own, is not an acceptable technique in terms of the failure rate. This recommendation, although the opinion of experts, is not supported by scientific evidence and the relative efficacy of any one method of occlusion and efficacy probably depends most on the skill of the surgeon.

The 'no-scalpel' vasectomy (NSV), developed in China in 1974, is now quite widely used. It makes use of specially designed instruments for isolating and delivering the vas through the scrotal skin and substitutes a small puncture for the skin incision. Any of the standard methods of occlusion may be used. NSV is quick and associated with a lower incidence of infection and haematoma. A comparison between NSV and conventional vasectomy in Thailand reported a complication rate of 0.4% versus 3.1% (Nirapathpongporn et al 1990).

Percutaneous injection of sclerosing agents such as polyurethane elastomers or occlusive substances such as silicone is also being used in China. The technique avoids any skin incision, the silicone plug is said to be easily removed and pregnancy rates of 100% up to 5 years after vasectomy reversal have been claimed.

The rate at which azoospermia is achieved depends on the frequency of ejaculation. In the UK seminal fluid is examined after 12 and 16 weeks and if sperm are still present, usually monthly thereafter. When sperm are absent from two consecutive samples the vasectomy can be considered complete; until then an alternative method of contraception must be used. Around 3% of men do not become azoospermic and the vasectomy has to be redone.

Complications of vasectomy
Local complications. Wound infection will occur in up to 5% of men and scrotal bruising is unavoidable. Postoperative bleeding will be sufficient in 1–2% of men to cause a haematoma and perhaps 1% of these will require admission to hospital.

Sperm granulomas. Small lumps may form at the cut ends of the vas as a result of a local inflammatory response to leaked sperm. They can be painful and may need excising. Their presence may also increase the chance of failure.

Chronic intrascrotal pain and discomfort (post-vasectomy syndrome). Some men complain of a dull ache in the scrotum which may be exacerbated by sexual excitement and ejaculation. The symptoms are probably due to distension and granuloma formation in the epididymis and vas deferens. Pain may also result from scar tissue forming around small nerves. Chronic pain associated with progressive induration, tubular distension and granuloma formation in the epididymis may require excision of the epididymis and obstructed vas deferens.

Late recanalization. Failure can occur up to 10 years after vasectomy despite two negative samples of seminal fluid following the procedure. It is rare (1 in 2000).

Anti-sperm antibodies. Most men develop detectable concentrations of autoantibodies, presumably as a result of leakage of sperm, some time after vasectomy. Their presence may compromise fertility if reversal is attempted.

Cardiovascular and autoimmune disease. Concerns about a possible link between vasectomy and cardiovascular disease were raised in the 1970s following reports that vasectomy increased atherosclerosis in monkeys, perhaps as a consequence of increased levels of autoantibodies. Several large studies, including a cohort study in the USA of over 10 000 vasectomized men, failed to substantiate increased rates of 98 diseases (McDonald 1997).

Cancer. Two studies from the USA and Scotland suggested an increased risk of testicular cancer following vasectomy. However, a recent large cohort study of over 73 000 men in Denmark (Moller et al 1994) demonstrated no increase in the incidence of testicular cancer among men who had a vasectomy.

A number of reports from the USA have also suggested an increased risk of prostate cancer following vasectomy. No known biological mechanism can account for any association or causal relationship between vasectomy and prostate cancer. A 1998 systematic review of 14 studies published from 1985 to 1996 (Bernal-Delgado et al 1998) reported a summary risk estimate of 1.23 (95% CI 1.01–1.49) but the authors concluded that there was evidence against a causal relationship. An editorial from the US National Cancer Institute, commenting on a large US population-based study which found no effect of vasectomy on prostate cancer (Peterson & Howards 1998), concluded that vasectomy appeared either not to cause prostate cancer or that there is only a relatively weak relationship.

Reversal
Reversal of vasectomy is technically feasible in many cases with patency rates of almost 90% being reported in some series. Pregnancy rates are much less (up to 60%) perhaps as a result of the presence of anti-sperm antibodies.

ABORTION

After the Abortion Act was passed in 1967 in the UK there was a rapid rise in the number of abortions, which reached a plateau in the late 1980s. Since then there has been a gradual rise in the numbers each year, with 18 0,000 abortions being performed in England and Wales and 12,000 in Scotland in the late 1990s. The abortion rate in Britain (11.1 per 1000 women aged 15–45 years in Scotland in 1999) is relatively low compared with many other developed countries. Nevertheless, at least one-third of British women will have had an abortion by the age of 45. The rate of teenage pregnancy (including both childbirth and abortion) in Britain is one of the worst in Europe. For a useful review of the topic see Kane & Wellings (1999).

Legal aspects

It is illegal in the UK to induce an abortion except under specific indications as defined by law. The conditions of the 1967 Abortion Act state that abortion can be performed if two registered medical practitioners, acting in good faith, agree that the pregnancy should be terminated on one or more of the following grounds.

1. The continuance of the pregnancy would involve risk to the life of the pregnant woman greater than if the pregnancy were terminated.
2. The termination is necessary to prevent grave permanent injury to the physical or mental health of the pregnant woman.
3. The pregnancy has NOT exceeded its 24th week and the continuance of the pregnancy would involve risk, greater than if the pregnancy were terminated, of injury to the physical or mental health of the pregnant woman.
4. The pregnancy has NOT exceeded its 24th week and the continuance of the pregnancy would involve risk, greater than if the pregnancy were terminated, of injury to the physical or mental health of the existing child(ren) of the family of the pregnant woman.
5. There is a substantial risk that if the child were born it would suffer from such physical or mental abnormalities as to be seriously handicapped.

In 1990 the law was amended to reduce the upper limit from 28 to 24 weeks' gestation reflecting the lowering of the limits of fetal viability resulting from advances in neonatal care. An exception was made in the case of a fetus with severe congenital abnormality incompatible with life (e.g. anencephaly) in which case there is no upper limit.

The 1967 Abortion Act does not apply to Northern Ireland where abortion is only legal under exceptional circumstances, e.g. to save the life of the mother.

The law recognizes that some doctors have ethical objections to abortion. Doctors who do have objections are obliged to refer women to another colleague who does not hold similar views.

Over 98% of induced abortions in Britain are undertaken on the grounds that the continuance of the pregnancy would involve risk to the physical or mental health of the pregnant woman.

Provision of services

In Scotland and north-east England over 90% of abortions are performed in NHS hospitals while in other areas of England, the majority are carried out in private clinics or by charities. In Scotland abortion accounts for over 22% of the inpatient gynaecological workload and it is thus a major issue for gynaecologists. Some hospitals have dedicated services which are quite separate from the general gynaecological service and which are staffed by experts who are more sensitive and sympathetic. While this has obvious advantages for individual patients and is recommended as best practice by the RCOG (RCOG 2000), the approach risks separating abortion from other aspects of reproductive healthcare and removing if from general gynaecological training. Without exposure during their training to the issue and to women who are seeking abortion, doctors may become increasingly reluctant to be involved with the provision of services as they are in the USA.

Counselling

Faced with the news of an unintended pregnancy, many women are emotionally devastated and the decision to have a pregnancy terminated is never an easy one. In the UK the Committee on the Working of the Abortion Act (the Lane Committee), reporting in 1974, recommended that every woman should have the opportunity to have adequate counselling before deciding to have her pregnancy terminated. Abortion counselling should provide opportunities for discussion, information, explanation and advice in a manner which is non-judgemental and non-directional.

By the time most women see a gynaecologist they have already seen one doctor (usually their GP) and are certain of their decision. However, in order to satisfy themselves that there are grounds for termination, gynaecologists should none the less discuss the reasons why the pregnancy is unwanted and whether the woman is absolutely certain about her decision since uncertainty may be more likely to lead to regret. The woman should be encouraged to think of the practical and emotional consequences of all the possible options of abortion, continuing with the pregnancy and adoption.

Not all doctors are sympathetic and women who are seen to have conceived because of a true method failure are more likely to get a sympathetic hearing. Many women feel that they have to 'make the case' to the gynaecologist for having their pregnancy terminated and some will claim method failure even when they have not been using contraception. One in five women who have had an abortion will present for another at some time in their lives. Women who seem to use abortion as a method of contraception and present again and again probably need psychiatric help and not a punitive approach from the gynaecologist.

In the UK around 1% of women will present too late for legal abortion. These, and some of those who choose to have the baby, will need information about adoption and benefits and sometimes referral to social services.

The gynaecologist should provide information about the procedure involved, offering where available and appropriate a choice of surgical or medical methods to women below 9 weeks' gestation. The possible complications and long-term side-effects of the abortion should also be discussed, together with the implications for future pregnancies. Verbal discussions should be supported by written information and confidentiality should be emphasized.

Future contraceptive plans are usually discussed before the abortion is carried out. Although this may not be the best time, it may be one of the few opportunities to discuss contraception as many patients do not attend for follow-up.

Assessment

After it has been decided that there are grounds for abortion, it is important to make a careful medical assessment of the woman.

- The medical history should pay particular attention to conditions such as asthma which may influence the choice of method of abortion.
- The stage of gestation should be determined by menstrual history and pelvic examination. A pelvic ultrasound scan is not essential unless there is real doubt about the gestation or if ectopic pregnancy is suspected.
- Whether the service chooses to screen for genital tract infection, particularly chlamydia, or simply to treat everyone with prophylactic antibiotics will depend on the background incidence of infection in the local population but one or other is essential. If screening is chosen, it is emphasized that antibiotic therapy should be started before abortion is performed.
- Women considered to be at high risk of hepatitis B or HIV should be offered screening with appropriate counselling. Women who refuse screening should be treated as high risk during the abortion procedure.
- Cervical screening should be offered in accordance with national screening policies.
- Blood should be collected for measurement of haemoglobin concentration and the group determined. All women who are rhesus negative should be injected with anti-D immuno-globulin prior to or within 48 hours of the abortion to prevent the development of rhesus isoimmunization.

Techniques of abortion

In general, the earlier the abortion is done, the safer it is. Mortality and morbidity associated with the procedure increase with the gestation of the pregnancy at the time of termination. The risk of major complications doubles when termination is carried out at 15 as compared with 8 weeks' gestation.

The method of choice depends on gestation, parity, medical history and the woman's wishes. The RCOG guidelines (2000) state that as a minimum all services must be able to offer abortion by one of the recommended methods for each gestation band but that ideally services should be able to offer a choice.

Early first trimester (up to 9 weeks)
Surgical.   Vacuum aspiration has been the method of choice for early surgical termination of pregnancy in industrialized countries for over 20 years. Dilatation and curettage requires more cervical dilatation and is associated with a significantly higher complication rate, including uterine injury, and a higher incidence of retained products of conception and adverse future reproductive outcome (Henshaw & Templeton 1993).

Vacuum aspiration can be performed under either local paracervical block or general anaesthesia. Some evidence suggests that the use of general anaesthesia increases the risk of the procedure. In the USA the mortality rate is 2–4 times greater when general rather than local anaesthesia is used for first-trimester abortion. Preoperative treatment with a cervical priming agent has been shown to reduce the risk of haemorrhage and genital tract trauma associated with vacuum aspiration. Prostaglandins, bougies and mifepristone are all effective but prostaglandins (gemeprost 1 mg vaginally or misoprostol 400 mg vaginally, both 3 hours before surgery) probably achieve their effect more quickly. Pretreatment of the cervix adds to the cost of the procedure and may be difficult to organize when abortion is performed as a day case. As cervical trauma is commoner in women under the age of 17 years and uterine perforation is associated with increasing parity and increasing gestation, efforts to arrange cervical ripening should be concentrated on young women (aged under 18), highly parous women and those presenting at a gestation of greater than 10 weeks.

A curette of up to 10 mm internal diameter is passed through the cervix and the contents of the uterus aspirated using negative pressure created by a pump. It is advisable to use the smallest diameter curette which is adequate for the gestation; most gynaecologists use an 8 mm curette at 8 weeks, 10 mm at 10 weeks and so on.

Vacuum aspiration at this stage of pregnancy is extremely safe and effective. Failure is more likely to occur before 7 weeks' gestation when it is possible to miss the fetus with the curette. For this reason medical methods or a rigorous protocol for early surgical abortion are recommended. The mortality from vacuum aspiration in the first trimester in less than about 1 per 100 000, considerably less than the maternal mortality from continuing pregnancy.

Medical.   Medical abortion is available to women in the UK up to 63 days of amenorrhoea (9 weeks' gestation) using a combination of the antiprogesterone mifepristone and a prostaglandin. The licensed regimen comprises mifepristone 600 mg orally followed 36–48 hours later by gemeprost 1 mg vaginally. Mifepristone is a synthetic steroid which blocks the action of progesterone by binding to its receptor. It also binds to the glucocorticoid receptor and blocks the action of cortisol. When mifepristone is used alone, complete abortion only occurs in around 60% of pregnancies. The rate of complete abortion rises to over 95% if a prostaglandin is given 36 or 48 hours after the administration of mifepristone. The antiprogesterone itself stimulates some uterine contractility but mainly works by greatly enhancing the sensitivity of the myometrium to the tocolytic effect of prostaglandins. 200 mg mifepristone is as effective as 600 mg and, with 36–48 hours later an oral prostaglandin misoprostol (which is not licensed for abortion) 800 µg vaginally, makes for a much cheaper and now commonly used regimen.

Offered the choice of method, in France and in the UK around 20–25% prefer medical abortion. Women often choose the medical method because it avoids an anaesthetic in most cases and because they feel more in control of the situation. It is, however, a two-stage procedure which other women find a

Box 30.2 Contraindications to medical abortion

Absolute contraindications	Adrenal insufficiency
	Ectopic pregnancy
	>9 weeks' gestation
	Asthma
	Cardiac disease
	Heavy smoker, older than 35 years
	On anticoagulants or bleeding disorder
Relative contraindications	Heavy smoker
	>35 years
	Obesity
	Hypertension (diastolic >100 mmHg)

disadvantage. The incidence of serious complications is probably similar to that associated with surgical abortion, but because 95% of women need neither anaesthesia nor instrumentation of the uterus, large randomized trials may eventually show medical abortion to be safer. Not all women are suitable for medical abortion; the contraindications are shown in Box 30.2.

There are very few side-effects following administration of mifepristone. The fetus is usually passed within 4 hours of prostaglandin administration and this is accompanied by bleeding and pain. The bleeding is usually described as being like a very heavy period although rarely (<1%) there may be very heavy bleeding requiring resuscitation. Nulliparous women and those with a history of dysmenorrhoea are more likely to experience severe pain and 10–20% of women may need opiate analgesia. The rest will cope with paracetamol. Prostaglandin synthetase inhibitors, such as aspirin or mefanamic acid, should be avoided for obvious reasons. A few women will abort at home in response to mifepristone with variable amounts of bleeding and discomfort.

Bleeding can continue for up to 20 days after the abortion although most women have usually stopped after 10 days. The total amount of blood lost is similar to that occurring at the time of vacuum aspiration.

All women should be given an appointment for follow-up about 2 weeks after administration of the prostaglandin. This visit is absolutely essential for those (about 30%) who have not passed an identifiable fetus and/or placental tissue while in hospital. Although ongoing pregnancy occurs in only 1% of cases, evacuation of the uterus will be necessary in about 2–5% because of incomplete or missed abortion. These figures are no different from those associated with surgical abortion.

The risk of fetal malformation following mifepristone alone or in combination with prostaglandins is not known. Women should be clearly advised that medical abortion is a two-stage procedure and that it is not possible to have a change of heart after taking mifepristone and before prostaglandin administration. Women who seem even remotely uncertain about abortion should certainly not be offered the medical method. In the event of failed medical abortion and therefore ongoing pregnancy the patient must be strongly advised to have vacuum aspiration, although babies born to the few women who have chosen to continue with the pregnancy after medical abortion has failed have been normal.

Late first trimester (9–14 weeks)

At this stage of pregnancy the method of choice is vacuum aspiration. Although abortion can be induced by anti-gestagens and prostaglandins, the incidence of incomplete abortion is high and hence, many women require surgical evacuation of the uterus. The cervix should be pretreated.

Although vacuum aspiration is an extremely safe operation, blood loss and other complications rise as gestation advances. It is important, therefore, to refer the woman for abortion promptly after the decision to terminate the pregnancy has been made.

Mid-trimester abortion

Second-trimester abortion accounts for 10–15% of all legal abortions in the UK. While many are done because of fetal malformation, it is often the women who are least able to cope with an unwanted pregnancy, particularly the very young, who first present at this time.

It is possible to induce abortion at this stage of pregnancy either medically or surgically. Surgical dilatation and evacuation (D&E) is the method of choice in the USA but in the UK its use is confined largely to gynaecologists in private practice. It may be necessary to dilate the cervix up to a diameter of 20 mm before the fetal parts can be extracted. In skilled hands, D&E is a safe procedure but if complications such as haemorrhage and perforation of the uterus are to be avoided surgeons should be adequately trained. D&E should be preceded by cervical preparation, as described earlier.

Medical abortion for women presenting at greater than 15 weeks' gestation can be performed with mifepristone 600 or 200 mg orally followed 36–48 hours later by either gemeprost 1 mg vaginally every 3 hours, up to a maximum of five pessaries, or by misoprostol 800 µg vaginally then 400 µg orally 3 hourly to a maximum of four oral doses.

Most women find the procedure painful and distressing and require opiate analgesia. Evacuation of the uterus is necessary in around 30% of women who retain all or part of the placenta.

Abortion beyond 18 weeks' gestation is rare and is usually for pregnancies complicated by severe fetal malformation. Particularly distressing for both the mother and the staff, these late abortions are often effectively managed with vaginal prostaglandins in combination with mifepristone with intra-amniotic urea or fetal intracardiac injection of potassium to minimize the chances of a live birth.

Follow-up

Anti-D IgG should be given to all non-sensitized RhD-negative women following any therapeutic abortion. Written advice about possible post-treatment symptoms, particularly those associated with infection, together with advice about what action to take should be given to patients before discharge home. All women should receive contraceptive advice and, if appropriate, supplies before going home. Ovulation can return within 20 days following abortion and contraception should be started early. All should be given a follow-up appointment within 2 weeks, either with the clinic which carried out the abortion or with a suitable alternative doctor. At follow-up, a pelvic examination should confirm complete abortion and the absence of infection. Discussion should include contraceptive advice and post-abortion counselling if required.

Complications

Although maternal mortality is fortunately extremely rare following abortion, the incidence of major complications, haemorrhage, thromboembolism, operative trauma (uterine perforation and cervical trauma) and infection is around 2%. The main factors affecting the incidence of complications in the RCGP study (Frank 1985) undertaken in the early 1980s were the place of operation (complications were less common when the abortion was done in a private hospital), gestation, method of abortion, sterilization at the time of operation and smoking habits.

Incomplete abortion
The commonest complication following abortion is the persistence of placental and/or fetal tissue. Up to 5% of women undergoing first-trimester medical abortion will require surgical evacuation of the uterus within the first month. The incidence of incomplete abortion and ongoing pregnancy after vacuum aspiration rises as the gestation increases.

The occurrence of bleeding at 2 weeks after a medical or surgical abortion is not in itself an indication to evacuate the uterus. Ultrasound scans often show residual trophoblastic tissue even in women who have stopped bleeding. Although an ultrasound scan of the uterus and the measurement of hCG in plasma may be helpful in diagnosing an ongoing pregnancy, the decision to evacuate the uterus should be made on clinical grounds, i.e. continued heavy or persistent bleeding from a bulky uterus in which the cervix is still dilated. The majority of women with an incomplete or missed abortion will pass the residual tissue with time if they are prepared to be patient. The belief that all women with an incomplete abortion had a high risk of intrauterine infection until the uterus was evacuated probably stemmed from the time when illegal abortion was common.

Minor complications
Some 10% of women undergoing abortion present to their GP during the 3 weeks following the procedure with a variety of complaints related to the abortion. Lower abdominal pain, vaginal bleeding and passage of clots or trophoblastic tissue are relatively common and usually only require reassurance. It is, however, important to exclude infection. Established pelvic inflammatory disease with pyrexia, abdominal pain and offensive vaginal discharge occurs in around 1% of women whatever method of abortion is used.

Cervical and vaginal lacerations
Lacerations to the vagina and cervix are rare and the risk of the latter can be reduced by pretreatment of the cervix in selected cases, as discussed earlier.

Late complications
There are very few late complications from abortion if the women have been carefully counselled.

Psychological sequelae
Many women feel tearful and emotional for a few days following the abortion. However, many studies have demonstrated a significant improvement in psychological well-being by 3 months after compared with before abortion (Adler et al 1990). There is no evidence of an increase in the incidence of serious psychiatric disease following abortion although relapse can occur in those with pre-existing psychiatric disease. In contrast, the incidence of depression, suicide and child abuse is higher in women who have continued with the pregnancy because abortion was refused (Matejcek et al 1985).

Infertility
Postabortion infection is a significant cause of tubal disease and infertility following illegal abortion. However, with modern methods performed under optimal conditions, the incidence of infection is very low, particularly where preoperative screening and treatment of infection are routine.

Subsequent pregnancy
Although damage to the cervix or perforation of the uterus can predispose to cervical incompetence, preterm delivery and/or uterine rupture there is no significant increase in adverse outcome of any subsequent pregnancy.

KEY POINTS

1. Lack of contraceptive use continues to be a major problem in many developing countries.
2. The combined oral contraceptive pill is still very widely used in the United Kingdom and is extremely safe.
3. The risks of myocardial infarction and stroke in association with the combined oral contraceptive pill have been exaggerated and in women with no other risk factors, particularly smoking and hypertension, are minimal.
4. The relative risk of VTE is increased in women taking the COC and appears to be higher among women using third- compared with second-generation pills. However, the absolute risk of VTE is very small.
5. The combined pill is associated with a highly significant reduction in the risk of ovarian and endometrial cancer but current and recent users (within 10 years) have an increased risk of having breast cancer diagnosed.
6. The efficacy of long-acting progestogen-only methods (implants, injectables, IUS) rivals that of sterilization.
7. The copper IUD is a very cheap and effective method of contraception which is underused.
8. The levonorgestrel-releasing intrauterine system significantly reduces menstrual blood loss and has increased the popularity of the IUD as a method of contraception.
9. Emergency contraception is safe and is now available without prescription.
10. Anti-hormones, particularly anti-gestogens, show great promise for the development of new contraceptives.
11. There is a variety of ways of inducing therapeutic abortion and women should be offered a choice of method within the context of a high-quality service which meets national standards.

REFERENCES

Adler NE, David HP, Major BN, Roth SH, Russo NF, Wyatt GE 1990 Psychological responses after abortion. Science 268:41–44

Akerlund M, Rode A, Westergaard J 1993 Comparative profiles of reliability, cycle control and side effects of two oral contraceptive formulations containing 150 µg desorgestrel and either 30 µg or 20 µg ethinyl oestradiol. British Journal of Obstetrics and Gynaecology 100:832–838

Andersson JK, Rybo G 1990 Levonorgestrel-releasing intrauterine device in the treatment of menorrhagia. British Journal of Obstetrics and Gynaecology 97:690–694

Archer D, Kovacs L, Landgren BM 1998 Implanon, a new single-rod contraceptive implant. Presentation of the clinical data. Contraception 58(6)(suppl)

Audet MC, Moreau M, Koltun WD et al for the ORTHO EVRA/EVRA 004 Study Group 2001 Evaluation of contraceptive efficacy and cycle control of a transdermal contraceptive patch vs an oral contraceptive. A randomized controlled trial. JAMA 285:2347–2354

Baird DT 1993 Antigestogens. British Medical Bulletin 49:73–87

Baird DT, Glasier A 2000 Science, medicine and the future: contraception. British Medical Journal 319:969–972

Beral V, Hermon C, Kay C, Hannaford P, Darby S, Reeves G 1999 Mortality associated with oral contraceptive use: 25 year follow up of a cohort of 46,000 women from Royal College of General Practitioners' oral contraception study. British Medical Journal 318:96–100

Bernal-Delgado E, Latour-Perez J, Pradas-Arnal F, Gomez-Lopez LI 1998 The association between vasectomy and prostate cancer: a systematic review of the literature. Fertility and Sterility 70:191–20

Bloemenkamp KWM, Rosendaal FR, Helerhorst FM, Buller HR, Vandenbroucke JP 1995 Enhancement by factor V Leiden mutation of risk of deep-vein thrombosis associated with oral contraceptive containing a third-generation progestagen. Lancet 364:1593–1596

Bonnar J, Flynn A, Freundl G, Kirkman R, Royston R, Snowden R 1999 Personal hormone monitoring for contraception. British Journal of Family Planning 24:128–134

Bounds W, Guillebaud J, Newman GB 1992 Female condom (Femidom). A clinical study of its use, effectiveness and patient acceptability. British Journal of Family Planning 18:36–41

Celentano DD, Klassen AC, Weisman CS, Rosenheim NB 1987 Role of contraceptive use in cervical cancer. American Journal of Epidemiology 126:592–604

Chang CL, Donaghy M, Poulter N and WHO Collaborative Study of Cardiovascular Disease and Steroid Hormone Contraception 1999 Migraine and stroke in young women: a case control study. British Medical Journal 318:13–18

Collaborative Group on Hormonal Factors in Breast Cancer 1996 Breast cancer and hormonal contraceptives: collaborative re-analysis of individual data on 53,297 women with breast cancer and 100,239 women without breast cancer from 54 epidemiological studies. Lancet 347:1717–1727

Cundy T, Evans M, Roberts H, Wattie D, Ames R, Reid IR 1991 Bone density in women receiving depot medroxyprogesterone acetate for contraception. British Medical Journal 303:13–16

Cundy T, Cornish J, Evans MC, Roberts H, Reid IR 1994 Recovery of bone density in women receiving depot medroxy progesterone acetate for contraception. British Medical Journal 308:247–248

Division of Reproductive Health 1998 Unsafe abortion. Global and regional estimates of incidence and of mortality due to unsafe abortion with a listing of available community data. WHO, Geneva

Dunn N, Thorogood M, Faragher B et al 1999 Oral contraceptives and myocardial infarction: results of the MICA case control study. British Medical Journal 318:1579–1584

Frank PI 1985 Sequelae of induced abortion. In: Porter R, O'Connor M (eds) Abortion: medical progress and social implications. Ciba Foundation Symposium 115. Pitman, London

Fraser HM 1993 GnRH analogues for contraception. British Medical Bulletin 49:62–72

Fraser IS 1983 A survey of different approaches to the management of menstrual disturbances in women using injectable contraceptives. Contraception 28:385–397

Fraser IS, Tiitinen A, Affandi B et al 1998. Norplant® consensus statement and background review. Contraception 57:1–9

Gbolade B, Ellis S, Murby B, Randall S, Kirkman R 1998 Bone density in long term users of depot medroxyprogesterone acetate. British Journal of Obstetrics and Gynaecology 105:790–794

Gentile GP, Kaufman SC, Helbig DW 1998 Is there any evidence for a post-tubal sterilization syndrome? Fertility and Sterility 69:179–186

Glasier A 2000 Emergency contraception. British Medical Bulletin 56(3):729–738

Grimes DA 2000 Intrauterine device and upper genital tract infection. Lancet 356:1013–1019

Henshaw RC, Templeton AA 1993 Methods used in first trimester abortion. Current Obstetrics and Gynaecology 3:11–16

Hieu DT, Tan TT, Tan DN, Nguyet PT, Than P, Vinh DQ 1993 31 781 cases of non-surgical female sterilization with quinacrine pellets in Vietnam. Lancet 342:213–217

Hillis SD, Marchbanks PA, Taylor LR, Peterson HB 1998 Higher hysterectomy risk for sterilized than nonsterilized women: findings in the U.S. Collaborative Review of Sterilization. The U.S. Collaborative Review of Sterilization Working Group. Obstetrics and Gynecology 91:241–246

Jick H, Jick SS, Gurewich V, Wald Myers M, Vasilakis C 1995 Risk of idiopathic cardiovascular death and nonfatal thromboembolism in women using oral contraceptives with differing progestagen components. Lancet 346:1589–1593

Kane R, Wellings K 1999 Reducing the rate of teenage conceptions. Health Education Authority, London

Kasonde JM, Bonnar J 1976 Effect of sterilization on menstrual blood loss. British Journal of Obstetrics and Gynaecology 83:572–577

Labbok M, Koniz-Booher P, Cooney K, Shelton J, Krasovec K 1990 Guidelines for breastfeeding in family planning and child survival programs. Institute for Studies in Natural Family Planning, Washington DC

Matejcek Z, Dytrych Z, Schüller V 1985 Follow up study of children born to women denied abortion. In: Porter R, O'Connor M (eds) Abortion: medical progress and social implications. Ciba Foundation Symposium 115. Pitman, London

McDonald SW 1997 Is vasectomy harmful to health? British Journal of General Practice 47:381–386

Medicines Commission 1999 Combined oral contraceptives containing desogestrel or gestodene and the risk of venous thromboembolism. Current Problems in Pharmacovigilance 25:12

Moller H, Knudsen LB, Lynge E 1994 Risk of testicular cancer after vasectomy: cohort study of over 73 000 men. British Medical Journal 309:295–299

Nirapathpongporn A, Huber DH, Krieger JN 1990 No-scalpel vasectomy at the King's birthday vasectomy festival. Lancet 335:894–895

O'Brien PA 1999 The third generation oral contraceptive controversy. British Medical Journal 319:795–796

Oddens BJ, Visser AP, Vermer HM, Everaerd W, Lehart P 1994 Contraceptive use and attitudes in Great Britain. Contraception 49:73–86

Orr-Walker BJ, Evans M, Ames R, Clearwater JM, Cundy T, Reid IR 1998 The effect of past use of the injectable contraceptive depot medroxyprogesterone acetate on bone mineral density in normal women. Clinical Endocrinology 49:615–618

Perez A, Labbok M, Queenan J 1992 Clinical study of the lactational amenorrhoea method for family planning. Lancet 339:968–969

Peterson HB, Howards SS 1998 Vasectomy and prostate cancer: the evidence to date. Fertility and Sterility 70:201–203

Peterson HB, DeStefano F, Rubin GL, Greenspan JR, Lee NC, Ory HW 1983 Deaths attributable to tubal sterilisation in the United States 1977–1981. American Journal of Obstetrics and Gynecology 146:131–136

Peterson HB, Xia Z, Hughes JM, Wilkox LS, Tylor LR, Trussel J for the U.S. Collaborative Review of Sterilization Working Group 1996 The risk of pregnancy after tubal sterilization: findings from the U.S. Collaborative Review of Sterilization. American Journal of Obstetrics and Gynecology 174:1161–1170

Peterson HB, Xia Z, Hughes JM, Wilkox LS, Tylor LR, Trussel J for the U.S. Collaborative Review of Sterilization 1997 The risk of ectopic pregnancy after tubal sterilization. New England Journal of Medicine 336:762–767

Rebar AW, Zeserson K 1991 Characteristics of the new progestogens in combination oral contraceptives. Contraception 44:1–10

Rosing J, Middeldorp S, Curves J et al 1999 Low-dose oral contraceptives and acquired resistance to activated protein C: a randomised cross-over study. Lancet 354:2036–2040

Royal College of Obstetricians and Gynaecologists 1999a The management of menorrhagia in secondary care. Evidence-based clinical guidelines no. 5. RCOG, London

Royal College of Obstetricians and Gynaecologists 1999b Male and female sterilisation. Evidence-based clinical guidelines no. 4. RCOG, London

Royal College of Obstetricians and Gynaecologists 2000 The care of women requesting abortion. Evidence-based guidelines no. 7. RCOG, London

SIGN Scottish Intercollegiate Guidelines Network 2000 Management of genital chlamydia trachomatis infection. SIGN publication no. 42. Royal College of Physicians, Edinburgh

Skegg DCG 2000 Third generation oral contraceptives. British Medical Journal 321:190–192

Spitzer W, Lewis MA, Hainemann LAJ, Thorogood M, MacRae KD 1996 Third generation oral contraceptives and risk of venous thromboembolic disorders: an international case-control study. British Medical Journal 312:83-88

Task Force on Postovulatory Methods of Fertility Regulation 1998 Randomised controlled trial of levonorgestrel versus the Yuzpe regimen of combined oral contraceptives for emergency contraception. Lancet 353:428–433

Task Force on Postovulatory Methods of Fertility Regulation 1999 Comparison of three single doses of mifepristone as emergency contraception: a randomised trial. Lancet 353:697–702

Templeton AA, Cole S 1982 Hysterectomy following sterilization. British Journal of Obstetrics and Gynaecology 89:845–848

Trussel J 1998 Contraceptive efficacy. In: Hatcher RA, Trussel J, Stewart F et al (eds) Contraceptive technology, 17th edn. Ardent Media, New York

Ursin G, Peters RK, Henderson BE, d'Ablaing III G, Monreo KR, Pike MC 1994 Oral contraceptive use and adenocarcinoma of cervix. Lancet 344:1390–1394

Van Damme L, Chandeying V, Ramjee G et al 2000 Safety of multiple daily applications of COL-1492, a nonoxynol-9 vaginal gel, among female sex workers. AIDS 14:85–88

Weiss N 1995 Third-generation oral contraceptives: how risky? Lancet 346:1570

Wildemeersch D, Batar D, Webb A et al 1999 Gynefix. The frameless intrauterine implant – an update. For interval, emergency and, postabortal contraception. British Journal of Family Planning 24:149–159

World Health Organization Task Force on Long-Acting Systemic Agents for Fertility Regulation 1990a Microdose intravaginal levonorgestrel contraception: a multicentre trial I. Contraceptive efficacy and side effects. Contraception 41:105–124

World Health Organization Task Force on Methods for the Regulation of Male Fertility 1990b Contraceptive efficacy of testosterone-induced azoospermia in normal men. Lancet 336:955–959

World Health Organization 1992 Oral contraceptives and neoplasia. WHO Technical Report Series 817. WHO, Geneva

World Health Organization Collaborative Study of Cardiovascular Disease and Steroid Hormone Contraception 1995 Effect of different progestagens in low oestrogen oral contraceptives on venous thromboembolic disease. Lancet 346:1582–1588

World Health Organization Scientific Group 1998 Cardiovascular disease and steroid hormone contraception. WHO Technical Report Series 877. WHO, Geneva

World Health Organization Collaborative Study of Cardiovascular Disease and Steroid Hormone Contraception 1998 Cardiovascular disease and use of oral and injectable progestogen-only contraceptives and combined injectable contraceptives. Contraception 57:315–324

31

Psychosexual medicine

Susan V. Carr

INTRODUCTION

Human sexuality is important because it is inherent in everyone. It is an integral part of every human being and it is up to every individual to deal with their own sexuality in whichever way they choose. Although so fundamental to human existence, scientific documentation of sexuality is relatively recent. Historically there was a persistent refusal to recognize that women could enjoy sex. In 1857 Acton stated that 'Happily for society the majority of women are not much troubled with sexual feelings of any kind'. At the beginning of the 20th century, Havelock Ellis, an English doctor, gave scientific voice to the idea that sexual activity was important in its own right, not just as a means of procreation. He wrote that 'Reproduction ... is not necessarily connected with sex, nor is sex necessarily concerned with reproduction'. Freud's revolutionary theories of psychoanalysis put sex and the subconscious firmly on the scientific agenda, but it was not until some decades later that Kinsey published his ground-breaking study on male sexual behaviour (Kinsey et al 1948) followed by his report on females (Kinsey et al 1953). These reports led to the ever-increasing interest in female sexuality from the scientific point of view.

THE ROLE OF THE GYNAECOLOGIST

The gynaecologist has a major role to play in the field of psychosexual problems, in both their prevention and detection. Gynaecology is the branch of medicine which focuses on a woman's sexual and reproductive system, which forms an essential essence of her femaleness and her perception of herself as a complete woman. Gynaecology is concerned with the area of the woman's body that is involved in sexual activity. Sexual activity and emotions are closely linked and it is therefore important to be aware of the effect that any gynaecological problem may have on the woman's sexuality and indeed, that of her partner if she has one.

Modern medical teaching tends to recognize the emotional needs of patients but unfortunately, some everyday gynaecological situations may unwittingly set the scene for psychosexual problems in the future. Psychosexual therapy concentrates on individual cases, interpreting each doctor–patient interaction as unique. None the less, there are patterns of aetiologies which emerge in practice, such as a history of gynaecological procedures. Women may often trace their problem back to what may seen a minor gynaecological procedure, such as sterilization, termination of pregnancy or even vaginal examination, which is thus of crucial importance not only from a gynaecological but also from a psychosexual perspective.

HUMAN SEXUALITY

Human sexuality can be divided into different components, for ease of understanding.

Gender identity

The first of these is gender identity or who you are. Just under 50% of the population are diagnosed at birth as being female.

They are biologically and legally female and most tend to follow female biopsychosocial pathways throughout their lifetimes. Similarly, a male gender identity is experienced by the other 50% of the population, who are diagnosed at birth to be male. There is a tiny proportion of the population, however, who are transsexual. These are individuals whose biological sex and gender identity do not match. They are, in effect, born into the wrong body and may spend many difficult years undergoing a gender reassignment process. As all transsexuals are female at some stage in their lives, they may come into contact with gynaecology services so it is therefore important to have an awareness of this condition. A postoperative male-to-female transsexual presents on gynaecological examination as a hysterectomized female.

Sexual orientation

Sexual orientation is the definition of sexual attraction – the people to whom one's sexual desire is directed. About 93% of the population are heterosexual; that is, attracted to individuals of the opposite sex. Between 5% and 10% of the population are homosexual – men who are sexually attracted to men. A further 0.5–2% of women are lesbian – women who are sexually attracted to women. Seven per cent of the population are bisexual and are attracted to both men and women. In the UK national survey of sexual attitudes and lifestyles, over half of the men who had a male sexual partner in the previous 5 years also had a female partner and for females the figure was higher, at 75.8% (Wellins et al 1994).

Sexual orientation has particular relevance in well woman healthcare. Lesbians may be reluctant to discuss their sexual orientation with the clinician (Carr et al 1999) but as the majority have experienced heterosexual sexual intercourse or had vaginal penetrative sexual activity with fingers or sex toys, they are at risk of cervical dysplasia and sexually transmitted infection. Lesbians should be included in national cervical screening programmes and have the same well woman checks as the rest of the female population.

Sexual response

The human physiological sexual response is dependent not only on intact endocrine, vascular and neurological input but also on sensory input. This was described as the psychosomatic circle of sex (Bancroft 1989). Female sexual responsiveness is a result of sensory input through the peripheral nerves of the somatic and autonomic nervous system as well as through the cranial nerves and psychogenic stimulation. Precisely where and how afferent information is processed within the spinal cord and brain is unknown (Yang 2000). The frontal and temporal lobes and anterior hypothalamus are all shown to have some function in mediating the sexual response but it is still unclear to what extent. Genital motor responses include pelvic vasocongestion and vaginal lubrication. During sexual intercourse the vagina lengthens, the labia increase in size, the uterus draws back and the clitoris retracts and at orgasm there is also contraction of the uterine and pelvic muscles.

Clinical clarification of the human sexual response was based on the model of four phases: excitement, plateau, orgasm and resolution (Masters & Johnson 1970). This description was then modified to a triphasic model of desire, arousal and orgasm (Kaplan 1974). These concepts provide the working models on which behavioural therapies for sexual problems are based. Recent scientific arguments are now proposing that sexual desire is, in fact, the first early stage of arousal, triggered by a stimulus which has sexual meaning and is modified by situational and partner variables (Janssen et al 2000).

Most human sexuality is non-problematic and will not be within the domain of the clinician. It is only when something goes wrong with the patient's sexual response that they may come to seek professional help.

SEXUAL PROBLEMS IN GENERAL

Population prevalence

The majority of the population at any one time have a trouble-free sex life. There is, however, a substantial minority for whom dealing with and expressing their sexuality is problematic. These problems may only be temporary or situational. If they persist and become increasingly distressing, then the individual will seek professional help. The population prevalence of some degree of sexual dysfunction is estimated to be about 20%. In the National Health and Social Life Survey (Laumann et al 1999) one-third of the women reported loss of libido. Almost 25% did not experience orgasm. Around 20% had problems with vaginal lubrication and a similar number did not enjoy sex. This study suggested that there was a substantial co-morbidity of sexual problems. For males, the prevalence of some degree of erectile dysfunction has been described as 30% of all males between the ages of 40 and 70. Premature ejaculation occurs in 10–30% of men during their lifetime (Laumann et al 1994, Spector & Carey 1990). In a control group of 591 of the general population in a Dutch study, 8.7% of men and 14.9% of women reported a sexual dysfunction unrelated to age (Diemont et al 2000), which is lower than that reported in other countries.

Having a sexual dysfunction does not necessarily mean that the individual has a sexual problem. This will depend on the effect, if any, that the dysfunction has on the life of the individual in terms of their feelings, relationships and lifestyle. Conversely, restoration of sexual function may not solve the sexual problem; in fact, it may serve to highlight an underlying emotional or relationship discord. Individuals with psychosexual problems usually have no organic sexual dysfunction whatsoever.

Problems of function or desire

Sexual disorders can be divided into problems of function or desire. They are often interlinked. For example, impaired sexual function, such as some degree of erectile problem, can result in the man protecting himself from the distress of failure by emotionally shutting himself off from coitus altogether. This results in loss of libido. If a woman is experiencing loss of function such as dyspareunia she may subconsciously employ the same defensive mechanisms and loss of desire develops.

Most common presenting problems

The most common female sexual problems are vaginismus, loss of libido, dyspareunia and inorgasmia. There will be differences in the frequency of presenting sexual complaints in different clinical settings. An American gynaecology clinic sample showed loss of libido (87.2%) with inorgasmia (83%) and dyspareunia (72%) (Nusbaum et al 2000). In a community-based setting such as a family planning clinic, however, loss of libido, dyspareunia and vaginismus are the most common presenting complaints, with a low incidence of lack of orgasm.

In males erectile dysfunction, ejaculatory disorders and loss of libido are the most frequent presenting complaints, all of which will affect the partner to some degree.

Problems relevant to gynaecology

There are many gynaecological conditions which may predispose to sexual problems. Anything which results in alteration of the genitalia may cause functional sexual difficulties. These conditions may range from trauma during delivery to gynaecological malignancy. Trauma or disease, however, may cause an alteration in the woman's perception of herself, such as distorted body image causing sexual problems. This may or may not be directly related to physical reality. An exceptionally high rate of sexual dissatisfaction was found in a gynaecology clinic sample in the United States. Over 98.8% of the sample reported one or more sexual concerns and body image concerns were reported by 68.5% of the 1480 women who attended (Nusbaum et al 2000). A study of Dutch gynaecologists found that 1 in 14 of their patients presenting in the previous week had problems of a sexual nature, mainly dyspareunia or lack of sexual desire (Frenken & van Tol 1987). A significant degree of deterioration of sexual function was described in a study of 41 women who had undergone vulvectomy, attributed to disturbed body image rather than physical impairment (Green et al 2000).

Once any gynaecological treatment is completed, the treatment approach for the sexual problem is the same as for any other patient.

SEXUAL PROBLEMS IN THE FEMALE

Vaginismus

Vaginismus is a condition in which nothing is able to enter the vagina. This means that penetrative sexual intercourse does not take place. It is caused by psychogenically mediated involuntary spasm of the vaginal muscles. Vaginismus can be primary or secondary. In primary vaginismus, nothing has ever entered the woman's vagina. A useful diagnostic question is 'Have you ever used a tampon?'. In a case of primary vaginismus the answer will always be 'no'. Secondary vaginismus can appear at any time in a woman's life, sometimes after childbirth or any other life-changing event.

The vagina is physiologically intact in a case of vaginismus. There is no stenosis or organic disorder. This is a psychogenic condition for which the treatment is psychosexual, never surgical.

Presentation

Vaginismus is a condition which usually has a masked presentation. One of the most common presentations is the avoidance of cervical smears. No woman likes having a vaginal examination or smear. The alert clinician, however, will observe a patient's persistent avoidance of examination or a fear of being examined which is in excess of that usually observed by the clinician. If vaginismus is suspected, a forced vaginal examination should not be done. This is the equivalent of medical rape, which can have a long-lasting traumatic effect on the woman.

It can present initially as dyspareunia or painful sexual intercourse. In this case the couple are not really having sex but as the erect penis attempts vaginal entry, the vaginal muscles contract and the interaction becomes painful. Vaginismus can also be a co-factor in loss of libido, although more commonly the woman has a strong desire to have sex, 'just like everybody else'.

Vaginismus may present as infertility. It is essential to ask the infertile couple whether or not they are having vaginal intercourse. Patients still reach tertiary referral centres for assisted conception, where it is discovered that sexual intercourse has never taken place and vaginismus is the primary diagnosis.

Treatment

There are two different approaches to the treatment of vaginismus. There are no data to suggest either method is superior and to date there has been no randomized controlled trial comparing methods of treatment. Treated by a skilled clinician, the reported cure rate is 90%.

Psychodynamic methods The trained clinician helps the patient to understand the basis for her problem and to recognize the barriers to sex. This method can take up to 2 years to cure the vaginismus but deals with the root causes of the problem as well as offering practical solutions.

Behavioural methods A more didactic approach is taken. The woman is taught to insert vaginal trainers, which are plastic 'pseudopenises' made in graduated sizes, into her own vagina. The same effect can be gained by using fingers. This teaches her that she can be in control of what enters her body.

Either treatment is acceptable but should be undertaken by trained individuals. There is no organic basis for the condition so the use of equipment such as this is essentially as an adjunct to psychosexual methods. Supplying vaginal trainers without supportive therapy is unlikely to show sustained benefit.

Surgery has no place in the treatment of vaginismus.

Inorgasmia

Inorgasmia is the lack of ability to experience orgasm. There are two main areas of innervation in the female genital region that can produce orgasmic symptoms if stimulated. The main area is the clitoris and there is another inside the vagina, about two-thirds of the way up, close to the urethra. This is known as the G-spot.

Presentation

The woman will either complain of inability to experience orgasm or may say that she doesn't know whether or not the feelings she is having constitute orgasm. Presentation at a clinic with this complaint will usually have been prompted by the acquisition of a new partner or by popular media interest in the topic.

Treatment

Often discussion of female genital anatomy and physiology will help. Encouraging masturbation is very rewarding. If this is combined with psychodynamic input, the patient usually responds.

There are some women, however, who have no feelings at all in the clitoral area. Drug therapies have been tried for this condition but have not proved successful, except for women with SSRI-induced loss of sensation (Nurnberg et al 1999). Combined oestrogen and androgen therapy may improve sexual sensation in menopausally triggered inorgasmia.

Loss of libido

Loss of libido is loss of sexual desire. It is generally associated with loss of self-esteem due to a multitude of underlying causes. There may be a traumatic event in the past which has not been dealt with emotionally and which may cause problems such as loss of libido at a later stage in the woman's lifetime. Examples of this are rape, sexual or emotional abuse, or a loss such as bereavement or redundancy leading to loss of status and loss of self-esteem.

There is much interest in hormonal influences on libido and current research is trying to answer some of these questions (Lunsen & Laan 1997).

Presentation

Loss of libido may present as depression or as a relationship problem. The woman may be uncomfortable at broaching the subject but if prompted by an empathetic clinician, may disclose the problem. In areas of gynaecological healthcare where body image becomes problematic, such as oncology, menopause and continence, loss of libido may be an overlooked complaint.

Treatment

The core treatment for loss of libido is psychosexual therapy, which deals with the underlying psychogenic origin of the problem. Counselling before procedures can allow women to explore their feelings in relation to these procedures. A past history of abortion is not uncommon in women with loss of interest in sex. Pre-termination of pregnancy counselling is, of necessity, information based and time limited. After termination of pregnancy, however, there is an opportunity for the woman to come to terms with what has happened, thus preventing the development of sexual problems later in life and hopefully preventing repeat unwanted pregnancy. After sterilization there will be some women who suffer loss of libido. Even if they have no regrets over the procedure, they may not have realized the emotional impact of losing their fertility as they have not understood the difference between choosing not to have a child, and not being able to conceive.

In cases where the loss of libido can be clearly linked to a hormonal trigger, such as starting a different combined oral contraceptive, changing contraception can improve the problem.

There is some evidence for the addition of androgens to

oestrogen replacement therapy for menopausal loss of libido (Sarrel 1999, Sherwin 1999). Hormonal therapy alone, however, can only return a woman to her premenopausal status and cannot change any underlying emotional blocks to sexual desire. The menopause is a time of major social and emotional upheaval for many women, which can be as overwhelming as adolescence, so psychosexual therapy combined with appropriate HRT would seem to be best practice.

Dyspareunia

Dyspareunia is painful sexual intercourse. It may be described as deep or superficial. There are organic causes for this, such as post delivery, after gynaecological operations, genital infections and in any condition which causes vaginal dryness, such as menopause. Vulval pain syndrome, or vulvodynia, is a complex condition which causes severe dyspareunia.

Vaginal dryness can be physiological, caused by lack of sufficient sexual stimulation during intercourse.

Presentation

Dyspareunia is a common presenting complaint to the gynaecologist. Some women (and doctors!) find it easier to discuss than some other sexual problems, as it seems more likely than other sexual complaints to have an organic origin. Post-delivery dyspareunia is frequently reported. An American study showed that on average women resumed sexual intercourse at 7 weeks post partum (Byrd et al 1998). Although in most of these cases sexual discomfort will resolve spontaneously, the opportunity to discuss the symptom may be helpful to the patient.

Treatment

If there is an underlying cause it should be treated. Common examples are persistent monilia, for which an antifungal regime should be given, and vaginal dryness due to menopause, which will improve with appropriate HRT. Recommended therapy for vulval pain syndromes is multidisciplinary with psychosexual input in co-ordination with gynaecological treatment (Nunns 2000).

If dyspareunia persists despite clinical evidence of cure of the underlying condition, then psychosexual therapy should be considered. Sometimes the memory of a painful condition may lead to expectation of pain on intercourse. This can produce involuntary vaginal muscle spasm, causing secondary vaginismus and thereby perpetuating the dyspareunia despite treatment of the original cause.

Physiological dyspareunia is caused by vaginal dryness due to lack of sufficient and appropriate sexual stimulation. It is treated by helping the woman understand the cause of the problem. Discussion of sexual technique may help, emphasizing foreplay. Enabling the woman to gain insight into the nature of her relationship with her partner is an essential part of this process.

Sexual problems of lesbians

Gynaecologists should remember that not all women are heterosexual. Lesbians have similar sexual problems to other women but, as they find it difficult to disclose their sexual orientation to doctors (Carr et al 1999), it may be even harder for them to discuss sexual problems than it is for heterosexuals. Women complaining of loss of libido, inorgasmia or dyspareunia may be in same-sex relationships. Vaginal penetration, as with all women, may occur with fingers and sex toys. Once organic causes have been excluded, psychosexual therapy should be offered. Synchronicity of menstruation in women living together, possibly due to pheromonal influence, has been documented (Mcclintock 1998). This is not universal but where it exists the coincidence of severe premenstrual symptoms can trigger domestic violence in lesbian couples, which can be an underlying cause of sexual problems.

Further issues related to gynecological and specific health problems of lesbians are dealt with in Chapter 66.

SEXUAL PROBLEMS IN THE MALE

Gynaecologists are unlikely to be in the front line when dealing with male sexual problems but as many of their female patients have male partners, it is important to have an overview of this area. If her partner has sexual problems, the woman can feel hurt and rejected and will frequently blame herself, presenting at a clinic for help in solving the problem.

Erectile dysfunction

Erectile dysfunction is the inability to sustain a penile erection sufficient to achieve satisfactory penetrative sexual intercourse. According to the Massachusetts Male Aging Study (Johannes et al 2000), the incidence of erectile dysfunction in men 40–69 years old is 25.9 cases per 1000 man-years; 60% is organic in origin, 15% is psychogenic and 25% of mixed origin.

Aetiology

Erectile dysfunction can be caused by any disruption of the neurological, endocrine or vascular supply to the genitalia. It can also occur for entirely psychogenic reasons. Associated factors are age, diabetes, alcohol intake, hypertension and the side-effects of many medications. Erectile dysfunction reduces quality of life and may lead to other associated sexual problems such as loss of libido.

Presentation

The man with erectile dysfunction may present to a doctor himself, although it is not unusual for the woman partner of a male with a sexual problem to present herself as the patient. She may say that she is experiencing either loss of sexual interest or painful sex. The couple themselves may not recognize where the problem lies.

Treatment

The treatment depends on the cause and falls into three basic categories: mechanical, chemical and psychosexual.

The simplest, non-invasive treatments are vacuum devices. A constriction ring is first applied to the base of the flaccid penis, then a vacuum is created, causing engorgement of the corpora cavernosa which is maintained by the constriction ring. This method creates a slightly blue, cold erection, which may be sufficient for intercourse, but is suitable for some men who prefer non-chemical treatment methods. Surgery is required if a venous shunt has been demonstrated or to insert a prosthesis, if there are no other options for treatment.

Chemical treatments have been widely used over the last few years. Locally acting alprostadil, which is prostaglandin E, can be injected into the base of the penis, causing smooth muscle relaxation and resulting in an erection. Success rates for this treatment are around 70% (Linet & Neff 1994). It can also be introduced by a tiny pellet into the urethra, with penile erection rates reaching 70% (Padma-Nathan et al 1997). Success rates with this urethral medication have been improved by the use of a penile constriction band which augments local retention (Lewis 1998). A newer combination of alprostadil and an α-adrenergic antagonist enhances erection rates (Costabile et al 1998). This causes smooth muscle relaxation, leading to engorgement of the corpora cavernosa and erection of the penis. Although there can be some local discomfort there are few contraindications to this therapy. It does, however, require manual dexterity and a willingness to inject or to insert medication into the penis. Unsurprisingly, there are fairly high discontinuation rates for this type of invasive therapy.

Oral therapy is now available which has revolutionized treatment of this distressing condition. Sildenafil (Viagra) inhibits phosphodiesterase type 5, a cyclic GMP inhibitor. It is therefore a facilitator, not initiator, of erections. This oral medication has reported efficacy rates of 69% for sexual intercourse (Goldstein et al 1998). It has a vasodilatory effect and must not be used for patients with coronary insufficiency on nitrates. Some cases of myocardial infarction were reported when sildenafil was used in these situations. The use of amyl nitrate 'poppers', employed to facilitate anal intercourse, is also strongly contra-indicated with sildenafil.

Psychosexual therapy is an important therapy to consider in cases of erectile dysfunction, either on its own or as an adjunct to physical therapy, as 40% of erectile dysfunction has a psychogenic element. This form of treatment allows the man to explore all the issues surrounding his problem and also allows him to include his partner in treatment if he wishes. It also takes a whole-person approach, rather than merely focusing on the genitalia.

Premature ejaculation

Premature ejaculation is a condition where the male comes to orgasm and ejaculates very rapidly, before satisfactory sexual intercourse has taken place. It is commonly a complaint of young men but may present at any time.

Presentation

The man suffering from premature ejaculation will ask for clinical help if it is affecting his relationships.

Treatment

A psychodynamic approach will help the man to understand and cope with his anxieties related to the problem.

The 'squeeze' technique can be used. If the thumb and forefinger are used to squeeze firmly at the base of the glans penis at the point of ejaculation, ejaculation will be delayed. This technique, however, requires a good degree of co-ordination. Antidepressant medication, such as clomipramine and the newer serotonin reuptake inhibitors, have been shown to increase ejaculation latency (Rowland & Burnett 2000).

Delayed ejaculation

Delayed ejaculation is a condition which is usually psychogenic in origin. It can be extremely distressing to the female partner and if penetrative, thrusting sexual intercourse becomes prolonged due to a failure of the man to become orgasmic, it can lead to dyspareunia. The male may be able to ejaculate when masturbating but is unable to do so intravaginally. This could be for various subconscious reasons, some of which are fear of losing control, fear of causing pregnancy or unwillingness to make a commitment to his partner (Thexton 1992).

Treatment

Psychosexual therapy is the treatment of choice. This problem may take a prolonged course of therapy before positive outcomes are achieved.

Loss of libido

This can affect men as well as women. Rarely, lack of testosterone may be implicated but the cause is usually emotional and will frequently be linked to some cause of loss of self-esteem in the man.

TREATMENTS

Most problems of a sexual nature have a psychogenic origin. Even sexual problems with clear organic origins tend to have some degree of psychogenic overlay, as sexual activity, or the lack of it, has emotional impacts.

There are three main treatment modalities for sexual problems.

Psychodynamic methods

Psychodynamic medicine is concerned with understanding how emotional factors interfere with sexual activity and enjoyment. These emotional factors may not be at the conscious level. The aim of treatment is to enable the patient to resolve the problem by removing the psychological blocks to satisfactory sexual activity and relationships (Skrine 1989). This is achieved by taking a 'mind–body' approach to the patient and their sexual problem. The psychosexually trained clinician will explore the problem with the patient by interpreting the doctor–patient interaction and feeding back these observations to the patient in order to elicit their response.

An important part of this treatment is the psychogenic genital examination. Many of the patient's underlying attitudes, fears and fantasies related to their sexual problem may be revealed in relation to this part of the consultation.

The philosophy of treatment is that the patient is 'whoever presents' at the consultation. This mode of treatment is suitable for individuals whether or not they are in a relationship. It is also appropriate for couples regardless of gender identity or sexual orientation.

Not all psychosexual problems require prolonged specialist treatment. A single consultation with a suitably trained doctor is sufficient help for some patients.

Behavioural methods

Behavioural methods involve a more didactic, 'hands-on' approach to treatment. This philosophy of treatment was developed through the work of Masters & Johnson (1970) and Helen Singer Kaplan (1974). Patients are given practical tasks in order to learn or relearn how to experience and enjoy sexual activity. This approach maintains that the many causes of sexual dysfunction can be effectively treated by a programme combining education, homework assignments and counselling (Hawton 1995). A staged approach to re-establishing healthy sexual contact can be a useful therapeutic tool when dealing with couples and has been modified to treat single individuals although it is felt to be of most use for people with partners.

Drug treatments

Drug treatment of male erectile dysfunction has been shown to have high success rates and there is some evidence for improvements in premature ejaculation with antidepressants such as SSRIs or anticholinergics such as clomipramine. Medication may restore genital function but associated emotional and relationship issues should also be appropriately addressed.

For women there has been increased interest in the possibility of drug treatment for sexual dysfunction. Despite much research, the only evidence-based conclusion is that appropriate hormone replacement therapy with the addition of androgen will improve sexual functioning in some postmenopausal women. Research has shown an influence of adrenergic compounds on physiological sexual arousal but not on the woman's subjective sexual experience (Everaerd & Laan 2000), which is in fact what matters most in sexual functioning. To date, compounds used to increase male penile blood flow have not been shown to be successful in women, except in very defined circumstances (Nurnberg et al 1999). As there are many medications associated with loss of libido, such as some hormonal contraceptives, antiepileptics and psychotropic drugs, a change of medication may help.

The mainstay of treatment for sexual problems, however, particularly for women, is therapy which deals with the emotional and interpersonal blocks to satisfactory sexual activity. Sensitivity to the emotional aspects of the consultation and possible sexual sequelae of the gynaecological condition or its treatment may prevent the onset of sexual problems in the future.

SERVICE PROVISION

Most localities have some provision of service for the treatment of psychosexual problems. Family planning and reproductive healthcare services usually have an attached sexual problems clinic, which provides treatment in a non-threatening and non-judgemental, community-based environment. Other sexual problem clinics may be based in psychiatric settings.

Many people find it very embarrassing to disclose a sexual problem to anyone and a self-referral facility for making appointments can encourage patients to come forward for treatment.

CONCLUSION

With such a large minority of women experiencing some form of sexual difficulty in their lifetime right through from adolescence to menopause and beyond, it is vital for the gynaecologist to be aware of these conditions and to allow the woman to voice her concerns in a non-threatening environment. It could be sufficient to listen to her and acknowledge her concerns in an empathetic and non-judgemental manner. If she wishes, referral can be made to the appropriate sexual problems service, which is usually attached to local family planning or psychiatry services. With suitable training, however, it is possible to employ brief focused analytic techniques within the context of a routine gynaecological appointment. This allows the gynaecologist to assess the psychosexual element of the situation and enhances quality of care for the patient.

KEY POINTS

1. Patients find it difficult to disclose problems of a sexual nature – increased awareness by the gynaecologist and a willingness to introduce the topic is helpful.
2. Sexual problems have either an organic, emotional or mixed origin – the mode of treatment depends on the cause.
3. A gynaecologist trained in psychosexual techniques can provide help to the patient within the context of the gynaecology clinic setting.
4. Sexual problems may be situational. They may occur in one context, but not in another.
5. Dyspareunia presenting to the gynaecologist with negative clinical findings may have a psychogenic origin.
6. Primary vaginismus is of psychogenic origin and surgery has no place in its treatment.
7. Loss of libido is mostly of emotional origin, but in some menopausal women testosterone addition to hormone replacement therapy is beneficial.

REFERENCES

Bancroft J 1989 Human sexuality and its problems. Churchill Livingstone, Edinburgh

Byrd JE, Hyde JS, de Lamater JD, Plant E, Ashby MS 1998 Sexuality during pregnancy and the year postpartum. Journal of Family Practice 47(4):305–308

Carr SV, Scoular A, Elliott L, Illett R, Meager M 1999 A community based lesbian sexual health service – clinically justified or politically correct? British Journal of Family Planning 25:93–95

Costabile R, Spevak M, Fishman I et al 1998 Efficacy and safety of transurethral alprostadil in patients with erectile dysfunction following radical prostatectomy. Journal of Urology 160(4):1325–1328

Diemont WL, Wruggink P, Meuleman E, Doesburg W, Lemmens W, Berden J 2000 Sexual dysfunction after renal replacement therapy. American Journal of Kidney Diseases 35:845–851

Everaerd W, Laan E 2000 Drug treatments for women's sexual disorders. Journal of Sex Research 37:195–204

Frenken J, van Tol P 1987 Sexual problems in gynaecological practice. Journal of Psychosomatic Obstetrics and Gynaecology 6:143–155

Goldstein I, Lue TF, Padma-Nathan H, Rosen RC, Steers WD, Wicker PA, 1998 Oral sildenafil in the treatment of erectile dysfunction. New England Journal of Medicine 338:1397–1404

Green MS, Naumann R, Elliott M, Hall J, Higgins R, Grigsby J 2000 Sexual dysfunction following vulvectomy. Gynaecologic Oncology 77:73–77

Hawton K 1995 Treatment of sexual dysfunctions by sex therapy and other approaches. British Journal of Psychiatry 167(3):307–314

Janssen E, Everaerd W, Spiering M, Janssen J 2000 Automatic processes and the appraisal of sexual stimuli. Journal of Sex Research 37:8

Johannes CB, Araujo AB, Feldman HA, Derby CA, Kleinmann KP, Mckinlay JB 2000 Incidence of erectile dysfunction in men 40 to 69 years old: longitudinal results from the Massachusetts male ageing study. Journal of Urology 163(2):460–463

Kaplan HS 1974 The new sex therapy. Baillière Tindall, London

Kinsey AC, Pomeroy WB, Martin CF 1948 Sexual behaviour in the human male. WB Saunders, Philadelphia

Kinsey AC, Pomeroy WB, Martin CF, Gebhard PH 1953 Sexual behaviour in the human female. WB Saunders, Philadelphia

Laumann E, Michael R, Gagnon J 1994 A political history of the National Sex Survey of adults. Family Planning Perspective 26(1):34–38

Laumann EO, Paik A, Rosen RC 1999 Sexual dysfunction in the United States: prevalence and predictors. Journal of the American Medical Association 281:537–544

Lewis RW 1998 Combined use of transurethral alprostadil and an adjustable penile constriction band in men with erectile dysfunction: results from a multi-centre trial (abstract). Journal of Urology 159:237

Linet OI, Neff LL 1994 Intracavernous prostaglandin E1 in erectile dysfunction. Clinical Investigations 72:139–149

Lunsen RHW, van Laan E 1997 Sex, hormones and the brain. European Journal of Contraception and Reproductive Health Care 2:247–251

Masters W, Johnson V 1970 Human sexual inadequacy. Little, Brown, Boston

Mcclintock M 1998 Whither menstrual synchrony? Annual Review of Sex Research II:77–95

Nunns D 2000 Vulval pain syndromes. British Journal of Obstetrics and Gynaecology 107:1185–1193

Nurnberg HC, Hensley PL, Lauriello J, Parker LM, Keith SJ 1999 Sildenafil for women patients with anti-depressant induced sexual dysfunction. Psychiatric Services 50(8):1076–1078

Nusbaum M, Gamle G, Skinner B. Heiman J 2000 The high prevalence of sexual concerns among women seeking routine gynaecology care. Journal of Family Practice 49:229–232

Padma-Nathan H, Hellstrom WJ, Kaiser FE et al 1997 Treatment of men with erectile dysfunction with transurethral alprostadil. Medicated urethral system for erection (MUSE) study group. New England Journal of Medicine 336:1–7

Rowland DL, Burnett AL 2000 Pharmacotherapy in the treatment of male sexual dysfunction. Journal of Sex Research 37:226–243

Sarrel PM 1999 Psychosexual effects of menopause: role of androgens. American Journal of Obstetrics and Gynecology 180:319–324

Sherwin BB 1998 Use of combined estrogen-androgen preparations in the post-menopause: evidence from clinical studies. International Journal of Fertility and Women's Medicine 43:98–103

Skrine R (ed) 1989 Introduction to psychosexual medicine. Chapman and Hall, London

Spector I, Carey M 1990 Incidence and prevalence of the sexual dysfunctions. Archives of Sexual Behaviour 19(4):389–408

Thexton R 1992 Ejaculatory disturbances. In: Lincoln R (ed) Psychosocial medicine: a study of underlying themes. Chapman and Hall, Boston

Wellins K, Field J, Johnson A, Wadsworth J 1994 Sexual behaviour in Britain. Penguin, London

Yang C 2000 Female sexual function in neurologic disease. Journal of Sex Research 37:205–212

FURTHER READING

Further reading materials can be obtained from:

Institute of Pyschosexual Medicine
Cavendish Square
12 Chandos Street
London W1G 9BR

The Association of Marital and Relationship Therapy
PO Box 13686
London SW20 9ZH

32

Menstruation and menstrual disorder

Mary Ann Lumsden   Jay McGavigan

INTRODUCTION

Menstrual abnormality is a frequent reason for women to present at gynaecological outpatient clinics and menorrhagia is one of the commonest causes of iron deficiency anaemia in Western women (Cohen & Gibor 1980). The average woman now experiences approximately 400 cycles in contrast to the 40 or so she would have experienced 50 years ago and with the advent of effective contraception, disorders of menstruation have become a significant public health issue. However, before discussing the aetiology of menstrual abnormality, the mechanism of normal menstruation will be reviewed.

MENSTRUATION

At the end of the ovarian cycle, a major portion of the endometrium in primates undergoes periodic necrosis and sloughing associated with blood loss. This is at a time when the gonadal steroids reach their lowest levels. The nature of the supportive effect on the endometrium is unknown, although possible mechanisms will be discussed later.

Anatomy of the uterus

The uterus is a muscular, pear-shaped organ consisting of a fundus, body and cervix. The uterus receives the fallopian tubes at the cornua whilst the cervix protrudes and opens into the vaginal vault.

The wall of the uterus consists of three layers: the serous coat, myometrium and endometrium. The serous coat is firmly adherent to the myometrium which consists of smooth muscle fibres, the main branches of the blood vessels and the nerves of the uterus and connective tissue. The endometrium consists principally of glandular and stromal cells, although its structure does vary spatially within the uterus and temporally with the stage of the menstrual cycle.

The blood supply of the uterus

The blood supply of the uterus (Fig. 32.1) is by the uterine artery, a branch of the internal iliac artery. It passes medially across the pelvic floor above the ureter, reaching the uterus at the supravaginal part of the cervix. Giving a branch to the cervix and vagina, the vessel turns upwards between the leaves of the broad ligament to run alongside the uterus as far as the entrance of the fallopian tube, where it anastomoses with the tubal branch of the ovarian artery. In its course it gives off branches that penetrate the walls of the uterus. Within the myometrium the uterine and ovarian arteries form the arcuate arteries. These in turn give rise to the radial arteries which, after passing through the endometrial–myometrial

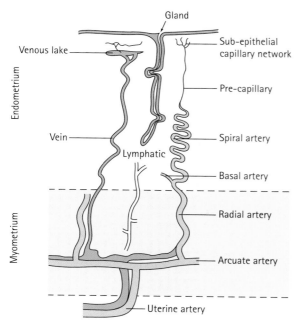

Fig. 32.1 Schematic representation of the blood supply of the uterus.

junction, branch into the basal arterioles, supplying the basal endometrium, and the spiral arterioles, supplying the superficial layer of the endometrium. Spiral arterioles are end arterioles and are present only in species that menstruate. Each supplies an area of 4–9 mm². Branching of the spiral arterioles occurs throughout the superficial layer of the endometrium. Just below the surface epithelium they break up into a prominent subepithelial plexus that drains into venous sinuses.

The endometrial vasculature is unlike any other vascular bed owing to its cyclic remodelling and regression during the menstrual cycle. These vessels are sensitive to changes in gonadal steroid levels and at menstruation the capillaries are shed with the glands and stroma (Rogers et al 1998).

The histology of the uterus

The endometrium

The endometrium is composed of heterogeneous cell types that undergo cyclic synchronized waves of proliferation and differentiation in response to the rise and fall of oestrogen and progesterone. Histologically it is divided into a superficial or functional layer, which lies adjacent to the uterine cavity, and a basalis, or deeper layer.

In the uterus, the superficial endometrial layer is characterized by rapid proliferation during the follicular phase of the cycle followed by secretory transformation of the glandular epithelium, predecidualization of the stromal compartment and influx of uterine natural killer (NK) cells in the luteal phase of the cycle (King et al 1998).

During the proliferative phase, the short, straight epithelial glands elongate and become tortuous (Fig.32.2a). Changes occur in the position of the nuclei and the number of mitoses. During the secretory phase, the glands increase in diameter and tortuosity and vacuoles appear in the cellular cytoplasm (Fig.32.2b). The tissue also becomes markedly oedematous.

These morphological events are controlled by a highly co-ordinated activation of certain gene sets essential for regulating uterine function. For instance, after ovulation the sequential expression of progesterone-dependent genes defines a limited period of uterine receptivity or, in the absence of pregnancy, maintains vascular integrity prior to menstruation (Lockwood et al 1998, Tabibzadeh & Babaknia 1995).

In contrast, the basal endometrium shows no 'classic' sex steroid hormone response and is characterized by low proliferative activity, absence of glandular secretory transformation and lack of a predecidualization reaction in the late luteal phase. This absence of the 'classic' sex steroid hormone response does not, however, imply refractoriness to ovarian hormones. The basal layer is an important source of uterotonins and the site of active metaplasia of basal endometrial stromal cells into myofibroblasts and vice versa. The basal layer of the endometrium is further characterized by the presence of resident CD-3-positive T-lymphocyte aggregates.

The microvascular blood supply of the endometrium undergoes the unique process of benign angiogenesis and is under the control of ovarian steroids during reproductive life. Following cessation of menstruation, they are simple in form, extending just into the endometrium. The secretory phase is characterized by growth of arterioles. In the late secretory phase coiling occurs due to proliferation and extension of the arterioles (Fig. 32.2c). With the fall in steroid concentrations, menstrual shedding of the functional layer of the endometrium occurs (Fig. 32.2d). Dramatic changes occur in the spiral arterioles at menstruation. These changes were described by Markee (1948) after experiments involving the transplantation of endometrium into the anterior chamber of the eye of the rhesus monkey. This work was the cornerstone of current concepts of menstruation. On observing the bleeding process, Markee suggested that the arteriolar coiling caused constriction of the vessel lumen with vascular stasis and leucocytic infiltration. About 24 hours premenstrually intense vasoconstriction led to ischaemic damage which was then followed by vasodilatation with haemorrhage from both arterial and venous vessels: 75% of the loss was arteriolar, 15% venous and 10% diapedesis of erythrocytes (Markee 1940). This work has never been repeated although some support comes from experiments where endometrium was implanted into hamster cheek pouch (an immunologically privileged site) and changes observed through a plastic window. Bleeding was observed although no hormonally induced changes in the blood vessels occurred.

The myometrium

The human myometrium is structurally and functionally polarized during the reproductive years. Compared with the outer myometrium, the subendometrial layer or junctional zone (JZ) is characterized by higher cell density, lower cellular nucleocytoplasmic ratios and the expression of different extracellular matrix components (Brosens et al 1998, Campbell et al 1998). Additionally, evidence from ³¹P nuclear magnetic resonance spectroscopic studies has demonstrated biochemical heterogeneity between both myometrial layers (Xu et al 1997).

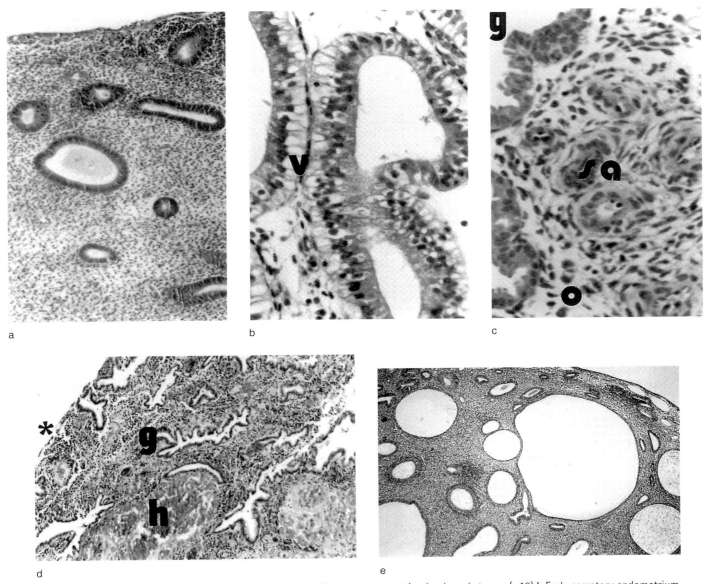

Fig. 32.2   a Proliferative endometrium showing tubular glands. Mitoses are present in glands and stroma (×10) b Early secretory endometrium showing subnuclear vacuolation (v) and the presence of secretions. There are now few mitoses (×40). c Midsecretory endometrium (day 23) characterized by 'saw-toothed' glands (g), convoluted spiral arterioles (sa) and stromal oedema (o) (×40). d Menstruating endometrium. The glands (g) are now thin and show little secretory activity. There are lakes of haemorrhage (h) and the endometrium is beginning to break up (*). There is infiltration with white blood cells (×10). e Cystic glandular hyperplasia (×4).

The differentiation of the myometrium into two distinct layers is strictly under ovarian hormonal control. In premenarchal girls and postmenopausal women the zonal anatomy is often indistinct. Ovarian suppression with gonadotrophin-releasing hormone analogues leads to an MRI appearance of the uterus mimicking that of postmenopausal women whilst hormone replacement therapy in postmenopausal women results in the reappearance of myometrial zonal anatomy (Demas et al 1985).

Further evidence for hormone responsiveness of the JZ is provided by the work of Wiczyk et al (1988) who demonstrated changes in JZ thickness throughout the menstrual cycle in conjunction with endometrial thickness.

MECHANISMS OF NORMAL MENSTRUATION AND THE CONTROL OF BLOOD LOSS

The tissue components of the endometrium are a surface epithelium and associated glands with a connective tissue stroma in which is embedded an elaborate vascular tree. The endometrial surface area is large (10–45 cm^2), indicating that haemostasis during menstruation is usually very efficient.

Withdrawal of progesterone from an oestrogen-primed endometrium results in menstrual shedding. Shedding arises because of the induction of matrix metalloproteinases (MMPs) from the endometrium, in particular MMPs 1, 2 and 9 (Jeziorska et al 1996, Marbaix et al 1996). This arises through a mechanism of upregulation of transforming growth factor-beta

461

(TGF-β) (Bruner et al 1995). The blood vessels are thus denuded of their support. Spiral arterioles and venules are then cleaved at the level of the junctional zone between the endometrial functionalis and basalis with subsequent bleeding.

Factors involved in the control of menstrual blood loss are:

- haemostasis
- vasoconstriction
- endometrial repair.

Derangement of any of these mechanisms is likely to lead to excessive menstrual loss.

Haemostasis

Coagulation occurs in the distal endometrium and platelets found within the endometrial cavity are deactivated and do not respond to collagen, as they would elsewhere. Once clinical bleeding and tissue shedding has started, haemostatic plug formation occurs, but less rapidly and less completely than is observed in human skin wounds (Christiaens et al 1982). Certain haemorrhagic conditions (e.g. thrombocytopenic purpura) are associated with an increased incidence of menorrhagia, suggesting that abnormalities of platelet structure may be important.

The coagulation cascade operates in the uterus and endometrium as in other tissues. Platelet accumulation, platelet degranulation and fibrin deposition occur within hours of the onset of menstruation, sealing endometrial vessels. The platelet count in menstrual discharge is only a tenth of that seen in peripheral blood. This is probably due to the consumption of platelet aggregates in endometrial blood vessels early in the haemostatic processes of menstruation (de Merre et al 1967). Additionally these platelets have been found to be devoid of granules and fail to aggregate when challenged with aggregating stimuli such as adenosine diphosphate and collagen. Compared with peripheral blood platelets, those in menstrual fluid do not produce appreciable cyclo-oxygenase products from arachadonic acid (Christiaens et al 1981, Rees et al 1984, Sheppard et al 1983).

Since prevention of clot formation is necessary to deter scarring and obliteration of the endometrial cavity, there appears to be an active fibrinolytic system in the endometrium mediated by plasmin through proteolytic cleavage of plasminogen by the activators urokinase-type plasminogen activator (μ-PA) and tissue-type plasminogen activator (t-PA) These activators are regulated by plasminogen activator inhibitor 1 (PAI-1) and PAI-2, both of which are expressed in the endometrium. The presence of these fibrinolytic agents would suggest that coagulation occurs but is rapidly reversed. Estradiol stimulates whilst progesterone inhibits u-PA (Casslen et al 1986). Further, progesterone inhibits production of tissue plasminogen activator, and this effect is amplified by production of PAI. Blood coagulation products have also been found to be severely depleted in menstrual fluid, suggesting consumption during menstruation (Hahn 1980).

Whilst early studies suggested that blood clots, commonly found in the vagina during menstruation, are devoid of fibrin and are actually red cell aggregations to mucoid substances,

ultrastructural studies showed that fibrin formation occurs during the process of menstruation (Beller 1971, Sheppard et al 1983). The high levels of fibrin degradation products in menstrual fluid are not solely due to direct digestion. There is general agreement that although menstrual blood contains high levels of fibrin and FDPs, it contains no fibrinogen. Similar levels of protein C_1 inactivator, α_2-macroglobulin and α_2-antitrypsin have been found in peripheral and menstrual blood (Daly et al 1990). However, compared with peripheral plasma lower levels of activated prothrombin, antithrombin, antiplasmin, plasminogen, protein C and factors V, VII, VIII and X have been reported in menstrual fluid (Daly et al 1990, Rees et al 1985).

Compared with peripheral plasma, menstrual blood has a marked increase in the levels of t-PA antigen with reduced levels of PAI. Levels of fibrinolytic enzymes in menstrual fluid vary according to cycle stage. Throughout the cycle, higher levels of t-PA are found in the myometrium than endometrium in the normal menstrual cycle (Sheppard 1992), whilst during the late secretory phase, several studies have demonstrated a significant increase in endometrial t-PA levels (Shaw et al 1980).

The above mechanisms ensure that during menstruation, as progesterone falls and estradiol rises, plasminogen activator levels increase to prevent uterine adhesions. There is increased fibrinolytic activity in the endometrium of women with increased menstrual blood loss. The endometrium also generates factors that inhibit platelet aggregation and platelet adhesion. Such factors include prostacyclin (PGI_2), nitric oxide (NO) and platelet-activating factor (PAF) (Alecozay et al 1991, Kelly et al 1984).

Vasoconstriction

In the menstruating uterus, haemostatic events are strikingly different from the rest of the body (Christiaens et al 1980). At the onset of menstruation, damaged blood vessels are sealed by intravascular thrombi of platelets and fibrin. However, as menstruation progresses, the functional endometrium is shed and so these haemostatic thrombi are lost. Subsequently, during the first 20 hours of menstruation intense vaso-constriction of the spiral arterioles occurs and assures haemostasis until regeneration of the endometrial surface is complete.

The role of prostaglandin $F_{2\alpha}$ ($PGF_{2\alpha}$) in vasoconstriction is well established. The effects of the vasoconstricting $PGF_{2\alpha}$ are balanced by those of the vasodilating prostaglandin E_2 (PGE_2). Concentrations of both these prostaglandins are increased in the luteal phase. Overproduction of the vasodilatory prostaglandins or reduced production of the vasoconstrictors is likely to lead to excessive blood loss at the time of menstruation. This is confirmed by work showing an elevated $PGE_2/PGF_{2\alpha}$ ratio, increased endometrial PGE_2 or increased PGE_2 receptor concentrations in women with menorrhagia (Adalantado et al 1988, Smith et al 1981). Steroid hormones influence endometrial prostaglandin synthesis and the highest levels of the latter are found during menstruation. This is particularly true for $PGF_{2\alpha}$, the synthesis of which rises significantly during the secretory phase of the menstrual cycle under the influence of progesterone.

Other vasoconstrictors which have attracted recent interest are the endothelins and PAF. Endothelins are powerful vasoconstrictors which are found in various tissues, including human endometrium (Cameron et al 1992). They belong to a family of small 21-amino acid peptides. The family is composed of three members of structurally related isoforms–endothelin 1 (ET-1), ET-2 and ET-3–which act on two distinct receptors, the endothelin A receptor (ETA) and the endothelin B receptor (ETB). In the human endometrium, immunoreactive endothelin has been localized to vascular endothelium, glandular and luminal epithelium and the stromal compartment where it is thought to be involved in paracrine regulation of a number of endometrial functions such as the induction of vascular and myometrial smooth muscle contractions, fibroblast mitogenesis and the release of other paracrine agents (Ohbuchi et al 1995). Recent evidence suggests that endothelins in the endometrium can induce $PGF_{2\alpha}$ and further endothelin release, in a paracrine and autocrine fashion. It has been proposed that as endometrial glandular epithelium breaks down during menstruation, stored endothelin gains access to the spiral arterioles, causing long-lasting vasoconstriction (Cameron & Davenport 1992).

PAF is present in the endometrium in the luteal phase and has an ambiguous effect on spiral arteriolar tone: PAF itself is a vasoconstrictor but stimulates production of the vasodilator PGE_2 (Bjork & Smedegard 1983, Smith & Kelly 1988).

Endometrial repair

Vasculature

Seventy per cent of menstrual loss arises from the spiral arterioles and most of this bleeding occurs within the first 3 days of menses (Haynes et al 1977). Concordantly vessel repair begins within the first 2–3 days of the onset of bleeding. As might be expected, the endometrium is a rich source of angiogenic growth factors (Smith 1998). The fibroblast growth factor (FGF) and the vascular endothelial growth factor (VEGF) families are the best known.

Vascular endothelial growth factor VEGF is a heterodimeric angiogenic growth factor expressed and secreted by a variety of endometrial cells including macrophages and large decidualized cells that cluster around the spiral arterioles during the late luteal phase (Charnock-Jones et al 1993, Gospodarowicz et al 1989). The variants of VEGF differ in their cellular localization.

Steroids and hypoxia regulate VEGF with steroid regulation being around two orders of magnitude lower than that of hypoxia. VEGF mRNA is abundant in the endometrium at the time of menstruation (Charnock-Jones et al 1993). This up-regulation probably follows the hypoxia induced by spiral arteriole vasoconstriction (Sharkey et al 2000). Its expression is followed by rapid angiogenesis when the functional endometrium is lost.

Vascular smooth muscle cells (VSMCs) in endometrium also express certain VEGF receptors. This provides a direct link between development of spiral arterioles and VEGF-A expression. The finding of reduced proliferation of VSMCs in menorrhagic patients could be explained by altered VEGF-A expression.

Fibroblast growth factor The FGF family consists of at least eight members some of which are expressed in the endometrium and are hormone dependent with expression during the proliferative phase and a reduction during the secretory phase (Basilico & Moscatelli 1992, Ferriani et al 1993). FGF synergizes with VEGFs in inducing angiogenesis (Pepper et al 1992). Inhibition of FGF action does not fully inhibit angiogenesis but this is possible when anti-VEGF agents are used. VEGFs promote the release of FGF from the extracellular matrix. Their role in menstruation is unclear.

Angiopoietins The angiopoietins are another family of molecules which influence vascular development and maintenance by stabilizing the endothelial cell–vascular smooth muscle structure (Suri et al 1998). It is possible that this may alter the function of the VSMCs that are essential for controlling the blood loss at menstruation.

Epithelium

Given its dynamic nature, growth factors and cytokines are especially important in the development of the endometrium. In addition, tissue remodelling is dependent on the integrity of the extracellular matrix (ECM). Profound hormone-dependent tissue remodelling is seen in the endometrium though currently there is no direct evidence linking disorders of tissue regeneration with menorrhagia. Proliferation of the endometrium is most active during menstruation. The proliferation starts at day 2 in the basal glands and is complete by day 5, leaving a completely re-epithelialized endometrial surface. Various agents regulate this process, the best known being epidermal growth factor (EGF). EGF is expressed in human epithelial cells throughout the cycle and stimulates endometrial epithelial proliferation (Haining et al 1991, Zhang et al 1995). Oestradiol induces the expression of EGF and its receptor EGF-R. However, during menstruation when the concentration of oestradiol is at its lowest there are sufficient amounts of residual EGF remaining in the epithelial cells as growth continues before oestradiol levels increase during the proliferative phase. Additionally, EGF has been shown to mimic the proliferative effect of oestradiol in the endometrium of transgenic mice lacking the oestradiol receptor (Ignar Trowbridge et al 1992). Numerous other growth factors (insulin-like growth factor, IGF; fibroblast growth factor, FGF) and their binding proteins are expressed in the endometrium and all promote cell proliferation. The complexities of tissue remodelling suggest that altered wound healing may be a factor in the aetiology of menorrhagia and its role warrants further investigation.

Matrix

The extracellular matrix is a dynamic structure composed of collagens, fibronectin, laminin, gelatins, entactins, hyaluronic acid and proteoglycans, all of which provide the tissue with structural integrity.

Integrins are the agents which link the ECM with epithelial cells of the endometrium (Hynes 1987, Lessey et al 1992). The matrix metalloproteinases (MMPs) are a highly regulated family of calcium and zinc endopeptidases which are able to degrade most components of the ECM in the activated state. These enzymes are active in normal and pathological processes involving tissue remodelling. MMP activity is greatest during days 1–4 of the cycle. Progesterone withdrawal and migratory leucocytes activate some MMPs. Abnormalities in the dynamic

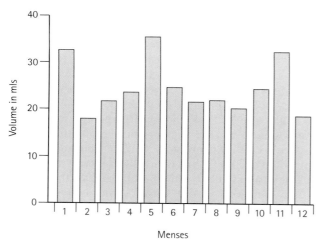

Fig. 32.3 The variability in menstrual blood loss in a single individual: values for 12 consecutive periods. Adapted from Hallberg & Nilsson (1964).

turnover of collagen production are likely to be important in menstrual upset given their importance in other vascular and fibrotic processes.

THE NORMAL MENSTRUAL CYCLE

The majority of cycles lie between 24 and 32 days and a normal cycle is considered to be 28 days. Menstrual cycle length varies during reproductive life, being most regular between the ages of 20 and 40 years. It tends to be longer after the menarche and shorter as the menopause approaches. The mean menstrual blood loss per menstruation in a healthy Western European population ranges between 37 and 43 ml; 70% of the loss occurs in the first 48 hours. Despite the large interpatient variability, loss between consecutive menses in the same woman does not vary to a great extent (Fig. 32.3). Only 9–14% of women lose more than 80 ml per period and 60% of these women are actually anaemic. The upper limit of normal menstruation is thus taken as 80 ml per menses (Rybo 1966). However, total fluid loss (mucus, tissue, etc.) may be considerably more than the blood loss alone and amounts vary.

During the first day or two of the menses, uterine contractility is at its greatest. This may aid expulsion of the degenerating endometrium from the uterus. Activity is extremely variable between women although it is remarkably constant between menses in the same woman. There is no objective method of separating normal and abnormal contractility; normal contractility is considered to be that which causes no debility to a woman although mild discomfort may occur.

The pattern of spontaneous myometrial contractions varies during the menstrual cycle (Lumsden et al 1983). Time-lapse ultrasound studies have shown that propagated myometrial contractions in the non-pregnant uterus emanate from the junctional zone. The frequency and direction of these contractions depend on the phase of the cycle. In the follicular and periovulatory phases cervicofundal subendometrial contractions can be seen, the amplitude and frequency of which increase notably towards ovulation. Short, asymmetrical

myometrial waves are present during the luteal phase but propagated fundocervical subendometrial contraction waves are noted during menstruation (Chalubinski et al 1993, de Vries et al 1990).

Kunz demonstrated the role of preovulatory cervicofundal contractions in assisting the rapid transport of sperm through the female reproductive tract (Kunz et al 1996). Others have postulated that the asymmetrical myometrial peristalsis during the luteal phase serves to maintain the developing blastocyst within the uterine fundus. The role of fundocervical contractions during menstruation is likely to be important in controlling menstrual flow and limiting retrograde menstruation (Chalubinski et al 1993).

ABNORMAL MENSTRUATION

This chapter will consider abnormalities of menstrual bleeding including menorrhagia, with particular reference to dysfunctional uterine bleeding (DUB), and dysmenorrhoea. Those defects most usually associated with infertility, e.g. oligo- or amenorrhoea, will not be discussed further.

Menorrhagia

The causes of menorrhagia fall into four categories:

- coagulation disorders
- dysfunctional uterine bleeding (DUB)
- pelvic pathology
- medical disorders.

Coagulation disorders

Although certain haemorrhagic conditions, e.g. thrombocytopenic purpura and von Willebrand's disease, are associated with an increased incidence of menorrhagia, coagulation disorders have a variable effect overall. There is no impairment of systemic coagulation in those with excess menstrual loss, nor are fibrin degradation products elevated in the menstrual fluid of those with heavy menstrual loss (Bonnar et al 1983). In women with thrombocytopenia, menstrual blood loss correlates broadly with platelet count at the time of the menses. Splenectomy has been known to reduce dramatically the menstrual blood loss in these patients.

Dysfunctional uterine bleeding

Disturbances in the pattern of menstruation are a common clinical presentation for abnormalities of the hypophyseal–pituitary–ovarian axis. DUB is defined as heavy and/or irregular menses in the absence of recognizable pelvic pathology, pregnancy or general bleeding disorder. It commonly occurs at the extremes of reproductive life (adolescence and perimenopausally). The abnormalities of ovarian activity may be classified as follows.

1. Anovulatory:
   - inadequate signal, e.g. in polycystic ovarian disease or premenopausally
   - impaired positive feedback, e.g. in adolescence
2. Ovulatory

Anovulatory DUB Occasionally anovulatory cycles occur in all women. Chronic anovulation, however, is associated with an irregular and unpredictable pattern of bleeding ranging from short cycles with scanty bleeding to prolonged periods of irregular heavy loss. Normal bleeding occurs in response to withdrawal of both progesterone and oestradiol. If ovulation does not occur then the absence of progesterone results in an absence of secretory changes in the endometrium, accompanied by abnormalities in the production of steroid receptors, prostaglandins and other locally active endometrial products. Unopposed oestrogen gives rise to persistent proliferative or hyperplastic endometrium and oestrogen withdrawal bleeding is characteristically painless and irregular. It tends to occur at the extremes of reproductive life but is rare at other times. Only 20% of those cycles with excessive menstrual blood loss are anovulatory (Haynes et al 1979); this same study fails to demonstrate any abnormalities in gonadotrophin or circulating steroid concentrations. In anovulatory cycles, the endometrium is unable to produce factors whose synthesis is controlled by progesterone, e.g. prostaglandin $F_{2\alpha}$ (Smith et al 1982). This may account for the painless nature of the bleeds. Ovulation occurs in response to the midcycle surge of luteinizing hormone. If this fails to occur due to insufficient estradiol secretion or impaired positive feedback, ovulation will not occur.

Failure of follicular development Follicular development which is insufficient to produce an oestrogen signal strong enough to induce a luteinizing hormone surge is one of the common reasons for the irregularities in menstrual cycle pattern in premenopausal women. This occurs perimenopausally and in the polycystic ovarian syndrome. (The aetiology and treatment of the latter are dealt with in Ch. 19.)

Anovulatory bleeding may be associated with cystic glandular hyperplasia of the endometrium (see Fig. 32.2e). This occurs in some older women and also in peripubertal girls where unopposed oestrogen secretion occurs. The first few cycles after the menarche are commonly anovulatory. However, if anovulation persists, a long period of amenorrhoea is accompanied by endometrial hyperplasia. This is probably a result of multiple follicular development (multicystic ovaries) with failure of antral follicle formation. Endometrial hyperplasia may cause excessive bleeding, anaemia, infertility and even cancer of the endometrium.

Ovulatory DUB: idiopathic bleeding As described above, an important factor in the control of menstrual blood loss is vasoconstriction. It appears that there are a number of endometrial products, which alter the degree of vasoconstriction and thus may affect the volume of menstrual blood lost. In the mid-1970s, a relationship between prostaglandin production and menorrhagia was suggested by work showing that total endometrial prostaglandin content was proportional to menstrual loss. It appears that a shift in endometrial conversion of endoperoxide from the vasoconstrictor prostaglandins ($PGF_{2\alpha}$) to the vasodilator prostaglandins (PGE_2 or prostacyclin) occurs. However, it is likely that it is not only prostaglandins that are of importance and work is now being performed on the role of endothelin in heavy menstrual loss. Endothelins are very potent vasoconstrictors that are produced within the endometrial vessels; their receptors are also present although it is not yet clear whether either of these two factors differs in those women with heavy menstrual loss. Although studies to date are limited, Marsh's group showed reduced immunostaining for endothelin in the endometrium of women with menorrhagia, implicating this peptide in the pathophysiology of increased menstrual blood loss (Marsh 1996). This is a rapidly changing area of knowledge and it is likely that other elements will come to light, which will be significant.

It is still uncertain why there is a difference in production of local factors in those with heavy menstrual loss compared with those with normal loss. Interest has centred on the role of steroid hormones, but it has been impossible to demonstrate either a difference in the circulating levels of estradiol and progesterone or in the receptor concentration within the endometrium (Critchley et al 1994). It is possible that there is a genetic difference altering the production of local hormones and growth factors or that there is a multifactorial aetiology. Reference has been made above, in discussion of the control of menstrual blood loss, to areas of research which may throw new light on the mechanism of menorrhagia.

Menorrhagia in the presence of pathology

Menorrhagia is thought to be associated with uterine fibroids, adenomyosis, pelvic infection, endometrial polyps and the presence of a foreign body such as an intrauterine contraceptive device (IUCD). Also, the rare conditions of myometrial hypertrophy and vascular abnormality may be associated with severe, even life-threatening menorrhagia. However, objective evidence of menorrhagia in most of these situations is remarkably limited. In women with menstrual blood loss greater than 200 ml, over half will have fibroids, although only 40% of those with adenomyosis actually have menstrual blood loss in excess of 80 ml per menses. Whether chronic pelvic inflammatory disease or endometrial polyps are associated with above average loss is unclear.

Although vasoactive peptides may contribute to menorrhagia associated with pathology, the non-steroidal anti-inflammatory agents are less effective in menorrhagia associated with IUCD presence than in DUB, making it likely that other factors are also important.

Medical problems

Menorrhagia is associated with various endocrine disorders such as hypothyroidism (thyrotoxicosis is more commonly associated with cycle disturbance) and Cushing's disease, although the mechanism is unknown. Thyroid disease is often considered to be a common cause for menorrhagia. However, it is rare for thyroid disease to present in this way without other associated symptoms, e.g. weight gain, hair loss, constipation, etc.

DYSMENORRHOEA

Dysmenorrhoea comes from Greek and means 'difficult monthly flow' but is now taken to mean painful menstruation. It is a symptom complex, with cramping lower abdominal pain radiating to the back and legs, often accompanied by gastrointestinal and neurological symptoms as well as general malaise. As with menorrhagia, it may be associated with pathology or may be idiopathic in origin.

Idiopathic (primary) dysmenorrhoea

There are many different theories as to why women suffer from dysmenorrhoea. The following factors may be of importance.

Uterine hyperactivity

The significance of uterine hyperactivity in women with dysmenorrhoea was first proposed in 1932. Since then there has been much research which suggests that those with dysmenorrhoea have increased uterine activity during menstruation (Filler & Hall 1970, Novak & Reynolds 1932). Patients often describe the pain as 'labour-like' and an increase in uterine contractility can be demonstrated by measuring the intrauterine pressure in those with dysmenorrhoea compared with women without (Lumsden & Baird 1985). The increased uterine contractility also appears to be related to uterine blood flow and the presence of pain (Åkerlund & Anderssen 1976).

During the reproductive years the myometrium is structurally and functionally polarized (see The Myometrium, above). Using transvaginal ultrasound scanning or magnetic resonance imaging it is possible to delineate between the myometrial zones (Brosens et al 1998, Lesny 1999).

Patients with endometriosis and adenomyosis have been found to have structural and functional abnormalities of the JZ (Brosens et al 2000). Leyendecker's group demonstrated marked hyperperistalsis of the JZ during the early and mid-follicular phase in women with endometriosis associated with a marked increase in the transport of inert particles from the vaginal depot to the peritoneal cavity (Leyendecker et al 1996).

Dysmenorrhoeic patients have been found to exhibit profound structural changes in the JZ, including irregular thickening, smooth muscle hyperplasia characterized by closely packed smooth muscle fibres which are poorly oriented and less vascular than the smooth muscle of normal inner myometrium (Brosens et al 1998, Togashi et al 1989). Consequently the term 'junctional zone hyperplasia' was coined for this disorder (Brosens et al 1998).

Dysperistalsis and hyperactivity of the uterine JZ are important mechanisms of primary dysmenorrhoea and possibly menstrual pain associated with adenomyosis and endometriosis (Brosens et al 2000).

Endothelins

Endothelins are potent uterotonins in the non-pregnant uterus. They are thought to be involved in the induction of myometrial smooth muscle contraction in a juxtacrine fashion. The greatest density of endothelin-binding sites is found on glandular epithelium in the endo-myometrial junction and recent evidence suggests that endothelins in the endometrium can induce $PGF_{2\alpha}$ and further endothelin release in a paracrine and autocrine fashion (Bacon et al 1995). Local ischaemia could further increase the expression of endothelins and prostaglandins which could further aggravate uterine dysperistalsis.

Prostaglandins

It has been shown that dysmenorrhoeic women have increased endometrial synthesis of $PGF_{2\alpha}$ and enhanced concentrations of $PGF_{2\alpha}$ and PGE_2 in menstrual blood compared with asymptomatic women (Lumsden et al 1983, Lundstrom & Green 1978). Prostaglandin $F_{2\alpha}$ is a potent oxytocic and vasoconstrictor. When administered into the uterus, it will give rise to dysmenorrhoea-like pain and occasionally menstrual bleeding. Menstrual fluid prostaglandin $F_{2\alpha}$ concentrations also correlate with uterine work during the menses in those with dysmenorrhoea (Lumsden et al 1983). These properties of prostaglandin $F_{2\alpha}$ could thus lead to 'angina' of the myometrium. The role of prostaglandin E_2 is less clear, although its administration may increase the sensitivity of nerve endings.

The reason for the abnormal prostaglandin levels is unknown. Primary dysmenorrhoea occurs almost exclusively in ovulatory cycles and steroid hormones affect both uterine prostaglandin concentration and myometrial contractility. However, no consistent abnormality of the hormone levels has been demonstrated in those with dysmenorrhoea. Treatment with prostaglandin synthetase inhibitors reduces uterine $PGF_{2\alpha}$ production, uterine activity and dysmenorrhoea.

Vasopressin

There are other stimulants of the non-pregnant uterus, such as vasopressin, a vasoconstrictor that also stimulates uterine contractility. On the first day of menstruation, circulating vasopressin levels are higher in those with dysmenorrhea than those without (Åkerlund et al 1979). Infusion of hypertonic saline results in increased uterine contractility and pain in women with dysmenorrhoea as a result of stimulation of endogenous vasopressin release, as well as a reduction in concentrations of $PGF_{2\alpha}$ metabolites. Preliminary studies also indicate that vasopressin analogues may have a place in treating dysmenorrhoea.

Other factors

Platelet-activating factor (PAF) is present in greater concentration in women with dysmenorrhoea (Migram et al 1991). This is somewhat surprising as PAF inhibits $PGF_{2\alpha}$ production, although it does stimulate overall phospholipid metabolism and other factors, which have not been measured, may be elevated.

Another factor of potential importance is the destruction of nerve endings in the myometrium and cervix by pregnancy. This may explain the observation that primary dysmenorrhoea is relieved by the birth of a baby. The literature suggests that psychological and physical causes for dysmenorrhoea are mutually exclusive. The evidence for physical factors is strong, treatment is very effective and it is unlikely that psychological problems would be removed simply by tablet taking. However, a recurring, debilitating pain may well cause depression and anxiety in women of any age.

Secondary dysmenorrhoea

As with menorrhagia, this may be associated with uterine and pelvic pathology such as fibroids, the presence of an IUCD,

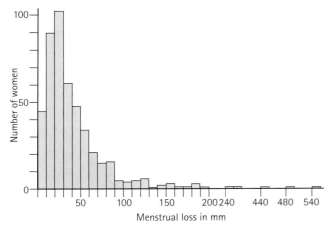

Fig. 32.4 The distribution of menstrual blood loss for a population of women who did not consider they had any menstrual abnormality. From Hallberg & Nilsson (1964) with permission.

pelvic inflammatory disease, adenomyosis, endometriosis or cervical stenosis. The cause of the pain is not always clear. Abnormal uterine contractility has been observed in those with fibroids and prostaglandins may be involved when dysmenorrhoea is associated with an IUCD, pelvic inflammatory disease, adenomyosis and possibly endometriosis. However, the use of prostaglandin synthetase inhibitors is less effective in the presence of pathology, making it likely that there are also other factors.

THE EPIDEMIOLOGY OF MENSTRUAL ABNORMALITY

The distribution of blood loss for a normal population shows a positively skewed distribution, as mentioned above (Fig. 32.4) (Cole et al 1971). Age per se does not influence the menstrual blood loss until the sixth decade. This may be due to an increased incidence of pathology (e.g. fibroids or perimenopausal endocrine abnormalities). A hereditary influence has been demonstrated following twin studies and parity is also thought to be an important factor: parous women have a greater menstrual blood loss than nulliparous women. Uterine pathology, particularly fibroids, is a well-documented cause for menorrhagia, although endometrial pathology is rather uncommon in menorrhagic women; it is found as a reasonable cause for menorrhagia in only about 6%.

The variation between menses for an individual (intramenses) is between 20% and 40%. About 90% of blood is lost during the first 3 days of the menses in both normal and menorrhagic women. These studies are based on objective measurement of menstrual blood loss, which is rarely done except for research purposes (Hallberg & Nilsson 1964). New methods of measuring menstrual symptoms are being designed in order to allow for better objective assessment with consideration given to the variety of symptoms that contribute to the overall complaint such as irregularity, menorrhagia, pain and premenstrual syndrome.

The results of epidemiological studies performed over the last 50 years give a variable incidence for dysmenorrhoea. This is due to the fact that pain is a subjective symptom and cannot be assessed accurately by an outsider. Different women will react to the same pain in different ways and how each woman perceives the pain will vary with altered circumstances. Also, the definition and diagnosis allow different interpretations by different workers. Severe dysmenorrhoea, which causes disruption of daily routine with time off work or study, occurs in 3–10% of 19-year-olds (Andersch & Milsom 1982), while mild discomfort occurs in a majority of women. The relative risk of dysmenorrhoea in those who have smoked for 10–20 years is up to six times the risk in non-smokers (Parazzini et al 1994). Its incidence is inversely correlated with age and parous women are less likely to report the condition. There is no correlation between the incidence of emotional stress factors and dysmenorrhoea.

PRESENTATION

Clinical history

Menstrual problems are a common cause for presentation to both the general practitioner and the gynaecologist. In 1998 the Royal College of Obstetricians and Gynaecologists released evidence-based guidelines for clinical evaluation and management of menorrhagia. A history of heavy, regular, cyclical menstrual blood loss over several consecutive cycles without additional irregular bleeding suggests dysfunctional uterine bleeding. A detailed history may suggest other underlying pathology; for example, heavy painful periods and dyspareunia might suggest endometriosis whilst heavy bleeding with a vaginal discharge and abdominal pain points to pelvic inflammatory disease.

Risk factors for endometrial carcinoma should be carefully noted in the history (Box 32.1, Fig. 32.5).

Examination

General examination may reveal signs of hypothyroidism, anaemia or blood clotting disorders. Abdominal and pelvic examination is mandatory in all women complaining of menorrhagia. Clues to diagnosis are often revealed on pelvic examination. A tender fixed uterus may suggest endometriosis or pelvic inflammatory disease whilst fibroids can often be palpated. Anaemia may also be present since menorrhagia is the commonest cause of iron deficiency anaemia in the Western world. Menorrhagia may arise as a consequence of disorders of the haemopoietic system, as described above.

INVESTIGATION

Haemoglobin concentration should be determined in all women with menorrhagia and iron supplementation given if required. Although thyroid disease is a cause of menstrual derangement in some women, screening TSH and T4 measurements are not justified unless there are other features in the history suggestive of thyroid disease (Fraser et al 1986). Similarly, routine screening for bleeding diatheses is not appropriate.

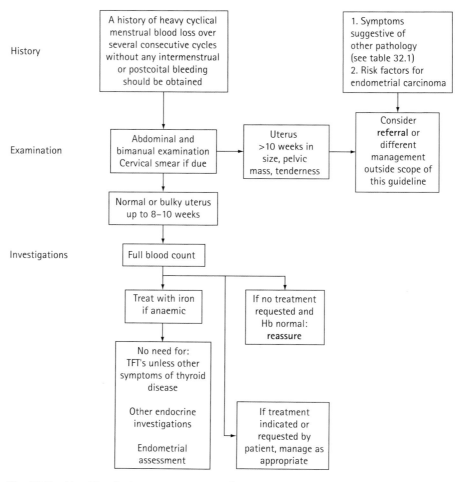

Fig. 32.5 Algorithm for heavy menstrual loss (from RCOG 1998 The initial management of menorrhagia. RCOG Press, London).

Box 32.1 Clinical history

Symptoms suggestive of other pathology
- Irregular bleeding
- Sudden change in blood loss
- Intermenstrual bleeding
- Postcoital bleeding
- Dyspareunia
- Pelvic pain
- Premenstrual pain

Risk factors for endometrial cancer
- Tamoxifen
- Unopposed oestrogen treatments
- Polycystic ovary syndrome
- Obesity

Assessment of the uterine cavity

The main indication for assessment of the uterine cavity is to exclude sinister pathology, most often seen in women over 45 years of age with anovulatory cycles. A history of irregular bleeding or the presence of risk factors for endometrial cancer will determine the need for endometrial assessment.

A wide array of methods are available for endometrial assessment including:

- dilatation and curettage
- hysteroscopy and endometrial sampling
- endometrial sampling
- ultrasonography – for evaluation of uterine architecture and endometrial thickness.

Dilatation and curettage

Dilatation and curettage (D&C) is a very commonly performed procedure. However, it is rarely indicated in women less than 40 years with a history of regular, heavy menses, as significant pathology is unlikely to be present (Grimes 1982, Vessey et al 1979). The work of Vessey et al showed that 3000–4000 D&Cs need to be performed to detect one endometrial carcinoma in women less than 35 years. Grimes (1982) compared D&C with Vabra aspiration and concluded that D&C, although safe, is associated with a higher risk of complications, including perforation and infection. Additionally the sensitivity and specificity of D&C are unknown and endometrial lesions may be undetected in up to 10 cases per 100 whilst only 50% of the uterine cavity is actually sampled (Grimes 1982, Stock &

Kanbour 1975). As many as 5% of cases of endometrial carcinoma may be missed by D&C alone (Schild & Kutta 1992).

Hysteroscopy

With the realization that hysteroscopy facilitates intrauterine surgical procedures such as endometrial ablation, it has now been accepted into UK gynaecological practice for diagnostic purposes. Given that D&C rarely samples the entire uterine cavity, it is not surprising that hysteroscopy and directed biopsy appear to be superior in identifying *benign* endometrial pathology (Gimpleson & Rappold 1988, Loffer 1989). More pertinently, in a significant minority of women with endometrial carcinoma, the diagnosis is missed when conventional curettage is used (Stovall et al 1989) and although large randomized studies are yet to be performed, it appears that hysteroscopy and directed biopsy is more sensitive in the diagnosis of this condition. Several authorities have suggested, therefore, that hysteroscopy and directed biopsy should replace D&C for the investigation of endometrial pathology (Lewis 1990, 1994).

The development of a narrow diameter (4 mm) scope allowed this investigation to be performed in the outpatient setting in a carefully selected patient group following counselling (Taylor & Hamou 1983). Patient selection is important to maximize success of the procedure; for example, women with a previous cervical cone biopsy or Manchester repair may have cervical stenosis, making passage of the hysteroscope through the internal os difficult.

Hysteroscopy should always be combined with an endometrial biopsy. It should be avoided during menstruation as blood in the cavity obscures the view. The cavity is distended with either gas or fluid. In addition, hysteroscopy enables detection of polyps, submucous fibroids and uterine synechiae in women who have previously had multiple previous 'negative' curettages.

These studies provide increasing evidence that hysteroscopy and endometrial sampling in combination is a superior diagnostic tool and is likely to replace D&C as the investigation of choice in menstrual disorders.

Endometrial sampling

In 1882, Moriche obtained the first endometrial sample using a catheter and endometrial biopsy has been performed in an outpatient setting since 1935. The 1970s saw the introduction of the Vabra curette followed by the Pipelle sampler in the 1980s. The Pipelle is simpler to use and more comfortable for the patient but only samples 4% of the endometrium compared with the Vabra aspirator which samples approximately 40%. The main disadvantage of blind sampling of the uterine cavity is that pathology such as polyps or submucous fibroids may be missed.

The risk of endometrial carcinoma in women with perimenopausal menorrhagia is approximately 1%; hence all women aged 40 and beyond need endometrial assessment. Although women less than 40 years have a lower risk of developing endometrial carcinoma, further investigation is needed if heavy, regular bleeding has not improved with medical management and/or intermenstrual bleeding is present (RCOG 1994).

Ultrasonography

Ultrasonography allows evaluation of the uterine architecture and endometrial thickness and is an important adjunct to endometrial sampling. Transvaginal ultrasound (TVU) scanning is a useful tool allowing better resolution than abdominal scanning because of the close proximity of the ultrasound probe with the pelvic organs. It has a specificity of 96% and a sensitivity of 89%. Endometrial thickness of 5 mm or less over the whole cavity is said to exclude endometrial carcinoma (Goldstein et al 1990), but this is really only of value after the menopause. Ultrasound assessment should be combined with endometrial biopsy when endometrial thickness exceeds 5 mm.

Abnormalities on pelvic examination should be investigated by ultrasound, with laparoscopy if required. The investigation of women presenting with heavy menstrual loss is summarized in Figure 32.5.

QUANTIFICATION OF MENSTRUAL BLOOD LOSS

The objective assessment of menstrual blood loss is rarely made except for research purposes. However, menstrual blood loss can be assessed either in a semi-quantitative manner, relying on the patient's assessment of the bleeding, or by the use of pictorial aids (Higham et al 1990). Attention is being given to the development of aids, including the use of hand-held computers, to assess the menstrual complaint as a whole, which consists of more than heavy bleeding. Many women also complain of pain and premenstrual syndrome. Again, these are not yet available for general use.

Anovulatory menorrhagia

In the younger patient (<40 years of age) assessment of the hypothalamic–pituitary–ovarian axis is indicated. The diagnosis of polycystic ovarian disease has increased over recent years with the finding of altered luteinizing hormone/follicle-stimulating hormone ratios in the follicular phase of the cycle and the identification of micro- and macro-cystic disease by vaginal ultrasound.

Dysmenorrhoea

Those women presenting with dysmenorrhoea who have no other complaints or abnormalities on examination can be safely treated without further investigation. Laparoscopy is indicated for those with a provisional diagnosis of endometriosis or pelvic inflammatory disease. D&C and examination under anaesthetic are required only if uterine abnormality is suspected. The standard treatment for dysmenorrhoea (prostaglandin synthetase inhibitors and the oral contraceptive pill) is so effective that laparoscopy in treatment failures will often demonstrate previously unsuspected abnormalities such as mild endometriosis, even in teenage girls.

TREATMENT

Women require rapid, safe and effective treatment for their menstrual problems. First-line treatment should always be medical in those with no obvious pathology.

Medical treatment

Current medical therapy falls into two broad groups: non-hormonal (prostaglandin synthetase inhibitors, antifibrinolytics and ethamsylate) and hormonal (progestogens, oral contraceptives, hormone replacement therapy, danazol, gestrinone, GnRH analogues). Non-hormonal treatment may be taken during menstruation, which avoids teratogenicity and is therefore suitable for women who wish to conceive. Some women, once reassured that there is no major pathology, will require no further treatment.

Non-hormonal treatment

Antifibrinolytics   As discussed previously, the endometrium possesses an active fibrinolytic system, which is more active in the endometrium of women with menorrhagia than in those without. Antifibrinolytic agents such as tranexamic acid reduce menstrual loss by about 50%. This is greater than following administration of prostaglandin synthetase inhibitors (Milsom et al 1991, Ylikorkala & Viinikka 1983).

The incidence of adverse effects is dose dependent. A third of women experience gastrointestinal side-effects following treatment with tranexamic acid 3–6 g daily. As 90% of menstrual blood is lost in the first 3 days of full flow, dose-related side-effects can be reduced by limiting the number of days on which the drug is taken to the first 3 or 4 days of the period. Serious side-effects are uncommon. No increase in the incidence of thromboembolic disease has been seen in women of reproductive age in Scandinavia, where tranexamic acid has been used since the early 1970s as a first-line treatment for menorrhagia (Rybo 1991). Antifibrinolytic agents therefore represent a relatively effective first-line treatment to reduce the degree of menstrual bleeding.

Prostaglandin synthetase inhibitors   Non-steroidal anti-inflammatory drugs (NSAIDs) remain a popular choice for the treatment of menorrhagia (Coulter et al 1995). Their principal mechanism of action is to decrease endometrial prostaglandin (PG) concentrations. The endometrium is a rich source of PGE_2 and $PGF_{2\alpha}$ and a number of studies have shown that PG concentrations are greater in the endometrium of women with menorrhagia than they are in the endometrium of women with normal blood loss (Cameron & Norman 1995).

There are four groups of prostaglandin synthetase inhibitors of which the fenemates are the most widely used. These are unique amongst the PG synthetase inhibitors in that in addition to inhibition of prostaglandin synthesis, they also bind and block the prostaglandin receptor (Rees et al 1988). Menstrual blood loss is reduced by a median of 25–40% in three-quarters of women with menorrhagia (Fig. 32.6). The beneficial effect of mefenamic acid on menstrual blood loss (and other symptoms including dysmenorrhoea, headache, nausea, diarrhoea and depression) persists for several months. Side-effects, mainly gastrointestinal (dyspepsia, nausea and diarrhoea), are mild and not frequently reported.

In summary, mefenamic acid and related compounds may be an effective first-line medical treatment for some women with menorrhagia. The mean reduction of menstrual blood loss is not as great as it is with antifibrinolytic agents, but the

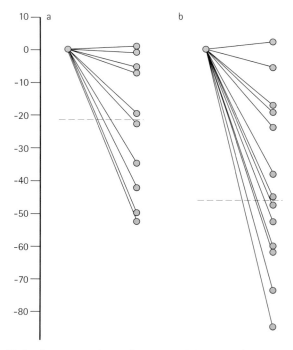

Fig. 32.6   Percentage change in menstrual blood loss (mean of two cycles) of women receiving: **a** norethisterone (5 mg bd, days 19–25), and **b** mefenamic acid (250 mg tds, days 1–5).

Box 32.2   Hormonal treatment for menorrhagia

Progestogens	• Norethisterone
	• Medroxyprogesterone acetate
	• Dydrogesterone
Intrauterine progestogens	• Levonorgestrel intrauterine system
	• Progestasert intrauterine system
Combined oestrogen/	• Oral contraceptives
progestogens	• Hormone replacement therapy
Others	• Danazol
	• GnRH analogues
	• Gestrinone

NSAIDs have a lower side-effect profile in otherwise healthy women and are more effective for treatment of pain.

Ethamsylate   Ethamsylate is believed to reduce endometrial capillary fragility. Trials of efficacy have shown inconsistent results and for this reason it is not widely used to treat menorrhagia (Chamberlain et al 1991).

Hormonal treatment

Hormonal treatments for menorrhagia are summarised in Box 32.2.

Progestogens   Synthetic progestogens are widely used to treat menorrhagia. They have an endometrial suppressive effect resulting in small depleted glands lined with a thin epithelium and decidualized transformation of the stroma.

Cyclical progestogens   It has been shown that low-dose, short-duration therapy of oral progestogens during the luteal phase is ineffective in reducing menstrual loss (Fig. 32.6) (Cameron et al 1990). However, they may be successful if given at a dose of 5 mg three times daily from days 5 to 26 of the cycle. On this regime, menstrual loss can be reduced by up to 30% (Irvine et al 1998). Cyclical progestogens can be used to regulate the onset of bleeding and are useful for those with an irregular, unpredictable cycle.

Continuous progestogens   Various continuous preparations are available including oral tablets, long-acting intramuscular injections and subdermal implants. Irregular bleeding and oligomenorrhoea (in many cases amenorrhoea) are common consequences. Progestogen-only contraceptive pill users may also report a decrease in their menstrual loss.

Intrauterine progestogens   The most recently described medicated device is the levonorgestrel intrauterine system (LNG IUS; Mirena). This delivers 20 µg of levonorgestrel to the endometrium every 24 hours in a sustained-release formulation that can last up to 5 years (Luukkainen et al 1986). Direct administration of the progestogen to the uterus results in minimal systemic absorption (Andersson & Rybo 1990), giving a good side-effect profile (Cheng Chi 1991).

The efficacy of the LNG IUS for the treatment of menorrhagia compares well with transcervical resection of the endometrium (TCRE) at 12 months after treatment (Crosignani et al 1997). It has also been suggested that it might be an acceptable alternative to hysterectomy (Lahteenmaki et al 1998).

The LNG IUS has a local effect on the endometrium causing endometrial glandular atrophy, stromal decidualization and epithelial cell inactivation. This is seen within 1 month of insertion and occurs independently of ovarian activity (Silverberg et al 1986). When removed, the endometrium recovers quickly and biopsies taken at 1–3 months show no signs of progesterone administration regardless of duration of treatment. The LNG IUS has a weak effect on ovarian function with ovulation continuing in about 75% of women.

Oestrogen/progestogen regimes   The combined oral contraceptive pill is widely used to treat menorrhagia. It causes endometrial atrophy and in this way reduces endometrial prostaglandin synthesis and fibrinolysis. Menstrual loss can be reduced by as much as 50% (Fraser & McCarron 1991). Although the use of the low-dose oestrogen pill in the management of menorrhagia has been affected by adverse publicity associated with its use in older women, it is now felt to be quite safe in women up to and over the age of 40 who are not obese, do not smoke and are not hypertensive. It has the added advantage of providing a regular menstrual cycle and also being effective in the treatment of dysmenorrhoea (Ekstrom et al 1989). The limiting factor is that many of the women will have been sterilized and are therefore reluctant to continue with something they see as a contraceptive agent. Hormone replacement therapy can be used in perimenopausal women with excessive menstrual bleeding (Rees & Barlow 1991).

Danazol   Danazol, a derivative of testosterone, causes endometrial atrophy by inhibiting the release of the pituitary gonadotrophins and can reduce menstrual loss by as much as 50% (Chimbira et al 1980, Dockeray et al 1989). The use of danazol is limited by its androgenic side-effects, which include weight gain, acne, depression and other long-term metabolic sequaelae all of which reduce compliance. This drug is probably best restricted to women awaiting surgery.

GnRH analogues   These act by causing pituitary down-regulation and subsequent inhibition of cyclical ovarian activity, resulting in amenorrhoea. Nevertheless, their use is limited to less than 6 months because of problems related to the hypo-oestrogenic state. These include hot flushes, dry vagina and decreased bone mineral density. 'Add-back' oestrogen/progestogen therapy used concurrently can minimize these effects. Additionally, GnRH analogues are costly. These factors preclude them from being a first-line option for treatment but they are useful in a minority of women (Shaw & Fraser 1984).

Surgical treatment

Hysterectomy
Hysterectomy is an effective treatment for menstrual problems. However, it is a major operation and is not without risk in terms of both mortality and morbidity. The incidence of hysterectomy is gradually increasing in the Western world as a whole but it varies considerably from one country to another, reflecting differences in the attitude of both patients and gynaecologists rather than a variation in pathology. Women in Scotland have a 20% chance of losing their uterus before the age of 60 years whereas in California this figure is 50%.

Hysterectomy may be performed by the abdominal or vaginal route. Abdominal hysterectomy involves a laparotomy incision that is transverse or longitudinal. A vaginal hysterectomy involves an incision through the vaginal wall. For many surgeons, vaginal hysterectomy is only performed on women with some degree of uterine descent and where the uterus is not excessively large. Abdominal hysterectomy allows better visualization of the pelvic cavity should there be pathology or where difficulty is anticipated. Non-randomized studies indicate that the complication rate for abdominal hysterectomy is greater than that for vaginal hysterectomy and women having vaginal procedures are able to go home quicker than those having abdominal operations (Clinch 1994, Dicker et al 1982).

Recently it has become possible to convert an abdominal to a vaginal hysterectomy using endoscopic techniques. The laparoscope allows visualization of the pelvic cavity and all or part of the hysterectomy may be performed using specially designed laparoscopic instruments. A laparoscopically assisted vaginal hysterectomy (LAVH) allows tissues accessible through the vagina to be ligated and the uterus to be removed by the vaginal route. This method facilitates the removal of ovaries and also aids the operation when there is no uterine descent. It allows for dissection of adhesions and the treatment of pelvic pathology, such as endometriosis, prior to the hysterectomy. Published complication rates are low but recovery does not appear to be quicker than after hysterectomy by the abdominal route (Lumsden et al 2000) although patients return home from hospital sooner (Boike et al 1993).

Endometrial ablation techniques
Attempts at endometrial destruction in cases of abnormal menstruation, with the aim of producing a therapeutic Asherman's syndrome, have been made by a variety of techniques. Early trials involved the intrauterine application of cytotoxic chemicals, intracavity radium, steam and cryosurgery.

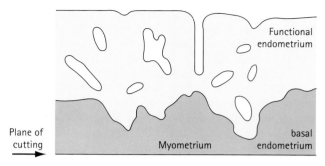

Fig. 32.7 A diagram of the uterine wall.

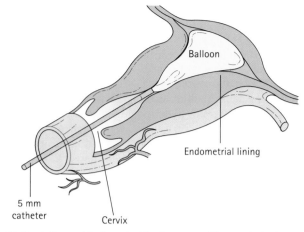

Fig. 32.8 A thermal balloon inside the uterus (Thermachoice®, Gynecare, Edinburgh).

However, these were either ineffective or had unacceptable side-effects. They were also carried out blindly and since the endometrium has remarkable powers of regeneration, any missed areas resulted in failure.

More recently, hysteroscopic techniques have been developed. These allow visualization of the uterine cavity, allowing the endometrium to be ablated under direct vision. Since regeneration of the endometrium occurs from the basal layer it is essential to destroy all the endometrium and as the endometrial–myometrial border is irregular, the superficial layer of myometrium must also be included (Fig. 32.7). There are a number of methods of achieving this, including vaporization of the tissue using laser, removal of the tissue using a cutting loop or coagulation.

Laser ablation Yttrium-aluminium-garnet (Nd:YAG) laser is optimal for intrauterine surgery since it can be delivered along a flexible fibre through a liquid medium and the depth of tissue penetration can be controlled. The beam produces warming, coagulation, evaporation and carbonization. Tissue destruction typically occurs to a depth of 4–5 mm. Heat transmission through the myometrium is minimized by the continuous flow of cold irrigation fluid.

Endometrial resection The technique of performing transcervical resection of the endometrium is essentially similar to that of transurethral prostatectomy in men and is performed through a continuous-flow resectoscope. The endometrium is systematically excised throughout the uterine cavity. It is important to destroy all the endometrium, otherwise regeneration will occur and the operation will fail.

Other methods

Transcervical endometrial resection requires considerable skill if it is to be effective and safe. Women who have a normal uterine cavity can be effectively treated using newer techniques to achieve destruction of the endometrium that require minimal skill. Popular examples of this type of treatment are destruction by thermal balloon and microwave endometrial ablation.

Thermal balloon (Fig. 32.8) This involves the blind insertion of a balloon through the cervix which is then filled with fluid until a pressure of 160–180 mmHg is reached. The fluid is then heated to between 75° and 90° (average 87°). Endometrial destruction occurs over the next 8 minutes. The diameter of the insertion tube is very small and no cervical dilatation is required. This means that the procedure is particularly appropriate for women who are not suitable or who do not wish to have a general anaesthetic. It is uncomfortable but pain relief can be improved by prior administration of a preparation such as diclofenac. Some sedation may be useful in certain instances. The success rate of this procedure appears to be similar to TCRE. One of the main advantages would appear to be that no pretreatment with GnRH agonist is required. Since the procedure is done in the outpatient setting in a number of units and has even been performed in general practice, it is likely to be a cheap and popular modality in the future.

Microwave endometrial ablation Microwave endometrial ablation (MEA) requires the insertion of a probe into the uterus that emits microwaves. The probe is then slowly moved across the fundus and down through the uterine cavity, destroying the endometrium. Provided the probe is in the cavity of the uterus, this is a very safe procedure as the temperature rises as the endometrium is treated and the probe moved to another area. Randomized comparisons of this technique with TCRE suggest that it is equally effective but like TCRE, it requires pretreatment with a GnRH agonist. In addition, since it requires dilatation of the cervix to 9 mm, it is unusual to perform this procedure under a local anaesthetic. However, it is likely that smaller probes will be developed in order to achieve this result.

These procedures make attractive alternatives to endometrial resection although they are less valuable in the presence of uterine fibroids, particularly if the cavity is enlarged.

Success rates

There is little variation in success rates between the different methods. Overall approximately 30% of women will be amenorrhoiec and a further 45–50% will have significantly decreased loss, giving a satisfaction rate of approximately 75% (Cooper et al 1999, Magos et al 1991, Scottish Hysteroscopy Audit Group 1995). Careful counselling is essential in that if a woman is keen to have amenorrhoea then this will not be the treatment of choice for her. Some women also experience relief from symptoms of dysmenorrhoea and premenstrual tension.

Complications

The most significant complications are those of uterine perforation and fluid absorption. Uterine perforation occurs in less than 1% and is not usually associated with major problems unless the electrode is activated within the abdominal cavity, when bowel or blood vessels may be damaged. Fluid absorption is rare since surgeons have become aware of the risk and stop the operation if absorption becomes excessive. Infection may also occur and most surgeons routinely give prophylactic antibiotics.

Comparison of endometrial resection with hysterectomy

Endometrial resection was developed as an alternative to hysterectomy. However, it appears that the number of hysterectomies being performed is continuing to rise, suggesting it is not serving this purpose. There have been a number of randomized comparisons between endometrial ablation and hysterectomy, which show that satisfaction with both procedures is high (Pinion et al 1994). Also, the operation can be performed on a day-case basis and recovery time is short, making it a cheap alternative to hysterectomy. However, it does appear that 20% of patients will require further surgical treatment and there is still uncertainty as to whether the number of failures will increase with time.

Guidelines

The operation is most likely to be successful in women over 40 who have a normal-sized uterus and no intrauterine pathology. Its use in dysmenorrhoea is equivocal since it appears to make women worse in approximately 12% of cases, which may be due to the formation of haematometra. However, approximately 40% will improve so the presence of dysmenorrhoea is not an absolute contraindication. The menstrual cycle length will not be changed by the procedure and in women with very irregular bleeding, hysterectomy may be an appropriate alternative (Lewis 1994).

Dysmenorrhoea

In young women dysmenorrhoea is frequently the only menstrual abnormality. Prostaglandin synthetase inhibitors and the oral contraceptive pill are very effective (Anderson 1981) but in a minority, even in the absence of disease, these measures are insufficient. Calcium channel blockers (e.g. nifedipine) have been used in Scandinavia and are effective, although their use is limited by cardiovascular side-effects.

In the past, presacral neurectomy was performed but this involved major abdominal surgery and was effective in only about 50% of cases. Recently neurectomy has been performed using intra-abdominal lasers. The long-term effect of this treatment has not been reported and it is only available in a few UK centres.

In older women where child bearing is completed, hysterectomy is often the solution since dysmenorrhoea in this group is frequently associated with other menstrual problems.

CONCLUSIONS

Menstrual dysfunction remains one of the commonest reasons for women to seek medical advice, yet the process of menstruation is poorly understood. Strategies to improve the investigation and management of this problem are likely to arise from two directions. First, a thorough investigation of the medico-sociological factors is required. Second, the role of vasoactive substances in the endometrium needs to be further investigated, as well as determination of the factors that control endometrial proliferation. At present, the diagnosis of menorrhagia is inadequate and medical treatment is disappointing. Gynaecologists need to address these problems if significant improvements in management are to be achieved.

KEY POINTS

1. Menorrhagia is the commonest cause of iron deficiency anaemia in Western women.
2. The menstrual cycle consists of a proliferative and a secretory phase.
3. Menstruation is initiated by a withdrawal of progesterone and oestrogen support to the endometrium.
4. Menstrual loss is dependent upon the degree of platelet plug formation, vasoconstriction and endometrial repair. Abnormality in these mechanisms can result in menstrual dysfunction. Paracrine factors are also thought to play a role in control of menstruation.
5. The mean menstrual blood loss is 37–43 ml per menses. Loss in excess of 80 ml per menses is considered to be menorrhagia.
6. Abnormal menstrual loss may arise from pelvic pathology, clotting disorders, medical disorders or dysfunctional uterine bleeding.
7. Dysfunctional uterine bleeding is defined as heavy or irregular bleeding in the absence of pelvic pathology, pregnancy or clotting disorder.
8. Anovulatory cycles may be associated with cystic glandular hyperplasia. This can occur in both older women and peripubertal girls and may result in excessive menstrual loss.
9. Primary dysmenorrhoea occurs almost exclusively in ovulatory cycles and prostaglandin secretion is strongly implicated in its aetiology.
10. Subjective and objective assessments of menstrual loss are poorly correlated. Medical treatment of menorrhagia is less effective if the blood loss is within normal limits unless there are other associated symptoms which are relieved.
11. Hysteroscopy may be more sensitive than endometrial curettage in the diagnosis of endometrial abnormality.
12. Hysterectomy is a very effective remedy for menstrual dysfunction but is associated with postoperative morbidity and mortality. It is the only treatment that is guaranteed to lead to amenorrhoea.
13. Laparoscopically assisted vaginal hysterectomy allows conversion of an abdominal to a vaginal hysterectomy. It is associated with a shorter hospital stay but recovery time is similar to that for abdominal hysterectomy.
14. Endometrial ablation is a useful alternative to medical treatment or hysterectomy in cases of dysfunctional uterine bleeding and can be performed under local anaesthesia.
15. Medical treatment of menorrhagia may result in good symptomatic relief and is safe but does not result in long-term cure.

REFERENCES

Adalantado JM, Rees MCP, Bernal AL, Turnbull AC 1988 Increased intrauterine prostaglandin E receptors in menorrhagic women. British Journal of Obstetrics and Gynaecology 95:162

Akerlund M, Anderssen KE 1976 Vasopressin response and turbutaline inhibition of the uterus. Obstetrics and Gynecology 48:528–536

Åkerlund M, Stromberg P, Forsling ML 1979 Primary dysmenorrhoea and vasopressin. British Journal of Obstetrics and Gynaecology 86:484–487

Alecozay AA, Harper MJK, Schenken RS, Hanahan DJ 1991 Paracrine interactions between platelet-activating factor and prostaglandins in hormonally-treated human luteal phase endometrium in vitro. Journal of Reproduction and Fertility 91:301–312

Andersch B, Milsom I 1982 An epidemiologic study of young women with dysmenorrhoea. American Journal of Obstetrics and Gynecology 144:655–660

Anderson A 1981 The role of prostaglandin synthetase inhibitors in gynaecology. Practitioner 225:1460–1470

Andersson K, Rybo G 1990 Levonorgestrel-releasing intrauterine device in the treatment of menorrhagia. British Journal of Obstetrics and Gynaecology 97:690–694

Bacon CR, Morrison JJ, O'Reilly G, Cameron IT, Davenport AP 1995 ETA and ETB endothelin receptors in human myometrium characterised by the subtype selective ligands BQ123, BQ3020, FR139317 and PD15142. Journal of Endocrinology 144:127–134

Basilico C, Moscatelli D 1992 The FGF family of growth factors and oncogenes. Advances in Cancer Research 59:115–165

Beller FK 1971 Observations on the clotting of menstrual blood and clot formation. American Journal of Obstetrics and Gynecology 11:535–546

Bjork J, Smedegard G 1983 Acute microvascular effects of PAF-acether, as studied by intravital microscopy. European Journal of Pharmacology 96:87

Boike GM, Elfstrand EP, Del Priore G et al 1993 Laparoscopically assisted vaginal hysterectomy in a university hospital: report of 82 cases and comparison with abdominal and vaginal hysterectomy. American Journal of Obstetrics and Gynecology 168:1690–1701

Bonnar J, Sheppard BL, Dockeray CJ 1983 The haemostatic system and dysfunctional uterine bleeding. Research and Clinical Forums 5:27–36

Brosens JJ, Barker FG, deSouza NM 1998 Myometrial zonal differentiation and uterine junctional zone hyperplasia in the non-pregnant uterus. Human Reproduction Update 4:496–502

Brosens JJ, Mak I, Brosens I 2000 Mechanisms of dysmenorrhoea. In: O'Brien S, Cameron IT, MacLean A (eds) Disorders of the menstrual cycle. RCOG Press, London, pp 113–132

Bruner KL, Rodgers WH, Old LI et al 1995 Transforming growth factor beta mediates progesterone suppression of an epithelial metalloproteinase by adjacent stroma in the human endometrium. Proceedings of the National Academy of Science USA 92:7362–7366

Cameron IT, Davenport AP 1992 Endothelins in reproduction. Reproductive Medicine Review 1:99–113

Cameron IT, Norman JE 1995 Endometrial biochemistry in menorrhagia. In: Studd J, Asch R (eds) Progress in reproductive medicine, volume II Parthenon Publishing Group, London, pp 267–279

Cameron IT, Haining R, Lumsden MA, Reid-Thomas V, Smith SK 1990 The effects of mefenamic acid and norethisterone on measured menstrual blood loss. Obstetrics and Gynecology 76:85–88

Cameron IT, Davenport AP, van Papendorp CL et al 1992 Endothelin-like immunoreactivity in human endometrium. Journal of Reproduction and Fertility 95:623–628

Campbell S, Young A, Stewart CJR et al 1998 Laminin beta 2 distinguishes inner and outer myometrial layers of the human myometrium. 22:12

Casslen B, Andersson A, Nilsson IM, Astedt B 1986 Hormonal regulation of the release of plasminogen activators and of a specific activator inhibitor from endometrial tissue in culture (42360). Proceedings of the Society for Experimental Biology and Medicine 182:419–424

Chalubinski K, Deutinger J, Bernaschek G 1993 Vaginosonography for recording of cycle-related myometrial contractions. Fertility and Sterility 59:225–228

Chamberlain G, Freeman R, Price F, Kennedy A, Green D, Eve L 1991 A comparative study of ethamsylate and mefenamic acid in dysfunctional uterine bleeding. British Journal of Obstetrics and Gynaecology; 98:707–711

Charnock-Jones DS, Sharkey AM, Rajput-Williams J et al 1993 Identification and localization of alternately spliced mRNAs for vascular endothelial growth factor in human uterus and estrogen regulation in endometrial carcinoma cell lines. Biology of Reproduction 48:1120–1128

Cheng Chi I 1991 An evaluation of the levonorgestrel-releasing IUD: its advantages and disadvantages when compared to the copper-releasing IUDs. Contraception 44:573–587

Chimbira TH, Anderson ABM, Turnbull AC 1980 Relation between measured menstrual blood loss and patients' subjective assessment of loss, duration of bleeding, number of sanitary towels used, uterine weight and endometrial surface area. British Journal of Obstetrics and Gynaecology 87:603–609

Christiaens G, Sixma JJ, Haspels AA 1980 Morphology of haemostasis in menstrual endometrium. British Journal of Obstetrics and Gynaecology 87:425–439

Christiaens G, Sixma JJ, Haspels AA 1981 Fibrin and platelets in menstrual discharge before and after the insertion of an intrauterine contraceptive device. American Journal of Obstetrics and Gynecology 140:793–798

Christiaens G, Sixma JJ, Haspels AA 1982 Haemostasis in menstrual endometrium: a review. Obstetrical and Gynecological Survey 37:281–303

Clinch J 1994 Length of hospital stay after vaginal hysterectomy. British Journal of Obstetrics and Gynaecology 101:253–254

Cohen BJB, Gibor Y 1980 Anaemia and menstrual blood loss. Obstetrical and Gynecological Survey 35:597–618

Cole SK, Billewicz WZ, Thomson AM 1971 Sources of variation in menstrual blood loss. Journal of Obstetrics and Gynaecology of the British Commonwealth 78:933–939

Cooper KG, Parkin DE, Garrett AM, Grant AM 1999 Two year follow-up of women randomised to medical management or transcervical resection of the endometrium for heavy menstrual loss; clinical and quality of life outcomes. British Journal of Obstetrics and Gynaecology 106:258–265

Coulter A, Kelland J, Peto V, Rees M 1995 Treating menorrhagia in primary care: an overview of drug trials and a survey of prescribing practice. International Journal of Health Technology Assessment in Health Care 11:456–471

Critchley H, Abberton KM, Taylor NH, Healy DL, Rogers AW 1994 Endometrial sex steroid receptor expression in women with menorrhagia. British Journal of Obstetrics and Gynaecology 101:428–434

Crosignani PG, Vercellini P, Mosconi P, Oldani S, Cortesi, de Giorgi O 1997 Levonorgestrel-releasing intrauterine device versus hysteroscopic endometrial resection in the treatment of dysfunctional uterine bleeding. Obstetrics and Gynecology 90:257–263

Daly L, Sheppard BL, Carroll E, Hennelly B, Bonnar J 1990 Coagulation and fibrinolysis in menstrual and peripheral blood in dysfunctional uterine bleeding. Irish Journal of Medical Science 159:24–25

de Merre LJ, Moss JD, Pattison OS 1967 The haematological study of menstrual discharge. Obstetrics and Gynecology 30:830–833

de Vries K, Lyons EA, Ballard G, Levi CS, Lindsay DJ 1990 Contractions of the inner third of the myometrium. American Journal of Obstetrics and Gynecology 162:679–682

Demas BE, Hricak H, Jaffe RB 1985 Uterine MR imaging: effects of hormonal stimulation. Radiology 159:123–126

Dicker RC, Greenspan JR, Strauss LT et al 1982 Complications of abdominal and vaginal hysterectomy among women of reproductive age in the United States. American Journal of Obstetrics and Gynecology 144:841–848

Dockeray CJ, Sheppard BL, Bonnar J 1989 Comparison between mefenamic acid and danazol in the treatment of established menorrhagia. British Journal of Obstetrics and Gynaecology 96:840–844

Ekstrom P, Juchnicka E, Laudanski T, Åkerlund M 1989 Effect of an oral contraceptive in primary dysmenorrhoea – changes in uterine activity and reactivity to agonists. Contraception 40:39–47

Ferriani RA, Charnock-Jones DS, Prentice A, Thomas EJ, Smith SK 1993 Immunohistochemical localization of acidic and basic fibroblast growth factors in normal human endometrium and endometriosis and the detection of their mRNA by polymerase chain reaction. Human Reproduction 8:11–16

Filler WW, Hall WC 1970 Dysmenorrhoea and its therapy: a uterine contractility study. American Journal of Obstetrics and Gynecology 106:104–109

Fraser IS, McCarron G 1991 Randomised trial of two hormonal and two prostaglandin-inhibiting agents in women with a complaint of menorrhagia. Australian and New Zealand Journal of Obstetrics and Gynaecology; 31:66–70

Fraser IS, McCarron G, Markham R, Resta T, Watts A 1986 Measured menstrual blood loss in women with menorrhagia associated with pelvic disease or coagulation disorder. Obstetrics and Gynecology 68:630–633

Gimpleson RJ, Rappold HO 1988 A comparative study between panoramic hysteroscopy with directed biopsies and dilatation and curettage. American Journal of Obstetrics and Gynecology 158:489–492

Goldstein SR, Nachtigall M, Snyder JK, Nachtingall L 1990 Endometrial assessment by vaginal ultrasonography before endometrial sampling in patients with post menopausal bleeding. American Journal of Obstetrics and Gynecology 163:119–123

Gospodarowicz D, Abraham JA, Schilling J 1989 Isolation and characterization of a vascular endothelial cell mitogen produced by pituitary-derived follicular stellate cells. Proceedings of the National Academy of Sciences USA 86:7311–7315

Grimes DA 1982 Diagnostic dilatation and curettage: a reappraisal. American Journal of Obstetrics and Gynecology 142:1–6

Hahn L 1980 Composition of menstrual blood. In: Diczfalusy E, Fraser IS, Webb FTG (eds) Endometrial bleeding and steroidal contraception. Pitman Press, Bath, pp 107–137

Haining REB, Cameron IT, van Papendorp CL et al 1991 Epidermal growth factor in human endometrium: proliferative effects in culture and immunocytochemical localisation in normal and endometriotic tissues. Human Reproduction 6:1200

Hallberg L, Nilsson L 1964 Consistency of individual menstrual blood loss. Acta Obstetrica et Gynecologica Scandinavica 43:352–359

Haynes P, Hodgson H, Anderson A, Turnbull A 1977 Measurement of menstrual blood loss in patients complaining of menorrhagia. British Journal of Obstetrics and Gynaecology 84:763–768

Haynes P, Anderson ABM, Turnbull AC 1979 Patterns of menstrual blood loss in menorrhagia. Research and Clinical Forums 1:73–78

Higham JM, O'Brien PMS, Shaw RW 1990 Assessment of menstrual blood loss using a pictorial chart. British Journal of Obstetrics and Gynaecology 97:734–739

Hynes RO 1987 Integrins: a family of cell surface receptors. Cell 48:549–554

Ignar Trowbridge DM, Teng CT, Ross KA, Parker MG, Korach KS, McLachlan JA 1993 Peptide growth factors elicit estrogen receptor-dependent transcriptional activation of an estrogen-responsive element. Molecular Endocrinology 7:992–998

Irvine GA, Campbell-Brown MB, Lumsden MA, Heikkila A, Walker JJ, Cameron IT 1998 Randomised comparative trial of the levonorgestrel intrauterine system and norethisterone for treatment of idiopathic menorrhagia. British Journal of Obstetrics and Gynaecology 105:592–598

Jeziorska M, Nagase H, Salamonsen LA, Woolley DE 1996 Immunolocalisation of the matrix metalloproteinase gelatinase B and stromelysin 1 in human endometrium throughout the menstrual cycle. Journal of Reproductive Fertility 107:43–51

Kelly RW, Lumsden MA, Abel MH, Baird DT 1984 The relationship between menstrual blood loss and prostaglandin production in the human: evidence for increased availability of arachidonic acid in women suffering from menorrhagia. Prostaglandins, Leukotrienes and Medicine 16:69–78

King A, Burrows T, Vernas S, Hiby S, Loke YW 1998 Human uterine lymphocytes. Human Reproduction Update 5:480–485

Kunz G, Beil D, Deininger, Wildt L, Leyendecker G 1996 The dynamics of rapid sperm transport through the female genital tract: evidence from vaginal sonography of uterine peristalsis and hysterosalpingoscintigraphy. Human Reproduction 11:627–632

Lahteenmaki P, Haukkamaa M, Puolakka J et al 1998 Open randomised study of use of levonorgestrel releasing intrauterine system as an alternative to hysterectomy. British Medical Journal 316:1122–1126

Lesny P, Killick SR, Tetlow RL et al 1999 Ultrasound evaluation of the uterine zonal anatomy during in-vitro fertilization and embryo transfer. Human Reproduction 14:1593–1598

Lessey BA, Castelbaum AJ, Buck CA, Lei Y, Yowell CW, Sun J 1992 Integrin adhesion molecules in the human endometrium. Correlation with the normal and abnormal menstrual cycle. Journal of Clinical Investigation 90:188–195

Lewis BV 1990 Hysteroscopy for the investigation of abnormal uterine bleeding. British Journal of Obstetrics and Gynaecology 97:283–284

Lewis BV 1994 Guidelines for endometrial ablation. British Journal of Obstetrics and Gynaecology 101:470

Leyendecker G, Kunz G, Wildt L, Beil D, Deiniger H 1996 Uterine hyperperistalsis and dysperistalsis as dysfunctions of the mechanism of rapid sperm transport in patients with endometriosis and infertility. Human Reproduction 11:1542–1551

Lockwood CJ, Krikun G, Hausknecht VA, Papp C, Schatz F 1998 Matrix metalloproteinase and matrix metalloproteinase inhibitor expression in endometrial stromal cells during progestin-initiated decidualisation and menstruation. Endocrinology 139:4607–4613

Loffer FD 1989 Hysteroscopy with selective endometrial sampling compared with D&C for abnormal uterine bleeding: the value of a negative hysteroscopic view. Obstetrics and Gynecology 73:16–20

Lumsden MA, Baird DT 1985 Intrauterine pressure in dysmenorrhoea. Acta Obstetrica et Gynecologica Scandinavica 64:183–186

Lumsden MA, Kelly RW, Baird DT 1983 Is prostaglandin F_2 involved in the increased myometrial contractility of primary dysmenorrhoea? Prostaglandins 25:683–692

Lumsden MA, Twaddle S, Hawthorn R et al 2000 A randomised comparison and economic evaluation of laparoscopic-assisted hysterectomy and abdominal hysterectomy. British Journal of Obstetrics and Gynaecology 107(11):1386–1391

Lundstrom V, Green K 1978 Endogenous levels of prostaglandin $F_{2\alpha}$ and its main metabolites in plasma and the endometrium of normal and dysmenorrhoeic women. American Journal of Obstetrics and Gynecology 130:640–646

Luukkainen T, Allonen H, Haukkamaa M, Lahteenmaki P, Nilsson CG, Toivonen J 1986 Five years experience with levonorgestrel-releasing IUCDs. Contraception 33:139–148

Magos AL, Baumann R, Lockwood GM, Turnbull AC 1991 Experience with the first 250 endometrial resections for menorrhagia. Lancet 337:1074–1078

Marbaix E, Kokorine I, Moulin P, Donnez J, Eeckhout Y, Courtoy PJ 1996 Menstrual breakdown of human endometrium can be mimicked in vitro and is selectively and reversibly blocked by inhibitors of matrix metalloproteinases. Proceedings of the National Academy of Science USA 93:9120–9125

Markee JE 1940 Menstruation in intraocular endometrial transplants in the rhesus monkey. Contributions to Embryology, Carnegie Institute 28:219–308

Markee JE 1948 Morphological basis for menstrual bleeding. Relation of regression to the initiation of bleeding. Bulletin of the New York Academy of Medicine 24:253–270

Marsh M 1996 Endothelin and menstruation. Human Reproduction 11:83–89

Migram S, Benedetto C, Zonka M, Leo Rosscerg I, Lubbert H, Hammerstein J 1991 Increased concentrations of eicosanoids and platelet-activating factor in menstrual fluid in women with primary dysmenorrhoea. Eicosanoids 4:137–141

Milsom I, Andersson K, Andersch B, Rybo G 1991 A comparison of flurbiprofen, tranexamic acid, and a levonorgestrel-releasing intrauterine contraceptive device in the treatment of idiopathic menorrhagia. American Journal of Obstetrics and Gynecology 164:879–883

Novak E, Reynolds SRM 1932 The cause of primary dysmenorrhoea with special reference to hormonal factors. Journal of the American Medical Association 99:1466–1472

Ohbuchi H, Nagai K, Yamaguchi M et al 1995 Endothelin-1 and big endothelin-1 increase in human endometrium during menstruation. American Journal of Obstetrics and Gynecology 173:1483–1490

Parazzini F, Tozzi L, Mezzopane R, Luchini L, Marchini M, Fedele L 1994 Cigarette smoking, alcohol consumption, and risk of primary dysmenorrhoea. Epidemiology 5:469–472

Pepper MS, Ferrara N, Orci L, Monteano R 1992 Potent synergism between vascular endothelial growth factor and basic fibroblast growth factor in the induction of angiogenesis in vitro. Biochemical and Biophysics Research Communications 189:824–831

Pinion SB, Parkin DE, Abramovich DR et al 1994 Randomised trial of hysterectomy, endometrial laser ablation and transcervical endometrial resection for dysfunctional uterine bleeding. British Medical Journal 309:979–983

Rees MCP, Barlow DH 1991 Quantitation of hormone replacement induced withdrawal bleeds. British Journal of Obstetrics and Gynaecology; 98:106–107

Rees MCP, Demers LM, Anderson ABM, Turnbull AC 1984 A functional study of platelets in menstrual fluid. British Journal of Obstetrics and Gynaecology 91:667–693

Rees MCP, Cederholm-Williams SA, Turnbull AC 1985 Coagulation factors and fibrinolytic proteins in menstrual fluid collected from normal and menorrhagic women. British Journal of Obstetrics and Gynaecology 92:1164–1168

Rees MCP, Canete-Soler R, Lopez-Bernal A, Turnbull A 1988 Effect of fenamates on prostaglandin E receptor binding. Lancet ii:541–542

Rogers PAW, Lederman F, Taylor N 1998 Endometrial microvascular growth in normal and dysfunctional states. Human Reproduction Update 4:503–508

Royal College of Obstetricias and Gynaecologists 1994 Inpatient treatment 1–1 D&C in women aged 40 or less. Guideline no. 3. RCOG, London

Rybo G 1966 Plasminogen activator in the endometrium. II. Clinical aspects. Acta Obstetrica et Gynecologica Scandinavica 45:97–118

Rybo G 1991 Tranexamic acid therapy: effective treatment in heavy menstrual bleeding. Clinical update on safety. Therapeutic Advances 4:1–8

Schild R, Kutta T 1992 Ranking of cervical cytology and uterine curettage in diagnosis of endometrial carcinoma. Geburtshilfe und Frquenheilkunde 52:467–470

Scottish Hysteroscopy Audit Group 1995 A Scottish audit of hysteroscopic surgery for menorrhagia–complications and follow up. British Journal of Obstetrics and Gynaecology 102(3):249–254

Sharkey AM, Day K, McPherson A et al 2000 Vascular endothelial growth factor expression in human endometrium is regulated by hypoxia. Journal of Clinical Endocrinology and Metabolism 85:402–409

Shaw RW, Fraser HM 1984 Use of a superactive luteinizing hormone-releasing hormone (LHRH) agonist in the treatment of menorrhagia. British Journal of Obstetrics and Gynaecology 91:913–916

Sheppard BL 1992 Physiology of dysfunctional uterine bleeding. In: Lowe D, Fox H (eds) Advances in gynaecological pathology. Churchill Livingstone, Edinburgh, pp 191–204

Sheppard BL, Dockeray CJ, Bonnar J 1983 An ultrastructural study of menstrual blood in normal menstruation and dysfunctional uterine bleeding. British Journal of Obstetrics and Gynaecology 90:259–265

Silverberg SG, Haukkamaa M, Arko H, Nilsson CG, Luukkainen T 1986 Endometrial morphology during long-term use of levonorgestrel-releasing intrauterine devices. International Journal of Gynecological Pathology 5:235–241

Smith SK 1998 Angiogenesis, vascular endothelial growth factor and the endometrium. Human Reproduction 4:519

Smith SK, Kelly RW 1988 Effect of platelet-activating factor on the release of PGF_{2a} and PGE_2 by separated cells of human endometrium. Journal of Reproduction and Fertility 82:271–276

Smith SK, Abel MH, Kelly RW, Baird DT 1981 Prostaglandin synthesis in the endometrium of women with ovular dysfunctional uterine bleeding. British Journal of Obstetrics and Gynaecology 88:434–442

Smith SK, Abel MH, Kelly RW, Baird DT 1982 The synthesis of prostaglandins from persistent proliferative endometrium. Journal of Clinical Endocrinology and Metabolism 55:284–289

Stock RJ, Kanbour A 1975 Prehysterectomy curettage. Obstetrics and Gynecology 45:537–541

Stovall TG, Solomon SK, Ling FW 1989 Endometrial sampling prior to hysterectomy. Obstetrics and Gynecology 73:405–408

Suri C, McClain J, Thurston DM et al 1998 Increased vascularization in mice overexpressing angiopoietin-1. Science 282:468–471

Tabibzadeh S, Babaknia A 1995 The signals and molecular pathways involved in implantation, a symbiotic interaction between blastocyst and endometrium involving adhesion and tissue invasion. Molecular Human Reproduction 1:1579–1602

Taylor PJ, Hamou J 1983 Hysteroscopy. Journal of Reproductive Medicine 28:359–389

Togashi K, Ozasa H, Konishi I et al 1989 Enlarged uterus: differentiation between adenomyosis and leiomyoma with MR imaging. Radiology 171:531–534

Vessey M, Clark J, MacKenzie I 1979 Dilatation and curettage in young women. Health Bulletin 39:59–62

Wiczyk HP, Janus CL, Richards CJ et al 1988 Comparison of magnetic resonance imaging and ultrasound in evaluating follicular and endometrial development throughout the normal cycle. Fertility and Sterility 49:969–972

Xu S, Yang Y, Gregory CD et al 1997 Biochemical heterogeneity in hysterectomised uterus measured by 31P NMR using SLIM localisation. Magnetic Resonance in Medicine 37:736–743

Ylikorkala O, Viinikka L 1983 Comparison between anti-fibrinolytic and anti-prostaglandin treatment in the reduction of increased menstrual blood loss in women with intrauterine contraceptive devices. British Journal of Obstetrics and Gynaecology 90:78–83

Zhang L, Rees MCP, Bicknell R 1995 The isolation and long term culture of normal human endometrial epithelium and stroma. Journal of Cell Science 108:323–331

SUGGESTED READING

Cameron IT 1993 Medical treatment of menorrhagia. In: Yearbook of the RCOG. RCOG Press, London, pp 55–64

Cameron IT, Fraser IS, Smith SK (Eds) 1998 Clinical disorders of the endometrium and menstrual cycle. Oxford University Press, Oxford

Fraser IS, Jansen RPS, Lobo RA, Whitehead M (eds) 1998 Estrogens and progestogens in clinical practice. Churchill Livingstone, London

O'Brien S, Cameron I, Machean A (eds) 2000 Disorders of the menstrual cycle. RCOG Press, London

Sheth S, Sutton C 1999 Menorrhagia. Isis Medical Media, Oxford

Vollenhover B 1998 Uterine fibroids. Bailliére's Clinical Obstetrics and Gynaecology 12:2

33

Uterine fibroids

David L. Healy   Beverley Vollenhoven   Gareth Weston

INTRODUCTION

Uterine fibroids are the most common tumour in women. These benign tumours arise from the uterine myometrium or, less commonly, from the cervix. They are composed not only of smooth muscle but of various amounts of elastin, collagen and extracellular matrix proteins. They are classified as leiomyomata and are also known as myomas.

Thus even the term fibroids is inaccurate by histological criteria. It is extraordinary that a tumour present in the uterus of up to 77% of patients requiring hysterectomy (Cramer & Patel 1990) has not been given higher priority in medical research. Uterine fibroids have been a low-priority area when compared with cancer research and poorly funded – surprisingly given that they are the most common neoplasm which any woman is likely to develop.

CLASSIFICATION AND PATHOPHYSIOLOGY

Macroscopically, fibroids are round or oval-shaped tumours, usually firm in consistency, with a characteristic white whorled appearance on cross-section. They may be single but are more commonly multiple and of varying sizes and present in multiple sites (Fig. 33.1). Tiny 'seedling' fibroids are commonly seen in association with larger tumours and surgical removal of over 120 individual fibroids from a patient has been recorded in the literature! Four clinical subgroups are recognized: subserosal, intramural, submucous and cervical.

Subserosal fibroids

These project outward from the uterine surface, covered with peritoneum. They may attain a very large size. Many fibroids in this site become pedunculated (Fig. 33.2) and torsion is a potential although rare complication. Sessile subserosal fibroids projecting from the fundal region may become adherent to omentum or bowel, particularly if there has been coincidental inflammatory disease. Fibroids rarely become attached to the omentum and if they develop an alternative blood supply, may become separated from the uterus, forming a so-called 'parasitic' fibroid. Subserosal fibroids arising from the lateral uterine wall may lie between the layers of the broad ligament where large tumours may displace the ureters or bulge between the layers of the sigmoid mesocolon. Broad ligament fibroids arising from the lateral uterine wall differ from true broad ligament fibroids, which have no attachment to the uterus but have their origin in smooth muscle fibres within the broad ligament, for example from the round ligament, ovarian ligament or perivascular connective tissue.

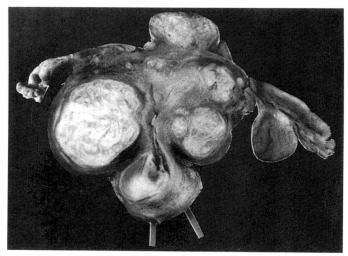

Fig. 33.1   Uterus enlarged by multiple fibroids. The patient presented at 43 years with menorrhagia; she had a 13-year history of primary infertility. Septate vagina and double cervix (marked with rods).

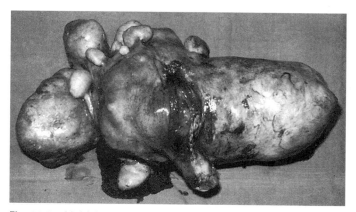

Fig. 33.2   Multiple subserous fibroids, some pedunculated. Specimen width 350 mm.

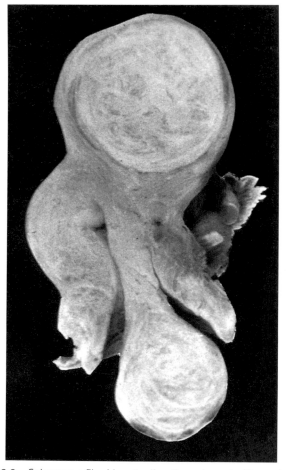

Fig. 33.3   Submucous fibroid protruding through cervix. The patient, aged 44 years, presented with a 3-week history of continuous bleeding; her haemoglobin level was 6.9 g/dl.

Intramural fibroids

These lie within the wall of the uterus. They are separated from the adjacent normal myometrium by a thin layer of connective tissue which forms the so-called pseudocapsule or false capsule. This pseudocapsule is of great help when performing the operation of myomectomy, as it provides a plane of easy cleavage to enucleate the fibroid tumour but to leave the remainder of the uterus.

Small nutrient arteries penetrate this capsule although a single larger artery usually provides the major blood supply. The vasculature of the fibroid, which is central to uterine artery embolization, one of the newer treatments, has received little attention. Although the perfusion of the vascular plexus around the fibroid is increased, the perfusion within the fibroid appears to be decreased. Forssman used ^{133}Xe injection intra-arterially and locally to demonstrate reduced blood flow in myomatous compared with normal uteri and reduced blood flow in the myomas compared with adjacent normal myometrium (Forssman 1976a,b). One study has shown reduced vascular area and microvascular density in fibroids compared with myometrium by immunostaining (Casey et al 2000). There is no explanation for the reduced vascular supply of the fibroid at present. A difference in angiogenesis-promoting factors may be the cause, but vascular endothelial growth factor (VEGF) is not the candidate, expression levels being the same as normal myometrium (Harrison-Woolrych et al 1995).

Submucous fibroids

These are less common, comprising around 5% of all leiomyomata. By definition they project into the uterine cavity, are covered by endometrium and may cause abnormal uterine bleeding and infertility. Uterine enlargement is not usually evident unless other fibroids are also present. Submucous fibroids, in which more than 50% of the size of the tumour projects into the uterine cavity, are regarded as suitable for hysteroscopic resection. Pedunculated submucous fibroids on a long stalk may prolapse through the cervix (Fig. 33.3) where they may cause intermenstrual bleeding or become ulcerated and infected. The author will long remember an 18-year-old who presented to casualty with 4 weeks of vaginal haemorrhage and a haemoglobin concentration of 1.9 g/dl. The fibroid in this patient was thought by casualty staff to be a fetal head.

Cervical fibroids

These are relatively uncommon but give rise to greatest surgical difficulty by virtue of their relative inaccessibility and close proximity to the bladder and ureters. Enlargement causes upward displacement of the uterus and the fibroid may become impacted in the pelvis, causing urinary retention and ureteric obstruction.

COMPLICATIONS

Fibroids have a characteristically firm fibrous texture, from which the clinical term 'fibroid' is presumably derived, with a typically whitish, whorled cut surface. They undergo a variety of degenerative changes, some of which can be detected on macroscopic appearance. They frequently become calcified; rarely, they become ossified so that they are rock hard. Areas of cystic degeneration or mucinous change may be seen and the most dramatic change is that of 'red' degeneration. This occurs classically during pregnancy, but may occur after gonadotrophin normone-releasing hormone (GnRH) agonist treatment, after menopause or after uterine artery embolization. Red degeneration is a form of coagulative necrosis resulting in a haemorrhagic, meaty, cut surface.

Microscopic appearances

Microscopically, fibroids are composed of smooth muscle cell bundles, also arranged in whorl-like patterns (Fig. 33.4a), admixed with a variable amount of connective tissue, although the latter rarely predominates. The relatively poor blood supply to individual fibroids may result in degenerative changes, particularly within large tumours. Hyaline degeneration (Fig. 33.4b) is the most common, resulting in a smoother and more homogeneous consistency, which may become cystic if liquefaction occurs. Much more rarely fatty change may develop. This is distinct from the true lipoma of the uterus, which is extremely uncommon. Calcification (Fig. 33.5) is a later consequence of degeneration secondary to circulatory impairment. It characteristically occurs after the menopause although it may occur earlier in subserosal fibroids with narrow pedicles.

There are a number of recognized histological variants of the usual microscopic appearance of uterine leiomyomata. The term 'cellular leiomyoma' is used when the density of the smooth muscle cells is significantly greater than usual, but there are no other atypical features such as increased mitotic activity or abnormal mitoses. Some pathologists use the term 'neurilemmoma-like leiomyoma' when there is a striking lining up or palisading of the tumour nuclei. This resembles nerve sheath tumours. Sometimes, fibroids are composed of polygonal cells rather than spindle cells. This type of nuclear pleomorphism is associated with giant cell formation and such tumours are called symplasmic, bizarre or atypical leiomyomas.

One differential diagnosis to uterine fibroids is the diagnosis of adenomyosis. Adenomyosis of the uterus may have a similar macroscopic appearance to uterine fibroids. However, in

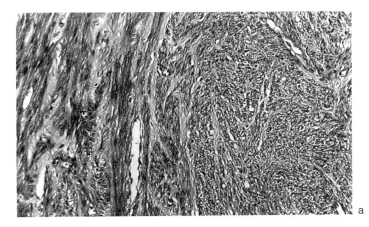

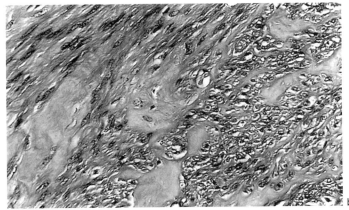

Fig. 33.4 Leiomyoma of uterus. **a** Bundles of elongated smooth muscle cells in both longitudinal (left) and transverse planes (×160). **b** Focal hyalinization. Smooth muscle bundles are separated by dense hyalinized connective tissue (×320) (courtesy of Dr K. Maclaren).

adenomyosis, there is no clear demarcation from the adjacent normal tissue. Leiomyosarcoma is a malignant tumour of the smooth muscle of the uterus. The macroscopic appearance of leiomyosarcoma shows an irregular invasive margin and a variegated cut surface. The microscopic appearance of leiomyosarcoma shows high cellularity, nuclear pleomorphism, a high mitotic rate with abnormal mitoses and areas of necrosis with infiltrating margins. Typically, the number of mitoses per 10 high-power fields in leiomyosarcoma is greater than 10, in contrast to standard leiomyoma where the number of mitoses per 10 high-power fields is below 5.

Finally, there are rare groups of uterine tumours having histological features intermediate between fibroids and leiomyosarcomas. These are termed smooth muscle tumours of uncertain malignant potential. Other rare tumours include endometrial stromal nodule, diffuse leiomyomatosis and endometrial stromal sarcoma.

Crow and colleagues (1995) have examined the microscopic appearances of uterine fibroids after treatment with GnRH agonists. They showed considerable variation from one fibroid to the next after a course of treatment and subsequent myomectomy or hysterectomy. Decreases in extracellular matrix, in particular, causes extreme crowding of tumour nuclei, resulting in a densely cellular appearance on microscopic

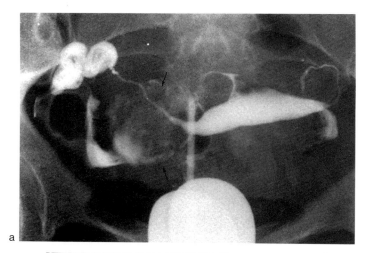

a

b

Fig. 33.5   a Calcified fibroid seen on hysterosalpingogram (courtesy of Dr B. Muir). b Ultrasound appearance of the uterus: *top:* two fibroids seen in transverse plane with calcified fibroid to left; *bottom:* calcified fibroid shown in longitudinal plane.

examination of such fibroids. For the inexperienced pathologist, this will be worrying in terms of possible malignancy. There should not, however, be mitotic activity, cytological atypia or coagulative necrosis.

AETIOLOGY

The aetiology of uterine fibroids is unknown. It appears that fibroid growth is dependent on ovarian hormones since fibroids do not occur prior to the menarche and normally show a reduction in size after the menopause or after a course of treatment with GnRH agonists. Moreover, there is no evidence that women developing uterine fibroids have any abnormality of circulating serum estradiol or progesterone concentrations.

Early studies based on the enzyme glucose-6-phosphate dehydrogenase (G-6-PD) electrophoresis (Townsend et al 1970) demonstrated that fibroids are derived from single myometrial cells: fibroids are monoclonal. The G-6-PD type may vary between individual fibroids within the same uterus.

A major impediment to the easy understanding of uterine fibroid growth is that there are no obvious animal models. Leiomyoma-like lesions can be induced in the myometrium of guinea pigs, rats and rabbits but in these species oestrogen appears to be a mitogen, in contrast to women, in whom progesterone appears to be the major mitogen for uterine fibroids (Kawaguchi et al 1989). Although estradiol is mitogenic for the endometrium, the available information in vitro shows that estradiol does not appear to be mitotic to human myometrial cells or uterine fibroid cells, in contrast to progesterone.

There is evidence emerging that progesterone plays an important role in fibroid growth. Progesterone receptor has been shown to be increased in fibroids relative to myometrium (Brandon et al 1993) and to upregulate the levels of some proteins which influence cell proliferation, such as the anti-apoptotic protein Bcl-2 (Matsuo et al 1999). Oncogenes and tumour suppressor genes may have a role in fibroid development. This may in part be regulated by the increased sensitivity of fibroid tissue to ovarian steroids. The secreted tumour suppressor mac25 is reduced in large fibroids (Kim et al 2000), while MCP-1, a chemokine with anti-tumour effects, is increased compared with normal myometrium (Sozen et al 1998). Oncogenes investigated in fibroids include *c-fos*, *c-jun* and *c-myc*, but their role in the aetiology of fibroids remains unclear. There is more evidence that they may play a role in leiomyosarcoma (Gustarson et al 2000).

In addition to the classic steroid sex hormones, estradiol and progesterone, peptide hormones are now recognized as important for local growth of tumours in many parts of the body. Extracellular matrix molecules such as collagen and fibronectin serve to confine peptide growth hormones to local areas by binding tightly to them and preventing them from dispersing. Peptide growth factors bind to specific membrane-bound receptors on the cell surface. This initiates a cascade of signals within the cell that is called signal transduction. In particular, the insulin-like growth factors IGF-1 and IGF-2 have been shown to stimulate the mitotic activity of leiomyoma cells in culture and to be present within fibroids in higher concentrations than in normal uterine smooth muscle (Vollenhoven et al 1993).

Uterine fibroids are not a single gene disorder. Non-random chromosomal changes such as translocations, duplications and deletions can be identified in almost 50% of fibroids. The most frequent cytogenetic changes are translocations involving chromosomes 7, 12 and 14 and deletions in chromosomes 7. The critical region affected in chromosome 7 appears to be on the long-arm (7Q21–22). Several known genes are coded in this apparently critical region. These include genes for collagen type 1α 2, the MET proto-oncogene and the cytochrome P450 gene.

EPIDEMIOLOGY

There has been considerable effort over the past several years in the application of clinical epidemiology, public health medicine principles and evidence-based approaches to medical care. Relevant articles from the Cochrane Library can be accessed to investigate the quality of the evidence on which the management and treatment of patients with uterine fibroids are based. In general, this approach shows that there is almost no high-quality evidence on which to base the treatment of uterine fibroids. It is a disgrace that there is so little evidence for patients to use in making decisions about the management of their tumours. We have many more cohort studies, case control studies and randomized control trials for rare diseases than for a condition which affects at least half of women during their reproductive years and is the leading indication for the most common major operation in women.

Evidence-based gynaecology can be accessed through the Cochrane Library. This library includes the Cochrane Controlled Trials Register, the Cochrane Database of Systematic Reviews and the Cochrane Database of Abstracts of Reviews of Effectiveness. These are powerful sources of published and unpublished randomized trials. A search of such an extensive library unfortunately indicates that there are very few randomized controlled trials regarding uterine fibroids. Conversely, the strongly held opinion of an individual patient or an individual clinician has just as much evidence going for it as that from expert panels or authors of chapters in learned textbooks! This does not occur in other areas of medicine.

At another epidemiological level, there appear to be consistent differences between women of different race regarding their uterine fibroids. The best of this information comes from the USA and suggests that there appear to be consistent differences between African Americans on the one hand and white, Hispanic and Asian Americans on the other. These last three groups have results which are statistically indistinguishable from each other (Marshall et al 1997).

The incidence for uterine fibroids among African American women appears to be approximately three times higher than among whites. Moreover, black women have uterine fibroids diagnosed earlier than white women and these tumours are larger and more numerous at diagnosis and treatment. In the USA, hysterectomy or myomectomy appears to be more frequent in black women.

There is very little information about the effect of age or menopausal status on the risks or benefits of treatment for symptomatic uterine fibroids. GnRH agonists, hysteroscopic myomectomy and uterine artery embolization all appear more likely to induce prolonged amenorrhoea in perimenopausal women. There are no data which allow prediction of which perimenopausal women would be most likely to respond to conservative treatment.

It is a myth that fibroids increase in size during pregnancy. The studies which actually examine this natural history contradict this notion (Aharoni et al 1988). By contrast, there is strong evidence that the presence of uterine fibroids is associated with pregnancy complications. These include first trimester bleeding, placental abruption with submucosal fibroids and increased risks of inco-ordinate uterine action or caesarean section. No study has had enough statistical power to prove whether fibroids increase the risk of premature delivery. Similarly, although it has been widely believed that women should undergo elective caesarean section for delivery after a myomectomy, especially when the uterine cavity has been entered, there are no data to support this recommendation.

Care of the infertile woman with uterine fibroids provides most evidence with submucosal fibroids. These tumours, which distort the uterine cavity, were shown from our group to significantly decrease implantation and pregnancy rates (Eldar-Geva et al 1998). The effectiveness of myomectomy to remove any other type of uterine fibroids in the infertile woman remains unproven. There have been no studies comparing the efficacy of open abdominal myomectomy versus laparoscopic myomectomy, nor of laparoscopic myomectomy versus hysteroscopic myomectomy. The reported pregnancy and delivery rates for infertile patients for all these procedures seem statistically similar. There is a great need for future clinical research to explicitly state the criteria being used to define infertility, as well as the precise location and size of the leiomyomata. Otherwise, operation for removal of uterine fibroids will remain a hobby for gynaecologists but with no benefit to the care of their patients.

PRESENTATION

The clinical presentation of uterine fibroids is dependent in part on the reproductive status of the woman and the site of the fibroids. The symptomatology has been reviewed in detail by Buttram & Reiter (1981). Many fibroids, possibly in excess of 50%, are asymptomatic and discovered at routine pelvic or abdominal examination or during pregnancy.

Menorrhagia

It is uncertain what proportion of women with fibroids have excessive menstrual loss although estimates vary between 30% and 50%. Investigation of women presenting with menorrhagia has shown the presence of fibroids in only 10% of those with moderately heavy menstrual blood loss (80–100 ml), compared with 40% of those with loss in excess of 200 ml (Rybo et al 1985). Menorrhagia attributable to fibroids may therefore be very heavy, causing significant anaemia. It is important to appreciate that fibroids are not usually a cause of irregular or intermenstrual bleeding and that any disruption of normal cyclicity should not be attributed to the presence of fibroids without first excluding other causes.

The mechanism of the menorrhagia remains a subject of debate. Theories include ulceration and haemorrhage of the

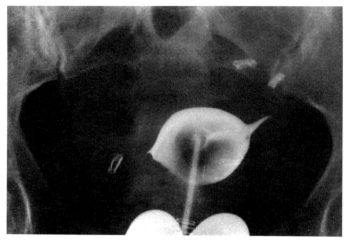

Fig. 33.6 Hysterosalpingogram showing enlargement of uterine cavity and filling defect from intramural fibroid. Extensive endometriosis had complicated laparoscopic sterilization (hence the two clips on the left tube) (courtesy of Dr B. Muir).

endometrium overlying submucous fibroids, enlargement of the total surface area of the endometrium due to mechanical distortion by submucous and intramural fibroids (Fig. 33.6) and stasis and dilatation of the venous plexuses draining the endometrium, due to mechanical compression of the venous drainage by fibroids at any site. All these mechanisms may be important and it is now clear that, contrary to some opinions, menorrhagia is not confined only to women with submucous fibroids and that while these may be associated with menorrhagia of greatest severity, they are sometimes asymptomatic.

Pelvic pain and pressure symptoms

Fibroids do not usually give rise to pain. Exceptionally, their presentation may be acute on account of torsion or degeneration. Attempted expulsion of a large submucous fibroid through the cervix causes uterine cramp associated with bleeding and may be mistaken for spontaneous abortion, particularly with the clinical finding of a dilated cervix and a protruding mass. This situation has been described as a complication of treatment with GnRH analogues. Rarely it can result in uterine inversion. Torsion or painful degeneration presents with an acute abdomen and is commonly confused with complications of ovarian neoplasia. Distinction between these conditions is particularly important in pregnancy complicated by red degeneration of a fibroid, in order to avoid subjecting the woman to unnecessary laparotomy.

It is surprising that even in the presence of multiple fibroids menstruation may be painless. They are more often associated with pelvic discomfort and urinary symptoms, attributed to pressure from large fibroids, particularly those arising from the cervix or low down on the anterior uterine wall. Cervical fibroids may present with acute retention of urine (Fig. 33.7), although this in uncommon.

Infertility

The effect of uterine fibroids on fertility is still subject to controversy. Impaired gamete transport, distortion of the

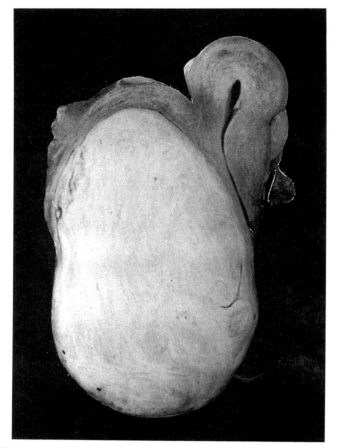

Fig. 33.7 Cervical fibroid growing anteriorly in the supravaginal cervix. Presentation was with frequency of micturition followed by acute urinary retention.

endometrial cavity, impairment of blood supply to the endometrium as well as atrophy and ulceration might be responsible for reduced implantation in patients carrying these tumours. There have been series indicating postoperative pregnancy rates of 50–60% in women after myomectomy but these studies have usually been uncontrolled or poorly controlled.

We examined the impact of uterine fibroids in a group of patients requiring assisted reproductive technology (ART) treatment (Eldar-Geva et al 1998). We found that the treatment outcome after ART was not influenced by the presence of subserosal fibroids. However, it was considerably impaired in patients with either intramural or submucosal fibroids, even when there was no deformation of the uterine cavity. Although our series was small (88 patients) these results beg the question of whether surgical or medical treatment should be considered in infertile patients with intramural or submucosal fibroids before resorting to in vitro fertilization – IVF/ART treatments. Our result also begs the question of whether shrinkage of uterine fibroids with GnRH agonist treatment would improve the prospect of pregnancy in patients undergoing these ART treatments.

INVESTIGATIONS

The range of investigations appropriate to each case of fibroids will vary according to the nature of the individual problem

Transvaginal ultrasound is particularly helpful in elucidating the nature of small lesions and in demonstrating the presence of submucosal fibroids.

Ultrasound assessment should include examination of the ovaries and it is important to look for the presence or absence of free peritoneal fluid as well as to study the nature and consistency of the mass itself. Serial ultrasound examination is of value in monitoring fibroid size during medical or conservative treatment. The volume of individual fibroids or of the whole uterus (Fig. 33.8) can be calculated by measuring the diameter in three planes at right angles and using the formula $4/3\pi r^3$, where r is the radius.

Magnetic resonance imaging (MRI)

Until proven otherwise, MRI has no place in the routine investigation of a patient suspected of uterine fibroids. Cost and issues of access are the major problems with using MRI for the typical patient. Excellent visualization and localization of tumours can be obtained and MRI is an excellent investigation to show the proximity of the fibroid to the endometrial cavity.

Hysteroscopy

Hysteroscopy and laparoscopy as investigational procedures are often merged into treatment. Whilst for individual patients this can be very effective and satisfactory, for many women with uterine fibroids there is the risk of unnecessary or ineffective surgery when there is no clear distinction made by the doctor between using these operations for investigation as opposed to using them as a proven treatment.

Hysteroscopy is an invasive procedure and, for diagnosis, has recently been compared to transvaginal ultrasound techniques although not in randomized controlled trials to our knowledge. Transvaginal ultrasonography for suspected uterine fibroids is made by demonstrating their patchy echogenicity. Saline contrast hysteroscopy increases the diagnostic capability by ultrasound of submucosal fibroids. The saline distends and acts as a contrast medium within the uterine cavity. Such a technique may show a submucosal uterine fibroid or fibroid polyp. Such leiomyomata up to a diameter of even 4–5 cm can then be considered for hysteroscopic resection, especially if more than 50% of the volume of the tumour is projecting into the uterine cavity. In individual patients, endometrial sampling by direct biopsy or one of the commercially available endometrial sampling instruments can also be undertaken at office or outpatient hysteroscopy (Healy & Petrucco 1998).

Laparoscopy

Diagnostic laparoscopy can be of clinical value if the uterus is not larger than a 12-week gestation size and there is associated infertility or pelvic pain. It may reveal the presence of co-incidental endometriosis, pelvic adhesions or other tubal pathology. Laparoscopy will also differentiate between a pedunculated fibroid and an ovarian neoplasm if there is an individual patient where this diagnosis is unclear on the basis of clinical and ultrasound findings.

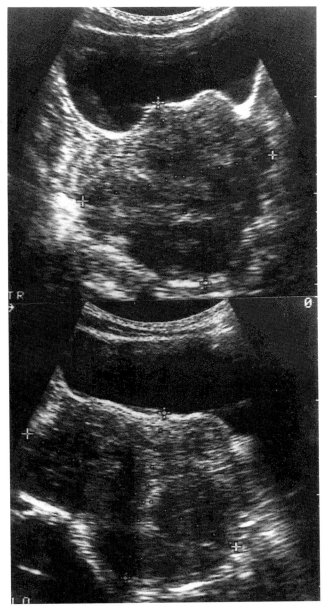

Fig. 33.8 Ultrasound appearance of uterus enlarged by multiple fibroids, showing patchy echogenicity (courtesy of Dr B. Muir).

and the proposed plan of management. General assessment should always include a full blood count, as many patients with fibroids do not complain of excessive menstruation even when this is present. Use of the available imaging techniques has been reviewed (Karasick et al 1992).

Ultrasound

Ultrasound should always be used to confirm or clarify the nature of a pelvic mass. Even in relatively unskilled hands it will diagnose pregnancy and differentiate between cystic and solid lesions (Fig. 33.8). With appropriate training and experience, the site and nature of a pelvic mass may be predicted with accuracy in over 80% of cases; difficulty mainly arises in the differentiation of pedunculated fibroids from solid ovarian lesions.

TREATMENT METHODS

Management of uterine fibroids is bedevilled by considerable practice variation and controversy, especially regarding the introduction of a variety of techniques typically reported as individual patient reports or as small case series. Cohort studies, case control studies and randomized controlled trials are few in this area of gynaecology and the management of uterine fibroids is the poorer for it.

There is no evidence to support the use of either hysterectomy or myomectomy for management of asymptomatic uterine fibroids. There are very few data to allow direct comparison of the risks and benefits comparing myomectomy and hysterectomy. Compared with other areas of medicine, the published data from the management of uterine fibroids are insufficient to allow conclusions about the most appropriate therapy for a given type of woman with uterine fibroids.

The incidence of recurrence of symptoms is unclear after conservative management of fibroids as well as the likelihood of increased morbidity associated with treatment for recurrent or persistent fibroid symptoms. Reported recurrence rates range up to 20% at 5 years after myomectomy with up to 8% of patients undergoing hysterectomy. For medical treatment, there is a similar remarkable lack of randomized trial data demonstrating any effectiveness of oral contraceptive pills, progestogens and GnRH agonists in the management of women with uterine fibroids.

Expectant management

Fibroids are frequently asymptomatic and provided that their nature can be determined with reasonable certainty using the diagnostic methods described above, active treatment is unnecessary. Surgical removal has traditionally been advocated when the uterine size exceeds that of a 12-week pregnancy but this policy has been challenged (Reiter et al 1992). Most pelvic swellings can be confidently diagnosed with the use of ultrasound. Similarly, the risk of sarcomatous change in fibroids if left is a myth. We know of no data proving this risk. Furthermore, the mere presence of a fibroid uterus is not known to carry any long-term detrimental effects: spontaneous regression after the menopause may be anticipated.

Leiomyosarcoma from fibroids: where is the evidence?

For the 'worried well', the diagnosis of a uterine fibroid naturally raises the issue 'Can it become cancer, doctor?'. It seems that a common reason for removing the uterus in a woman with uterine fibroids or undertaking myomectomy is 'to be certain', 'just in case' the uterine fibroid(s) 'grows' into a uterine sarcoma. Gard & colleagues (1999) have recently reviewed uterine leiomyosarcoma in Australia. These authors conducted a retrospective survey at major teaching hospitals in Melbourne and Sydney. They identified 49 patients treated over 28 years at these two hospitals. For the population involved, this equates to approximately one leiomyosarcoma of the uterus in one million Australian women each year. On this basis, removing each and every uterine fibroid from all women

cannot be justified. Until proven otherwise, sarcomatous 'change' in a fibroid is a myth.

In the above article, the mean age of presentation was postmenopausal – 55 years. The range was 17–82 years. The most common presentation was abnormal bleeding, usually postmenopausal bleeding. A preoperative diagnosis was more likely in those patients who presented with postmenopausal bleeding, where 43% had a uterine curettage, which showed a histological diagnosis of leiomyosarcoma. Seventy-six per cent of patients underwent hysterectomy for symptoms assumed to be related to uterine fibroids.

There are many types of uterine sarcomas. These all differ in their biological behaviour. The clinical benefits of oophorectomy, lymphadenectomy and cytotoxic chemotherapy remain controversial for these various types of leiomyosarcoma, not least because they are rare even in the clinical experience of gynaecological oncologists.

Hysterectomy

Hysterectomy is the time-honoured treatment for symptomatic uterine fibroids. The decision to perform hysterectomy should not be undertaken without due consideration of the alternatives: for women who wish to preserve reproductive function, myomectomy or medical treatment must be considered.

The route selected for hysterectomy will depend on the size of the uterus, the situation of the fibroids and the history of any previous surgical procedures. Abdominal hysterectomy with ovarian conservation (Fig. 33.9) will be the procedure of choice where fibroids are very large. For gynaecologists who favour vaginal hysterectomy, consideration should be given to preoperative shrinkage with a GnRH agonist as described below. Similarly, a reduction in volume and vascularity may facilitate removal of a very large uterus by the abdominal route. Abdominal hysterectomy is rendered difficult in the presence of large fibroids arising from the cervix or situated in

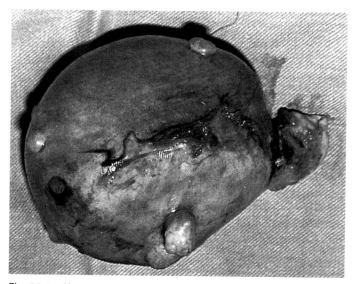

Fig. 33.9 Hysterectomy specimen from uterus enlarged to 16-week gestation size by single intramural fibroid and several small seedling fibroids. Uterine volume was 575 ml.

the broad ligament. It is also more complicated if there are adhesions from previous myomectomies or from associated endometriosis or pelvic inflammatory disease. Difficult access to the pelvis during hysterectomy for large fibroids will be rendered easier by prior enucleation of the fibroids. The ureters may be vulnerable during an operation to remove a broad ligament fibroid and their pathway must always be identified. Regardless of the direction of displacement, they are always extracapsular. In the case of a large cervical fibroid an alternative approach is hemisection of the uterus, followed by enucleation of the fibroid in order to gain access to the uterine arteries and cervix. These techniques are described in detail elsewhere (Monaghan 1986).

The increasing popularity of minimal access surgery has led to the use of laparoscopically assisted methods of vaginal hysterectomy in women with large fibroids, usually following prior shrinkage with a GnRH agonist. The evidence base of this approach currently remains unclear. The use of the laparoscope will facilitate oophorectomy, as well as allowing the surgeon to inspect and achieve meticulous haemostasis at the vaginal vault, in conjunction with vaginal hysterectomy.

Myomectomy

Removal of individual fibroids was first reported in the middle of the 19th century although current surgical techniques are largely attributable to Victor Bonney who described a personal series of 403 cases. Since then there have been several large published series, reviewed in detail elsewhere (Buttram & Reiter 1951, Verkauf 1992).

Enucleation of intramural fibroids from their false capsule can be a rapid and simple procedure but may also be associated with considerable technical difficulties, major haemorrhage and a greater postoperative morbidity and mortality than hysterectomy. It is therefore an operation which should be restricted to women who have completed child bearing. It is most satisfactory where fibroids are solitary or few in number. Although removal of as many as 125 individual tumours from one uterus was described by Bonney, such a procedure is tedious and modern outcome in terms of reproductive function must be in considerable doubt. In a woman presenting with infertility, it is sometimes difficult to establish the extent to which the fibroids are interfering with conception and full investigation of both the woman and her partner is indicated.

Because of difficulty to access to submucous fibroids at laparotomy, consideration should be given to hysteroscopic methods of removal. Subserous fibroids are easily removed with minimal morbidity, particularly if pedunculated (Fig. 33.10), but such fibroids are the least likely to give rise to problems. Some authorities would advise their removal if they are large because of the risk, albeit rare, of acute torsion in pregnancy.

Potential problems with myomectomy

The major problems associated with myomectomy are heavy operative blood loss and postoperative adhesion formation, reducing the chance of successful conception and rendering future surgery more difficult. It is therefore most important that the decision to perform a myomectomy is carefully

considered. If operative haemorrhage is very heavy the surgeon may have to resort to hysterectomy and should be reluctant to embark upon surgery if the patient is not willing to consent to the latter alternative.

Various methods have been advocated to reduce intra- and postoperative complications. Postoperative adhesions are usually a consequence of difficulties with haemostasis and oozing from incision lines. Adhesions are increased where there are multiple incisions over the uterine body. We try for minimal tissue handling and meticulous haemostatis at all myomectomies. We not only keep the pelvis moist by continuous irrigation, but also regularly add a large volume of fluid by a suction/irrigator to check for haemostasis 'under water'.

Adhesions after incisions on the posterior uterine wall are potentially more serious because of involvement of the uterine tubes and ovaries. To minimize adhesion formation, as many fibroids as possible should be removed through a single incision (Fig. 33.10). Some authorities recommend removal of posterior wall fibroids via the uterine cavity through an incision on the anterior uterine wall. Others avoid opening the uterine cavity unless submucous fibroids are known to be present because of the risk of intrauterine adhesions.

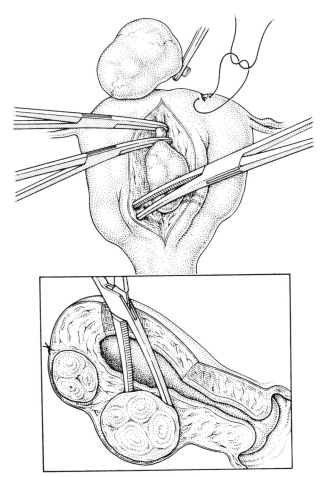

Fig. 33.10 Removal of subserous, intramural, submucous and posteriorly located intramural fibroids through a single anterior incision (with permission of the American Society for Reproductive Medicine, formerly the American Fertility Society).

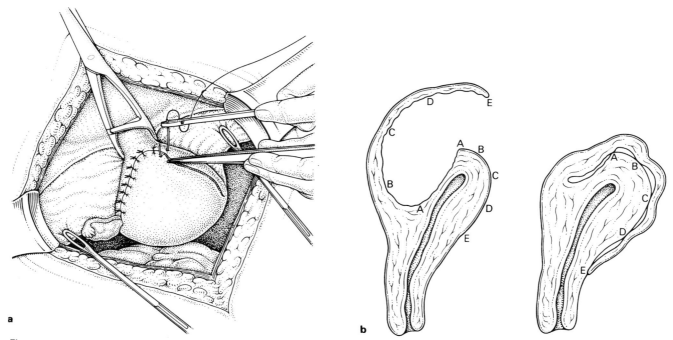

Fig. 33.11 **a** Closure of myomectomy through transverse posterior incision using Bonney's 'hood', showing final anterior suture line and Bonney's clamp in place. **b** Construction of Bonney's hood showing the capsule after enucleation (*left*) and the hood in place (*right*) (with permission of Chapman and Hall).

Careful obliteration of large cavities left by enucleation of fibroids is very important and opinions vary as to whether redundant myometrium should be removed or preserved. Bonney (Monaghan 1986) described a 'hood' method of closure of the cavity left after enucleation of a very large single posterior tumour (Fig. 33.11), suturing the redundant flap of serosal-covered myometrium over the fundus and low down on to the anterior wall to avoid adhesion formation. Plication of the round ligaments at the end of the procedure to hold the uterus forward in anteversion, the instillation of concentrated solutions of dextran and the use of oxidized regenerated cellulose have also been recommended to reduce the risk of postoperative adhesions.

Both mechanical and medical methods have been described to reduce operative blood loss. One such method is the use of the Bonney's myomectomy clamp which is placed across the lower uterus to occlude the uterine arteries (see Fig. 33.11a). It can be used in conjunction with ring forceps to occlude the ovarian blood supply. An alternative is the use of a rubber tourniquet or catheter, placed around the uterus through an incision in the broad ligament at the level of the lower segment. Occlusion of the arterial blood supply for prolonged intervals of time may cause ischaemic damage to tissues and release of histamine-like substances into the general circulation has been reported (Monaghan 1986). During a long operation, intermittent release of the clamp or catheter at 10–20-minute intervals is recommended. Such occlusive methods are unsuitable for use where there are large cervical or broad ligament fibroids and these are the very tumours which may give rise to greatest difficulty.

Pretreatment with GnRH agonists has also been used to reduce the vascularity of the uterus (see below) and this has the advantage of also reducing by approximately 50% the size of the fibroids. It is our standard preoperative treatment for 3 months prior to myomectomy. Some gynaecologists have found enucleation more difficult because the false capsule plane of cleavage between the fibroid and the surrounding myometrium becomes less well defined. This has not been our experience.

Endoscopic surgical methods

Hysteroscopy

Most submucous fibroids which are protruding through the cervix (see Fig. 33.3) can be removed vaginally with cautery or ligation of the pedicle. If the fibroid is very large, piecemeal removal has been described. Such procedures might be facilitated by preoperative treatment with a GnRH agonist. Diagnostic and therapeutic hysteroscopy (Siegler & Vaue 1988) is gaining popularity in the UK and submucous fibroids (such as those illustrated in Fig. 33.12) are amenable to hysteroscopic removal. Such procedures can be combined with endometrial ablation for the relief of menorrhagia if the woman has completed child bearing.

Techniques of hysteroscopic myomectomy are described (Drews & Reyniak 1992) and have been used for removal of lesions measuring up to 7 cm in diameter although many authorities would set a maximum of 3–4 cm. Prior shrinkage with a GnRH analogue is advantageous in this context. Small pedunculated lesions may be removed with scissors after coagulation of the base while larger broad-based lesions that are predominantly submucosal are resected using electrocautery. The neodymium:YAG laser can be used for ablation of small fibroids or alternatively, larger lesions can be cut off at their base and if small, extracted whole, or if larger, quartered and

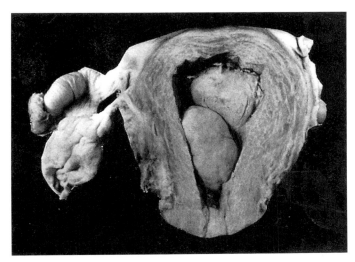

Fig. 33.12 Submucous fibroids (subtotal hysterectomy specimen).

removed piecemeal. Postoperative bleeding can be controlled by tamponade with the balloon of a Foley catheter.

For fibroids with an intramural extension, Donnez and colleagues (1990) describe a two-stage removal procedure using the neodymium:YAG laser, after prior shrinkage with a GnRH analogue. They advocate leaving individual fibroids, once enucleated, in the uterine cavity where eventual expulsion during menstruation is anticipated.

Hysteroscopic surgery of this type requires considerable experience and training in order to optimize results and minimize complications, which include uterine perforation (immediate or pregnancy related), haemorrhage, infection and excessive systemic absorption of the fluid distending medium. However, these techniques have the advantage of being performed as outpatient procedures with avoidance of major surgery.

Laparoscopy

Laparoscopy is a standard investigation for infertility and inevitably many women thus investigated will be found to have small asymptomatic uterine fibroids. Laparoscopic methods of removal of both subserous and small intramural fibroids have been described (Drews & Reyniak 1992) but as these are unlikely to be interfering with fertility it is not clear whether their removal will carry any long-term advantage for the patient. In theory, it may prevent the growth of larger, potentially symptomatic tumours and avoid more major surgical intervention, but these advantages have yet to be proven. It is also unlikely that intramural seedlings can be removed by this method.

Recently laparoscopic techniques have been applied to the enucleation of larger intramural as well as subserosal fibroids, which are then morcellated or removed by colpotomy. Such procedures are very time consuming and as yet there is no evidence that they offer any advantages over conventional laparotomy.

Medical management

There are two main objectives in the medical treatment of uterine fibroids, namely relief of symptoms and reduction in

fibroid size. The ideal end-point of medical treatment would be complete regression but to date this has not been described. For this reason, medical methods have in the past had a limited role in the management of fibroids. However, with recent advances in diagnostic and therapeutic techniques, enabling a more conservative approach to management, there is a greater role for medical therapies, both for symptomatic treatment of fibrids and also as adjuncts to surgery. The role of medical therapies in the relief of fibroid-associated menorrhagia has been reviewed (van Eijkeren et al 1992, West & Lunsder 1989).

Oestrogen–progestogen combinations

The role of the oral contraceptive pill in women with fibroids is unclear. Since an early report of enlargement of fibroids during oral contraceptive therapy, its use has been avoided in this situation although a modest reduction in menstrual blood loss was reported (Nilsson & Rybo 1971). The relevance of early studies to modern contraceptive practice must, however, be questioned as they related to much higher dose formulations than those in current use. In women known to have fibroids, there seems to be no clear contraindication to the use of the pill for contraceptive purposes, provided that uterine volume is monitored and there is no deterioration in its size or in any fibroid-related symptoms. For women without fibroids, long-term use of the oral contraceptive pill may be protective against their development (Ross et al 1986) although not all authors have reported similar findings.

The influence of the oestrogen–progestogen combinations used for hormone replacement therapy is also unclear, although re-enlargement of fibroids might be expected. This has not been confirmed in studies of the addition of low-dose hormone replacement therapy to GnRH analogues for the shrinkage of fibroids. Because of the ease of monitoring fibroid size with ultrasound, the use of low-dose oral hormone replacement therapy should not be contraindicated in postmenopausal women with fibroids, particularly if these have been asymptomatic, unless there is any suspicion of co-existing endometrial pathology.

Antiprogesterones

There have been reports (Reinsch et al 1994) of shrinkage of uterine fibroids in response to continuous therapy with the antiprogesterone RU486, mifepristone, given continuously at a dose of 25–50 mg daily. Shrinkage is similar to that observed during therapy with a GnRH agonist and is associated with amenorrhoea but less profound oestrogen suppression, levels being maintained in the early to midfollicular phase range. Although preliminary, these results may indicate an exciting new approach to the medical management of uterine fibroids.

GnRH analogues

GnRH agonists Analogues of GnRH significantly reduce the size of uterine fibroids, thus relieving pressure symptoms as well as menorrhagia. GnRH agonists should be commenced in the midluteal phase of the ovarian cycle for most rapid pituitary gonadotrophin downregulation. Bleeding in response to oestrogen withdrawal occurs during the initial treatment cycle but amenorrhoea is usual thereafter. The shrinkage of fibroids is therefore a consequence of gonadal suppression and women are likely to experience side-effects, in particular vasomotor symptoms and vaginal dryness. Uterine volume, assessed by ultrasound or MRI, shrinks by an average of 35% after 3 months of administration and 50% after 6 months, with little further change thereafter. The effects of treatment persist only for the duration of administration. This makes GnRH agonist treatment most effective preoperatively or in the premenopausal woman. Cessation of therapy is usually followed by rapid regrowth of the fibroids to their pretreatment size in younger patients (West 1993)

If such treatment is to be used prior to surgery, its optimum duration is 3 months, which should be sufficient to correct any associated anaemia. Appropriate doses of currently available GnRH agonists include goserelin 3.6 mg or leuporelin 3.75 mg, by monthly subcutaneous depot injection, and buserelin 900–1200 μg or nafarelin 800 μg daily in divided doses by intranasal spray. Therapy should be commenced in the midluteal phase of the cycle with no sexual intercourse that month to avoid accidental initiation during early pregnancy. Compliance may be a problem with the nasal spray and as erratic usage may result in stimulation rather than suppression of pituitary–ovarian function, administration by subcutaneous depot is preferable.

For women who are keen to avoid surgery, particularly those approaching the age of the natural menopause or those with contraindications to surgery, the use of GnRH agonists in combination with hormonal 'add-back' therapy is an option. Such therapy comprises oestrogen-progestogen combinations, equivalent to low-dose hormone replacement therapy, given with the object of reducing vasomotor side-effects and protecting against bone loss. This is commenced once initial uterine shrinkage has been obtained with 3 months of GnRH agonist alone. The add-back therapy may be given cyclically or as continuous combined therapy, the latter having the potential advantage of sustained amenorrhoea. Results (Friedman 1993, West 1993) indicate that fibroid shrinkage and symptomatic relief can be maintained in a proportion of patients with such regimens. Use of progestogens alone as add-back therapy appears to be less effective compared with oestrogen–progestogen combinations. Regimens of this nature are very costly and some women very near the natural menopause gain sustained relief of their symptoms following 6 months of treatment with a GnRH agonist alone.

There have been reports of spontaneous pregnancy immediately following GnRH agonist-induced shrinkage of small submucous fibroids which had caused tubal obstruction. This is a relatively unusual situation and one in which hysteroscopic myomectomy may offer a more long-term solution in skilled hands. Currently, it is not clear whether medical therapies have a role in the management of younger women with larger symptomatic fibroids who wish to preserve their reproductive function but to delay child bearing. Here, early myomectomy may not be desirable because of the risk of recurrence of fibroids and the need for a second operation. In theory, interim therapy with a GnRH agonist, either alone or in combination, may control symptoms and prevent further significant enlargement of the fibroids, enabling surgery to be delayed. It is not clear whether such therapy would inhibit the initiation of new lesions or simply mask their presence, making early recurrences more prevalent.

GnRH antagonists The antagonist analogues directly inhibit the action of GnRH on the pituitary, resulting in immediate gonadal suppression and avoidance of the stimulatory phase seen with the agonists. Cetrorelix and ganirelix are becoming widely available for clinical use. An early study (Kertel et al 1993) with one antagonist, given by daily subcutaneous injection, demonstrated a rapid reduction in uterine volume. The overall shrinkage was equivalent to that seen with agonists but was more rapidly achieved and with immediate onset of amenorrhoea.

RESULTS OF TREATMENT

Application of an evidence-based approach to the treatment of uterine fibroids indicates that there is almost no high-quality evidence on which to base treatment. Given this lack of evidence, it is not surprising that individual patients and individual doctors decide treatment on their own wishes and personal experiences.

Results of myomectomy

There is no evidence to support the use of myomectomy for management of asymptomatic fibroids. Typically, studies of abdominal or laparoscopic myomectomy do not carefully report the effects of the operation on relieving a patient's symptoms. Studies of hysteroscopic myomectomy also typically report symptomatic relief but the methods and their validity for determining the severity of symptoms are usually unreliable. Blood loss resulting in blood transfusion is usually the most commonly reported short-term complication of all myomectomy procedures, by any method, with ranges typically 2–10%.

Removal of a single fibroid seems less likely to result in short-term complications or long-term recurrence and appears to be associated with higher pregnancy rates. Unfortunately, variations in the methods of reporting prevent a clear conclusion to this question. It is unclear whether the risks associated with a single fibroid myomectomy represent differences in surgical success rate or in the underlying biology in a given woman.

Recurrent fibroids

Reported cumulative recurrence rates after myomectomy range up to 50% at 5 years, with approximately 20% of women undergoing hysterectomy. It is not clear whether 'recurrent' fibroids after conservative treatment represent regrowth of existing tumours or de novo development of additional fibroids. The literature is of poor quality with inconsistent reports regarding the definition of 'recurrence', the length of follow-up, the percentage of women lost to follow-up and why, and the use of other treatments which might affect recurrence. From the literature which is available, a larger preoperative fibroid size, an increased number of fibroid tumours, increasing fibroid penetration into the myometrium and any residual tissue at the completion of the procedure were all associated with increased recurrence risk. These factors, leading to the development of further symptomatic fibroids after treatment, seem to occur with medical therapies, uterine artery embolization or myomectomy.

GnRH agonists

At present, it is only possible to comment on the results of treatment with GnRH agonist analogues although the antagonists are likely to give rise to similar or improved results in the future. Randomized controlled studies (Friedman 1993, West 1993) have demonstrated that treatment with a GnRH analogue prior to hysterectomy results in significant improvements in preoperative haemoglobin concentrations as well as reduced operative blood loss and fewer blood transfusions. Particular benefits for the patients are greater use of low transverse rather than midline surgical incisions and of the vaginal rather than the abdominal route. Reduced blood loss at myomectomy has also been reported in cases where initial uterine volume exceeded 600 ml, but there is no evidence that pregnancy rates are improved following pretreatment. Benefits for hysteroscopic myomectomy have been confirmed in non-randomized studies (Perino et al 1993) with significant reductions in operating time, blood loss and in the volume of distension medium infused.

Specific complications may be associated with the use of GnRH agonists for fibroids (West 1993). Failure of menstrual suppression, with continued irregular bleeding, occurs in 20–30% of women. This may be related to the presence of submucosal fibroids and several cases of acute prolapse associated with severe haemorrhage have been reported. Opponents of the use of GnRH agonists argue that this treatment delays the achievement of a definitive tissue diagnosis and thus cases of uterine sarcoma may be missed. Such cases are extremely rare but their reported occurrence does emphasize the need to adequately monitor the response to medical therapy of women with known fibroids and to consider further investigation or surgical intervention should symptoms not respond adequately and promptly.

The use of GnRH analogues as adjuncts to surgery thus remains a subject of debate. Few countries have granted product licences as yet for fibroid-related indications and there is agreement that the additional costs do not justify their routine use. Specific indications would include severe preoperative anaemia, to facilitate vaginal hysterectomy and for preoperative shrinkage of particularly large or awkwardly situated fibroids. For myomectomy, opinions vary and in the absence of large randomized studies with long-term follow-up, gynaecologists must weigh up the merits of such therapy for their individual patients. As an adjunct to endoscopic myomectomy, the current consensus is in favour of their use.

Uterine artery embolization (UAE)

Transarterial embolization for the successful treatment of obstetric and gynaecological haemorrhage has been practised for over 20 years (Heaston et al 1979). It has been used subsequently in various situations ranging from postpartum and post-caesarean haemorrhage, haemorrhage following gynaecological surgery (benign and malignant) and arteriovenous malformation.

The initial report of the use of UAE as a therapy for symptomatic uterine fibroids appeared in 1995 and the same group then reported a larger series of 88 patients (Ravina et al 1997). A mean percentage fibroid shrinkage as measured by ultrasound of 69% was reported. Nine patients underwent subsequent hysterectomy, eight for pain, one for bleeding associated with a submucous fibroid. A number of other series have now been reported with variable results of percentage shrinkage of fibroids (Goodwin et al 1999, Spies et al 1999).

Technique

The date of last menses should be assessed and a urine pregnancy test done to exclude pregnancy. The objective of the procedure is to occlude both uterine arteries with particulate emboli and hence induce ischaemic necrosis of the uterine fibroids whilst having no adverse effect in the long term on the normal uterus.

UAE should only be carried out in a specialist angiographic suite by experienced interventional radiologists. The normal approach is a transfemoral one most commonly via the right side. A guidewire is manipulated until it engages in the uterine artery and allows the catheter to be advanced. Embolization is then performed, most commonly utilizing polyvinyl alcohol (PVA) of a variety of particulate sizes (150–1000 microns) suspended in a contrast solution (Fig. 33.13).

Complications

Complications of the technique include failure to cannulate the relevant artery (8–11%); local haematoma formation or thrombosis and femoral arterial damage; severe pain (due to infarction of fibroid), often requiring narcotic analgesia for 24–36 hours; borderline pyrexia and persistent vaginal discharge.

Fibroid expulsion occurs in up to 10% of cases and larger fibroids may cause pain at expulsion or become obstructed in the cervix. Such a complication is more common with submucous fibroids.

Following the procedure serious infection associated with the necrotic process in the fibroid occurs in 1–2% of patients. Such an infection has been associated with a patient's death following UAE (Vashist et al 1999). Single-dose prophylactic antibiotic therapy is reasonable at the time of the procedure to try and reduce the risk of infection. However, when a patient presents with late infection associated with an offensive discharge, urgent gynaecological care is needed with intensive antibiotic therapy and assessment of the need for surgical intervention.

Amenorrhoea may follow the procedure and be either permanent or temporary, with a frequency of not more than 1%.

Indications for UAE

UAE offers an alternative conservative treatment approach. Early results are encouraging but long-term follow-up data on efficacy of controlling symptoms, complications and recurrence rates are required.

Accurate pretreatment diagnosis is essential and the patient should be warned of the possible need for a hysterectomy,

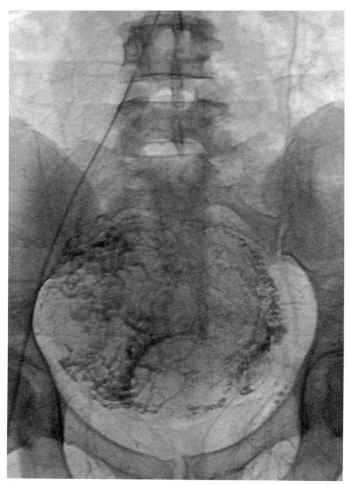

Fig. 33.13 Catheter inserted via right femoral artery. The contrast medium clearly shows marked vasculature around a fibroid prior to embolization.

blood transfusion or failure to be able to perform UAE. Women who are infertile or who may wish to become pregnant subsequently present particular problems. They should be warned that treatment may not result in a subsequent pregnancy and that there is little evidence on subsequent pregnancy outcomes although one report of a small series of cases is encouraging (Ravina et al 2000).

The technique of UAE is not available in every hospital and requires radiologists with the relevant interventional radiology skills. UAE looks a promising technique for which further long-term data are required but may well prove to be another alternative to myomectomy in appropriately selected patients.

FUTURE DIRECTIONS

It is astonishing that uterine fibroids affect at least half of women during their reproductive years, are the most common reason for the most common gynaecological major operation performed in women, exhibit consistent epidemiological differences between racial groups and result in major hospital charges in all developed countries and yet there is almost no high-quality evidence on which to base treatment. One future direction may be for national and internatinal societies interested in women's health to develop standardized reporting measures for uterine fibroids. Standardized measures of the severity of uterine fibroids and the outcome of whatever treatment is chosen would help comparison between studies. For example, standardized reporting of excessive bleeding or dysmenorrhoea or non-cyclical pelvic pain would be useful. Perhaps thought should be given to the validation of a staging system similar to that used for gynaecological cancer.

Another future direction could be to carefully plan randomized controlled trials about the effectiveness of medical therapy. Proving or disproving the effectiveness of commonly used medical agents such as oral contraceptives or NSAIDs should increase their use or eliminate these agents from medical treatment. Long-term follow-up studies are urgently required for this common tumour. Appropriate statistical methods and clinical trial methods are performed for other diseases and would be certainly possible for uterine fibroids. For example, long-term follow-up of cohorts of women, if performed carefully, would give a body of information on patients who had myomectomy and patients who had, say, UAE, which would at least provide enough information to help design a randomized trial. Appropriate statistical tests such as survival analysis could then be undertaken.

Future lab-based research will undoubtedly make use of recently developed tools for gene expression and protein analysis, such as the microarray and proteomics, to identify differences in gene expression between fibroids and normal uterine muscle. Such work is already under way in several centres. In time, data should emerge from such studies that will improve our understanding of the molecular basis of fibroids and their progression. The inevitable aim will be to identify new targets for drugs, as either stand-alone or adjuvant therapies.

Future directions in uterine fibroid research might also look at the question of the prevalence of fibroids in asymptomatic women. How many, if followed up, will develop symptoms? What outpatient management of symptomatic uterine fibroids occurs and what percentage of women proceed to surgery? Do the differences apparently observed between uterine fibroids in black and white women arise because the biology of the fibroids or uterus is different in black women or because of difference in ages at pregnancy or cultural differences in terms of severity or socioeconomic factors affecting when the patient seeks medical care?

KEY POINTS

1. Uterine fibroids are common, benign tumours of the uterus affecting approximately 20% of women of reproductive age.
2. Uterine fibroids are more common in black women in whom they present at an earlier age.
3. Many cells within the fibroid are chromosomally abnormal, which may result in their abnormal cell division.

KEY POINTS (*CONTINUED*)

4. Uterine fibroids seem to be hormone sensitive. They do not occur until the menarche and reduce in size at the menopause. Progesterones may play a major role in fibroid growth.

5. Fibroids may undergo hyaline or fatty degeneration, calcification and red degeneration.

6. Fibroids may adversely affect reproductive function by enlargement and distortion of the uterus and disturbance of uterine blood flow.

7. Asymptomatic fibroids may be managed conservatively without harmful effects, with regression at the time of menopause to be expected.

8. Medical management of fibroids may control patient symptoms but does not result in complete fibroid regression.

9. GnRH analogues may be used to shrink fibroids prior to hysterectomy or myomectomy.

10. Sarcoma (leiomyosarcoma) occurs in one in one million women each year and presents as, typically, postmenopausal bleeding. Fear of sarcoma is not an indication for removal of a fibroid.

11. When using GnRH analogues to limit or shrink fibroid growth, the vasomotor and oesteoporotic side-effects may be reduced by addition of hormone replacement therapy.

12. Hysteroscopic and laparoscopic management of fibroids can provide good symptomatic relief and may reduce postoperative morbidity. The gynaecologist should undergo adequate training before embarking on such procedures.

13. Myomectomy may result in conception in women who were previously infertile. The spontaneous abortion rate is reduced but remains above that of the general population.

REFERENCES

Aharoni A, Reiter A, Golan D et al 1988 Patterns of growth of uterine leiomyomas during pregnancy. A prospective longitudinal study. British Journal of Obstetrics and Gynaecology 95:510–513

Brandon DD, Bethea CL, Strawn EY et al 1993 Progesterone receptor messenger ribonucleic acid and protein are overexpressed in human uterine leiomyomas. American Journal of Obstetrics and Gynecology 169(1):78–85

Buttram VC, Reiter RC 1981 Uterine leiomyomata: etiology, symptomatology and management. Fertility and Sterility 36:433–445

Casey R, Rogers PAW, Vollenhoven BJ 2000 An immunohistochemical analysis of fibroid vasculature. Human Reproduction 15(7):1469–1475

Cramer SF, Patel A 1990 The frequency of uterine leiomyomas. American Journal of Clinical Pathology 94:435–438

Crow J, Gardner RL, McSweeney G et al 1995 Morphological changes in uterine leiomyomas treated by GnRH agonist goserelin. International Journal of Gynaecological Pathology 14:235–248

Donnez J, Gillerot S, Bougonjon D et al 1990 Neodymium:YAG laser hysteroscopy in large submucous fibroids. Fertility and Sterility 54:999–1003

Drews MR, Reyniak JV 1992 Surgical approach to myomas: laparoscopy and hysteroscopy. Seminars in Reproductive Endocrinology 10:367–377

Eldar-Geva T, Meagher S, Healy DL et al 1998 Effect of intramural, subserosal and submucosal uterine fibroids on the outcome of assisted reproductive technology treatment. Fertility and Sterility 70:687–691

Forssman L 1976a Blood flow in myomatous uteri as measured by intra-arterial 133Xenon. Acta Obstetrica et Gynecologica Scandinavica 55(1):21–24

Forssman L 1976b Distribution of blood flow in myomatous uteri as measured by locally injected 133Xenon. Acta Obstetrica et Gynecologica Scandinavica 55(2):101–104

Friedman AJ 1993 Treatment of uterine myomas with GnRH agonists. Seminars in Reproductive Endocrinology 11:154–161

Gard GB, Mulvany NJ, Quinn MA 1999 Management of uterine leiomosarcoma in Australia. Australia and New Zealand Journal of Obstetrics and Gynaecology 39:93–98

Goodwin SC, McLucas B, Lee M, Chen G, Perrela R, Vedantham S 1999 Uterine artery embolisation for the treatment of uterine leimyomata – mid term results. Journal of Vascular Interventional Radiology 10:1159–65

Gustavson I, Englund K, Faxen M et al 2000 Tissue differences but limited sex steroid responsiveness of *c-fos* and *c-jun* in human fibroids and myometrium. Molecular Human Reproduction 6(1):55–59

Harrison-Woolrych ML, Sharkey AM, Charnock-Jones DS, Smith SK 1995 Localization and quantification of vascular endothelial growth factor messenger ribonucleic acid in human myometrium and leiomyomata. Journal of Clinical Endocrinology and Metabolism 80(6):1853–1858

Healy DL, Petrucco O 1998 Effective gynecological day surgery. Chapman and Hall Medical, London

Heaston DK, Mineau DE, Brown BJ, Miller FJ 1979 Trans-catheter arterial embolisation for control of persistent massive puerperal haemorrhage after bilateral surgical hypogastric artery ligation. American Journal of Roentgenology 133:152–154

Karasick S, Lev-Toaff AS, Toaff ME 1992 Imaging of uterine leiomyomas. American Journal of Roentgenology 158:799–805

Kawaguchi K, Fujii S, Konishi I et al 1989 Mitotic activity in uterine leiomyomas during the menstrual cycle. American Journal of Obstetrics and Gynecology 160:637–641

Kettel LM, Murphy AA, Morales AJ et al 1993 Rapid regression of leiomyomas in response to daily administration of gonadotrophin releasing hormone antagonist. Fertility and Sterility 60:642–646

Kim JG, Kim MH, Kim IS et al 2000 Decreased expression of mac25 mRNA in uterine leiomyomata compared with adjacent myometrium. American Journal of Reproductive Immunology 43(1):53–57

Marshall LM, Spiegelman D, Barbieri R et al 1997 Variation in the incidence of uterine leiomyoma among premenopausal women by age and race. Obstetrics and Gynecology 90:967–973

Matsuo H, Kurachi O, Shimomura Y et al 1999 Molecular bases for the actions of ovarian sex steroids in the regulation of proliferation and apoptosis of human uterine leiomyoma. Oncology 57(suppl 2):49–58

Monaghan JM 1986 Bonney's gynaecological surgery, 9th edn. Baillière Tindall, London

Nilsson L, Rybo G 1971 Treatment of menorrhagia. American Journal of Obstetrics and Gynecology 110:713–720

Perino A, Chianchiano N, Petronio M et al 1993 Role of leuprolide acetate depot in hysteroscopic surgery: a controlled study. Fertility and Sterility 59:507–510

Ravina JH, Bouret JM, Ciraru-Vigneron N, Repiquet D, Herbreteau D, Aymard A 1997 Recourse to particulate arterial embolisation in the treatment of some uterine leimyomata. Bulletin of the Academy of National Medicine 191:233–46

Ravina JH, Ciraru-Vigneron N, Aynard A, Le Def O, Merland JJ 2000 Pregnancy after embolisation of uterine myoma: report of 12 cases. Fertility and Sterility 73:1241–1243

Reinsch RC, Murphy AA, Morales AJ et al 1994 The effects of RU 486 and leuprolide acetate on uterine artery blood flow in the fibroid uterus: a prospective, randomised study. American Journal of Obstetrics and Gynecology 170:1623–1628

Reiter RC, Wagner PLG, Ambone JC 1992 Routine hysterectomy for asymptomatic uterine fibroids: a reappraisal. Obstetrics and Gynecology 79:481–484

Ross RK, Pike MC, Vessey MP et al 1986 Risk factors for uterine fibroids: reduced risk associated with oral contraceptives. British Medical Journal 293:359–362

Rybo G, Leman J, Tibblin R 1985 Epidemiology of menstrual blood loss. In: Baird DT, Michie EA (eds) Mechanisms of menstrual bleeding. Raven Press, New York, pp 181–193

Siegler AM, Valle RF 1988 Therapeutic hysteroscopic procedures. Fertility and Sterility 50:685–701

Sozen I, Olive DL, Arici A 1998 Expression and hormonal regulation of monocyte chemotactic protein-l in myometrium and leiomyomata. Fertility and Sterility 69 (6):1095–1102

Spies JB, Scialli AR, lha RC, Imaoka I, Ascher SM, Fraga VM 1999 initial results from uterine fibroid embolisation for symptomatic leimyoma. Journal of Vascular Interventional Radiology 10:1149–57

Townsend DE, Sparkes RS, Baluda MC et al 1970 Unicellular histogenesis of uterine leiomyomas as determined by electrophoresis of glucose-6-phosphate dehydrogenase. American Journal of Obstetrics and Gynecology 107:1168–1173

Van Eijkeren MA, Christiaens GCML, Scholten N et al 1992 Menorrhagia. Current concepts. Drugs 43:201–209

Vashist A, Studd J, Carey A 1999 Fatal septicaemia after fibroid embolisation. Lancet 354:307–308

Verkauf BS 1992 Myomectomy for fertility enhancement and preservation. Fertility and Sterility 58:1–15

Vollenhoven BJ, Herington AC, Healy DL 1993 Messenger ribonucleic acid expression of the insulin-like growth factors and their binding proteins in uterine fibroids and myometrium. J Clin. Endocrin. Metabol 76:1106–1110

West CP 1993 GnRH analogues in the treatment of fibroids. Reproductive Medicine Reviews 2:1–97

West CP, Lumsden MA 1989 Fibroids and menorrhagia. Baillière's Clinical Obstetrics and Gynaecology 3:357–374

34
Endometriosis
Robert W. Shaw

INTRODUCTION

Endometriosis is one of the most common benign gynaecological conditions. It is second only to uterine fibroids as the most common reason for major surgical procedures in women under 45. It has been estimated that it is present in between 10% and 25% of women presenting with gynaecological symptoms in the UK or USA (Tyson 1974). These figures are based on the findings of patients who have undergone laparoscopy for diagnostic indications such as pelvic pain or infertility or in patients undergoing laparotomy. Although it is such a widespread condition, it is true to say that little is understood regarding its aetiology and pathogenesis and the condition still arouses much controversy with regard to its treatment and management.

DEFINITION

Endometriosis is defined as a disease characterized by the presence of tissue that is morphologically and biologically similar to normal endometrium and contains functional endometrial glands and stroma in ectopic locations outside the uterine cavity. This ectopic endometrial tissue responds to hormones and drugs in a generally similar manner to ectopic endometrium undergoing cyclical changes. Cyclical bleeding from the endometriotic deposit appears to contribute to the induction of a local inflammatory reaction, fibrous adhesion, formation and, in the case of deep ovarian implants in the ovary, leads to the formation of an endometrioma or chocolate cyst. Endometrial tissue deep within the myometrium of the uterine wall is termed adenomyosis. This condition is

Box 34.1 Prevalence of endometriosis through various presentations

Unexplained infertility	70–80%[1]
Infertile women (all causes)	15–20%[1]
At diagnostic laparoscopy	0–53%[2]
At treatment laparoscopy	0.1–50%[2]
Women undergoing sterilizations	2%[3]
In women with diagnosed 1° relatives	7%[4]

[1]Kistner 1977; [2]Houston 1984; [3]Strathy et al 1982; [4]Simpson et al 1980

Table 34.1 Frequency of the more common symptoms in endometriosis patients

Symptom	Likely frequency (%)
Dysmenorrhoea	60–80
Pelvic pain	30–50
Infertility	30–40
Dyspareunia	25–40
Menstrual irregularities	10–20
Cyclical dysuria/haematuria	1–2
Dyschesia	1–2
Rectal bleeding (cyclic)	<1

increasingly being viewed as a separate pathological entity to that of endometriosis since it affects a different population of women and probably has a different aetiology.

PREVALENCE

Continued growth of endometriotic tissue, as with that of the endometrium, is dependent on ovarian steroid hormones, particularly oestrogen. Thus endometriosis is prevalent in the reproductive years with a peak incidence between 30 and 45 years of age, although it is increasingly being diagnosed in much younger women as the threshold for investigation of gynaecological symptoms utilizing diagnostic laparoscopy has altered. Endometriosis is thus primarily a disease of the reproductive years and is only rarely described in adolescence, when it is associated with obstructing genital tract abnormalities or in postmenopausal women where it has been reactivated because of hormone replacement therapy.

No racial differences in the incidence of the disease have been found except for Japanese women who have been reported to have twice the incidence of Caucasian women (Miyazawa 1976).

The exact prevalence of endometriosis is unknown since precise diagnosis depends on observation of implants predominantly at the time of laparoscopy or laparotomy and until simple non-invasive screening tests are developed, the true prevalence will remain unknown. Current prevalence therefore depends upon identification in women who are either symptomatic or undergoing various operative procedures (Box 34.1). The incidence is markedly variable as the data in Table 34.1 show. Endometriosis commonly affects women during their child-bearing years. In the main this is reflected in deleterious sexual, reproductive and social consequences as a result of its associated painful symptoms and often associated infertility. Symptomatology may extend over several decades of a patient's life because of its often late diagnosis and the recurrent nature of the disease. For individual patients and healthcare systems it represents a major call upon resource use.

AETIOLOGY

The precise aetiology of endometriosis still remains unknown. Indeed, it is often called the disease of theories because of the many mechanisms postulated to explain its pathogenesis (Fig. 34.1). It is likely that no one of these theories would

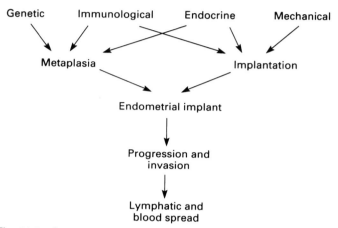

Fig. 34.1 Suggested aetiological factors in the pathogenesis of endometriotic implants.

explain all forms of endometriosis and in an individual a combination of factors is necessary to allow endometriosis to develop fully. The two major theories of causation of endometriosis are:

- implantation of endometrial fragments which reach the pelvic cavity by retrograde menstruation
- metaplasia of the coelomic epithelium.

Menstrual regurgitation and implantation (metastatic theory)

As early as 1927 Sampson proposed the metastatic theory, postulating that retrograde menstrual flow transported desquamated endometrial fragments through the fallopian tubes into the peritoneal cavity. Once there, the still viable cells subsequently implanted and began growth and invasion. In support of this theory, experimental endometriosis has been induced in animals with replacement of menstrual fluid or endometrial tissue to the peritoneal cavity. Supporting this theory in humans is the finding that in young girls with associated abnormalities in the genital tract causing obstruction to the outflow of menstrual fluid, endometriosis is commonly found (Schifrin et al 1973). Halme et al (1984) observed bloody fluid at the time of menstruation in the pelvis during laparoscopic assessment but as this finding occurs in up to 90% of all women it is regarded as a physiological phenomenon. The high incidence of retrograde menstruation suggests that this phenomenon alone does not give rise to endometriosis but that some other factor(s) must be involved in the development of the disease. These factors could include some alteration in the (uterine) endometrium; altered immune response to retrograde menstruation (hence failure to clear the peritoneal cavity of debris efficiently); or alternatively a more favourable peritoneal environment which may stimulate the growth and implantation of ectopic endometrium within the peritoneal cavity itself.

Further support of the metastatic theories comes from the observation of endometriotic foci in a laparotomy scar after uterine surgery or caesarean section or within episiotomy scars following delivery. In addition, lymphatic or vascular spread is postulated to explain the presence of endometriosis in extragenital locations such as the lung, skeletal muscle, joints, skin and kidney.

Metaplasia theory

This theory, first described by Meyer (1919), postulated the possibility of differentiation by metaplasia towards an endometrial-like tissue of the original coelomic membrane following prolonged irritation and oestrogen stimulation. It is proposed that these adult cells undergo de-differentiation back to their primitive origin and then transform to endometrial cells. This theory has many attractions which could explain the occurrence of endometriosis in nearly all the ectopic sites in the presence of aberrant müllerian cells. What induces this transformation – whether it is hormonal stimuli, inflammatory irritation or other processes – is uncertain. If coelomic metaplasia is similar to metaplasia elsewhere the frequency of the disorder should increase with advancing age. The clinical pattern of endometriosis is distinctly different from this with an abrupt halt in the disease with the cessation of menses at the menopause and reduced oestrogen production, thus raising some questions over this theory.

Genetic and immunological factors

Many studies indicate that there may be a genetic factor related to endometriosis since the disease is more prevalent in certain families. It has been shown that there is a seven times higher risk of developing endometriosis, which may be severe, in women with an affected first-degree relative (Halme et al 1986, Simpson et al 1980). Endometriosis is also more common in monozygotic twin sisters than dizygotic twins, but no association was found with specifically identified tissue types (Simpson et al 1984). Whilst Dmowski et al (1981) demonstrated a decreased cellular immunity to endometriotic tissue in women with endometriosis, no clinically significant immune system abnormality has been observed in women with the disease; hence, the precise genetic or immune components increasing an individual's potential to develop this disorder are yet to be defined.

Conclusion

The conclusion reached from the above theories is that pelvic endometriosis is probably a consequence of transplantation of viable endometrial cells regurgitated at the time of menstruation from the fallopian tubes into the peritoneal cavity. In addition, transport of endometrial cells may occur by other routes (some iatrogenic). It is unclear whether endometriotic implants are derived from in situ pluripotential cells generated by metastatic seeding, but it is known that endocrine and immunological factors allow the growth and spread within the pelvis and neighbouring organs. Delayed child bearing, either by choice or infertility, has been implicated as risk factor for the development of endometriosis. The risk of developing endometriosis also corresponds with cumulative menstruation, menstrual frequency and volume. Women with shorter menstrual cycles of less than 27 days and longer flows (more than 7 days) are twice as likely to develop the disease than those with longer cycles and short numbers of days of blood loss.

PERITONEAL FLUID ENVIRONMENT IN ENDOMETRIOSIS

It has been suggested that peritoneal fluid volume and its contents may be adversely affected by the presence of endometriotic tissue in the pelvis, with possible consequent interference with tubo-ovarian function and/or fertilization and early implantation. Peritoneal fluid is an ultrafiltrate of plasma and in normal women the volumes are very low. Endometriosis may alter the peritoneal fluid volume by increasing fluid production in the ovary, altering mesothelial permeability or increasing the hydrostatic pressure as a result of altered protein content.

Peritoneal macrophages

Normal peritoneal fluid contains approximately 10^6 cells per ml of which 90% are macrophages, the remainder being lymphocytes and desquamated mesothelial cells. The role of peritoneal macrophages in women with endometriosis has been the source of much interest and women with endometriosis associated with infertility have been reported as having significantly higher concentrations of macrophages in peritoneal fluid than either fertile women or infertile women without endometriosis. Macrophages in patients with endometriosis appeared to be highly phagocytic against spermatozoa in vitro, compared with those from fertile women or infertile women without endometriosis (Muscato et al 1982). In addition, they are also able to survive better in vitro than those from fertile controls (Halme et al 1986). Peritoneal fluid from patients with endometriosis has also been shown to have a cytotoxic effect on in vivo cleavage of mouse embryos. These findings on the quantitative and qualitative properties of macrophages in peritoneal fluid may partially explain the mechanisms of infertility in patients with endometriosis.

Prostaglandins and prostanoids

The role of prostaglandins and their metabolites in peritoneal fluid in the pathogenesis and symptomatology of endometriosis is controversial. It has been reported that increased levels of prostaglandin $F_{2\alpha}$ ($PGF_{2\alpha}$) are found in peritoneal fluid patients with the disease (Meldrum et al 1977); also increased peritoneal fluid volume and increased concentrations of the prostaglandin metabolites thromboxane B_2 and 6-keto $PGF_{2\alpha}$ have been noted. Other investigators have found no increase in either the volume of peritoneal fluid or its concentrations of prostaglandins or metabolites (Rock et al 1982). These conflicting reports may reflect the timing of peritoneal fluid sampling and difficulties in assay measurement of the small quantities of substrates all of which have very short half-lives.

It has been appreciated in recent years that more subtle forms of endometriosis may be present with only minimal evidence of visual changes in the peritoneum. However, if there are changes in the peritoneal fluid prostaglandin content, the mechanisms by which these changes influence endometriosis or its association with infertility remain unclear.

Cytokines and growth factors

A large number of cells, including macrophages, lymphocytes, fibroblasts and epithelial cells, synthesize a wide range of polypeptides of high biological activity all within the cytokinine/growth factor group. They have multiple effects including the regulation of differentiation, growth and function of a wide variety of cell types. It was generally believed that cytokines were produced in increased amounts as part of the inflammatory process or as part of a response to infection or immune challenge. Cytokines are very potent and active at picogram to nanogram levels and are difficult to detect and identify. Research activity has been concentrated on the measurement of various cytokines including various interleukins, colony stimulating factors, human necrosis factor and transforming growth factors. No consistent changes between normal, infertile women with and without endometriosis and patients with endometriosis who are not infertile have to date been reported to satisfactorily explain the aetiology or pathogenesis of the disease.

Peritoneal environment: conclusions

Peritoneal macrophages play an important role in the peritoneal cavity where endometrial tissue fragments often arrive and are likely to adhere to the mesothelial lining. The adherence may be mediated by cell adhesion molecules and other factors produced by activated macrophages. Endometrial tissue will potentially adhere if the regurgitated amount of the tissue is too great or if the capacity of the intra-abdominal cells to clear the cellular debris is in any way impaired. Once an endometrial fragment has gained adherence, further tissue growth may be promoted by steroids, cytokines, growth factors and angiogenic factors present in peritoneal fluid in a paracrine and autocrine fashion.

SYMPTOMATOLOGY

The symptoms of endometriosis are variable and often unrelated to the extent of the disease process as currently quantified. The three most frequent complaints amongst women with endometriosis are: dysmenorrhoea, dyspareunia and pelvic pain. The pain symptoms are often cycle related and increased premenstrually. However, it must be stated that the finding of endometriosis may not conclusively link it with painful symptoms in an individual since the severity of symptoms is rarely correlated with the extent of the disease and endometriosis is often found coincidentally during surgery or investigation for other gynaecological conditions such as infertility to similar levels in patients not complaining of pain.

Atypical bleeding patterns are a leading symptom in a variety of gynaecological diseases but may also characterize endometriosis patients. Premenstrual spotting and menometrorrhagia are frequently noted (Wentz 1980). On the other hand cyclical rectal bleeding or haematuria is pathognomonic of the disease and although rarely observed (1–2% of cases), these symptoms give strong evidence for bowel or bladder involvement. Painful micturition or defaecation at the time of menstruation may be the first signs of progressing disease. Symptoms of endometriosis related to the sites of implants are outlined in Table 34.2.

Pelvic pain

Pelvic pain is arguably the symptom causing the most misery amongst endometriosis sufferers and is more distressing than infertility. Chronic pelvic pain, as with other forms of pain, often produces a serious long-term detrimental effect on the personality and affects working ability and social and marital life.

Dysmenorrhoea

Dysmenorrhoea often occurs with pelvic pain but patients commonly describe a background of constant dragging, aching pain which may be exacerbated by the menses but is often a different type of pain from the typical cramping nature of spasmodic dysmenorrhoea and often in a different site.

Table 34.2 Symptoms of endometriosis related to sites of implants

Symptoms	Site
Dysmenorrhoea Lower abdominal pain Pelvic pain Low back pain Menstrual irregularity Rupture/torsion endometrioma Infertility	Reproductive organs
Cyclical rectal bleeding Tenesmus Diarrhoea/cyclic constipation	Gastrointestinal tract
Cyclical haematuria Dysuria (cyclical) Ureteric obstruction	Urinary tract
Cyclical haemoptysis	Lungs
Cyclical pain and bleeding	Surgical scars/umbilicus
Cyclical pain and swelling	Limbs

The basis of the pelvic pain and dysmenorrhoea is uncertain but could reflect stretching of tissues by the menstrual process and an effect of the local production of prostaglandins within the endometriotic implants. The pain also relates to tissue damage and fixity of organs from scar and adhesion formation. What is immediately clear when reviewing patients with endometriosis is the huge variation in extent of symptomatic disease which does not correlate with the extent of the observed disease process. In addition, many patients who are asymptomatic are found to have endometriosis and in some of these patients, severe disease is discovered following laparoscopy during infertility investigations. One possible explanation for this is that in these individuals the disease may have disrupted the pelvic sensation altogether.

Dyspareunia

One of the common symptoms of endometriosis is deep dyspareunia resulting from stretching at intercourse of the involved pelvic tissues such as a fixed retroverted uterus, the uterosacral ligaments or rectovaginal septum or pressure on an involved enlarged ovary. The presence of endometriotic tissue within these areas, however, is not always associated with dyspareunia; perhaps less than half the patients who are coitally active admit to this symptom when deposits are found in these areas.

Whilst the symptoms of dysmenorrhoea, dyspareunia and pelvic pain can occur with other gynaecological pathologies, it is the cyclical, menstrually related component of several symptoms which should alert the clinician to the potential diagnosis of endometriosis.

Correlation between severity of endometriosis and severity of pain

There appears to be little correlation between sites involved in endometriosis and symptoms complained of. Various 'types' of symptoms can, however, to some degree be related to the system involved (see Table 34.2). However, these do not always correlate with the anatomy and type of pain innervation of the pelvis (for review, see MacLaverty & Shaw 1995).

One reason for this apparent lack of correlation between disease severity and symptom severity is that the classification systems for endometriosis so far developed have primarily been directed towards infertility prediction rather than pain symptom severity.

Deeply infiltrating endometriosis is very strongly associated with the presence and severity of pelvic pain (Koninckx et al 1991). In addition, superficial non-pigmented endometriosis has the capacity to produce more prostaglandin F (PGF) than pigmented classic powder burn lesions. PGF is implicated in pain causation (Vernon et al 1986). Thus in the early, less florid stages before it has become destructive and more easily recognized, endometriosis may be producing large quantities of PGF and hence possess a greater potential to increase severity of pain. The type of pain may alter with the disease progression, with constant pain and exacerbation at the menses present initially in the disease, but pain later becoming continuous due to scar formation and organ fixity.

Conclusions

The symptoms of endometriosis are similar to those of other common gynaecological conditions and may be similar to disorders of the gastrointestinal and urinary genital system. For this reason many women with endometriosis have delayed diagnosis of their condition and may well have been treated for other assumed disorders prior to the definitive diagnosis being made. One of the greatest sources of complaints amongst women with endometriosis is their perception of a delay in making the true diagnosis often because general practitioners and other specialists fail to consider it as a diagnostic possibility.

The aetiology of pain in endometriosis is uncertain given the poor correlation between the extent of endometriosis and the degree of pain symptoms. One could conclude that endometriosis does not cause pelvic pain and the finding of this disease process at laparoscopy in a patient complaining of pelvic pain symptoms is coincidental. Alternatively it could be postulated that endometriosis exists in many different forms, only some of which cause pain. However, in the absence of a universally accepted hypothesis that explains how endometriosis can cause pain, especially in the case of minimal/mild disease, many clinicians propose that women with endometriosis have an altered pelvic environment that interferes with infertility and provides the mechanism for pain which accumulates support for the role of macrophages in endometriosis and its symptomatology. Activated macrophages may release factors which interfere with reproduction and activate nociceptors. Fibrosis, a common finding associated with endometriosis itself, may lead to ischaemic changes in deep-seated disease, whilst direct invasion of nerve endings is a clear possible explanation of causation of pain.

ENDOMETRIOSIS AND INFERTILITY

It is accepted that endometriosis resulting in structural damage to the tubes and ovaries causes infertility. However, what is less clear is whether the milder forms of endometriosis are likewise the cause of infertility, in otherwise asymptomatic patients.

Endometriosis is one of the most frequently made diagnoses in couples undergoing infertility investigation, as routine use of laparoscopy for investigation of such couples has been employed in recent years. The assumption is made that the endometriotic implants are responsible for the patient's inability to conceive. Estimates of the incidence of endometriosis in the general population of reproductive age vary between 2% and 10% (Barbieri 1990). From retrospective studies in infertile patients the incidence has been reported as being between 20% and 40% (Mahmood & Templeton 1990). This increased incidence in infertile patients has led many clinicians to consider the endometriotic implants responsible, in some way, for the associated infertility. The question is how and a number of suggested mechanisms have been reported. These are summarized in Table 34.3.

Tubo-ovarian dysfunction

Increased levels of prostaglandins in peritoneal fluid have been reported in infertile women with endometriosis (Drake et al

Table 34.3 Possible mechanisms of causation of infertility with mild endometriosis

Problem area	Mechanism
Ovarian function	Endocrinopathies
	Anovulation
	LUF syndrome
	Altered prolactin release
	Altered gonadotrophin midcycle surge
	Luteolysis caused by $PGF_{2\alpha}$
	Oocyte maturation defects
Coital function	Dyspareunia causing reduced penetration and coital frequency
Tubal function	Alterations in tubal and cilial motility by prostaglandins
	Impaired fimbrial oocyte pick-up
Sperm function	Phagocytosis by macrophages
	Inactivation by antibodies
Endometrium	Interference by endometrial antibodies
	Luteal phase deficiency
Early pregnancy failure	Increased early abortion
	Prostaglandin induced or immune reaction

LUF, luteinized unruptured follicle; $PGF_{2\alpha}$, prostaglandin $F_{2\alpha}$.

1981). It has been suggested that these prostaglandins may have an adverse impact on fertility by causing tubal dysfunction which could alter sperm, oocyte or embryo transport. However, tubal transport of the oocyte in the distal tube is dependent primarily upon cilial action that is not known to be prostaglandin dependent.

Elevated peritoneal prostaglandin levels have also been invoked to explain altered luteal function but again there is little evidence to suggest that prostaglandins are luteolytic in primates.

Subtle alterations in the pattern of LH surges with increased prolactin secretion which may alter luteal progesterone synthesis have also been suggested, but with little confirmatory evidence when comparable studies have been repeated in other centres.

More recently, a variety of follicular phase defects have been observed in women with mild endometriosis, including a range of abnormal follicular growth patterns, shortened follicular phases and decreased follicular size. Such changes may cause an alteration to the maturation of oocytes and result in reduced potential for fertilization following oocyte release. However, experiences of workers in in vitro fertilization (IVF) have not added support that such features are likely to be relevant, since comparable fertilization rates are achieved in endometriosis patients as compared to other diagnostic groups (Chillik et al 1985).

Luteinized unruptured follicle (LUF) syndrome

Based upon the reports of altered peritoneal levels of gonadal steroids in the luteal phase, a lack of sonographic disappearance of the follicle at midcycle and an inability to visualize an ovulatory stigma during laparoscopy in the luteal phase, Koninckx et al (1980) developed the hypothesis of the luteinized unruptured follicle (LUF) syndrome. More widespread investigation has shown that the LUF syndrome can occur in a wide variety of infertility cases and does not appear to be a consistent feature of consecutive cycles. At present it is concluded that LUF syndrome is unlikely to be an important contributing factor to either infertility in general or endometriosis-associated infertility specifically.

Autoimmunity

The presence of ectopic endometrial implants in women with endometriosis has been postulated to lead to an autoimmune response resulting in implantation failure. Autoantibodies to endometrial tissue have been identified in both the serum and peritoneal fluid of some women with endometriosis, although many studies have failed to show consistent differences between endometriosis patients, other infertile women or fertile controls. The absence of any differences in implantation rates between patients with endometriosis and other infertility causes in women undergoing IVF treatment further suggests that the role of antibodies and the causal relationship between endometriosis and infertility is unlikely to be proven.

Habitual/recurrent abortion

A number of factors affect the rate of spontaneous abortion, including the likelihood that infertile women document pregnancies earlier than the general population and a relationship with increasing age. Such a relationship in endometriosis has been suggested, following the observation that treatment of endometriosis significantly reduced the spontaneous abortion rate. However, further controlled prospective trials have failed to confirm these earlier findings (Pittaway et al 1988), thus bringing this relationship also into question.

Peritoneal environment

In addition to the reported change in peritoneal prostaglandin levels discussed previously, it has been suggested that an increased number of macrophages in the peritoneum may increase the rate of sperm phagocytosis and that other secretory products from activated macrophages may also have toxic effects on the gametes. This is supported by Curtis et al (1993) who reported a degree of sperm toxicity with reduced sperm motility in the presence of peritoneal fluid in patients with endometriosis compared with fertile controls and other infertility subgroups.

Abnormal oocytes

Fertilization rates in vitro are a partial quantitative evaluation of oocyte and sperm function. The fertilization rates per oocyte and per couple when compared in women with minimal/mild endometriosis to those in unexplained infertility or tubal damage show lower rates in women with endometriosis (Wardle et al 1985). In addition, following treatment of the disease, improvement in the fertilization rates was found (Wardle et al 1986). Numerous studies in this area have been published and a meta-analysis comparing outcome of IVF in women with endometriosis and tubal fertility has shown significantly lower rates in the endometriosis group (26% versus 36%; $p > 0.05$) (Landazabal et al 1999). Analysis of the large HFEA database, however, indicates no difference in outcome (Templeton et al 1996). Overall, the evidence suggests that the presence of endometriosis does not influence success of IVF or gamete intrafallopian transfer unless there is accompanying damage to the tubal lining or fimbria.

Mechanisms of infertility: conclusions

A variety of mechanisms have been postulated to try to relate infertility to the presence of mild endometriosis, but none have been shown to occur consistently and there is as much evidence to disprove a relationship in any single case. When there is adhesion formation with the tube bound to the ovary, or the posterior surface of the ovary to the pelvic side wall, then in these circumstances the association between the presence of the endometriotic process and difficulty in conception can readily be explained. It is in such cases that appropriate treatment may be of value, but to date no trials of medical or surgical therapy of mild endometriosis have been proven to be beneficial by improving fecundity rates (for review see Ingamells & Thomas (1995)).

DIAGNOSIS

The diagnosis of endometriosis still presents several problems resulting from the similarities in clinical symptoms produced by endometriosis to other benign gynaecological disorders and to several non-gynaecological disorders, particularly related to the gastrointestinal system.

Symptomatic pointers

No single symptom is pathognomic of endometriosis but severe dysmenorrhoea (pain sufficient to require time off work and/or to interfere with normal everyday activity) is highly predictive. Dyspareunia and pelvic pain are less predictive in the absence of severe dysmenorrhoea (Overton & Kennedy 1993). These gynaecological symptoms may, however, be of diagnostic help in the suspicion of endometriosis which should be a differential diagnosis in any patient presenting with worsening dysmenorrhoea, pelvic pain and/or dyspareunia or with other cycle-associated symptoms relating specifically to the bowel, bladder or localized skin lesion (see Boxes 34.2, 34.3). In endometriosis the associated dysmenorrhoea extends to the pre- and postmenstrual phase and is typically of secondary onset and progressive rather than being present from the onset of the menarche. In women presenting with pelvic pain, a history of whether or not this relates to the menstrual cycle is helpful in differentiating other aetiological causes of pain. In those with associated marked bowel symptoms a trial of treatment for irritable bowel syndrome may be worthwhile before considering referral for diagnostic laparoscopy, although other pathologies may be present concurrently.

Clinical examination

Clinical abdominal examination may demonstrate local tender nodular lesions in a caesarean section or laparotomy scar or at

Box 34.2 Symptoms suggestive of the presence of endometriosis

Primary symptoms
- Dysmenorrhoea – secondary onset
- Pain not normally controlled by simple analgesics or OCP
- Pain severe enough to cause significant incapacitation

Plus two or more in addition
- Dyspareunia – deep
- Pelvic pain – worse in premenstrual phase
- Dysmenorrhoea/pain continues with postmenstrual days

Less common associated symptoms
- Infertility
- Bleeding from rectum coinciding with menstruation
- Pain at micturition or defaecation – worse or only at time of menses

Box 34.3 Differential diagnosis of endometriosis

Pelvic infection	Chronic
Adhesions	Postoperative or post pelvic inflammation
Ovarian cyst	Torsion or haemorrhage into a cyst
Haemoperitoneum	Ruptured corpus luteum or ectopic
Large bowel	Irritable bowel syndrome, diverticulitis, ulcerative colitis, obstruction
Small bowel	Crohn's disease, obstruction
Musculoskeletal	

the umbilicus or other site of a laparoscopy port. Gynaecological speculum examination may visualize endometriotic lesions as clear red or bluish cysts or nodules in the vagina, most commonly in the posterior fornix, or on the cervix. This visual diagnosis cannot substitute for histological confirmation even if bleeding occurs from the lesions at the time of menstruation.

Pelvic examination often reveals induration of the uterosacral ligaments or nodules in the pouch of Douglas or rectovaginal septum. Involvement of the ovaries can lead to the development of endometriotic cysts which eventually become large enough to be palpable. There may be fixation of the uterus in retroversion, with the immobilization of the ovaries by adhesion formation, and tenderness, most particularly when the patient is examined in the immediate premenstrual phase of the cycle. These clinical findings, whilst not specific to endometriosis, may add to the suspicion of the presence of the disease from the pointers obtained in the history.

Pelvic endometriosis

Diagnosis of pelvic endometriosis cannot be made with absolute certainty from symptoms or examination alone and laparoscopic examination may be required to confirm the initial clinical diagnosis. The role of laparoscopy is to:

- provide direct visualization of the endometriotic lesions
- present an opportunity to biopsy suspected areas, if desired
- stage the disease by extent, type and site of lesions

- evaluate the extent and type of adhesions present
- provide an opportunity for concomitant laparoscopic surgical treatment, if felt appropriate.

The laparoscopic features of pelvic endometriosis are many and varied and it is clear that a carefully undertaken laparoscopy by an experienced surgeon is essential if cases are not to be missed at this diagnostic opportunity. Whenever there is any doubt the need for biopsy confirmation is paramount.

Morphology of the typical black lesions

The typical peritoneal endometriotic lesion is described as a 'powder burn' which results from tissue bleeding and retention of blood pigments, producing a brown/black discoloration of the tissue. In the early stages these lesions may appear more pink, red and haemorrhagic and develop into brown/black lesions with increasing time. Eventually, discoloration disappears altogether and a white plaque of old collagen is all that remains of the endometriotic implant (Fig. 34.2).

Scarring in the peritoneum surrounding implants is also a typical finding. Apart from encapsulating an isolated implant, the scar tissue may deform the surrounding peritoneum, resulting in development of adhesions between adjacent pelvic structures. These adhesions are commonly found between the mobile pelvic structures, particularly the posterior leaf of the broad ligament and the ovary, and the dependent sigmoid colon and posterior aspect of the vagina and/or cervix.

Classification and morphology of subtle appearances

More recently, more subtle laparoscopic appearances have been reported which were confirmed on biopsy as being due to endometriosis (Donnez & Nisolle 1991, Jansen & Russel 1986). The subtle forms are more common and may be more active and more important than the puckered black lesions that represent the latter stages of the disease. These other peritoneal lesions include the following.

Red lesions

1. *Red flame-like lesions* on the peritoneum, with the appearance of red vascular excrescences in the broad ligament and uterosacral ligaments, largely due to the presence of active endometriosis surrounded by stroma.
2. *Glandular excrescences* which closely resemble the mucosa of the endometrium as seen at hysteroscopy; biopsy reveals the presence of numerous glandular elements (Figs 34.3, 34.4).

White lesions

1. *White opacification of the peritoneum* – these lesions contain an occasional retroperitoneal glandular structure, scanty stroma surrounded by fibrotic tissue and connective tissue (Fig. 34.5).
2. *Yellow-brown peritoneal patches* called 'café au-lait spots', found in the cul-de-sac, broad ligament or over the bladder. Histologically they are similar to findings of white opacification; the yellow-brown patches indicate the presence of haemosiderin.
3. *Circular peritoneal defects* of the pelvic peritoneum, uterosacral ligaments or broad ligament. Serial section has demonstrated the presence of endometrial glands in about 50% of these structures (Fig. 34.6).

Ovarian endometriosis

The ovary represents a unique site for implantation of endometrial fragments as levels of gonadal steroids are several times higher than those in the general circulation or peritoneal cavity (Figs 34.7, 34.8)

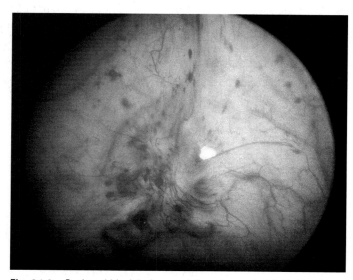

Fig. 34.2 Puckered black lesion overlying uterovesical fold. Classic 'power burn' lesions.

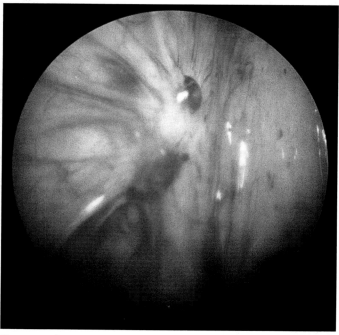

Fig. 34.3 Red papules in association with peritoneal puckering and scarring.

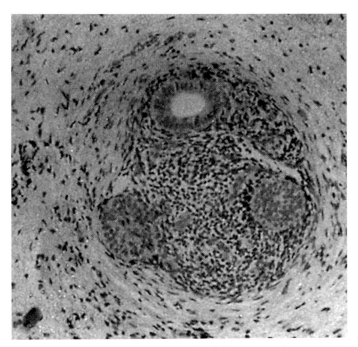

Fig. 34.4 Active endometriosis with glandular or stromal components in a biopsy specimen from a red lesion.

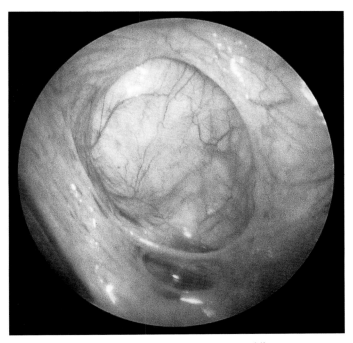

Fig. 34.6 Peritoneal pouches near right uterosacral ligament associated with endometriosis.

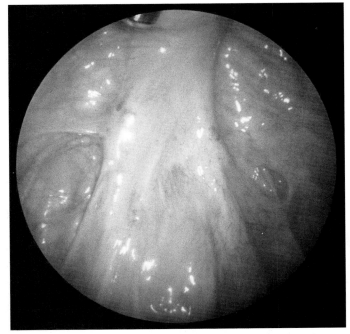

Fig. 34.5 Thickened white scarified lesion in the left uterosacral ligament.

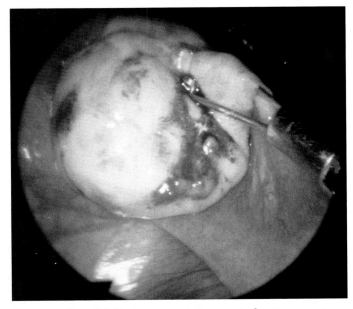

Fig. 34.7 Superficial lesions on posterior aspect of ovary.

Superficial endometriosis
Superficial implants on the ovary resemble implants in other peritoneal sites. Comparable features are typical black, red or white lesions as described (Fig. 34.7).

Subovarian adhesions
Subovarian adhesions may be confined to the peritoneum of the ovarian fossa, which are distinctive from adhesions charac-

teristic of previous salpingitis or peritonitis; this connective tissue often contains sparse endometrial glands.

Endometrioma
The pathogenesis of the typical ovarian endometriotic cyst or endometrioma has now been clarified. It is a process originating from a free superficial implant which is in contact with the ovarian surface and is sealed off by adhesions (Fig. 34.8). A pseudocyst is thus formed by accumulation of menstrual debris from shedding and bleeding of the small implant,

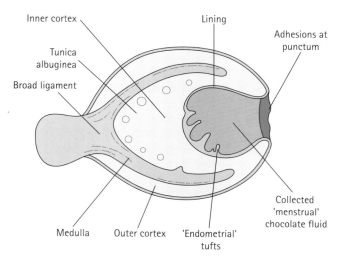

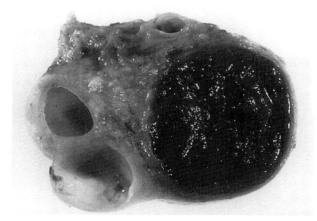

Fig. 34.8 Diagrammatic representation of endometriosis formation – beginning on serosal surface and invaginating into cortex.

Fig. 34.9 Classic chocolate cyst of ovary (endometrioma) in an ovary containing two other fibrotic walled smaller cysts previously filled with 'chocolate' material prior to section.

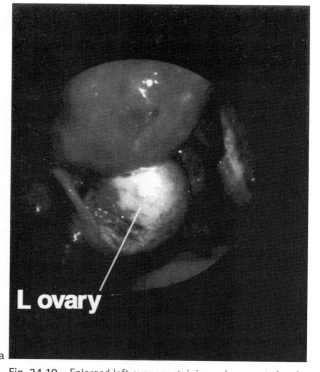

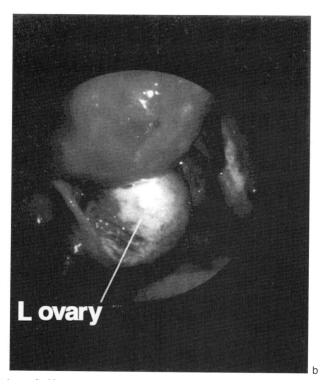

Fig. 34.10 Enlarged left ovary containing a deep-seated endometrioma *(left)* and another ovary with superficial deposits on the ovarian capsule, in addition to others on the peritoneal surface in the pouch of Douglas *(right)*.

resulting in fluid collection. Progressive invagination of the ovarian cortex occurs and the associated inflammatory reactive tissue progressively thickens the inverted cortex. Outgrowths through the endometrial epithelium, with or without stroma, extend over the surface or become embedded in the fibroreactive tissue covering the wall. This pathogenesis explains the typical features of an endometrium such as frequent location of the cyst, adhesions on the anterior side of the ovary opposing the posterior side of the parametrium or, when on the posterior aspect of the ovary, adhesions to the ovarian fossa. The contents of the cyst are, to a large extent,

fluid which represents the debris from cyclical menstruation (Fig. 34.9).

There is usually a well-defined separation between the normal adjacent ovarian stroma and the cyst wall but whilst the epithelial lining of the cyst may initially resemble the endometrium, with increasing time and size, pressure atrophy compresses the epithelium to a flat cuboidal pattern (Fig. 34.11)

Ovarian endometriomas rarely occur in the adolescent but incidence increases with age. Laparoscopic features of a typical endometrioma include ovarian cysts not greater than

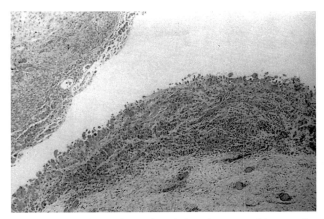

Fig. 34.11 Wall of an endometriomal chocolate cyst with extensive fibrosis and haemorrhage but no recognizable endometrial glands or stroma.

12 cm in diameter; adhesions to the pelvic side wall and/or the posterior broad ligament; powder burns; minute red or blue spots with adjacent puckering on the surface, and the presence of the characteristic tarry, thick, chocolate-coloured fluid content (Fig. 34.10).

Extrapelvic endometriosis

Pelvic endometriosis has been defined as endometriotic implants involving the peritoneum and anterior and posterior cul-de-sac and pelvic side walls and surface of uterus tubes and surface of the ovaries. Extrapelvic endometriosis is defined as endometriotic-like implants elsewhere in the peritoneal cavity or other body cavities.

Extrapelvic endometriosis has been reported in virtually every organ, system and tissue but far less frequently than pelvic endometriosis. Overall the incidence of extrapelvic disease represents less than 12% of reported cases of endometriosis (Rock & Markham 1987) and it would appear that the frequency of occurrence decreases with the distance from the pelvis.

Urinary tract endometriosis

Endometriotic implants can be found over the pelvic ureter and bladder with unilateral involvement of the ureter and potential obstruction to drainage of the kidney more common than bilateral involvement. The highest incidence of involvement of endometriosis of the urinary tract involves the bladder followed by the lower ureter, the upper ureter and the kidney itself being the least frequent site.

The common symptoms associated with bladder endometriosis are cyclical haematuria, dysuria, urgency and frequency. Ureteral endometriosis eventually induces partial or complete obstruction of the ureter which will always require surgical management, either segmental resection and re-anastomosis or reimplantation of the ureter. For temporary resolution of hydronephrosis the insertion of a ureteric stent may be necessary until definitive surgery is undertaken.

Gastrointestinal tract endometriosis

Extrapelvic endometriosis is most commonly found with involvement of the gastrointestinal tract. The commonest sites for involvement are the sigmoid colon followed by the rectum, ileocaecal area and appendix. The transverse colon and small bowel are infrequently involved.

When there is involvement of the gastrointestinal tract invariably endometriosis is not the first diagnosis in the majority of patients. Symptoms are non-specific and include abdominal pain, followed by distension, disturbed bowel function and rectal bleeding. The occurrence of cyclical rectal bleeding at the time of menstruation is the key pointer to endometriosis. Discomfort and pain at defaecation (dyschezia) is a hallmark of involvement of the rectosigmoid area. Besides rectal bleeding, there is often little to observe in the mucosal lining at endoscopy since involvement is deep within the smooth muscle wall. In advanced stages, a typical irregular stricture formation can be demonstrated on barium enema and the use of magnetic resonance imaging (MRI) demonstrates the extent of involvement in the rectovaginal septum. Superficial implants on the serosal surface of the bowel are not uncommon and can be treated by laser destruction or medical suppressive therapy. However, involvement of the smooth muscle of the bowel wall and evidence of stricture formation will require surgical excision by open or laparosopic approaches depending upon the localized site of involvement.

Involvement in surgical scars

Endometriosis in surgical scars has been reported in the umbilicus or other port sites following laparoscopy, in abdominal incisions following gynaecological surgery and caesarean section and the perineum within episiotomy scars following childbirth (Fig. 34.12). Such patients present with a painful, palpable swelling usually more symptomatic at the time of menstruation. Occasionally some women report discharge or cyclical bleeding occurring perimenstrually from the lesions. While medical treatment will control the symptoms with effective suppression of menstruation, in the long term surgical excision of the nodule will normally be necessary.

Vaginal endometriosis

Endometriosis of the vagina may occur following hysterectomy most commonly in patients with a past history of endometriosis and in whom an ovary has been conserved. It has also been reported in women who have undergone bilateral oophorectomy, but have been commenced on hormone replacement therapy soon after surgery.

However, endometriosis involving the posterior vaginal fornix is found in most instances as a continuance of deep infiltrating disease from the cul-de-sac and rectovaginal septum. Bimanual examination of these patients is essential as the small vaginal lesions do not represent the full extent of involvement and assessment at or near the time of menstruation may be the most informative.

Pulmonary and thoracic endometriosis

Cyclical haemoptysis and cyclical haemo/pneumothorax have been reported in patients in whom endometriosis has been found involving the lungs and thorax. Pulmonary thoracic

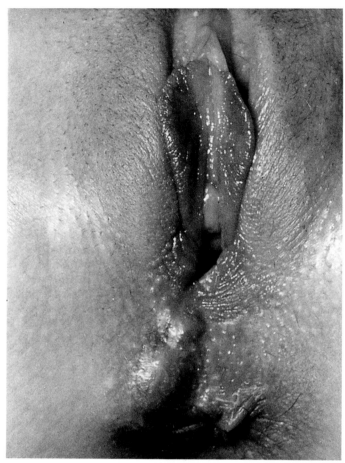

Fig. 34.12 Endometriosis in episiotomy scar. The patient presented with cyclic, tender swelling in the perineum.

endometriosis is uncommon. Hormone therapy is of value as an interim measure but as with other deep-seated extrapelvic endometriosis, recurrence is inevitable on cessation of medical treatment and surgical excision would be the eventual treatment of choice.

Non-invasive methods of diagnosis

It is an unsatisfactory situation that in order to diagnose endometriosis with certainty an invasive, albeit minor, surgical procedure in the form of laparoscopy needs to be performed. This can readily be justified for making the initial diagnosis, but if the nature of the disease is of recurrence for the majority of patients throughout their reproductive life, this may involve repeat laparoscopies on many occasions if one is to be certain that the disease process has returned. Attempts have therefore been made to provide a non-invasive test which is highly sensitive and specific for endometriosis. Currently such a test has eluded investigators although a number of adjunctive non-invasive tests may be contributory in the management of patients.

Serum markers: CA125
The most widely used serum marker for endometriosis has been the monoclonal antibody OC125, raised against a human ovarian cancer cell line containing the antigen designated CA125 (Bast et al 1986). CA125 is a high molecular weight glycoprotein found in over 80% of cases of epithelial ovarian carcinoma. Investigation leads to the conclusion that CA125 is possessed by many tissues present in the pelvis as well as the more distant sites, including the pericardium and the pleura. Moderate elevation of serum CA125 has been observed in endometriosis, particularly in patients with severe disease (Barbieri et al 1986, Pittaway & Douglas 1989). In these studies serum levels in excess of 35 u/ml were used as a cut-off point, but sensitivity and specificity have proved inadequate for the use of CA125 as a screening test for endometriosis. However, in individuals in whom the disease has been confirmed and treated, an increase in serum levels above 35 u/ml may well be a useful marker of recurrence of the disorder.

Imaging techniques
Ultrasound. Ultrasound examination of the pelvis may be useful in delineating the presence and aetiology of ovarian cystic structures. The characteristic pictures on ultrasound are different when there is a large proportion of blood, e.g. haemorrhagic corpus luteum cysts or endometriomas, which in a minority of cases may be echo free. However, the walls of an endometrioma are irregular as opposed to the smooth wall of the simple ovarian cyst. The commonest pattern is for the chocolate cyst to contain low-level echoes or lumps of dense high-level echoes representing blood clots. The picture may sometimes be confused if there are several cysts in different phases of evolution.

Computed tomography (CT) scans and magnetic resonance imaging (MRI). CT provides better definition than ultrasound in many situations, but it has not established a role in the assessment of pelvic endometriosis. MRI, which is even more expensive and currently has been used in only a limited number of patients with ovarian endometriomas, has not proved to be diagnostic since again there has been a significant overlap between endometriomas and cystic adenomas on MRI scanning appearances.

Ultrasound, CT and MRI scanning do not appear to be of any help in the diagnosis of peritoneal endometriosis, the deposits of which are too small to be detected by current technology although various strategies utilizing enhancement agents are being investigated.

Immunoscintigraphy. Efforts have been made to use immunoscintigraphic methods to detect deposits of endometriotic tissue on the grounds that these tissue deposits do express CA125 and if an isotopic labelled OC125 (FAB) 2 fragment has been injected then binding to sites of CA125 expression could be detected (Kennedy et al 1988). Using a gamma camera the sites where binding has occurred can be visualized but whilst results from this method are encouraging, there is still great overlap with binding in other conditions, particularly pelvic inflammatory processes and to adhesions.

In summary, whilst there are promising areas of investigations currently being pursued concerning non-invasive techniques, none at present can stand in place of laparoscopy for initial confirmatory diagnosis.

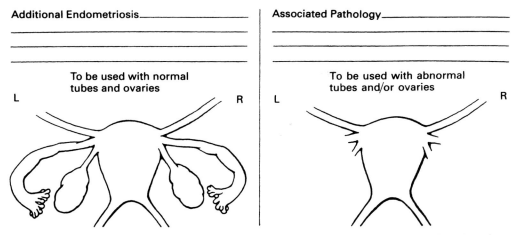

Additional Endometriosis_____

To be used with normal
tubes and ovaries

L   R

Associated Pathology_____

To be used with abnormal
tubes and/or ovaries

L   R

Fig. 34.13   Accurate charting of sites of endometrial deposits is helpful for re-evaluation following treatment or in suspected cases of recurrence. Modified from Revised American Fertility Society Classification of Endometriosis (1985).

CLASSIFICATION SYSTEMS

Over the last three decades various classification systems have been proposed which attempt to standardize criteria on which the severity of endometriosis could be based. Such a system, if available, would help in the critical assessment of performance of various forms of treatment and hopefully provide meaningful prognostic indicators. No classification system so far devised has received uniform acceptance; all have suffered from various pitfalls which make it difficult to compare treatment results. The most recent attempt to provide a standardized classification for uniform use has been the Revised American Fertility Society Classification of Endometriosis (1985) shown in Figure 34.13. This serves to record the sites of deposits accurately and makes some effort to differentiate between superficial and deep-seated disease, as well as the presence or absence of adhesions. Whilst it offers a differential weighting to the score given to different types of endometriosis, it must be appreciated that these scores are arbitrary. Classification of the extent of the disease as minimal, mild, moderate or severe is certainly helpful in explaining the problem to the patient and perhaps in determining whether a medical, surgical or combined medical and surgical approach is the most logical treatment step, at least in relation to fertility outcome.

In addition to the Revised American Fertility score it may be helpful to chart carefully the exact sites of all implants and their sizes, a method as used in the scheme of Additive Diameter of Implants (ADI score) described by Doberl et al (1984), which gives a simple quantitative valuation of alteration of the volume of endometriotic disease although not the activity. For each square millimetre of disease a score of 1 is given. The ADI helps to quantify the volume of disease and may be useful in evaluating response to treatment options.

The major pitfall of any scoring system has been the lack of correlation between the score, or severity of the disease, and the degree of symptoms experienced. What is most important for the patient management is an accurate record of the extent and site of each deposit.

With increasing understanding of the morphological changes of deposits and their relationship to ovarian steroid hormones and the precise colour and type of each lesion, more accurate selection of treatment options may become possible. Accurate records are vitally important to prevent needless repeat laparoscopies for patients referred to secondary and tertiary referral centres where previous laparoscopies have been performed. Too often the lack of this accurate information results in laparoscopies being undertaken which in many instances could have been avoided with accurate records.

Provided the above limitations are appreciated classification systems do have some value and are essential in any clinical trial of a new treatment for comparison with other published series with currently accepted therapies.

TREATMENT: GENERAL PRINCIPLES

Endometriosis is a particularly difficult disease to treat. Often response to therapy relies on recognition of the disease in its earliest possible stages. With most treatment modalities, there is eventual recurrence in up to 60% of cases. Thus there is no known permanent cure and eventually clinicians have to proceed to surgical oophorectomy in selected cases; this offers the most effective available treatment to date. In addition, in minimal and mild disease (according to Revised American Fertility Society classifications), particularly in asymptomatic cases presenting only with infertility, there exists a controversy as to whether treatment should be given, since no control studies have shown a significant increase in fertility rates following such ovarian suppression therapies. However, placebo-controlled studies in such cases have shown that endometriosis tends to be a progressive disease, at least for many patients (Thomas & Cooke 1987), and hence treatment may at least arrest progression or eradicate disease for significant intervals.

When endometriosis is associated with symptoms, particularly pain, then there can be no doubt that treatment is of benefit, at least in relieving those symptoms for a period of time.

The treatment should be individualized, taking into account the patient's age, wish for fertility, severity of symptoms and extent of disease. An important aspect of therapy is a sympathetic approach, with adequate counselling and explanation to the patient that will also ensure her compliance whilst on therapy. Current treatment is essentially surgical, medical or a combination of both approaches. A combined medical and surgical treatment might utilize medical therapy before, after or both before and following surgical intervention. This approach may be adopted in patients with moderate to severe disease in whom fertility prospects need to be improved or maintained.

MEDICAL TREATMENTS

Ectopic endometrial tissue does respond to endogenous and exogenous ovarian steroid hormones in a fashion sufficiently similar to that of normal endometrium. Thus a hormonal approach which suppresses oestrogen-progesterone levels and which prevents cyclical changes and menstruation should be beneficial in its treatment. In the hypo-oestrogenic state following the menopause, atrophy of the normal endometrium and atrophy and regression of endometriotic deposits occur. Administration of progestogens opposes the effect of oestrogen on endometrial tissue by inhibiting the replenishment of cytosolic oestrogen receptors. Progestogens also induce secretory activity in endometrial glands and decidual reaction in the endometrial stroma.

The success of various hormonal therapies depends to a large extent on the localization of the endometriotic lesions. Superficial peritoneal and ovarian serosal implants may respond better to hormone therapy than deep ovarian or peritoneal lesions or lesions within organs (e.g. bladder and rectum) which rapidly recur after medical therapy and require ultimate surgical excision.

The treatment of endometriosis has undergone a remarkable evolution in the last 40 years. In the past, testosterone, diethylstilboestrol and high-dose combination oestrogen-progestogen pill preparations were used with some success. However, therapies which induce decidualization (pseudo-pregnancy regimes) or suppress ovarian function (pseudo-menopausal regimes) appear to offer the best chance of inducing clinical remission of endometriosis (Table 34.4).

Prostaglandin synthetase inhibitors

An association with prostaglandin release and dysmenorrhoea has long been established. One might therefore expect that prostaglandin synthetase inhibitors (PGSIs) might have a beneficial effect in treating the symptoms of endometriosis. PGSIs are a heterogeneous group of non-steroidal inflammatory agents which act mainly by inhibiting the production of prostaglandins, though some (fenamates) also antagonize prostaglandins at the target level. These agents are perhaps beneficial in the early stages of initial or recurrent disease but when symptoms become more severe, they are usually inadequate by themselves to control symptomatology.

Gestagen and anti-gestagen treatment

A state of pseudopregnancy can be induced effectively by the continuous administration of progestogenic preparations. The

Table 34.4 Various hormonal states and their effects upon normal endometrium and ectopic endometrial deposits

Hormonal state	Effects on endometrium	Effects on endometriotic implants
Oestrogenic, e.g. exogenous oestrogens	Proliferative activity, hyperplasia	Proliferative activity, hyperplasia
Hypo-oestrogenic, e.g. postmenopause, pseudomenopause regimens postoophorectomy GnRH analogues	Atrophic changes	Atrophy, regression, resorption
Progestational, e.g. pregnancy, exogenous progestogens, pseudopregnancy treatment	Secretory activity, decidualization	Secretory activity, necrobiosis and resorption
Androgenic, e.g. danazol and its metabolites Gestrinone	Atrophy	Atrophy and regression

GnRH, gonadotrophin-releasing hormone.

progestogens used are derivatives of progesterone (dydogesterone or medroxyprogesterone acetate) or 19-nor-testosterone (norethisterone, norethisterone acetate, norgestrel, ethynodrel and lynoestrenol).

The use of progestogens induces a hyperprogestogenic/hypo-oestrogenic state. Treatments are available orally or injected as a depot formulation and are administered for 6–9 months. The results achieved appear to be comparable to those achieved with combined oral oestrogen-progestogen preparations in the past. The side-effects most commonly seen with progestogen usage include breakthrough bleeding, weight gain, abdominal bloating, oedema, acne and mood changes.

The adverse effects of some progestogens on circulating levels of low- and high-density lipoproteins may determine choice of progestogen if long-term administration is planned.

Combined oral contraceptive pill (COCP)

COCP reduces pain associated with endometriosis and is well tolerated and can be continued long term for the control of symptoms in healthy women without risk factors. One of a number of 'high-dose' COCPs may be administered and regimes often utilize COCPs prescribed continuously for three cycles to reduce the frequency of menstruation. If breakthrough bleeding occurs before planned interval bleeding, changing to another preparation with a higher progestogenic content is advocated.

Side-effects such as weight gain, headaches, breast enlargement and/or tenderness, nausea and depression may occur. The risk of thromboembolism is increased and a personal previous history or family history of venous thromboembolism may involve screening for risk factors, including factor-5 Leiden polymorphism, prior to administration.

Levonorgestrel–releasing intrauterine system

A small observational study of women with recurrent moderate or severe dysmenorrhoea utilizing a levonorgestrel-releasing intrauterine system has been reported (Vercellini et al 1999). Fifteen of the 20 women had significantly reduced menstrual pain and amenorrhoea or hypomenorrhoea, but in the other patients the device was expelled or symptoms were not significantly improved. Such an approach needs further studies and a properly conducted randomized controlled trial to determine its true role and in which group of patients such an approach is indicated.

Danazol

Danazol is an isoxazol derivate of 17-α-ethinyl testosterone. Because of its base structure it has both androgenic and anabolic properties. Danazol is currently one of the most widely used medical treatments for endometriosis. Its mechanism of action is complex and includes suppression of the hypothalamic-pituitary axis with interference in pulsatile gonadotrophin secretion and inhibition of the midcycle gonadotrophin surge, but with no change in basal gonadotrophin levels. It achieves a direct inhibition of ovarian steroidogenesis by inhibiting several enzymatic processes and by competitive blockage of androgen, oestrogen and progesterone receptors in the endometrium. An increase in free testosterone occurs because of a reduction in sex hormone-binding globulin and this explains many of danazol's androgenic side-effects. The increase in free testosterone may also contribute to its direct action in inducing endometrial atrophy. The degree of endocrine changes described above is dose related.

In the treatment of endometriosis, danazol is administered in a dose range of between 400 and 800 mg daily, titrated by the induction of amenorrhoea and tolerance. In the case of mild to moderate endometriosis there is a highly effective symptomatic improvement in over 85% of cases (Dmowski & Cohen 1978).

Objective resolution of endometriotic lesions has been observed at post-treatment laparoscopic evaluation in between 70% and 95% of patients, depending upon the stage of the disease (Barbieri et al 1982). However, recurrence rates of up to 40% have been reported in the 36 months after completion of a course of danazol; annual recurrences in the first, second and third years were 23%, 5% and 9% respectively (Dmowski & Cohen 1978).

Danazol therapy should be commenced in the early follicular phase of the menstrual cycle. It is recommended that the patient should use additional barrier methods of contraception in order to avoid the drug being administered during early pregnancy where continued use could lead to androgenization of a developing female fetus. The drug dosage should be related to the patient's clinical staging, response and severity of side-effects, starting with a dose of 400 mg/day in mild disease and 600–800 mg/day in moderate to severe cases, for a recommended treatment course of at least 6 months.

Danazol is associated with side-effects related to its androgenic and anabolic properties. These include weight gain, acne, oily skin, fluid retention, muscle cramps, hot flushes, depression and mood changes. Less commonly, hirsutism, skin rash and deepening of voice are noted. The incidence and severity of these side-effects are dose related. It is recommended that patients immediately discontinue treatment if they develop hirsutism, a skin rash or experience deepening of the voice.

Metabolic side-effects include elevation of low-density lipoproteins and reduction of high-density lipoproteins and cholesterol concentrations (Fahraeus et al 1984). These effects are quickly reversed after ceasing treatment. In addition, changes in liver enzymes are noted and danazol is contra-indicated in patients with liver disease.

Gestrinone

Gestrinone is a synthetic trienic 19-norsteroid (13 ethyl-17-α-ethinyl-17-hydroxy-gona-4, o, Il-triene-3-one). It has been shown in clinical trials to be another effective clinical treatment for endometriosis (Thomas & Cooke 1987). The drug exhibits mild androgenic and antigonadotrophic properties. The combined effect is to induce progressive endometrial atrophy. Gestrinone has a high binding affinity for progesterone receptors; it also binds to androgen receptors but not to oestrogen receptors (Azadian-Boulanger et al 1984). The combined endocrine effect of gestrinone therapy is similar to that of danazol in that the midcycle gonadotrophin surge is abolished, although basal gonadotrophin levels are not significantly reduced, together with inhibition of ovarian steroidogenesis and reduction of sex hormone-binding globulin levels. Gestrinone has a prolonged half-life and may be administered orally at a dosage of 2.5–5.0 mg twice weekly for a period of 6–9 months in patients with endometriosis. This dosage schedule effectively induces endometrial atrophy with 85–90% of patients becoming amenorrhoeic within 2 months.

Whilst gestrinone has only recently been introduced for the treatment of endometriosis, current controlled open studies appear to show that it compares favourably with danazol in terms of both symptomatic relief and resolution of endometrial deposits (Azadian-Boulanger et al 1984, Mettler & Semm 1984).

The side-effects, occurring in up to 50% of patients, include weight gain, breakthrough bleeding, reduced breast size, muscle cramps and, uncommonly, hirsutism, voice change and hoarseness.

Gonadotrophin–releasing hormone (GnRH) agonists

Surgical castration is known to be an effective therapy for severe endometriosis. Thus the possibility of inducing a reversible medical castration with the continued administration of GnRH agonists has been investigated as an alternative therapy in endometriosis. Modification of the native GnRH molecule with substitution, particularly in positions 6 and 10, with alternative amino acids, produces agonistic analogues with a reduced susceptibility to degradation and hence a prolonged therapeutic half-life (Fig. 34.14). Continued administration of these analogues induces pituitary gonadotrophin desensitization via downregulation of GnRH receptors and an eventual state of hypogonadotrophic hypogonadism. Reduced gonadotrophic stimulation of the ovaries leads to cessation of follicular growth

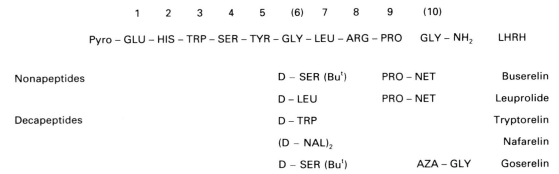

Fig. 34.14 Amino acid sequence of native luteinzing hormone-releasing hormone (LHRH) and some of the agonistic gonadotrophin-releasing hormone (GnRH) analogues used in the treatment of endometriosis.

Table 34.5 Principal side-effects experienced in patients randomized to receive buserelin or danazol for 6 months

	Buserelin	Danazol
Dose	400 µg tds intranasally	600–800 mg orally daily
Number of patients	39	18
Symptoms		
Hot flushes	74%*	22%
Breakthrough bleeding	23%	55%*
Headaches	20%	39%
Vaginal dryness	23%*	5.5%
Superficial dyspareunia	5.2%*	Nil
Weight gain (>3 kg)	Nil	66%*
Acne/oily skin	Nil	39%*

From Matta & Shaw (1987).
* $p \leq 0.05$ between treatments.

and reduction in ovarian steroidogenesis with circulating 17β-oestradiol levels falling to those observed in the postmenopausal range (less than 100 pmol/l, typically).

A large amount of data has now appeared in the literature, from both controlled and randomized comparative trials of GnRH analogues and danazol (for review, see Shaw 1995). These trials have all confirmed the value of GnRH analogues for the treatment of endometriosis. Rapid and effective symptomatic relief is achieved with these agents as well as a marked degree of resolution of the endometrial deposits in the majority of patients. However, for both symptomatic relief and the resolution of endometrial deposits there is essentially no significant difference in comparative trials between the GnRH analogues and danazol. However, patient acceptability and the profile of side-effects may be slightly in favour of the GnRH analogues (Henzl et al 1988, Matta & Shaw 1987) (Table 34.5).

Side-effects of GnRH analogues include those which are predictable from induction of pseudomenopause. These include hot flushes (in virtually all patients), headaches and, less commonly, atrophic vaginitis, vaginal dryness and reduced libido.

Dosage varies depending on the analogue used and its formulation, but regimens include: nafarelin 200 µg twice daily intranasally; buserelin 300–400 µg three times daily intra-nasally; goserelin 3.6 mg subcutaneous depot monthly; and leuprorelin 3.75 mg intramuscular depot monthly.

Metabolic side-effects include (as in the menopause) increased excretion of urinary calcium. Over a 6-month period there is a 3–5% loss in the vertebral trabecular bone density of the lumbar spine as assessed by dual energy X-ray absorptiometry (DEXA). In most patients, the bone density changes induced following a 6-month course of therapy with GnRH analogues are reversed after 6 months' return of ovarian function (Henzl et al 1988, Matta et al 1987). However, the implications of such changes in calcium homeostasis with prolonged and repetitive treatment with GnRH analogues are being further investigated. This is likely to lead to the development of protective 'add-back' regimens, which ideally would also reduce the symptomatic effects of the GnRH agonist-induced hypo-oestrogenism but not result in reduced therapeutic effectiveness on symptom relief or implant resolution.

A new series of GnRH antagonists are currently being developed and these peptides contain multiple and complex substitutions of the GnRH molecule. There is little evidence on long-term use of GnRH antagonists in the treatment of endometriosis to date and their structural complexity and costs may make substitution of GnRH antagonists for the current widely used GnRH agonists unlikely. However, orally administered non-peptide GnRH receptor antagonists are being developed and may in future present alternative therapies.

SURGICAL TREATMENT

Many forms of severe endometriosis do not respond to drug treatment: deep-seated invasive disease, endometriomas, extrapelvic endometriosis of the bladder and bowel or within surgical scars. In these instances, surgery may be required to relieve the symptomatology and effect a longer term cure.

Conservative surgery

Endometriotic deposits may be excised, destroyed by electrocautery or evaporated utilizing CO_2 or KTP/YAG lasers or argon beam.

With the increasingly widespread availability of laparoscopic expertise, commonly improved instrumentation and experience of laser technology, minimal access surgery is becoming a more popular treatment option. There have been few appropriately conducted randomized trials, but one small double-blind placebo-controlled study measured pain relief following laser ablation and/or LUNA or placebo (no treatment). At 6-month follow-up 53% of those treated with laser compared with only 23% from the placebo diagnostic laparoscopy group had improvements in symptoms (Sutton et al 1994). It was of interest that in minimal disease only 38% of women had a reduction in pain so this approach appeared to be more effective in reducing pain symptoms in women with more severe disease.

Sutton et al (1997) published the results of a longer term follow-up of this cohort of patients. Sadly, 1 year after the initial treatment 44% had recurrence of pain requiring additional treatment. The reasons for failure of the surgical approach may result from missing lesions, incomplete resection and, of course, recurrence of the disease. It must also be considered, particularly in minimal disease, that pain symptoms may be due to other aetiologies.

Laparoscopic uterosacral nerve ablation (LUNA)

The uterosacral ligaments are a commonly affected site in patients suffering with endometriosis and infiltration of endometriotic deposits results in invasion, inflammation and fibrosis of the anterior extension of the inferior hypogastric nerve, the uterovaginal plexus (or Lee–Frankenhauser plexus). Ablation of the uterosacral ligaments, forming two small craters, can be performed at the time of laparoscopy. The risks of the procedure are haemorrhage from a vessel within the uterosacral ligaments and damage to the ureter which needs to be identified before laser treatment commences. The results of properly conducted randomized trials are awaited to determine the value of LUNA although it does seem beneficial at reducing the severity of central dysmenorrhoea-type pain.

Radical surgery

Radical surgery is reserved for those patients with severe symptoms, where there is no desired fertility potential and especially when other forms of treatment have failed. Total abdominal hysterectomy and bilateral salpingo-oophorectomy are performed along with resection of any endometriotic lesions as completely as possible. As the majority of these patients are relatively young, hormone replacement therapy (HRT) should be commenced but kept to a minimum to control oestrogen deficiency symptoms, as a small percentage of those patients may develop a recurrence of endometriosis when on such oestrogen replacement.

Combined oestrogen-testosterone implants may minimize the risk of recurrence as well as offering the beneficial effects of the androgens in maintaining libido in young women who are sexually active, but no data exist from randomized trials to define if one particular HRT regimen is superior to others. At present clinicians are advised to follow the type and route of HRT depending upon patient tolerance and symptoms control.

Surgical treatment of endometriomas

The definitive treatment of the typical endometrioma is the surgical release of the adhesions and fibrosis at the site of invagination and the eversion of the invaginated cortex. Simply puncturing and draining the endometrioma, whether this is followed by GnRH agonist therapy, or not, has no beneficial effects in the long term (Vercellini et al 1992). Medical treatment is highly effective for the destruction of active implants located on the surface of the normal ovarian cortex. However, when a definite endometrioma is present, surgery is necessary. This can be performed laparoscopically with smaller endometriomas, using laser destruction. With endometriomas larger than 3 cm diameter treatment may be facilitated to enable surgery to be performed laparoscopically if, following initial drainage, patients are pretreated for 3 months with a GnRH agonist prior to laser ablation (Donnez et al 1990).

On the other hand, fibrotic larger endometriomas have a thickened capsule which is more likely to be removed effectively by excisional techniques.

In many instances, however, because of other associated extensive adhesions and fixity of ovaries onto other structures, a laparotomy rather than laparoscopy may be necessary.

Whatever the surgical approach, be it minimal access or open laparotomy, if at the time of original surgery dense and extensive adhesions are present it is likely that such patients will have recurrence of adhesions with attendant problems of fixity of the ovary following such approaches (Shaw et al 2001).

Combination of medical and surgical therapy

There is perhaps more speculation as to the value of pre- or postoperative medical therapy than hard data. Individual gynaecologists have a 'belief' in one or the other, even though published data do not suggest advantages of one method over another.

It is the frequency of recurrent endometriosis after medical or surgical therapy, and the documentation of microscopic disease, together with differences in vascularity between various lesions that have encouraged the use of combination therapy.

Preoperative therapy might help to reduce the size of an endometrioma prior to surgical removal and will also reduce vascularity and may subsequently aid dissection of implants and adhesive processes. The role of postoperative medication is to eliminate any residual macro- or microscopic disease.

The duration of such therapies is uncertain since no true randomized comparative trials exist, but most gynaecologists prescribe a 3-month treatment course preoperatively and between 3 and 6 months postoperatively, depending upon the amount of macroscopic disease left following attempted surgical removal.

Infertility associated with endometriosis

It is now clear from several studies that medical treatment of endometriosis produces no improvement in pregnancy rates compared to expectant management (for review, see Ingamells & Thomas (1995)). The contrast surgical ablation of minimal to mild endometriosis in one study (Marcoux et al 1997) reported a significant improvement in pregnancy rates in a multicentred randomized controlled trial. In this study in the treated group 31% of patients became pregnant within 36 weeks compared to 18% in the diagnostic laparoscopy group. There have been a number of criticisms of the study regarding variations in treatment and alternative fertility/activity treatments. Another smaller randomized study (Parazzinni 1999) could show no differences in pregnancy rate within one year following laparoscopic laser treatment or in the control group – 19.6% versus 22.2%.

It is therefore unclear as to what treatment approaches should be used in infertile patients. What is apparent is that the age of the patient and the duration of infertility are perhaps of more relevance in determining appropriate treatment options in women with minimal/mild endometriosis who are infertile. Current evidence suggests that ovarian stimulation using exogenous gonadotrophins and intrauterine insemination are appropriate treatments and produce better results than expectant management or intrauterine insemination alone for such women (Tummon et al 1997).

RECURRENT ENDOMETRIOSIS

The natural course of the disease remains a mystery. It has been suggested that in only one-third of cases is the disease progressive, whilst in the remainder the endometriosis remains in a steady state or eventually even resolves spontaneously.

After medical suppression of the disease or after surgical destruction of all visible deposits, residual viable (microscopic) implants can regenerate once ovarian function is re-established. In other cases new disease develops at new sites, perhaps indicating the potential for an entire 'field change' within the pelvic peritoneum. The degree of differentiation of a lesion may also correlate with persistence of disease following medical therapy. Two-thirds of those lesions which were most highly differentiated disappeared following 6 months of medical therapy, whilst three-quarters of poorly differentiated lesions persisted (Schweppe 1984).

However, as far as therapeutic options are concerned, there is no essential difference between primary and recurrent endometriosis. The choice of treatment in a patient with recurrent disease is not determined by the manifestations of the disease as such but more by the extent of distortion of the pelvic anatomy and the severity of symptomatology. In many instances repeat medical therapy or repeat conservative surgery is appropriate, but when there are severe symptoms and repeated recurrence, a radical surgical approach may be the patient's best option to achieve long-standing relief of pain.

KEY POINTS

1. Endometriosis is one of the most common gynaecological conditions and is present in between 10% and 25% of women presenting with gynaecological symptoms.
2. Endometriosis is most commonly found inside the pelvis, but rarely it has been described in sites such as the urinary tract, bowel, lungs and umbilicus.

KEY POINTS (CONTINUED)

3. The growth of endometriotic tissue depends on oestrogen; thus endometriosis occurs almost exclusively in the reproductive years, with a peak incidence between 30 and 45 years of age.
4. The theories of aetiology of endometriosis include Sampson's theory of retrograde menstruation and implantation and Meyer's theory of transformation of coelomic epithelium. Genetic predisposition and immunological factors are also thought to be important in rendering individuals susceptible to the disease.
5. The peritoneal fluid in women with endometriosis contains higher concentrations of more active macrophages and prostaglandins than in normal women. These factors may be important in explaining the link between infertility, pain and endometriosis.
6. Endometriosis that is associated with tubal and ovarian damage and the formation of adhesions can compromise fertility. The link between mild endometriosis and infertility is more controversial.
7. The best means to diagnose endometriosis is by direct visualization at laparoscopy or laparotomy, with histological confirmation where uncertainty persists. Non-invasive tests are being developed and additional investigations are of value in diagnosing extrapelvic disease.
8. The typical blue-black peritoneal endometriotic lesion is described as a powder burn. Recently non-pigmented lesions and red lesions have been described together with many other visual appearances now recognized as hallmarks of the disease process.
9. The medical treatment of endometriosis involves suppressing oestrogen-progesterone levels to prevent cyclical changes and menstruation. Treatments include progestogens, gestrinone, danazol and gonadotrophin-releasing hormone analogues. Induction of complete amenorrhoea is the key to successful control of symptoms.
10. The surgical treatment of endometriosis is either minimally invasive, such as laparoscopic diathermy or laser vaporization, or radical, when total abdominal hysterectomy and bilateral salpingo-oophorectomy are performed. Extrapelvic and deep-seated endometriosis invariably requires a surgical approach.
11. The natural course of the disease is not clearly defined, but in perhaps a third of cases the disease is progressive whilst in the remainder the disease remains in a steady stage or may even resolve spontaneously. For many patients the disease is one of recurrent episodes of treatment cycles and recurrence throughout reproductive life.
12. There seems no justification to treat minimal/mild endometriosis where infertility and not pain is the predominant symptom. Such cases are best assessed for infertility treatment options based on the woman's age, duration of infertility and the presence/absence of other infertility factors.

REFERENCES

Azadian-Boulanger G, Secchi J, Tournemine C, Sakiz E, Vige P, Henrion R 1984 Hormonal activity profiles of drugs for endometriosis therapy. In: Raynaud JP, Ojasoo T, Martinin L (eds) Medical management of endometriosis. Raven Press, New York, pp 125–148

Barbieri RL 1990 Etiology and epidemiology of endometriosis. American Journal of Obstetrics and Gynecology 162(2):565–567

Barbieri RL, Evans S, Kistner RW 1982 Danazol in the treatment of endometriosis: analysis of 100 cases with a 4-year follow-up. Fertility and Sterility 37:737–749

Barbieri RL, Niloff JM, Bast RC, Shaetzl E, Kistner RW, Knapp RC 1986 Elevated serum concentrations of CA-125 in patients with advanced endometriosis. Fertility and Sterility 45:630–634

Bast RC, Feeney M, Lazarus H, Nadler LM, Colvin RB, Knapp RC 1986 Reactivity of a monoclonal antibody with human ovarian carcinoma. Journal of Clinical Investigation 68:1331

Chillik CF, Acosta AA, Cardcia JE et al 1985 The role of in vitro fertilisation in infertile patients with endometriosis. Fertility and Sterility 44:56–62

Curtis P, Lindsay P, Jackson AE, Shaw RW 1993 Adverse effects on sperm movement characteristics in women with minimal and mild endometriosis. British Journal of Obstetrics and Gynaecology 100:165–169

Dmowski WP, Cohen MR 1978 Antigonadotrophin (danazol) in the treatment of endometriosis: evaluation of post-treatment fertility and 3-year follow-up data. American Journal of Obstetrics and Gynecology 130:41–48

Dmowski WP, Steele RW, Baker GF 1981 Deficient cellular immunity in endometriosis. American Journal of Obstetrics and Gynecology 141:377–383

Doberl A, Bergquist A, Jeppson S, Koskimies AI, Ronnberg L, Segerbrand E 1984 Repression of endometriosis following shorter treatment with or lower dose of danazol. Acta Obstetricia et Gynecologica Scandinavica 123(suppl):51–58

Donnez J, Nisolle M 1991 Appearance of peritoneal endometriosis. In: Third Laser Surgery Symposium, Brussels

Donnez J, Nisolle M, Clerckx F et al 1990 The ovarian endometrial cyst: combined (hormonal and surgical) therapy. In: Brosens I, Jacobs HS, Runnebaum B (eds) LHRH analogues in gynaecology. Parthenon, Carnforth, pp 165–175

Drake TS, O'Brien WF, Ramwell P et al 1981 Peritoneal fluid thromboxane B$_2$ and 6-keto prostaglandin in F2$_\beta$ in endometriosis. American Journal of Obstetrics and Gynecology 140:401–404

Fahraeus L, Larsson-Cohn U, Ljungberg S, Wallentin I 1984 Profound alterations in the lipoprotein metabolism during danazol treatment in pre-menopausal women. Fertility and Sterility 42:52–57

Halme J, Beecher S, Wing R 1984 Accentuated cyclic activation of peritoneal macrophages in patients with endometriosis. American Journal of Obstetrics and Gynecology 148:85–90

Halme J, Becher S, Haskill S 1986 Altered life span and function of peritoneal macrophages: a new hypothesis for pathogenesis of endometriosis. Society of Gynecologic Investigation, Toronto, Abstract 48

Henzl MR, Corson SL, Moghissi K, Buttram VC, Bergquist C, Jacobson C 1988 Administration of nasal nafarelin as compared with oral danazol for endometriosis. New England Journal of Medicine 318:485–489

Houston DE 1984 Evidence for the risk of pelvic endometriosis by age, race and socioeconomic status. Epidemiologic Reviews 6:167–191

Ingamells S, Thomas EJ 1995 Infertility and endometriosis. In: Shaw RW (ed) Endometriosis – current understanding and management. Blackwell Science, Oxford, pp 147–167

Jansen RPS, Russel P 1986 Nonpigmented endometriosis: clinical laparoscopic and pathologic definition. American Journal of Obstetrics and Gynecology 155:1154–1159

Kennedy SH, Soper NDW, Mojiminiyi OA, Shepstone BJ, Barlow DH 1988 Immunoscintigraphy of ovarian endometriosis. A preliminary study. British Journal of Obstetrics and Gynaecology 95:693–697

Kistner RW 1977 In: Sciarra J (ed) Gynaecology and obstetrics, vol 1. Harper and Row, London

Koninckx PR, de Moor P, Brosens IA 1980 Diagnosis of the luteinizing unruptured follicle syndrome by steroid hormone assays in peritoneal fluid. British Journal of Obstetrics and Gynaecology 87:929–934

Koninckx PR, Meuleman C, Demeyere S, Lesaffre E, Cornillie F 1991 Suggestive evidence that pelvic endometriosis is a progressive disease whereas deeply infiltrating endometriosis is associated with pelvic pain. Fertility and Sterility 55:759–765

Landazabal A, Diaz I, Valbuena D 1999 Endometriosis and in vitro fertilisation: a meta-analysis. Human Reproduction 14:181–182

MacLaverty CM, Shaw RW 1995 Pelvic pain and endometriosis. In: Shaw RW (ed) Endometriosis – current understanding and management. Blackwell Science, Oxford, pp 112–146

Mahmood TA, Templeton A 1990 The impact of treatment on the natural history of endometriosis. Human Reproduction 5:965–970

Marcoux S, Maheux R, Berube S 1997 The Canadian collaborative group on endometriosis laparoscopic surgery in infertile women with minimal-mild endometriosis. New England Journal of Medicine 337:217–222

Matta WH, Shaw RW 1987 A comparative study between buserelin and danazol in the treatment of endometriosis. British Journal of Clinical Practice 41(suppl 48):69–73

Matta WM, Shaw RW, Hesp R, Katz D 1987 Hypogonadism induced by luteinizing hormone releasing hormone agonist analogues: effects on bone density in premenopausal women. British Medical Journal 294:1523–1524

Meldrum DR, Shamonki IM, Clarke KE 1977 Prostaglandin content of ascitic fluid in endometriosis: a preliminary report. 25th Annual Meeting of the Pacific Coast Fertility Society, Palm Springs, California

Mettler L, Semm K 1984 Three-step therapy of genital endometriosis in cases of human infertility with lynestrenol, danazol or gestrinone administration. In: Raynaud JP, Ojasoo T, Martini L (eds) Medical management of endometriosis. Raven Press, New York, pp 233–247

Meyer R 1919 Uber den Staude der Frage der Adenomyosites Adenomyoma in allegemeinen und Adenomyometitis Sarcomastosa. Zentralblatt für Gynäkologie 36:745–759

Miyazawa K 1976 Incidence of endometriosis among Japanese women. Obstetrics and Gynecology 48:407–409

Muscato JJ, Haney AF, Weinberg JB 1982 Sperm phagocytosis by human peritoneal macrophages: a possible cause of infertility in endometriosis. American Journal of Obstetrics and Gynecology 144:503–510

Overton C, Kennedy S 1993 Endometriosis and pelvic pain. Contemporary Reviews of Obstetrics and Gynaecology 5:94–97

Parazzinni F 1999 Ablation of lesions or no treatment in minimal-mild endometriosis in infertile women: a randomized trial. Human Reproduction 14:1332–1334

Pittaway DE, Douglas JW 1989 Serum CA-125 in women with endometriosis and chronic pelvic pain. Fertility and Sterility 51:68–70

Pittaway DE, Vernon C, Fayez JA 1988 Spontaneous abortions in women with endometriosis. Fertility and Sterility 50:711–715

Revised American Fertility Society 1985 Classification of endometriosis. Fertility and Sterility 43:351–352

Rock JA, Markham SM 1987 Extrapelvic endometriosis. In: Wilson EA (ed) Endometriosis. Alan R. Liss, New York, pp 185

Rock JA, Dubin NM, Ghodgaonkar RB, Bergquist CA, Erozan YS, Kimball AW Jr 1982 Cul-de-sac fluid in women with endometriosis: fluid volume and prostanoid concentration during the proliferative phase of the cycle – days 8–12. Fertility and Sterility 37:747–752

Sampson JA 1927 Perforating haemorrhagic (chocolate) cysts of the ovary, their importance and especially their relation to pelvic adenomas of endometrial type. Archives of Surgery 3:245–323

Schifrin BS, Erez S, Moore JG 1973 Teenage endometriosis. American Journal of Obstetrics and Gynecology 116:973–980

Schweppe KW 1984 Morphologie und Klinik der Endometriose. F.K. Schattauer Verlag, Stuttgart, pp 198–207

Shaw RW 1995 Evaluation of treatment with gonadotrophin-releasing hormone analogues. In: Shaw RW (ed) Endometriosis – current understanding and management. Blackwell Science, Oxford, pp 206–234

Shaw RW, Garry R, McMillan L et al 2001 A prospective randomized open study comparing goserelin (Zoladex) plus surgery and surgery alone in the management of ovarian endometriomas. Gynaecological Endoscopy 10:151–157

Simpson JL, Elias S, Malinak LR, Buttram VC Jr 1980 Heritable aspects of endometriosis I: genetic studies. American Journal of Obstetrics and Gynecology 137:327–331

Simpson JL, Malinak LR, Elias S, Carson SA, Redvary RA 1984 HLA associations in endometriosis. American Journal of Obstetrics and Gynecology 148:395–397

Strathy JH, Molgaard GA, Coulam CB, Molton LJ III 1982 Endometriosis and infertility: a laparoscopic study of endometriosis among fertile and infertile women. Fertility and Sterility 38:667–672

Sutton CJ, Ewen SP, Whitelaw N, Haines 1994 Prospective, randomized double blind, controlled trial of laser laparoscopy in the treatment of pelvic pain associated with minimal mild, and moderate endometriosis. Fertility and Sterility 62(4):696–700

Sutton CJ, Polley AS, Ewen SP, Haines P 1997 Follow-up report on a randomized controlled trial of laser laparoscopy in the treatment of pelvic pain associated with minimal to moderate endometriosis. Fertility and Sterility 68:1070–1074

Templeton A, Morris DJK, Parslow W 1996 Factors that affect the outcome of in vitro fertilisation treatment. Lancet 348:1402–1406

Thomas EJ, Cooke ID 1987 Impact of gestrinone on the course of asymptomatic endometriosis. British Medical Journal 294:272–274

Tummon IS, Asher LJ, Martin JSB, Tulandi T 1997 Randomized 'controlled' trial of superovulation and insemination for infertility associated with minimal or mild endometriosis. Fertility and Sterility 68:8–12

Tyson JEA 1974 Surgical consideration in gynecologic endocrine disorders. Surgical Clinics of North America 54:425–442

Vercillini P, Vendola N, Bocciolone L et al 1992 Laparoscopic aspiration of ovarian endometriomas: effect with postoperative gonadotropin releasing hormone agonist treatment. Journal of Reproductive Medicine 37:577–580

Vercillini P, Aimi G, Panazza S, de Giorgi O, Pesole A, Crosigniani PG 1999 A levo-norgestrel-releasing intrauterine system for the treatment of dysmenorrhoea associated with endometriosis: a pilot study. Fertility and Sterility 72:505–508

Vernon M, Beard J, Graves K, Wilson EA 1986 Classification of endometriotic implants in morphologic appearance and capacity to synthesize prostaglandin F. Fertility and Sterility 46:801–805

Wardle PG, McLaughlin EA, McDermott A, Mitchell JD, Ray BD, Hull MGR 1985 Endometriosis and ovulatory disorder. Reduced fertilisation in vitro compared with tubal and unexplained infertility. Lancet 2:236–239

Wardle PG, Foster PA, Mitchell JD et al 1986 Endometriosis and in vitro fertilisation: effect of prior therapy. Lancet 1:276–277

Wentz AC 1980 Premenstrual spotting: its association with endometriosis but not luteal phase inadequacy. Fertility and Sterility 33:605–607

Section 3
BENIGN AND MALIGNANT TUMOURS

35
Epidemiology of gynaecological cancer

Peter Sasieni   Jack Cuzick

INTRODUCTION

Epidemiology is the study of disease in populations as opposed to individuals. The scope ranges from the description of the incidence of disease at a national level, through analytic studies of disease causation, to interventions aimed at disease prevention and mortality reduction. Epidemiology has made significant contributions to our understanding of the causes and control of gynaecological cancers. Human papilloma virus is the primary cause of cervix cancer but requires other co-factors to cause malignancy. Obesity, nulliparity and use of unopposed oestrogens are major risk factors for endometrial cancer. Oral contraceptives are highly protective for ovarian cancer. Oestrogen exposure is the underlying factor for breast cancers although genetic factors are also important. Screening programmes have resulted in a substantial reduction in cervical cancer and breast screening is beginning to make an impact on the mortality rates of breast cancer.

GENERAL OVERVIEW

On a global basis, breast cancer and cervical cancer are the two most common female malignancies. The geographic distribution of these two cancers is complementary, with breast cancer being by far the most common cancer in industrialized countries and cervical cancer being the most common in developing countries. Cancer of the uterine corpus and ovarian cancer have, like breast cancer, higher incidence in industrialized countries. Indeed, in the presence of cervical screening, these cancers are more common than cervical cancer in most Western countries. Table 35.1 provides an overview of age-standardized incidence and mortality rates of these four cancers around the world. Other gynaecological cancers (principally cancer of the vulva) are relatively rare in all parts of the world. The age-standardized rates are about two per 100 000 in most countries, with lower rates (0.5–1.0 per 100 000) in China and Japan (Parkin et al 1997).

513

Table 35.1 Age-standardized rates (per 100 000 women-years) for cancer of the breast, cervix, corpus uterus and ovary (world standard population). Data from Ferlay et al (2001)

Region	Breast		Cervix		Corpus uterus		Ovary	
	Cases	Deaths	Cases	Deaths	Cases	Deaths	Cases	Deaths
E. Africa	20.2	9.2	44.3	24.2	3.4	1.1	9.0	5.6
M. Africa	13.5	6.2	25.1	14.2	3.0	0.9	2.9	1.6
N. Africa	28.3	12.8	16.8	9.1	2.2	0.7	3.2	1.9
S. Africa	31.8	14.5	30.3	16.5	4.6	1.7	3.9	2.4
W. Africa	24.8	11.3	20.3	10.9	1.6	0.6	3.1	1.8
Caribbean	33.8	12.5	35.8	16.8	8.6	3.1	5.6	3.3
C. America	36.2	11.6	40.3	17.0	15.8	4.3	7.0	4.8
S. America	45.1	14.8	30.9	12.0	14.3	2.5	7.3	3.8
N. America	90.4	21.4	7.9	3.2	15.5	2.0	10.7	6.2
E. Asia	18.1	4.9	6.4	3.2	2.4	0.6	3.7	1.8
S.E. Asia	25.6	11.5	18.3	9.7	4.3	1.3	7.1	4.2
S.C. Asia	22.2	10.8	26.5	15.0	2.2	0.8	5.2	3.1
W. Asia	27.9	11.8	4.8	2.5	4.9	1.6	5.9	3.5
E. Europe	49.4	17.2	16.8	6.2	10.7	2.7	10.3	5.0
N. Europe	73.2	24.6	9.8	4.0	11.1	2.1	12.6	8.2
S. Europe	56.2	19.1	10.2	3.3	13.8	2.3	8.7	4.5
W. Europe	78.2	23.5	10.4	3.7	10.9	2.2	11.1	6.9
Aust/NZ	82.7	20.8	7.7	2.7	10.8	1.7	9.6	5.5
Melanesia	21.7	9.7	43.8	23.8	7.1	2.2	7.1	4.2
World	35.7	12.5	16.1	8.0	6.4	1.5	6.5	3.8

The variation in the rates of gynaecological cancers around the world is enormous (Table 35.1). Breast cancer is seven times as common in North America as it is in Middle Africa. Cervical cancer rates in East Africa are nine times greater than in West Asia (the Middle East). The rates for cancer of the uterine corpus are nearly 10 times higher in Central America than in West Africa. And ovarian cancer is four times as common in Northern Europe than in Middle Africa. Some, but certainly not all, of these variations can be explained in terms of differences in lifestyle and public health interventions. Much current research is focused on new screening methods and vaccines to reduce cervical cancer rates in developing countries and on pharmacological interventions (chemoprevention) to reduce breast cancer rates in those at high risk.

CERVICAL CANCER

There are two main types of cervical cancer. The most common type is squamous cell carcinoma. Previously this accounted for around 90% of all cervical cancer. However, more recent data show that adenocarcinoma (including adenosquamous carcinoma) is becoming more common, particularly in younger women (Stockton et al 1997). As a result, squamous cell carcinoma now accounts for only about 75% of all cervical cancer in the US and the UK. The reasons for the increasing proportion of adenocarcinoma seem to be threefold: adenocarcinoma truly is becoming more common; it is being reported more often by pathologists because of the introduction of mucin staining and greater awareness; cytological screening is better able to prevent the development of squamous cancers than

adenocarcinomas and thus the relative incidence of the two types of cancer has changed.

Invasive squamous cervical cancer is preceded by preinvasive neoplasia variously referred to as high-grade squamous intraepithelial lesion (HSIL), cervical intraepithelial neoplasia (CIN) or carcinoma in situ (CIS). Epidemiological studies have focused not only on invasive cancer, but also on the more common preinvasive disease. A similar preinvasive phase has also been identified for adenocarcinoma.

Descriptive epidemiology

It is estimated that there are nearly half a million new cases of cervical cancer worldwide each year, accounting for about 10% of all female cancers (Parkin 2001). The cumulative rate of a cancer by the age of 74 years is the approximate probability of a woman developing cancer by the age of 74, assuming that she does not die first from some other cause. This cumulative rate for cervical cancer ranges from over 5% in parts of Latin America and in sub-Saharan Africa to around 0.5% in parts of the Middle East and in Finland. In most European countries it is under 2% (Parkin et al 1997). Rates also vary considerably between different ethnic populations within a given geographic area. Thus, for instance, the Maori population of New Zealand have nearly three times the risk of the non-Maori, and in Los Angeles, Hispanic women have more than twice the risk of non-Hispanic white women, who are in turn at nearly twice the risk of Japanese Americans (Table 35.2).

Incidence of cervical cancer in most countries has decreased

Table 35.2 Cumulative incidence of cancer of the cervix in different populations 1988–92 (Parkin et al 1997)

Population	Cumulative incidence (age 0–74) per 1000 women
New Zealand:	
Non-Maori	12
Maori	34
Los Angeles:	
Non-Hispanic white	8
Hispanic	18
Black	12
Japanese	4

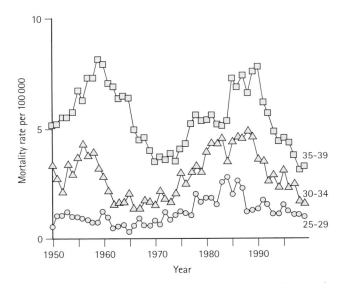

Fig. 35.1 Trends in age-specific mortality rates for cervical cancer in young women for England and Wales 1950–99.

significantly since the 1960s (Coleman et al 1993). In the UK, mortality from cervical cancer has been declining since 1950. However, in young British women (aged 20–39 years), mortality rates more than doubled between 1970 and the mid-1980s but have since declined to previous levels (Fig. 35.1).

In unscreened populations, incidence rates typically increase rapidly from age 25 to 40, more slowly until age 55 and then begin to decline. This characteristic relationship is often modified by birth cohort effects. The absolute rate of cervical cancer is determined by environmental exposure to the human papilloma virus, particularly in the late teens and 20s. The level of exposure is determined by sexual behaviour and will vary over time. Careful analysis shows that incidence and mortality rates can be modelled well by age and cohort effects until the 1980s. However, for more recent data, the addition of age-specific time trends corresponding to a beneficial effect of screening is required to provide a satisfactory model, particularly in younger women (Sasieni & Adams 2000). From a public health perspective it is important to note that women born in the 1960s are at 3–4 times the risk of cervical cancer compared to women born in the 1930s.

Risk Factors

Epidemiological evidence suggestive of a sexually transmitted agent being associated with cervical cancer has grown over the years. Traditional risk factors include number of sexual partners and age at first sexual intercourse (Brinton 1992). The behaviour of men is also important, as shown by increasing risk in women with just one partner, according to the number of their husband's partners (Buckley et al 1981). More recently, the causal sexually transmitted agent has been identified as certain high-risk anogenital types of the human papillomavirus (HPV) (IARC 1995).

There are over 90 types of HPV, only some of which infect the anogenital region. These can be split into low-risk types, which cause genital warts, and high-risk types (most commonly 16, 18, 31, 33, 35, 39, 45, 51, 52, 56, 58 and 68), which can lead to cervical cancer. It has been estimated that HPV is the most common sexually transmitted infection worldwide, with most people being exposed to the virus by the age of 30. Most infections with high-risk types are transitory and harmless. In only a minority of women does the infection become persistent. This may lead to high-grade cervical lesions with a potential for progression to cancer. Immune factors are certainly associated with persistence, but are poorly understood. Similarly, it is largely unknown why some women with persistent infection develop cervical cancer whereas others do not.

The association between high-risk HPV infection and cervical cancer is extremely strong. Case-control studies of both invasive cancer and high-grade preinvasive disease consistently find odds ratios of over 20 for high-risk HPV types detected by PCR (Table 35.3). In case series of invasive cervical cancer virtually all tumours have detectable HPV (Walboomers et al 1999). Longitudinal studies have shown that HPV infection precedes the development of cervical cancer (Dillner et al 1997) and that viral persistence is a key determinant of risk (Wallin et al 1999). A recent Dutch study (Nobbenhuis et al 1999) followed 353 women with low-grade cytology for a median of 33 months. Of 122 women with persistent HPV infection, 98 had CIN III by the end of the study. There were only five other cases of CIN III and four of these had HPV detected at least once during the study. The strong epidemiological evidence in favour of a causative role of HPV infection is supported by molecular studies, which have demonstrated that gene products from oncogenic HPV types block the action of cancer suppressor proteins. The HPV E6 protein binds the p53 gene product (Werness et al 1990) and the E7 protein forms complexes with pRb (Dyson et al 1989).

Other risk factors are less clearcut. Smoking is associated with cervical cancer, but it has been difficult to disentangle the confounding caused by the sociological link between smoking and increased numbers of sexual partners. Nevertheless, the accumulated evidence suggests smoking increases the risk of cervical cancer two- to threefold, probably by reducing the local immune response to HPV infection (Szarewski & Cuzick 1998). Immunosuppression certainly conveys an increased risk of cervical cancer, as shown in studies on renal transplant patients receiving immunosuppressive drugs (Birkeland et al 1995) and on women who are HIV positive (Wright 1997). Most studies find a weak association between oral contraceptive use

Table 35.3 Odds ratio of HPV and high-risk HPV detected in case-control studies of women with high-grade preinvasive disease or invasive cervical cancer

Reference	Country	No. cases	No. controls	OR HPV	OR HR-HPV
High-grade preinvasive disease of the cervix					
Becker 1994	US	201	337	20.8	
Bosch 1993	Spain	157	193	56.9	296
	Columbia	125	181	15.5	27
Cuzick 1995	England	81	1904		65
Schiffman 1993	US	50	453		180
van den Brule 1991	Netherlands	177	1762	68.1	136
Invasive cervical cancer					
Eluf-Neto 1994	Brazil	199	225	37.1	75
Munoz 1995b	Spain	250	238	46.2	
	Columbia	186	149	15.6	30
Peng 1991	China	101	146		33

Selected case-control studies of cervical neoplasia using PCR to test for HPV.
The first odds ratio is generally for a consensus primer detecting both high- and low-risk types and the second is either for a mixture of high-risk types or type 16 alone.

and cervical cancer (IARC 1999, Moreno et al 2002). Diet may play a role in the immune response to HPV, but studies on diet and cervical cancer are as yet inconclusive (Brinton 1992). It has been shown recently that cervical neoplasia (including carcinoma in situ) exhibits familial clustering and that the strength of association increases with increasing genetic relatedness (Magnusson et al 1999). Several groups have found an association between certain HLA class II antigens and cervical neoplasia (Odunsi et al 1995), but much more remains to be done in understanding the factors that determine why some women develop cervical cancer after infection with oncogenic HPVs, but the vast majority do not.

A recent case-control study considered factors associated with CIN III in women with a high-risk HPV and also factors associated with HPV infection in women with no evidence of cervical neoplasia (Deacon et al 2000). Comparison between the 181 HPV-positive controls and the 203 HPV-negative controls only found a significant association for HPV positivity with the number of sexual partners, a new sexual partner within the previous 2 years and a history of miscarriage. By contrast, the factors associated with CIN III when comparing the 181 HPV-positive controls to the 199 HPV-positive cases were early age at first sexual intercourse, a long time since starting a new sexual relationship and cigarette smoking.

Natural history

There are few data from studies that directly observe the entire natural history of cervical cancer development because it is generally felt to be unethical not to treat precancerous cervical disease. The situation is further complicated by the possibility that the process of taking a biopsy, required for definitive diagnosis of disease, may affect the natural history by stimulating the immune response to induce regression.

The first step in cervical carcinogenesis is exposure to HPV. The time from infection to the development of invasive cancer is many years; typically between 10 and 50. Longitudinal studies on young women show that the majority of HPV infections are transient (Hildesheim et al 1994, Moscicki et al 1998, Wheeler et al 1996, Woodman et al 2001) and that the virus is indeed sexually transmitted (Burk et al 1996, Dillner et al 1996). Persistence of infection is associated with the development of cervical lesions (Ho et al 1995, Koutsky et al 1992, Remmink et al 1995) and viral load can be used as an (imperfect) surrogate for persistence (Brisson et al 1996, Cuzick 1997). It is generally believed that integration of the viral DNA in the host genome is a key step in the development of cancer (Cullen et al 1991). However, some carcinomas only have episomal viral DNA and integration is uncommon in CIN III, suggesting that it is a late-stage event (Das et al 1992).

Cervical neoplasia appears to constitute a disease continuum ranging from cervical intraepithelial neoplasia (CIN) grades I–III to microinvasive and finally fully invasive cancer. More recent evidence shows that CIN I is frequently not associated with HPV infection and may therefore not be part of the continuum in all cases (Kiviat et al 1992) and that in some instances CIN III can develop extremely rapidly. CIN III rates rise rapidly with age, peaking at about age 30, and fall rather more slowly, being at about half their peak by age 40 and just 10–20% of their maximum by age 50. Follow-up studies have found that about 60% of CIN I and 33% of CIN III regress whilst 11% and 22% of CIN I and II, respectively, progress to CIN III (Ostor 1993). At most, about a third of high-grade CIN progresses to cancer over 15 years (McIndoe et al 1984).

Prevention and screening

Dramatic falls in cervical cancer rates following the introduction of screening have been seen in several countries. The age-standardized incidence of cervical cancer fell substantially between 1965 and 1980 in Denmark, Sweden and, in particular, in Finland following the introduction of mass screening in the mid to late 1960s (Hakama 1982). By contrast, rates in Norway, which was the only Nordic country without mass cervical screening, increased. UK rates have fallen by 50% in the last decade and this is primarily due to a high-quality screening programme with excellent population coverage (Quinn et al 1999).

Prevention of cervical cancer may one day be achievable by vaccination of teenagers (male as well as female) against oncogenic HPVs (Munoz et al 1995a). Until then, the most likely route to reducing cervical cancer morbidity is through the detection and treatment of precancerous cervical lesions. Screening by cytological analysis of cervical smears has proven to be effective in many industrialized countries but requires a great deal of skill and organization and has not been successful in reducing cancer rates in any developing country.

Case-control studies comparing the screening experience of women diagnosed with cervical cancer with that of healthy women conducted in eight countries demonstrated that cervical screening could be effective in identifying women at increased risk of developing cervical cancer (IARC 1986). Compared to women who had never been screened, women with two or more negative smears were 15 times less likely to develop cervical cancer within a year of having a negative test. The effect lasted several years but decreased with time since the negative smear, so that after 5–6 years women were 'only' three times less likely to develop cancer than those who had never been screened. A more recent study suggests a somewhat smaller effect and shorter duration of protection (Sasieni et al 1996).

Several new developments in cytology have been investigated in recent years and may be introduced (possibly in conjunction with some other technologies such as HPV testing) over the next decade. These include liquid-based slide preparation to produce a thin layer of cells (Payne et al 2000) and automatic or semi-automatic screening of slides (McGoogan 1997). Scientifically, the most interesting new development is the possibility of using HPV testing in screening. Although tests for high-risk HPV DNA are more sensitive than conventional cytology for detecting CIN III, there remains considerable uncertainty as to how HPV testing might best be utilized to improve cervical screening (Cuzick et al 1999, Sasieni 2000). Another option being considered in developing countries is visual inspection of the cervix after application of dilute acetic acid. Initial studies suggest that this may be a sensitive but non-specific screening tool (Sankaranarayanan et al 1999, University of Zimbabwe 1999) but there is a major question over whether inspections of sufficient quality could be established and maintained at a population level.

ENDOMETRIAL CANCER

Most cancers of the uterine corpus are adenocarcinomas of the endometrium (the lining of the womb). Sarcomas of the myometrium (muscle) are rare and are not considered in this chapter. Incidence rates of endometial cancer in Western countries are 5–7 times as great as mortality rates, reflecting the high cure rate for these cancers. Endometrial cancer is rare under the age of 40. Incidence increases steeply, particularly between the ages of 45 and 55, but levels off after the age of 60. Rates are highest in America (Latin America as well as North America) and lowest in Asia and Africa (see Table 35.1).

Although rates among blacks and Americans of Japanese descent in the US are lower than they are among US whites, they are much higher than in their ancestral countries (Parkin et al 1997). Rates among US whites are higher than those in Europe, possibly due to greater use of unopposed oestrogens.

When studying trends in endometrial cancer, it is important to look also at 'cancer of the uterus, site not specified' since in many countries the majority of those cancers will have originated in the endometrium. In both England (Sasieni et al 1997) and the US (Ries et al 2001) mortality rates have fallen steadily and substantially (~60%) since 1950 in all but the oldest age groups (80+). Incidence, by contrast, has been more stable. In England, there was an increase in incidence in the over-50s in the early 1970s and a further increase in the over-60s in the late 1980s (Sasieni et al 1997). For those under the age of 60, incidence has fallen slightly since the mid-1970s. Interpretation of trends is complicated by the prevalence of women who have had a hysterectomy, since obviously women without a uterus are not susceptible to uterine cancer.

Risk factors

The main aetiological factors are obesity, hormonal status and reproductive history. Obesity and unopposed oestrogen in hormone replacement therapy are the most important from a public health perspective. Nulliparity is consistently found to be associated with a 2–3-fold increase in risk and most case-control studies find that increasing parity reduces the risk still further. Late age at menopause is also associated with increased risk of endometrial cancer in most studies (Pike 1987).

Obesity is consistently found to be associated with endometrial cancer in both case-control and cohort studies and, because of the high prevalence of obesity in many populations, is likely to be responsible for a significant proportion of endometrial cancer in many countries. Typically, those who are most obese have 2–3 times greater risk than those who are least obese, but some studies have found much stronger effects (e.g. Henderson et al 1983). Obesity is likely to affect cancer rates by increasing the level of circulating oestrogens, particularly in postmenopausal women. This occurs both through peripheral aromatization of androstenedione to estrone and through decreased concentrations of sex hormone-binding globulin (Grady & Ernster 1996).

Oestrogen replacement therapy has been consistently found to be associated with an increase in endometrial cancer. A meta-analysis estimated a relative risk of 2.3 in ever-users compared to never-users and found that the risk remains elevated for several years after cessation of use (Grady et al 1995). The risk appears to increase both with increasing duration of use and increased dose of oestrogen (Weiderpass et al 1999b) with a relative risk of 10 associated with 10 years use (Grady et al 1995). However, newer preparations including a progestogen either as a continuous combined replacement or used sequentially for at least 10 days per month cause only minimal increased risk of endometrial cancer (Beresford et al 1997, Pike et al 1997).

Unusually, smoking has fairly consistently been associated

with a decreased risk of endometrial cancer of about 50% in case-control studies (Brinton et al 1993, Weiderpass & Baron 2001, Weiss et al 1980). The association remains after adjustment for obesity and is thought to be due to anti-oestrogenic effects of smoking and an earlier age at menopause in smokers. This is supported by those studies that find an association only in postmenopausal women.

The combined oral contraceptive (COC) pill reduces the risk of endometrial cancer (Schlesselman 1995, Vessey 1989). Four years use reduces the risk by about 50% and the effect lasts for 15 or more years (Pike et al 1997, Weiderpass et al 1999a, WHO 1988). Shorter duration of use results in a smaller reduction in risk.

Prevention and screening

Primary prevention of endometrial cancer could be aimed at weight loss and the use of the COC pill, both of which would have net benefits on women's health. Screening is unlikely to have a role in the foreseeable future.

OVARIAN CANCER

Ovarian cancer affects between 1% and 2% of women in the developed world. Survival is very poor, except when the tumour is detected early, which is rarely in most countries. Over 80% of ovarian cancers are adenocarcinomas of the epithelium, but germ cell tumours are the most common histological type in women under the age of 30. In both the US and England, germ cell tumours seem to have two peaks in incidence, the first in the late teens and the second (smaller peak) around age 70. The age distribution suggests that germ cell tumours have different epidemiology from adenocarcinomas but because they are so rare (the age-specific incidence in England peaks at about five cases per million) little is known about their aetiology.

Descriptive epidemiology

Variation in the rates of ovarian cancer around the world is less marked than for other gynaecological cancers (see Table 35.1). The highest rates are found in Northern Europe and in white women in North America and Western Europe. Women in Latin America tend to have lower rates, but Hispanic women in the US have rates similar to those of whites (Table 35.4). Similarly, rates tend to be lower in most Asian countries, but women of Japanese and Chinese descent in the US have rates that are higher than in their countries of origin.

Trends in ovarian cancer in England and Wales have been different in different age groups. Mortality rates in premenopausal women fluctuated somewhat between 1950 and 1970, but have fallen considerably since (Fig. 35.2). This is most likely due to the widespread use of oral contraceptives since 1972 (Villard-Mackintosh et al 1989). By 1999 the rates in women aged 30–44 were just half of what they had been in 1970. The picture for older women is dramatically different. Rates in the over-60s have increased and by 1999 the rates in women aged 70–84 were over 75% greater than they were in 1950.

Table 35.4 Cumulative incidence of cancer of the ovary in different populations 1988–92 (Parkin et al 1997)

Population	Cumulative incidence (age 0–74) per 1000 women
US, Puerto Rico	6
Japan, Osaka	6
Los Angeles:	
Non-Hispanic white	16
Hispanic	10
Black	10
Japanese	9

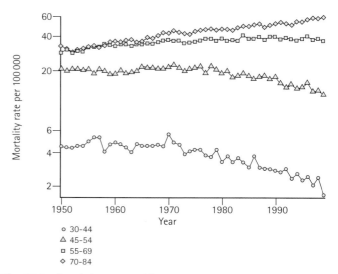

Fig. 35.2 Trends in age-specific mortality rates for ovarian cancer from data for England and Wales 1950–99.

Risk factors

The main factors affecting the risk of epithelial cancers of the ovary are reproductive history and contraceptive use, although a small proportion of women are at greatly increased risk due to inherited genetic susceptibility. Overall, the main risk factor appears to be the lifetime number of ovulatory cycles.

Reproductive history

One of the first observations relating reproductive history to ovarian cancer risk was that never-married women were at about 1.5 times the risk of ever-married women (Dorn & Cutler 1955). Subsequently, decreasing risk with increasing numbers of full-term pregnancies has been consistently shown in over a dozen case-control studies. Typically, one or two children are associated with about a 30% decreased risk and three or more with about a 60% decreased risk. In a recent US study of 563 cases and 523 controls, one child was associated with a 40% reduction in risk, two children with a 60% reduction in risk and five or more with a 80% reduction (Titus-Ernstoff et al 2001). A cohort study from Norway (Kvale et al 1988) yielding 445 cases found relative risks of 0.9 for parity 1, 0.6 for parity 2 and 0.5 for parity 3 or 4 compared to nulliparous women. The effect of parity does not appear to be attributable to confounding by age at first birth, age at last birth, age at menarche or age at menopause.

Menstrual factors have an effect on ovarian cancer risk, but are less important than parity. Age at menarche has been extensively investigated and tends to have a small effect on risk. It would appear that women with an early menarche (below age 12) are at about 25% greater risk than those with a late menarche (aged 15 or older) (Risch 1998). Women with irregular cycle lengths tend to have reduced risk of ovarian cancer (Parazzini et al 1991). The effect, if any, of early age at menopause is protective (Chiaffarino et al 2001, Franceschi et al 2001, Schildkraut et al 2001).

Infertility, however, does appear to have a small independent effect on ovarian cancer risk. In a pooled analysis of 12 US case-control studies (Whittemore et al 1992), nulliparous women who tried to conceive for at least 2 years were at slightly higher risk of ovarian cancer than those who had not tried to conceive for more than 1 year. Additionally, women who received fertility treatment had an increased risk compared to those who had never been treated with fertility drugs. However, recent case-control studies, while confirming the increased risk associated with infertility, find no increased risk associated with fertility drugs per se (Mosgaard et al 1997, Parazzini et al 2001).

Exogenous hormones

The protective effect of combined oral contraceptives on ovarian cancer risk has been demonstrated beyond any reasonable doubt (IARC 1999). Pooled estimates of the protection indicate that the risk is reduced by about 50% with 5 years use and that the protection increases with the duration of use (Hankinson et al 1992, Whittemore et al 1992). The protective effect of oral contraceptives persists for at least 15 years after cessation of use and is not confined to any particular formulation of the pill (Beral et al 1999). The length of persistence of the protective effect of oral contraceptives clearly has enormous public health implications in many countries, but there are as yet insufficient data to estimate the effect 20–40 years after last use.

Hormone replacement therapy has minimal effect on ovarian cancer (Whittemore et al 1992), but some studies have reported a moderate increase in risk (IARC 1999).

Family history

It is a well-known clinical observation that ovarian cancer tends to aggregate in families. Rarely such clustering can be extreme with increased risk of breast cancer (in BRCA1 and BRCA2 gene mutation carriers) and with colon and endometrium in other cancer family syndromes (Lynch et al 1991). Case-control studies generally find relative risk of around 3 associated with one affected family member and 7 with two affected relatives. More recently, the Swedish cancer family database reported a relative risk of 2.9 in women with an affected mother and 2.5 in women with an affected sister (Dong & Hemminki 2001). The high lifetime risk of ovarian cancer in BRCA1 mutation carriers (estimated by Risch et al (2001) to be 36%) has led many to consider prophylactic oophorectomy for those who have completed their families.

Other factors

Epidemiological evidence regarding diet is inconclusive. An effect of diet was originally suggested because of the correlation between ovarian cancer rates and dietary fat intake internationally. High intakes of meat and fats have been associated with ovarian cancer in case-control studies in both China (Shu et al 1989) and Italy (Bosetti et al 2001). In the latter study red meat increased the risk of ovarian cancer by up to 50% whilst fish and vegetables decreased the risk by a similar percentage. Coffee drinking appears to increase the risk of ovarian cancer, but the evidence is primarily from case-control studies and one cannot exclude recall bias and confounding as explanations (IARC 1991, Kuper et al 2000).

There has been great interest in whether talcum powder applied to the perineal area increases the risk of ovarian cancer. Despite the lack of any animal evidence to support such a relationship, it has been investigated by many case-control studies. A recent study (Cramer et al 1999) found an adjusted relative risk of 1.6 associated with use of talc in genital hygiene. The authors also included a meta-analysis of 14 case-control studies and provided a summary (unadjusted) relative risk with a 95% confidence interval of 1.24–1.49. Despite this finding, we suggest caution because the majority of studies fail to observe a dose–response relationship and there is the possibility of recall bias differentially affecting cases and controls.

Prevention and screening

There are two screening tools that may potentially lead to reduced mortality through early detection of ovarian cancer. Serum levels of CA125, a tumour marker, are raised in 80% of women with epithelial ovarian cancer, but they are raised in only about 50% of women with early tumours. CA125 levels are also raised in women with a variety of other conditions such as endometriosis, benign ovarian neoplasms and fibroids. Thus the test is neither sensitive nor specific for pre-symptomatic ovarian cancer. Screening for enlarged ovaries using transvaginal ultrasound is more sensitive, but lacks specificity because it is unable to differentiate benign cysts from malignant disease. Colour Doppler ultrasound can be used to study blood flow in an attempt to distinguish benign from malignant lesions (Bourne et al 1993), but it is unclear whether this will be sufficiently discriminative to make population screening viable. There is much interest in combining ultrasound with CA125 testing and in monitoring changes in CA125 levels over time, but it has not yet been demonstrated whether such an approach will reduce the mortality from ovarian cancer. The results of large randomized trials will not be available for some time.

CANCERS OF THE VULVA AND THE VAGINA

In England and Wales, vulval cancer accounts for about 6% of female genital cancer and vaginal cancer for 1.5%. Over 95% of deaths due to other female genital sites (ICD9:184) are due to either cancer of the vulva (ICD9:184.1–184.4) or the vagina (ICD9:184.0). They are both uncommon malignancies in all parts of the world with rates that increase almost exponentially with age. Over 80% are squamous in origin, with 5–10% of vulva cancers being melanomas.

Mortality rates from both cancers have fallen considerably in England and Wales since 1958 (Fig. 35.3). By 1994, age-standardized rates fell by 43% for vulval cancer (from 2.5 to 1.4 per 100 000) and by 66% in vaginal cancer (from 0.9 to 0.3 per 100 000). Analysis of age-specific trends shows that rates have declined by a similar percentage in all ages (Sasieni et al 1997). Trends in incidence rates for cancers of the vulva and vagina show no clear patterns.

Little is known for certain about the aetiology of these cancers because they are quite rare. Vulva cancer tends to be associated with similar risk factors as cervical cancer. For instance, it is more common in women of lower social class (Berg & Lampe 1981, Peters et al 1984). Brinton et al (1990) found that 15% of 209 women with vulval cancer reported a history of genital warts compared to 1.4% of 348 community controls. Hording and colleagues (1993) used PCR to detect HPV in 62 vulval cancer specimens and 101 blocks of normal vulval tissue. They found HPV types 16, 18 or 33 in 19 (31%) of the cancer specimens and none of the normal material. Thus, although there is a significant association between HPV infection and vulval cancer the relationship is nowhere near as strong as it is with cervical cancer and the majority of cases of

vulval cancer are not caused by HPV infection. It has been suggested that vulval cancer is two distinct diseases with HPV-related type primarily affecting women under the age of 65 and a second type of unknown pathogenesis affecting older women (Crum 1992, Lee et al 1994). Smoking also appears to be a risk factor (Brinton et al 1990, Daling et al 1992, Madeleine et al 1997), but the data are far from conclusive. The one risk factor that has been consistently associated with cancer of the vulva is immunosuppression: invasive vulval cancer is significantly more common in women with renal transplants (Blohme & Brynger 1985) and vulval intraepithelial neoplasia has an increased incidence in HIV-positive women (Chiasson et al 1997). Now that women in developed countries are surviving much longer after HIV infection, it remains to be seen whether they will have an appreciable risk of vulval cancer. Currently, however, women with identified immunosuppression account for only a very small proportion of those with vulval cancer.

Even less is known about the aetiology of vaginal cancer. The one exception is that vaginal cancer in adolescents has been attributed to in utero exposure to diethylstilboestrol (DES), a synthetic oestrogen used to prevent spontaneous abortions between 1940 and 1970 (Bornstein et al 1988, Greenwald et al 1971, Herbst et al 1971). Teenage vaginal cancer is almost never diagnosed in cohorts who could not have been exposed to DES in utero (either because they were born prior to 1945 or because DES was never prescribed in that country). But vaginal cancer is still rare even in those who were exposed. One study estimated the risk to be about 1 in 1000 by the age of 30 (Melnick et al 1987).

BREAST CANCER

It is not possible to provide more than a superficial overview of breast cancer epidemiology within a chapter covering the epidemiology of all gynaecological cancers. The estimated number of cases worldwide in 2000 was just over a million, accounting for around 22% of female cancers (Parkin 2001). In North America, the lifetime risk of breast cancer is over 10%. Endogenous hormones play a key role in the aetiology of disease and there is currently much interest in preventing the disease by use of selective oestrogen receptor modulators (SERMs) such as tamoxifen.

Breast cancer is rare before the age of 30, but increases rapidly up to age 50 and then more slowly in postmenopausal women. Pike and co-workers (1983) introduced the notion of 'breast tissue age' to explain the age–incidence curve. Plotted against breast tissue age, rather than actual age, breast cancer rates follow a power law typical of other cancers. The advantage of this model is that it can incorporate the known reproductive and endocrine risk factors.

In England and Wales mortality from breast cancer had been steadily increasing from 1950 to 1989 but has recently fallen dramatically (Fig. 35.4). The substantial reduction in mortality is probably mostly due to greater use of tamoxifen, but better management of early tumours, as a result of an organized screening programme, may also be a factor. Similar but less dramatic effects have been seen in the US and elsewhere. Incidence figures are difficult to interpret due to the

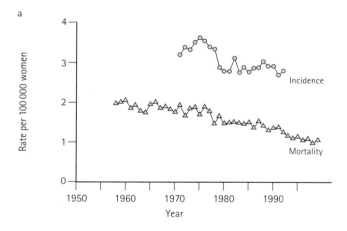

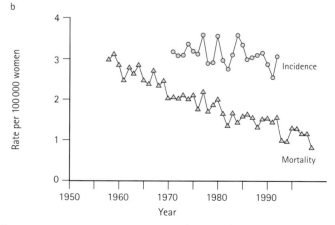

Fig. 35.3 Age-standardized mortality (1958–99) and incidence (1971–92) rates for cancer of the (a) vulva and (b) vagina.

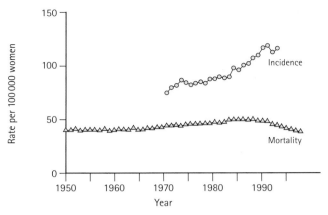

Fig. 35.4   Age-standardized mortality (1950–99) and incidence (1971–94) rates for cancer of the breast.

influence of screening, which leads to a substantial increase in cancer detection amongst screened women.

Risk factors

Family history

A positive family history of breast cancer is associated with an increased risk of breast cancer especially when there is a history of early onset or bilateral disease. Women with a mother or sister who developed breast cancer have at least a twofold risk and higher risks are found for early onset or multiply affected individuals (Pharoah et al 1997). Highly penetrant mutations in two genes, BRCA1 and BRCA2, are responsible for the majority of cancers in families with four or more cases under the age of 60, but account for only a small fraction of less extreme familial clustering of the disease. Individuals with these mutations in affected families have about a 70–80% lifetime risk of developing breast cancer. The penetrance in unselected individuals appears to be lower (40–60%).

Age at menarche and menopause

Early age of menarche and late age at menopause are both associated with an increased risk of breast cancer. Women with early menopause (before age 45) have just half the risk of those with late menopause (after 55). Artificial menopause (bilateral oophorectomy) also has a marked protective effect on breast cancer risk similar in magnitude to that of a natural menopause. Late menarche is also protective, but the effects are smaller. Further, case-control studies have found that, on average, women with breast cancer have shorter menstrual cycles (and therefore more cycles in a fixed length of time) than controls (La Vecchia et al 1985, Olsson et al 1983). Thus the cumulative number of ovulatory cycles appears to be an important determinant of breast cancer risk. In this respect, it is interesting to note that several authors have found a modest protective effect of lactation, especially for women who have a cumulative time of breast feeding in excess of 5 years (Newcomb et al 1999, Ross & Yu 1994, Zheng et al 2000, 2001).

Pregnancy

Nulliparity increases the risk of breast cancer. However,

MacMahon et al (1970) found that the risk is more to do with the age at first birth than nulliparity per se. Breast cancer risk approximately doubled with 15 years increase in age at first birth, with nulliparous women having similar risk to those whose first birth was at age 30. In that study, subsequent births had little effect on breast cancer risk, but more recent studies tend to find a small residual benefit of increasing numbers of children after taking into account the age at first birth. It may be that early childbirth is the protective factor and subsequent births have a smaller effect because of their later age.

Exogenous hormones

A meta-analysis of 54 epidemiological studies found that current users of oral contraceptives have a small increased risk of breast cancer (around 25%), but that the risk approaches background rates 5 years after cessation (CGHFBC 1996). Cancers diagnosed in women taking the pill are less likely to be advanced clinically and there is no significant increase in risk associated with duration of use or with dose or type of hormone within the pill. Thus, there must be some concern that effects of this magnitude could be due to bias in case-control studies. Nevertheless, it is clear that oral contraceptives do not have a major impact on the lifetime risk of breast cancer, since the majority of diagnoses are made more than 10 years after oral contraceptive use has stopped.

The effect of hormone replacement therapy (HRT) is also somewhat unclear. A recent overview (CGHFBC 1997) found that the risk of breast cancer increased by about 12% for every 5 years of use and there was little evidence of risk for use of less than 5 years. This is roughly in keeping with the effect of a delayed menopause. Once again, breast cancers in women taking HRT tend to be less advanced and there is no evidence of an increase in breast cancer mortality among women taking HRT (O'Meara et al 2001). Any increased risk seems to disappear quite rapidly after cessation of HRT use.

Weight and height

Increased weight is consistently associated with increased risk of postmenopausal breast cancer (Friedenreich 2001). Each kilogram is associated with about a 1% increase in relative risk with the heaviest quartile of postmenopausal women being at about 25% increased risk compared to the lightest quartile. By contrast, in most studies, very heavy pre-menopausal women (over 80 kg) are at a decreased risk of breast cancer (Friedenreich 2001). The increase in post-menopausal women is consistent with the fact that their oestrogen is derived primarily from aromatization of peripheral fat. In premenopausal women, obesity may lead to anovulatory menstrual cycles which in turn would result in decreased levels of estradiol and progesterone and hence to a decreased risk of breast cancer.

Height increases the risk of breast cancer by about 1% per centimetre, so that tall women are at about 25% greater risk than short women (van den Brandt et al 2000). It should be noted that the association of breast cancer with weight in postmenopausal women is seen after adjusting for height, for instance by using body mass index. More convincingly, weight gain in adult life is consistently found to be associated with increased risk (Friedenreich 2001).

Diet

Although international comparisons show that breast cancer rates are correlated with fat intake, such a relationship has not been found consistently at an individual level. Epidemiological studies have examined a variety of dietary factors from total fat intake to dietary fibre and phyto-oestrogens (as found in soy), but no clear picture emerges.

Meta-analyses suggest that heavy drinkers (three or more alcoholic drinks per day) have about 50% greater risk of breast cancer than non-drinkers (Longnecker et al 1988) with smaller increases associated with more modest drinking (Smith-Warner et al 1998), but the magnitude of the increase varies considerably between studies.

Mammographic density

Mammographically dense breasts have been found to increase the risk of breast cancer in over two dozen studies, beginning with the initial work of Wolfe (1976). Wolfe's original classification has been slightly modified to more fully use the extent of the breast covered by dense parenchymal patterns. These studies have been reviewed by Oza & Boyd (1993). Based on the Canadian screening programme (Boyd et al 1995), we estimate a relative risk of 3.1 and an attributable fraction of 21% due to densities covering more than 50% of the breast in women aged 50–59. Using US data, Byrne et al (1995) found similar, but slightly smaller risks. In both studies the relative risks were smaller in pre-menopausal women, although dense breasts are more common in that age group and the attributable fraction is similar.

Prevention and screening

Mammography

Eight trials have reported on mortality reductions from breast cancer screening (Table 35.5). These data have been subjected to several overviews (Elwood et al 1993, Hendrick et al 1997, Nystrom et al 1996). Overall there is clear evidence for a mortality reduction of around 30% for women aged 50–70. Much controversy still exists regarding younger women, but a recent overview suggests an 18% mortality reduction, although there is considerable heterogeneity between trials (Hendrick et al 1997). Case-control studies are also supportive of these general results but tend to provide larger estimates of benefit, which are to some extent affected by the higher mortality amongst those who do not take up screening than found in the general population (Duffy et al 2002).

Chemoprevention

Four trials using tamoxifen have been performed (Table 35.6). The largest trial (NSABP-P1) shows about a 50% reduction in breast cancer incidence and the IBIS trial found but the two smaller trials are not so favourable. A review of trial parameters does not clearly explain this difference but a meta-

Table 35.5 Randomized trials of breast screening: age at entry, follow-up and relative risks for breast cancer death. Modified from Andersson & Ryden (2001)

Study	Age at entry (years)	Relative risks (95% CI)	
		All ages	Age under 50 years
HIP	40–46	0.71 (0.55–0.93)	0.77 (0.53–1.11)
Kopparberg (W)	40–74	0.68 (0.52–0.89)	0.57 (0.37–1.22)
Östergötland (E)	40–74	0.82 (0.64–1.05)	1.02 (0.59–1.77)
Malmö	45–69	0.81 (0.62–1.07)	0.64 (0.45–0.89)
Stockholm	40–64	0.80 (0.53–1.22)	1.01 (0.51–2.02)
Gothenburg	40–49	0.86 (0.54–1.37)	0.95 (0.31–0.96)
Edinburgh	45–64	0.84 (0.63–1.12)	0.88 (0.55–1.41)
Canada 1	40–49	–	1.14 (0.83–1.56)
Canada 2	50–59	0.97 (0.62–1.52)	–

Table 35.6 Numbers of women randomized, follow-up times and breast cancers detected (including in situ lesions). Updated from Cuzick (2000)

	Total randomized	Median follow-up (months)	Cancers			
			Total	Tamoxifen/ raloxifene	Placebo	Relative Risk
Royal Marsden	2471	70	70	34	36	0.94
NSABP-P1	13 388	57	368	124	244	0.51
Italian	5408	46	41	19(11)‡	22(19)‡	0.91
IBIS	7139	50	170	69	101	0.68
MORE (raloxifene)	7705	40	74	31/2†	43	0.36

‡ Tamoxifen >1 year
† 2:1 ratio of SERM:placebo in MORE study

analysis indicates that all results are compatible with a 40% reduction in short-term incidence (Cuzick 2000). A fifth trial using raloxifene found a 65% reduction in breast cancer incidence. Several important questions remain about the clinical implication of these results, including the effect on mortality, the appropriate risk groups for chemoprevention and the long-term effects on incidence. Continued follow-up of these trials is crucial for resolving these issues.

KEY POINTS

1. Breast cancer and cervical cancer are the two most common female malignancies in the world.
2. Breast cancer is by far the most common cancer in industrialized countries and cervical cancer is the most common in developing countries.
3. The variation in the rates of gynaecological cancers around the world is enormous.
4. Well organised cytological screening has had a dramatic effect on the incidence and mortality rates of cervical cancer.

KEY POINTS (*CONTINUED*)

5. HPV infection is very common but only a tiny minority of women infected with HPV develop cervical cancer. The development of cancer depends on persistence of HPV infection.
6. HPV testing offers potential for improving the effectiveness and feasibility of cervical screening particularly in the developing world.
7. In the long term, vaccination against HPV may eliminate cervical cancer all together.
8. The incidence of endometrial cancer has remained stable but the mortality rate has fallen slowly in the UK.
9. Obesity and oestrogens are the main factors associated with endometrial cancer.
10. The oral contraceptive pill has reduced the incidence of ovarian cancer in women aged 30–44. The rate has risen in older women.
11. Mortality from breast cancer in the UK has recently fallen dramatically after a period of gradual increase.
12. Two rare high-penetrance genes, BRCA1 and BRCA2, have been identified that are linked with familial breast and ovarian cancer.
13. Most of the familial clustering of breast cancer is due to genes that are yet to be identified.
14. Mammographic screening can reduce the mortality from breast cancer.
15. Tamoxifen reduces the risk of breast cancer by 30–40%, but has side-effects, and the overall risk-benefit ratio is still unclear.

REFERENCES

Andersson I, Ryden S 2001 Early detection and prevention: benefits, costs and limitations of screening. In: Tobias JS, Houghton J, Henderson IC (eds) Breast cancer: new horizons in research and treatment. Arnold, London, pp 105–117

Becker TM, Wheeler CM, McGough NS et al 1994 Sexually transmitted diseases and other risk factors for cervical dysplasia among southwestern Hispanic and non-Hispanic white women. JAMA 271(15):1181–1188

Beral V, Hermon C, Kay C et al 1999 Mortality associated with oral contraceptive use: 25 year follow up of cohort of 46 000 women from Royal College of General Practitioners' oral contraception study. British Medical Journal 318(7176):96–100

Beresford SAA, Weiss NS, Voigt LF et al 1997 Risk of endometrial cancer in relation to use of oestrogen combined with cyclic progestagen therapy in postmenopausal women. Lancet 349:458–461

Berg JW, Lampe JG 1981 High-risk factors in gynecologic cancer. Cancer 48(suppl 2):429–441

Birkeland SA, Storm HH, Lamm LU et al 1995 Cancer risk after renal transplantation in the Nordic countries, 1964–1986. International Journal of Cancer 60(2):183–189

Blohme I, Brynger H 1985 Malignant disease in renal transplant patients. Transplantation 39(1):23–25

Bornstein J, Adam E, Adler-Storthz K et al 1988 Development of cervical and vaginal squamous cell neoplasia as a late consequence of in utero exposure to diethylstilboestrol. Obstetric and Gynecological Survey 43(1):15–21

Bosch FX, Munoz N, de Sanjose S et al 1993 Human papillomavirus and cervical intraepithelial neoplasia grade III/carcinoma in situ: a case-control study in Spain and Colombia. Cancer Epidemiology, Biomarkers and Prevention 2(5):415–422

Bosetti C, Negri E, Franceschi S et al 2001 Diet and ovarian cancer risk: a case-control study in Italy. International Journal of Cancer 93(6):911–915

Bourne TH, Campbell S, Reynolds KM et al 1993 Screening for early familial ovarian cancer with transvaginal ultrasonography and colour blood flow imaging. British Medical Journal 306(6884):1025–1029

Boyd NF, Byng JW, Jong RA et al 1995 Quantitative classification of mammographic densities and breast cancer risk: results from the Canadian National Breast Screening Study. Journal of the National Cancer Institute 87(9):670–675

Brinton LA 1992 Epidemiology of cervical cancer – overview. In: Muñoz N, Bosch FX, Shah KV et al (eds) The epidemiology of cervical cancer and human papillomavirus. International Agency for Research on Cancer, Lyon, pp 3–23

Brinton LA, Nasca PC, Mallin K et al 1990 Case-control study of cancer of the vulva. Obstetrics and Gynecology 75:859–866

Brinton LA, Barrett RJ, Berman ML et al 1993 Cigarette smoking and the risk of endometrial cancer. American Journal of Epidemiology 137(3):281–291

Brisson J, Bairati I, Morin C et al 1996 Determinants of persistent detection of human papillomavirus DNA in the uterine cervix. Journal of Infections Diseases 173(4):794–799

Buckley JD, Harris RW, Doll R et al 1981 Case-control study of the husbands of women with dysplasia or carcinoma of the cervix uteri. Lancet 2(8254):1010–1015

Burk RD, Ho GY, Beardsley L et al 1996 Sexual behavior and partner characteristics are the predominant risk factors for genital human papillomavirus infection in young women. Journal of Infections Diseases 174(4):679–689

Byrne C, Schairer C, Wolfe J et al 1995 Mammographic features and breast cancer risk: effects with time, age, and menopause status. Journal of the National Cancer Institute 87(21):1622–1629

CGHFBC (Collaborative Group on Hormonal Factors in Breast Cancer) 1996 Breast-cancer and hormonal contraceptives – collaborative reanalysis of individual data on 53297 women with breast-cancer and 100239 women without breast-cancer from 54 epidemiologic studies. Lancet 347 (9017):1713–1727

CGHFBC (Collaborative Group on Hormonal Factors in Breast Cancer) 1997 Breast cancer and hormone replacement therapy: collaborative reanalysis of data from 51 epidemiological studies of 52,705 women with breast cancer and 108,411 women without breast cancer. Lancet 350 (9084):1047–1059

Chiaffarino F, Pelucchi C, Parazzini F et al 2001 Reproductive and hormonal factors and ovarian cancer. Annals of Oncology 12(3):337–341

Chiasson MA, Ellerbrock TV, Bush TJ et al 1997 Increased prevalence of vulvovaginal condyloma and vulvar intraepithelial neoplasia in women infected with the human immunodeficiency virus. Obstetrics and Gynecology 89:690–694

Coleman MP, Esteve J, Damiecki P et al 1993 Trends in cancer incidence and mortality. IARC scientific publications no. 121 IARC, Lyon.

Cramer DW, Liberman RF, Titus-Ernstoff L et al 1999 Genital talc exposure and risk of ovarian cancer. International Journal of Cancer 81(3):351–356

Crum CP 1992 Carcinoma of the vulva: epidemiology and pathogenesis. Obstetrics and Gynecology 79:859–866

Cullen AP, Reid R, Campion M et al 1991 Analysis of the physical state of different human papillomavirus DNAs in intraepithelial and invasive cervical neoplasm. Journal of Virology 65(2):606–612

Cuzick J 1997 Viral load as a surrogate for persistence in cervical human papillomavirus infection. In: Franco ELF, Monsonégo J (eds) New developments in cervical cancer screening and prevention. Blackwell Science, Oxford, pp 373–378

Cuzick J 2000 A brief review of the current breast cancer prevention trials and proposals for future trials. European Journal of Cancer 36(10):1298–1302

Cuzick J, Szarewski A, Terry G et al 1995 Human papillomavirus testing in primary cervical screening. Lancet 345(8964):1533–1536

Cuzick J, Sasieni P, Davies P et al 1999 A systematic review of the role of human papillomavirus testing within a cervical screening programme. Health Technology Assessment 3(14):1–204

Daling JR, Sherman KJ, Hislop TG et al 1992 Cigarette smoking and the risk of anogenital cancer. American Journal of Epidemiology 135(2):180–189

Das BC, Sharma JK, Gopalakrishna V et al 1992 Analysis by polymerase chain reaction of the physical state of human papillomavirus type 16 DNA in cervical preneoplastic and neoplastic lesions. Journal of General Virology 73(pt 9):2327–2336

Deacon JM, Evans CD, Yule R et al 2000 Sexual behaviour and smoking as determinants of cervical HPV infection and of CIN3 among those infected: a case-control study nested within the Manchester cohort. British Journal of Cancer 83(11):1565–1572

Dillner J, Kallings I, Brihmer C et al 1996 Seropositivities to human papillomavirus types 16, 18, or 33 capsids and to Chlamydia trachomatis are markers of sexual behavior. Journal of Infective diseases 173(6):1394–1398

Dillner J, Lehtinen M, Bjorge T et al 1997 Prospective seroepidemiologic study of human papillomavirus infection as a risk factor for invasive cervical cancer. Journal of the National Cancer Institute 89(17):1293–1299

Dong C, Hemminki K 2001 Modification of cancer risks in offspring by sibling and parental cancers from 2,112,616 nuclear families. International Journal of Cancer 92(1):144–150

Dorn HF, Cutler SJ 1955 Morbidity from cancer in the United States. US Department of Health, Education and Welfare. US Government Printing Office, Washington DC

Duffy SW, Cuzick J, Tabar L et al 2002 Correcting for non-compliance bias in case-control studies to evaluate cancer screening programmes. Applied Statistics 51(2):235–243

Dyson N, Howley PM, Munger K et al 1989 The human papilloma virus-16 E7 oncoprotein is able to bind to the retinoblastoma gene product. Science 243(4893):934–937

Eluf-Neto J, Booth M, Munoz N et al 1994 Human papillomavirus and invasive cervical cancer in Brazil. British Journal of Cancer 69(1):114–119

Elwood JM, Cox B, Richardson AK 1993 The effectiveness of breast cancer screening by mammography in younger women. Online Journal Current Clinical Trials Feb 25; doc no 32: para 1–195

Ferlay J, Bray F, Pisani P et al 2001 GLOBOCAN 2000: cancer incidence, mortality and prevalence worldwide, Version 1.0. IARC CancerBase No. 5. IARC Lyon Press,

Franceschi S, La Vecchia C, Booth M et al 1991 Pooled analysis of 3 European case-control studies of ovarian cancer: II. Age at menarche and at menopause. International Journal of Cancer 49(1):57–60

Friedenreich CM 2001 Review of anthropometric factors and breast cancer risk. European Journal of Cancer Prevention 10(1):15–32

Grady D, Ernster VL 1996 Endometrial cancer. In: Schottenfeld D, Fraumeni JF (eds) Cancer epidemiology and prevention. Oxford University Press, Oxford, pp 1058–1089

Grady D, Gebretsadik T, Kerlikowske K et al 1995 Hormone replacement therapy and endometrial cancer risk: a meta-analysis. Obstetrics and Gynecology 85:304–313

Greenwald P, Barlow JJ, Nasca PC et al 1971 Vaginal cancer after maternal treatment with synthetic estrogens. New England Journal of Medicine 285:390–392

Hakama M 1982 Trends in the incidence of cervical cancer in the Nordic countries. In: Magnus K (ed) Trends in cancer incidence. Hemisphere, New York

Hankinson SE, Colditz GA, Hunter DJ et al 1992 A quantitative assessment of oral contraceptive use and risk of ovarian cancer. Obstetrics and Gynecology 80:708–714

Henderson BE, Casagrande JT, Pike MC et al 1983 The epidemiology of endometrial cancer in young women. British Journal of Cancer 47(6):749–756

Hendrick RE, Smith RA, Rutledge JH 3rd et al 1997 Benefit of screening mammography in women aged 40–49: a new meta-analysis of randomized controlled trials. Journal of the National Cancer Institute 22:87–92

Herbst AL, Ulfelder H, Poskanzer DC 1971 Adenocarcinoma of the vagina: association of maternal stilbestrol therapy with tumour appearance in young women. New England Journal of Medicine 284:878–881

Hildesheim A, Schiffman MH, Gravitt PE et al 1994 Persistence of type-specific human papillomavirus infection among cytologically normal women. Journal of Infectious Diseases 169(2):235–240

Ho GY, Burk RD, Klein S et al 1995 Persistent genital human papillomavirus infection as a risk factor for persistent cervical dysplasia. Journal of the National Cancer Institute 87(18):1365–1371

Hording U, Kringsholm B, Andreasson B et al 1993 Human papillomavirus in vulvar squamous-cell carcinoma and in normal vulvar tissues: a search for a possible impact of HPV on vulvar cancer prognosis. International Journal of Cancer 55(3):394–396

IARC Working Group on Evaluation of Cervical Cancer Screening Programmes 1986 Screening for squamous cervical cancer: duration of low risk after negative results of cervical cytology and its implication for screening policies. British Medical Journal 293(6548):659–664

IARC 1991 IARC monographs on the evaluation of carcinogenic risks to humans, vol. 51, coffee, tea, mate, methylxanthines and methylglyoxal. IARC, Lyon

IARC 1995 IARC monographs on the evaluation of carcinogenic risks to humans, vol. 64, human papillomaviruses. IARC, Lyon

IARC 1999 IARC monographs on the evaluation of carcinogenic risks to humans, vol. 72, hormonal contraception and post-menopausal hormonal therapy. IARC, Lyon

Kiviat NB, Critchlow CW, Kurman RJ 1992 Reassessment of the morphological continuum of cervical intraepithelial lesions: does it reflect different stages in the progression to cervical carcinoma? In: Munoz N, Bosch FX, Shah KV, Meheus A (eds) The epidemiology of cervical cancer and human papillomavirus (IARC scientific publications no. 119). IARC, Lyon, pp 59–66

Koutsky LA, Holmes KK, Critchlow CW et al 1992 A cohort study of the risk of cervical intraepithelial neoplasia grade 2 or 3 in relation to papillomavirus infection. New England Journal of Medicine 327(18):1272–1278

Kuper H, Titus-Ernstoff L, Harlow BL et al 2000 Population based study of coffee, alcohol and tobacco use and risk of ovarian cancer. International Journal of Cancer 88(2):313–318

Kvale G, Heuch I, Nilssen S et al 1988 Reproductive factors and risk of ovarian cancer: a prospective study. International Journal of Cancer 42(2):246–251

La Vecchia C, Decarli A, di Pietro S et al 1985 Menstrual cycle patterns and the risk of breast disease. European Journal of Cancer and Clinical Oncology 21(4):417–422

Lee YY, Wilczynski SP, Chumakov AC et al 1994 Carcinoma of the vulva: HPV and p53 mutations. Oncogene 9:1655–1659

Longnecker MP, Berlin JA, Orza MJ et al 1988 A meta-analysis of alcohol consumption in relation to risk of breast cancer. Journal of the American Medical Association 260(5):652–656

Lynch HT, Conway T, Lynch J 1991 Hereditary ovarian cancer. Pedigree studies, Part II. Cancer Genetics and Cytogenetics 53(2):161–183

MacMahon B, Cole P, Lin TM et al 1970 Age at first birth and breast cancer risk. Bulletin of the World Health Organisation 43(2):209–221

Madeleine MM, Daling JR, Carter JJ et al 1997 Cofactors with human papillomavirus in a population-based study of vulvar cancer. Journal of the National Cancer Institute 89(20):1516–1523

Magnusson PK, Sparen P, Gyllensten UB 1999 Genetic link to cervical tumours. Nature 400(6739):29–30

McGoogan E 1997 Automation and cervical cytopathology: an overview. In: Franco ELF, Monsonégo J (eds) New developments in cervical cancer screening and prevention. Blackwell Science, Oxford pp 265–273

McIndoe WA, McLean RW, Jones RW et al 1984 The invasive potential of carcinoma in situ of the cervix. Obstetrics and Gynecology 64:451–458

Melnick S, Cole P, Anderson D et al 1987 Rates and risks of diethylstilbestrol-related clear-cell adenocarcinoma of the vagina and cervix. An update. New England Journal of Medicine 316(9):514–516

Moreno V, Bosch FX, Munoz N et al 1995 Quantitative classification of mammographic densities and breast cancer risks: results from the Canadian National Breast Screening Study. Journal of the National Cancer Institute 87(9):670–5

Moscicki AB, Shiboski S, Broering J et al 1998 The natural history of human papillomavirus infection as measured by repeated DNA testing

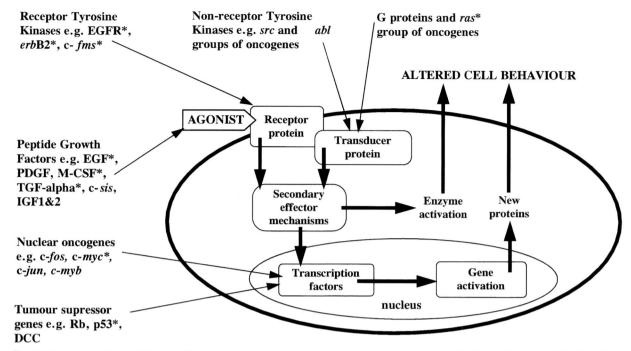

Fig. 36.2 An overview of the role of oncogenes and tumour suppressor genes in the control of cell growth and proliferation. The purpose of this figure is to emphasize that the genetic abnormalities in cancer are a result of alterations to or abnormal expression of genes which are normally involved in cell regulation. Genes which are implicated in ovarian carcinogenesis are marked*. Note that many aspects of the figure are oversimplified for clarity, e.g. although a function of p53 and retinoblastoma is transcriptional regulation this is not true of all tumour suppressor genes.

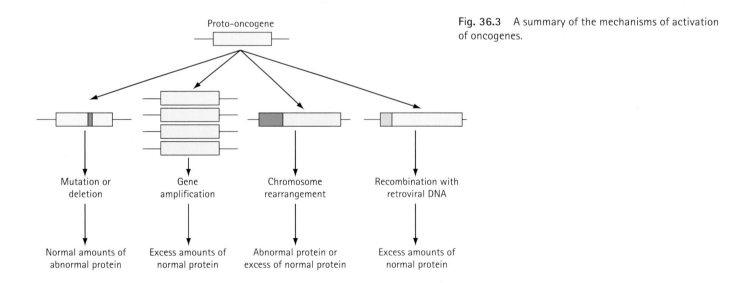

Fig. 36.3 A summary of the mechanisms of activation of oncogenes.

human cancer cell lines (Krontiris & Cooper 1981) and found that some of the transforming oncogenes identified were mutated versions of the protooncogenes identified by the retroviral approach (Santos et al 1982). Subsequently it was demonstrated that chromosome translocations such as the Philadelphia chromosome in chronic myeloid leukaemia involved known oncogenes (DeKlein et al 1982).

Approximately 100 protooncogenes have been identified and many can be assigned to the groups of functions summarized in Figure 36.2. The mutation resulting in conversion of a protooncogene into an oncogene may occur in several different ways (Fig. 36.3) and may result in an abnormal protein produced in normal quantity, a normal protein produced in excessive amount or a normal protein produced inappropriately due to loss or alteration of control regions of the gene.

529

Tumor suppressor genes

The existence of tumour suppressor genes was suggested by cell fusion studies of transformed cells and non-transformed cells which resulted in a non-transformed hybrid cell (Harris et al 1969). The subsequent identification of the first tumour suppressor gene followed from the study of retinoblastoma, a rare childhood cancer which may occur in a hereditary and sporadic form. On the basis of epidemiological and statistical analysis Knudson (1971) suggested that development of the cancer required two events. He postulated that in the hereditary form the first event was a germline mutation present in every cell of the individual and that a second event in any of the many million retinoblasts could result in tumour formation. The rarity, later onset and unilateral nature of the sporadic form could be attributed to the need for two events in a single retinal cell in the absence of a germline mutation. When the Rb (retinoblastoma) gene was mapped to chromosome 13q and cloned it was confirmed that in both familial and sporadic retinoblastoma, the two copies of the gene were inactivated in tumour cells consistent with Knudson's 'two-hit' hypothesis (Cavanee et al 1983). Subsequently a number of other tumour suppressor genes have been identified including p53 (Baker et al 1989), APC (Kinzler et al 1991) and DCC (Fearon et al 1990).

At a cellular level there is a fundamental difference in the mode of action of tumour suppressor genes and oncogenes (Fig. 36.4). Mutations creating oncogenes result in a gain of function and will have an effect even in the presence of a remaining normal copy of the gene, i.e. they are dominant at a cellular level. In contrast, tumour suppressor genes involve a loss of function and act recessively at a cellular level. In general both copies of a tumour suppressor gene must be lost or inactivated for an effect on cellular regulation to occur.

Multistep carcinogenesis

Although the spontaneous mutation rate of a gene is low (approximately 10^{-6} per gene per cell division), the total number of cell divisions in the lifetime of an individual is high (approximately 10^{16}) and consequently each gene is likely to have undergone at least 10^{10} spontaneous mutations (Cairns 1975). Mutations affecting genes involved in carcinogenesis are therefore likely to be manyfold more frequent than the observed rates of malignancy.

Clearly a single mutation of a single gene cannot generally be sufficient to cause cancer and several lines of evidence support the concept of carcinogenesis as a multistep process. First, the relationship of cancer incidence and age is logarithmic and consistent with a requirement of 4–7 separate steps (Armitage & Doll 1954). Second, in vitro studies of fibroblasts and studies of transgenic mice indicate that transformation requires at least two complementing oncogenes, e.g. ras and myc (Land et al 1983). Third, animal studies of chemical

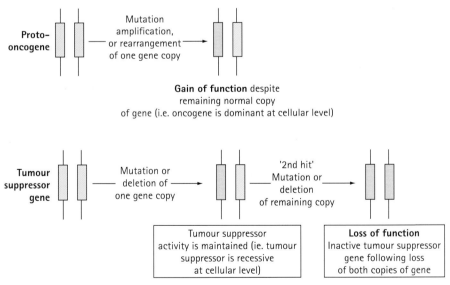

Fig. 36.4 A summary of the fundamental difference between oncogenes and tumour suppressor genes. Oncogenes are dominant at a cellular level and mutation of only one of the two gene copies is required for activation. Tumour suppressor genes are recessive at a cellular level. Both copies of the gene must usually be inactivated for loss of suppressor activity. An important exception to these general principles occurs when the product of a mutant copy of a tumour suppressor gene can interfere with the function of the product of the remaining wild-type copy of the gene. If this occurs both copies of the gene will be functionally inactive even though a normal wild-type copy of the gene remains. This is known as a dominant–negative effect and an example is the p53 gene. The p53 protein functions as a dimer and dimers formed by wild-type and mutant protein are inactive. Loss of p53 tumour suppressor activity therefore seems to occur in some tumours following mutation of just one copy of the gene.

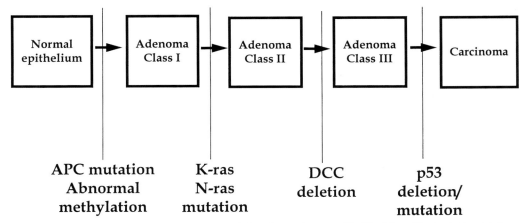

Fig. 36.5 The multistep model of carcinogenesis in colorectal cancer. Modified from Kinzler & Vogelstein (1993).

induction of tumours have revealed three stages in carcinogenesis: initiation which is irreversible, promotion which is reversible and progression. Most recently, direct evidence has been obtained for some cancers of the specific set of genetic alterations involved in carcinogenesis. One of the best examples of multistep carcinogenesis involving a common cancer is colorectal cancer (Fearon et al 1990) which is illustrated in Figure 36.5.

Germline and somatic genetic alterations

An important distinction must be made between germline and somatic mutations. Somatic mutations are found in the tumour cells but not the normal cells of an individual with cancer and cannot therefore be passed on to descendants of the patient. Germline mutations predisposing to cancer involve all the cells of the individual as well as the tumour, can be passed on to descendants of the individual and can be identified in DNA obtained from normal cells, such as a peripheral blood sample. The same genetic abnormalities frequently occur as both germline and somatic mutations in different individuals. For example, mutations of the p53 gene are one of the commonest genetic changes found in human cancer. In most cancers mutation of p53 occurs as a somatic event but germline p53 mutations have been identified in some families with the rare Li–Fraumeni syndrome characterized by sarcomas, breast cancer and other malignancies occurring at a young age. Another example is germline mutations of the APC gene which is responsible for familial adenomatous polyposis (FAP) (Kinzler et al 1991). Somatic mutations of APC have been detected in over 80% of sporadic colorectal cancers and appear to be one of the earliest events in colorectal carcinogenesis.

Most of the familial cancer syndromes identified to date have an autosomal dominant pattern of inheritance. Individuals inheriting the germline abnormality are at high risk of developing malignancy as the penetrance of most of these genes is of the order of 80%. It is possible that another class of genetic predispositions to cancer will be identified which increase susceptibility to cancer but with a low penetrance (i.e. a relatively small proportion of individuals with the genetic abnormality develop cancer). Such individuals would not be easy to identify by familial studies because of the low penetrance but may account for a significant proportion of cancer cases.

GENETICS OF FAMILIAL GYNAECOLOGICAL CANCER

Although there are anecdotal reports of more than one case of vulval and cervical cancer occurring in close relatives there is no good evidence of inherited predisposition to these cancers. Well-defined cancer family syndromes with an autosomal dominant inheritance pattern have, however, been described for ovarian and endometrial cancers. Pedigree studies of families with a high incidence of cancer have revealed three main syndromes associated with ovarian cancer. Hereditary site-specific ovarian cancer without an excess of breast or colorectal cancer is the least common familial ovarian cancer syndrome. The most common hereditary form of ovarian cancer occurs in association with breast cancer. A large number of hereditary breast/ovarian cancer families have now been described in which there is a high frequency of both cancers and an association with an early age of onset. Less frequently ovarian cancer occurs in hereditary non-polyposis colorectal cancer families (HNPCC). Women in HNPCC families most frequently develop colorectal or endometrial cancer. Some families have recently been described with an apparently high risk of site-specific endometrial cancer. It is important to recognize that all these families combined probably account for less than 5% of cases of ovarian cancer and a smaller proportion of cases of endometrial cancer.

The BRCA1 and BRCA2 genes

Identification of families at high risk of breast and ovarian cancer along with the development of polymorphic DNA markers made it possible to perform detailed linkage analysis with the aim of locating genes involved in familial cancer. A major step forward was the report of linkage of early-onset breast cancer to the polymorphic marker CMM86 located on chromosome 17q (Hall et al 1990). Subsequently, linkage to 17q was confirmed by a consortium of 13 research groups from Europe and the USA which analysed linkage data on six genetic markers on 17q in 214 families (Easton et al 1993). Almost all breast/ovarian cancer families and 40% of the families with breast cancer alone were found to have linkage to the BRCA1 (*Breast Cancer 1*) gene on chromosome 17q and the consortium data localized the gene to a 2cM region on 17q. Intensive efforts were then made in a number of research units in Europe and the USA to further localize and clone the BRCA1 gene. Eventually, in 1994 a group in Utah described a large gene on 17q within which they had identified mutations in five affected families (Miki et al 1994). Subsequent work by other research groups has confirmed that this gene is the BRCA1 gene and over 300 distinct mutations have now been described in breast/ovarian cancer.

BRCA1 is a large gene with 22 exons which encode a protein of 1863 amino acids. There are no specific hotspots for mutation in the gene and only a small proportion of mutations are recurrent. Overall the penetrance of a BRCA1 mutation for ovarian cancer appears to be 40–50% and for breast cancer 80% (Ford et al 1994, 1998). However, there is evidence that penetrance may be modified by both environmental factors and other genetic influences. Furthermore, the location of a mutation within the BRCA1 gene may influence both the overall risk of cancer and the type of cancer. Gayther et al (1995) reported a correlation between mutations toward the 3′ end of the gene and a greater risk of ovarian than breast cancer. Well-defined founder mutations have been described in BRCA1. Mutations at 185delAG and 5382insC have been documented in approximately 1% of the Ashkenazi Jewish cancers and in some studies up to 40% of Ashkenazi Jewish women with ovarian cancer or early-onset breast cancer. Identification of BRCA2 closely followed the cloning of BRCA1. Wooster et al (1995) identified the gene following studies involving high-risk families in which the disease pattern was not linked to BRCA1.

BRCA2 is also a large gene with 26 coding exons encoding a protein with 3418 amino acids. Over 100 mutations have been described to date and, just like BRCA1, there are no hotspots for mutation although there are founder mutations in some ethnic groups such as Ashkenazi Jews (Levy-Lahad et al 1997, Thorlacius et al 1997). Although the penetrance for breast cancer is approximately 80% the penetrance for ovarian cancer seems to be lower than for BRCA1 mutations and is approximately 25% (Ford et al 1998). There is a suggestion that mutations in exon 11 confer a higher risk of ovarian cancer than mutations in other areas (Gayther et al 1997). Overall BRCA1 and BRCA2 are believed to account for over 95% of hereditary cases of ovarian cancer and over 80% of hereditary breast cancers.

The function of the BRCA1/2 genes is still unclear. Most of the mutations of BRCA1 are small insertions or deletions which result in loss of protein synthesis or production of a truncated protein. This observation supports the concept that BRCA1 functions as a tumour suppressor gene. In this 'two-hit' model, although one copy of the gene is inherited as an inactive mutant form, the development of cancer requires somatic mutation of the other wild-type ('normal') gene copy.

Analysis of tumours from familial breast/ovarian cancer families has demonstrated that loss of heterozygosity in these tumours involves the wild-type gene, thus providing further evidence that the BRCA1 gene is a tumour suppressor (Smith et al 1992). Both BRCA1 and BRCA2 are expressed in largest amounts in the testis and thymus and at lower levels in the breast and ovary. Although the genes have limited sequence homology they do have similarities including being A-T rich, a large exon 11 and start of translation at codon 2. The presence of a zinc finger motif in BRCA1 has suggested a role as a transcription factor whilst BRCA2 has homology with known transcription factors. Association of BRCA1 and BRCA2 with the DNA repair gene RAD51 suggests that they may be involved in RAD51 repair of DNA double strand breaks.

HNPCC–associated gynaecological cancer and DNA repair genes

HNPCC is associated with autosomal dominant inheritance of colorectal cancer in those who do not have the multiple adenomas which occur in FAP. The identification of the genetic basis of Lynch II syndrome is a notable example of the power of molecular technology. HNPCC was classified by Henry Lynch into site-specific hereditary colon cancer (Lynch I syndrome) and families with a predisposition to non-polyposis colorectal cancer in association with other cancers including stomach, small bowel, ureter, renal pelvis and brain as well as ovarian and endometrial cancer (Lynch II syndrome) (Lynch 1985). The identification of the genes responsible for HNPCC was a result of several developments which showed that HNPCC is associated with hereditary defects in one of five DNA mismatch repair genes (MSH2, MLH1, PMS1, PMS2 and MSH6/GTBP). Over 200 mutations have been identified in these five genes in HNPCC families, making mutation testing a difficult challenge in these families (Lynch & de la Chapel 1999). Available evidence suggests that these genes function as tumour suppressor genes in a manner consistent with Knudson's 'two-hit' model. The inherited germline mutation inactivates one copy of the mismatch repair gene but inactivation of the remaining wild-type copy by a second somatic mutation is required prior to tumour formation. The secondary, acquired mutations which result from loss of DNA repair gene function include defects of APC, K-ras, DPC4 and p53 (Huang et al 1996, Kinzler & Vogelstein 1996). The penetrance for colorectal cancer in mutation carriers is in excess of 80% in men and 30% in women and HNPCC accounts for approximately 5% of colorectal cancers (Aarnio et al 1999, Dunlop et al 1997, Salovaara et al 2000). Endometrial cancer is the second most common cancer in HNPCC families, female carriers having a 42% risk by age 70 (Dunlop et al 1997). The penetrance for ovarian cancer is less, with a reported lifetime risk of 9% (Marra & Roland 1995).

MANAGEMENT OF FAMILIAL GYNAECOLOGICAL CANCER

Risk assessment

At present risk assessment is based largely upon information derived from a detailed family tree. Important information includes the number of cases of cancer relative to the number of people at risk, the pattern of cancers of different types and the age at diagnosis of cancer. For a number of reasons, risk assessment should ideally be undertaken in the setting of a multidisciplinary specialist familial cancer clinic run by a geneticist working with a team of genetic counsellors and with close links to specialists in areas such as gynaecological, colorectal and breast cancer. Obtaining a detailed family history and confirming the history with clinical and histopathological information is time consuming and requires an organization and resources specifically established for this pupose. The interpretation of family histories is not always straightforward, particularly when there are a variety of different primary sites in the family. Specialist training is required to counsel patients about the implications and consequences of genetic testing. Particular expertise is also required to provide the patient with sound advice about methods of prevention and screening.

Although it is difficult to define precisely the minimum family history necessary to satisfy the description of a familial cancer syndrome involving a gynaecological cancer, some broad guidelines can be outlined:

- families in which two first-degree relatives have ovarian cancer
- families in which first-degree relatives have breast cancer at less than 50 years of age and ovarian cancer
- families in which two first-degree relatives have breast cancer at less than 60 years of age and a third relative with ovarian cancer.

The likelihood that high frequency of cancer in such families is due to an inherited predisposition rather than a change event is in excess of 60%. Families in which one relative has ovarian or endometrial cancer and two or more first-degree relatives cancer of the colon/rectum, at least one at less than 50 years of age, can be classified as HNPCC families. Although the BRCA1 gene and DNA repair genes have now been identified analysis of these genes for mutations in the clinical setting remains challenging. The genes are large and the mutations are not localized to specific regions of the gene. Using currently available techniques mutation detection is still a lengthy, time-consuming and often expensive process. Nevertheless, mutation testing is now widely available for high-risk families via clinical genetics centres in the UK after thorough counselling about the implications of testing.

Prevention of familial cancer

Use of the oral contraceptive pill may be suggested for HNPCC and breast/ovary family members on the basis of case-control studies in the general population which indicate a protective effect against ovarian and endometrial cancer. While one study has suggested a protective effect of the oral contraceptive pill in BRCA1/2 carriers, this was not confirmed in a second study and the situation remains unclear (Modan et al 2001). Furthermore, there is concern in breast/ovary families that a reduction in risk of ovarian cancer may be offset by an increased risk of breast cancer.

Prophylactic salpingo-oophorectomy and hysterectomy as a primary procedure is justifiable in women from breast/ovarian and HNPCC families after completion of their family and after thorough counselling. However, there is evidence that women in breast/ovarian families are at risk of primary peritoneal cancer as part of a field change involving the peritoneal mesothelium as well as the ovarian epithelium which share a common embryological origin. For this reason some doubts have been raised about the efficacy of oophorectomy as a preventive strategy. Available data suggest that intra-abdominal carcinomatosis following oophorectomy in women with a strong family history of ovarian cancer is a real entity (Piver 1994) but that oophorectomy does reduce substantially the cancer risk (Struewing et al 1995). Women undergoing prophylactic surgery should be counselled that the procedure will prevent ovarian cancer but that they may still be at risk of primary peritoneal cancer.

It should also be noted that cases of intra-abdominal carcinomatosis following oophorectomy have been reported in which subsequent review of the oophorectomy specimen revealed a small focus of ovarian cancer (Chen et al 1985). Surgery should therefore include a careful inspection of the abdomen and pelvis and thorough histological examination of the ovary. Fallopian tube cancer does seem to be more common in BRCA1/2 families, so prophylactic surgery should include salpingectomy. Hysterectomy should be advised for women from HNPCC families but women in breast/ovarian families do not appear to be at increased risk of endometrial cancer and the decision about hysterectomy will depend on other factors.

Screening for familial cancer

The efficacy of ovarian cancer screening is unproven to date although a survival benefit was noted in a pilot randomized trial in the general population (Jacobs et al 1999). A larger randomized trial involving 200 000 postmenopausal women from the general population will not yield definitive data until 2010 (UK Collaborative Trial of Ovarian Cancer Screening – UKCTOCS). Although the value of ovarian cancer screening is unclear there is a consensus that it is reasonable to screen women in breast/ovarian families with transvaginal ultrasonography and serum CA125 measurement in view of their level of risk. Screening is usually performed on an annual basis from the mid 30s or 5 years prior to the earliest age of onset of ovarian cancer in the family.

It should be noted that both CA125 and ultrasound are associated with a substantial risk of false-positive results leading to unnecessary surgery (Campbell et al 1993, Jacobs et al 1993). It is essential to warn women clearly about this risk. The false-positive rate for both CA125 and ultrasonography is approximately 1–2% in postmenopausal women and more in premenopausal women. It is therefore likely that a 30-year-old woman undergoing annual screening for up to 50 years will have a false-positive result at some stage with consequent anxiety and the risk of unnecessary surgery.

Women in breast/ovarian cancer families may be advised to commence screening with mammography from the mid 30s or 5 years prior to the earliest age of onset of breast cancer in their family, although the value of mammography in premenopausal women is controversial. Women in HNPCC families should be advised to undergo regular colonoscopy and mammography in addition to ovarian cancer screening. Ultrasound screening for endometrial cancer is not useful because of the very high number of false-positive results but can be justified in this group of women because of the particularly high risk. Ultrasound measurement of endometrial thickness can be performed at the time of screening for ovarian size and morphology. It is reasonable to add an outpatient form of endometrial sampling such as pipelle aspiration. It should be emphasized that these screening strategies are currently recommended on a pragmatic basis in view of the high risk of cancer rather than on the basis of clear evidence concerning their efficacy.

Women with a family history not consistent with a familial syndrome

Most of the women who seek advice about a family history of gynaecological cancer have one affected first-degree relative and do not fall into a familial syndrome. Requests for advice from this group of women have increased dramatically following recent media publicity about screening for ovarian cancer and the identification of the BRCA1/2 genes. Although women with a first-degree relative with ovarian cancer are at increased risk compared to the general population, the absolute risk remains small. They should be reassured that although their risk of ovarian cancer may be increased several fold it remains low (lifetime risk of 4–5% vs 1% in the general population). Screening with either CA125 or ultrasound should not routinely be offered to these women for two reasons. First, an improvement in prognosis for ovarian cancer through detection by screening has not been demonstrated. Second, because the incidence of ovarian cancer in this population is relatively low, the risk of a false-positive result resulting in surgical investigation is likely to be more than 10 times that of a true positive result (i.e. the positive predictive value of screening is <10%). The value of screening for women in this group and for those without a family history awaits evaluation in the UKCTOCS trial. Oophorectomy should not be recommended as a primary procedure but may be considered as a secondary procedure at the time of surgery for benign disease (e.g. hysterectomy).

THE MOLECULAR GENETICS OF SPORADIC GYNAECOLOGICAL CANCER

Cervical cancer

The histopathological progression of cervical neoplasia from mild to increasingly severe dysplasia and ultimately invasive cervical cancer is well described, as is the evidence for an association with human papillomavirus infection. During recent years important progress has been made in understanding the mechanism of papillomavirus-induced carcinogenesis and incorporating these findings with the principles of multistep carcinogenesis. Human papillomaviruses form a group of more than 80 viruses most of which give rise to benign tumours such as wart infections. Risk of cervical neoplasia is associated with particular HPV types (HPV 16 and

18) (Vousden 1989). The genomes of all HPVs have a similar organization which encodes eight major open reading frames encoding early (E1–7) and late (L1–2) viral proteins. It is the early proteins E6 and E7 which are responsible for the transforming activity of the virus (Vousden 1991). The E6 and E7 proteins of high-risk HPV types (16 and 18) but not those of low-risk types cause in vitro changes which parallel the changes in CIN (Hudson et al 1990).

During a normal viral infection resulting in production and release of new virus the viral genome exists episomally without integration in the nucleus of the infected cell. In tumour cells the viral DNA is integrated with the DNA of the host cell. Although the sites of integration of viral DNA are random in cancer cell lines and many of the viral genes are lost, the E6 and E7 viral ORFs are always conserved and are the most abundant viral transcripts in such cell lines (Shirashawa et al 1987). Furthermore, integration of E6 and E7 usually occurs in a manner which disrupts the normal viral regulation of expression of these proteins (Durst et al 1985). These observations suggest that the E6 and E7 proteins have an important role in cervical carcinogenesis and are supported by recent evidence that these proteins can interact with and inactivate several important cellular proteins. E7 protein binds to the product of the retinoblastoma tumour suppressor gene, interfering with normal protein complex formation and disrupting the normal function of Rb protein. E6 protein interacts with the protein product of the p53 tumour suppressor gene, causing rapid breakdown of the protein and loss of normal p53 function. The overall effect of E6 and E7 expression in the cell is therefore equivalent to loss of the Rb and p53 tumour suppressor genes. This is consistent with the observation that p53 mutation is uncommon in cervical cancer but is found in HPV 16 and 18 negative cervical cancer cell lines (Crook et al 1992).

Clinical and experimental evidence suggests that in common with other mechanisms of carcinogenesis, HPV infection alone is not sufficient to cause cervical cancer but requires other factors which may influence local immune responses or result in other genetic alterations. First, only a small proportion of women with HPV infection develop cancer and there is a long latent period before this occurs. Second, epidemiological studies suggest that other factors such as smoking and herpes simplex infection may play a role. Third, a number of genetic abnormalities have been identified in cervical cancers. These include amplification or overexpression of c-myc, mutation of c-H-ras and loss of heterozygosity at a number of chromosomal loci.

As tumour suppressor genes inhibit cell proliferation, both copies of the gene must be inactivated for neoplastic effect (i.e. they act recessively at a cellular level). The first 'hit' is frequently a point mutation whilst the second 'hit' inactivating the remaining wild-type copy of the gene is often a larger event involving loss of a portion or the whole of a chromosome. The relatively large losses associated with the second 'hit' are easier to identify than point mutations and have been exploited as a method of mapping the location of tumour suppressor genes by loss of heterozygosity (LOH) analysis.

In cervical carcinogenesis three major events have been identified. First, the oncogenic effects of E6 and E7 proteins. Second, integration of viral DNA in chromosomal material.

Some of these viral integrations occur frequently at specifc loci, such as chromosome 8 and 12 (Lazo 1999), harbouring HPV18 and HPV16. Third, other genetic alterations not related to HPV. Recurrent LOH is identified in chromosome regions 3p14-22, 4p16, 5p15, 6q21-22, 11q23, 17p, 18q12-22 and 19q13. All these regions may harbour potential tumour suppressor genes. Several studies reported amplification of chromosome 3q24-28 in up to 90% of cervical cancers. Comparative genomic hybridization (CGH) is a powerful molecular tool which allows screening of the entire genome of a tumour for genetic alterations, by highlighting regions of altered DNA sequence copy numbers. CGH from preinvasive (dysplastic) cervical cells reveals several chromosomal imbalances. Most frequent gains were found on chromosomes 1p, 2q, 4 and 5, whereas losses could be found on chromosome 13q (Aubele et al 1998). Another study revealed a comparable recurrent pattern of chromosomal aberrations between preinvasive and invasive lesions; however, more aberrations were found in the invasive lesions (Kirchhoff et al 1999). The most consistent chromosomal gain was found on chromosome 3q, for both preinvasive (35%) and invasive lesions (72%). In cervical cancer, frequent gains were found on chromosome arms 1q, 5p, 8q, 15q and Xq, whereas losses were mapped on 3p, 4p, 6q, 11q and 13q.

Ovarian cancer

The majority of cases of ovarian cancer are not associated with familial predisposition. There is good evidence from epidemiological studies that the risk of sporadic ovarian cancer is associated with factors which influence the frequency of ovulation (e.g. parity, breastfeeding, oral contraceptive use). Ovulation results in disruption of the ovarian epithelium which is repaired by proliferation of ovarian epithelial cells exposed to growth factors present in follicular fluid. The proliferation of ovarian epithelium at the time of ovulation may provide the opportunity for mutations resulting in somatic activation of oncogenes and tumour suppressor genes. The genetic abnormalities in ovarian cancer involve genes at each step in the complex pathway of cell regulation which are summarized in Figure 36.1. These include involving growth factors (M-CSF, TGF-β), growth factor receptors (fms, EGFR, Her-2/neu), genes involved in signal transduction (ras), genes involved in transcriptional regulation (myc, p53) and LOH at various loci, which occur in a proportion of epithelial ovarian cancers. Recent LOH studies in ovarian cancer demonstrated a relationship between losses at specific chromosomal loci and tumour grade and stage. For example, loss of chromosome 4 occurs more frequently in poorly differentiated tumours, and gains of 3q26-qter, 8q24-qter and 20q13-qter occur more frequently in well-differentiated and early-stage tumours and thus may be early events in ovarian carcinogenesis (Suzuki et al 2000).

Oncogenes in sporadic ovarian cancer
Over 60 different oncogenes have been identified and they are categorized according to their cellular location and function.

Growth factors There is good evidence that the response of ovarian cancer cells to growth factors is altered compared to

normal ovarian epithelial cells. The proliferative response of ovarian cancer cells in culture to epidermal growth factor (EGF) and transforming growth factor alpha (TGF-α) is variable but usually less than normal ovarian epithelium (Berchuck et al 1990) whilst the inhibitory effect of TGF-β is less marked in ovarian cancer cell lines than in normal ovarian epithelium (Berchuck et al 1992). TGF-β appears to function as an autocrine inhibitory factor in normal ovarian epithelial growth and the loss of this regulatory loop may represent a step in the process of ovarian carcinogenesis. The macrophage colony stimulating factor (M-CSF) is a ligand for a cell surface receptor encoded by the c-fms proto-oncogene. Normal ovarian epithelium does not express fms whereas the majority of ovarian cancer cells do express the receptor (Kacinski et al 1990). M-CSF is a potent attractant for macrophages and can stimulate the invasiveness of cancer cell lines that express fms. It is possible that M-CSF regulates ovarian cancer cells via an autocrine pathway in cells expressing fms as well as by a paracrine pathway through attraction of macrophages and consequent release of cytokines such as IL-1, IL-6 and TNF.

Growth factor receptors The growth factor receptors are a family of cell membrane tyrosine kinases which act as receptors for the growth factors discussed above and are involved in signal transduction via autophosphorylation and phosphorylation of intracellular proteins. The EGF receptor (EGFR also referred to as erbB) and HER-2/neu (also referred to as erbB2) are structurally similiar and both have been shown to be overexpressed in human cancers. EGFR is expressed by most advanced-stage ovarian cancers and there is some evidence that EGFR-positive tumours have a worse prognosis than tumours not expressing the receptor (Berchuck et al 1991). Her-2/neu is overexpressed in approximately a third of ovarian cancers (Slamon et al 1989) and overexpression is associated with gene amplification.

Oncogenes involved in signal transduction Although mutations of the ras oncogene occur in ovarian cancer they are relatively less frequent than in some other epithelial cancers. Ki-ras (G protein) mutations in ovarian tumours almost exclusively involve codon 12 and are more frequent in border-line (33–63%) and invasive tumours (5–13%) of mucinous type than serous tumours.

Chromosome 3q26 is found to be increased in copy number in approximately 40% of ovarian cancers. This region contains a recently identified oncogene, PIK3CA, which encodes the p110-α subunit of phosphatidylinositol 3-kinase (P13-kinase). P13-kinase mediated signalling is involved in a broad range of cancer-related functions, including glucose transport, catabolism, apoptosis, cell adhesion, RAS signalling and oncogenic transcription.

Nuclear oncogenes Little is known about the role of most nuclear oncogenes in ovarian cancer. Amplification of c-myc and increased expression of the protein product has been described in approximately a third of ovarian cancers. Over-expression of c-myc is found in 38% of ovarian tumours (Tashiro et al 1992).

Tumour suppressor genes in sporadic ovarian cancer Mutations of the p53 gene are the most frequent genetic alteration in cancer and occur most frequently in regions of the gene which show the greatest degree of conservation between p53 proteins of different species. Immunohisto-chemical studies have revealed overexpression of the p53 protein in 50% of advanced-stage ovarian cancers (Marks et al 1991). Sequencing of p53 from ovarian cancers over-expressing the p53 protein has in most cases confirmed point mutations in conserved regions of the gene (Marks et al 1991). In most of these tumours LOH studies have revealed that the second copy of the gene is inactivated through deletion of the gene. Mutation of p53 is less common in stage I disease than advanced-stage disease and clonal analysis suggests that the occurrence of p53 mutation precedes but is temporally associated with metastases (Jacobs et al 1992). No clear relationship between p53 mutation and histological grade or prognosis has been established. The location and nature of the p53 mutations in ovarian cancer have now been reported in 149 tumours. Over 100 different mutations involving approximately 60 different codons have been identified and most occur in the highly conserved exons 5–8 of the gene. The codons most frequently involved in p53 mutations are the same as those described in other cancers. The pattern of mutations suggests that most p53 alterations in ovarian cancer arise due to endogenous mutagenic processes rather than exposure to a carcinogen.

Several novel potential candidate tumour suppressor genes have recently been reported for ovarian cancer and their role in ovarian carcinogenesis has yet to be elucidated. For example, chromosome 17p13.3 maps OVCA1 and OVCA2 (Schultz et al 1996). Other suggested candidates are nm23, on chromosome 17q, and SPARC (Mok et al 1996, Srivatsa et al 1996). Recent evidence suggests that inactivation of the PTEN gene, a tumour suppressor gene commonly mutated in endometrial cancer, is an early event in the carcinogenesis of both clear cell and endometrioid ovarian carcinoma (Sato et al 2000).

Loss of heterozygosity   Studies of LOH in ovarian cancer have revealed a number of regions with high frequencies of loss. The reported frequency of LOH for each chromosome arm is summarized in Figure 36.6. Losses have been observed on almost all chromosome arms and the background 'random' rate of loss in ovarian cancer is high (in the range 15–25%). A high frequency of allelic deletion (>33%) based upon more than 50 tumours in at least three separate studies has been documented for seven chromosome arms: 6p, 6q, 13q, 17p (possibly associated with p53), 17q, 18q and Xp. A number of other chromosome arms have frequencies of loss in the range 25–33% which may be above background rates: 4p, 8p, 9p, 9q, 11p, 14q, 16q, 19p and 21q, 22q (McCluskey & Dubeau 1997). Some of these allelic deletions have been correlated with clinicopathological parameters. Recent studies have shown a distinct relationship between allelic imbalance at 8p12-p21 and 8p22-pter in ovarian cancer and tumour grade, stage and histological subtype. Poorly differentiated tumours, advanced-stage cancers and serous tumours were more prone to allelic imbalance at these regions (Lassus et al 2001, Pribill et al 2001).

Further localization of putative tumour suppressor genes in regions with a high rate of LOH requires detailed analysis with a panel of polymorphic markers for the relevant chromo-

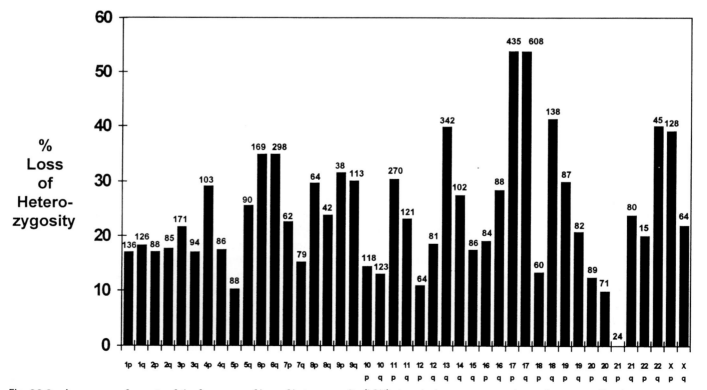

Fig. 36.6   A summary of reports of the frequency of loss of heterozygosity (LOH) at each chromosome arm in ovarian cancer. The data represent the number of tumours with LOH for the chromosome arm/the number of informative tumours for each chromosome arm. The number of tumours studied at each chromosome arm is shown at the top of each bar.

some arm. Available data suggest that a number of as yet unidentified tumour suppressor genes are involved in ovarian carcinogenesis and recent reports have defined deletion units on chromosome arms with the highest rates of LOH including 6p, 6q, 11p, 13q, 17q and Xp. The nature of specific chromosomes affected by LOH can influence tumour biological aggressiveness, as losses on certain chromosomes such as 13q and Xq are strongly associated with poorly differentiated tumours (Cheng et al 1996). LOH in chromosomes 6q or 17 is more frequently found in well-differentiated tumours.

Comparative genomic hybridization (CGH) The application of this technique recently revealed that 53–69% of human ovarian cancers demonstrate amplifications on chromosomes 1q, 3q, 8q, 13q, 19p and 20q (Kiechle et al 2001). Under-representations were found for chromosomes 4q, 13q and 18q in approximately 50% of ovarian cancers. Undifferentiated tumours were found to correlate significantly with under-representation of 11p and 13q as well with amplification of 7p and 8q.

BRCA1 The high rate of LOH on chromosome 17q in sporadic ovarian cancers was reported when the BRCA1 gene was mapped to 17q and raised the exciting possibility that the same gene may be of importance in sporadic as well as familial ovarian. When the cloning of the BRCA1 gene was reported considerable effort was therefore invested in searching for somatic BRCA1 mutations in sporadic breast and ovarian cancers. Alongside the report of the cloning of BRCA1, mutational analysis of a series of apparently sporadic breast and ovarian cancers from individuals without a known family history of ovarian cancer but with LOH on 17q was described (Futreal et al 1994). None of the cancers had somatic BRCA1 mutations although some had germline mutations. However, more recently two groups have described a total of five somatic mutations in 64 cancers (Hosking 1995, Merajver et al 1995). The current state of knowledge suggests that BRCA1 mutations do occur in sporadic disease but are relatively uncommon. It is still possible that the spectrum of mutations is different in sporadic tumours from that in familial cancer and that the full story will be rather more subtle than is now apparent. The pattern of LOH on chromosome 17 suggests that, in addition to BRCA1, several unidentified tumour suppressor genes on the long arm of 17q are involved in ovarian carcinogenesis.

cDNA microarrays The development of cancer is the result of a series of molecular changes at DNA level and these events lead subsequently to changes in gene expression (mRNA) levels of numerous genes resulting in different phenotypic characteristics of tumours. cDNA microarray analysis enables the identification of differences in gene expressions between normal and malignant tissues by analysing thousands of genes at the same time. A recent study comparing 5766 different gene expressions between normal and malignant ovarian tissue revealed that several genes were under- or overexpressed (Wang et al 1999). Several genes were highly overexpressed in ovarian cancer such as epithelial glycoprotein (GA733), PUMP1 (MMP7) and cytokeratin 8, and some of these have also been shown to be overexpressed in other cancers such as colorectal cancer. This illustrates that phenotypical similarity between different types of tumours is also reflected at molecular level.

Another study, using a DNA microarray of 9121 genes,

identified 55 genes commonly upregulated and 48 genes downregulated in ovarian cancer specimens when compared to the corresponding normal ovarian tissues (Ono et al 2000). The 55 genes that were often upregulated in the nine adenocarcinomas analysed represent candidates for stimulating cell growth and preventing apoptosis. Serial analysis of gene expression (SAGE) has recently been introduced to generate global gene expression profiles from various ovarian cell lines and tissues including primary ovarian cancers, ovarian surface epithelial cells and cystadenoma cells. More than 56 000 gene expressions (10 different libraries) were generated (Hough et al 2000). Interestingly, ovarian cancer cell lines showed high levels of similarity to libraries from other cancer cell lines such as colorectal cancer, indicating that these cell lines had lost many of their tissue-specific expression patterns. Many of the genes upregulated in ovarian cancer represent surface or secreted proteins such as mucin-1, HE4, epithelial cellular adhesion molecule, mesothelin and several keratins (e.g. keratin 18 and 19).

Endometrial cancer

A small proportion of endometrial cancers occur as part of the Lynch II syndrome and it is possible that site-specific hereditary endometrial cancer exists as a distinct entity (Sandles et al 1992). The majority of cases of endometrial cancers are, however, sporadic. Although it is known that unopposed oestrogens are important in the aetiology of sporadic endometrial cancer there is limited information about the molecular basis of this disease. Oestrogen and progesterone receptors are frequently expressed by endometrial cancers and loss of expression is correlated with poor prognosis. In contrast to ovarian cancer, the majority of endometrial cancers have a diploid DNA content but approximately 25% are aneuploid and this feature is associated with aggressive disease and poor prognosis.

A number of recent studies have identified mutations of known oncogenes and tumour suppressor genes in endometrial cancer but no genetic alterations specific to this cancer have been documented. Kohler et al (1992) reported immunohistochemical evidence of p53 mutations in 21% of a series of 107 endometrial cancers. The results suggested that p53 mutations were more frequent in advanced-stage than early-stage disease and were associated with non-endometrioid histology, positive peritoneal cytology and metastatic disease. These findings are consistent with other studies of p53 in endometrial cancer. Approximately 20% of endometrial cancers studied have p53 mutations, usually in conserved regions of the gene with a similiar distribution to p53 mutations in ovarian cancer. Kohler et al (1993) also studied a series of 117 endometrial hyperplasias, none of which were found to have p53 mutations suggesting that p53 mutation is a relatively late event in endometrial carcinogenesis.

A number of studies of ras mutations in endometrial cancer have been reported. Overall Ki-ras mutations have been documented in approximately 20% of endometrial cancers analysed. Of the mutations reported, the majority are in codon 12 and the remainder in codon 13. The relationship of prognostic factors to Ki-ras mutation is not yet clear. In contrast to p53 mutation, Ki-ras mutation appears to be a relatively early event in endometrial carcinogenesis. The frequency of Ki-ras mutation in endometrial hyperplasia is similiar to that in invasive disease (Enomoto et al 1993, Sasaki et al 1993). When Ki-ras mutations are present in areas of invasive endometrial cancer they are also in adjacent areas of atypical hyperplasia but not simple or complex hyperplasia without atypia. Thus Ki-ras mutation appears to be involved in progression to atypical hyperplasia. Both overexpression and amplification of the ErbB2 oncogene have been reported to occur in endometrial cancer. Small studies also suggest endometrial cancer may be associated with amplification of c-myc and alteration of the retinoblastoma gene. Fewer candidate tumour suppressor genes have been associated with endometrial cancer, compared to ovarian cancer.

Forty per cent of endometrial cancers have mutations in the *PTEN* tumour suppressor gene (chromosome 10q23) and 21% of endometrial hyperplasias have mutations (Cass et al 1999). It has been suggested that *PTEN* inactivation may be an early event in the development of certain endometrial cancer types, such as endometrioid cancers. Some mutations in DNA mismatch repair genes, such as *MSH3* and *MSH6*, have been described in endometrial cancer.

Vulval cancer

Neoplasia of the vulva are rare malignancies accounting for <5% of all female genital tract cancers. However, in recent years the incidence of vulval intraepithelial neoplasia (VIN), precursor of vulval cancer, has increased in young women, generating considerable interest in its molecular pathogenesis.

CGH has recently been used to study alterations (losses or gains) on all chromosomes in vulval cancer (Jee et al 2001). Frequent chromosomal losses were found on 3p, 4p13-pter and 5q; less frequent on 6q, 11q and 13q. Most frequent chromosomal gains were observed on 3q and 8p and less frequent on 9p, 14, 17 and 20q. The pattern of chromosomal imbalance in vulval cancer detected by CGH was revealed to be very similar to that in cervical cancer. These results suggest that the molecular pathways in vulval and cervical carcinomas may be similar. However, it is not clear whether HPV-positive and -negative vulval cancers have similar or different molecular pathways.

Vulval squamous cell carcinomas (VSCCs) exhibit a broad range of allelic losses irrespective of HPV status, with high frequencies of LOH on certain chromosomal arms. High frequencies of LOH are found on 1q, 2q, 3p, 5q, 8p, 8q, 10p, 10q, 11p, 11q, 15q, 17p, 18q, 21q and 22q (Pinto et al 1999). This suggests that despite their differences in pathogenesis, both HPV-positive and -negative VSCCs share similarities in type and range of genetic losses during their evolution. Another recent study observed a greater number of molecular alterations in HPV-negative vulval cancers compared with HPV-positive tumours (Flowers et al 1999). Allelic losses at 3p are common early events in vulval carcinogenesis in HPV-negative cancers and detected at a high rate in the corresponding high-grade precursor lesions (VIN II/III). TP53 gene mutations with associated 17p13.1 LOH are also more common in HPV-negative cancers. Fractional regional loss index (FRL), an index of total allelic loss at chromosomal regions 3p, 13q14 and 17p13.1, is greater in HPV-negative vulval cancers than in HPV-positive tumours (Flowers et al 1999). Similar observations have been found in HPV-negative high-grade VINs compared with HPV-positive lesions. Overall, LOH at any 3p region is frequent (80%) in both groups of cancers and in their associated VIN lesions. Although TP53 gene mutations are present in a minority of VCs (20%), allelic losses at the TP53 locus are frequently present, especially in HPV-negative VCs, as compared with the HPV-positive tumours.

Fallopian tube cancer

Histologic features, biological and clinical behaviour are similar to ovarian cancer. In addition, there is recent evidence that similar genetic alterations occur with the same frequency between fallopian tube and ovarian cancer when considering the same histological subtype. This suggests a common molecular pathogenesis between these cancer types (Pere et al 1998). Recent molecular genetic analyses using CGH reveals that different histological subtypes differ in respect to their genomic alterations but similar subtypes of different cancers have similar patterns of genomic abnormalities. For example, frequency and the pattern of chromosomal changes detected in serous tubal carcinoma, 95% of all fallopian tube carcinomas, are strikingly similar to those observed in serous ovarian carcinoma, suggesting common molecular pathogenesis. In fallopian tube carcinoma frequent gains are found on chromosome 3q and 8q and frequent losses on chromosome 4q, 5q, 8q and 18q (Pere et al 1998). There is also evidence that fallopian tube cancers are similar to ovarian cancer with respect to the proportion of tumours with abnormal expression of her-2/neu and p53 (Lacy et al 1995). The prognostic significance and predictive drug response of these two genes need to be explored in fallopian tube cancer.

CLINICAL ASPECTS OF THE GENETICS OF GYNAECOLOGICAL CANCER

Cancer prevention

Genetic approaches may help in the identification of pre-malignant conditions amenable to conventional therapy. For example, in contrast to cervical cancer, there is no well-documented precursor lesion in ovarian carcinogenesis. The possibility has been raised that ovarian epithelial atypia, inclusion cysts and benign or borderline ovarian tumours may represent steps in the pathway of ovarian carcinogenesis (Puls et al 1992). Genetic studies may establish the relationship between these histopathological features and ovarian cancer and consequently provide new opportunities for prevention. Where there are known abnormalities conferring a high risk of cancer it may be possible to design strategies to correct the abnormality. In familial cancer syndromes it may ultimately be possible to transfer normal copies of the abnormal gene (e.g. p53, BRCA1) to the tissue at risk using tissue-specific viral vectors.

In cervical cancer work is in progress to develop a vaccine directed against the HPV types associated with the disease. It may be possible to generate an immune response to viral coat particles (L1 and L2) or to viral transforming proteins (E6 and E7) using either a protein vaccine or a presentation of these antigens in a viral or bacterial vector. Although cervical cytology is the established method of screening for preinvasive change in cervical neoplasia the sensitivity of this methodology is no greater than 50%. Recent evidence suggests that greater sensitivity for detection of cervical dysplasia may be achieved by using a sensitive PCR-based assay to detect HPV in cervical smears (Cusick 1995). In addition, recent reports suggest that women who have consistently high viral loads of HPV 16 in their normal cervical smears, over a long period, are more likely to develop cervical carcinoma in situ than those who have a low viral load or are negative for HPV 16 (Josefsson et al 2000, Ylitalo et al 2000).

Early detection of cancer

Knowledge of specific genetic alterations associated with cancer along with the high sensitivity of molecular techniques such as the polymerase chain reaction may provide new methods for detection of cancer. As direct sampling of the ovary requires an invasive procedure any screening test for ovarian cancer based upon genetic markers will be directed toward identification of a gene product in peripheral blood. The protein product of the M-CSF gene is detectable at elevated levels in the serum of ovarian cancer patients. It is possible that the products of other genes coding for secreted and cell surface proteins produced in abnormal forms or increased amounts in cancer will be markers for early-stage disease.

The opportunities may be even greater for cancers arising from accessible tissues such as the endometrium. Using techniques such as the polymerase chain or ligase chain reaction, it is possible to identify a small proportion of mutated copies of a gene in a background of many thousand-fold excess normal copies of the gene. Since it is a relatively simple outpatient procedure to obtain an endometrial sample, it may be possible to detect mutation of a gene associated with endometrial cancer at a very early stage of the disease. This approach has been used to detect mutations of p53 and K-ras in urine, sputum and stool specimens in cancers of the bladder, lung and colon (Sidransky et al 1991).

Microsatellite DNA alterations are an integral part of neoplastic transformation and are valuable as markers for the detection of human cancers. In head and neck cancers, micro-satellite alterations can be found in blood DNA of patients with advanced-stage disease and adverse prognosis (Nawroz et al 1996). A recent study showed the ease with which tumour-specific chromosomal alterations can be detected in serum and peritoneal samples from ovarian cancer patients (Hickey et al 1999). Molecular detection methods could therefore be used to identify early-stage disease, minimal residual disease and the early stages of recurrent disease as well as monitoring of the disease. PCR-based methods are able to detect one cancer cell in a background of a million normal cells. Quantitative reverse transcriptase PCR is even able to quantify accurately specific gene expressions present in tumour cells and this method has recently been introduced to quantify the burden of micro-metastases in apparently normal lymph nodes on histology (Van Trappen et al 2001). Efforts to define the biological

behaviour and clinical importance of micrometastases are under way. This approach might be of particular importance in early-stage cancers and may identify patients at high risk for recurrence and decreased survival.

Prognostic indicators

The behaviour of a malignancy is a consequence of the complex interaction of all the genetic alterations which have accumulated during the process of carcinogenesis. Since different genetic alterations have different effects and the set of genetic changes leading to a particular malignancy is not fixed, it is reasonable to infer that genetic analysis will provide important prognostic information. Evidence for this is emerging from studies of ovarian cancer. Several molecular markers including oncogene products (her-2/neu, k-ras, c-myc, p21), tumour suppressor gene products (p53, p16, pRB) and drug sensitivity markers (GST, BAX, Pgp, LRP, MRP) have been investigated as independent prognostic markers. However, due to contradictory results, it is not clear which of these markers may contribute to the clinical management of ovarian cancer. There is some recent evidence that the expression of the apoptosis-related proteins BAX and Bcl-2 combined is of independent prognostic significance in advanced ovarian cancer (Baekelandt et al 2000).

Several authors have investigated the relationship between LOH and tumour characteristics. Correlations with frequency of LOH in ovarian cancer have been reported for (i) histological type on chromosome 6q, 13q, 17q and 19q, LOH being more frequent in serous than other histological types; (ii) FIGO stage of disease on 17q, with LOH more frequent in advanced-stage disease and (iii) tumour grade. Zheng et al (1991) found a correlation between tumour grade and frequency of LOH at all loci analysed on nine chromosomes. On the basis of the results it was hypothesized that LOH on chromosomes 3 or 11 results in high-grade malignancy whilst LOH on chromosome 6 is consistent with a well-differentiated phenotype. Dodson et al (1993) found the average fractional allelic loss in high-grade tumours to be greater than that in low-grade tumours (39.5% vs 16%). Chromosome arms 6p, 17p, 17q and 22q were frequently lost in low- and high-grade tumours whilst LOH on 13q and 15q was more common in high-grade tumours and LOH on 3p more common in low-grade tumours. These data raise the possibility that pattern of LOH is an independent prognostic indicator for ovarian cancer.

Although p53 mutation does not appear to correlate with prognosis there is evidence that erbB2 amplification is associated with decreased survival. A recent report using two different molecular techniques, DNA sequence analysis and oligonucleotide microarray, for assessment of TP53 mutations demonstrated that women with mutations in loop 2, loop 3 or the loop-sheet-helix domain have significantly shorter survival than women with other mutations or women with no mutations (Wen et al 2000).

Recent studies suggest that her-2/neu overexpression in ovarian cancer may be associated with chemotherapy resistance, thus raising important implications for potential therapeutic strategies. Concomitant administration of anti-her-2/neu antibodies and cisplatin is shown to have a synergistic cytotoxic effect in ovarian cancer cell lines. Based on the recent promising results of anti-her-2/neu antibodies in metastatic breast cancer (Pegram & Slamon 1999, Shak 1999), a phase II study is under way for patients with recurrent ovarian cancers that overexpress the oncogene. Taxol and platinum chemotherapy may be more effective in ovarian cancers expressing mutant TP53 that causes more p53-independent apoptosis (Lavarino et al 2000). Certain chromosome breakpoints within specific, non-randomly involved chromosome regions (1p1, 1q2, 1p3, 3p1, 6p2, 11p1, 11q1, 12q2 and 13p1) are associated with impaired survival in ovarian carcinoma (Taetle et al 1999). Tumour grade is a better indicator of the extent of genomic progression than stage (Suzuki et al 2000). Loss of chromosome 16q24 and a total number of independent genome copy number aberrations >7 are associated with reduced survival.

Chromosomal regions that are frequently abnormal and associated with altered survival are strong candidates for more detailed analysis and gene discovery and may be useful markers for prediction of clinical outcome. Genome-wide detection of allelic imbalance using high-density DNA microarrays and human single nucleotide polymorphisms (SNPs) may identify specific gene profiles or polymorphisms associated with poor clinical outcome (Lindblad-Toh et al 2000, Ono et al 2000). It may also provide information on drug resistance and the development of novel (gene) therapies individualized to the tumour. The application of CGH recently revealed some specific chromosomal changes in cisplatin-resistant ovarian cancer. Gains in chromosomal region 1q21-q22 and 13q12-q14 were found to be related to drug-resistant phenotype in ovarian cancer (Kudoh et al 2000). These regions contain several oncogenes, cell cycle regulators, regulators of the apoptotic pathway and transcription factors.

Strategies for gene therapy

The increase in understanding of carcinogenesis at a molecular level has raised the possibility that cancer can be treated by selectively targeting cells with specific genetic abnormalities. A broad range of different methods for gene therapy have been suggested and numerous clinical trials are in progress.

Ex vivo approaches to gene therapy

Ex vivo techniques involve removal of cells from the individual, manipulation of the cells in vitro and reinjection of altered cells. One approach is to remove tumour cells from a patient, insert genes in vitro which increase their immunogenicity and reinject them into the patient in order to stimulate a systemic immune response that will recognize and destroy tumour cells. Suitable genes for this approach include cytokines which activate the immune system such as the interleukins and genes for MHC class I antigens. An alternative approach is to transfer a gene that activates a pro-drug to become cytotoxic. For example, transfer of the thymidine kinase gene of the herpes simplex virus results in phosphorylation of the anti-herpes drug ganciclovir and cell death due to inhibition of DNA polymerase. The potential of this approach is enhanced by the observation that adjacent cells which do not have the gene are also affected, presumably due to diffusion of the phosphorylated drug (Culver 1992). A trial of intraperitoneal therapy using this strategy is under way in stage III ovarian cancer (Freeman 1993).

In situ approaches to gene therapy

An exciting possibility is the correction of specific molecular genetic abnormalities responsible for carcinogenesis by replacing a normal copy of a tumour suppressor gene such as p53 or by suppressing expression of an oncogene product such as K-ras. There is evidence that insertion of wild-type p53 and antisense K-ras into tumour cells with abnormalities of these genes suppresses tumorigenicity (Harris & Hollstein 1993, Zhang 1993). It may also be possible to target genes involved in metastasis. Decreased expression of the nm23 gene is associated with increased metastatic potential in some cancers and transfection of nm23 into melanoma cells decreases metastatic potential (Leone et al 1991). The technical limitations of corrective gene therapy are currently twofold. First, in order to control a cancer in vivo the gene must be transferred to all tumour cells. The most hopeful method of gene transfer is the use of a recombinant virus since viral replication and spread may overcome the difficulty of targeting tumour cells with a poor vascular supply which limits other therapeutic approaches such as the use of monoclonal antibodies. Second, the vector used for gene transfer must be targeted to tumour but not normal cells of the individual. It may be possible to construct viral vectors which will bind to cell surface proteins expressed preferentially on tumour cells or which require a transcription factor expressed in tumour cells but not normal cells. Ultimately a highly sophisticated therapeutic approach may involve a viral vector modified to contain a therapeutic gene, to recognize tumour cell surface antigens and require tumour-specific factors for transcription.

KEY POINTS

1. Oncogenes result in a gain in function which will take effect even in the presence of the remaining normal copy of the gene; tumour suppressor genes involve a loss of function that requires inactivation or deletion of both copies of the gene before cellular regulation is affected.
2. Several mutations (4–7) are required to cause cancer.
3. The genetic changes required for cancer usually occur in the somatic cells and are random events. However, some individuals develop oncogenic mutations in their germ cells which can then be passed on to their progeny.
4. Among gynaecological cancers inherited malignancies occur only in the ovary, endometrium and breast. These are rare, accounting for less than 5% of ovarian or endometrial cancers.
5. Two genes, termed BRCA1 and BRCA2, have been identified. BRCA1 is found in almost all families with both breast and ovarian cancer and in 40% of families with breast cancer alone.

KEY POINTS (*CONTINUED*)

1. Oncogenes result in a gain in function which will take effect even in the presence of the remaining normal copy of the gene; tumour suppressor genes involve a loss of function that requires inactivation or deletion of both copies of the gene before cellular regulation is affected.
2. Several mutations (4–7) are required to cause cancer.
3. The genetic changes required for cancer usually occur in the somatic cells and are random events. However, some individuals develop oncogenic mutations in their germ cells which can then be passed on to their progeny.
4. Among gynaecological cancers inherited malignancies occur only in the ovary, endometrium and breast. These are rare, accounting for less than 5% of ovarian or endometrial cancers.

REFERENCES

Aarnio M, Sankila R, Pukkala E et al 1999 Cancer risk in mutation carriers of DNA-mismatch-repair genes. International Journal of Cancer 12:214–218

Alberts B, Bray D, Lewis J, Raff M, Roberts K, Watson JD 1989 Molecular biology of the Cell, 2nd edn. Garland Publishing, New York

Ames BN, Durston WE, Yamasaki E, Lee FD 1973 Carcinogens are mutagens: a simple test system combining liver homogenates for activation and bacteria for detection. Proceedings of the National Academy of Sciences USA 70:2281–2285

Armitage P, Doll R 1954 The age distribution of cancer and a multi-stage theory of carcinogenesis. British Journal of Cancer 8:1–12

Aubele M, Zitzelsberger H, Schenck U, Walch A, Hofler H, Werner M 1998 Distinct cytogenetic alterations in squamous intraepithelial lesions of the cervix revealed by laser-assisted microdissection and comparative genomic hybridization. Cancer 84:375–379

Baekelandt M, Holm R, Nesland JM, Trope CG, Kristensen GB 2000 Expression of apoptosis-related proteins is an independent determinant of patient prognosis in advanced ovarian cancer. Journal of Clinical Oncology 18:3775–3781

Baker SJ, Fearon ER, Nigro JM et al 1989 Chromosome 17 deletions and p53 gene mutations in colorectal carcinomas. Science 244:217–221

Berchuck A, Rodriguez G, Kamel A et al 1990 Expression of epidermal growth factor receptor and HER-2/neu in normal and neoplastic cervix, vulva, and vagina. Obstetrics and Gynecology 76:381

Berchuck A, Rodriguez GC, Kamel A et al 1991 Epidermal growth factor receptor expression in normal ovarian epithelium and ovarian cancer. I. Correlation of receptor expression with prognostic factors in patients with ovarian cancer. American Journal of Obstetrics and Gynecology 164:669

Berchuck A, Rodriguez G, Olt G et al 1992 Regulation of growth of normal ovarian epithelial cells and ovarian cancer cell lines by transforming growth factor-beta. American Journal of Obstetrics and Gynecology 166:676

Cairns J 1975 Mutation selection, and the natural history of cancer. Nature 255:197–200

Campbell S, Bourne T, Bradley E 1993 Screening for ovarian cancer by transvaginal sonography and colour Doppler. European Journal of Obstetrics, Gynecology and Reproductive Biology 49:33

Cass I, Baldwin RL, Karlan BY 1999 Molecular advances in gynaecologic oncology. Current Opinion in Oncology 11:394–400

Cavenee WK, Dryja TP, Phillips RA et al 1983 Expression of recessive alleles by chromosomal mechanisms in retinoblastoma. Nature 305:779–784

Chen KT, Schooley JL, Flam MS 1985 Peritoneal carcinomatosis after prophylactic oophorectomy in familial ovarian cancer syndrome. Obstetrics and Gynecology 66:93

Cheng PC, Gosewehr JA, Kim TM 1996 Potential role of the inactivated X chromosome in ovarian epithelial tumor development. Journal of the National Cancer Institute 88:510–518

Crook T, Wrede D, Tidy JA, Mason WP, Evans DJ, Vousden KH 1992 Clonal p53 mutation in primary cervical cancer: association with human-papillomavirus-negative tumours. Lancet 339:1070–1073

Culver KW, Ram Z, Wallbridge S et al 1992 In vivo gene transfer with retroviral vector-producer cells for treatment of experimental brain tumors. Science 256:1150–1152

Cuzick J, Szarewski A, Terry G et al 1995 Human papillomavirus testing in primary cervical screening. Lancet 345(8964):1533–1536

DeKlein A, van Kessel AG, Grosveld G et al 1982 A cellular oncogene is translocated to the Philadelphia chromosome in chronic myelocytic leukemia. Nature 300:765–767

Dodson MK, Hartmann LC, Cliby WA et al 1993 Comparison of loss of heterozygosity patterns in invasive low-grade and high-grade epithelial ovarian carcinomas. Cancer Research 53:4456–4460

Dunlop MG, Farrington SM, Carothers AD et al 1997 Cancer risk associated with germline DNA mismatch repair gene mutations. Human Molecular Genetics 6:105–110

Durst M, Kleinheinz A, Hotz M 1985 The physical state of human papillomavirus type 16 DNA in benign and malignant genital tumours. Journal of General Virology 66:1515–1522

Easton DF, Bishop DT, Ford D, Crockford GP 1993 Genetic linkage analysis in familial breast and ovarian cancer: results from 214 families. The Breast Cancer Linkage Consortium. American Journal of Human Genetics 52:678

Enomoto T, Fujita M, Inoue M et al 1993 Alterations of the p53 tumor suppressor gene and its association with activation of the c-K-ras-2 protooncogene in premalignant and malignant lesions of the human uterine endometrium. Cancer Research 53:1883

Fearan ER, Hamilton SR, Vogelstein B 1987 Clonal analysis of human colorectal tumors. Science 238(4824):193–197

Fearon ER, Cho KR, Nigro JM et al 1990 Identification of a chromosome 18q gene that is altered in colorectal cancers. Science 247:49–56

Flowers LC, Wistuba II, Scurry J et al 1999 Genetic changes during the multistage pathogenesis of human papillomavirus positive and negative vulvar carcinomas. Journal of the Society for Gynecologic Investigation 6:213–221

Ford D, Easton DF, Bishop DT et al 1994 Risks of cancer in BRCA1-mutation carriers. Breast Cancer Linkage Consortium. Lancet 343:692–695

Ford D, Easton DF, Stratton M et al 1998 Genetic heterogeneity and penetrance analysis of the BRCA1 and BRCA2 genes in breast cancer families. The Breast Cancer Linkage Consortium. American Journal of Human Genetics 62:676–689

Freeman SM, McCune C, Robinson W et al 1993 The treatment of ovarian cancer with a gene-modified cancer vaccine: a phase I study. Cancer Reserach 53:5274–5283

Futreal PA, Liu Q, Shattuck-Eidens D et al 1994 BRCA1 mutations in primary breast and ovarian carcinomas. Science 266:120–122

Gayther SA, Warren W, Mazoyer S et al 1995 Germline mutations of the BRCAI gene in breast and ovarian cancer families provide evidence for a genotype-phenotype correlation. Nature Genetics, 11:428–433

Gayther SA, Mangion J, Russell P et al 1997 Variation of risks of breast and ovarian cancer associated with different germline mutations of the BRCA2 gene. Nature Genetics 15:103–105

Hall JM, Lee MK, Newman B et al 1990 Linkage of early-onset familial breast cancer to chromosome 17q21. Science 250:1684–1689

Harris CC, Hollstein M 1993 Clinical implications of the p53 tumor-suppressor gene. New England Journal of Medicine 329:1318–1327

Harris H, Miller OJ, Klein G, Worst P, Tachibana T 1969 Suppression of malignancy by cell fusion. Nature 223:363–368

Hickey KP, Boyle KP, Jepps HM, Andrew AC, Buxton EJ, Burns PA 1999 Molecular detection of tumour DNA in serum and peritoneal fluid from ovarian cancer patients. British Journal of Cancer 80:1803–1808

Hosking L 1995 A somatic BRCA1 mutation in an ovarian tumour. Nature Genetics 9:343–344

Hough CD, Sherman-Baust CA, Pizer ES et al 2000 Large-scale serial analysis of gene expression reveals genes differentially expressed in ovarian cancer. Cancer Research 60:6281–6287

Huang J, Papadopoulus N, McKinley AJ et al 1996 APC mutations in colorectal tumours with mismatch repair deficiency. Proceeding National Academy of Sciences USA 93:9049–9054

Hudson JB, Bedell MA, McCance DJ, Laimins LA 1990 Immortalisation and altered differentiation of human keratinocytes in vitro by the E6 and E7 open reading frames of human papillomavirus type 18. Journal of Virology 64:519–526

Jacobs IJ, Kohler MF, Wiseman RW et al 1992 Clonal origin of epithelial ovarian carcinoma: analysis by loss of heterozygosity, p53 mutation, and X-chromosome inactivation. Journal of the National Cancer Institute 84: 1793

Jacobs I, Davies AP, Bridges J et al 1993 Prevalence screening for ovarian cancer in postmenopausal women by CA 125 measurement and ultrasonography [see comments]. British Medical Journal 306:1030

Jacobs IJ, Skates SJ, MacDonald N et al 1999 Screening for ovarian cancer: a pilot randomized controlled trial. Lancet 353(9160):1207–1210

Jee KJ, Kim YT, Kim KR, Kim HS, Yan A, Knuutila S 2001 Loss in 3p and 4p and gain of 3q are concomitant aberrations in squamous cell carcinoma of the vulva. Modern Pathology 14:377–381

Josefsson AM, Magnusson PK, Ylitalo N et al 2000 Viral load of human papilloma virus 16 as a determinant for development of cervical carcinoma in situ: a nested case-control study. Lancet 355:2189–2193

Kacinski BM, Carter D, Mittal K et al 1990 Ovarian adenocarcinomas express fms-complementary transcripts and fms antigen, often with coexpression of CSF-1. American Journal of Pathology 137:135

Kiechle M, Jacobsen A, Schwarz-Boeger U, Hedderich J, Pfisterer J, Arnold N 2001 Comparative genomic hybridization detects genetic imbalances in primary ovarian carcinomas as correlated with grade of differentiation. Cancer 91:534–540

Kinzler KW, Vogelstein B 1996 Lessons from hereditary colorectal cancer. Cell 87:159–170

Kinzler KW, Nilbert MC, Su L-K et al 1991 Identification of FAP locus genes from chromosome 5q21. Science 253:661–665

Kirchhoff M, Rose H, Petersen BL et al 1999 Comparative genomic hybridization reveals a recurrent pattern of chromosomal aberrations in severe dysplasia/carcinoma in situ of the cervix and in advanced-stage cervical carcinoma. Genes, Chromosomes and Cancer 24:144–150

Knudson AG 1971 Mutation and cancer: statistical study of retinoblastoma. Proceeding National Academy Science USA 68:820–823

Kohler MF, Berchuck A, Davidoff AM et al 1992 Overexpression and mutation of p53 in endometrial carcinoma. Cancer Research 52:1622

Kohler MF, Nishii H, Humphrey PA et al 1993 Mutation of the p53 tumor-suppressor gene is not a feature of endometrial hyperplasias. American Journal of Obstetrics and Gynaecology 169:690

Krontiris TG, Cooper GM 1981 Transforming activity of human tumour DNAs. Proceeding National Academy Science USA 78:1811–1184

Kudoh K, Takano M, Koshikawa T et al 2000 Comparative genomic hybridization for analysis of chromosomal changes in cisplatin-resistant ovarian cancer. Human Cell 13:109–116

Lacy MQ, Hartmann LC, Keeney GL et al 1995 erbB-2 and p53 expression in fallopian tube carcinoma. Cancer 75:2891–2896

Land H, Parada LF, Weiberg RA 1983 Tumorigenic conversion of primary embryo fibroblasts requires at least two cooperating oncogenes. Nature 304:596–602

Lassus H, Laitinen MP, Anttonen M et al 2001 Comparison of serous and mucinous ovarian carcinomas: distinct pattern of allelic loss at distal 8p and expression of transcription factor GATA-4. Laboratory Investigation 81:517–526

Lavarino C, Silvana Pilotti S, Oggionni M et al 2000 p53 gene status and response to platinum/paclitaxel-based chemotherapy in advanced ovarian carcinoma. Journal Clinical Oncology 18:3936–3945

Lazo PA 1999 The molecular genetics of cervical carcinoma. Br J Cancer 80:2008–2018

Leone A, Flatow U, King CR et al 1991 Reduced tumor incidence, metastatic potential, and cytotine responsiveness of nm23-transfected melanoma cells. Cell 65:25–35

Levy-Lahad E, Catane R, Eisenberg S et al 1997 Founder BRCA1 and BRCA2 mutations in Ashkenazi Jews in Israel: frequency and differential penetrance in ovarian cancer and in breast-ovarian cancer families. American Journal Humanity Genetics 60:1059–1067

Lindblad-Toh K, Tanenbaum DM, Daly MJ et al 2000 Loss of heterozygosity analysis of small-cell lung carcinomas using single nucleotide polymorphism arrays. Nature Biotechnology 18:1001–1005

Lynch HT, de la Chapelle H 1999 Genetic susceptibility to non-polyposis colorectal cancer. Journal of Medical Genetics 36:801–808

Lynch HT, Kimberling W, Albano WA et al 1985 Hereditary nonpolyposis colorectal cancer (Lynch syndromes I and II). Cancer 15:938–938

Marks JR, Davidoff AM, Kerns BJ et al 1991 Overexpression and mutation of p53 in epithelial ovarian cancer. Cancer Research 51:2979

Marra G, Boland CR 1995 Hereditary nonpolyposis colorectal cancer. Journal National Cancer Institute 87:1114–1125

McCluskey LL, Dubeau L 1997 Biology of ovarian cancer. Current Opinion in Oncology 9:465–470

Merajver SD, Pham TM, Caduff RL et al 1995 Somatic mutations in the BRCA1 gene in sporadic ovarian tumours. Nature Genetics 9:439–443

Miki Y, Swensen J, Schattuck-Eidens D et al 1994 Isolation of BRCA1, the 17q linked breast and ovarian cancer susceptibility gene. Science 266:66–71

Modan B, Hartge P, Hirsh-Yechezkel G et al for the National Israel Ovarian Cancer Study Group 2001 Parity, oral contraceptives, and the risk of ovarian cancer among carriers and noncarriers of a BRCA1 or BRCA2 mutation. New England Journal of Medicine 345(4):235–240

Mok SC, Chan WY, Wong KK, Muto MG, Berkowitz RS 1996 SPARC, an extracellular matrix protein with tumor-suppressing activity in human ovarian epithelial cells. Oncogene 12:1895–1901

Nawroz H, Koch W, Anker P, Stroun M, Sidransky D 1996 Microsatellite alterations in serum DNA of head and neck cancer patients. Nature Medicine 2:1035–1037

Ono K, Tanaka T, Tsunoda T et al 2000 Identification by cDNA microarray of genes involved in ovarian carcinogenesis. Cancer Research 60:5007–5011

Pegram MD, Slamon DJ 1999 Combination therapy with trastuzumab (Herceptin) and cisplatin for chemoresistant metastatic breast cancer: evidence for receptor-enhanced chemosensitivity. Seminars in Oncology 26:89–95

Pere H, Tapper J, Seppala M, Knuutila S, Butzow R 1998 Genomic alterations in fallopian tube carcinoma: comparison to serous uterine and ovarian carcinomas reveals similarity suggesting likeness in molecular pathogenesis. Cancer Research 58:4274–4276

Pinto AP, Lin MC, Mutter GL, Sun D, Villa LL, Crum CP 1999 Allelic loss in human papillomavirus-positive and -negative vulvar squamous cell carcinomas. American Journal of Pathology 154:1009–1015

Piver MS, Jishi MF, Tsukada Y et al 1993 Primary peritoneal carcinoma after prophylactic oophorectomy in women with a family history of ovarian cancer. A report of the Gilda Radner Familial Ovarian Cancer Registry. Cancer 71(9):2751–2755

Pribill I, Speiser P, Leary J et al 2001 High frequency of allelic imbalance at regions of chromosome arm 8p in ovarian carcinoma. Cancer Genetics and Cytogenetics 129:23–29

Puls LE, Powell DE, DePriest PD et al 1992 Transition from benign to malignant epithelium in mucinous and serous ovarian cystadenocarcinoma. Gynecologic Oncology 47:53

Rous P 1911 A sarcoma of the fowl transmissible by an agent separable from the tumour cells. Journal of Experimental Medicine 13:396–411

Salovaara R, Loukola A, Kristo P et al 2000 Population-based detection of hereditary nonpolyosis colorectal cancer. Journal Clinical Oncology 18:2193–2200

Sandles LG, Shulman LP, Elias S et al 1992 Endometrial adenocarcinoma: genetic analysis suggesting heritable site-specific uterine cancer. Gynecologic Oncology 47:167

Santos E, Tronick SR, Aaronson SA, Pulciani S, Barbacid M 1982 T24 human bladder carcinoma oncogene is an activated form of the normal human homologue of BALB- and Harvey-MSV transforming genes. Nature 298:343–347

Sasaki H, Nishii H, Takahashi H et al 1993 Mutation of the Ki-ras protooncogene in human endometrial hyperplasia and carcinoma. Cancer Research 53:1906

Sato N, Tsunoda H, Nishida M et al 2000 Loss of heterozygosity on 10q23.3 and mutation of the tumor suppressor gene PTEN in benign endometrial cyst of the ovary: possible sequence progression from benign endometrial cyst to endometrioid carcinoma and clear cell carcinoma of the ovary. Cancer Research 60:7052–7056

Schultz DC, Vanderveer L, Berman DB, Hamilton TC, Wong AJ, Godwin AK 1996 Identification of two candidate tumor suppressor genes on chromosome 17p13.3. Cancer Research 56:1997–2002

Shak S 1999 Overview of the trastuzumab (Herceptin) anti-HER2 monoclonal antibody clinical program in HER2-overexpressing metastatic breast cancer. Herceptin Multinational Investigator Study Group. Seminars in Oncology 26:71–77

Shirashawa J, Tomita Y, Sekiya S, Takamizawa H, Simizu B 1987 Integration and transcription of human papillomavirus type 16 and 18 sequences in cell lines derived from cervical carcinomas. Journal of General Virology 68:583–591

Sidransky D, von Eschenbach A, Tsai Y et al 1991 Identification of p53 mutations in bladder cancers and urine samples. Science 252:706–709

Slamon DJ, Godolphin W, Jones LA et al 1989 Studies of the HER-2/neu proto-oncogene in human breast and ovarian cancer. Science 244:707

Smith SA, Easton DF, Evans DG, Ponder BA 1992 Allele losses in the region 17q12-21 in familial breast and ovarian cancer involve the wild-type chromosome. Nature Genetics 2:128

Srivatsa PJ, Cliby WA, Keeney GL et al 1996 Elevated nm23 protein expression is correlated with diminished progression-free survival in patients with epithelial ovarian carcinoma. Gynecologic Oncology 60:363–372

Stehelin D, Varmus HE, Bishop JM, Vogt PK 1976 DNA related to the transforming gene(s) of avain sarcoma viruses is present in normal avain DNA. Nature 260:170–173

Struewing JP, Watson P, Easton DF et al 1995 Prophylactic oophorectomy in inherited breast/ovarian cancer families. Journal National Cancer Institute 17:33–35

Suzuki S, Moore DH 2nd, Ginzinger DG et al 2000 An approach to analysis of large-scale correlations between genome changes and clinical endpoints in ovarian cancer. Cancer Research 60:5382–5385

Taetle R, Aickin M, Panda et al 1999 Chromosome abnormalities in ovarian adenocarcinoma: II. Prognostic impact of nonrandom chromosome abnormalities in 244 cases. Genetics, Chromosomes and Cancer 25:46–52

Tashiro H, Miyazaki K, Okamura H, Iwai A, Fukumoto M 1992 c-myc over-expression in human primary ovarian tumours: its relevance to tumour progression. International Journal of Cancer 50:828

Thorlacius S, Sigurdsson S, Bjarnadottir H et al 1997 Study of a single BRCA2 mutation with high carrier frequency in a small population. American Journal of Human Genetics 60:1079–1084

Van Trappen PO, Gyselman VG, Lowe DG et al 2001 Molecular quantification and mapping of lymph-node micrometastases in cervical cancer. Lancet 357:15–20

Vousden KH 1989 Human papillomaviruses and cervical cancer. Cancer Cells 1:43–49

Vousden KH 1991 Human papillomavirus transforming genes. Seminars in Virology 2:307–317

Wang K, Gan L, Jeffery E et al 1999 Monitoring gene expression profile changes in ovarian carcinomas using cDNA microarray. Genetics 229:101–108

Wen WH, Bernstein L, Lescallett J et al 2000 Comparison of TP53 mutations identified by oligonucleotide microarray and conventional DNA sequence analysis. Cancer Research 60:2716–2722

Wooster R, Bignell G, Lancaster J et al 1995 Identification of the breast cancer susceptibility gene BRCA2. Nature 378:789–792

Ylitalo N, Sorensen P, Josefsson AM et al 2000 Consistent high viral load of human papillomavirus 16 and risk of cervical carcinoma in situ: a nested case-control study. Lancet 355:2194–2198

Zhang Y, Mukhopadhyay T, Donehower LA et al 1993 Retroviral vector-mediated transduction of K-ras antisense RNA into human lung cells inhibits expression of the malignant phenotype. Human Gene Therapy 4:451–460

Zheng JP, Robinson WR, Ehlen T, Yu MC, Dubeau L 1991 Distinction of low grade from high grade human ovarian carcinomas on the basis of losses of heterozygosity on chromosomes 3, 6, and 11 and HER-2/neu gene amplification. Cancer Research 51:4045

37

The principles of radiotherapy and chemotherapy

Bleddyn Jones   Hilary Thomas

RADIOTHERAPY

Radiotherapy is the therapeutic use of ionizing radiation. It is used primarily for treating malignant tumours, including gynaecological cancers, and has an important curative role in carcinoma of the cervix.

Radiation physics

Ionizing radiation used for medical treatment is either electromagnetic or particulate. Ionization is usually the result of radiation energy ejecting one or more electrons from an atom and, in the case of biological molecules, can result in significant biochemical, cellular and tissue changes.

Electromagnetic radiation

Megavoltage X-rays and γ-rays (gamma rays) are similar types of electromagnetic radiation, the former produced artificially by machine and the latter from naturally occurring or artificially manufactured radio-isotopes. X-rays for treatment purposes are produced by a linear accelerator, which accelerates electrons to a high kinetic energy and onto a target of tungsten or gold. Part of the kinetic energy of the electrons is converted to energetic X-rays. γ-Rays are emitted naturally by radio-active isotopes such as ^{60}Cobalt or ^{192}Iridium as they decay to reach a stable form.

X-rays and γ-rays are characterized by a very short wavelength and high frequency. They consist of a stream of photons (packets of energy) which are capable of tissue ionization that can result in chemical bond breakage. The higher the energy imparted to the X-rays, the greater is the penetration of the beam within tissues (see Fig. 37.2). Treatment of pelvic tissues requires megavoltage therapy greater than 4 million electron volts (MeV or megavolts) but usually in the 6–12 MeV range. At lower energies there may be greater variations of dose within the patient. Very obese patients require the use of higher X-ray (or photon) energies for an adequate dose at the centre of the pelvis, which is at a relatively long distance from the skin surface.

Particulate radiation

This consists of atomic subparticles: electrons (negative charges), protons (positive charges), neutrons (no charge) and negative π-mesons. At present only electrons are commonly used in radiotherapy, having been accelerated to high energy in a linear accelerator from which the tungsten target has been removed so that X-rays are not produced. Electron particles react more rapidly with tissue such that the dose–depth profile follows a plateau for a distance that is determined by the energy of the particles followed by a rapid fall-off of dose. In this way tissues such as the vulva may be irradiated by a direct field without appreciable dose to deeper structures such as the bladder.

The gray

Radiation energy absorbed in tissue is measured in grays (Gy). One gray is the equivalent of 1 J/kg. Previously radiation energy was measured in rads, 1 Gy being equivalent to 100 rad. Particulate radiation causes ionization directly and X-rays and γ-rays indirectly by giving up their energy to eject fast-moving electrons from atoms.

Radiobiology

The study of the effects of ionizing radiation on living matter is called radiobiology. The initial ionization event is usually within water molecules with secondary ionization of surrounding macromolecules depending on the partial pressure of oxygen present. Total hypoxia will result in a dose reduction of a factor of 2–3 in most biological systems. The principal critical target in a cell is DNA. When this is damaged, cell metabolism and reproduction are affected. Death of the cell may result from apoptosis at low doses. More frequently, death occurs at a subsequent mitotic division. The onset of the latter will depend on the cellular turnover time of the tissue. More rapidly dividing systems such as the intestinal epithelium will show the effects of radiation earlier than in slowly dividing systems such as the central nervous system or bone.

Ionizing radiation will act on both normal and cancer cells and the problem for radiotherapy is to eliminate cancer cells without permanently damaging vital tissues. Recovery of normal tissue is usually better than that of malignant tissue, as long as the overall dose is not too large and it is given over a period of time. It is therefore the practice to fractionate the dose of radiation over several days or weeks to allow:

- DNA repair in normal tissues
- multiple exposures during more radiosensitive phases of the cell cycle
- normal tissue cellular repopulation
- time for the process of reoxygenation in hypoxic tumours that have outgrown their own blood supply.

Scheduling and dose of radiotherapy

Dose fractionation

Fractionated external beam therapy is usually given once daily five times a week. To attempt to improve cure rates, particularly in rapidly growing tumours, treatment can be accelerated by giving larger doses per fraction over a shorter time. This will increase the cell kill per fraction but will also interfere with normal cellular repair. Acceleration may also be carried out using normal-sized fractions twice daily, separated by at least 6 hours. Hyperfractionation, in which three or more small fractions are given each day, is also being examined in clinical trials. The theoretical reason for increasing the number of daily fractions is to allow sufficient time for normal tissue to regenerate but insufficient for tumour cells.

Dose prescription

The radiation dose prescribed includes the total dose to be given, the total number of fractions, the total time and the dose per fraction, for example 50 Gy in 25 fractions given five times weekly in 5 weeks at 2 Gy per fraction. For radical curative treatment, the greater the tumour volume, the higher the radiation dose necessary to eliminate the cancer. For example, 50 Gy in 5 weeks is sufficient for microscopic foci in 90% of patients but 6570 Gy in 6.5–7 weeks is needed to destroy a 2 cm mass. When there is no likelihood of cure but the patient is symptomatic, palliative radiotherapy has a valuable role in relieving pain. Doses are smaller and treatment time is reduced. If radiation fails, repeat treatment is of no value and will cause severe injury to normal tissues.

For normal tissues the concept of tissue tolerance is important. There are accepted tolerance ranges of total dose which result in an acceptably low incidence of radiation side-effects. Tolerance is itself adversely influenced by other factors including concomitant medical conditions such as diabetes, hypertension, vascular or inflammatory disorders or degenerative conditions. It is inversely related to the volume of tissue and may depend on other factors such as previous surgery and previous exposure to cytotoxic agents.

Radiotherapy techniques

Several techniques are used in the management of gynaecological cancer.

- Teletherapy is external irradiation where the tumour is a 'long' distance, usually 100 cm, from the source of ionizing radiation.
- Brachytherapy is either intracavitary or interstitial (inserted directly into tissues) irradiation where there is a 'short' distance between source and tumour (e.g. in the vagina and cervical canal).
- Instillation of radioactive fluids into the pleural and peritoneal cavity or, more rarely, by intra-arterial infusion to the tumour site.

Teletherapy: external irradiation

Teletherapy is used to treat large volumes, such as in carcinoma of the cervix where the volume includes the tumour itself, the parametria and the regional lymph nodes. The size of the treatment volume and the overall dose will be influenced by the age and general condition of the patient. For example, arteriosclerosis and bowel disease such as diverticulitis both reduce bowel tolerance. The small bowel tolerates only relatively low doses of radiation but its mobility enables it to move in and out of the treatment area, thus reducing the dose it receives. Damage to the small bowel can result from surgical adhesions which immobilize it. Care must also be taken with the rectum and pelvic colon, which will be partly in the treatment volume.

Treatment planning The aim of planning is to deliver a homogeneous dose to the tumour volume while giving only a low dose to surrounding normal tissues. The volume is measured in three dimensions: superior–inferior, anterior–posterior and right to left laterally. The dose of radiation which will be tolerated by normal tissues within the tumour volume must be known. Particular attention must be given to critical organs, such as the kidney or spinal cord, which tolerate only low doses of radiation. Accurate tumour localization is essential and is assessed by both clinical and surgical findings, with additional information from X-rays, ultrasound and computed tomography (CT) scanning and magnetic resonance imaging (MRI) when appropriate.

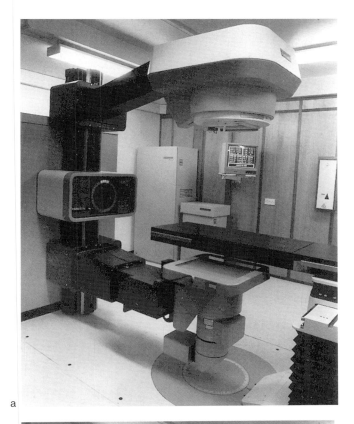

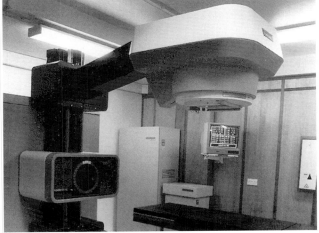

Fig. 37.1 **a** A Ximatron simulator with couch (manufactured by Varian TEM). **b** The gantry rotated.

Planning procedure The patient is placed on a mobile couch beneath a simulator – a diagnostic X-ray machine connected to a television screen which emulates a treatment machine (Fig. 37.1). The simulator defines the limits of the treatment volume, using a beam of light in place of the X-rays of the treatment machine. It will also take X-ray films for a permanent record.

The patient is positioned carefully with the help of a laser beam to ensure accurate replication at each treatment session. Cross-wires mounted in the light beam from the simulator define the size of the area to be treated (Fig. 37.2). This is marked on the patient with a semipermanent dye, usually

gentian violet, which will not wash off easily during the treatment period or the patient accepts a permanent tattoo mark at the centre of the beam entry points. The body contour at the volume centre is measured using pliable wire or more accurately with CT. On to this contour the tumour volume will be drawn, either on paper or by using a CT planning computer.

For the tumour to receive an adequate dose without overdosing the skin or other tissues, several fields arranged at different entry points to the body are used (Fig. 37.3). A planning computer (Fig. 37.4) calculates field sizes, the dose from each field and the angles of the treatment machine to give a homogeneous distribution to the tumour. The computerized plan of the final radiation dose delivered to the pelvis for carcinoma of the cervix by a three-field arrangement is shown in Figure 37.5.

The most usual field arrangement is 2–4 fields, but a rotational or moving field and conformal techniques may also be used (but not usually for gynaecological cancers). In the former the radiation source rotates around the tumour centre to provide an even dose throughout the tumour volume, while reducing the total dose given to the normal tissues. This is time-consuming and is less used today with the advent of high-energy machines. In the latter technique the field is shaped around the tumour volume, again with the aim of reducing the dose to normal tissues. This is particularly useful where large radiation fields are needed, as in the combined irradiation of the pelvis and para-aortic nodes.

Lead compensators may be placed in the path of the radiation beam to absorb unnecessary radiation. The most frequently used compensators are wedge-shaped (Fig. 37.6). The wedges are made with angles from $15°$ to $60°$ to vary the amount of radiation absorbed. Sometimes compensators need to be designed specially for individual patients. The most modern linear accelerators contain multiple leaf collimators that can shape the beam to better conform with carefully defined clinical targets that are often defined directly on CT scanning units linked to radiotherapy treatment planning software. The ultimate form of radiotherapy envisaged is that of intensity modulated radiotherapy (IMRT) where these collimators move during the treatment to further enhance the degree of treatment conformity to the target.

Choice of machine The intensity of a beam of radiation decreases with depth in tissue, but high-energy machines spare skin by delivering more radiation below the skin surface at the same time as reaching deeply situated tumours. Such machines have included those with a ^{60}Co source releasing γ-rays of 1.3 meV energy, but it is more usual today to use linear accelerators which deliver X-rays of 4–8 meV.

Implementation of the plan Treatment is carried out in a specially protected room with thick concrete walls, preventing radiation of personnel outside. The patient lies on the treatment couch in the same position as established with the simulator (Fig. 37.7). The machine angle, size of field and the use of wedges are carefully prepared for each treatment field. Radiographers, who set up and treat patients, use a control console outside the treatment room to start and stop the radiation and to set the dose and the time. Treatment time for each field is short, usually less than 1 minute. As the patient has to be alone during this time, she is supervised using

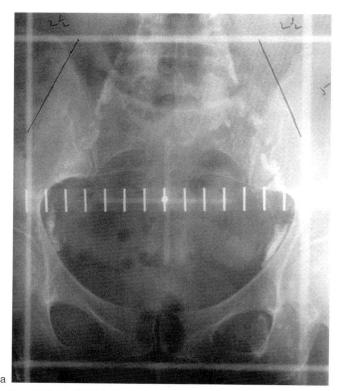
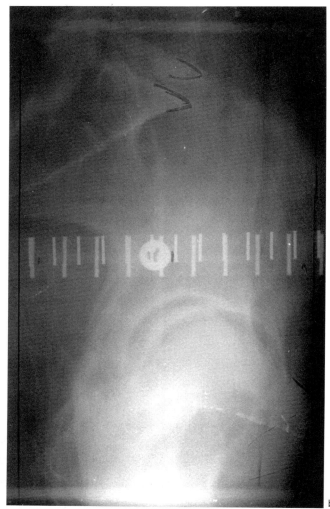

Fig. 37.2 **a** Anteroposterior X-ray of the treatment area (the pelvis) showing the superior, inferior and lateral margins. The triangular areas are protected from the beam. The patient has had a lymphangiogram. **b** Lateral X-ray of the treatment area.

a television camera. A microphone enables patients to talk to staff and if they are distressed the treatment is stopped immediately, so the radiographers can re-enter the room. There are many safety precautions to prevent accidental overdosage and treatment machines are checked frequently.

Brachytherapy

Brachytherapy gives a very high dose of radiation from a source close to the tumour. Because radiation dose decreases with the square of the distance travelled, there is a very rapid fall-off of radiation around the source and less damage to normal tissues. For the same reason, this method is suitable only for treating small tumour volumes. In the past, the energy source used was radium-226, but because of its long half-life, approximately 1600 years, and because it produces a radio-active gas, radon, it has been replaced by other radio-active isotopes such as caesium-137 (^{137}Cs), which has a half-life of 33 years and produces no toxic gases, and iridium-192 (half-life 74 days).

Direct insertion The commonest method of giving intra-cavitary radiation for gynaecological tumours is the Manchester system, in which a single uterine tube containing ^{137}Cs is passed through the cervix into the uterine cavity so that the inferior margin is flush with the external cervical os. Smaller tubes, containing ^{137}Cs in plastic vaginal ovoids, are inserted into the lateral vaginal fornices. The tumour volume treated by these three radio-active sources is shown in Figure 37.8. This is a low-dose rate treatment lasting for several days.

Afterloading Most radiotherapy centres have replaced the direct insertion of radio-active sources into a patient with an afterloading system. This system allows time to be taken over the positioning of source trains without hazard to the operator. Only after the accuracy of their placement has been verified with X-ray films are the radio-active sources inserted. In manual afterloading systems (Fig. 37.9), the active sources are inserted after the patient has returned to the ward, so eliminating radiation risk to theatre staff.

Remote afterloading systems are preferred as they allow complete staff protection. The patient is treated in a protected room for approximately 20 hours in the case of the Selectron, which uses ^{137}Cs, or for a few minutes with high dose rate systems such as the High Dose Selectron, which uses ^{60}Co

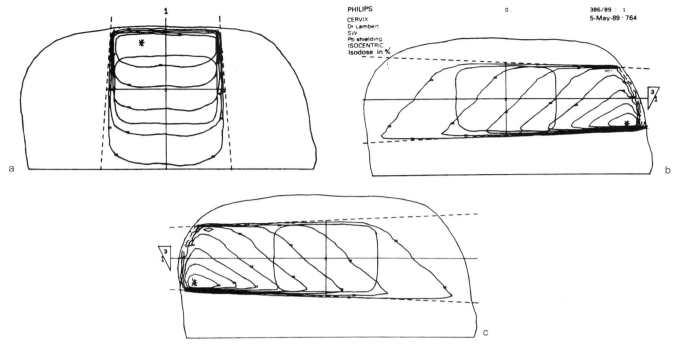

Fig. 37.3 Computer simulations of the isodose pattern of **a** the anterior field, **b** the left lateral field, **c** the right lateral field.

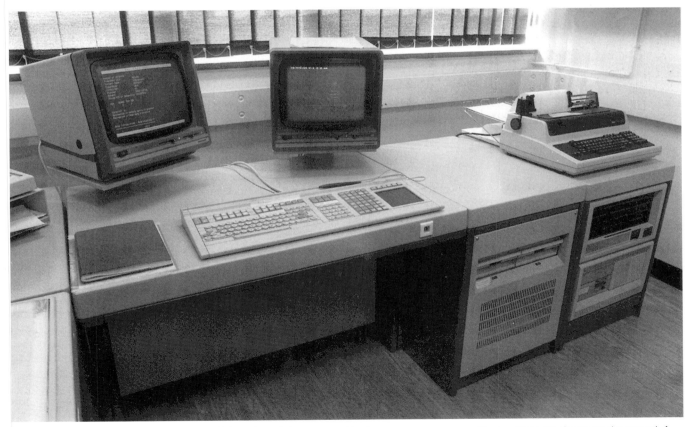

Fig. 37.4 The planning computer. A plan of the volume being prepared is shown on one screen and instructions are shown on the second. A permanent record is produced as in Figures 37.3 and 37.5.

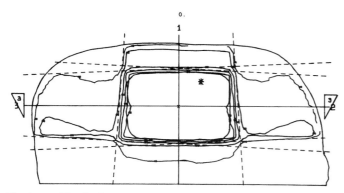

Fig. 37.5 The final tumour volume is shown derived from the summation of the isodoses from all three fields.

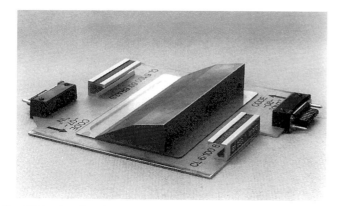

Fig. 37.6 A 60° wedge compensator.

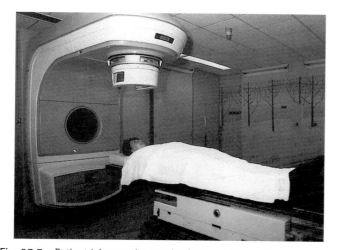

Fig. 37.7 Patient lying on the couch of a 6 meV Varian linear accelerator.

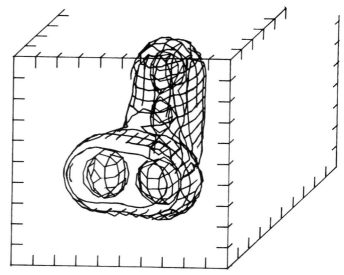

Fig. 37.8 The volume from the summation of three brachytherapy sources, an intrauterine tube and two vaginal ovoids. This shows the limits of the treatment volume and the rapid fall-off of the dose.

length measured with a sound to ascertain the length of the uterine tube required. The width of the vaginal vault is assessed to decide on the size of applicator or applicators to be inserted. The uterine tube is inserted first and then the vaginal applicators. A gauze pack keeps the sources in place and away from the rectum to reduce the rectal dose, which can be checked with a dosimeter. A computer using information from X-rays is a better way of measuring the doses given to both the treatment volume and to normal tissues (see Fig. 37.8).

For carcinoma of the cervix the dose can be calculated at reference point A, which in theory estimates the normal tissue dose where the ureter crosses the uterine artery. It is 2 cm lateral to the cervical canal and 2 cm superior to the lateral fornix. In practice this point is measured from the X-rays as 2 cm lateral to the centre of the uterine radio-active source and 2 cm superior to its inferior margin. A newer method of describing the given dose recommended by the International Commission on Radiation Units and Measurements (ICRU) measures the size of the tumour volume receiving full radiation dose. If the sole method of treatment is by low dose rate intracavitary radiation, 80 Gy are given in two fractions. After external irradiation only one fraction of 20–30 Gy is required.

Interstitial brachytherapy In some areas, treatment of small tumours with sparing of normal tissues can best be carried out by the insertion directly into the tumour of radio-active sources as needles, wires or seeds. An example is the insertion of radio-active needles for early cases of vaginal carcinoma. One such technique is to use a template (Fig. 37.12), which allows the insertion of guide tubes which can be afterloaded with active sources once X-rays have confirmed the correct position of the guides. Templates increase the accuracy of implants by ensuring that the sources are distributed in a regular fashion, giving a uniform dose to the treatment volume without 'hot' or 'cold' spots. The isotopes commonly used for this procedure are ^{192}Ir, ^{137}Cs and ^{125}I. For

(Figs 37.10, 37.11). With high dose rates severe damage to normal tissues is avoided by reducing and fractionating the total dose. All the techniques described are equally effective.

Intracavitary brachytherapy The procedure is carried out under general anaesthetic. A pelvic examination, including cystoscopy and proctoscopy, is performed. For cervical cancer the bladder is catheterized, the cervix is dilated and the uterine

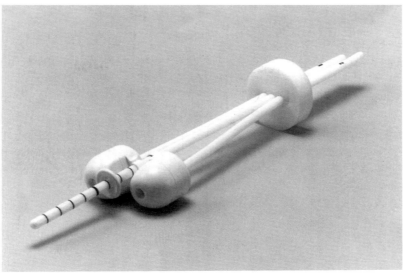

Fig. 37.9 The Amersham manual afterloading system for treating carcinoma of the cervix. There are three trains, a central one for the uterine tube and two lateral trains for the vaginal ovoids.

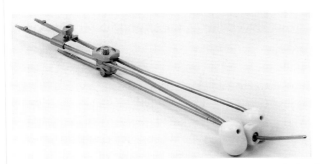

Fig. 37.10 Source train for Microselectron high dose rate afterloading therapy. This shows a central uterine tube and two lateral vaginal ovoids.

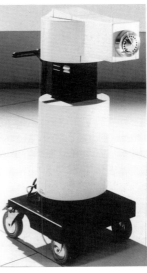

Fig. 37.11 The safe containing the radiation sources for the Microselectron.

a radical course of treatment, doses such as 60 Gy are given in 6 days.

Instillation of radio-isotopes in solution

Radiotherapy for small-volume disease in the peritoneal, pleural or pericardial spaces can be given as a solution of radio-isotopes. Early ovarian cancers have been treated using radio-active isotopes of either gold or phosphorus linked to carrier colloids. This gives a high dose of radiation but only to a depth of 4–6 mm, limiting therapy to small deposits on the pleural or peritoneal surfaces. Radio-active labelled monoclonal antibodies have been used in the same way in the hope that the antibody will target the radiotherapy to the tumour site.

Radiation damage

The dose of radiation is limited by the tolerance of normal tissue. Large single fractions of radiation cause more damage than multiple small fractions for the same total dose. Normal tissue reactions occur both early and late. Early reactions take place during or immediately after a course of radiotherapy, but recovery is usually rapid. Late reactions occur from 1 year onwards, are permanent and usually slowly progressive. Skin, bowel and bone marrow proliferate rapidly and so are particularly susceptible to acute reactions during treatment. Tissues which divide slowly, such as kidney, show late reactions because the damage to the DNA only becomes apparent when cells divide.

Early reactions

Skin Except when the vulval or anal region is included, radiation damage to skin is largely avoided when treating pelvic tumours because megavoltage machines deliver their maximum dose below the skin surface and the use of multiple treatment fields reduces the dose to any particular area of skin.

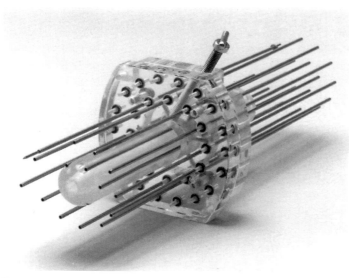

Fig. 37.12 A template (the 'Hammersmith hedgehog') for the interstitial treatment of carcinoma of the vagina.

Epidermal cells turn over in 2–3 weeks, so any damage becomes apparent after that time. Erythema may be followed by dry desquamation or, with more severe damage, by moist desquamation. The basal cells are usually spared, allowing the skin to regrow.

Bowel   Cells in the intestinal mucosa are replaced every 3–6 days, leading to diarrhoea when bowel is included in the treatment volume. Most patients also complain of nausea and anorexia.

Bone marrow   The bone marrow is very sensitive to radiation and frequent blood counts are essential when large volumes of marrow are included in the treatment fields, as for example in whole abdominal radiotherapy for ovarian carcinoma. The white blood count and platelet count are affected early, but anaemia occurs later because of the longer lifespan of red blood cells.

Late complications

Bowel   Late but uncommon complications to both small and large bowel include bleeding, stenosis and malabsorption. These may require special diets and nutritional support with vitamin supplements. Exceptionally, surgical intervention such as excision of damaged bowel with or without a stoma is necessary. The poor blood supply after radiation damage makes surgery difficult and the security of bowel anastamoses uncertain.

Bladder and ureter   Bladder changes, including telangiectasiae, are common and occasionally cause haemorrhagic cystitis. Ureteric damage and vesicovaginal fistulae are rare.

Other organs   Late damage to liver and kidneys owing to damage to the vascular supply may cause cirrhosis or loss of renal function. The ovaries are particularly sensitive to radiation and even small doses can cause ovarian failure.

It is important to note that the endometrium is very resistant to radiotherapy and may well persist after radiotherapy for cervical cancer (Habeshaw & Pinion 1992). Hormone replacement therapy may cause withdrawal bleeding or haematometra and should include progestogens to avoid the risk of inducing endometrial carcinoma.

Conclusion

Ionizing radiation is a sophisticated technique used for the treatment of cancer. It requires both highly technical machinery and expertise from specially trained personnel – engineers, physicists, doctors and radiographers. Side-effects are usually slight and the incidence of severe complications can be markedly reduced by individualization of the treatment (Tan et al 1997). However, complications can occur even after ideal treatment.

CHEMOTHERAPY

Cytotoxic chemotherapy developed from the realization that the effects on bone marrow cells of mustard gas used in World War I could be extended to the treatment of cancer. In the 1940s methotrexate and other antimetabolite drugs were discovered and since that time many drugs have been found that are of potential use in cancer therapy. In the past decade a number of new drugs have been developed, several of which are important in the treatment of gynaecological malignancies.

Drug evaluation

Before cytotoxic drugs can be used to treat cancer in humans they must first be tested for both their efficiency and their toxicity in animals. A promising drug is then studied in patients with advanced cancer to obtain pharmacological information (phase I trials). Sensitive tumours are identified in phase II trials, before a large number of patients with responsive tumours are treated to further define the drug's role (phase III trials).

Pharmacology

When considering the pharmacology of a drug, the following aspects must be investigated: absorption, distribution, metabolism and excretion. Drugs can only be taken orally if they are well absorbed from the alimentary tract. Parenteral administration – intravenous, intramuscular or intra-arterial – is the optimal route for most cytotoxic drugs. Although new drug development is starting to focus on orally bioavailable agents, many of these are not yet widely used in gynaecological cancer and the mainstay of treatment is given via the intravenous route.

The metabolism of drugs within the body is often unknown but several, including 5-fluorouracil, are metabolized in the liver. Most drugs are excreted in urine but a few are excreted in the alimentary tract via the bile duct. Only a very few drugs, such as the nitrosoureas and etoposide, cross the blood–brain barrier. This barrier can be overcome by intrathecal administration and methotrexate is given this way in the treatment of lymphatic leukaemia (Table 37.1).

Table 37.1 Cytotoxic drugs: dosage, routes of administration and excretion

Drug	Route of administration	Dose (as a single agent)	Excretion
Alkylating agents			
Chlorambucil	Oral	10 mg/day or 10–14 days per month	Urine
Cyclophosphamide	Oral or i.v.	Oral 100–200 mg/day i.v. 500–1000 mg/week High dose 20–40 mg/kg	Bile Urine
Ifosfamide	i.v.	$8–10 \text{ g/m}^2 \times 5$ days 2–4 weekly	Urine
Melphalan	Oral	$0.2 \text{ mg/kg/day} \times 5$ days 4-weekly	Urine
Treosulphan	i.v. or oral	i.v. 5 g/m^2 3-weekly	Urine
Platinum compounds			
Cisplatin	i.v.	$50–120 \text{ mg/m}^2$ weekly to 4-weekly	Urine
Carboplatin	i.v.	400 mg/m^2 or $5 \times$ (EDTA clearance +25) mg 3–4 weekly	Urine
Antimetabolites			
Methotrexate	Oral, i.m. or i.v.	e.g. $100–1000 \text{ mg/m}^2$ with folinic acid rescue or 2.5–5 mg/day orally	Urine Bile
5-Fluorouracil	Oral or i.v.	Loading dose $12 \text{ mg/kg/day} \times 3$ Maintenance 3–15 mg/kg/week	Urine
Vinca alkaloids			
Vincristine	i.v.	1–2 mg weekly	Bile
Vinblastine	i.v.	0.1–0.2 mg/kg weekly	Bile
Vindesine	i.v.	$3–4 \text{ mg/m}^2$ weekly	Bile
Anthracyclines			
Doxorubicin (Adriamycin)	i.v.	$60–75 \text{ mg/m}^2$ 3-weekly Total dose $<450 \text{ mg/m}^2$	Bile
Epirubicin	i.v.	$75–90 \text{ mg/m}^2$ 3-weekly	Bile
Mitozantrone	i.v.	14 mg/m^2 3-weekly	Bile
Other antibiotics			
Actinomycin D	i.v.	$0.5 \text{ mg/day} \times 5$ 4-weekly	Bile
Mitomycin	i.v.	4–10 mg 6-weekly	Urine
Bleomycin	i.m., i.v., i.p. Malignant effusions	10–60 mg weekly 60 mg i.p. Maximum total dose 300 mg	Urine
Miscellaneous			
Dacarbazine (DTIC)	i.v.	$250 \text{ mg/m}^2/\text{day} \times 5$ 3-weekly	Urine
Etoposide (VP 16)	Oral or i.v.	$60–120 \text{ mg/m}^2/\text{day} \times 5$ 4-weekly	Urine
Lomustine (CCNU)	Oral	120 mg/m^2 6–8-weekly	Urine
Paclitaxel (Taxol)	i.v.	175 mg/m^2 over 3 h after premedication 3–4 weekly	Bile
Docetaxel (Taxotere)	i.v.	$75–100 \text{ mg/m}^2$	Bile?

The doses shown are for general information only. The appropriate dose will vary in different circumstances and specific protocols should be consulted for detailed guidance.

Classification

The most common classification of cytotoxic drugs is one based on their biochemistry. Drugs are divided into alkylating agents, antimetabolites, vinca alkaloids, antibiotics, topoisomerase inhibitors, tubulin binding agents and others.

Cytotoxic drugs commonly used in gynaecology

Alkylating agents

These drugs cross-link DNA strands by forming covalent bonds between highly reactive alkylating groups and nitrogen groups on the DNA helix. This either prevents division of the helix at mitosis or results in an imperfect division and cell death.

The most frequently used alkylating agents are cyclophosphamide, chlorambucil and melphalan. Newer agents include treosulfan and ifosfamide. Many alkylating agents may be taken orally. Cyclophosphamide is inactive until it is converted into its active metabolite in the liver (Table 37.1).

The toxic effects of alkylating agents are listed in Table 37.2. In particular, they can cause vomiting if given in large doses, but this is seldom intractable. Most cause significant myelotoxicity, which can be cumulative. Alopecia is most marked with cyclophosphamide and ifosfamide. Both these last drugs are excreted in the urine in the form of active metabolites, which can cause a severe chemical cystitis when given in high doses unless mesna (sodium 2-mercaptoethanesulphonate) is administered at the same time to protect the bladder mucosa. In addition, ifosfamide may cause a fatal encephalopathy and must be given only after reference to a treatment nomogram.

Platinum agents Cisplatin and carboplatin both contain platinum. They act in a similar way to alkylating agents, forming DNA adducts. Both are given intravenously but, because of its potential nephrotoxicity, cisplatin requires a forced diuresis.

Cisplatin causes severe nausea and vomiting which require potent antiemetic therapy. Peripheral neuropathy can be disabling and is usually dose related. Cisplatin has little myelotoxicity except for anaemia, which frequently has to be corrected with blood transfusion.

Carboplatin has very little nephrotoxicity or neurotoxicity and is less emetogenic. It may be given to outpatients, as it only requires a half-hour infusion unless vomiting is severe. Carboplatin is myelotoxic, a particular problem being thrombocytopenia. Impaired renal function increases thrombocytopenia and so the drug is now usually given in a dose related to renal function, 'area under the curve' (AUC; Table 37.1) rather than surface area (Calvert et al 1989).

Antimetabolites

These compounds closely resemble metabolites essential for the synthesis of nucleic acids and proteins. They are incorporated into natural metabolic pathways and enzyme systems and disrupt the cellular mechanism. Each antimetabolite acts at different sites in the pathway of nucleic acid synthesis.

Methotrexate Methotrexate is a folic acid antagonist. It inhibits the enzyme dihydrofolate reductase, which reduces dihydrofolate to tetrahydrofolate, the precursor of co-enzymes essential for the formation of purines and pyrimidines, the nitrogen bases of DNA. These effects are bypassed by giving folinic acid. Folinic acid rescue is given from about 12 hours after the methotrexate dose to all patients receiving 100 mg or more. The commonest complication with methotrexate is oral ulceration. Because it is excreted in urine, the dose must be reduced in women with renal impairment or with large fluid collections such as ascites which delay excretion (Tables 37.1, 37.2).

5-Fluorouracil 5-Fluorouracil is a pyrimidine analogue which blocks thymidine synthesis and inhibits the incorporation of uracil into DNA. Myelosuppression and mucositis are the most common toxic effects, but unless very high doses are given they are not usually severe (Table 37.2).

Vinca alkaloids

Vincristine, vinblastine, vindesine and vinorelbin are derived from the periwinkle plant *Vinca rosea*. They act during the metaphase of mitosis, probably through toxicity to the microtubules of the mitotic spindle.

Peripheral and autonomic neuropathy are particular problems with vinca alkaloids, particularly vincristine. In addition, they are very irritant and are best injected into a fast-flowing drip. Vincristine is one of the very few chemotherapeutic drugs that is not myelotoxic.

Etoposide

Etoposide is a semisynthetic derivative of podophyllotoxin that acts on cells in G2 in the cell cycle. Toxicity is shown in Table 37.2.

Antibiotics

Many antibiotics inhibit tumour cell division. Actinomycin D and doxorubicin (Adriamycin) form irreversible complexes with DNA. Bleomycin breaks up DNA chains, thus interfering with DNA replication.

Doxorubicin (Adriamycin) Doxorubicin is a widely used anthracycline but causes marked alopecia and is myelosuppressive. It should always be given as a fast-running infusion as it is very irritant and will cause a necrotic ulcer if injected subcutaneously. Cardiomyopathy results from high cumulative doses unless the total dose is limited to $450\,mg/m^2$. As it is excreted in bile, an elevated bilirubin is an indication to reduce the dose. Newer anthracycline drugs epirubicin and mitozantrone appear to be as effective as doxorubicin but are much less cardiotoxic (Tables 37.1, 37.2).

Bleomycin Bleomycin is commonly included in multidrug regimens. It is not myelotoxic but sometimes causes a febrile reaction. Increased pigmentation of flexures is common. The most important toxic effect is a pulmonary fibrosis, which is dose related and not often seen at a cumulative dose less than $300\,mgm^2$. There is evidence to suggest that an infusion duration of 6 hours or more dramatically reduces the incidence of pulmonary fibrosis in comparison with shorter infusion times.

Taxanes

Paclitaxel (Taxol) was the first of the taxanes to be identified and tested. It was first derived from the bark of the Pacific yew tree, so production was very expensive, but production is now semi-synthetic which has improved the availability and cost of the drug. It has a unique cytotoxic action, preventing depolymerization of microtubules. It is active in ovarian and breast cancer and in many other tumours (Spencer & Faulds 1994). Hypersensitivity reactions were common until a premedication cocktail of antihistamines, H_2 antagonists and steroids was devised. The vast majority of patients develop total alopecia. Otherwise nausea and vomiting are mild and peripheral neuropathy is uncommon. With appropriate premedication it is very well tolerated. It is now usually given as a 3-hour infusion in a non-PVC system by the manufacturers. More recently it has become available in a plastic bag which

Table 37.2   The major toxic effects of some commonly used cytotoxic agents

Agent	Nausea & vomiting	Myelosuppression	Urological toxicity	Neuropathy	Others
Alkylating agents					
Chlorambucil	–	Moderate	–	–	Stomatitis, pulmonary fibrosis, hepatitis – all rare
Cyclophosphamide	Moderate	Moderate	Haemorrhagic cystitis	–	Alopecia; rare cardiomyopathy; very rare pulmonary fibrosis
Ifosfamide	Severe	Mild	Haemorrhagic cystitis	Confusion, tonic–clonic spasm, coma (rare)	Alopecia
Melphalan	Mild–moderate	Moderate	–	–	Rare pulmonary fibrosis
Treosulphan	Oral-moderate i.v. nil	Moderate	–	–	Very rare pulmonary fibrosis
Platinum agents					
Cisplatin	Very severe	Mild	Severe nephropathy	Moderate	Ototoxicity; hypomagnesaemia
Carboplatin	Moderate	Moderate–severe	Mild	Rare	Mild ototoxicity
Antimetabolites					
Methotrexate	Mild	Mild–moderate	Severe with high doses	–	Stomatitis; hepatitis with high doses
5-Fluorouracil	Mild	Moderate	–	–	Mucositis; dermatitis; alopecia with high doses
Vinca alkaloids					
Vincristine	–	–	Rare bladder atony	Severe: constipation, paralytic ileus, rare convulsions	Alopecia
Vinblastine	Mild	Moderate	–	Mild	Alopecia
Vindesine	Mild	Mild	–	Moderate: constipation, rare convulsions	Alopecia; stomatitis
Anthracyclines					
Doxorubicin	Severe	Moderate	–	–	Severe alopecia; severe cardiomyopathy if dose >450 mg/m^2
Epirubicin	Moderate	Moderate	–	–	Alopecia; mucositis; moderate cardiomyopathy
Mitozantrone	Mild	Moderate	Mild	–	Mild cardiomyopathy
Other antibiotics					
Actinomycin D	Moderate	Moderate–severe	–	–	Alopecia; mucositis; diarrhoea; fever; myalgia
Bleomycin	–	–	–	–	Fever; skin changes; pulmonary fibrosis and interstitial pneumonia
Mitomycin	–	Severe delayed	–	–	Stomatitis
Miscellaneous					
Dacarbazine (DTIC)	Severe	Severe	–	–	Photosensitivity; rare fever; alopecia; hepatitis
Etoposide (VP 16)	Moderate	Severe	–	–	Alopecia
Lomustine (CCNU)	Moderate	Severe delayed	Rare	–	–
Paclitaxel (Taxol)	Mild	Mild–moderate	–	Only at higher doses	Alopecia; hypersensitivity
Docetaxel (Taxotere)	Mild	Moderate–severe	–	Mild	Alopecia; hypersensitivity skin rash; oedema

makes administration more straightforward and significantly more convenient. When combined with a platinum agent, Taxol should be administered first to reduce toxicity and increase synergism. The reverse is the case for combination with Adriamycin.

Docetaxel (Taxotere) is a synthetic molecule with a structure similar to paclitaxel. It was introduced after paclitaxel and has a slightly different side-effect profile and at a dose of 100 mg/m^2 it does cause marked skin toxicity and oedema. Neutropenia seems to be more common at this dose than with paclitaxel at

$175\,mg/m^2$ and some patients experience a sensory neuropathy and fatigue. A Japanese study using a dose of $75\,mg/m^2$ did not report these problems. Docetaxel appears to have greater activity than paclitaxel as a single agent but it is not as suitable for combination therapy as a result of myelosuppression. Although it also causes alopecia this can be protected with use of scalp cooling more effectively than with paclitaxel. This may be due to the shorter infusion times.

The only direct comparison of paclitaxel and docetaxel in ovarian cancer is the SCOTROC trial. The toxicity findings in this trial have recently been reported but no difference in efficacy has been measured as yet since the trial was only recently closed to recruitment. It appears that paclitaxel causes more neurotoxicity and docetaxel causes a greater degree of bone marrow suppression and is associated with more sepsis and hospital admissions.

Gemcitabine

Gemcitabine (2′2′-diflurodeoxycytidine (dFdC)) is a new antineoplastic agent which is active against ovarian carcinoma, non-small cell lung cancer, head and neck squamous cell carcinoma. It has mechanisms of action which may be complementary with platinum analogues and there is some in vitro evidence to suggest synergy.

The potential synergy between gemcitabine and platinum analogues makes it a prime candidate for investigation with the use of concurrent radiotherapy in the treatment of carcinoma of the cervix. At doses lower than those which achieve cytotoxicity it has been demonstrated in vitro and in vivo to have radio-sensitizing properties.

The role of gemcitabine in the treatment of ovarian cancer and squamous cell carcinoma of the cervix is increasing. There are now a number of combination studies involving paclitaxel, carboplatin and gemcitabine which show very promising results in phase I and phase II studies and may add benefit in triple combination studies. This work is currently being pursued by an international collaborative group including the Gynae Oncology Group in the US.

Hormones

Progestins such as medroxyprogesterone acetate are used in endometrial cancer. There is little evidence that doses higher than 200 mg twice daily are more effective. Although widely regarded as free of side-effects and toxicity, many patients do complain of fluid retention and there is some concern that prolonged use may increase the risk of cardiovascular disease. Tamoxifen, an anti-oestrogen widely used in breast cancer, may have a role in endometrial cancer (see Ch. 42). Glucocorticoids are often useful as antiemetics and in terminal care.

Biological agents

Biological therapy includes methods of altering the host response to cancer and treatment with natural substances normally produced by the body but synthesized in the laboratory. Such treatment includes the use of vaccines, antibodies, activated lymphocytes or cytokines such as interleukin, interferon or tumour necrosis factor.

Interferons consist of a large family of molecules with similar but diverse and complex actions on the immune system, but with marked side-effects which are dose limiting. Different members of the family have been used with varying success in leukaemias and renal cell carcinomas. They have been used in genital warts and cervical intraepithelial neoplasia with limited success. Low response rates have been reported in ovarian cancer. A place has yet to be defined for any of these agents in gynaecological cancer.

Route of administration

Most cytotoxic drugs are given orally or intravenously. The intramuscular and intra-arterial routes are sometimes used and drugs are also instilled into the peritoneal or pleural cavities.

Oral chemotherapy

The alkylating agents are among the few drugs well absorbed by the oral route. Administration may be continuous on a daily basis, but is usually intermittent. For example, chlorambucil is often given 10 mg daily for 14 days every 28 days, to allow normal cells to recover.

Systemic chemotherapy

With intravenous and intramuscular administration drugs are normally given at intervals of 1–4 weeks. This pulsed treatment allows the bone marrow to recover and although some cancer cells will also recover, there is a net loss of cancer cells in every cycle.

Intrapleural and intraperitoneal chemotherapy

Chemotherapy can be given into both the pleural and peritoneal cavities. Bleomycin has been used in this way for recurrent ascites or pleural effusions, but it acts mainly by stimulating an inflammatory reaction and forming adhesions. Tetracycline is equally effective. Cytotoxic drugs given systemically are far more effective at dealing with ascites and do not cause 'pocketing' from adhesions.

Use of the intraperitoneal route has been explored as a way of giving high concentrations of drugs into the peritoneal cavity, which acts as a reservoir, releasing the drugs slowly into the systemic circulation. This results in very high and prolonged local concentrations of drug. However, absorption of cytotoxic drugs directly into tumour nodules is limited as penetration will be only 3–6 cells deep. Some agents are unsuitable because they cause a severe local chemical peritonitis. Cisplatin can be given by this route, but if the dose is too high systemic complications ensue. There is currently no firm evidence that intraperitoneal chemotherapy is superior to intravenous therapy. There may be some benefit in a very select group of patients with microscopic or a very small amount of residual disease, i.e. less than 1 cm in diameter. However, there is no doubt that further randomised trials are required.

Single-agent and combination chemotherapy

Drugs can be used alone or in combination. Combination chemotherapy in conditions such as Hodgkin's disease or germ cell ovarian tumours can be curative and is much more effective than single-agent regimens. However, combination

38

Premalignant disease of the genital tract

Pat Soutter   Roberto Dina

THE CERVIX

Terminology of cervical premalignancy

The terminology used to classify squamous cell lesions on the cervix has changed over the years in an attempt to reflect changing views of their nature (Table 38.1). Scheme 1 represents the original terms in use until Richart (1967) suggested scheme 2, incorporating the term 'cervical intraepithelial neoplasm' (CIN) to indicate the concept of cervical premalignancy as a continuum of change. Later, milder lesions thought to be due to human papillomavirus (HPV) infection were identified. The Bethesda terminology attempts simplification by grouping CIN I with HPV as a lesion with low potential for malignant change. The Bethesda terminology does not have wide support in the UK.

Table 38.1   Different terminologies for squamous cell cervical lesions

Scheme 1	Scheme 2	Bethesda scheme
	HPV changes	Low-grade lesions
Mild dysplasia	CIN I	
Moderate dysplasia	CIN II	
Severe dysplasia	CIN III	High-grade lesions
Carcinoma-in-situ		

HPV = Human papilloma virus; CIN = cervical intraepithelial neoplasia

Adenocarcinoma in situ is recognized more frequently than before. It has become relatively more important where screening has reduced the numbers of squamous cancers without affecting the incidence of adenocarcinoma.

Pathology of cervical premalignancy

Cervical intraepithelial neoplasia

The diagnosis of CIN is based upon the architectural and cytological appearances of the cervical epithelium.

Architectural features include differentiation, stratification and maturation, terms which are closely related but not synonymous. The proportion of the thickness of the epithelium showing differentiation is a useful feature to be taken into account when deciding the severity of a CIN. It is not the most important criterion despite the fact that it is one of the easiest to assess. In CIN I (Fig. 38.1) at least the upper half of the epithelium usually shows good differentiation and stratification whereas in CIN III differentiation may be very slight or even absent (Fig. 38.2).

Nuclear abnormalities are the most important combination of features to be taken into account when assessing CIN. The nuclei are examined using similar criteria to those employed by the cytologist in assessing a cervical smear: nuclear cytoplasmic ratio, hyperchromasia, nuclear pleomorphism and variation in size of nuclei. Both the overall number of mitotic figures and their height in the epithelium are assessed. The more

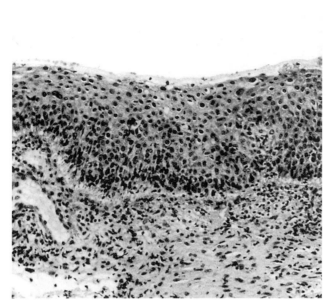

Fig. 38.1 CIN I. Haematoxylin and eosin ×170 (by kind permission of Dr MC Anderson).

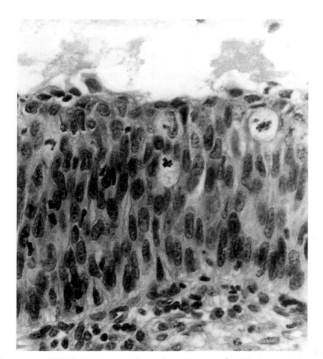

Fig. 38.2 CIN III. Haematoxylin and eosin ×170 (by kind permission of Dr MC Anderson).

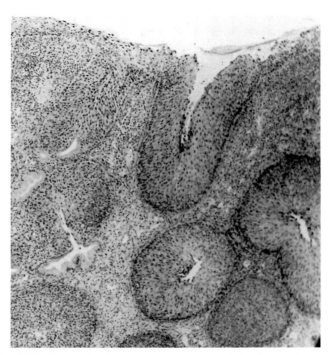

Fig. 38.3 CIN in gland crypts. The morphology of the abnormal epithelium in the involved crypts is similar to that on the surface. Normal columnar epithelium is recognizable in some crypts. Haematoxylin and eosin ×90 (by kind permission of Dr MC Anderson).

1.25 mm and that the mean plus 3 standard deviations (taking in 99.7% of the population) was 3.8 mm. These figures suggested that treatment to a depth of 5 mm into the stroma would be sufficient to eradicate most CIN; however, practical experience has shown that treatment to 10 mm gives much better results without increasing morbidity (Soutter et al 1986a).

Adenocarcinoma in situ (AIS)

This underdiagnosed lesion is characterized by columnar cells with large hyperchromatic nuclei and prominent nucleoli (Fig. 38.4). The nuclei may be stratified and show abnormal mitotic figures. There is often gland budding and a 'back-to-back' arrangement. In some cases, the whole of a gland may be involved but often the lesion occurs as a sharply demarcated area in the deep portions of the glands. It may be multifocal. Early invasion is said to have occurred when these lesions are seen lying more deeply in the stroma than the normal glands.

The vast majority of women with AIS are detected by abnormal cytology although in only half of these is an abnormality of the glandular cells recognized. In the remainder, the smear contains a squamous abnormality (Andersen & Arffmann 1989). In two-thirds of cases there is associated CIN or invasive squamous cancer and it is usually only the squamous lesion which is recognized. There are no specific colposcopic features which identify AIS. It is often not detected until a cone biopsy or hysterectomy is performed.

In the great majority of cases, the lesion lies in the transformation zone, close to the squamocolumnar junction (SCJ). Isolated AIS high in the endocervical canal some distance from

superficially the mitotic figures are found, the more severe the CIN is likely to be. Abnormal configurations (three-group metaphases and multipolar mitotic figures) are more likely to be found in severe forms of CIN.

CIN may affect the gland crypts as well as the surface epithelium (Fig. 38.3). Anderson & Hartley (1980) showed that the mean depth of crypt involvement in women with CIN III was

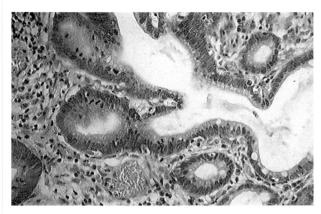

Fig. 38.4 A focal area of AIS showing gland budding, large hyperchromatic nuclei and nuclear stratification (by kind permission of Dr J Pryse Davies).

the SCJ is uncommon in young women. It follows that a cone biopsy with a good margin of excision in the endocervical canal ought to be adequate treatment for most young women with AIS.

Diagnostic precision

The histological diagnosis of these lesions is based largely upon subjective criteria. It is not surprising to find substantial inter- and intra-observer variation in the grading of CIN and the identification of AIS (Robertson et al 1989). Although the variation is greatest at the mild end of the spectrum there is still a considerable amount of disagreement over severe lesions.

The scope for disagreement is inevitably increased when comparing two samples from the same lesion. In a study performed at Hammersmith Hospital, London, there were substantial differences between the colposcopically directed punch biopsy diagnosis and that based on a laser cone biopsy (Skehan et al 1990). This relative imprecision of histological grading of CIN makes it virtually impossible invariably to distinguish by punch biopsy a woman with CIN I from one with CIN III. This should be borne in mind when considering any discussion of the natural history of different grades of CIN and different treatment policies.

Malignant potential of CIN

Progression from CIN III to invasion

The malignant potential of CIN III is amply demonstrated by McIndoe et al (1984) in a crucial paper. A group of 131 patients who had been treated for CIN III and who continued to produce abnormal cytology for more than 2 years after the initial treatment were followed for 4–24 years. After 20 years' follow-up, 36% of these women had developed invasive disease. There was no evidence that the rate of conversion to invasive disease was slowing towards the end of this period.

Progression from CIN I to CIN III or invasion

Studies of progression from CIN I to CIN III are blighted by the difficulty in accurately determining the grade of the initial lesion. Those reports that relied upon cytology only to determine the initial diagnosis and to document progression or

regression are invalidated by the poor correlation between the grade of cytologic abnormality and that of the histology (Soutter et al 1986b). Basing the diagnosis of CIN I upon a colposcopic assessment without punch biopsy, progression to CIN III was observed in 26% of women within 2 years (Campion et al 1986).

Which lesions to treat?

Given the clear malignant potential of untreated CIN III, the difficulty in identifying CIN I accurately and the high progression rate in women whose CIN I was not treated, it seems to be prudent to treat all women with CIN when they first present regardless of the grade of abnormality. There is no justification for treating subclinical HPV lesions. More caution is needed before treating what seems to be recurrent or residual CIN I after treatment. This is often just a post-treatment effect and second treatment increases the risks of pregnancy complications.

Screening for cervical premalignancy

The objective of cervical screening is to reduce the incidence and the mortality from cervical cancer. When the screening programme detects early invasive disease it can be said to have been only partly successful since the treatment of these early lesions carries a substantial morbidity, is not universally successful and is expensive. The objectives of cervical screening can only be achieved by detecting cervical premalignancy.

Cervical cytology

Cervical cytology is the only well-established screening method. When a properly organized programme is implemented, substantial reductions in both incidence and mortality from cervical cancer are achieved (Anderson et al 1988). The vital elements of a successful programme are obtaining wide cover of the population at risk and taking effective action when a cytological abnormality is discovered (Fig. 38.5).

To achieve wide cover, the confidence of the target population must be won. They must know about the programme, what it aims to achieve and how, and they must be convinced that the programme will be successful. If the quality of a cytology service is high, 3-yearly smears are virtually as effective as annual

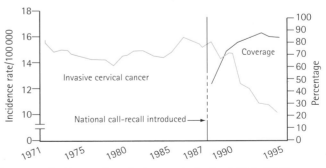

Fig. 38.5 Incidence of cervical cancer in England 1971–95. The incidence has fallen sharply since the national call and recall scheme was introduced in 1988 and coverage of the population has increased from 40% to over 80%.

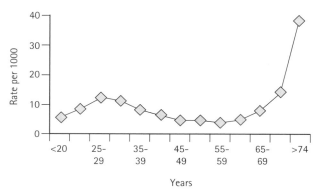

Fig. 38.6 Rate of severely dyskaryotic smears per 1000 women compared with age. The increasing rates after 65 years of age are due to smears being taken in women with symptoms. (Cervical Screening Programme, England 2000–01, Statistical Bulletin, Department of Health.)

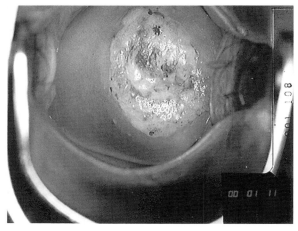

Fig. 38.7 Cervigram showing CIN III. A strongly staining aceto-white lesion with well-demarcated, regular edges is seen.

smears (IARC Working Group 1986). In the UK, the proportion of a screened population with positive smears (moderate-severe dyskaryosis) is highest in women aged 25–35 years (Fig. 38.6). A rational programme would therefore recommend 3-yearly smears for all at-risk women between 20 and 60 years of age. Indeed, the falling rate of positive smears in asymptomatic women over 50 years and data from Dundee (Wijngaarden & Duncan 1993) and Aberdeen suggest that screening might be stopped safely at 50 years of age in well-screened women.

The standard method of preparing material for cytological examination is to spread it directly upon a glass slide. A variety of liquid-based methods have been developed in which the collecting device is rinsed or broken off into a vial of preservative fluid. The suspended cells are then treated to remove unwanted material and a thin layer of cells is deposited upon a slide and stained as usual. There seems little doubt that this reduces the number of inadequate samples and there is some evidence that the sensitivity is improved (NICE 2000). The results of pilot studies in UK are awaited before a decision is taken on the introduction of this methodology.

In spite of the success achieved by cervical cytology, it is not without its shortcomings. A satisfactory sample must include cells from the relevant part of the cervix. The screener must scan the whole slide carefully to detect one of what may be a small number of abnormal cells. The assessment and definition of cytologic abnormality are subjective with considerable interobserver variation. The process is laborious and tiring with considerable scope for operator error, especially when the workload is high. Furthermore, cytology screening has little effect on the incidence of adenocarcinoma of the cervix (Nieminen et al 1995).

The imprecision of cervical cytology is evident from the many studies which report CIN II–III or invasive disease in about 50% of women with smears showing only mild dyskaryosis (Soutter et al 1986b, Flannelly et al 1994). The high risk associated with a mildly dyskaryotic smear is confirmed by a meta-analysis that showed an annual incidence of invasive cancer of 208 per 100 000 women in patients with mild dyskaryosis followed up cytologically (Soutter & Fletcher 1994). This should be compared with the annual incidence of

cervical cancer of 9 per 100 000 women in UK women of a similar age at that time.

There have been few satisfactory investigations of the accuracy of cervical cytology. Although false-negative rates from 2.4% to 26% have been estimated by a variety of different types of study, there have been few in which a large asymptomatic population has been screened by cytology and the results of cytology corroborated by an alternative test like colposcopy. In studies of this sort, the sensitivity of cytology was low (44–52%) but the specificity high (91–94%) (Kesic et al 1993, University of Zimbabwe 1999). There is clearly scope for a more accurate and less labour-intensive screening method.

Cervicography

Cervicography is a method of detecting cervical pathology which uses the same principles as colposcopy. The cervix is visualized, 5% acetic acid is applied and, after allowing 1 minute for the effect of the acetic acid to become apparent, two photographs are taken of the cervix using a specially designed camera (Fig. 38.7). The film is developed as 35 mm slides and these are projected and interpreted by an experienced reviewer. Slides from between 30 and 50 patients can be reported in an hour. The sensitivity of this method is high (89%; Kesic et al 1993) but initial reports suggested low specificity. With increased experience and minor modifications to the reporting technique, the specificity can become more satisfactory (92%; Kesic et al 1993). This promising technique might be taken up first in countries which have no established cervical cytology service or where it can be added to an established cytology screening programme either as an additional primary screening method or as a secondary screen of women with equivocal cytology.

Visual inspection with acetic acid

This technique has been investigated enthusiastically in parts of the developing world in the search for an effective, low-cost screening method. The method relies upon the naked-eye inspection of the cervix for whitened epithelium after the application of acetic acid – colposcopy without a colposcope. One very large study reported a sensitivity of 76.7% but this was accompanied by a false-positive rate of 35.9% that makes this unusable (University of Zimbabwe 1999).

Other new methods

HPV testing has been utilized as an adjunct to cytology screening but 5–15% of women, depending on their age, have evidence of HPV infection using sensitive techniques. A variety of semi-quantitative tests have become available, the Hybrid Capture II being one of the most widely studied. These all have high sensitivity but poor specificity, making this a poor test for identifying women with CIN. However, the negative predictive value of Hybrid Capture II is very high indeed, making this potentially very valuable as a means of identifying those who do not have CIN. Using this as the first-line test on a sample collected into a liquid medium would allow the cytologists to concentrate their efforts on those women with positive HPV results.

Using a very different approach, measurements of the electrophysical characteristics of cervical epithelium have been investigated with promising results (Coppleson et al 1994, Brown et al 2000). The positive predictive value was a very encouraging 89% in the more recent of these two studies but the negative predictive value and the specificity were both disappointingly low at 45% and 71% respectively. A major disadvantage of both these techniques is that they depend upon contact between the probe and the lesion itself. The whole diameter of the 5.5 mm probe must be in contact with an area of abnormal epithelium to register an abnormal value. Consequently, several careful measurements must be taken at different sites on the cervix to ensure that an abnormality is not missed.

Colposcopy of the cervix

The basis of colposcopy

Eversion of the cervix   At puberty, during pregnancy or when the combined oral contraceptive pill is taken, the cervix enlarges. As it does so, there is a tendency to eversion and to the exposure of columnar epithelium on the ectocervix (Fig. 38.8). The thin columnar epithelium appears red and the result is what is so often erroneously referred to as a 'cervical erosion'.

Squamous metaplasia   The columnar epithelium on the ectocervix is gradually replaced by a process of squamous metaplasia spreading from the SCJ towards the cervical canal. The normal end-result of this transformation is the replacement of the ectopic columnar epithelium with mature squamous epithelium (Fig. 38.8c). If squamous epithelium now covers the entrance to a cervical crypt and the columnar cells continue to secrete mucus in the crypt, a nabothian follicle results. This is the only clinical evidence of the prior existence of columnar epithelium in that area. When the cervix shrinks in the months and years following pregnancy and after the menopause, it gradually inverts, drawing the new SCJ up the endocervical canal (Fig. 38.8d).

The transformation zone   The region of the cervix in which this process of metaplasia occurs is called the transformation zone. In some women the transformation zone may extend on to the vaginal walls. A common source of confusion

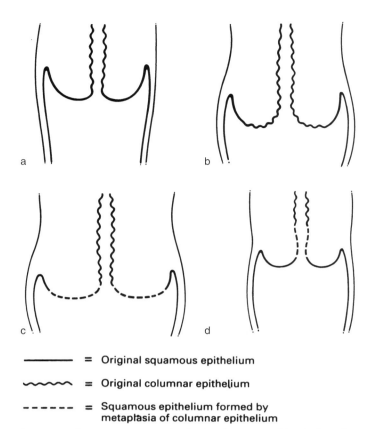

————	= Original squamous epithelium
∿∿∿∿∿	= Original columnar epithelium
- - - - -	= Squamous epithelium formed by metaplasia of columnar epithelium

Fig. 38.8   The different stages in the development and involution of the cervix. **a** Before puberty the ectocervix is covered with squamous epithelium and columnar epithelium is usually confined to the endocervical canal. **b** The cervix enlarges and everts when oestrogen levels rise. This exposes columnar epithelium on the ectocervix. **c** The columnar epithelium on the ectocervix is replaced with squamous epithelium by a process of metaplasia. **d** Following the climacteric when oestrogen levels fall, the cervix shrinks, drawing the squamocolumnar junction up the canal.

in colposcopy is the loose use of the term 'transformation zone' when referring to that part of the true transformation zone where metaplastic or dysplastic epithelium can be seen colposcopically.

The genesis of squamous cervical neoplasia   Squamous neoplasia results from a disruption of the normal metaplastic process. Thus, CIN develops as a confluent lesion confined to an area of the cervix contiguous with the SCJ. It is this characteristic localization which enables the colposcope to be used in the assessment of CIN.

Referral for colposcopy

Prior to the advent of colposcopy, cytologists recommended referral to a gynaecologist only after two successive severely dyskaryotic smears were obtained. The reason for this delaying policy was because a knife cone biopsy would be required to determine whether or not there was a premalignant lesion on the cervix and this operation had potentially serious consequences for the future obstetric prospects of the young women in whom these abnormalities were most often found.

That conservative policy is no longer justifiable. With colposcopy, the women who require treatment can be identified and those who do not can be reassured. In addition, the treatment can be carefully tailored to remove only the minimum of cervical tissue. Most women with CIN can be treated in the outpatient clinic with methods that do not prejudice their future fecundity. With the recognition that mild cytological abnormalities are associated with a high prevalence of significant histological abnormalities, it is apparent that the indications for referral need to be revised (Table 38.2). Nowadays, no woman with abnormal cytology should be treated without prior colposcopy.

Although the majority of women sent for colposcopy have abnormal smears, a suspicious-looking cervix is sufficient reason for referral even if the smear is negative. Such women sometimes have invasive cancer. Similarly, worrying symptoms such as postcoital bleeding should always be investigated by colposcopy even if the smear is normal. About 4% of women with postcoital bleeding have invasive cancer of the cervix, vagina or endometrium, and 17% have CIN (Rosenthal et al 2001). Cervical cancer is found in 1.3% of women with postmenopausal bleeding (Gredmark et al 1995).

The colposcopic method

A detailed description of the author's personal method may be found elsewhere (Soutter 1993). Space permits only an outline description here.

Bimanual examination and the smear   A bimanual examination is essential to aid detection of frank invasive

Table 38.2   Management of abnormal cervical cytology. This differs from the guidelines issued by the National Co-ordinating Network in 1997 in which a repeat smear was recommended for women with mild dyskaryosis unless the woman was unlikely to comply with cytological surveillance. That was a controversial recommendation taken in the knowledge that the results of all prospective studies have supported immediate colposcopy

Papanicolaou class	Histology	Action
I Normal	0.1% CIN II–III	Repeat 3 years (unless clinical suspicion)
II Inflammatory	6% CIN II–III	Repeat in 6 months (colposcopy after 3 abnormal)
Borderline nuclear changes	20–37% CIN II–III	Repeat in 6 months (colposcopy after 2 abnormal)
III Mild dyskaryosis	50% CIN II–III	Colposcopy
Moderate dyskaryosis	50–75% CIN II–III	Colposcopy
IV Severe dyskaryosis 'Positive' 'Malignant cells'	80–90% CIN II–III 5% Invasion	Colposcopy
V Invasion suspected	50% Invasion	Urgent colposcopy
Abnormal glandular cells	? Adenocarcinoma of the cervix or endometrium	Urgent colposcopy

disease of the cervix, a uterine or an ovarian mass. A bivalve speculum is then introduced and a smear is taken. Deferring the smear until after the colposcopic inspection may reduce the risk of removing the epithelium one wishes to study (see below) but unfortunately it provides a less satisfactory sample for the cytologist (Griffiths et al 1989). Only if the os is narrowed or the SCJ out of sight up the canal is an endocervical brush used.

Pre-acetic acid examination   If the view of the cervix is obscured by a discharge this should be removed gently with saline. The preliminary inspection should include both the cervix and upper vagina. At this stage of the examination there are three objectives: to identify leucoplakia; to exclude obvious evidence of invasive disease; and to identify viral condylomata.

Leucoplakia must be identified prior to the application of acetic acid after which it may be impossible to differentiate from aceto-white epithelium. Because the hyperkeratinization of leucoplakia may conceal invasive disease, biopsy is mandatory.

Invasion is often obvious from the bizarre appearances of the surface of the cervix, which may appear grossly irregular, either raised or ulcerated (Fig. 38.9). This disorganization of the surface is usually recognizable even when atypical vessels cannot be identified or the area subsequently fails to turn white after the application of acetic acid. The atypical vessels seen on invasive lesions run a bizarre course and are often corkscrew- or comma-shaped (Fig. 38.10). They are large in diameter, abruptly appearing on and disappearing from the surface. They do not branch dichotomously like normal vessels.

Condylomata are usually obvious from their regular frond-like surface (Fig. 38.11) but biopsies should be taken, especially when they are located within the active part of the transformation zone where it is more difficult to be sure of their benign nature.

Acetic acid examination

A low-power inspection   Having completed the first inspection of the cervix, 5% acetic acid should be applied liberally and gently. This turns abnormal epithelium white, producing the so-called 'aceto-white' changes of CIN. It is important to allow sufficient time to elapse for faintly staining areas to show up. While waiting for any colour changes to occur, the cervix and vaginal fornices are inspected under low power in order to have the widest field of view possible so that areas of faint aceto-white may be observed against the contrasting background of normal epithelium. After about 30 seconds it is usually possible to proceed. If a lesion has become visible, its outer limits should be determined first.

Identifying the SCJ   Next, the position of the SCJ must be ascertained to define the upper limits of the abnormality. Failure to identify the SCJ correctly is one of the main pitfalls in colposcopy. It is important to note that the SCJ is marked by the lower limit of normal columnar epithelium, not the upper limit of squamous, as these do not always lie at the same level. The higher the SCJ appears to lie in the canal, the more difficult it becomes to assess the lesion accurately and, except when the cervix is very patulous, 5 mm represents the limit above which colposcopic evaluation becomes unsafe.

Determining the nature of the lesion   It is necessary only to decide whether or not a lesion with malignant potential

Fig. 38.9   A cervigram of a stage Ib cervical cancer showing the irregular surface.

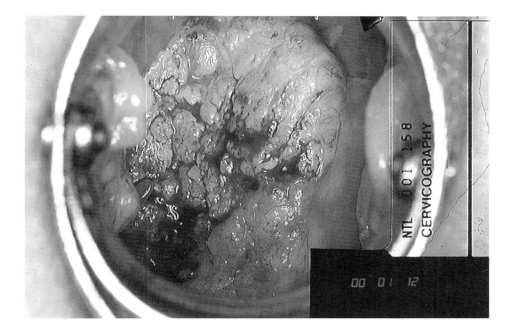

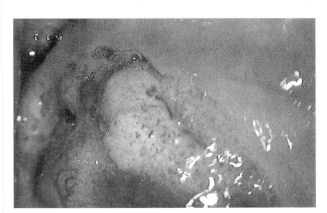

Fig. 38.10   This high-power view of a cervical tumour shows some short atypical vessels in the lower centre of the picture and longer stretches of atypical vessels above this area. Note also the irregular surface.

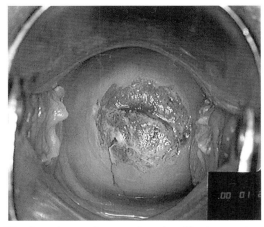

Fig. 38.12   A cervigram of a normal cervix with a large ectropion. The central portion of the cervix around the os is covered with normal columnar epithelium.

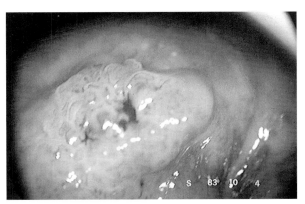

Fig. 38.11   A high-power view of a large cervical condyloma prior to the application of acetic acid. Note the regular form and the microvilli with looped capillaries on the top of the condyloma.

is indeed present and whether invasion may have already occurred. It is preferable to adopt a very conservative approach to the latter objective and to regard cases of severe CIN III as being potentially invasive. When determining the significance of a lesion, the colposcopist assesses the colour, the margins and the vascular markings.

Non-malignant epithelium that becomes aceto-white
Not all areas of aceto-white change are abnormal. Columnar epithelium will blanch briefly after exposure to acetic acid. It may be identified by its villous or furrowed surface (Fig. 38.12). Squamous metaplasia has a glassy white appearance but can be hard to distinguish from CIN I (Fig. 38.13). After any form of treatment, the cervix may develop areas of aceto-white, subepithelial fibrosis. This can be recognized by the radial arrangement of lines of fine punctation.

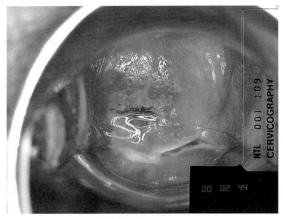

Fig. 38.13 This cervigram shows an area of faintly aceto-white epithelium around the cervical os; however, it is seen most clearly on the anterior lip in this photograph.

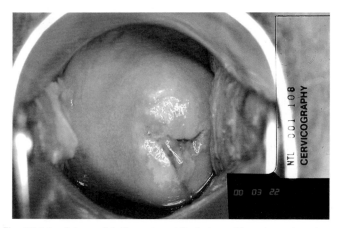

Fig. 38.14 A large, faintly aceto-white lesion with an irregular edge is visible on both lips of the cervix. Two satellite lesions are visible on the posterior lip at 6 o'clock below the main lesion.

Wart virus lesions Considering the difficulties the histopathologist has in differentiating CIN from wart virus lesions, it is no surprise that flat viral lesions are difficult to identify with certainty colposcopically. In general, they have faint, very irregular margins and isolated satellite lesions (Fig. 38.14). In early condylomata, looped capillaries may be seen in small villi (Fig. 38.11). The delicate fronds of fully formed condylomata are usually easy to identify but all raised lesions on the active transformation zone must be biopsied lest they be invasive cancer.

Features of CIN CIN are usually distinct aceto-white lesions with clear margins (Fig. 38.7). They often show a mosaic vascular pattern with patches of aceto-white separated by vessels like red weeds between white flagstones. Where the vessels run perpendicular to the surface, punctation is seen as the vessels are viewed end-on. This appears as red spots on a white background. In general, the more quickly and strongly the aceto-white changes develop, the clearer and more regular the margins of the lesion, and the more pronounced the mosaic or punctation, the more severe is the lesion likely to be.

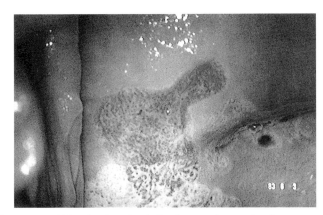

Fig. 38.15 This microinvasive lesion is a good example of coarse punctuation.

However, not all features will be equally marked and many CIN III lesions show only a strong matt-white colour.

Features of invasion Frank, early invasion is often obvious before acetic acid is applied (see above) but microinvasion may not become apparent until after the application of the acid. Although atypical vessels may be seen, the only indication of invasion is often a very marked mosaic pattern or coarse punctation: large-diameter, widely separated red spots (Fig. 38.15).

Because even expert colposcopists will fail to identify correctly every case of early invasion (Bekassy et al 1983), excisional treatment which removes the whole lesion for histological assessment merits wide use to avoid the risk of undertreating invasive disease.

Pitfalls in colposcopy

The first pitfall: the false SCJ caused by an abrasion The SCJ should be identified by observing the lower limit of normal columnar epithelium, not the upper limit of squamous. The reason for this is the ease with which CIN and metaplastic epithelium can be detached from the underlying stroma, particularly at the SCJ where the unwary may mistakenly regard the upper limit of aceto-white change as synonymous with the SCJ. Careful inspection of the red epithelium at this junction will reveal a flat surface covered by spidery and often whorled blood vessels characteristic of exposed stroma. This can be distinguished from columnar epithelium which has a soft, velvety-looking surface and blanches briefly when exposed to acetic acid.

The second pitfall: the SCJ in the canal When the SCJ lies within the endocervical canal, if the upper part of the lesion is inspected from too acute an angle, the assessment of both the length of the endocervical canal involved with CIN and the severity of the lesion becomes unreliable.

The third pitfall: the previously treated cervix When a cervix has been treated previously for any reason, the topography of the transformation zone will have been altered. Areas of metaplasia, CIN or invasive disease in the canal or in cervical glands may have escaped destruction and may persist as isolated iatrogenic skip lesions surrounded by columnar epithelium or covered by new squamous epithelium

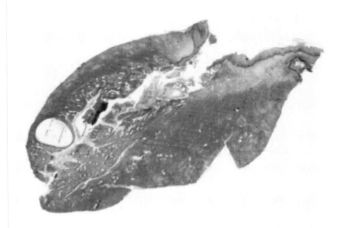

Fig. 38.16 An iatrogenic skip lesion can be seen in this cone biopsy performed in spite of normal, satisfactory colposcopy because of severe dyskaryosis in a woman who had previously been treated with cervical electrodiathermy. The ectocervical end of this cone biopsy to the top and right is covered with normal squamous epithelium. The SCJ is near the external os and the lower canal is lined by columnar epithelium but halfway up the canal, near the nabothian cyst on the left, is an isolated area of CIN III. In deeper sections this was shown to be an invasive tumour.

(Fig. 38.16). Such patients should always be treated by an excisional method.

The fourth pitfall: glandular lesions It cannot be assumed that the rules of colposcopy apply to women with adenocarcinoma or AIS. AIS and small adenocarcinomas cannot be identified colposcopically, so a cone biopsy is an essential investigation in the management of a patient with abnormal glandular cells in her smear. Older women also require an endometrial biopsy. Many of these patients also have CIN which requires treatment in its own right.

Treatment of CIN and AIS

Detailed descriptions of the techniques discussed may be found elsewhere (Soutter 1993). CIN was originally treated by radical hysterectomy but it soon became evident that this was unnecessary and simple hysterectomy became the method of choice. In time, it was realized that cone biopsy was just as effective and now hysterectomy is reserved for those with difficult-to-treat recurrent disease or who have additional indications for hysterectomy. The introduction of colposcopy and a better appreciation of the limited location of CIN led to the introduction of more conservative methods of treatment.

Ablative methods

A large number of ablative methods are available (Table 38.3). The chief advantage of these (with the exception of radical electrodiathermy) is that general anaesthesia is not required. Cryotherapy is the one method most often associated with unsatisfactory results. A 24% failure rate was described in one recent prospective trial (Mitchell et al 1998).

A disadvantage common to all these techniques is that they depend heavily upon the exclusion of invasion by colposcopy

Table 38.3 Methods of ablative treatment of CIN: in chronological order, with the longest established methods first.

Method	Anaethesia	Restrictions
Radical electrodiathermy	GA	Vaginal extension of CIN?
Cryotherapy	None	CIN III; large lesions
Laser vaporization	LA	None
'Cold' coagulation	None	Vaginal extension of CIN

GA = general anaesthesia; LA = local anaesthesia

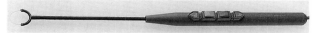

Fig. 38.17 One of the varieties of large wire loops used for LLETZ. (Figure supplied by Valleylab UK.)

and directed biopsy. In addition, they are not applicable to all patients – some will always require an excisional treatment. The indications for excisional treatment of CIN are listed below:

- Any suspicion of invasive disease.
- Any suspicion of a glandular abnormality.
- SCJ not clearly visible.
- History of any previous cervical surgery.
- Elective method of treating any case of CIN.

Excisional methods

Knife cone biopsy was supplanted as the standard treatment by ablative techniques partly because of the complications and partly because of the need for general anaesthesia. Complications are listed below.

- Intraoperative haemorrhage
- Secondary haemorrhage
- Pelvic infection
- Cervical stenosis
- Cervical incompetence.

The complications of laser cone biopsy are fewer than those of knife cone biopsy, the technique is far more precise (Larsson et al 1983) and the distortion of the cervix that results is much less, suggesting that there will be fewer problems in any subsequent pregnancies. In addition, laser cone biopsy can very often be performed under local anaesthesia (Partington et al 1987).

The ability to perform laser cone biopsy under local anaesthesia, the observation that the complications were no greater than in laser vaporization (Partington et al 1989) and anxieties about invasive cancer being missed led to a widening of the indications for excisional therapy and to the suggestion that laser excision should replace vaporization for most patients. The advent of large loop electrodiathermy excision of the transformation zone (LLETZ) made excisional treatment quicker and reduced the cost of the equipment required (Prendiville et al 1989). This technique employs a blended diathermy current and a loop of very thin stainless steel wire (Figs 38.17, 38.18). It has become the most widely used treatment for CIN in the UK but the recurrent costs are much

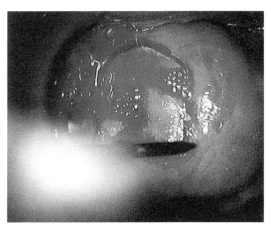

Fig. 38.18 A cone biopsy being taken with LLETZ. (Figure supplied by Valleylab UK.)

higher than for the laser. In addition, it is becoming apparent that the incomplete excision rate and the failure rate is unacceptably high in some hands (Robinson et al 1998).

A diathermy loop is a rather inflexible instrument in that the amount of tissue removed and the shape of the sample is largely predetermined by the shape and size of the loop. In addition, it is not possible to see the deep cutting edge of the loop during the procedure, so excision may be more shallow than intended. As a result, loop diathermy gives poorer results when dealing with disease inside the cervical canal. The lesions are often removed in multiple fragments, making orientation of the specimen and assessment of completeness of excision impossible.

Needle diathermy excision of the transformation zone (NETZ) is a modification of loop diathermy in which a straight tungsten wire electrode is used like a knife (Basu et al 1999). This means that the volume of tissue removed and the shape of the sample are not dictated by the shape and size of the instrument. In contrast, the amount and location of tissue removed by needle diathermy are under precise control at all times and a cone biopsy is fashioned in the same way as one might previously have used a cold knife or a laser beam but with the added advantage of good control of haemostasis. NETZ has replaced cold knife cone biopsy in my practice and is the treatment of choice when the SCJ is not visible in the canal or the lesion is large or when AIS is suspected.

Choice of technique

None of the different methods of treating CIN is more effective than any of the others when used appropriately by a well-trained and experienced operator. Each has particular advantages of cost or ease of use or speed or precision. The particular method chosen will depend upon local circumstances. It seems sensible to choose a method which will allow abnormalities to be excised under local anaesthesia. In spite of its greater capital cost, the laser does have the advantage that it may be used both to excise and to vaporize lesions when it is appropriate to do so. An example of the latter are large lesions which extend on to the sides of the cervix or beyond the cervix into the fornices. However, NETZ and LLETZ have largely replaced the

laser because of the reduced capital cost, greater simplicity in the maintenance of the instrument and more rapid treatment with less blood loss.

Treatment of adenocarcinoma in situ (AIS)

It is often said that a cone biopsy with free margins is adequate treatment for most women with AIS (Cullimore et al 1992). However, some 20% of women managed in this way required further treatment for suspected recurrence within 4 years (Soutter et al 2001). Moreover, only 46% of women with AIS had clear margins on the cone biopsy, 21% were treated by simple hysterectomy after invasive disease had been excluded and 8% were treated radically for invasive cervical cancer.

In addition, LLETZ is associated with a very much higher recurrence rate than knife cone biopsy and should probably not be used knowingly in a case of AIS (Widrich et al 1996). These problems with LLETZ in the treatment of AIS are probably due to removing too little of the endocervical canal. This problem does not occur with NETZ.

In summary, many women thought to have AIS will actually have invasive disease. Free margins are obtained in only half of the cone biopsies. When the margins are not free of disease, a simple hysterectomy is probably the safest treatment, provided that invasive disease has been excluded. A further cone biopsy as definitive treatment would be acceptable management for young women who want more children. If the margins are clear, close observation with 6-monthly cervical smears is reasonable management provided that both patient and physician are aware of the relatively high likelihood of the need for further treatment for suspected recurrence.

See and treat

'See and treat' means different things to different people. To some it means offering treatment at the first visit to women who meet certain criteria, including the colposcopy findings at that visit. To others it means treating all women referred to the clinic with certain cytological abnormalities, regardless of the colposcopy findings.

There are advantages to the hospital and to the women themselves in being able to deal with an abnormality in one visit. The disadvantage is the extent of overtreatment that will result depending on the criteria that are used to select women for immediate treatment (Brady et al 1994). Because the referral population differs greatly between clinics, it is not possible to define a set of rules that would be suitable for all clinics. Each centre must audit its own data and adjust its criteria accordingly. Unfortunately, cytology, colposcopy and histopathology are all subjective and prone to observer error so that not even a pretreatment punch biopsy can be relied upon to identify accurately those who do not require treatment (Skehan et al 1990).

My own practice remains one of selective treatment, based upon the referral cytology, my colposcopic impression, a selective punch biopsy from lesions I am unsure about and the result of the smear which I have taken in the clinic. To these factors I add the patient's age, being less conservative in older women, and the patient's own viewpoint: is she particularly anxious to be treated or would she prefer a more conservative approach if it is warranted? Provided I can see the SCJ clearly and the cytological abnormality is not glandular, I would rarely treat in the absence of a colposcopic abnormality. The only common exception would be a woman with a persistent moderate or severe dyskaryosis, especially if she had been treated before (Soutter 1993).

Results of treatment

Treated adequately, some 5% of patients treated for CIN will have recurrent disease within 2 years (Paraskevaidis et al 1991, Soutter et al 1986a). Thereafter, the number of recurrences is small. However, long-term follow-up is necessary as these women remain at a higher risk of CIN or invasive cervical cancer than the general population (Burghardt & Holzer 1980). In that study, the prevalence of invasive cancer in 1219 women treated by cone biopsy after colposcopic assessment was 574 per 100 000 during a follow-up of 4–20 years. All the cancers were detected within 11 years. A further 2.21% were found to have recurrent CIN but the authors did not specify how long after the initial treatment these were discovered. In addition, recurrent vaginal intraepithelial neoplasia was found in 3.8% of the 183 women in the 11 years after hysterectomy following incomplete excision by cone biopsy. All but one of these was treated with radiotherapy.

A study combining the experience of four UK centres provided data on 36 435 woman-years of follow-up with 896 women still under observation in the 8th year (Soutter et al 1997). The cumulative rate of invasion after 8 years was 0.76% and the annual incidence of invasive cancer during this period was 85 per 100 000 women. The rates for women treated for CIN III were 1.31% and 142 per 100 000 women respectively. Although most of the cancers were diagnosed in the first 5 years following treatment, because fewer women had been followed longer than that, the risk of developing a cancer remained broadly similar throughout the 8 years.

In the light of the results of this and other similar studies, annual cytological follow-up up of patients treated for CIN by any method would seem to be prudent for at least 10 years.

Complications of diathermy excision

Moderate to severe intraoperative haemorrhage may occur in 4.5–8.5%, with sutures required for 0.5% (Luesley et al 1990, Murdoch et al 1991). Secondary haemorrhage may occur in up to 4.3% of cases, usually after a deep excision. Most women note a vaginal discharge but this usually lasts less than 2 weeks but can go on for over 6 weeks. Severe cervical stenosis may be seen after 1.3% of treatments. These are nearly all deep treatments. There is no evidence of reduced fertility after diathermy excision and little evidence of premature delivery (Cruickshank et al 1995). However, the risk of premature delivery is likely to be increased if the biopsy is deep and the effective length of the remaining cervix is reduced substantially (Raio et al 1997). This will apply particularly if treatment has to be repeated.

THE VAGINA

Terminology and pathology of vaginal intraepithelial neoplasia

The terminology and pathology of vaginal intraepithelial neoplasia (VAIN) are analogous to that of CIN (VAIN I–III). The

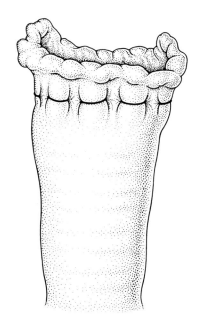

Fig. 38.19 Sutures in the vaginal vault isolate a cuff of the vagina above the suture line.

main difference is that vaginal epithelium does not normally have crypts so the epithelial abnormality remains superficial until invasion occurs. The common exception to this is found following surgery, usually hysterectomy, when abnormal epithelium can be buried below the suture line or in suture tracks.

Natural history of VAIN

VAIN is seldom seen as an isolated vaginal lesion. It is more usual for it to be a vaginal extension of CIN. In most cases it is diagnosed colposcopically prior to any treatment during the investigation of an abnormal smear. However, it may not be recognized until after a hysterectomy has been performed. When this happens, abnormal epithelium is likely to be buried behind the sutures used to close the vault. Consequently a portion of the lesion will remain invisible and unevaluable (Fig. 38.19). In the series reported by Ireland & Monaghan (1988), 28% of those treated surgically proved to have unexpected invasive disease. Untreated or inadequately treated VAIN may progress to frank invasive cancer (Woodman et al 1984). Very rarely, VAIN may be seen many years after radiotherapy for cervical carcinoma when it is probably a new lesion. Care must be taken in these women to ensure that postradiotherapy changes are not being misinterpreted as VAIN.

Colposcopy of the vagina

Colposcopy of the vagina is more difficult than the cervix, partly because of the greater area of epithelium to be examined, partly because the surface of the vaginal epithelium is very irregular and partly because it is very difficult to view the vaginal walls at right angles. If the patient has had a hysterectomy it is very difficult to see into the angles of the vagina and impossible to visualize epithelium that lies above the suture line or vaginal

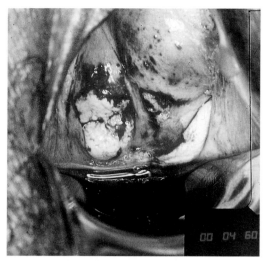

Fig. 38.20 VAIN after a hysterectomy. A patch of dense aceto-white epithelium is easily visible in the centre of the figure in the left vaginal angle. A second area of VAIN can be seen just above the speculum, spreading out of the right angle.

adhesions. The colposcopic features of VAIN are very similar to those of CIN except that mosaic is seen less often (Fig. 38.20).

Treatment of VAIN

Carbon dioxide laser

Provided invasive disease has been excluded, laser vaporization is a satisfactory way of treating VAIN in women who have not undergone previous surgery. However, the report of invasive disease developing in two out of 14 post-hysterectomy patients treated with the laser illustrates the dangers of overlooking disease buried above the suture line (Woodman et al 1984). Thus, although the laser may be useful in reducing the size of a lesion or in treating women who have not had a hysterectomy, it should not be used as the sole method of treatment in VAIN of the vaginal vault following hysterectomy. The same applies to the use of topical 5-fluorouracil.

Partial or total vaginectomy

Surgical excision of VAIN gives far more satisfactory results (Ireland & Monaghan 1988) and is the only effective option available to patients previously treated with radiotherapy. The patients in Ireland & Monaghan's series were treated by an abdominal operation or by a combined abdominal and vaginal approach. This necessitates extensive pelvic dissection which can be avoided by a vaginal approach (Fig. 38.21). While the latter procedure is often very straightforward, it can prove to be extremely taxing in patients with a narrow introitus and no laxity of the vaginal vault.

Where the lesion involves a large area of the vagina there may be a place for laser vaporization to reduce the size of the lesion. The entire lesion is vaporized under general anaesthesia and some months later when the effect of the laser treatment can be assessed, the vault of the vagina is excised. When this approach is unsuccessful and in older patients, total vaginectomy or radiotherapy is required.

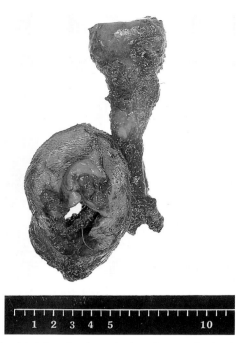

Fig. 38.21 A total vaginectomy, hysterectomy and vulvectomy performed by the vaginal route in an elderly woman with severe irritation from extensive VAIN and VIN 20 years after radiotherapy for cervical cancer (units in cm).

Radiotherapy

There can be no doubt that intracavitary radiotherapy is a highly effective treatment for VAIN (Hernandez-Linares et al 1980, Woodman et al 1988). The two major concerns about this form of therapy are the possibility of radiation-induced cancer and the effects it may have upon coital function. Radiation-induced second cancer in the vaginal vault may occur but it is probably an extraordinarily rare event (Boice et al 1985, Choo & Anderson 1982). Brachytherapy to the vault of the vagina is unlikely to cause major coital problems if the patient and her partner are encouraged to resume normal sexual relations as soon as possible (Woodman et al 1988). Where the area of disease is more extensive, no method of therapy is likely to be free of the risk of inducing sexual dysfunction.

Conclusions

The management of VAIN after hysterectomy in a young woman is likely to be surgical. If the lesion is extensive, prior laser therapy may be helpful in reducing the extent of disease. In older patients, especially when access is difficult, surgery offers few additional benefits but carries a potential for greater morbidity. Radiotherapy is therefore likely to be the treatment of choice. Whatever the circumstances, it would be sensible for such patients to be evaluated and treated by those with experience of this unusual but troublesome condition.

THE VULVA

Vulval intraepithelial neoplasia (VIN) are seen more commonly than was the case 10–20 years ago. It is not certain whether this represents a real increase or is simply the result of a greater awareness of the problem. Bowen's disease, Bowenoid papulosis and erythroplasia of Queyrat are all terms for different clinical manifestations of VIN.

Pathology of premalignant disease of the vulva

Both squamous VIN and AIS (Paget's disease) occur on the vulva. The latter is very rare. The histological features and terminology of VIN are analogous to those of CIN and VAIN. In the same way, the histological appearance of Paget's disease is similar to the lesion seen in the breast. In a third of cases of Paget's disease, there is an associated invasive cancer, often an adenocarcinoma in underlying apocrine glands, and these carry an especially poor prognosis (Creasman et al 1975, Parker et al 2000).

Vaginal intraepithelial neoplasia

Natural history of VIN

Forty per cent of women with VIN are younger than 41 years (Buscema et al 1980). Although histologically very similar to CIN and often occurring in association with it, VIN is said not to have the same malignant potential (Buscema et al 1980, Kaufman & Gordon 1986b). However, this opinion is based largely on studies of women who have been treated by excision biopsy or vulvectomy. This may not be true of untreated or inadequately treated patients; seven of eight such women progressed to invasive cancer within 8 years (Jones & Rowan 1994). Three of these were under 40 years of age.

Diagnosis and assessment of VIN

Intraepithelial disease of the vulva often presents as pruritus vulvae but 20–45% are asymptomatic and are frequently found after treatment of preinvasive or invasive disease at other sites in the lower genital tract, particularly the cervix (Jones & McLean 1986, Kaufman & Gordon 1986a).

These lesions are often raised above the surrounding skin and have a rough surface. The colour is variable: white, due to hyperkeratinization; red, due to thinness of the epithelium; or dark brown, due to increased melanin deposition in the epithelial cells (Figs 38.22, 38.23). They are very often multifocal.

However, the full extent of the abnormality is often not apparent until 5% acetic acid is applied (Fig. 38.24a). After 2 minutes, VIN turns white and mosaic or punctation may be visible. While these changes may be seen with the naked eye in a good light, it is much easier to use a hand lens or a colposcope. Toluidine blue is also used as a nuclear stain but areas of ulceration give false-positive results and hyperkeratinization gives false negatives.

Adequate biopsies must be taken from abnormal areas to rule out invasive disease. This can usually be done under local anaesthesia in the outpatient clinic using a disposable 4 mm Stiefel biopsy punch or a Keyes punch.

Treatment of VIN

The treatment of VIN is difficult. Uncertainty about the malignant potential, the multifocal nature of the disorder and

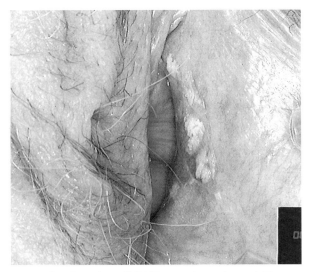

Fig. 38.22   Small patches of VIN III appearing as leucoplakia.

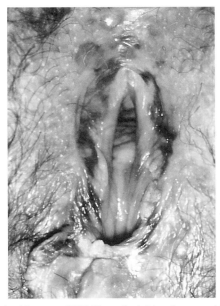

Fig. 38.23   A wide area of VIN III on the labia minora and the perineum seen as slightly raised, red lesions anteriorly, whitish lesions posteriorly and extensive dark brown lesions.

the discomfort and mutilation resulting from therapy suggest that recommendations should be cautious and conservative in order to avoid making the treatment worse than the disease. The youth of many of these patients is a further important consideration. Spontaneous regression of VIN III in women with the variant known as Bowenoid papulosis is well known (Friedrich 1972). These women are young, often present in pregnancy, have dark skin and the lesions are usually multifocal, papular and pigmented. However, progression to invasion does occur in young women (Planner et al 1987).

The documented progression of untreated cases of VIN III to invasive cancer underlines the potential importance of these lesions (Jones & Rowan 1994). If the patient has presented with symptoms, therapy is required. Asymptomatic patients,

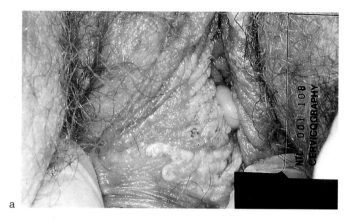

a

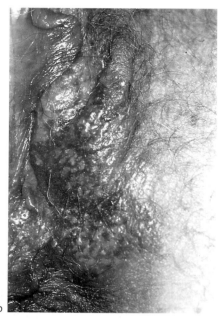

b

Fig. 38.24   a A patch of VIN III on the labium minorum after the application of acetic acid. b Paget's disease of the vulva. Note the crusted surface and clear margins.

particularly under the age of 50 years, may be observed closely with biopsies repeated if there are any suspicious changes.

Medical therapy   The main role for medical treatment is in relieving symptoms in women for whom surgery may be avoided.

Provided invasion has been excluded as far as possible, topical steroids provide symptomatic relief for many women. A strong, fluorodinated steroid is usually required. This may be applied twice daily for not more than 6 months because of the thinning of the skin which can result. Frequent review is necessary initially.

Topical 5-fluorouracil is painful and ineffective. Topical α-interferon produced promising results in one small series (Spritos et al 1990).

Surgery   If the lesion is small, an excision biopsy may be both diagnostic and therapeutic. If the disease is multifocal or covers a wide area, a skin graft may improve the cosmetic result of a skinning vulvectomy (Caglar et al 1986). However,

the donor site is often very painful and a satisfactory result can be obtained in most patients without grafting.

Carbon dioxide laser   An alternative approach is to vaporize the abnormal epithelium with the carbon dioxide laser. Careful control of the depth of destruction is essential for good cosmetic results (Reid 1985). Given the very irregular surface of the vulva, it is very difficult to achieve a uniform depth of destruction. Moreover, the depth of treatment required for VIN is still unclear (Dorsey 1986). In some cases hair follicles may be involved for several millimetres below the surface (Mene & Buckley 1985) but it may not always be necessary to destroy the whole depth of involved appendages (Dorsey 1986). In any case, treatment of the whole vulva to such a depth would result in a third-degree burn which would need skin grafting. In practice, laser vaporization has proved to be disappointing in UK practice and is now seldom used (Shafi et al 1989).

Results   Assessment of the results of treatment should include a consideration of the length of follow-up. Surgical excision is associated with crude recurrence rates of 15–43% (Jones & McLean 1986, Shafi et al 1989). Short-term results from patients treated by laser were very promising (Leuchter et al 1984) but longer follow-up showed a recurrence rate similar to surgery (Shafi et al 1989). Close observation and rebiopsy are essential to detect invasive disease among those who relapse. Early invasion was detected in three (14%) of 21 patients with persisting signs of disease (Shafi et al 1989). Repeated treatments are commonly required.

Conclusions

VIN is becoming more common, especially in young women. The treatment must be carefully tailored to the individual to avoid mutilating therapy whenever possible.

In view of the mutilating nature of treatment, the high recurrence rate and the uncertainty about the risk of invasion, there is a place for careful observation, especially of young women without severe symptoms. However, some of these untreated patients will develop vulval cancer so the importance of close follow-up must be emphasized to the patient and her general practitioner.

Paget's disease

This is an uncommon condition, similar to that found in the breast. Pruritus is the presenting complaint. It often presents as a red, crusted plaque with sharp edges (Fig. 38.24b). Multiple erosions may be seen. The diagnosis must be made by biopsy.

Associated malignancies

In approximately one-third of patients there is an adenocarcinoma in the apocrine glands (Boehm & Morris 1971, Creasman et al 1975, Parker et al 2000). This has a poor prognosis if the groin lymph nodes are involved with no women surviving 5 years (Boehm & Morris 1971). Excluding underlying adnexal carcinomas, concomitant genital malignancies are found in 15–25% of women with Paget's disease of the vulva (Degefu et al 1986, Parker et al 2000). These are most commonly vulval or cervical, but transitional cell carcinoma

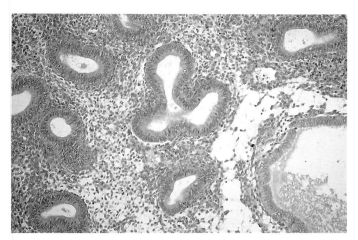

Fig. 38.25 Simple cystic hyperplasia. Haematoxylin and eosin ×100 (by kind permission of Dr Thomas Krausz).

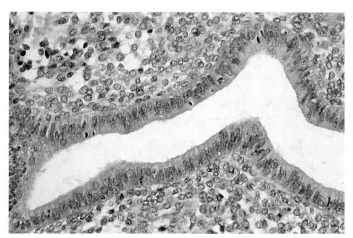

Fig. 38.26 Simple cystic hyperplasia. Haematoxylin and eosin ×250 (by kind permission of Dr Thomas Krausz).

of the bladder (or kidney), and ovarian, endometrial, vaginal and urethral carcinomas have all been reported (Degefu et al 1986).

Treatment

The treatment of Paget's disease is very wide local excision, usually involving total vulvectomy because of the propensity of this condition to involve apparently normal skin (Creasman et al 1975). The specimen must be examined histologically with great care to exclude an apocrine adenocarcinoma.

ENDOMETRIUM

Premalignant disease of the endometrium is less well characterized than the equivalent lesions in the squamous epithelium of the cervix, vagina and vulva. This is partly because these lesions cannot be identified clinically and their detection is largely dependent on blind biopsy which required general anaesthesia until recently.

Pathology of endometrial hyperplasia

Endometrial hyperplasia may be subdivided into:

- cystic (simple) hyperplasia
- adenomatous (complex) hyperplasia
- Atypical hyperplasia.

Simple glandular hyperplasia

In this condition the endometrium is increased in volume and the glands show marked variations in shape, with many cystically dilated forms and pseudostratified lining epithelium that may show mitoses but lacks cytological atypia (Figs 38.25, 38.26). This is the most common hyperplasia (Table 38.4).

Complex hyperplasia

In adenomatous hyperplasia, the glands have very irregular outlines showing marked structural complexity and glandular proliferation. In addition, the glands show 'back-to-back' crowding with little intervening stroma (Figs 38.27, 38.28).

Table 38.4 Frequency of endometrial hyperplasia and endometrial carcinoma in curettage specimens not associated with pregnancy (after Sherman 1978, Wentz 1974)

Histology	Detection rate
Cystic hyperplasia	5.1%
Adenomatous hyperplasia	2.6%
Atypical hyperplasia	1.3%
Carcinoma	2.6%

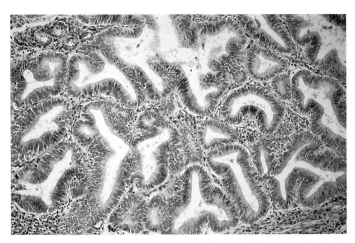

Fig. 38.27 Adenomatous hyperplasia without significant cytological atypia. Haematoxylin and eosin ×100 (by kind permission of Dr Thomas Krausz).

Atypical hyperplasia

Atypical hyperplasia is defined by the presence of glands showing nuclear atypia (Figs 38.29, 38.30). Loss of nuclear polarization, enlarged rounded nuclei with hyperchromatism, chromatin clumping and enlarged nucleoli are seen. Abnormal mitotic figures are often visible. These appearances may be accompanied by structural complexity. In severe cases, it may be impossible to differentiate from carcinoma (Figs 38.31, 38.32).

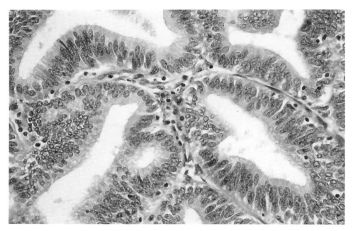

Fig. 38.28 Adenomatous hyperplasia without significant cytological atypia. Haematoxylin and eosin ×250 (by kind permission of Dr Thomas Krausz).

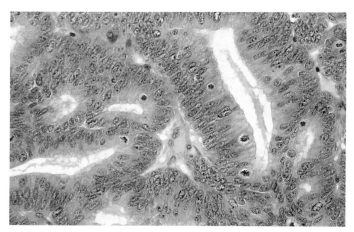

Fig. 38.29 Moderate atypical hyperplasia. Haematoxylin and eosin ×250 (by kind permission of Dr Thomas Krausz).

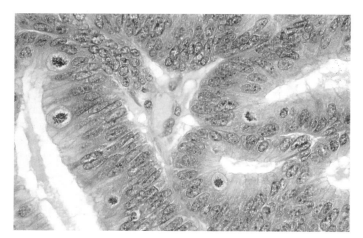

Fig. 38.30 Moderate atypical hyperplasia. Note the pseudostratification of the cells and the mitotic figures. The nuclei are plump with some irregularity of the nuclear membrane and prominent nucleoli. Haematoxylin and eosin ×400 (by kind permission of Dr Thomas Krausz).

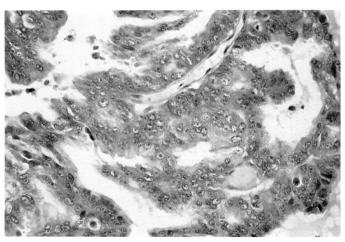

Fig. 38.31 Severe atypical hyperplasia. It is impossible to exclude invasive carcinoma from this material. Haematoxylin and eosin ×250 (by kind permission of Dr Thomas Krausz).

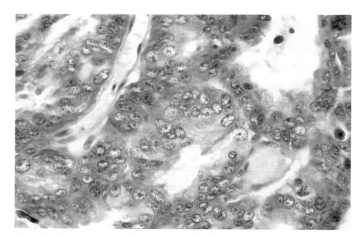

Fig. 38.32 Severe atypical hyperplasia. The nuclei are rounded, vesicular with prominent nucleoli. Haematoxylin and eosin ×400 (by kind permission of Dr Thomas Krausz).

Unfortunately, the diagnosis of atypical hyperplasia depends upon subjective criteria so there is substantial interobserver variability in the diagnosis. So far no special techniques, such as ploidy, histochemistry or molecular biology, have demonstrated reproducible differences between atypical hyperplasia and well-differentiated adenocarcinoma, rather supporting the unifying concept of an endometrial intraepithelial neoplasm.

Approximately 10–20% of all cases with atypia will have an underlying carcinoma present and invasive cancer will develop later in up to 50% of cases. These figures are higher in the case of complex atypical than in simple atypical hyperplasia (47% vs 7.4%) (Silverberg 2000).

Aetiology of endometrial hyperplasia

- Ideopathic
- Anovulation
- Exogenous oestrogens

- Tamoxifen
- Oestrogen-secreting tumour.

The majority of endometrial hyperplasias occur without any obvious predisposing cause. The most commonly recognized causes result from excessive oestrogen stimulation, unopposed by progesterone. This may arise from an endogenous source such as anovulatory cycles or an oestrogen-secreting tumour but exogenous, unopposed oestrogen administration and the oestrogenic effects of tamoxifen are more common causes.

Natural history of endometrial hyperplasia

The important, practical considerations in the natural history of endometrial hyperplasias are:

- co-existing endometrial carcinomas
- co-existing ovarian carcinomas
- risk of progression to endometrial carcinoma.

Cystic hyperplasia

Cystic hyperplasia is a common finding in postmenopausal women and anovulatory teenagers. It is not often seen in association with endometrial carcinoma or other pathology and the risk of progression to endometrial carcinoma is 0.4–1.1% (Kurman et al 1985, Lindahl & Willen 1994b, McBride 1959).

Adenomatous hyperplasia

Adenomatous hyperplasia is not always identified separately in studies of endometrial hyperplasias and mixed patterns with atypical changes are common. Thus there is little agreement in the literature about the rates of co-existent carcinoma or progression to invasion.

Estimates of the rate of progression to carcinoma in five studies range from none to 26.7% (Table 38.5). The highest rate came from a study of women with persistent abnormalities, after two curettages more than 8 weeks apart. The low estimates in more recent studies in which the lesions were more clearly defined on the basis of the cytological features are more likely to reflect the level of risk for these lesions as defined currently.

Atypical hyperplasia

Co-existent carcinoma rates range from 25% to 50% (Tavasolli & Kraus 1978, Widra et al 1995). Clearly, this rate will depend

upon the definition of the lesions included – no cancers were found in women without nuclear atypia (Widra et al 1995). It will also depend upon the readiness with which invasion is diagnosed in early cases without myometrial invasion. Only one of the 12 cases in one series invaded the myometrium and that was very superficial (Tavasolli & Kraus 1978). However 17 of the 19 cases of cancer in another study did invade the myometrium (Janicek & Rosenshein 1994). Some women will have a concurrent, endometrioid ovarian cancer.

The estimates of the risk of progression to endometrial carcinoma range from 22.6% to 88.9% (Table 38.5). Again, the highest rate comes from a study of women with persistent, untreated atypical hyperplasia.

Morphometry may help to some extent in predicting the behaviour of these lesions (Baak et al 1994, Colgan et al 1983) but DNA ploidy is not useful.

Presentation of endometrial hyperplasia

- Abnormal uterine bleeding
- Infertility
- Postmenopausal bleeding.

Premenopausal women will usually present with abnormal bleeding. Simple hyperplasia is most often found in women with infrequent, heavy periods but complex and atypical hyperplasia do not give a characteristic pattern of bleeding. Some of these lesions are discovered in the course of infertility investigations. The largest group are women with postmenopausal or perimenopausal bleeding.

Investigation of endometrial hyperplasia

The main objectives of investigation of a woman found to have endometrial hyperplasia are to exclude invasive endometrial cancer or ovarian cancer and to rule out an endogenous aberrant source of oestrogen secretion.

If endometrial hyperplasia has been diagnosed using an outpatient biopsy instrument, a formal examination under anaesthesia, hysteroscopy and curettage are required to palpate the adnexae and explore the endometrial and endocervical cavities. An ultrasound examination of the ovaries would be a sensible precaution, as would serum CA125 and estradiol estimations.

Management of endometrial hyperplasia

The management will depend upon the severity of the abnormality and upon the patient's wishes for further children. The first step would be to discontinue oestrogen therapy or remove an oestrogen-secreting ovarian tumour.

Cystic hyperplasia

Cystic hyperplasia does not require special follow-up and may be managed on the basis of subsequent symptoms. Recurrent postmenopausal bleeding would require further investigation.

Adenomatous hyperplasia

Given the low risk of progression to carcinoma, there is no indication for hysterectomy or for progestin therapy in these

Table 38.5 Frequency of progression to carcinoma after diagnosis of hyperplasia

Author	Cystic (%)	Adenomatous (%)	Atypical (%)
McBride 1959	0.4		
Gusberg & Kaplan 1963		10.4	
Wentz 1974		26.7	88.9
Sherman 1978		19.8	57.1
Kjorsted et al 1978			31.0[+]
Colgan et al 1983			33.3[+]
Kurman et al 1985	1.1	3.4	22.9
Lindahl & Willen 1994a	0.8	0	31.4
Baak et al 1994			22.6

[+] Some of these patients were treated with progestins

Table 38.6 Studies of treatment of atypical hyperplasia with progestins

Author	Lesion & no. of cases	Drug & dose	Short/long term	Persistence %	Recurrence %	Cancer %	Length of follow-up
Eichner & Abelerra 1971	Adenomatous & atypical 16 cases	Megestrol 20 mg qid MPA 80 mg/day	Short term (6–9 weeks)	6	38	0	Up to 4 yrs
Kjorstad et al 1978	Atypical 29 cases	Hydroxyprogesterone caproate 500 mg IM weekly	Short term (12 weeks)	24	31	31	3–10 yrs
Wentz 1985	Atypical 50 cases	Megestrol 20–40 mg qid	Short term (6–8 weeks)	0	0	0	1–5 yrs Mean >4 yrs
Gal 1986	Atypical 32 cases	Megestrol 20–40 mg daily continuous	Long term	6	6*	0	$2\frac{1}{2}$–12 yrs Mean 5 yrs
Ferenczy & Gelfand 1989	Atypical 20 cases	MPA 20 mg/day continuous	Long term	50	25	25 mean 5.5 yrs	2–12 yrs Mean 7 yrs
Lindahl & Willen 1994b	Atypical 10 cases	Medroxyprogesterone acetate 500 mg IM twice weekly	Short term (3 months)	0	10	0	5 yrs

* Both women who stopped megestrol recurred 10–18 months later.

women. Like women with cystic hyperplasia, subsequent management can probably be decided on the basis of further symptoms.

Atypical hyperplasia

Most women with atypical hyperplasia should have a hysterectomy and bilateral salpingo-oophorectomy because of the high risk of co-existent carcinoma. However, younger women who wish to preserve their fertility may be managed with medical therapy and repeated curettage. The data on medical treatment are scanty. While both danazol and tamoxifen have been used in 52 women, only four had atypical hyperplasia. Similarly, a study of the use of a progesterone-containing IUCD included only four women with atypical hyperplasia.

Most data relate to the use of various progestins given for short-term courses or as continuous therapy for many years (Table 38.6). Most of the studies include only carefully selected cases and the results of the different studies are not really comparable because of the selection criteria applied. The best results were obtained with moderately high doses of progestins – at least 20 mg/day of megestrol. If an adequate dose has been given, it is probably safe to stop after 8–12 weeks but Gal's experience of recurrence in both his patients who stopped indicates that there is not enough information to be sure of the optimum duration of therapy (Gal 1986). One thing is clear: long-term follow-up is essential because recurrences may not appear for many years (Ferenczy & Gelfand 1989, Gal 1986).

One long-term study of 19 women said to have atypical hyperplasia investigated the use of 500 mg norethisterone acetate weekly for 3 months and a monthly injection of a GnRH analogue (triptorelin) for 6 months (Perez-Medina et al 1999). The women were followed up with 6-monthly hysteroscopy and directed endometrial biopsy. Regression occurred in 84%. Others obtained similar results in women with complex hyperplasia without atypia but none of the three women with atypia responded (Grimbizis et al 1999). Some report apparently good results with progestin therapy of atypical hyperplasia or well-differentiated adenocarcinoma (Randall & Kurman 1997) although the treatment delay was associated with the development of metastatic disease in the obturator lymph nodes in a patient who relapsed after an apparent response (Kaku et al 2001).

What is inexplicable is that treatment that has failed in the past is now said to be highly effective. This raises questions about the definition of the pathology being treated (Kaku et al 2001) as does a report of regression in 55% of what was described as complex hyperplasia with atypia (Tabata et al 2001). These uncertainties suggest that these results should be regarded with considerable caution.

KEY POINTS

1. Both squamous (CIN) and glandular (AIS) premalignant lesions are seen on the cervix.
2. The diagnostic precision of small biopsies is not good. Invasive disease is not always detected and CIN II–III may be substantially undercalled.
3. After 20 years, about one-third of untreated women with CIN III will develop invasive disease.
4. Progression of CIN I to CIN III or worse may occur in 26% of women within 2 years.
5. A well-organized cervical cytology screening programme which reaches a large proportion of the population at risk and which includes effective action when abnormal smears are detected will reduce the incidence and mortality of cervical cancer.
6. The four pitfalls in colposcopy are: the false SCJ caused by an abrasion; the SCJ in the canal; the previously treated cervix; glandular lesions.
7. The majority of women with CIN can be treated in the outpatient department.
8. Excisional methods provide the whole lesion for histology without increasing the discomfort or complications for the patient.
9. Most cases of VAIN are seen after hysterectomy.
10. VAIN hidden above the vaginal suture line cannot be evaluated and early invasive cancer is common.

KEY POINTS (*CONTINUED*)

11. Surgical excision (preferably by the vaginal route) and intracavitary radiotherapy are the most effective treatments.
12. The malignant potential of VIN is uncertain but untreated cases can progress to invasion.
13. Treatment of VIN is mutilating and should be limited for the most part to symptomatic patients and those in whom invasion is suspected.
14. Atypical hyperplasia is the only form of endometrial hyperplasia with a significant risk of progression to malignancy and the only one which merits surgical treatment.

REFERENCES

Andersen ES, Arffmann E 1989 Adenocarcinoma in situ of the uterine cervix: a clinico-pathologic study of 36 cases. Gynecologic Oncology 35:1–7

Anderson CH, Boyes DA, Benedet JL et al 1988 Organisation and results of the cervical cytology screening programme in British Columbia, 1955–85. British Medical Journal 296:975–978

Anderson MC, Hartley RB 1980 Cervical crypt involvement by intraepithelial neoplasia. Obstetrics and Gynecology 55:546–550

Baak J, Kuik DJ, Bezemer PD 1994 The additional prognostic value of morphometric nuclear arrangement and DNA-ploidy to other morphometric and stereological features in endometrial hyperplasias. International Journal of Gynecological Cancer 4:289–297

Basu PS, D'Arcy T, McIndoe A, Soutter WP 1999 Is needle diathermy excision of the transformation zone a better treatment for cervical intraepithelial neoplasia than large loop excision? Lancet 353:1852–1853

Bekassy Z, Alm P, Grundsell H, Larsson G, Astedt B 1983 Laser miniconisation in mild and moderate dysplasia of the uterine cervix. Gynecologic Oncology 15:357–362

Boehm F, Morris JM 1971 Paget's disease and apocrine gland carcinoma of the vulva. Obstetrics and Gynecology 38:185–192

Boice JD, Day NE, Andersen A et al 1985 Second cancers following treatment for cervical cancer. An international collaboration among cancer registries. Journal of the National Cancer Institute 74:955–975

Brady JL, Fish A, Woolas RP, Brown CL, Oram DH 1994 Large loop diathermy of the transformation zone: is 'see and treat' an acceptable option for the management of women with abnormal cervical smears? Journal of Obstetrics and Gynecology 14:44–49

Brown BH, Tidy JA, Boston K, Blackett AD, Smallwood RH, Sharp F 2000 Relation between tissue structure and imposed electrical current flow in cervical neoplasia. Lancet 355:892–895

Burghardt E, Holzer E 1980 Treatment of carcinoma-in-situ: evaluation of 1609 cases. Obstetrics and Gynecology 55:539–545

Buscema J, Stern J, Woodruff JD 1980 The significance of histologic alterations adjacent to invasive vulvar carcinoma. American Journal of Obstetrics and Gynecology 137:902–909

Caglar H, Delgado G, Hreshchyshyn MM 1986 Partial and total skinning vulvectomy in treatment of carcinoma in situ of the vulva. Obstetrics and Gynecology 68:504–507

Campion MJ, McCance DJ, Cuzick J, Singer A 1986 The progressive potential of mild cervical atypia: a prospective cytological, colposcopic and virological study. Lancet ii:237–240

Choo YC, Anderson DG 1982 Neoplasms of the vagina following cervical carcinoma. Gynecologic Oncology 14:125–132

Colgan TJ, Norris HJ, Foster W, Kurman RJ, Fox CH 1983 Predicting the outcome of endometrial hyperplasia by quantitative analysis of nuclear features using a linear discriminant function. International Journal of Gynecological Pathology 1:347–352

Coppleson M, Reid BL, Skladnev VN, Dalrymple JC 1994 An electronic approach to the detection of pre-cancer and cancer of the uterine cervix: a preliminary evaluation of Polarprobe. International Journal of Gynaecological Cancer 4:79–83

Creasman WT, Gallacher HS, Rutledge F 1975 Paget's disease of the vulva. Gynecological Oncology 3:133–148

Cruickshank ME, Flannelly G, Campbell DM, Kitchener HC 1995 Fertility and pregnancy outcome following large loop excision of the cervical transformation zone. British Journal of Obstetrics and Gynaecology 102:467–470

Cullimore JE, Luesley DM, Rollason TP et al 1992 A prospective study of conisation of the cervix in the management of cervical intraepithelial glandular neoplasia (CIGN) – a preliminary report. British Journal of Obstetrics and Gynaecology 99:314–318

Degefu S, O'Quinn AG, Dhurandhar HN 1986 Paget's disease of the vulva and urogenital malignancies: a case report and review of the literature. Gynecological Oncology 25:347–354

Dorsey JH 1986 Skin appendage involvement and vulval intraepithelial neoplasia. In: Sharp F, Jordan JA (eds) Gynaecological laser surgery. Perinatology Press, New York, pp 193–195

Eichner E, Abellera M 1971 Endometrial hyperplasia treated by progestins. Obstetrics and Gynecology 38:739–742

Ferenczy A, Gelfand M 1989 The biologic significance of cytologic atypia in progestogen-treated endometrial hyperplasia. American Journal of Obstetrics and Gynecology 160:126–131

Flannelly G, Anderson D, Kitchener HC et al 1994 Management of women with mild and moderate cervical dyskaryosis. British Medical Journal 308:1399–1403

Friedrich EG 1972 Reversible vulvar atypia. Obstetrics and Gynecology 39:173–181

Gal D 1986 Hormonal therapy for lesions of the endometrium. Seminars in Oncology 13(Suppl 4):33–36

Gredmark T, Kvint S, Havel G, Mattson LA 1995 Histopathological findings in women with post menopausal bleeding. British Journal of Obstetrics and Gynaecology 102:133–136

Griffiths M, Turner MJ, Partington CK, Soutter WP 1989 Should smears in a colposcopy clinic be taken after the application of acetic acid? Acta Cytologica 33:324–326

Grimbizis G, Tsalikis T, Tzioufa V, Kasapis M, Mantalenakis S 1999 Regression of endometrial hyperplasia after treatment with the gonadotrophin-releasing hormone analogue triptorelin: a prospective study. Human Reproduction 14:479–484

Gusberg SB, Kaplan AL 1963 Precursors of corpus cancer. American Journal of Obstetrics and Gynecology 87:662–678

Hernandez-Linares W, Puthawala A, Nolan JF, Jernstrom PH, Morrow CP 1980 Carcinoma in situ of the vagina: past and present management. Obstetrics and Gynecology 56:356–360

IARC Working Group on Evaluation of Cervical Cancer Screening Programmes 1986 Screening for cervical squamous cancer: duration of low risk after negative results of cervical cytology and its implication for screening policies. British Medical Journal 293:659–664

Ireland D, Monaghan JM 1988 The management of the patient with abnormal vaginal cytology following hysterectomy. British Journal of Obstetrics and Gynaecology 95:973–975

Janicek M, Rosenshein NB 1994 Invasive endometrial cancer in uteri resected for atypical endometrial hyperplasia. Gynecologic Oncology 52:373–378

Jones RW, McLean MR 1986 Carcinoma in situ of the vulva: a review of 31 treated and five untreated cases. Obstetrics and Gynecology 68:499–503

Jones RW, Rowan DM 1994 Vulval intraepithelial neoplasia III: a clinical study of the outcome in 113 cases with relation to the later development of invasive vulvar carcinoma. Obstetrics and Gynecology 84:741–745

Kaku T, Yoshikawa H, Sakamoto A et al 2001 Conservative therapy for adenocarcinoma and atypical hyperplasia of the endometrium in young women: central pathologic review and treatment outcome. Cancer Letters 167:39–48

Kaufman R, Gordon A 1986a Squamous cell carcinoma in situ of the vulva. Part I. British Journal of Sexual Medicine 13:24–27

Kaufman R, Gordon A 1986b Squamous cell carcinoma in situ of the vulva. Part II. British Journal of Sexual Medicine 13:55–58

Kesic VI, Soutter WP, Sulovic V, Juznic N, Aleksic M, Ljubic A 1993 A comparison of cytology and cervicography in cervical screening. International Journal of Gynaecological Oncology 3:395–398

Kjorstad KE, Welander C, Halvorsen T, Grude T, Onsrud M 1978 In: Brush MG, King R, Taylor RW (eds) Endometrial cancer. Baillière Tindall, London, pp 188–191

Kurman RJ, Kaminski PF, Norris HJ 1985 The behaviour of endometrial hyperplasia: a long-term study of 'untreated' hyperplasia in 170 patients. Cancer 56:403–412

Larsson G, Gullberg B, Grundsell H 1983 A comparison of complications of laser and cold knife conisation. Obstetrics and Gynecology 62:213–217

Leuchter RS, Townsend DE, Hacker NF, Pretorius RG, Lagasse LD, Wade ME 1984 Treatment of vulvar carcinoma in situ with the CO2 laser. Gynecologic Oncology 19:314–322

Lindahl B, Willen R 1994a Spontaneous endometrial hyperplasia. A prospective, 5 year follow up of 246 patients after abrasion only, including 380 patients followed up for 2 years. Anticancer Research 14:2141–2146

Lindahl B, Willen R 1994b Spontaneous endometrial hyperplasia. A 5 year follow up of 82 patients after high dose gestagen treatment. Anticancer Research 14:2831–2834

Luesley DM, Cullimore J, Redman C et al 1990 Loop diathermy excision of the cervical transformation zone in patients with abnormal cervical smears. British Medical Journal 300:1690–1693

McBride JM 1959 Premenopausal cystic hyperplasia and endometrial carcinoma. Journal of Obstetrics and Gynaecology of the British Empire 66:288–296

McIndoe WA, McLean MR, Jones RW, Mullins PR 1984 The invasive potential of carcinoma in situ of the cervix. Obstetrics and Gynecology 64:451–458

Mene A, Buckley CH 1985 Involvement of the vulval skin appendages by intraepithelial neoplasia. British Journal of Obstetrics and Gynaecology 92:634–638

Mitchell MF, Tortolero-Luna G, Cook E, Whittaker L, Rhodes-Morris H, Silva E 1998 A randomised clinical trial of cryotherapy, laser vaporisation and loop electrosurgical excision for treatment of squamous intraepithelial lesions of the cervix. Obstetrics and Gynecology 92:737–744

Murdoch JB, Grimshaw RN, Monaghan JM 1991 Loop diathermy excision of the abnormal transformation zone. International Journal of Gynecological Cancer 1:105–111

National Institute for Clinical Excellence 2000 Guidance on the use of liquid based cytology for cervical screening. Technology Appraisal Guidance No. 5. NICE, London

Nieminen P, Kallio M, Hakama M 1995 The effect of mass screening on incidence and mortality of squamous and adenocarcinoma of cervix uteri. Obstetrics and Gynecology 85:1017–1021

Paraskevaidis E, Jandial L, Mann EMF, Fisher PM, Kitchener HC 1991 Pattern of treatment failure following laser for cervical intraepithelial neoplasia: implications for follow-up protocol. Obstetrics and Gynecology 78:80–83

Parker LP, Parker JR, Bodurka-Bevers D et al 2000 Paget's disease of the vulva: pathology, pattern of involvement and prognosis. Gynecologic Oncology 77:183–189

Partington CK, Soutter WP, Turner MJ, Hill AS, Krausz T 1987 Laser excisional biopsy under local anaesthesia: an outpatient technique? Journal of Obstetrics and Gynaecology 9:48–52

Partington CK, Turner MJ, Soutter WP, Griffiths M, Krausz T 1989 Laser vaporisation versus laser excision conisation in the treatment of cervical intraepithelial neoplasia. Obstetrics and Gynecology 73:775–779

Perez-Medina T, Bajo J, Folgueira G, Haya J, Ortega P 1999 Atypical endometrial hyperplasia treatment with progestins and gonadotrophin-releasing hormone analogues: long-term follow up. Gynecologic Oncology 73:299–304

Planner RS, Andersen HE, Hobbs JB, Williams RA, Fogarty LF, Hudson PJ 1987 Multifocal invasive carcinoma of the vulva in a 25 year old with Bowenoid papulosis. Australian and New Zealand Journal of Obstetrics and Gynaecology 27:291–295

Prendiville W, Cullimore J, Norman S 1989 Large loop excision of the transformation zone (LLETZ). A new method of management for women with cervical intraepithelial neoplasia. British Journal of Obstetrics and Gynaecology 96:1054–1060

Raio L, Ghezzi F, di Naro E, Gomez R, Luscher K 1997 Duration of pregnancy after carbon dioxide laser conisation of the cervix: influence of cone height. Obstetrics and Gynecology 90:978–982

Randall TC, Kurman RJ 1997 Progestin treatment of atypical hyperplasia and well differentiated carcinoma of the endometrium in women under the age of 40. Obstetrics and Gynecology 90:434–440

Reid R 1985 Superficial laser vulvectomy 11. The anatomic and biophysical principles permitting accurate control over the depth of dermal destruction with the carbon dioxide laser. American Journal of Obstetrics and Gynecology 152:261–271

Richart RM 1967 Natural history of cervical intraepithelial neoplasia. Clinics in Obstetrics and Gynecology 10:748–784

Robertson AJ, Anderson JM, Swanson Beck J et al 1989 Observer variability in histopathological reporting of cervical biopsy specimens. Journal of Clinical Pathology 42:231–238

Robinson WR, Lund ED, Adams J 1998 The predictive value of LEEP specimen margin status for residual/recurrent cervical intraepithelial neoplasia. International Journal of Gynecological Cancer 8:109–112

Rosenthal AN, Panoskaltsis T, Smith T, Soutter WP 2001 The frequency of significant pathology in women attending a general gynaecological service who complain of post-coital bleeding. British Journal of Obstetrics and Gynaecology 108:103–106

Shafi M, Luesley DM, Byrne P et al 1989 Vulval intraepithelial neoplasia – management and outcome. British Journal of Obstetrics and Gynaecology 96:1339–1344

Sherman AI 1978 Precursors of endometrial cancer. Israel Journal of Medical Science 14:370–378

Silverberg S 2000 Problems in the differential diagnosis of endometrial hyperplasia and carcinoma. Modern Pathology 13:309–327

Skehan M, Soutter WP, Lim K, Krause T, Pryse-Davies J 1990 Reliability of colposcopy and directed punch biopsy. British Journal of Obstetrics and Gynaecology 97:811–816

Soutter WP 1993 A practical guide to colposcopy. Oxford University Press, Oxford

Soutter WP, Fletcher A 1994 Invasive cancer of the cervix in women with mild dyskaryosis followed cytologically. British Medical Journal 308:1421–1423

Soutter WP, Brough AK, Monaghan JM 1984 Cervical screening for younger women. Lancet ii:745

Soutter WP, Wisdom S, Brough AK, Monaghan JM 1986a Should patients with mild atypia in a cervical smear be referred for colposcopy? British Journal of Obstetrics and Gynaecology 93:70–74

Soutter WP, Abernethy FM, Brown VA, Hill AS 1986b Success, complications and subsequent pregnancy outcome relative to the depth of laser treatment of cervical intraepithelial neoplasia. Colposcopy and Gynecologic Laser Surgery 2:35–42

Soutter WP, de Barros Lopes A, Fletcher A et al 1997 Invasive cervical cancer after conservative therapy for cervical intraepithelial neoplasia. Lancet 349:978–980

Soutter WP, Haidopoulos D, Gornall RJ et al 2001 Is conservative treatment for adenocarcinoma in situ of the cervix safe? British Journal of Obstetrics and Gynaecology 108:1184–1189

Spritos NM, Smith LH, Teng NNH 1990 Prospective randomised trial of topical α interferon (α interferon gels) for the treatment of vulval intraepithelial neoplasia III. Gynecologic Oncology 37:34–38

Tabata T, Yamawaki T, Yabana T, Ida M, Nishimura K, Nose Y 2001 Natural history of endometrial hyperplasia: a study of 77 patients. Archives of Gynecology and Obstetrics 265:85–88

Tavasolli F, Kraus FT 1978 Endometrial lesions in uteri resected for atypical endometrial hyperplasia. American Journal of Clinical Pathology 70:770–779

University of Zimbabwe/JHPIEGO Cervical Cancer Project 1999 Visual inspection with acetic acid for cervical cancer screening: test qualities in a primary-care setting. Lancet 353:869–873

Wentz WB 1974 Progestin therapy in endometrial hyperplasia. Gynecologic Oncology 2:362–367

Wentz WB 1985 Progestin therapy in lesions of the endometrium. Seminars in Oncology 12(Suppl 1):23–27

Widra EA, Dunton CJ, McHugh M, Palazzo JP 1995 Endometrial hyperplasia and the risk of carcinoma. International Journal of Gynecological Cancer 5:233–235

Widrich T, Kennedy AW, Myers TM, Hart WR, Wirth S 1996 Adenocarcinoma in situ of the uterine cervix: management and outcome. Gynecologic Oncology 61:304–308

Wijngaarden van WJ, Duncan ID 1993 Rationale for stopping cervical screening in women over 50. British Medical Journal 306:967–971

Woodman CBJ, Jordan JA, Wade-Evans T 1984 The management of vaginal intraepithelial neoplasia after hysterectomy. British Journal of Obstetrics and Gynaecology 91:707–711

Woodman CBJ, Mould JJ, Jordan JA 1988 Radiotherapy in the management of vaginal intraepithelial neoplasia after hysterectomy. British Journal of Obstetrics and Gynaecology 95:976–979

39
Malignant disease of the cervix

Roberto Dina   Bleddyn Jones   Henry Kitchener
Hilary Thomas

EPIDEMIOLOGY

Cervical cancer is the second most common female cancer (after breast cancer) worldwide, but in developed countries cytology screening has resulted in a very significant reduction in both incidence and deaths. In the UK, cervical cancer incidence is now well behind ovarian and endometrial cancer in terms of incidence, responsible for just 1500 deaths annually. When it presents or is discovered early, it has a high cure rate but advanced disease is frequently incurable with very unpleasant consequences. Prevention of cervical cancer is regarded as a very sensitive and important public health issue. Human papillomavirus (HPV) infection is widely regarded as the most important factor in cervical carcinogenesis and with prophylactic vaccines now in development, there is the potential that within 10–20 years HPV vaccines will be able to help prevent this disease.

Figure 39.1 shows the incidence and death rate from cervical cancer since 1971 and the effect of systematic coverage of the female population by screening after it began in earnest in 1988. Recently the incidence has been falling at a rate of around 7% per year.

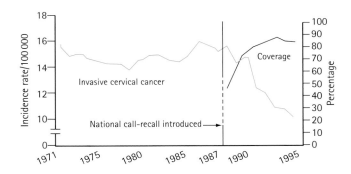

Fig. 39.1   Age-standardized incidence of cervical cancer in England 1971 to 1995 and screening coverage (after Quinn et al 1999).

ANATOMY

Origin of cervical neoplasia

The stratified squamous epithelium of the vagina and ectocervix meets the columnar epithelium of the uterine cavity at the squamocolumnar junction. In premenopausal women this squamocolumnar junction is usually situated just inside the external cervical os and can be readily visualized using a colposcope. The position of the squamocolumnar junction tends to lie inside the canal after the menopause. This is the site of origin of most preinvasive and invasive squamous cell cervical neoplasias.

Gross anatomy

The cervix lies partly in the upper vagina and partly in the retroperitoneal space behind the bladder and in front of the rectum. It is related on each side to the terminal portion of the ureters as they swing anteriorly and medially below the uterine arteries into the bladder. The cardinal ligaments laterally and the uterosacral ligaments posterolaterally are inserted into the cervix and provide the main supports of the uterus.

Lymphatic drainage

The regional lymph drainage of the female genital organs follows a relatively well-defined pattern. Cervical tumours spread via the parametrial lymphatics to the internal (hypogastric) and external iliac nodes, which surround the corresponding iliac vessels on the pelvic side wall, and to the obturator nodes. The lymph vessels ascend towards the network of nodes around the common iliac vessels on each side and amalgamate in a plexus surrounding the aorta and vena cava. The inferior margin of the aortic nodes is at the lower border of the fourth lumbar vertebra. The common iliac vessels commence to the right of the midline at the upper border of the same vertebra and pass in front of the sacroiliac joint on each side before bifurcating into external and internal branches.

AETIOLOGY

Human papillomavirus

During the 1980s it became clear that HPV, particularly types 16 and 18, is closely associated with cervical carcinogenesis. It emerged that HPV, which now includes over 80 types, includes high-risk oncogenic types, e.g. 16, 18, 31, 33, and low-risk types, e.g. 6 and 11. It became clear that high-grade CIN and cancer contained so-called high-risk HPV DNA, in a very high proportion of cases; indeed, with sufficiently sensitive testing, 100% of squamous cervical cancer contains HPV.

During the late 1990s a great deal was learned regarding the complex actions of HPV in the host cervical cell. For example, the E6 gene binds p53, a gene which helps to protect the cell from uncontrolled growth. Although the complex molecular biology of HPV is not fully understood, the scientific community believes that HPV infection is essential, but not solely sufficient to achieve cancerous development. In addition to understanding its role in carcinogenesis, there is considerable interest now in exploiting its close association with cervical neoplasia in a pragmatic way to use it as a marker in several settings, including population screening. Its most immediate role may be in triaging women with mildly abnormal smears

into high- and low-risk groups for the purpose of selecting those most likely to benefit from colposcopy.

It is thought that the majority of women have an HPV infection of the cervix at some time in their lives. The prevalence in women aged 20–25 is probably 20%. Indeed, 44% of young women will acquire HPV infection within 3 years of commencing sexual relations and 26% will show evidence of a second, different infection (Woodman et al 2001). The immune system clears the majority of infections so that by the age of 50 years the prevalence of HPV infection is only 5% or less. Longitudinal studies have revealed that in some women HPV infection may persist and after 2 years or more, the relative risk of developing CIN III is extremely high (Hopman et al 2000). It is known that in some of these women the HPV DNA is integrated into the host cell genome. These events are reflected in changes in the morphological appearance of the cells. In women with low-grade lesions there are often the classic features of koilocytosis but, in high-grade lesions, koilocytosis is often absent.

The immunological response to HPV infection is still incompletely understood, but it is known that type-specific neutralizing antibodies may be generated as well as type-specific, cytotoxic T cell lymphocytes (CTLs). This immune response is variable but is probably crucial in determining the natural history of the HPV infection in any given individual.

The length of time for lesions to transit from early events in precancer to invasive disease is obviously variable, but is said to be of the order of 10 years or more. The median age for women with CIN III is around 30 years compared with 40–45 years for invasive cancer. It used to be thought that there was an orderly progression from CIN I to CIN III but there is really very little evidence to support this hypothesis. It is now widely felt that many low-grade lesions will never progress and that many CIN III lesions may appear de novo.

Co-factors

If HPV is the necessary agent in inducing key early events in cervical carcinogenesis, what are the other co-factors that could be involved? It is well known that sexual activity is very important and while this may be largely accounted for by transmission of HPV, a number of studies over the past 20 years have implicated other STDs. Most prominent in the 1980s were seroepidemiological studies of herpes simplex virus (HSV), especially HSV-2. More recently, interest has focused on chlamydia and a recent study has reported a significant association (Anttila et al 2001).

It may be that STDs somehow render the cervical cells more susceptible to the carcinogenic potential of HPV infection. Early onset of sexual intercourse, multiple sexual partners and probably non-barrier contraception are therefore risk factors for developing CIN and cancer. A possible common factor is the immunosuppressant found in semen that inhibits the lymphocyte response to infection with Epstein–Barr virus (Turner et al 1990).

Recently the relationship between abnormal cervical cytology and HIV infection has come into the spotlight. HIV-positive women have a very high incidence of CIN III, though the increased risk for invasive cancer is not yet certain. HIV causes immunosuppression that is probably responsible for increased HPV-associated pathology. When immunosuppression is more marked, the incidence of CIN is greater (Davis et al 2001). Highly active antiretroviral therapy (HAART), which results in a rise in CD4 count and a reduction in HIV viral load, probably reduces the risk of HPV-associated pathology.

The other significant risk factor is smoking. Many epidemiological studies have indicated a higher prevalence of smokers among women who develop CIN and cancer and that this risk may increase with 'pack years' smoked. An intervention study indicated some evidence that stopping smoking could result in CIN lesion regression and a very recent report has shown that smoking increases the risk of treatment failure (Acladious et al 2001).

PREVENTION

The advent of exfoliative cervical cytology screening in the late 1940s rendered cervical cancer a largely preventable disease. Its long natural history and the relative accessibility of the cervix means that detection of abnormal cytology has enabled a strategy of preventing invasive disease by detection and treatment of preinvasive disease. The technique based on the work of Papanicolaou has remained largely unchanged for 50 years. It has stood the test of time and in countries where population coverage exceeds 80% and screening takes place at least 5 yearly there has been a large reduction in death from cervical cancer. Unfortunately, in many impoverished countries there is no cervical screening and, furthermore, there are usually inadequate facilities for treating the disease, which is often advanced at presentation. Therefore in poor countries there is a great burden of disease with a very high death rate and in developed countries the disease is becoming less frequent with overall cure rates around 60–70%. In the United Kingdom deaths are continuing to fall by several per cent per year.

Improvements in cervical screening, now the subject of intense interest, include liquid-based cytology and HPV testing. Liquid-based cytology, which is currently being piloted in the NHS Cervical Screening Programme, appears to result in far fewer inadequate smears and may increase sensitivity. Instead of a smear being made by smearing cells on a glass slide using the spatula, the cells are shaken off the sampling device into a vial of fluid and at the laboratory a thin layer preparation of cells is placed onto a glass slide for reading.

HPV testing is also being piloted to see whether it can effectively triage women with mildly abnormal smears. It is well established that the detection of HPV in women with borderline and mildly dyskaryotic smears makes underlying CIN far more likely and that HPV-negative women have a very low risk of underlying disease. This approach means that women at very low risk could avoid colposcopy, with its attendant anxiety and expense. The ALTS study in the United States suggests that HPV testing adds little to cervical cytology in women with smears suggesting low-grade squamous intraepithelial lesions (LSIL) because the HPV test was positive in 82.9% of these women (ALTS 2000). It may however be useful in borderline smears.

The close association between HPV and underlying cervical neoplasia means that HPV testing is also a strong candidate to increase the sensitivity of cervical screening. HPV can now be detected by convenient kit-based systems that make screening more feasible. There are very important questions that need to be addressed in large randomized trials before population screening can be advocated. These include the degree of increased sensitivity, the psychological consequences of HPV testing and economic considerations. Another major question as yet unanswered is how to manage a woman with a negative smear and a positive HPV test. We know that being HPV positive would increase risk but how is this best managed without resorting to colposcopy for all HPV-positive women?

In addition to HPV there are candidate markers of abnormal cellular proliferation that are being considered for cervical screening. These could have the major advantage of automation and avoidance of the need to examine manually thousands of cells on a smear.

PATHOLOGY

Malignant tumours of the cervix are usually of squamous or glandular type. The former has become less common as a result of screening but there has been little reduction in the numbers of adenocarcinomas so these now account for a much larger proportion of cervical tumours in the United Kingdom than in former years. Other, rare but highly lethal malignancies that affect the cervix are described below.

Squamous cell carcinoma

Microinvasive carcinoma
Squamous cell carcinomas that show only microscopically evident foci of invasion up to 3 mm are considered stage IA1 and those that are larger but do not exceed 5 mm in depth of invasion and 7 mm in a horizontal dimension are defined as stage IA2 by FIGO (FIGO 1998) (Fig. 39.2). Measuring the depth of invasion and determining the presence of vascular/lymphatic invasion accurately predicts the likelihood of lymph node metastasis.

Estimates of the frequency of microinvasion relative to all invasive cervical squamous cancers average approximately 8%. Microinvasion is manifested by the presence of irregularly shaped tongues of epithelium projecting from the base of an intraepithelial neoplasm into the stroma. The invasive cells usually contain more abundant eosinophilic cytoplasm and show features of keratinization. An accompanying fibrosis and inflammatory infiltrate may be evident. Involvement of the cone margin by invasive carcinoma or even by a high-grade CIN precludes a diagnosis of microinvasive carcinoma because deeper invasion may be present higher in the endocervix.

Invasive carcinomas
Macroscopically they may be exophytic, infiltrative or ulcerative and microscopically they can exhibit considerable heterogeneity, ranging from compact masses and nests of eosinophilic, large cell keratinizing to non-keratinizing atypical squamous cells. Keratinizing carcinomas show keratin pearls within the nests of neoplastic epithelium. Some tumours may

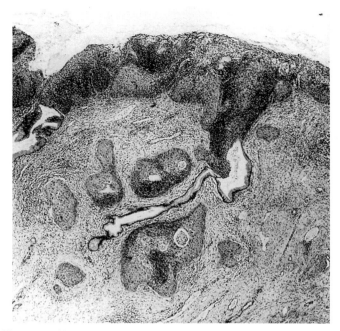

Fig. 39.2 Microinvasive carcinoma showing multiple foci of invasion arising from a gland crypt. The invasive islands are irregular in outline and partly show better differentiation than the overlying CIN. Haematoxylin and eosin ×42.

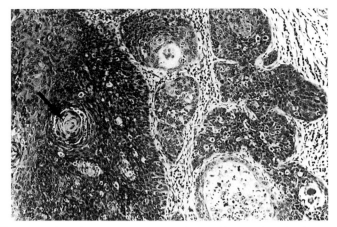

Fig. 39.3 Invasive squamous cell carcinoma. The invasive islands are composed of poorly differentiated cells, but an attempt at formation of a keratin pearl is marked by an arrow. Haematoxylin and eosin ×160.

be mostly composed of basaloid cells, only focally showing a more typical squamoid appearance. Such lesions should not be confused with the small cell carcinoma of neuroendocrine type, identical to the more frequent lung counterpart and associated with a very aggressive behaviour.

Well-differentiated squamous carcinomas (grade 1) show predominantly mature squamous cells, with abundant keratin and minimal mitotic activity, while moderately differentiated tumours (grade 2) are composed of cells with less abundant cytoplasm and greater nuclear pleomorphism. Poorly differentiated neoplasms (grade 3) show either nests of smaller, basaloid cells with scant cytoplasm and hyperchromatic nuclei with high mitotic activity or large, very atypical squamoid cells with bizarre highly pleomorphic nuclei (Fig. 39.3). In reporting all such tumours, the depth of invasion, the presence or absence of vascular invasion and the size of the tumour as well as the grading must be recorded. Tumour mass, as measured by MRI, is also a very significant predictor of outcome. Local extension may involve the adjacent vaginal mucosa, parametrial soft tissue and pelvic wall, lower uterine segment and corpus, and hypogastric, external iliac and sacral lymph nodes and, secondarily, the common iliac, inguinal and para-aortic nodes. Lymph node involvement occurs in 15–20% of stage IB, 25–40% of stage II and 50% of stage III and IV tumours.

Verrucous carcinoma

This is a distinctive type of very well-differentiated squamous carcinoma that tends to recur locally but does not metastasize. They have a warty, fungating appearance and the deep margin is always sharply demarcated. Microscopically they resemble condyloma acuminatum but the papillary hyperkeratotic projections characteristically lack fibrovascular cores. Nuclear atypia is only minimal and mitotic activity scarce.

Other squamous cell carcinomas

Papillary squamous (transitional) cell carcinoma is a rare variant of invasive squamous cell carcinoma. It has a superficial resemblance to transitional cell carcinoma of the urinary bladder, while lymphoepithelioma-like carcinoma is characterized by a circumscribed margin and by nests of undifferentiated cells with abundant cytoplasm and vesicular nuclei, surrounded by an intense inflammatory reaction consisting of lymphocytes, plasma cells and eosinophils. The prognosis of this tumour is better than that of glassy cell carcinoma, which is characterized by nests of undifferentiated cells with distinct cell borders, ground-glass cytoplasm, nuclei with prominent nucleoli and much higher mitotic activity.

Adenocarcinoma

Malignant tumours of glandular origin comprise 10–15% of cervical tumours. This figure is increasing, representing both an absolute increase in the number of cases of adenocarcinoma and an increase in the proportion of glandular tumour frequency. Microscopically, adenocarcinoma in situ generally retains the architectural pattern of the normal endocervical crypts, replacing the normal epithelium with an atypical epithelium showing loss of polarity, increased nuclear size, nuclear pleomorphism and anisokaryosis, mitotic activity, reduction in cytoplasmic mucin and, frequently, stratification (Fig. 39.4). The glandular abnormalities of the cervix appear to form a continuous spectrum of disease in exactly the same way as the squamous abnormalities. The less severe forms are referred to as glandular atypias, often divided into low- (L-CGIN) and high-grade (H-CGIN) glandular intraepithelial neoplasia. Precursor glandular lesions tend to progress to invasive carcinoma. There is a progressive increase in age of patients from L-CGIN to invasive disease, a span of approximately 10 years. There is a high association between H-CGIN

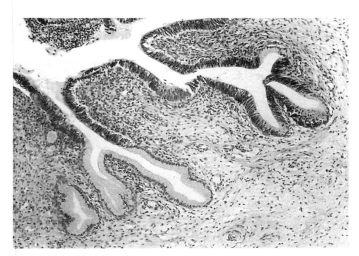

Fig. 39.4 Adenocarcinoma in situ. The abnormal epithelium follows the architecture of the normal crypts but the epithelium shows marked nuclear crowding, with loss of polarity and reduced mucin production. Haematoxylin and eosin ×160.

and invasive disease. In the management of such precursors, it is important to ensure adequate free margins of at least 3 mm.

A number of different histological patterns are found in invasive adenocarcinoma of the cervix and diverse cell types may form the actual lesion; if >10% of the tumour shows a different pattern from the main one, this is recorded. The endocervical type accounts for up to 90%. It is composed of crowded glands of variable size and shape, with budding and branching of the epithelium, somewhat resembling that of normal endocervical epithelium (Fig. 39.5).

Adenoma malignum or minimal deviation adenocarcinoma

These terms describe a carcinoma in which the glandular pattern is particularly well differentiated and there is virtually no atypia of the epithelial cells. Such tumours are only recognized by the presence of distorted glands with irregular outlines, deep in the cervical stroma.

Endometrioid adenocarcinoma

Cervical adenocarcinomas of endometrioid type should be distinguished from a primary endometrial adenocarcinoma; the latter usually also invades the myometrium by the time it involves the cervix.

Clear cell carcinoma

These have been associated with intrauterine exposure to diethylstilboestrol (DES) and may arise also in the vagina. Exposure to DES has been reported for 64% of these women. The DES medication was most often reported as having started before the 18th week of pregnancy. Cytopathologic examination was informative in 81% of the cases of CCAC of the cervix, but only in 41% of the cases of CCAC of the vagina (Hanselaar et al 1997). Most tumours are associated with vaginal adenosis or tubal metaplasia of the cervix. Differential diagnosis includes all those conditions associated with clear cells, such as microglandular hyperplasia, Arias–Stella reaction and mesonephric remnants.

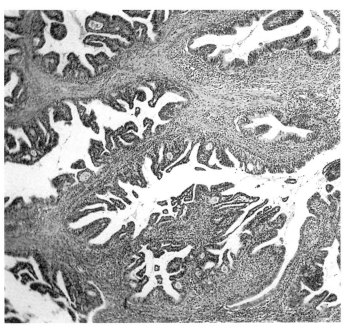

Fig. 39.5 Invasive adenocarcinoma of the cervix. Although the architectural pattern bears a superficial resemblance to normal cervical crypts, the pattern is excessively complex and papillary, with associated cellular abnormalities. Haematoxylin and eosin ×100.

Well-differentiated (papillary) villoglandular adenocarcinoma

These are usually found in young women and are composed of exophytic polypoid lesions with thick or thin papillae lined by endocervical, endometrial or intestinal-type epithelium showing mild cytologic atypia. All tumours are usually confined to the cervix and the prognosis is excellent (Jones et al 1993).

Mesonephric adenocarcinoma

This rare tumour arises from mesonephric remnants and is therefore deeply situated in the cervical stroma, without involvement of the endocervical mucosa. It may be confused with müllerian endometrioid adenocarcinomas (Silver et al 2001).

Adenosquamous carcinoma

This is defined as a tumour exhibiting both glandular and squamous differentiation, both components being malignant. It appears that when both components are poorly differentiated, the prognosis is worse than in ordinary squamous cell carcinomas or adenocarcinomas.

Cervical endocrine tumours

These are highly aggressive and can be subdivided into definable categories: small cell carcinoma (SCC), large cell neuroendocrine carcinoma (LCNC) and atypical or typical carcinoid tumours. Loss of heterozygosity (LOH) at 3p loci is a frequent finding, as is nuclear staining with a combined HPV-16/18 probe. LOH at 17p (TP53 locus) appears to be relatively uncommon, suggesting that p53 mutations may not be developmentally significant. Adenocarcinomas may contain neuroendocrine cells in different proportions, morphologically ranging from pure carcinoids to SCC. The presence of a neuroendocrine component in an otherwise classic adenocarcinoma makes it resistant to conventional therapy.

NATURAL HISTORY

Carcinoma of the cervix spreads predominantly by either direct invasion or lymphatic permeation. Some tumours are exophytic in nature and in other cases the tumour expands the endocervix in the shape of a barrel. The tumour may invade into the vaginal mucosa or into the myometrium of the lower uterine segment. Whereas spread into the parametrial tissues may occur as a continuous wave of infiltrating tumour, it is more common for there to be scattered foci of tumour in the parametrium, which only gradually become palpable as they coalesce.

Only 5% of small primary lesions that involve less than 20% of the cervix have histological evidence of parametrial disease, usually in parametrial nodes. In contrast, 48% of tumours invading more than 80% of the cervix are associated with parametrial extension, which is confluent in 23% (Burghardt et al 1988). If lymphatic spaces within the tumour are invaded, spread to the pelvic nodes may occur more often. The incidence of node involvement increases with the stage, grade and volume of the tumour (Table 39.1).

Survival following surgical treatment is closely related to the tumour volume (Burghardt et al 1992). The 345 women in this study with a tumour volume 2.5–10 cm^3 had a 5-year survival of 79.2%; 330 women with a tumour volume 10–50 cm^3 had a 5-year survival of 70.4%; and those with larger tumours had a 48% 5-year survival. In addition, involvement of the parametrium and lymph node metastases were associated with a worse prognosis.

Forty per cent of patients with carcinoma of the cervix die with uncontrolled pelvic disease leading to ureteric obstruction. Direct involvement of bone within the pelvis is common. Bloodstream metastases also occur, usually with poorly differentiated tumours and the higher stages of disease. The most common sites are the lungs, bones and liver.

STAGING

Because the most effective treatment of cervical cancer depends on the extent of disease, accurate staging is required. The extent of the disease is defined in three ways:

- the size of the tumour locally
- involvement of adjacent tissues, such as the parametrium or the bladder
- the presence of metastases.

The FIGO classification is the most widely used (Table 39.2; FIGO 1998). It is recommended that bimanual examination under anaesthesia should be performed by more than one examiner. The intravenous urogram findings should be included, as should cystoscopy, but neither special imaging techniques nor subsequent operative findings alter the staging.

Surgical staging has been advocated, particularly to assess involvement of the para-aortic nodes. However, this delays the commencement of radiotherapy. The transperitoneal approach to the nodes, combined with radiotherapy, increases the incidence of bowel damage and is not recommended. The postoperative risk is less with a retroperitoneal approach, but it is unlikely that the information gained will lead to changes in management that will improve the prognosis. If para-aortic nodes are enlarged on imaging, fine needle aspiration cytology

Table 39.2 The FIGO staging classification for cervical cancer (FIGO 1998)

Stage	Description
0	Preinvasive carcinoma (carcinoma in situ, CIN)
I	Carcinoma confined to the cervix (corpus extension should be disregarded)
Ia	Invasive cancer identified only microscopically. All gross lesions, even with superficial invasion, are stage Ib cancers. Depth of measured stromal invasion should not be greater than 5 mm and no wider than 7 mm*
Ia1	Measured invasion no greater than 3 mm in depth and no wider than 7 mm
Ia2	Measured depth of invasion greater than 3 mm and no greater than 5 mm and no wider than 7 mm
Ib	Clinical lesions confined to the cervix or preclinical lesions greater than Ia
Ib1	Clinical lesions no greater than 4 cm in size
Ib2	Clinical lesions greater than 4 cm in size
II	Carcinoma extending beyond the cervix and involving the vagina (but not the lower third) and/or infiltrating the parametrium (but not reaching the pelvic side wall)
IIa	Carcinoma has involved the vagina
IIb	Carcinoma has infiltrated the parametrium
III	Carcinoma involving the lower third of the vagina and/or extending to the pelvic side wall (there is no free space between the tumour and the pelvic side wall)
IIIa	Carcinoma involving the lower third of the vagina
IIIb	Carcinoma extending to the pelvic wall and/or hydronephrosis or non-functioning kidney due to ureterostenosis caused by tumour
IVa	Carcinoma involving the mucosa of the bladder or rectum and/or extending beyond the true pelvis
IVb	Spread to distant organs

* The depth of invasion should not be more than 5 mm from the base of the epithelium, either surface or glandular, from which it originates. Vascular space involvement, either venous or lymphatic, should not alter the staging.

Table 39.1 Increased incidence of nodal metastases with increasing FIGO stage

FIGO stage	% Positive nodes	
	Pelvic	Para-aortic
Ib	16	7
II	30	16
III	44	35
IV	55	40

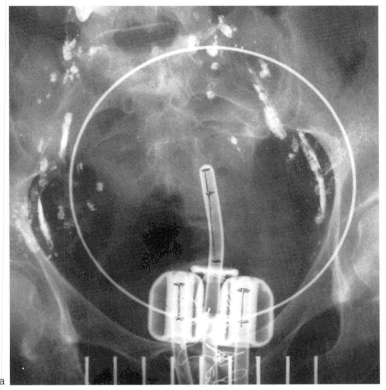
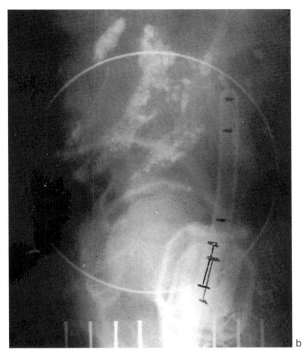

a

b

Fig. 39.9 These X-rays show an Amersham tube and ovoids in position. Contrast material can be seen in the lymph nodes from a previous lymphangiogram.

uterine canal and 2 cm above the external cervical os in most treatment centres. This point is considered to lie in the paracervical region close to the uterine artery and the ureter. Point B is 5 cm lateral to the central uterine canal and 2 cm above the cervical os. The dose to point B is usually about one-third of the dose given to point A, owing to the rapid fall-off in dosage with intracavitary insertions.

In the Manchester system, 6600–7600 cGy were prescribed to point A in two treatments each lasting 70 hours 4–7 days apart. Following external beam therapy to 40–50 Gy, a dose of 2000–2500 cGy is usually given to point A in a single insertion.

Patients with small-volume stage I tumours are treated by intracavitary treatment alone, but more advanced disease requires a combination of an intracavitary dose and external beam therapy. The rationale for the different techniques is that the risk of lymph node involvement increases with the size of the tumour. In some cases, external beam therapy may be poorly tolerated (e.g. patients who have inflammatory bowel disease, diabetes, previous endometriosis, surgical adhesions, etc.) and in such patients a greater proportion of intracavitary treatment rather than external beam radiotherapy is better tolerated.

Rapid computerized normal tissue dose estimation is now possible in individual patients. Bladder doses are estimated using a Foley catheter containing an X-ray contrast solution (Tan et al 1996a) and the anterior rectal wall dose by addition of 0.5 cm for vaginal mucosal thickness beyond the edge of the vaginal applicators (Tan et al 1997). Some departments use intrarectal markers to assess the intra luminal or mucosal doses, but these provide the dose in the lumen rather than the anterior rectal wall.

External Beam Therapy

External beam therapy is normally given first because it shrinks the tumour mass, allowing reoxygenation and also a more satisfactory dose distribution from the intracavitary sources. A homogeneous dose of radiation is given to the true pelvis through either three or four fields. The treatment volume usually extends from the junction between L4 and L5 to cover the common iliac nodes, to the lower border of the obturator foramen radiologically or the lower margin of the pubic symphysis by palpation. If the disease extends down the vagina the lower border must be taken to the introitus, which can be defined with a marker placed at a vaginal examination with the patient in the treatment position. The lateral margins of the field should lie at least 1 cm outside the bony margins of the pelvis.

The radiotherapy apparatus used is most commonly a linear accelerator of 6–10 million electron volts (MeV) or greater. The total dose to the rectum should not exceed 6400 cGy. The dose given to the pelvis varies depending upon the stage of the disease. Stage IIb–IVa patients receive 5000 cGy to the whole pelvis in 25 fractions in 5 weeks or in some centres 50.4 Gy in 28 fractions. If bulky disease is present in one parametrium, a further 500–600 cGy may be given in 3–4 fractions to this area. Following this an intracavitary insertion is performed and a further 2000 cGy given to point A. If an insertion is not possible, the central pelvic dose may be taken to 5500–6000 cGy using external beam therapy alone and a lower intracavitary dose may be given later. Alternatively, if the cancer is not fixed to pelvic bony structures, three cycles of platinum-based cytotoxic chemotherapy may be used to provide further tumour shrinkage, followed by the same intracavitary dose (Tan et al 1996b).

About 35% of stage III patients have involved para-aortic nodes. However, it is difficult to assess the nodes accurately and to treat involved nodes effectively. Piver & Barlow (1977) treated biopsy-positive para-aortic nodes with more than 5500 cGy; 20% of patients died of the complications of treatment, usually small bowel stenosis, so that lower doses are now given.

Patients with stage IVa cancers may have a fistula at presentation or develop this during radiotherapy. Such patients are sometimes best treated by urinary diversion followed by radical radiotherapy. In patients with disease outside the pelvis (stage IVb), the treatment should be directed to relieving symptoms. If pelvic symptoms such as bleeding or offensive discharge are predominant, palliative treatment may be given to a small volume using opposed fields and giving a 2500–3000 cGy midline dose in five or six treatments over 3 weeks. If pain is due to para-aortic node spread into the underlying vertebrae, cytotoxic chemotherapy and palliative radiotherapy can be given but a high dose (4500–5000 cGy midline dose in 5 weeks) is needed for control. If there is metastatic bone pain, a 1–2 week course of palliative radiotherapy may be given to a dose of 2000–3000 cGy in 5–10 treatments.

Results of radiotherapy

Tumour bulk and clinical stage are major predictors of the response to treatment, but squamous carcinomas and adenocarcinomas have a similar prognosis (Table 39.3). Substantial tumour regression during external beam therapy predicts a high chance of local tumour control and survival. If at the time of intracavitary treatment substantial tumour is still present, surgery or cytotoxic chemotherapy should be considered.

Radiotherapy complications

During radiotherapy most patients will develop diarrhoea. A low-residue diet is usually helpful and antidiarrhoeal medica-

tions such as codeine phosphate or loperamide are prescribed. The radiation reaction usually settles down within 2–3 weeks of completion of all therapy, but a minority of patients will continue to need antidiarrhoeal drugs. If severe diarrhoea is associated with severe colicky pain and nausea, the possibility of small bowel damage must be considered and the treatment suspended. Treatment may be restarted at a lower daily dose, but if the problem persists external beam radiotherapy may have to be abandoned.

Acute urinary symptoms are less common and co-existing infection must be excluded. Occasionally anticholinergic agents may be helpful.

Late complications are related to dose, fraction size and intracavitary dose rate and may be influenced by pre-existing medical problems that reduce pelvic radiotolerance (Barillot et al 2000). Depending on technique, some 1–10% of patients develop long-term problems (Denton et al 2000), which are usually related to the small or large bowel but may involve the urinary tract. These include subacute obstruction, diarrhoea due to radiation colitis and haematuria due to radiation cystitis. The symptoms are often quite mild. Patients at particularly high risk of developing radiation complications are those with poor nutritional status and recent weight loss, previous pelvic or abdominal surgery, severe vascular disease or pelvic inflammatory disease.

Late complications may develop at any time after treatment, but symptoms of bowel damage usually occur on average after 6 months and bladder symptoms after 1–2 years. Bowel and bladder symptoms should always be investigated and it must not be assumed that they are due to recurrent malignant disease.

Management of complications must be individualized and early detection is of the greatest importance. Multidisciplinary management may be required and a clinical oncologist/radiotherapist should remain involved in patient management. Small bowel obstruction following radiotherapy should be managed conservatively only in its initial stages. If prolonged or repeated episodes occur, surgical intervention is imperative. Rectosigmoid constriction can normally be diagnosed from the clinical history and readily confirmed by barium studies. It can be managed without the need for a permanent colostomy in the majority of patients.

Vesicovaginal fistulae will occasionally occur in patients who have been treated entirely appropriately. Repair of such fistulae involves the provision of an alternative blood supply to the area, by either omental or myocutaneous grafting.

CHEMOTHERAPY

Radiotherapy and surgery are the only modalities that can cure cervical cancer but chemotherapy can cause tumour regression. Single agents that have significant response rates include cisplatin, bleomycin and methotrexate. Combination regimens have been developed using these drugs and, as with ovarian cancer, cisplatin combinations appear to have the highest response rates.

The combination of 'neoadjuvant' chemotherapy and radiotherapy has not resulted in improved survival, as a good response to chemotherapy seems to occur only in women who also respond well to radiotherapy (Vermorken 1993).

Table 39.3 Results of treatment by radiotherapy

| FIGO stage | 5-year survival (%) | |
	Squamous carcinoma	Adenocarcinoma
I	79.9	81.8
II	61.9	65.9
III	39.9	29.8
IV	14.3	21.0
All stages	54.6	54.0

CHEMOIRRADIATION IN CERVICAL CANCER

Attempts have been made to find a role for chemotherapy in both primary treatment of cervical cancer (neoadjuvant treatment) or concurrently with radiotherapy. There is a large body of work in head and neck squamous cell carcinoma and in the West the difficulty in obtaining evidence for the effectiveness of chemoirradiation in cervical cancer is at least partly due to the diminishing incidence of the disease.

In February 1999 the National Cancer Institute in the US issued a clinical alert on the basis of three papers which were about to be published in the *New England Journal of Medicine*. These showed a consistent benefit of the addition of cisplatin chemotherapy to radiotherapy in a range of patients with cervical carcinoma requiring radiation therapy. A further two publications have since been published and a meta-analysis including a negative study from Canada still shows a small, statistically significant benefit for the addition of cisplatin to radiation (Green et al 2001).

It appears that this evidence will now change UK practice and most centres now treat women fit enough to receive cisplatin and radiation with the two modalities concurrently. The standard protocol of 40 mg/m^2 cisplatin once weekly has been widely adopted. The benefits of chemoirradiation include improved local control and survival but there is a potential risk as the dose of cisplatin used is comparable in dose intensity to the treatment of ovarian cancer without simultaneous irradiation. It undoubtedly causes myelotoxicity with anaemia, thrombocytopenia and neutropenia; it also has important implications for resources as the pre- and post hydration for cisplatin require the patient to spend much of the day in the chemotherapy unit at the hospital and treatment then has to be co-ordinated with radiotherapy. Over the next decade the use of other possible drugs in addition to or as an alternative to cisplatin is likely to be more widely explored.

SPECIAL TREATMENT PROBLEMS

Carcinoma of the cervical stump

Subtotal hysterectomy is now performed more often than in the recent past, so this problem may be seen more frequently in the future. Radical surgery may be employed for localized disease in younger women. Otherwise external beam radiotherapy to the usual dose should be given if bowel tolerance allows. To obtain a satisfactory dose, a medium caesium tube should be inserted together with ovoids. If this is not possible the external beam dose must be increased. The results are comparable with those in patients with an intact uterus.

Carcinoma after simple hysterectomy

Invasive carcinoma may be found after a hysterectomy for presumed preinvasive disease or when cervical pathology was not suspected. The management and prognosis depend on the true stage of disease before the operation. If the patient was carefully evaluated before surgery and the invasive lesion was a small Ib tumour, the prognosis is good (Heller et al 1986). In studies where the outcome is poor, it is likely that the original lesion extended outside the cervix (Bissett et al 1994, Kinney et al 1992).

A 5-year survival of 82% may be achieved with radical parametrectomy, upper vaginectomy and pelvic lymphadenectomy (Kinney et al 1992). Alternatively, pelvic irradiation may be given to a dose of 4500–5000 cGy in 5–5.5 weeks, followed by vault irradiation. Provided the lesion was originally stage Ib, this offers a 5-year survival of 78%, similar to that for patients treated with an intact uterus (Heller et al 1986).

Carcinoma of the cervix during pregnancy

Management will depend on the stage at diagnosis, the gestational age and the wishes and beliefs of the patient and her partner (Table 39.4). When fetal survival is desired, delivery should be delayed until the fetus is mature rather than just potentially viable. The prognosis does not seem to be affected adversely by the pregnancy in women with early-stage disease (van der Vange et al 1995).

Haemorrhage

If a patient presents with massive bleeding, bedrest, vaginal packing and the use of styptic solutions (such as hypoferric solutions) and tranexamic acid may arrest the haemorrhage. If this is not successful, treatment should begin with a low-dose intracavitary application giving 2000 cGy to point A or 7 Gy by HDR. Usually, however, the bleeding gradually reduces by daily use of external radiotherapy and adequate bedrest. The haemoglobin in such a patient, and in any other, should always be restored to above 12 g/dl, as patients with a haemoglobin of less than that have a poorer survival. In rare cases emergency radical surgery may be required.

RECURRENCE AFTER RADIOTHERAPY

The patient should be assessed jointly with a gynaecological oncologist to ensure that the possibility of surgical salvage is not overlooked. The prognosis for those few women with central pelvic recurrence alone is relatively good with exenterative procedures and such women should be carefully assessed and considered for such procedures in recognized gynaecological oncology units. In some instances it may be noted that the recurrent cancer is outside the previous high-dose region and may be amenable to further radiotherapy or chemoradiotherapy, although there are increased risks of serious complications (Jones & Blake 1999).

Table 39.4 The suggested management of cervical cancer during pregnancy

Trimester	Stage I	Stages II–IV
First	Wertheim's hysterectomy	Vaginal termination and radiation
Second	Termination of pregnancy by hysterotomy and Wertheim's hysterectomy	Prostaglandin termination and radiotherapy
Third	Caesarean at 34/52 and Wertheim's hysterectomy	Caesarean at 34/52; start radiotherapy after 10 days

FOLLOW-UP

The continuing follow-up of these patients is of great importance to evaluate results, provide reassurance and to give symptomatic relief to those whose treatment has failed. It is recommended that there should be 3-monthly follow-up for 3 years, 6-monthly follow-up for 2 years and annual visits thereafter.

Counselling and support should be provided throughout the patient's treatment and help her to cope with all aspects of readjustment, including prevention of the sexual problems that tend to develop in these women and their partners (see Chapter 48). Premenopausal patients will have suffered functional ovarian ablation and may be treated with hormone replacement therapy if they are troubled by menopausal symptoms. Younger patients with a good prognosis should be encouraged to take hormone replacement therapy to reduce the risk of osteoporosis and cardiovascular disease. Hormone therapy should always include progestins if the patient has been treated by radiotherapy and retains her uterus. The endometrium is very resistant to radiotherapy (Habeshaw & Pinion 1992), and endometrial carcinoma may develop if unopposed oestrogens are given. In some instances, endocervical canal stenosis may occur with the development of a haematometrium which can be relieved by dilatation.

Radiotherapy will cause the vagina to contract and it is important to remind patients who were sexually active to try and resume activity, often with the help of lubricants, within a couple of months of the completion of treatment. Dilators can be used to maintain vaginal patency. Patients need to be reassured that coitus will not cause the tumour to become active and that the cancer cannot be communicated to their partner.

KEY POINTS

1. In England and Wales the incidence and mortality of cervical cancer have been falling as a result of the introduction of organized screening. Cervical cancer remains the second most common cancer in women worldwide.
2. The cause remains unknown, but HPV infection is widely believed to be a key step. HPV infection is very common indeed in young people, implying that some other factors are necessary before cancer will develop.
3. Conservative treatment of microinvasive lesions should only be considered where invasion is not greater than 3 mm from the nearest basement membrane and lymphatic channel involvement is not seen.
4. Squamous cell carcinoma is the most common type and has a similar prognosis to adenocarcinoma. Undifferentiated tumours have a poor prognosis.
5. Metastatic spread is mainly lymphatic and involvement of the parametria is initially focal rather than confluent.
6. The volume of the primary tumour is one of the most important indications of prognosis after the status of the lymph nodes.

KEY POINTS (CONTINUED)

7. Magnetic resonance imaging with an endovaginal coil gives the best estimate of the volume of the tumour but MRI is not reliable in identifying nodal disease.
8. Overall, 42% of women with cervical cancer die within 5 years.
9. Surgery is most often performed on the younger patient with lower-volume stage Ib disease.
10. Radiotherapy is used for older and less fit patients, regardless of the size of the tumour, and for women with bulky stage Ib and IIa tumours or with more advanced disease.
11. Chemoradiation offers a small increase in cure rate but at the cost of increased immediate toxicity.

REFERENCES

Acladious N, Mandel, Kitchener HC 2001 Persistent human papillomavirus infection and smoking increase the risk of failure of treatment of cervical intraepithelial neoplasia. International Journal of Cancer (in press)

Anttila T, Saikku P, Koskela P et al 2001 Serotypes of Chlamydia trachomatis and risk for development of cervical squamous cell carcinoma. JAMA 285:47–51

ALTS 2000 Human papillomavirus testing for triage of women with cytologic evidence of low-grade squamous intraepithelial lesions: baseline data from a randomized trial. Journal of the National Cancer Institute 92:397–402

Bafna UD, Umadevi K, Savithi M 2001 Closed suction drainage versus no drainage following pelvic lymphadenectomy for gynaecological malignancies. International Journal of Gynecological Cancer 11:143–146

Barillot I, Horiot JC, Maingon P et al 2000 Impact on treatment outcome and late effects of customized treatment planning in cervix carcinomas: baseline results to compare new strategies. International Journal of Radiation Oncology, Biology, Physics 48:189–200

Basu PS, d'Arcy T, McIndoe A, Soutter WP 1999 Is needle diathermy excision of the transformation zone a better treatment for cervical intraepithelial neoplasia than large loop excision? Lancet 353:1852–1853

Bissett D, Lamont D, Nwabineli N, Brodie M, Symonds R 1994 The treatment of stage I carcinoma of the cervix in the west of Scotland 1980–1987. British Journal of Obstetrics and Gynaecology 101:615–620

Burghardt E, Haas J, Girardi F 1988 The significance of the parametrium in the operative treatment of cervical cancer. In: Burghardt E, Monaghan JM (eds) Operative treatment of cervical cancer. Baillière Tindall, London

Burghardt E, Baleer J, Tulusan AH, Haas J 1992 Results of surgical treatment of 1028 cervical cancers studied with volumetry. Cancer 70:648–655

d'Argent D, Martin X, Sacchetoni A, Mathevet P 2000 Laparoscopic raginal radical trachelectomy. Cancer 88:1877–1882

Davis AT, Chakraborty H, Flowers L, Mosunjac MB 2001 Cervical dysplasia in women infected with the human immunodeficiency virus (HIV): a correlation with HIV viral load and CD41 count. Gynecologic Oncology 80:350–354

Denton AS, Bond SJ, Matthews S, Bentzen SM, Maher EJ 2000 National audit of the management and outcome of carcinoma of the cervix treated with radiotherapy in 1993. Clinical Oncology 12:347–353

Elliott P, Coppleson M, Russell P et al 2000 Early invasive (FIGO stage IA) carcinoma of the cervix: a clinico-pathologic study of 476 cases. International Journal of Gynecological Cancer 10:42–52

FIGO 1998 Annual report on the results of treatment in gynaecological cancer. Twenty-third volume. Journal of Epidemiology and Biostatistics 3:5–7

Fuller A, Elliott N, Kosloff C, Lewis J 1982 Lymph node metastases from carcinoma of the cervix, Stages Ib and IIa: implications for prognosis and treatment. Gynecological Oncology 13:165–174

Gleeson N 1995 A modification of the Cherney incision in gynaecological oncology surgery. British Journal of Obstetrics and Gynaecology 102:925–926

Green JA, Kirwan JM, Tierney JF et al 2001 Survival and recurrence after concomitant chemotherapy and radiotherapy for cancer of the uterine cervix: a systematic review and meta-analysis. Lancet 358:781–786.

Habeshaw T, Pinion S 1992 The incidence of persistent functioning endometrial tissue following successful radiotherapy for cervical carcinoma. International Journal of Gynecological Cancer 2:332–335

Hanselaar A, van Loosbroek M, Schuurbiers O, Helmerhorst T, Bulten J, Bernhelm J 1997 Clear cell adenocarcinoma of the vagina and cervix. An update of the central Netherlands registry showing twin age incidence peaks. Cancer 79:2229–2236

Heller P, Barnhill D, Mayer A et al 1986 Cervical carcinoma found incidentally in a uterus removed for benign indications. Obstetrics and Gynecology 67:187–190

Hopman E, Rozendaal L, Voorhorst T, Walboomers J, Kenemans P, Helmerhorst Th 2000 High risk human papillomavirus in women with normal cervical cytology prior to the development of abnormal cytology and colposcopy. British Journal of Obstetrics and Gynaecology 107:600–604

Jones B, Blake PR 1999 Commentary: re-treatment of cancer after radical radiotherapy. British Journal of Radiology 72:1037–1039

Jones B, Tan LT, Blake PR, Dale RG 1994 Results of a questionnaire regarding the practice of radiotherapy for carcinoma of the cervix in the UK. British Journal of Radiology 67:1226–1230

Jones B, Pryce P, Blake PR, Dale RG 1999 High dose rate brachytherapy practice for the treatment of gynaecological cancers in the UK. British Journal of Radiology 72:371–377

Jones M, Silverberg S, Kurman R 1993 Well-differentiated villoglandular adenocarcinoma of the uterine cervix: a clinicopathological study of 24 cases. International Journal of Gynecological Pathology 12(1):1–7

Kinney W, Egorshin E, Ballard D, Podratz K 1992 Long-term survival and sequelae after surgical management of invasive cervical carcinoma diagnosed at the time of simple hysterectomy. Gynecologic Oncology 44:24–27

Landoni F, Maneo A, Colombo A et al 1997 Randomised study of radical surgery versus radiotherapy for stage Ib-IIa cervical cancer. Lancet 350:535–540

Landoni F, Maneo A, Cormio G et al 2001 Class II versus class III radical hysterectomy in stage IB–IIA cervical cancer: a prospective randomized study. Gynecologic Oncology 80:3–12

Morrow C, Shingleton H, Austin M et al 1980 Is pelvic radiation beneficial in the postoperative management of stage Ib squamous cell carcinoma of the cervix with pelvic node metastases treated by radical hysterectomy and pelvic lymphadenectomy? Gynecologic Oncology 10:105–110

Piver M, Barlow J Jr 1977 High dose irradiation to biopsy confirmed aortic node metastases from carcinoma of the uterine cervix. Gynecologic Oncology 3:168–175

Quinn M, Babb P, Jones J, Allen E on behalf of the United Kingdom Association of Cancer Registries 1999 Effect of screening on incidence of and mortality from cancer of cervix in England: evaluation based on routinely collected statistics. British Medical Journal 318:1–5

Shepherd TH, Mould T, Oram DH 2001 Radical trachelectomy in early stage carcinoma of the cervix: outcome as judged by recurrence and fertility rates. British Journal of Obstetrics and Gynaecology 108:882–885

Silver S, Devouassoux-Shisheboran M, Mezzetti T, Tavassoli F 2001 Mesonephric adenocarcinomas of the uterine cavity: a study of 11 cases with immunohistochemical findings. American Journal of Surgical Pathology 25(3):379–387

Tan LT, Warren J, Freestone G, Jones B 1996a Bladder dose estimation during intracavitary brachytherapy for carcinoma of the cervix using a single line source system. British Journal of Radiology 69:953–962

Tan LT, Jones B, Green JA, Kingston RE, Clark PI 1996b The treatment of carcinomas of the uterine cervix after initial external beam radiotherapy: a pilot study using integrated cytotoxic chemotherapy prior to brachytherapy. British Journal of Radiology 69:165–171

Tan LT, Jones B, Shaw JE 1997 Radical radiotherapy for carcinoma of the uterine cervix using a single line source brachytherapy technique: the Clatterbridge technique. British Journal of Radiology 70:1252–1258

Trimbos JB, Maas CP, Deruiter MC, Peters AAW, Kenter GG 2001 A nerve-sparing radical hysterectomy: guidelines and feasibility in Western patients. International Journal of Gynecological Cancer 11:180–186

Turner MJ, White JO, Soutter WP 1990 Human seminal plasma inhibits the lymphocyte response to infection with Epstein–Barr virus. Gynecologic Oncology 37:60–65

van der Vange N, Weverling G, Ketting B et al 1995 The prognosis of cervical cancer associated with pregnancy: a matched cohort study. obstetrics and Gynecology 85:1022–1026

Vermorken J 1993 The role of chemotherapy in squamous cell carcinoma of the uterine cervix: a review. International Journal of Gynecological Cancer 3:129–142

Woodman C, Collins S, Winter H et al 2001 Natural history of cervical human papillomavirus infection in young women: a longitudinal cohort study. Lancet 357:1831–1836

40

Benign disease of the vulva and the vagina

Alan MacLean   Roberto Dina

This chapter will be confined to discussion of benign conditions and mention of malignant or premalignant disease will be made only in relation to differential diagnosis or management. Premalignant disease is discussed in Chapter 38 and invasive disease in Chapter 41. Similarly, only passing mention is made of sexually transmitted diseases, which are described in Chapter 62. Space does not permit an exhaustive description of all of the many conditions which may affect the vulva. Instead, the emphasis is on common or important conditions (not always the same thing) with the intention of providing the reader with a sound framework upon which to build. More information may be obtained from the excellent books by Dr Marjorie Ridley (1988) and by the late Dr Eduard Friedrich (1983).

Patients with vulval symptoms are met frequently in gynaecological practice. The complaint is often long-standing and distressing and frequently induces a feeling of despair in both patient and doctor. A careful, sympathetic approach and a readiness to consult colleagues in other disciplines are essential. Even when it seems that no specific therapy can be offered, many patients are helped by the knowledge that there is no serious underlying pathology and by a supportive attitude.

DEVELOPMENT AND ANATOMY

The vulva and vagina develop in association with the urogenital sinus, the caudal end of the paramesonephric or müllerian ducts and the development of the anus posteriorly and bladder and urethra anteriorly. Debate continues as to how much of the lower vagina, hymen and vestibule originate from the ectoderm, the endoderm of the hindgut forming the urogenital sinus and the mesoderm of the paramesonephric ducts. Developmental abnormalities are not unusual and range from a single cloaca to variations in vaginal development, including agenesis or the presence of a transverse or midline septum.

The vulva consists of the labia majora, labia minora, mons pubis, clitoris, perineum and the vestibule. The labia join anteriorly at the anterior commissure and posteriorly merge into the perineum, the anterior margin of which is the posterior commissure. From puberty, the mons and lateral parts of the labia majora are covered in strong coarse hair and are distended with subcutaneous fat. In addition to hair follicles, they contain sebaceous and sweat (eccrine and apocrine) glands. The labia minora are two smaller, longitudinal, cutaneous, non-hair bearing folds medial to the labia majora and extending from the clitoris for a variable distance beside the vestibule to end before reaching the perineum. The labia majora and minora are separated from each other by the interlabial fold and during pregnancy and later life may contain prominent or tortuous veins. The labia minora contain numerous blood vessels, nerve endings and sebaceous glands. There is considerable variation in size and shape from woman to woman and sometimes gross enlargement or asymmetry. Anteriorly they fuse above the clitoris to form the prepuce and below the clitoris to form the frenulum.

The clitoris consists of a body formed of the two corpora cavernosa composed of erectile tissue enclosed in a fibrous membrane and attached to the puboischial ramus on each side by the crus. The body of the clitoris ends in the glans which also contains spongy tissue and nerve endings. The clitoris has a rich blood supply, which comes from the terminal branch of the pudendal artery.

The vagina consists of a non-keratinized squamous epithelial lining supported by connective tissue and surrounded by circular and longitudinal muscle coats. Vaginal epithelium has a longitudinal column on the anterior and posterior walls and from each column there are numerous transverse ridges or rugae extending laterally on each side. The squamous epithelium during the reproductive years is thick and rich in glycogen. It does not change significantly during the menstrual cycle. The prepubertal and postmenopausal vaginal epithelium is thin or atrophic.

CLASSIFICATION OF VULVAL DISEASE

Terminology of lesions and conditions of the vulva has caused confusion because of the many and complex names used, sometimes for similar changes. The International Society for the Study of Vulvovaginal Disease has circulated a classification of non-neoplastic disorders (Box 40.1). It is neither comprehensive nor absolute, but serves as a starting point to group some of the diseases described in this chapter.

PRESENTATION OF VULVAL DISEASE

The majority of women present with vulval pruritus (itch) and associated scratching. Others will present with pain, burning, soreness, rawness, stinging or irritation but without scratching. However, the symptoms do not necessarily imply a particular condition. Sometimes a lesion will be noted as white, red or pigmented or as raised or ulcerated. Some lesions will be asymptomatic.

The onset of symptoms will sometimes be associated with other life events such as following a course of antibiotics, a diagnosis of certain medical disorders, the introduction of certain therapeutic drugs or withdrawal of systemic corticosteroids. A full medical history will sometimes identify other conditions with vulval manifestations and dental details should not be overlooked. Some patients with vulvovaginal lichen planus will already have a diagnosis of oral lichen

Box 40.1 Revised ISSVD classification of vulval disease or non-neoplastic epithelial disorders

Infections
Parasitic, e.g. pediculosis, scabies
Protozoal, e.g. amoebiasis
Viral, e.g. herpes virus infection, condyloma acuminatum
Bacterial
Fungal, e.g. candidiasis, dermatophytosis
Others

Inflammatory skin disease

Spongiotic disorders
   Contact dermatitis
     Irritant
     Allergic
   Atopic dermatitis (acute and chronic)
   (Seborrhoeic dermatitis)
   Others

Psoriasiform disorders
   Psoriasis
   Lichenification (lichen simplex)[1]
Atrophic dermatitis (chronic)
Seborrhoeic dermatitis
Others

Lichenoid disorders
Lichen sclerosus
Lichen planus
Fixed drug eruption
Plasma cell vulvitis
Lichenoid reaction, not otherwise specified (focal or diffuse)
Lupus erythematosus
Others

Vesicobullous disorders
Pemphigoid
Pemphigus
Erythema multiforme
Stevens–Johnson syndrome
Others

Granulomatous disorders
Non-infectious
   Crohn's disease
   (Hidradenitis suppurativa)
   Sarcoidosis
   Others
Infectious
   Tuberculosis
   Granuloma inguinale
   Others

Vasculitis or related inflammatory disorders (vascular inflammatory condition)
Leucocytoclastic
Urticaria
Aphthous ulcer
Lymphoedema
Behçet's disease
Pyoderma gangrenosa

Box 40.1 *(Continued)*

(Fixed drug eruption)
(Erythema multiforme)
(Stevens–Johnson syndrome)
Others

Skin appendage disorders
Hidradenitis suppurativa
Fox–Fordyce disease
Disorders of sweating
Others

Hormonal disorders
Oestrogen
  Excess
    Precocious puberty
    Others
  Deficiency
    Physiological
    Lactation
    Postmenopausal
    Others
  Iatrogenic
Androgen
  Excess
    Physiological
    Iatrogenic

Functional disorders (debate on appropriateness of term)
Disorders of sensation
Dysaesthesia (includes pain and entities formally known as dysaesthetic vulvodynia and vestibulitis, see footnote 2)
Pain
Pruritus
Sexual disorders
  Arousal failure
  Vaginismus
  Anorgasmia
  Others

Ulcers and erosions
(Diseases that ulcerate and/or erode are listed according to histological findings)

Trauma
Obstetric
Surgical
Sexual
Accidental
Others (include fissures of the fossa navicularis)

Disorders of pigmentation
Hyperpigmentation
  Melanin
    Lentigo
    Melanosis vulvae
    (Postinflammatory hyperpigmentation)
  Haemosiderin
    (Postinflammatory hyperpigmentation)
  Vitiligo
  Others

Box 40.1 *(Continued)*

Hypopigmentation
  Vitiligo
  Postinflammatory hypopigmentation
  Others

This revised classification replaces the ISSVD classification of non-neoplastic epithelial disorders. It is not intended to be a comprehensive listing of all known dermatologic or pathologic disorders that may involve the vulva or vagina, but to include the more common disorders that involve the vulva.
[1]Lichenification encompasses the term lichen simplex (lichen simplex chronicus).
[2]What has been interpreted as vulval vestibulitis inflammation may represent, in some cases, findings considered as within normal.

planus. Many patients will bring a list or bag full of topical treatments previously used. A comprehensive list is useful because those drugs that have helped or caused deterioration can be identified and will also allow the prescribing with confidence of a preparation not yet tried.

EXAMINATION OF THE PATIENT

General examination of the patient should include inspection of the buccal and gingival mucosa and the skin of the face, hands, finger nails, wrists, elbows, scalp, trunk and knees. Evidence of systemic disease such as diabetes, hepatic, renal or haematological disease should be sought. Where appropriate, urinalysis or blood testing should also be performed.

A combined clinic conducted by gynaecologists, dermatologists and genitourinary physicians has considerable merit (McCullough et al 1987). Facilities should include adequate lighting, a tilting examination chair to obtain access to the posterior part of the pudendum, a colposcope and a camera for colpophotography and clinical photography.

Examination should consist of inspection of the vulva including the vestibule, urethral meatus, the perineum and perianal area. Patients with neoplastic disorders must also have the cervix and vagina examined but many older patients and those with lichen sclerosus will not tolerate a speculum examination and unless there is any specific symptom, it is unnecessary to include this as part of the examination. Cytology of vulval lesions is being reassessed because of some of the advantages of liquid-based preparation technology and cell collection with cytobrush (Bishop et al 2000).

Colposcopic assessment of the vulva is not essential if there is an obvious, readily diagnosed lesion and there are no suggestion of neoplastic change. However, colposcopy is valuable if the patient is symptomatic but no lesion can be seen, if there is difficulty in interpreting or defining the limits of the visible lesions and to select an appropriate site for biopsy. The techniques are described elsewhere (MacLean & Reid 1995). The vascular patterns can be complex and may be associated with neoplasia. Sometimes sites of previous biopsies will develop unusual vascular patterns associated with healing. Excessive applications of potent topical corticosteroids will exaggerate vascularity with prominent telangiectasia and thinned epidermis.

Once the vulva has been scanned with the colposcope, aqueous acetic acid solution should be applied. It is important to realize that the aceto-white changes will not be as dramatic as those seen on the cervix and may not be apparent in areas of abnormal keratinization. Aceto-white epithelium may represent VIN or viral changes with HPV and Epstein–Barr virus, as well as tissue repair with ulcers and erosions, scratch damage or coital trauma. It is incorrect to interpret the papillae seen in the vestibule as 'microwarts'; Jonsson et al (1997) showed aceto-white changes in the vulva were a poor predictor of viral presence.

In the past, histological diagnosis of the vulval lesions depended on inpatient biopsy performed under general anaesthesia. Very appropriate biopsy material can be obtained using a 4 mm diameter Stiefel disposable sterile biopsy punch performed as an outpatient procedure under local anaesthesia (Fig. 40.1) (McCullough et al 1987). A silver nitrate stick with a small plug of cotton wool or alternatively ferric subsulphate (Monsel's solution) is applied for haemostasis.

PREVALENCE OF VULVAL LESIONS

Box 40.2 shows the range of lesions seen in a combined vulva clinic (MacLean et al 1998). There may be some bias in these figures because the clinic received referrals from gynaecologists and because our research interests included vulval precancer and pain.

Infections included recurrent candidiasis, bacterial vaginosis, trichomoniasis, herpes simplex virus, condyomata acuminata, ulcers associated with human immunodeficiency virus, hidradenitis suppurativa, *Enterobius vermicularis* (threadworms), vulva lymphoedema secondary to filariasis and were not enumerated because they sometimes co-existed with other conditions.

Box 40.2 Prevalence of vulval lesion seen in 1000 women (MacLean et al 1998)

Lichen sclerosus	243
Lichen simplex/eczema	56
Lichen planus	23
Vulval vestibulitis syndrome	98
Dysaesthetic vulvodynia	32
Vulval intraepithelial neoplasia	82
Vulval carcinoma	23
Paget's disease of the vulva	4
Malignant melanoma	2
Psoriasis	25
Diabetic vulvitis	9
Vulval Crohn's disease	5
Benign mucous membrane pemphigoid	2
Acute contact dermatitis	2
Plasma cell vulvitis of Zoon	2

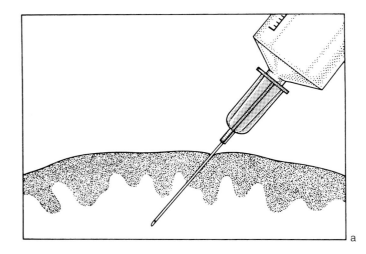
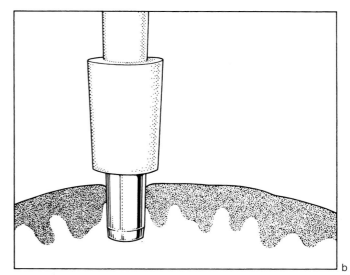
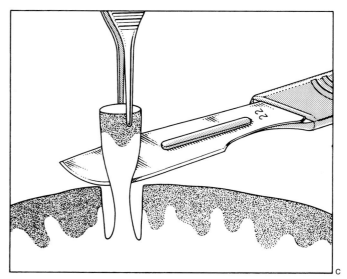

Fig. 40.1 Vulval biopsy under local anaesthesia.

USE OF TOPICAL CORTICOSTEROIDS

Because many gynaecologists are apprehensive about the use of topical corticosteroids in the vulval area, some basic information is desirable.

Topical steroids are effective in the management of inflammatory changes but are contraindicated in the presence of untreated infection. In some situations corticosteroids can be combined with an antifungal or antibacterial but care must be taken with the latter because an allergic contact dermatitis can develop.

Topical preparations are suspended in a vehicle, usually as a cream or ointment. Creams are miscible with skin secretions, easy to apply smoothly (and sparingly) but may contain additive to which the patient will become sensitized. Ointments are usually insoluble in water, greasy in texture and therefore more difficult to apply and more occlusive than creams. As they encourage hydration they are better suited for dry lesions. Pastes are stiffer but useful for localized lesions. They are less occlusive than ointments and can be used to protect excoriated or ulcerated lesions.

Topical corticosteroids are graded according to their potency, which reflects the degree of absorption or penetration through a lesion to be effective. A very potent steroid is necessary if there is lichenification or hyperkeratosis. These include clobetasol propionate 0.05% (Dermovate) and diflucortolone valerate 0.3% (Nerisone Forte). Potent preparations include betamethasone 0.1% (Betnovate) and triamcinolone acetonide 0.1% (Adcortyl); moderately potent include clobetasone butyrate 0.05% (Eumovate) and mild preparations include hydrocortisone 1%.

Patients will have anxieties about applying potent topical corticosteroids, particularly because some of the patient information with the packaging advises against their use in the genital area. This can be reduced by giving the patient written instructions on their use, either as an information sheet or in a letter with specific instructions for the patient.

Long-term use of potent corticosteroids does have side-effects which include the development of telangiectasia, striae, thinning of the skin, increased hair growth, mild depigmentation and a risk of worsening infection. Systemic absorption is rarely seen. Side-effects can be reduced by using less potent preparations where possible. However, it is better to use more potent steroids to gain relief and then either reduce the potency or the frequency of application to maintain control. Sudden cessation will often produce a rebound of symptoms. A 30 gram tube of Dermovate, if used appropriately, i.e. one application using a finger-tip length (or approximately 0.5 g) as squeezed from the tube, should last between 3 and 6 months.

On nights when topical steroids are not being applied or during the day, emollients can be applied to soothe and smooth the surface and to act as a moisturizer. Some emollients must be used with care as they can cause sensitization. Examples include aqueous cream BP, E45, Sudocrem, Ultrabase, Unguentum Merck (as creams), Diprobase (cream or ointment), emulsifying ointment BP, zinc and castor oil ointment BP (as ointments). Some of these are suitable as soap substitutes or preparations such as Alphakeri, Balneum or Oilatum can be added to the bath or shower (but can make the bath or shower dangerously slippery for the unsuspecting).

Gynaecologists often prescribe oestrogen creams for vulval conditions. The vulva has few oestrogen receptors (MacLean et al 1990) and the cream probably has only an emollient effect. Oestrogen cream has well-recognized indications for vaginal disorders and application to the vestibule may be helpful in vulval vestibulitis syndrome.

NON-NEOPLASTIC DISORDERS OF THE VULVA

Terms such as 'ichthyosis', 'leucoplakia', 'kraurosis' and 'lichen planus sclereux' have created confusion in describing vulval lesions (Ridley 1988). The current terminology is shown in Box 40.3

This terminology is not perfect and continues to have its critics MacLean 1991, Ridley 1988) even if only to recognize that non-neoplastic lesions such as lichen sclerosus may progress to neoplastic lesions.

Lichen sclerosus and squamous hyperplasia

These two conditions may occur separately or may be found together and may be seen at different times or stages in the same lesion. Ridley (1988) supports the concept of calling them all lichen sclerosus with or without lichenification.

The importance of lichen sclerosus is that it is common and is associated rarely with vulval carcinoma. It accounts for up to one-quarter of women seen in vulval clinics (MacLean et al 1998) and 0.3 to 1 per 1000 of all new patients seen in a

Box 40.3 Terminology of disorders of vulval skin and mucosa

Non-neoplastic disorders
Lichen sclerosus
Squamous cell hyperplasia (formerly hyperplastic dystrophy)
Other dermatoses

Vulval intraepithelial neoplasia (VIN)
Squamous VIN
  VIN I Mild dysplasia
  VIN II Moderate dysplasia
  VIN III Severe dysplasia or carcinoma in situ
Non-squamous VIN
  Paget's disease

1 Mixed epithelial disorders may occur. In such cases it is recommended that both conditions be reported. For example, lichen sclerosus with associated squamous cell hyperplasia (formerly classified as mixed dystrophy) should be reported as lichen sclerosus and squamous cell hyperplasia. Squamous cell hyperplasia with associated vulval intraepithelial neoplasia (formerly hyperplastic dystrophy with atypia) should be diagnosed as vulval intraepithelial neoplasia.
2 Squamous cell hyperplasia is used for those instances in which the hyperplasia is not attributable to another cause. Specific lesions or dermatoses involving the vulva (e.g. psoriasis, lichen planus, lichen simplex chronicus, candida infection, condyloma acuminatum) may include squamous cell hyperplasia, but should be diagnosed specifically and excluded from this category. From International Society for the Study of Vulvar Disease (1989)

general hospital (Wallace 1971). It occurs in men, where it is known as balanitis xerotica obliterans, but at approximately only one-tenth of the incidence in women. It occurs from age 5 to 94 years, with one-quarter under 50 years (MacLean et al 1998) and is not uncommon under the age of 5 years.

Lichen sclerosus involves the pudendum, either partially or completely as a figure-of-eight lesion encircling the vestibule and involving clitoris, labia minora, the inner aspects of the labia majora and the skin surrounding the anus. It is usually bilateral and symmetrical. It does not involve the vestibule or extend into the vagina or anal canal.

The lesions consist of thin, pearly, ivory or porcelain white crinkly plaques. Sometimes there is marked shrinkage and adsorption of the labia minora, coaptation of the labia across the clitoris to form a phimosis and narrowing of the introitus to obscure the urethra and make intercourse impossible. Scratching will produce lichenification or may produce epidermal erosion and ulceration. Areas of ecchymoses and subsequent pigmentation are common. Lichen sclerosus may also involve the trunk or limbs in 18% of patients (Meyrick-Thomas et al 1988).

The histological features of lichen sclerosus typically show epidermal atrophy, dermal oedema, hyalinization of the collagen and subdermal chronic inflammatory cell infiltrate. There is a correlation between clinical appearance and histology with the clinically thin area showing marked epidermal thinning with loss of rete ridges and vacuolation of the basal cells, while thick white fissured areas will histologically show hyperkeratosis, parakeratosis (abnormal keratinization) acanthosis, elongation, widening and blunting of the rete ridges (lichen sclerosus with lichenification; Ridley 1988). The inflammatory infiltrate may extend into the superficial dermis (Anderson 1991). These histological features are often modified secondary to trauma with the presence of red blood cells or haemosiderin. However, histological changes may be minimal and in some clinically obvious cases the histology may appear normal.

The cause of lichen sclerosus

The aetiology of lichen sclerosus remains unknown. The possibility of a hormonal cause has been examined without conclusive results (Friedrich & Kalra 1984, Kohlberger et al 1998). Some supportive evidence for a genetic cause has been described (Marren et al 1995). The suggestion that lichen sclerosus might be related to an autoimmune process (Goolamali et al 1974) has some tantalizing but inconclusive supportive evidence (Meyrick-Thomas et al 1988) as no circulating autoantibody has been identified. Other theories related to diet or infection have not gained support.

Relationship between lichen sclerosus and vulval squamous cell carcinoma

This relationship continues to be an area of debate and has been presented elsewhere (MacLean, 1993, 2000). Several authorities report a prevalence of carcinoma of 2.5–5% in women with lichen sclerosus (Friedrich 1985, Meyrick-Thomas et al 1988). Many vulval cancers have lichen sclerosus in the adjacent skin but the data are difficult to interpret. The changes in the adjacent epidermis have been studied for various alterations including changes in tumour suppressor

gene activity and increased expression of mutant p53 (Kagie et al 1997, Kohlberger et al 1995) and allelic imbalance with loss of heterozygosity or allelic gain (Pinto et al 2000). Our group have had several patients with lichen sclerosus plus hyperplasia progress to carcinoma and suggest that immunohistochemical staining of increased expression of p53 and Ki67 may be useful (Rolfe et al 2001).

Treatment of lichen sclerosus

Most dermatologists and gynaecologists use topical steroids like clobetasol and bland emollients to treat lichen sclerosus (Tidy et al 1996). However, it is only relatively recently, that the effectiveness of topical steroids has been confirmed (Dalziel et al 1989, Lorenz et al 1998, Sinha et al 1999). Most patients will respond to nightly applications within a few weeks, but treatment can be continued for up to 3 months. If patients do not improve, co-existing fungal infection, sensitization to the cream or co-existing carcinoma must be considered.

Patients with squamous hyperplasia are less likely to respond (Clark et al 1999) but longer use or very potent steroids might be more successful. There is no advantage in applying oestrogen cream or testosterone ointment to the vulva.

Physical destruction by cryotherapy or laser ablation of areas of lichen sclerosus no longer seems justified and nor is vulvectomy. Very occasionally, it may be necessary to divide labial or preputial adhesions.

Dermatoses

While dermatologists will have little difficulty in reaching a diagnosis with these lesions, most gynaecologists are likely to be less certain. Dermatitis is found in 64% of patients with chronic vulval symptoms (Fischer et al 1995). Many of these patients will have manifestations elsewhere and will be identified by history and examination. In some cases biopsy and histology will be diagnostic. Many lesions will respond to topical corticosteroids although the required potency will depend on the diagnosis.

Lichen simplex chronicus

Lichen simplex chronicus (previously known as neurodermatitis) occurs in normal skin which becomes dry, thick, scaly, white but sometimes pigmented and fissured in response to the trauma of constant scratching. Lichenification is a similar change which is superimposed on another pathology such as eczema. These lesions are usually not symmetrical and occur in areas accessible to scratching.

Treatment consists of the use of emollients or low-to-moderate potency topical corticosteroids. Sometimes sedation at night is useful to stop nocturnal scratching. Once control is gained, assessment for an underlying cause or lesion is often necessary.

Lichen planus

The lesions of lichen planus may be seen on mucous membrane or on cutaneous surfaces such as the inner surfaces of the wrists and lower legs. These cutaneous lesions are usually red or purple flat-topped nodules or papules with an overlying white lacy patterned appearance.

Involvement of the vulva is usually with white patterned areas that are sometimes elevated and thickened (hypertrophic lichen planus) or may appear red and raw with features of erosion. Changes in the mouth may be seen frequently. The vulval lesions may extend into the vagina where scarring, stenosis and adhesions make intercourse painful or impossible.

Histology will show liquefactive degeneration of the basal epidermal layer, long and pointed rete ridges, with parakeratosis and acanthosis and a dense dermal infiltrate of lymphocytes close to the dermal epidermal margin. Immunohistochemistry shows differences in the expression of interleukin-4 and interferon-α between lichen planus and lichen sclerosus (Carli et al 1997).

When the condition is severe treatment can be difficult, requiring systemic steroids, azathioprine or other immune-modifying agents. Lesser symptoms, particularly those externally on the vulva, can be managed with the application of topical corticosteroids; vaginal lesions can be managed with Colifoam (hydrocortisone) or Predfoam (prednisolone). Rarely, vulval cancer will arise in association with lichen planus (Dwyer et al 1995, Zaki et al 1996).

Contact dermatitis

Contact dermatitis occurs as an allergic response to various allergens including topical antibiotics, anaesthetic and anti-histamine creams, deodorants and perfumes, lanolin, azo-dyes in nylons, biological washing powders, spermicidals, latex of sheaths or diaphragms, etc. Sometimes the vulval lesion is a response to exposure to an allergen such as perfume or nickel jewellery elsewhere on the body.

Clinically there is a diffuse erythema and oedema with superimposed infection or lichenification. Patch testing may identify the allergen to allow removal or avoidance of the factor and moisturizing cream or mild steroids should provide local control.

Eczema

Vulval eczema will show similar appearances to those described for dermatitis but usually with no identifiable contact allergen. Usually there is evidence of eczema elsewhere such as in the flexures. Treatment is with moisturizing cream or mild steroids as above.

Psoriasis

Psoriasis may occur exclusively on the vulva but often there are lesions elsewhere and a family history. It affects about 2% of the population. Unlike psoriatic lesions elsewhere, they are unlikely to show the hyperkeratotic silvery scales as seen on knees and elbows but are often salmon pink in appearance with a sharp but irregular outline and with satellite lesions. Vulval psoriasis is treated with mild or moderately potent topical corticosteroids.

VULVAL PAIN

Many of the above will cause acute vulval pain; some will persist or become chronic but usually long-standing pain is due to different pathologies.

Chronic vulval discomfort, such as burning, stinging, irritation or rawness, is called vulvodynia (McKay et al 1991). This term replaces 'burning vulval syndrome' and describes a different set of problems to those that cause pruritus, although inevitably there is some overlap (McKay 1985). Vulval pain may be due to dermatoses, cyclical vulvitis, vulval vestibulitis syndrome or dysaesthetic vulvodynia.

Vulval dermatoses

These include many of the dermatological disorders that usually cause pruritus. McKay (1991) observed that a particular lesion will cause burning in some women and pruritus in others; this variation may be due to partial treatment with topical steroids or other local factors.

Cyclical or episodic vulvitis

This is characterized by recurrent symptoms associated with menstruation or coitus. Changes in vaginal pH are probably responsible and will be associated with recurrent candidiasis or bacterial vaginosis. Herpes simplex viral infection may also be episodic. Some suggest that cyclical vulvitis is a manifestation of atypical candidiasis.

Vulval vestibulitis syndrome

The vulvovaginal vestibule is the cleft between the labia minora and lies below the hymenal rim, is covered by non-keratinized squamous epithelium and contains the greater and lesser vestibular and periurethral glands. Vulval vestibulitis syndrome (VVS) is characterized by severe pain on touching the vestibule or on attempted vaginal entry and focal erythema involving the vestibule or around the gland openings. However, 43% of asymptomatic volunteers have vestibular erythema and 53% of these have a positive touch test (van Beurden et al 1997).

The pain or burning seems inappropriate and exaggerated and is essentially of neuropathic type, with stimuli that would normally or previously be tolerated being felt as marked pain (hyperalgesia). These sensations can be tested in VVS patients by touching or pressing the vestibule with a Q-tip or cotton bud or can be quantified using an algesiometer to measure pressure (Eva et al 1999).

The cause of VVS remains unknown but is probably multifactorial. These women are more likely to be Caucasian, from higher social classes (Furlonge et al 1991), nulliparous and under the age of 50 years. Most have had satisfactory relationships and pain-free intercourse in the past and there is no evidence that these patients have had sexual or physical abuse during childhood (Edwards et al 1997) or subsequently. However, some patients time the onset of symptoms to a change in partner. Infection, wearing certain clothing, condoms or spermicides, prolonged use of the oral contraception pill and diet have all been suggested causes. There may be some parallels between VVS and interstitial cystitis (Stewart & Berger 1997). Histopathology of biopsies in VVS has failed to show consistent features.

The management of VVS starts with a confident diagnosis and the reassurance to the patient that her problem is physical and not 'in her head'. An appropriate information sheet is helpful (Nunns 2000). Advice is given on avoiding additives in the bath, using soap substitutes, avoiding the use of soap powders containing biological enzymes and avoiding tight or constricting clothing. Some advocate a low-oxalate diet and calcium citrate supplements while others advise repeated and prolonged use of oral fluconazole or Trimovate (clobetasone plus oxytetracycline and nystatin) to the vestibule nightly for up to 3 months. Pelvic floor muscle relaxation, either under the supervision of physiotherapists or using biofeedback, may be helpful (Glazer et al 1995).

Persistent cases and those who find intercourse impossible may be considered for vestibulectomy using a procedure that involves excision of the whole vestibule, removing a horseshoe-shaped crescent from the peri urethral glands on one side around to the other. Surgery should only be performed on selected patients where all other treatment has been unsuccessful. Some would say it is never justified.

Vestibular papillomatosis

The presence of multiple papillae covering mucosal surfaces of the labia minora has been called vestibular papillomatosis. These were thought to be due to human papilloma virus (Boden et al 1988). However, papillae are often found in asymptomatic normal women and their presence is of uncertain clinical significance. It is possible that multiple, prominent papillae are the result of underlying irritation, not the cause.

Essential or dysaesthetic vulvodynia

In this condition the patient complains of diffuse or poorly localized, constant, unremitting burning of the vulva, buttocks or upper thighs but there is nothing abnormal in appearance on physical examination, because the changes occur in the nerve endings and not the skin. These patients are usually postmenopausal but do not respond to topical or systemic oestrogens. There are similarities between this condition and trigeminal neuralgia, postherpetic neuralgia or glossodynia (burning tongue) and pain is neuropathic in type, with light touch or pressure inducing pain (allodynia) and prolonged stimulus such as contact with clothing or on sitting producing a build-up of pain which persists after cessation of the stimulus (hyperpathia) (Galer 1995, Woolf & Mannion 1999). Sometimes the apparent localization to one side or to the perineum and the diagnosis of 'pudendal neuralgia' have led to investigation of the pudendal nerve along its course within the pelvis by magnetic resonance imaging but this is usually unrewarding.

Management requires exclusion of possible pelvic pathologies and then control of pain with an anticonvulsant or anti-depressant drug. Gabapentin is effectve in post herpetic neuralgia when increased incrementally to 3.6 g daily and used for 8 weeks. The alternative is amitriptyline, starting at 25 mg at night (10 mg in older women) increased to a maximum of 150 mg. One-third of patients will experience drowsiness or dry mouth and some patients will refuse to take this medication because they misbelieve they are being treated for depression. A simple explanation of the effect of lower doses on the peripheral nerves, compared to the bigger doses required to have a central effect and treat depression, is usually reassuring. There is no evidence that the newer antidepressants are more effective, but selective serotonin reuptake inhibitors (fluoxetine and paroxetine) have a lower incidence side-effects than tricyclics and therefore may be worth trying if tricyclics are not tolerated (McQuay & Moore 1997).

Inevitably, some patients with features of vulvodynia will not fall into any of the above groups. The temptation to remove the vulva by knife or laser should be resisted. In some cases, there will be underlying psychosexual reasons, such as childhood sexual abuse, and appropriate psychiatric assessment will provide insight into the problem and relief for the patient. Reassurance of normality, exclusion of infection and prevention of any topical applications may be valuable.

VULVAL ULCERATION

Vulval ulceration may be infective, aphthous or associated with Behçet's syndrome, Stevens–Johnson syndrome, dermatitis artefacta, benign mucous membrane pemphigoid, familial benign chronic pemphigus (Hailey-Hailey disease), pyoderma gangrenosum, Crohn's disease, histiocytosis X and toxic epidermal necrolysis (Lyell's syndrome). These conditions are uncommon although may be serious or even fatal. Sometimes the diagnosis can be made clinically or with a good history but occasionally biopsy will be necessary and may require immuno-fluorescent techniques.

VULVAL INFECTION

Some lesions will be due to primary infection, while in others a lesion has become secondarily infected. The commensal flora of the vulva consists of staphylococci, aerobic and anaerobic streptococci, Gram-negative bacilli and yeasts. Increased temperature, humidity and lower pH of vulval skin make it more susceptible to infection compared to skin elsewhere.

Fungal infections

Genital candida infection is caused by the yeast *Candida albicans* in the majority of cases. This organism is frequently found within the vagina but its incidence is increased with pregnancy, the use of oral contraceptives, the concurrent use of broad-spectrum antibiotics, the presence of glucosuria or diabetes mellitus and in association with the wearing of nylon underwear and tights. Infection produces acute vulval pruritus associated with a crusting discharge and white plaques will be seen within the vagina and on the vulva. With more extensive infection the vulva will become acutely erythematous with oedema and superficial maceration. Culture on appropriate medium or direct microscopy will demonstrate the presence of fungus or hyphae.

Treatment of simple infection may be with topical nystatin or an imidazole preparation. More extensive or recurrent infections can be treated with fluconazole 150 mg capsule as a single dose and repeated 1–2 weeks later or itraconazole 200 mg morning and evening for one day.

Tinea cruris is relatively uncommon in females, but may be transmitted from a partner and appropriate enquiry may be rewarding.

The lesions of pityriasis versicolor are due to *Malassezia furfur*, are small, circular and pigmented, involving the trunk and/or proximal limb but occasionally the vulva. They may cause pruritus. The fungus will be identified in skin scrapings or an adhesive tape preparation and will respond to imidazole cream, e.g. clotrimazole.

Genital warts

These are known as condylomata acuminata and are caused by human papillomavirus (HPV). There are now at least 60 types of HPV virus, those involving the genital area including HPV 6, 11, 16, 18, 31, 32, 33 and 35. Such lesions may involve not only vulval skin but also the vagina and the cervix and may extend around the perianal area or out onto non-genital skin. Typical lesions are elevated with epithelial proliferation, usually discrete but sometimes confluent and covering large areas. The typical lesion shows koilocytosis in the upper third of the epithelium, acanthosis, parakeratosis, dyskeratosis and basal hyperplasia. The majority of condylomata acuminata are diploid and only 10% may show nuclear atypia of various degrees, requiring differentiation from VIN with associated viral changes. The transmission of this virus is usually by sexual contact. The diagnosis is usually made on clinical appearance.

The treatment of single or small numbers of condylomata consists of the application of 25% trichloracetic acid followed by 25% podophyllin, at weekly intervals. This combination should be applied to the lesion and the patient asked to bathe some 6–8 hours later to remove any excess. Prolonged application can lead to excessive skin excoriation. Podophyllin should not be used during pregnancy. Those condylomata that are resistant to such treatment can be treated with imiquimod or some form of physical therapy. Atypical or resistant condylomata should be biopsied in order to exclude verrucous carcinoma (Partridge et al 1980).

Because of the widespread distribution of papillomavirus and the difficulty in eradicating this virus from genital skin, it may not always be appropriate to apply repeated, painful treatments that damage the vulval skin.

Herpes simplex

Vulval herpes lesions are usually associated with type 2 herpes simplex virus rather than type 1. The primary episode is associated with an incubation period of some 2–20 days with an average of 1 week. There is often an associated prodromal illness before a localized area of vulval skin becomes erythematous, followed by the appearance of blisters and subsequent ulceration. These lesions are usually acutely painful and may be associated with inguinal lymphadenitis. Vulval discomfort associated with micturition may cause urinary retention. Secondary bacterial infection can occur. Resolution of discomfort and healing occurs some 7–14 days after the onset of symptoms. Frequently the primary infection is much less dramatic. Following the primary episode the virus enters the dorsal ganglia where it becomes dormant or latent.

Reactivation may occur and a secondary episode results. Recurrences are less painful than primary lesions and rarely last more than 48 hours.

The diagnosis of herpes simplex virus can be made on history and inspection of the lesions. Specimens can be taken for viral culture or demonstration of virus using transmission electron microscopy or fluorescent antibody techniques.

The treatment of herpes simplex is specifically with aciclovir which interferes with viral DNA replication via thymidine kinase. The drug is poorly absorbed orally and therefore needs to be taken 200 mg five times daily or by topical application to the vulval area. Patients who have multiple recurrences can use 400 mg of aciclovir twice daily for 3–6 months and then less frequently to see if further episodes occur. Occasionally HIV-positive patients will be seen with large ulcers, probably due to herpes simplex which has become resistant to aciclovir.

Other viral infections

Herpes zoster may affect the vulval skin if dermatomes S1 to S4 are involved. The lesions are similar to those seen elsewhere on the body, with the formation of blisters which will coalesce to give large bullae with eventual crusting and resolution. Management consists of sedation, analgesia and control of secondary bacterial infection. Occasionally and more commonly in older patients, post-herpes zoster neuralgia can occur.

Molluscum contagiosum is caused by pox virus. The lesions are hard, pearly papules with central umbilication, that appear on the mons, buttocks or inside of the thighs. Diagnosis is usually made on the appearance but on squeezing the lesion a cheesy white material can be expressed and light microscopy will demonstrate the presence of rounded molluscum bodies. Treatment is usually by excoriation with a needle and the application of phenol, silver nitrate or an antiseptic paint repeated as necessary.

Bacterial infections

Bartholinitis

This is the commonest bacterial infection of the vulva. It is usually found between menarche and menopause, but not necessarily associated with sexual activity. It results from infection of the duct leading from the gland. Obstruction of the duct will produce an abscess in the acute situation or a cyst if infection is low grade or recurrent. Causative organisms may be from the vulval flora or may be sexually transmitted.

The management of bartholinitis requires appropriate swabs for bacteriology, analgesia, antibiotics and surgical drainage of a cyst or abscess by marsupialization. In women aged over 40 years, the edges of the cyst should be sent for histological examination to exclude carcinoma.

Staphylococcal infection

This may take the form of perifolliculitis, involving the hair follicles and adjacent glandular structures within the dermis, or furunculosis which are larger, deeper lesions involving subcutaneous tissue that eventually discharge through multiple sinuses. Occasionally staphylococcal impetigo is seen. Management consists of the application of povidone iodine washes or

607

mupirocin ointment or use of an anti-staphylococcal antibiotic such as flucloxacillin. Occasionally surgical drainage of the pus is required.

Hidradenitis

Similar features of recurrent staphylococcal infection are seen with hidradenitis suppurativa, a chronic inflammatory disease involving the apocrine glands (Thomas et al 1985). This condition is more likely to involve the axilla but occasionally will involve the vulva or perianal areas or the genitofemoral fold. These abscesses are deep and may often involve anaerobic organisms. Acute cases will require intravenous antibiotics such as flucloxacillin and metronidazole and may require surgical deroofing of the abscess. Long-term antibiotic treatment may be combined with hormone control of apocrine gland activity. This appears to be best achieved using a combination of oestrogen and cyproterone. There is a small risk of carcinoma developing in areas of chronic scarring.

Other bacterial infections

Streptococcal infection of the vulva may be relatively superficial or localized, as in erysipelas. This will be associated with sharply defined erythema, oedema and pain. Streptococci may cause deeper infection involving tissue down to the fascia or periostium. Gangrene of the skin (necrotizing fasciitis) may complicate any form of vulval surgery, especially in diabetic women. High doses of penicillin are required. In cases with deep infection other aerobic and anaerobic organisms are often involved and a combination of antibiotics and very wide surgical excision is required. Infection of the vulva with *Neisseria gonorrhoeae* is rare in adults. The urethra, however, will be infected in about 75% of cases of gonorrhoea and this may lead to infection of periurethral glands. Involvement of the duct of Bartholin's gland is described above. Gonococcal vulvitis can occur in children.

Erythrasma is due to *Corynebacterium minutissimum* and causes areas of red-brown scaling on the vulva or in the groin. These areas will fluoresce with Wood's light (ultraviolet light). The diagnosis can be confirmed with bacteriology and treatment is with erythromycin.

Trichomycosis is also due to corynebacteria and is not fungal, as its name would suggest. Asymptomatic yellow, red or black nodules are present on hair shafts and they produce staining on underclothing. They can be seen with Wood's light and are treated with antiseptic washing.

Vulval tuberculosis (lupus vulgaris) is seen infrequently in women and is usually associated with pelvic tuberculosis. A vulval lesion may follow sexual contact with an infected male.

Syphilis

A single painless indurated ulcer of the vulva associated with painless inguinal lymphadenopathy is the primary lesion. The lesions may be multiple at the points of sexual contact and trauma and heal slowly without any treatment. If there is any clinical suspicion the patient should be referred to a genito-urinary medicine clinic. Secondary syphilis appears some 2 or 3 months after the initial lesion and may have various manifestations. The skin may have a macular, papular or maculopapular rash, while the vulval mucosa may have soft, moist, velvety condylomata lata, painless eroded mucous patches or these latter may coalesce and then ulcerate to form snail-track ulcers. These lesions are highly infectious and contain many of the causative *Treponema pallidum* organisms. Involvement of the vulva with tertiary lesion or gumma is unusual.

If the diagnosis of early syphilis is certain the woman should be treated with Bicillin (a mixture of procaine penicillin and benzylpenicillin) or doxycyline or erythromycin if she is allergic to penicillin.

Chancroid

This is caused by *Haemophilus ducreyi*. The initial lesions are small but tender papules which break down to form tender non-indurated ulcers involving the labia, fourchette, perineum and perineal areas. Inguinal lymphadenitis will develop, with progression to abscess formation and subsequent discharge. This infection, like granuloma inguinale and lymphogranuloma venereum (below), is uncommon outside tropical and subtropical developing countries.

Granuloma inguinale

This is also known as donovanosis and is due to Donovania or *Calymmatobacterium granulomatis*. Lesions start as papules or nodules, followed by soft, slowly enlarging ulcers; they may eventually involve extensive areas. The inguinal lymph nodes do not become involved.

Lymphogranuloma venereum

This is caused by certain serovars of *Chlamydia trachomatis*, causing a rather unimpressive vulval lesion which heals rapidly but is followed by progressive inguinal lymphadenopathy which eventually suppurates through the skin. Lymphatic obstruction is followed by vulval elephantiasis and hypertrophy.

Protozoal and parasitic infections

Trichomonas vaginalis

This involves the vagina initially although the patient may present with vulval symptoms. This infection is due to *Trichomonas vaginalis*, a flagellated protozoan, and is associated with vaginal discharge (which is often frothy and brown or green), vaginal irritation and dyspareunia. The organisms may be identified in a wet film by their motility or may be recognized in cervical smears. Colposcopic assessment of the vagina shows characteristic double-looped coarse punctation of the vagina and cervix which may be diffuse and extensive or patchy and localized (strawberry vagina). Treatment of this infection is with metronidazole 200 mg three times a day for 7 days or a single 2 g dose. The partner should be treated concurrently and both should be warned not to take alcohol with this antibacterial agent.

Pediculosis

This condition (crabs) is caused by the pubic louse *Phthirus pubis* and both the insect and its eggs are visible to the unaided eye. It is usually spread by sexual contact but sometimes from clothing or bedding. It involves the hair-bearing areas of the vulva and causes itching. Treatment is with topical malathion or carbaryl.

Scabies

This is caused by the mite *Sarcoptes scabiei*, is spread by direct body contact and is associated with intense itching which is worse at night or after a hot bath. It commonly involves the hands, including the interdigital webs, axillae, buttocks and the genital skin in men but not in women. The typical burrows are diagnostic but sometimes a generalized papular rash, due to hypersensitivity reaction, is seen. Treatment is with γ-benzene hexachloride (Lindane) or benzyl benzoate applications.

Threadworms

Enterobius vermicularis live in the large bowel, lay eggs on the anal margins and cause pruritus ani; vulval irritation may also occur. The ova can be recognized on microscopy of a sellotape strip left in position overnight. Treatment is with piperazine or mebendazole.

Amoebiasis

Entamoeba histolytica occasionally causes vulval or perineal lesions, either secondary to intestinal involvement or by sexual contact. Painful serpiginous ulcers follow the development of cutaneous lesions; there is an associated lymphadenopathy. Diagnosis is by microscopy and treatment is with oral metronidazole plus iodochlorohydroxy-quinolone pessaries.

Schistosomiasis (bilharzia)

The fluke responsible for this condition enters the skin from water during swimming or wading, reaches the circulation for maturation of the parasite and can cause chronic granulomata or lesions resembling warts in the skin, including the genitalia, following blood spread. The lesions ulcerate and produce scarring of the vulva. Diagnosis is by microscopy for ova and praziquantel is the treatment.

Filariasis

This is due usually to the worm *Wuchereria bancrofti* which is spread by mosquitoes. The parasite reproduces in the lymphatics, producing swelling and lymphoedema. If the inguinal nodes are involved this will produce vulval swelling and elephantiasis.

Leishmaniasis

The protozoon *Leishmania tropica* is transmitted by sandfly bites. Vulval lesions occur, usually consisting of a nodule initially which later ulcerates.

Vulval lesions due to entamoeba, schistosoma, filarial worms and leishmania are uncommon in Western countries. They should be considered in anyone returning from overseas and may cause diagnostic difficulties if considering a 'tropical' venereal infection or even syphilis.

BENIGN TUMOURS OF THE VULVA

Lipomas and fibromas are the commonest benign tumours of the vulva which arise from other than the epithelial tissues.

Haemangiomas are benign tumours composed of blood vessels, the capillary type (strawberry haemangioma) being most commonly encountered in infants and young children. A variety of site-specific stromal tumours can occur in the vulvo-vaginal area, including aggressive angiomyxoma, angiomyo-fibroblastoma and cellular angiofibroma. Fibroepithelial stromal polyps (FSP) occur in young to middle-aged women more frequently in the vagina, but also in the vulva or cervix. They are benign and are lined by normal squamous epithelium, which may be keratinized, depending on the location; the stroma varies from bland to cellular and pleomorphic, especially in pregnancy-associated cases. There is potential for local recurrence, particularly if incompletely exicsed.

Angiomyofibroblastoma (AMF) is a well-circumscribed lesion which occurs almost exclusively in the vulvovaginal region and is often clinically thought to be a Bartholin's gland cyst. The stromal cells may have an epithelioid appearance and tend to cluster around vessels; they show reactivity for desmin and are actin negative. Cellular angiofibroma occurs exclusively in the vulva and behaves in a benign fashion; it is composed of spindle cells arranged in short fascicles in a meshwork of thick-walled vessels. The cells express vimentin but not desmin or actin. Aggressive angiomyxoma is a locally infiltrative tumour that in 30–40% of cases recurs if incompletely excised. It occurs most commonly in the reproductive years and usually has a gelatinous appearance. Histologically it is a myxoid, poorly cellular neoplasm composed of bland spindle cells which merge imperceptibly into the surrounding stroma. Superficial angio-myxoma arises in the dermis and subcutaneous tissue and therefore often appears polypoid. If multiple lesions also involving other sites are present Carney's complex may be suspected and further investigations to exclude a cardiac myxoma are warranted.

Smooth muscle tumours of vulva are much rarer than the uterine counterpart; the presence of mitotic activity, nuclear pleomorphism or an infiltrative margin is associated with locally recurrent potential (atypical smooth muscle tumours), while tumours with any three of the following features are considered sarcomas: >50 mm in size, infiltrative margins, >5 mitoses/10 HPFs, moderate to severe atypia.

Granular cell tumours are of peripheral nerve sheath origin and arise in the vulva of children or adults as painless subcutaneous nodules of the mons pubis, labia majora or clitoris. They are often associated with pseudoepitheliomatous hyperplasia of the overlying epithelium and are composed of epithelioid, granular cells infiltrating the stroma and typically exhibiting S-100 protein. Wide local excision is the treatment of choice. Neurofibromas may affect the vulva as part of the von Recklinghausen disease. Benign angiokeratoma may be difficult to distinguish from a melanoma, especially if the initial red colour has given way to the later brown or black hue and the lesion has begun to bleed due to trauma.

Squamous papillomata and 'skin tags' are common, benign and similar in appearance. They may be solitary or multiple (vestibular or squamous papillomatosis, microwarts). They lack significant correlation with HPV-DNA and histology may overestimate viral changes.

Seborrhoeic keratosis may also occur on the hair-bearing skin of the vulva of elderly women. The rare keratoacanthoma might well be mistaken for invasive squamous cancer because of its rapid growth over a matter of weeks. Spontaneous involution usually begins after about 6 months. The centre of this well-demarcated, regular dome contains a plug of keratin, which may suggest the diagnosis, but complete excision of the lesion is required for histological confirmation.

Folliculitis – infection of hair follicles – may be caused by shaving or depilatory creams. Infestation with lice may present in this way. Any precipitating cause should be dealt with. Topical antiseptics or even systemic antibiotics may be required.

VAGINAL INFECTION

Between puberty and the menopause the presence of lactobacilli maintains a vaginal pH of between 3.8 and 4.2; this protects against infection. Before puberty and after the menopause, the higher pH and urinary and faecal contamination increase the risk of infection. Normal physiological vaginal discharge consists of transudate from the vaginal wall, squames containing glycogen, polymorphs, lactobacilli, cervical mucus, residual menstrual fluid and a contribution from the greater and lesser vestibular glands.

Vaginal discharge varies with hormonal levels and does not automatically mean infection. Non-specific vaginitis may be associated with sexual trauma, allergies to deodorants or contraceptives or the chemical irritation of topical antimicrobial therapy. Infection may be aggravated by the presence of foreign bodies, continuing use of tampons and the presence of an intrauterine contraceptive device.

Vaginal infection may produce vulval symptoms and the descriptions above of genital candidiasis, trichomoniasis, herpes simplex and human papilloma viruses and syphilis are relevant to vaginal lesions. *Neisseria gonorrhoeae* will not infect the vaginal epithelium except in prepubertal girls or postmenopausal women. If there is suspicion of sexual abuse in a young girl, an appropriate vaginal swab should be taken.

Bacterial vaginosis

Bacterial vaginosis is now believed to be due to a vibrio or comma-shaped organism named Mobiluncus. Other organisms, including anaerobes, may have a contributory role. These organisms are believed to be sexually transmitted although the condition may be due to imbalance in the vaginal ecosystem. Usually the vagina is not inflamed and therefore the term 'vaginosis' is used rather than 'vaginitis'. Nearly half of 'infected' patients will not have symptoms (Thomason et al 1990) while others will complain of increased or unpleasant discharge, soreness and irritation.

Examination will reveal a thin, grey-white discharge and a vaginal pH greater than 5 and a Gram stain of the discharge will show 'clue cells' which consist of vaginal epithelial cells covered with micro-organisms. The absence of lactobacilli will be confirmed if a characteristic fishy amine smell is released when a drop of vaginal discharge is added to saline on a glass slide, along with one drop of 10% potassium hydroxide. The diagnosis is made if three of these four criteria are met.

There are claims that bacterial vaginosis is associated with increased risk of preterm labour (Hay et al 1994), pelvic inflammatory, disease and postoperative pelvic infection (Eschenbach et al 1988, Paavonen et al 1987). The treatment of bacterial vaginosis is metronidazole, either as 400 mg two or three times a day for 7 days or as a single 2 g dose. Alternatively clindamycin 2% can be used as a vaginal cream but, unlike metronidazole, this is active against lactobacilli and will delay the restoration of normal vaginal flora.

Toxic shock syndrome

This topic has been included here because it is associated with the use of vaginal tampons during menstruation or less frequently in the puerperium (Shands et al 1980). Although there is a link between this syndrome and certain organisms found within the vagina of affected women, it is not a vaginal infection.

The characteristics of the syndrome are an abrupt onset of pyrexia greater than 38.8°C, myalgia, diffuse skin rash with oedema and blanching erythema like sunburn and subsequent (1–2 weeks later) desquamation of the skin of the palms and soles. Less commonly, vomiting and diarrhoea and symptomatic hypotension are seen. Leucocytosis, thrombocytopenia and increased serum bilirubin, liver enzymes and creatine phosphokinase may be observed. *Staphylococcus aureus* can be identified frequently from the vagina but blood cultures are usually negative. It is believed that the syndrome is due to the systemic effects of a toxin and subsequent release of bradykinin, tumour necrosis factor or other biological response mediators. Group A β-haemolytic streptococci have also been implicated because they can release a similar toxin (erythrogenic toxin A) (Sanderson 1990).

Removal of super-absorbent brands of tampons from the market in the USA and greater care in tampon use and insertion reduced the frequency of the syndrome from 17 per 100 000 menstruating women to only one per 100 000.

Early effective treatment of hypovolaemia in severe cases is essential. Treatment is the same as for septicaemia and includes intravenous fluids and inotropic support where necessary. The cause should be eliminated where possible and a β-lactamase resistant penicillin given parenterally. Further attacks can occur and it is recommended that tampons should not be used until *Staphylococcus aureus* has been eradicated from the vagina.

OTHER VAGINAL PATHOLOGY

Atrophy

This is seen following the menopause, but can also occur prior to puberty and during prolonged lactation. Examination shows loss of rugal folds and prominent subepithelial vessels, sometimes with adjacent ecchymoses. The patient may present with vaginal bleeding, vaginal discharge or vaginal dryness and dyspareunia. Superficial infection, with Gram-positive cocci or Gram-negative bacilli, may be associated.

Treatment requires oestrogen to restore the vaginal epithelium and pH. This is usually by topical oestrogen cream or pessary. Systemic absorption will increase blood levels of oestrogen. Alternatively, hormone replacement therapy can be used.

Trauma

A torn hymen following a first attempt at intercourse may result in profuse, frightening haemorrhage. Transfusion may be indicated. Suture of the bleeding vessel under general anaesthesia should be accompanied by one or more radial incisions in the hymen to prevent a recurrence.

Trauma is usually the result of falling astride a sharp object like a fence. It may result from sexual abuse, sometimes self-inflicted. It may also occur following normal sexual intercourse, particularly in a postmenopausal woman who has not had intercourse for some time. In these cases the laceration is usually at the vault of the vagina in the posterior fornix.

An indwelling catheter may be necessary and ice packs will give some comfort. Damage to the vagina, rectum, urethra, bladder or ureter may also occur. Pain relief with opiates and replacement of blood loss may be needed urgently. Examination under anaesthesia is often required to determine the extent of the damage. A closed haematoma is best managed conservatively but bleeding lacerations will require suture. Devitalized tissues will need to be excised and tears in bowel or bladder must be repaired in layers. Occasionally a hysterectomy must be performed.

SEMINAL FLUID ALLERGY

Occasionally, patients will present with a history of dyspareunia, with itching, burning or swelling but occasionally more wide-spread symptoms, with urticaria or even anaphylaxis, after intercourse. The allergic reaction appears to be due to sensitization to seminal fluid (Halpern et al 1967, Poskitt et al 1995). Symptoms may arise following first coitus or after exposure to several sexual partners.

Treatment has included long-term immunotherapy following skin testing (Friedman et al 1984). Treatment with desensitization may be helpful and antihistamines and intravaginal cromo-glycate are described (Poskitt et al 1995).

SJOGREN'S SYNDROME

Patients with vaginal dryness and pain may have Sjogren's syndrome if there is ocular or oral dryness. They may have arthralgia, myalgia or Raynaud's phenomenon. The diagnostic criteria include ocular and oral symptoms, ocular signs, salivary gland histology, other evidence of salivary gland involvement and the presence of autoantibodies. Vaginal symptoms may predate the oral or ocular symptoms.

BENIGN TUMOURS OF THE VAGINA

Tumours in the vagina are uncommon. Condyloma acuminata are by far the commonest seen (Fig. 40.2). The frond-like surface is usually characteristic but it is wise to await the result of a biopsy before instituting treatment.

Endometriotic deposits may be seen in the vagina. They are most common in an episiotomy wound and may lie deep to the epithelium.

Simple mesonephric (Gartner's) or paramesonephric cysts may be seen, especially high up near the fornices. If asympto-matic, they are best not treated. If treatment is required,

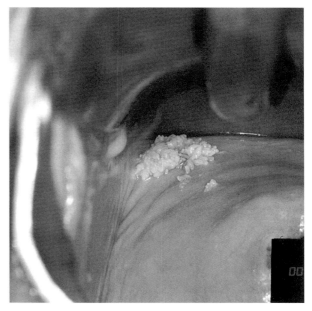

Fig. 40.2 These vaginal condylomata have turned bright white after the application of 5% acetic acid.

marsupialization is effective and safer than excision. Similarly, management of anterior wall cysts must include the exclusion of a bladder or urethral diverticulum.

Adenosis (multiple mucus-containing vaginal cysts) is a rare condition which even more rarely gives rise to symptoms. A variety of abnormalities are reported in the daughters of women who took diethylstilboestrol during their pregnancy. Most of these are of no significance (see Chapter 39).

Vaginal neoplasia

VIN are discussed in Chapter 38 and vaginal cancer in Chapter 41.

KEY POINTS

1. A multidisciplinary team approach to vulval disease is helpful.
2. The presenting symptoms will not indicate the nature of the pathology.
3. Topical steroids are effective and safe in the treatment of many vulval disorders.
4. Topical oestrogens have little to offer the woman with a vulval disorder.
5. There is no place for vulvectomy in the management of lichen sclerosus.

REFERENCES

Anderson MC 1991 Systemic pathology, vol 6, 3rd edn. Churchill Livingstone, Edinburgh

Bishop JW, Marshall CJ, Bentz JS 2000 New technologies in gynaecologic cytology. Journal of Reproductive Medicine 45:701–719.

Boden E, Eriksson A, Rylander E et al 1988 Clinical characteristics of papillomavirus vulvovaginitis. Acta Obstetricia Gynecologica Scandinavica 67:147–151.

Borgno G, Micheletti L, Barbero M et al 1988 Epithelial alterations adjacent to 111 vulvar carcinomas. Journal of Reproductive Medicine. 33:500–502.

Bornstein J, Zarfati D, Goldik Z, Abramovici H 1995 Perineoplasty compared with vestibuloplasty for severe vulvar vestibulitis. British Journal of Obsetrics and Gynaecology 102:652–5.

Carli P, Moretti S, Spallanzani A et al 1997 Fibrogenic cytokines in vulvar lichen sclerosus. Journal of Reproductive Medicine 42:161–165.

Clark T J, Etherington IJ, Luesley DM 1999 Response of the vulvar lichen sclerosus and squamous cell hyperplasia to graduated topical steroids. Journal of Reproductive Medicine 44(11):958–962.

Dalziel K, Millard P, Wojnarowska F 1989 Lichen sclerosus et atrophicus treated with a potent topical steroid (clobetasol dipropionate 0.05%). British Journal of Dermatology 121 (suppl 34):34–35

Dwyer CM, Kerr RE, Millan DW 1995 Squamous cell carcinoma following lichen planus of the vulva. Clinical and Experimental Dermatology 20:171–172

Edwards L, Mason M, Phillips M et al 1997 Childhood sexual and physical abuse. Incidence in patients with vulvodynia. Journal of Reproductive Medicine 42:135–139

Eschenbach DA, Hillier S, Critchlow C 1988 Diagnosis and clinical manifestations of bacterial vaginosis. American Journal of Obstetrics and Gynecology 158:819–828

Eva LJ, Reid WMN, MacLean AB, Morrison GD 1999 Assessment of response to treatment in vulvar vestibulitis syndrome by means of the vulvar algesiometer. American Journal of Obstetrics and Gynecology 181:99–102

Fischer G, Spurett B, Fischer A 1995 The chronically symptomatic vulva: aetiology and management. British Journal of Obstetrics and Gynaecology 102:773–779

Friedman SA, Bernstein IL, Enrione M et al 1984 Successful long-term immunotherapy for human seminal plasma anaphylaxis. JAMA 251:2684–2687

Friedrich EG 1983 Vulva disease, 2nd edn. WB Saunders, Philadelphia

Friedrich EG 1985 Vulvar dystrophy. Clinical Obstetrics and Gynecology 28:178–187

Friedrich EG, Kalra PS 1984 Serum levels of sex hormones in vulvar lichen sclerosus and the effect of topical testosterone. New England Journal of Medicine 310:488–491

Furlonge CB, Thin RN, Evans BE, McKee PH 1991 Vulvar vestibulitis syndrome: a clinico-pathological study. British Journal of Obstetrics and Gynaecology 98:703–706

Galer BS 1995 Neuropathic pain of peripheral origin: advances in pharmacologic treatment. Neurology 4 (suppl 9): S17–S25

Glazer HI, Rodke G, Swencionis C et al 1995 Treatment of vulvar vestibulitis syndrome with electromyographic biofeedback of pelvic floor musculature. Journal of Reproductive Medicine 40:283–290

Goolamali SK, Barnes EW, Irvine WJ et al 1974 Organ-specific antibodies in patients with lichen sclerosus. British Medical Journal ii:78–79

Halpern BN, Ky T, Robert B 1967 Clinical and immunological study of an exceptional case of reaginic type sensitization to human seminal fluid. Immunology 12:247–258

Hay PE, Lamont RF, Taylor-Robinson D et al 1994 Abnormal bacterial colonisation of the genital tract and subsequent preterm delivery and late miscarriage. British Medical Journal 308:295–298

International Society for the Study of Vulva Disease 1989 New nomenclature for vulvar disease. American Journal of Obstetrics and Gynecology 73:769

Jonsson M, Karlsson R, Evander M 1997 Acetowhitening of the cervix and vulva as a predictor of subclinical human papillomavirus infection: sensitivity and specificity in a population based study. Obsetric Gynecology 90:744–747

Kagie MJ, Kenter GG, Tollenaar RAE et al 1997 p53 protein overexpression, a frequent observation in squamous cell carcinoma of the vulva and in various synchronous vulva epithelia, has no value as a prognostic parameter. International Journal of Gynecological Pathology 16:124–130

Kohlberger PD, Joura EA, Bancher D et al 1998 Evidence of androgen receptor expression in lichen sclerosus: an immunohistological study. Journal of the Society for Gynecological Investigation 5:331

Kohlberger PD, Kainz CH, Breitenecker ?? et al 1995 Prognostic value of immunohistochemically detected p53 expression in vulvar carcinoma. Cancer 76:1796–1889

Lorenz B, Kaufman RF, Kutzner SK 1998 Lichen sclerosus. Therapy with clobetasol propionate. Journal of Reproductive Medicine 43:790–794

MacLean AB 2000 Are 'non-neoplastic' disorders of the vulva premalignant? In: Huesley D (Ed) Cancer and precancers of the vulva. Arnold, London

MacLean AB, 1991 Vulval dystrophy – the passing of a term. Current Opinion in Obstetrics and Gynaecology 1:97–102

MacLean AB, 1993 Precursors of vulval cancers. Current opinion in Obstetrics and Gynaecology 3:149–156

MacLean AB, Nicol LA, Hodgins MB 1990 Immunohistochemical localisation of estrogen receptors in the vulva and vagina. Journal of Reproductive Medicine 35:1015–1016

MacLean AB, Reid WMN 1995 Benign and premalignant disease of the vulva. British Journal of Obstetics and Gynaecology 102:359–363

MacLean AB, Roberts DT, Reid WMN 1998 Review of 1000 women seen at two specially designated vulval clinics. Current Opinion in Obstetrics and Gynaecology 8:159–162

Marren P, Yell J, Charnock FM et al 1995 The association between lichen sclerosus and antigens of the HLA system. British Journal of Dermatology 132:197–203

McCullough AM, Seywright M, Roberts DT, MacLean AB 1987 Outpatient biopsy of the vulva. Journal of Obstetrics and Gynaecology 166–169

McKay M 1985 Vulvodynia versus pruritus vulvae. Clinical Obstetrics and Gynaecology 28:123–133

McKay M 1991 Vulvitis and vulvovaginitis: cutaneous considerations. American Journal of Obstetrics and Gynecology 165:1176–1182

McKay M, Frankman O, Horowitz BJ et al 1991 Vulvar vestibulitis and vestibular papillomatosis. Report of the ISSVD Committee on vulvodynia. Journal of Reproductive Medicine 36:413–415

McQuay HJ, Moore RA 1997 Antidepressants and chronic pain. British Medical Journal 314:763–764

Meyrick-Thomas RH, Ridley CM, MacGibbon DH et al 1988 Lichen sclerosus and autoimmunity – study of 350 women. British Journal of Dermatology 118:41–46

Nunns D 2000 Vulval pain syndromes. British Journal of Obstetrics and Gynaecology 107:1185–1193

Paavonen J, Teisala K, Heinonen PK et al 1987 Microbiological and histopathological findings in acute pelvic inflammatory disease. British Journal of Obstetrics and Gynaecology 94:454–460

Partridge EE, Murad T, Shingleton HM et al 1980 Verrucous lesions of the female genitalia. American Journal of Obstetrics and Gynecology 137:412–424

Pinto AP, Lin MC, Sheers EE et al 2000 Allelic imbalance in lichen sclerosus, hyperplasia and intraepithelial neoplasia of the vulva. Gynecologic Oncology 77:171–176

Poskitt BL, Wojnarowska FT, Shaw S 1995 Semen contact urticaria. Journal Royal Society of Medicine 88:108–109

Ridey CM 1988 The vulva. Churchill Livingstone, London

Rolfe KJ, Eva LJ, MacLean AB et al 2001 Cell cycle proteins as molecular markers of malignant change in lichen sclerosus. International Journal of Gynecological Cancer (in press)

Sanderson P 1990 Do streptococci cause toxic shock? British Medical Journal 301:1006–1007

Shands KN, Schmid GP, Dan BB 1980 Toxic shock syndrome in menstruating women. Association with tampon use and Staphylococcus aureus, and clinical features in 52 cases. New England Journal of Medicine 303:1436–1442

Sinha P, Sorinola O, Luesley DM 1999 Lichen sclerosus of the vulva. Long-term steroid maintenance therapy. Journal of Reproductive Medicine 44:621–624

Stewart EG, Berger BM 1997 Parallel pathologies? Vulvar vestibulitis and interstitial cystitis. Journal of Reproductive Medicine 42:131–134

Thomas R, Barnhill D, Bibro M 1985 Hidradenitis suppurativa: a case presentation and review of the literature. Obstetric Gynecology 66:592–595

Thomason JL, Gelbart SM, Anderson B et al 1990 Statistical evaluation of diagnostic criteria for bacterial vaginosis. American Journal of Obstetrics and Gynecology 162:155–60

Tidy JA, Soutter WP, Luesley DM et al 1996 Management of lichen sclerosus and intraepithelial neoplasia of the vulva in the U.K. Journal of the Royal Society of Medicine 89:699–701

van Beurden M, van der Vange N, de Craen AJM et al 1997 Normal findings in vulvar examinations and vulvoscopy. British Journal of Obstetrics and Gynaecology 104:320–324.

Wallace HJ 1971 Lichen sclerosus et atrophicus. Transactions of St John's Dermatology Society 57:9–30

Woolf CJ, Mannion RJ 1999 Neuropathic pain: aetiology, symptoms, mechanisms and management. Lancet 353:1959–1964

Zaki l, Dalziel KL, Solomonsz FA et al 1996 The under reporting of skin disease in association with squamous cell carcinoma of the vulva. Clinical and Experimental Dermatology 21:334–337

41

Malignant disease of the vulva and the vagina

Roberto Dina   Pat Soutter   Hilary Thomas

CANCER OF THE VULVA

Introduction

Invasive vulvar cancer is an uncommon and unpleasant but potentially curable disease even in elderly, unfit women if referred early and managed correctly from the outset. If mismanaged, the patient with vulvar cancer is condemned to a miserable, degrading death. The surgical treatment appears deceptively simple, but few gynaecologists and their nursing colleagues acquire sufficient experience of this disease to offer the highest quality of care for these women. All too often, an inadequate initial attempt at surgery is made and the patient referred for specialist care only after recurrent disease is evident. There are about 800 new cases of carcinoma of the vulva each year in England and the annual incidence is approximately 3.2/100 000, making it about three times less common than cervical cancer (OPCS 2001). The majority of these women are elderly (Fig. 41.1). With increased life expectancy this cancer will be seen more frequently.

Aetiology

Little is known of the aetiology of vulvar cancer. A viral factor has been suggested by the detection of antigens induced by herpes simplex virus type 2 (HSV2) and of DNA from type 16/18 human papillomavirus (HPV) in vulval intraepithelial neoplasia (VIN) and also by the association of a history of genital warts with vulvar cancer (Brinton et al 1990). The

significance of this viral association remains uncertain. The majority of genital condylomata contain HPV 6/11, not now considered to have any oncogenic potential, and very few contain HPV 16, the type found in invasive lesions (Bergeron et al 1987). There seem to be two distinct types of vulval carcinoma: one which occurs predominantly in older women, is typically a well-differentiated keratinizing tumour unassociated with VIN or HPV infection but which often shows adjacent squamous hyperplasia and/or lichen sclerosus; and a second type which occurs mostly in young women, is associated with VIN, shows evidence of HPV infection and may be associated with synchronous or metachronous squamous preneoplastic or neoplastic lesions of cervix, vagina and anal canal. Smoking may be an important co-factor involved in the aetiology of HPV-related vulvar tumours (Hildesheim et al 1997).

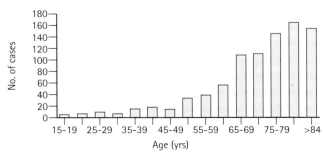

Fig. 41.1   The age-specific distribution of vulval carcinoma (OPCS 1994).

Anatomy

The gross anatomy is discussed in Chapters 2 and 40.

Lymphatic drainage

The lymph drains from the vulva to the inguinal and femoral glands in the groin and then to the external iliac glands. Drainage to both groins occurs from midline structures – the perineum and the clitoris – but some contralateral spread may take place from other parts of the vulva (Iversen & Aas 1983). Direct spread to the pelvic nodes along the internal pudendal vessels occurs only very rarely and no direct pathway from the clitoris to pelvic nodes has been demonstrated consistently.

Pathology

Most invasive cancers (95%) are squamous. The mean age is between 60 and 74 years. Some 5% are melanomas and the remainder are made up of carcinomas of Bartholin's gland, other adenocarcinomas, basal cell carcinomas and the very rare verrucous carcinomas, rhabdomyosarcomas and leiomyosarcomas. In a third of cases of Paget's disease there is an adenocarcinoma in underlying apocrine glands; these carry an especially poor prognosis (Boehm & Morris 1971, Creasman et al 1975). Squamous carcinomas can be divided into microinvasive and frankly invasive squamous cell carcinomas. The depth of invasion should be assessed by measuring the tumour from the epithelial–stromal junction of the adjacent most superficial dermal papilla to the deepest point of invasion. The thickness of the tumour is defined as the measurement from the surface to the deepest point of invasion and is used by some in preference to depth as being easier to measure and more reproducible (Wilkinson 1991).

Natural history

Microinvasive disease

The definition of microinvasion of the vulva has proved extremely problematical. The purpose is to identify a group of women with invasive carcinoma who could safely be treated without inguinofemoral lymphadenectomy. The potential for disaster if lymphadenectomy is wrongly omitted is all too clear (Table 41.1).

Although it was initially suggested that up to 5 mm invasion into the stroma might be acceptable (Rutledge et al 1970, Wharton et al 1974), subsequent reports have suggested lower limits. Some have suggested 2 mm (Friedrich & Wilkinson 1982), others preferred 1 mm (Iversen et al 1981) and further reports emphasize the importance of lymphatic or vascular invasion and the degree of differentiation (Parker et al 1975) or confluence (Hoffman et al 1983). However, all these have been retrospective studies and most of the subjects were women in whom invasive disease was not suspected initially but found in a specimen removed in the treatment of vulval intraepithelial disease.

The Gynecological Oncology Group undertook a prospective study of women with vulval cancer treated with radical vulvectomy and groin node dissection between November 1977 and February 1984. Superficial vulval cancer was identified in 272 of 558 women (Sedlis et al 1987). The group chose tumour thickness rather than depth of stromal invasion, which they found impracticable in their material. They found positive nodes even in women with tumours less than 1 mm thick (Table 41.2). They concluded that the risk of nodal disease was best assessed by a combination of factors. A later study of the whole group of 558 patients concurred that several factors were independent predictors of positive groin nodes (Homesley et al 1993). It was not possible to define a group free of risk. Finally, it is important to remember that prognostic factors worked out on one population must be tested against a second population to confirm their general applicability. This has never been done in this disease. It seems that the safest course is to perform groin node dissection in all cases of clinical carcinoma, regardless of the depth of invasion or the thickness of the tumour.

Frank invasion

Typical invasive disease is a keratinizing squamous carcinoma and involves the labia majora in about two-thirds of cases and the clitoris, labia minora or posterior fourchette and perineum in the remainder (Cavanagh et al 1985). Microscopic variants comprise a non-keratinizing carcinoma with multinucleated giant cells, a spindle cell squamous carcinoma and an acantholytic variant, the latter showing non-cohesive cells which may be arranged in an alveolar pattern, mimicking adenocarcinoma. The histopathologic report should include the site, size (in three dimensions), associated features (such as the presence of VIN or condylomata), the tumour type, depth of invasion, maximum horizontal measurement, whether the tumour is completely excised and the margins are free, presence or absence of vascular invasion, the nature of the adjacent non-malignant squamous epithelium, the number of

Table 41.1 Groin recurrences in women who did not undergo any form of groin node surgery. None had clinically suspicious lesions in the groin, all were regarded as 'low-risk cases'. In many, groin node surgery was omitted because of associated medical problems

Reference	Depth of lesion (mm)	Diameter of lesion (cm)	Number evaluable	Groin recurrence	DoD with groin disease
Magrina et al 1979	≤ 5	≤ 2	35	4	3
Hacker et al 1984a	> 1	≤ 2	23	2	2
Bryson et al 1991	NK	≤ 2	27	6	NK
Sutton et al 1991	≤ 1	≤ 2	10	0	0
Kelly et al 1992	≤ 1	≤ 2	13	0	0
Lingard et al 1992	NK	NK	20	7	7
			128	19 (14%)	

Table 41.2 Tumour thickness and positive groin nodes (Modified from Sedlis et al 1987)

Tumour thickness (mm)	Number of cases	% with positive nodes
< 1	32	3.1
1–2	56	8.9
2–3	59	18.6
3–4	68	30.9
4–5	57	33.3

Table 41.3 The FIGO staging of vulvar cancer (1995)

Stage	Definition
Stage Ia	Confined to vulva and/or perineum, 2 cm or less maximum diameter. Groin nodes not palpable. Stromal invasion no greater than 1 mm
Stage Ib	As for Ia but stromal invasion greater than 1 mm
Stage II	Confined to vulva and/or perineum, more than 2 cm maximum diameter. Groin nodes not palpable
Stage III	Extends beyond the vulva, vagina, lower urethra or anus; or unilateral regional lymph node metastasis
Stage IVa	Involves the mucosa of rectum or bladder; upper urethra; or pelvic bone; and/or bilateral regional lymph node metastases
Stage IVb	Any distant metastasis, including pelvic lymph node

lymph nodes lymph and the node status. The grading of the tumour is based on the percentage of undifferentiated cells, grade 1 having no undifferentiated cells, grade 2 having less than half undifferentiated cells and in grade 3 more than half consisting of poorly differentiated cells.

The tumour usually spreads slowly, infiltrating local tissue before metastasizing to the groin nodes. Spread to the contralateral groin occurs in about 25% of those cases with positive groin nodes, so bilateral groin node dissection is required in all cases with metastatic disease in the groin lymph nodes (Monaghan 1985a). Pelvic node involvement is not common (1.4–16.1%; Cavanagh et al 1985) and haematogenous spread to bone or lung is rare. Death is a long, unpleasant process and is often due to sepsis and inanition or haemorrhage. Uraemia from bilateral ureteric obstruction may supervene first. Such is the abject misery of this demise that all patients with resectable vulvar lesions should be offered surgery regardless of their age and general condition.

Clinical staging

The FIGO classification is shown in Table 41.3. In spite of the apparent limitations of this classification, it does give a reasonable guide to the prognosis. The main drawback was reliance on clinical palpation of the groin nodes, which is notoriously inaccurate (Monaghan 1985a). Now that the surgical findings are incorporated in the staging evaluation, the prognostic value of staging is greatly improved.

Diagnosis and assessment

Most patients with invasive disease (71%) complain of irritation or pruritus and 57% note a vulvar mass or ulcer (Monaghan 1985a). It is usually not until the mass appears that medical advice is sought. Bleeding (28%) and discharge (23%) are less common presentations. One of the major problems in invasive vulvar cancer is the delay between the first appearance of symptoms and referral for a gynaecological opinion. This is only partly due to the patient's reluctance to attend. In many cases the doctor fails to recognize the gravity of the lesion and prescribes topical therapy, sometimes without examining the woman. Delays of over 12 months are common, occurring in 33% of a large series collected in Florida (Cavanagh et al 1985).

Because of the multicentric nature of female lower genital tract cancer (Hammond & Monaghan 1983), the investigation of a patient with vulvar cancer should include inspection of the cervix and cervical cytology. The groin nodes must be palpated carefully and any suspicious nodes sampled by fine needle aspiration. A chest X-ray is always required and intravenous pyelography or lymphangiography may sometimes be helpful. Thorough examination under anaesthesia and a full-thickness generous biopsy are the most important investigations. The examination should note particularly the size and distribution of the primary lesion, especially the involvement of the urethra or anus, and secondary lesions in the vulval or perineal skin must be sought. The groins should be re-examined under general anaesthesia when the diagnostic biopsies are taken, as previously undetected nodes may be palpated at that time.

Ultrasound and fine needle aspiration cytology of the groins

It is possible to detect metastatic disease in groin nodes with the combination of ultrasound and fine needle aspiration for cytology (Moskovic et al 1999). The smallest metastasis detected was about 3 mm in diameter. The authors suggest that, if their findings are confirmed in a larger study, it may be possible to defer groin node dissection in those with no apparent disease. Their proposal is that such women would be followed up with ultrasound and fine needle aspiration at regular intervals for a number of years in order to detect progression of metastases that are initially below the threshold of detection of this technique. The most recent results suggest false-positive and false-negative results of around 10%. More false-negative results may become apparent with longer follow-up of those women who declined lymphadenectomy.

The frequency of scans will be determined by how long it would take the metastatic focus to grow from the limit of detection to the largest size that remains readily curable. For example, the limit of detection may be about 3 mm in diameter ($14\,mm^3$) and the largest, easily curable metastasis might be 5–7 mm in diameter (65–$180\,mm^3$). Such data as are available suggest that these tumours may double in volume every 6 weeks, implying that an undetected metastasis 3 mm in diameter might grow to 5–7 mm in diameter in 14–21 weeks.

The duration of follow-up will be determined by how long it takes the smallest, viable, undetected metastasis to grow to a detectable size. The smallest, viable metastasis is approximately $1000\,\mu^3$ so the tumour would need to double in volume 24 times to reach a diameter of 3 mm. The upper 95% confidence value for volume doubling time for these tumours is about 9 weeks, so it might take up to 216 weeks (4 years) before a tiny metastatic focus had grown sufficiently to be detected.

Given that some 35% of women with carcinoma of the vulva are found to have metastatic disease in their groin lymph nodes, it might seem that this technique might spare 65% an unnecessary lymphadenectomy. However, many of these apparently negative nodes will have undetected micrometastases. Occult metastases are found by serial sectioning or by immunohistochemistry in the axillary nodes of 9–17% of women with breast cancer (Cote et al 1999) and in 39% of women with stage I endometrial cancer (Yabushita et al 2001) and the presence of such metastases confers a worse prognosis. It is likely that even smaller metastases remain undetected. While no such studies have been undertaken in groin nodes from women with vulval cancer, these data would suggest that undetected micrometastases might affect at least 25% of apparently node-negative women. These metastases would be detected during follow-up but would reduce the proportion of women who are spared lymphadenectomy to 40%.

Avoidance of unnecessary inguinofemoral lymphadenectomy is a worthwhile objective. Ultrasound and fine needle aspiration may provide a way of achieving this but the technique is unproven. The calculations above suggest that follow-up ultrasound and fine needle aspiration of the most medial lymph node would need to be performed every 3 months for 4 years and might allow 40% of women with vulval carcinoma to avoid inguinofemoral lymphadenectomy. While this innovative technique offers the hope of sparing many women groin node dissection, its success will depend upon a very high level of ultrasound expertise and a rigorous follow-up regimen.

Treatment

Surgery

Surgery is the mainstay of treatment. The introduction of radical vulvectomy reduced the mortality from 80% to 40% (Taussig 1940, Way 1960). However, these techniques removed large areas of normal skin from the groins to control lymphatic spread and primary wound closure was rarely achieved. Modifications of this en bloc excision were devised to allow primary closure and to reduce the considerable morbidity (Fig. 41.2; Cavanagh et al 1990, Monaghan 1986). Although these variations did reduce the rate of wound breakdown without any apparent loss of efficacy, the morbidity remained high and impaired psychosexual function was common (Andersen & Hacker 1983). Much work in the past decade has aimed at reducing the morbidity still further without compromising the efficacy of the treatment.

Separate groin incisions In pursuit of an effective treatment with lower morbidity, the en bloc dissection of the groin nodes in continuity with the vulva was replaced by an operation using three separate incisions. This technique was originally suggested by Taussig (1940) and depended on the principle that lymphatic metastases developed initially by embolization. Therefore, in the early stages of spread there would be no residual tumour in the lymphatic channels between

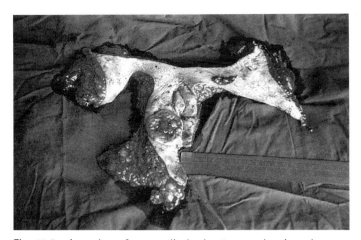

Fig. 41.2 A specimen from a radical vulvectomy and groin node dissection en bloc using a modified incision removing a minimum of skin from the groins. This operation would now only be used in women with clinical involvement of the groin nodes. Note the large amount of subcutaneous tissue removed from the vulva seen on the right.

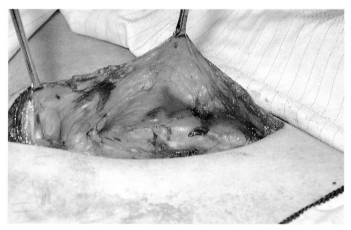

Fig. 41.3 The superficial plane deep to Camper's fascia is defined carefully, thus preserving sufficient subcutaneous fat to provide an adequate blood supply to the skin flap.

the tumour and the local lymph nodes in the groin. Many studies have since attested to the reduced morbidity of this method without loss of efficacy (Ballon & Lamb 1975, Byron et al 1962, Cavanagh et al 1990, Grimshaw et al 1993, Hacker et al 1981, Helm et al 1992). However, care needs to be taken in undercutting the skin edges so as to leave sufficient subcutaneous fat to provide a blood supply for the skin without, on the other hand, leaving superficial nodes in situ (Fig. 41.3). The inguinal nodes are removed from over the medial two-thirds of the inguinal ligaments and anterior to the cribriform fascia. The deep femoral nodes are removed by incising the cribriform fascia close to its medial margin over the femoral vessels and removing the fat and nodes medial to the vessels in the femoral triangle in the manner described by Micheletti et al (1990) (Fig. 41.4). The linear incision closes without tension and usually heals well (Fig. 41.5). Recurrent tumour in the bridge of skin between the groin and the vulva has been reported occasionally (Grimshaw et al 1993, Hacker

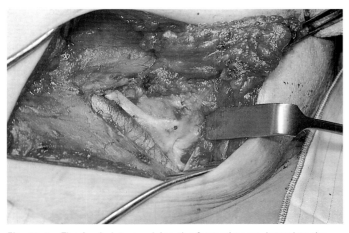

Fig. 41.4 The fascia lata overlying the femoral nerve, lateral to the femoral artery, has been preserved, but the femoral artery and the triangle medial to it have been meticulously dissected down to the surface of the adductor longus muscle posteriorly.

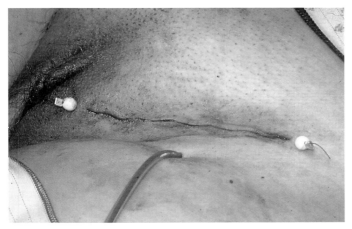

Fig. 41.5 The linear incision heals by first intention in the majority of cases, with greatly reduced morbidity.

et al 1981, Schulz & Penalver 1989, Sutton et al 1991). This is most likely to occur when the lymph nodes are extensively involved and such women are better treated with an en bloc technique.

Ipsilateral lymphadenectomy Spread to the contralateral groin from a lesion placed on one side of the vulva is very unusual without the ipsilateral nodes being involved (Grimshaw et al 1993, Homesley et al 1991, Table 41.4). This has led to the suggestion that, in the absence of clinical suspicion of groin node involvement, ipsilateral lymphadenectomy is sufficient to detect lymph node disease *provided the lesion is not centrally placed or bilateral*. If nodal disease is found in one groin, the opposite groin must also be explored.

Superficial inguinal lymphadenectomy A further modification of groin node lymphadenectomy, applied to women without clinical evidence of nodal disease, was the limitation of the dissection to the superficial nodes lying anterior to the cribriform fascia (DiSaia et al 1979). The rationale for this suggested change was the belief that lymphatic drainage from

Table 41.4 Inguinal node metastases in women with carcinoma of the vulva (Modified from Homesley et al 1991)

Nodal status	Midline lesions (n = 301)	Unilateral lesions (n = 287)	Total (n = 588)
Negative	61%	70%	65%
Bilateral	15%	6%	11%
Unilateral	24%	24%	24%
Ipsilateral		21%	
Contralateral		3%	
All positive	39%	30%	35%

the vulva passes first to the superficial inguinal nodes before subsequently going to the femoral nodes deep to the cribriform fascia (Borgno et al 1990, Parry-Jones 1960, Way 1948). The superficial nodes were sent for frozen section. Femoral lymphadenectomy was performed only if the pathologist identified lymphatic metastases. This placed a great responsibility upon the pathologist, who would have to identify and examine rapidly an average of 19 nodes from each groin (Helm et al 1992). Inevitably mistakes will occur, with tragic consequences (Berman et al 1989). It is unlikely that postoperative radiotherapy will prove an adequate substitute for complete surgical clearance of the groin in this situation. While superficial lymphadenectomy does reduce still further the risk of troublesome lymphoedema and wound breakdown (DiSaia et al 1979, Helm et al 1992) several authors have commented upon an apparent increase in nodal recurrences (Table 41.5).

The only prospective study of conservative surgery has been performed by the Gynecological Oncology Group (Stehman et al 1992a). This examined the role of ipsilateral superficial inguinal lymphadenectomy and modified radical hemivulvectomy in 121 women with primary carcinoma of the vulva, 2 cm or less in maximum diameter, 5 mm or less in thickness, without vascular space invasion and with no suspicious groin nodes. Patients found to have positive lymph nodes at primary surgery were withdrawn. Although this was a highly selected, low-risk group of patients, invasive disease recurred in 19 women (15.6%). There were nine (7.3%) groin and 10 (8.3%) vulval recurrences. Six of the groin recurrences occurred on the same side as the lymphadenectomy. At the time of the report, five of the nine women with recurrence in the groin had died, as had two of the 10 with vulval recurrences. These results were compared with a historical group of 96 similar patients who had been treated with radical vulvectomy and bilateral inguinofemoral lymphadenopathy. Six (6.3%) of these developed a vulval recurrence, one (1.0%) developed a pelvic recurrence, but none recurred in the groin. The recurrence-free survival was significantly better in the historical controls ($p = 0.0028$). The authors expressed concern at the high rate of recurrent disease and noted especially the groin recurrences. They speculated very reasonably that this might be due to undetected disease in the femoral nodes. This combined experience of superficial lymphadenectomy is not very reassuring. Even when applied to a low-risk population, it seems to be associated with an unacceptably high risk of recurrent disease in the groin, which is ultimately fatal in most cases.

Table 41.5 Groin recurrence after superficial inguinal lymphadenectomy. None had clinically suspicious groin nodes

Reference	Depth of lesion (mm)	Diameter of lesion (cm)	Other criteria	Vulval surgery	Number evaluable	Groin recurrence	DoD with groin disease
DiSaia et al 1979	≤ 5	≤ 1	Non-clitoral, nodes negative	WLE	16	0	0
Hacker et al 1984a	≤ 5	≤ 2	No suspicious nodes	WLE	3	1	1
Berman et al 1989	< 5	≤ 2	No suspicious or positive nodes	WLE	50	1	1
Burke et al 1990	> 1	0.5–6.5	No suspicious nodes	WLE	32	1	0
Sutton et al 1991	1–5	≤ 2	No suspicious nodes	MRV	36	1	1
Kelly et al 1992	< 1	≤ 2	No suspicious nodes	Various	11	1	0
Stehman et al 1992a	≤ 5	≤ 2	No suspicious or positive nodes	WLE	121	9	5
Helm et al 1992			All Stages	Various	32	3	1
					301	17 (5.7%)	9 (3.0%)

DoD, died of disease; WLE, wide local excision; MRV, modified radical vulvectomy

Sentinel node biopsy Sentinel node biopsy is a new technique which aims to avoid unnecessary lymphadenectomy. The data available on its use in breast disease are of interest to gynaecologists contemplating its potential value in vulval cancer.

Sentinel node biopsy began to be investigated in the management of breast cancer as an alternative to axillary lymph node dissection after initial work in melanoma (Querci della Rovere & Bird 1998). This depends upon the assumption that lymph drains from a specific area of the body into a single sentinel node before spreading on to other regional nodes and that this node can be identified by the injection of dye or radio-active isotope or both together into the skin adjacent to the tumour. The sentinel node is then dissected out and identified by the accumulation of dye or radio-activity. The node removed is then sent for detailed analysis by step section, immuno-histochemistry and PCR for epithelial or tumour-specific genes. If tumour is found, the patient undergoes lymph-adenectomy 1 or 2 weeks later.

This technique has not yet been tested in a randomized trial and its safety remains unproven. It is not always possible to identify a sentinel node and the dissection is often difficult and time consuming (Krag et al 1998). There is often more than one sentinel node (Veronesi et al 1997) and maybe as many as eight (Turner et al 1997) and the sentinel node may not be in the most superficial nodal group (Krag et al 1998).

It is the potential for false-negative results which is the most worrying aspect of this method. This is partly a failure of conventional techniques to identify metastatic disease in the lymph nodes removed. In one study, using immunostains for cytokeratin added 10 patients to the 33 identified by haematoxylin and eosin stain (Turner et al 1997). However, a residual problem is the presence of tumour in non-sentinel nodes. Different authors use different definitions for the false-negative rate, making rapid comparison of studies very difficult. Defining the false-negative rate as the number of women with a falsely negative result divided by the total number of women with nodal disease, multiplied by 100, the false-negative rates for four studies were 2.3%, 4.7%, 11% and 11.5% (Kapteijn et al 1997, Krag et al 1998, Turner et al 1997, Veronesi et al 1997). While most breast surgeons appear to be prepared to accept a false-negative rate of 1% and some would accept 5%, women appear not to be prepared to

accept any risk of false-negative results (Rozenberg et al 1999). Thus, none of the studies above has achieved a standard of safety which would be acceptable to the women interviewed by Rozenberg and his colleagues and two have false-negative rates well above the level regarded as acceptable by most of the surgeons.

Attempts to apply sentinel node biopsy to vulval carcinoma have proved even more disappointing (Ansink et al 1999). Even those who have expressed enthusiasm were unable to identify a sentinel node in 15% of groins dissected even after 2 years experience (Levenback et al 2001). In vulval carcinoma, effective lymphadenectomy clearly improves survival. This is probably not the case for melanoma and remains controversial in breast cancer. It is therefore particularly important to evaluate very carefully any new technique for vulval carcinoma because of the disastrous results which would ensue if metastatic disease was left untreated. At the moment, there is no place for the use of sentinel node biopsy in the management of vulval carcinoma outwith a clinical trial.

Deep femoral lymphadenectomy with preservation of the cribriform fascia A study in Turin has suggested that the deep femoral nodes may be excised without removing the fascia lata or the cribriform fascia (Micheletti et al 1990). An earlier study of 50 female cadavers confirmed that these nodes lie medial to the femoral vein and can be seen through the fossa ovalis (Borgno et al 1990). The altered technique suggested by this anatomical information was used in 42 women with vulval cancer. An average of nine nodes were removed from each groin, a number similar to cadaver studies. The 5-year survival rates of 91.4% and 86.7% in 14 and 18 women with stages I and II respectively are comparable to those reported in the literature. However, the wound complication rate remained high owing to retention of the 'butterfly' incision in the first 25 patients. This technique allows the radical removal of superficial and deep groin lymph nodes with reduced morbidity and has become our standard technique.

Pelvic lymphadenectomy There is little value in performing a pelvic node dissection, as this probably has no therapeutic value (Shimm et al 1986) and as radiation therapy to the groins and pelvis gives superior results when the groin nodes are involved (Homesley et al 1986).

Modified radical vulvectomy The major cause of psychosexual morbidity and of damage to body image comes from vulvectomy, particularly the removal of the clitoris and mons pubis. This has led some surgeons to devise more limited operations on the primary tumour when this has been small and unifocal (DiSaia et al 1971, Hacker et al 1984a). In all of these, the objective has been to obtain a margin of apparently healthy tissue of 2–3 cm all round the lesion. This is often impossible with lesions adjacent to the urethra or anus, but every effort must be made to maximize the margins even if this means sacrificing the lower 1–2 cm of the urethra or parts of the anus. The latter will sometimes make a colostomy necessary.

The risk of local recurrence is related to the size of the tumour-free margin (Heaps et al 1990). These authors recommended aiming for a tumour-free margin of only 1 cm, but the lesion may extend much further than is obvious to naked-eye inspection, so obtaining a wider zone of healthy tissue would be prudent. Not only are wide lateral margins required, but the dissection must be taken down to the deep fascia in exactly the same way as a traditional radical vulvectomy. These 'wide local excisions', 'hemivulvectomies' or 'modified radical vulvectomies' are very radical operations indeed, but in suitable cases do permit preservation of the clitoris and part of the vulva. The effect on psychosexual function has not been studied in depth, but it does seem likely that these procedures are less damaging (DiSaia et al 1979).

The reported vulval recurrences following radical local excision are shown in Table 41.6. The recurrence rate of 6.3% is a little disappointing for what are generally small, low-risk tumours. However, very few of these women subsequently died of their disease because vulval recurrences are fairly readily treated (Piura et al 1993, Tilmans et al 1992). A retrospective comparison of radical vulvectomy with modified radical vulvectomy found no difference in recurrence rates or cancer deaths in a small study with 45 patients in each group (Hoffman et al 1991). However, there were differences between the groups, not least in the length of follow-up, which

was much shorter in the modified vulvectomy patients. More importantly, it was impossible to say why the women had been assigned to a particular form of treatment. There must be a substantial risk of an undetected bias in any study of this sort.

A similar, but much larger, study was undertaken at the MD Anderson Centre (Rutledge et al 1991), consisting of an analysis of the records of 365 women with carcinoma of the vulva treated between 1944 and 1990. A Cox proportional hazards model was used to identify factors which predicted recurrence and death. This technique allows the effect of all known variables to be evaluated individually and together. An analysis of the 176 stage I–II lesions treated with curative intent showed no difference in the disease-free survival or the survival corrected for death from intercurrent disease between women treated with radical vulvectomy and those who underwent radical local excision. Although this is reassuring, it should be noted that only 27 women were treated with radical local excision and few of these had been followed for more than 2 years (Mitchell, personal communication).

Complications The complication rate depends on the surgical method, but all share common problems. The most common complication is wound breakdown and infection. With the triple incision technique this is seldom more than a minor problem. Conservative therapy with liquid honey packs is all that is required for the occasional dehiscence. Osteitis pubis is a rare but very serious complication that requires intensive and prolonged antibiotic therapy. Thromboembolic disease is always a greatly feared complication of surgery for malignant disease, but the combination of perioperative epidural analgesia to ensure good venous return with subcutaneous heparin begun 12–24 hours before the operation seems to reduce this risk. Secondary haemorrhage occurs from time to time. Chronic leg oedema may be expected in 14–21% of women (Grimshaw et al 1993, Hacker et al 1981). Numbness and paraesthesia over the anterior thigh are common owing to the division of small cutaneous branches of

Table 41.6 Vulval recurrences and deaths following conservative vulval surgery

Reference	Depth of lesion (mm)	Diameter of lesion (cm)	Other criteria	Vulval surgery	Groin surgery	Number evaluable	Vulval recurrence	DoD with vulval disease
DiSaia et al 1979	≤ 5	≤ 1	Non-clitoral, nodes negative	WLE	SIL	16	0	0
Hacker et al 1984a	9/10<1	≤ 2	No suspicious nodes	WLE	None	11	1	1
Hacker et al 1984a	≤ 5	≤ 2	No suspicious nodes	WLE	SIL	3	0	0
Hacker et al 1984a	≤ 5	≤ 2	No suspicious nodes	WLE/MRV	IFL	14	0	0
Burrell et al 1988	> 1	0.7–4.5	Included suspicious nodes	MRV	IFL	28	0	0
Berman et al 1989	< 5	≤ 2	No suspicious or positive nodes	WLE	SIL	50	4	0
Burke et al 1990	> 1	0.5–6.5	No suspicious nodes	WLE	SIL	32	2	0
Hoffman et al 1991	> 1	≤ 6	Included suspicious nodes	MRV	Various	45	1	0
Sutton et al 1991	≤ 1	≤ 2	No suspicious nodes	WLE	None	10	0	0
Sutton et al 1991	1–5	≤ 2	No suspicious nodes	MRV	SIL	36	3	0
Kelly et al 1992	> 1	≤ 2	No suspicious nodes	WLE	Various	18	3	0
Stehman et al 1992a	≤ 5	≤ 2	No suspicious or positive nodes	WLE	SIL	121	10	2
						384	24 (6.3%)	3 (0.8%)

DoD, died of disease; WLE, wide local excision; MRV, modified radical vulvectomy; SIL, superficial inguinal lymphadenectomy; IFL, inguinofemoral lymphadenectomy the femoral nerve. Loss of body image and impaired sexual function are common after surgery but 72% of those who were sexually active before surgery continue with sexual activity after surgery (Green et al 2000). The extent of surgery is not related to the degree of sexual dysfunction.

Conclusions The current emphasis of research in the surgical treatment of vulval carcinoma is on reducing morbidity, especially for the young women in whom the disease appears to be becoming more common. However, reduced morbidity must not be gained at the cost of increased recurrence and mortality. There is little solid evidence on which to base a decision as to the best practice. Whereas most agree that an en bloc dissection of the inguinofemoral nodes and the vulva remains the optimum treatment for women with clinically suspicious nodes, there is no general agreement as to the best management for early invasive disease.

Groin node dissection Given the available evidence, the lack of consistent results and the very high mortality associated with groin recurrences, it seems that the safest course is to perform a groin node dissection in all cases with more than 1 mm stromal invasion and to remove both superficial and deep nodes en bloc. A possible exception might be women with what appears to be VIN III in whom a small, superficial focus of invasion is found histologically. These might not require lymphadenectomy. It certainly does not make sense to omit groin node dissection in elderly women, because they have a higher incidence of nodal disease (Homesley et al 1993). Individual women with selected stage I–II lesions may prefer to take the risk of unilateral lymphadenectomy, but very careful pathological and clinical assessment would be necessary to advise on the degree of risk. Separate incisions in the groin are recommended in cases without clinically suspicious nodes, but en bloc excision with the vulva is probably required in other cases. The technique of deep femoral lymphadenectomy which preserves the cribriform fascia appears to reduce morbidity without any loss of efficacy.

Vulval dissection Because recurrent disease on the vulva does not carry such a high risk of mortality, and because it is the vulval surgery which has the greatest impact upon a woman's body image and sexuality, there is more to be gained and less to lose from conservative vulval surgery. Although the evidence supporting radical local excision is far from conclusive it would seem to offer a reasonable approach, provided the principles of wide lateral and deep margins are observed. The benefits will be far less in anterior and clitoral lesions. Large or multicentric lesions will still require radical vulvectomy to achieve adequate local control. Such tumours may benefit from preoperative irradiation (see below).

The role of radiotherapy

The three major roles for radiotherapy in the treatment of vulval cancer are in preoperative, postoperative and palliative therapy. Research continues into the use of radiotherapy and chemotherapy as alternatives to surgery. Just as surgery has evolved to reduce morbidity, so radiotherapy has been modified to minimize morbidity without compromising the outcome. Modern treatment machines mean that this is an easier objective and the severe late radiation reactions, including vulva fibrosis, atrophy and even necrosis, are now largely

things of the past. Similarly, more conservative regimens are being adopted in parallel with more conservative surgery.

Technique Hyperfractionation, giving two fractions per day at least 6 hours apart, has been used in order to complete treatment prior to the development of acute toxicity. The use of chemoirradiation either alone or as an adjunct to surgery has been advocated by GM Thomas who dominates the literature in this area. Giving radiotherapy both pre- and postoperatively can be difficult depending on the local reaction which may interfere with the surgery subsequently or delayed healing which may be seen when giving postoperative radiotherapy.

Where surgical management is not possible interstitial radiotherapy may be used. This can involve an isotope such as iridium-192, which is often delivered using needles. The procedure is carried out under general anaesthesia. For small lesions when interstitial therapy is used alone, the total dose should be no higher than 65 Gy given over 6–7 days to prevent serious morbidity.

Primary radical radiotherapy Radiotherapy is considered as primary radical treatment only for patients who are unfit for surgery. In general, this is a limited number of cases and more usually a combined approach of radiotherapy, chemotherapy and conservative surgery is used.

Preoperative radiotherapy to the vulva Patients with large tumours which extend very close to or involve the urethra, vagina or anus may benefit from preoperative radiotherapy alone or with chemotherapy to facilitate subsequent surgery and reduce morbidity. Preoperative radiotherapy can be given to the vulva without serious complications and substantially reduces the size of the lesions (Acosta et al 1978, Boronow et al 1987, Hacker et al 1984b, Rotmensch et al 1990). However, postoperative wound breakdown is common and very debilitating. Healing may take many months.

Postoperative radiotherapy to the vulva Heaps et al (1990) concluded that a surgical disease-free margin of less than 8 mm was associated with a 50% chance of recurrence. If further surgery is not going to be possible, postoperative radiotherapy to the vulva should be considered. The radiotherapy field may not always need to cover the whole vulva but can be confined to the site of disease in early lateral lesions (Thomas et al 1991).

Radiotherapy for groin node disease Some 20% of women with positive groin nodes will have metastatic disease in the pelvic lymph nodes. Radiotherapy to the groin and pelvic nodes is more effective than pelvic lymphadenectomy in the management of women with positive groin nodes if given after a complete inguinofemoral lymphadenectomy (Homesley et al 1986) and is now given to all women with more than microscopic disease of one groin node. A total dose of 45–50 Gy in 1.8–2.0 Gy fractions is administered to the midplane of the pelvis in opposed anterior and posterior fields, using a midline block to protect the vulva. In addition, 45–50 Gy, measured 2–3 cm from the anterior surface, is given to the centre of the inguinal and femoral nodes. Using this technique, both the time to recurrence and the survival are improved.

Preoperative radiotherapy to the groins and pelvis may be of value in women with clinically detectable disease in the nodes (Boronow et al 1987). Only one of seven had residual disease at surgery following radiotherapy, compared with seven of nine to whom radiotherapy was not given. Some authors have even suggested radiotherapy as an alternative to inguinofemoral lymphadenectomy (Perez et al 1993). However, this opinion was based upon a retrospective review of a highly selected group of 37 women treated over a period of 22 years. In contrast, the Gynecological Oncology Group prematurely terminated a prospective randomized controlled trial comparing radiotherapy with inguinofemoral lymphadenectomy in a group of women with clinically non-involved nodes because of the higher recurrence rate ($p = 0.033$) and mortality ($p = 0.035$) in the radiation group (Stehman et al 1992b). The 20% of those who were found to have positive nodes at surgery received postoperative radiotherapy to the groin and pelvis. Five (18.5%) groin relapses occurred in the radiation-only group, compared to none in the groin dissection regimen. Although radiation is a useful supplement to inguinofemoral lymphadenectomy, it is not an effective substitute and preoperative radiotherapy is associated with substantial wound problems.

Multimodality therapy for carcinoma of the vulva

Given the very promising results seen in carcinoma of the cervix, it is likely that concurrent chemoradiation will be more widely investigated in the treatment of carcinoma of the vulva. The data from carcinoma of the cervix suggest that the most important drug is cisplatin and therefore this is most likely to be the candidate drug in chemoradiation protocols for carcinoma of the vulva. The aim of such treatment would be to decrease tumour bulk prior to surgery and therefore improve outcome and lower the morbidity of surgery. Unfortunately, the morbidity is often increased by the high rate of wound problems.

Preoperative chemoradiation for very advanced disease in the groin nodes or the vulva does produce complete responses in up to 30% of patients and reduces the radicality of surgery required in many (Montana et al 2000, Moore et al 1998). The results seem to be superior to radiation alone (Han et al 2000). However, these regimens are very toxic, many patients are unable to complete the therapy, wound complications are considerable and the treatment-related death rate is around 5%. In spite of promising initial responses, the recurrence rate remains high. There is no doubt that such multimodality protocols require close co-operation of oncologist and gynaecologists in both the design and implementation of trials.

Conclusion Surgery remains the mainstay of treatment, but radiotherapy has a proven role in the treatment of groin node disease after inguinofemoral lymphadenectomy. It may also prevent local recurrence in the vulva when there is an insufficient tumour-free margin. Radiotherapy may be used for the preoperative treatment of advanced disease. Chemotherapy may add to the efficacy of radiotherapy when used concurrently, but this has not yet been demonstrated by randomized studies.

Recurrent disease

Although most women with recurrence in the groin die in spite of treatment, surgical excision of a vulval recurrence can be effective, especially if the recurrence is delayed for more than 2 years (Grimshaw et al 1993, Shimm et al 1986). However, in many patients only palliative treatment

is possible and this is usually radiotherapy, either external or interstitial.

Chemotherapy may be given with the radiotherapy or alone. As well as regimens using 5-fluorouracil, other cytotoxic combinations have been assessed. The EORTC used a continuous low-dose regimen designed for elderly women consisting of bleomycin, methotrexate and CCNU given as a 6-week cycle repeated three times, depending on response and toxicity (Durrant et al 1990). Although 60% of 28 women with inoperable or recurrent tumours showed a response, toxicity was unacceptably high, particularly stomatitis and infection secondary to myelosuppression. Single-agent chemotherapy using bleomycin or cisplatin can give a few partial responses, but is usually ineffective (Deppe et al 1979, Thigpen et al 1986).

Results of treatment

Corrected survival rates from two large studies are shown in Table 41.7 (Grimshaw et al 1993, Homesley et al 1993). These use the 1988 FIGO staging which includes the surgical findings, so stages I and II do not have groin lymph node involvement. However, stages III and IV are more heterogeneous. The overall 5-year corrected survival in the British study was 74.6% (Grimshaw et al 1993).

Uncommon tumours of the vulva

Melanoma

Approximately 9% of melanomas in women occur on the vulva where they occur more commonly than in any other location. Melanoma is the second most common vulval malignancy (Monaghan & Hammond 1984, Morrow & DiSaia 1976). Melanin production is variable and the lesions range from black to completely amelanotic in 27% of patients, predominantly in glabrous skin (Ragnarsson-Olding et al 1999). The most usual presenting complaint is of a lump or an enlarging mole. Pruritus and bleeding are less common. Vulval melanomas are divided into mucosal lentiginous (57%), nodular (22%) and superficial spreading types (4%). Staging and tumour thickness are independent predictors of survival.

Local invasion occurs in an outward direction as well as downward, so excision margins must be very wide, 3–5 cm being suggested for all but the most superficial lesions (White & Polk 1986). Approximately one-third of patients have inguinal lymph node metastases at presentation and 2.6% have distant spread (Morrow & DiSaia 1976). When the nodes are negative, the 5-year survival is approximately 56%, falling to 14% when

Table 41.7 Survival by FIGO Stage (1988) (Homesley et al 1993, Grimshaw et al 1993)

FIGO Stage	Corrected 5-year survival (%)	
	Grimshaw et al (1993)	Homesley et al (1993)
I	97	98
II	85	85
III	46	74
IV	50	31

the nodes are positive (Morrow & DiSaia 1976). Involvement of urethra or vagina, or the presence of satellite lesions, all worsen the prognosis.

It is probable that the minimum therapy should be wide local excision (this usually requires a radical vulvectomy) without lymphadenectomy unless there is clinical evidence of groin disease (Davidson et al 1987, White & Polk 1986). If the groin nodes are removed, the operation should be performed en bloc rather than through separate incisions because of the melanoma's propensity to spread unseen by lateral intradermal infiltration (Karlen et al 1975). Radiation therapy is ineffective (White & Polk 1986) and adjuvant chemotherapy and immunotherapy have no proven value. Chemotherapy has not proved effective in the treatment of recurrent disease (Seeger et al 1986).

Verrucous carcinoma

This slowly growing neoplasm is seen rarely on the vulva (Gallousis 1972, Isaacs 1976). Both macroscopically and histologically it resembles condyloma acuminata and the diagnosis can be difficult. Generous biopsies are required to provide sufficient material for the pathologist. The lesion is a very well-differentiated squamous carcinoma showing prominent acanthosis with a pushing tumour–dermal interface. The treatment is surgery, usually a radical vulvectomy but very occasionally wide local excision. The place of lymphadenectomy is debatable, as lymph node metastases are uncommon. Radiotherapy is ineffective and may result in anaplastic transformation (Kraus & Perez-Mesa 1966).

Basal cell carcinoma

This tumour is rarely found on the vulva (2–4%). Wide local excision gives excellent results in most cases.

Bartholin's gland carcinoma

The criteria for the diagnosis of Bartholin's gland tumour are that it must arise at the site of Bartholin's gland and not be metastatic. Usually an adenocarcinoma, this tumour may be squamous, transitional cell type or even mixed squamous and adenocarcinoma (Cavanagh et al 1985). It has often spread widely to pelvic and groin nodes before the diagnosis is made. It must be distinguished from adenoid cystic carcinoma, which is similar to the tumour found in salivary glands and which seldom gives rise to metastatic disease (Cavanagh et al 1985, Webb et al 1984). The treatment is surgery but because of its deep origin, part of the vagina, levatores ani and the ischiorectal fat must be removed.

Sarcomas

This is a heterogeneous group of rare tumours arising from soft tissue. Leiomyosarcomas are the most frequent and may be difficult to distinguish from their benign counterpart histologically. Features of malignancy are tumour size 5 cm or more in greatest dimension, infiltrative margins, five or more mitotic figures per 10 high-power fields and moderate to severe cytologic atypia. Tumours that have only one of these characteristics should be diagnosed as leiomyoma; those that exhibit only two of these features are considered benign but atypical leiomyomas. The sarcomas should be excised with wide margins. Leiomyomas and the atypical leiomyomas are excised more conservatively, with long-term follow-up (Nielsen et al 1996). In contrast, rhabdomyosarcomas are rapidly growing, aggressive tumours. A radical vulvectomy and groin node dissection is the usual treatment, but local recurrence is common and haematogenous spread is unaffected by this treatment (Cavanagh et al 1985, DiSaia et al 1971).

Conclusions

The main problems with carcinoma of the vulva are delay in presentation and diagnosis and inadequate initial therapy. Surgery remains the cornerstone of treatment but, in carefully selected cases, this can be made less extensive than in the past. Even when radical surgery is necessary, new techniques have reduced the morbidity enormously. Radiotherapy has an important role to play in the treatment of patients with metastatic groin node disease.

CANCER OF THE VAGINA

Introduction

Invasive vaginal cancer is rare. With 184 cases in England and Wales in 1997, the incidence was 0.7/100 000 women (OPCS 2001). However, like the cervix, the vagina has a range of premalignant lesions, many of which may be previously unrecognized extensions of cervical abnormalities. Coincident with the rise in prevalence of cervical intraepithelial neoplasia (CIN) is an increase in the frequency with which vaginal intraepithelial neoplasia (VAIN) is seen.

Aetiology

Irritation, immunosuppression, infection

There is little firm evidence on aetiological agents. The irritation caused by procidentia and vaginal pessaries has been suggested but this is an infrequent association (Al-Kurdi & Monaghan 1981, Benedet et al 1983). A field effect in the lower genital tract has been suggested by the observation of multicentric neoplasia involving cervix, vagina and vulva (Hernandez-Linares et al 1980, Weed et al 1983), and both immunosuppression and infection with HPV have been suggested (Carson et al 1986, Weed et al 1983).

Radiation-induced vaginal cancer

The aetiological role of radiotherapy is hard to determine, but is no longer simply a theoretical question in view of the proposal that preinvasive disease of the vaginal vault after hysterectomy should be treated by radiotherapy (Woodman et al 1988).

Evidence for radiation-induced vaginal cancer Three studies have raised a concern that women less than 40 years old treated with radiotherapy for cervical cancer may be at a high risk of subsequently developing vaginal cancer 10–40 years later. A high proportion of those women who developed a primary vaginal cancer after radiotherapy for cervical cancer were less than 40 years of age when treated for their first cancer (Barrie & Brunschwig 1970, Choo & Anderson

1982). Futoran & Nolan (1976) reported the appearance of a primary vaginal cancer in eight of 42 women treated with radiotherapy for stage I cervical cancer when less than 40 years of age and followed for 10 years or more.

Evidence for the defence However, only 50 (1.54%) of 3239 patients treated for cervical cancer, most with radiotherapy, subsequently developed a primary vaginal neoplasm and only 29 of these had invasive lesions (Choo & Anderson 1982). Furthermore, an international collaborative study of cancer registers recorded only 48 cancers of the vagina or vulva (ICD7–176) in 25 995 women treated with radiotherapy for cervical cancer and followed for 10 or more years (Boice et al 1985). The proportion of women treated with surgery and followed for 10 or more years and who were recorded as developing a vaginal or vulval cancer was similar (seven of 5125) to that seen following radiotherapy. These data suggest that if vaginal cancer is induced by radiotherapy, it is a very rare event.

Diethylstilboestrol

For some time the prevalence of clear cell adenocarcinoma of the vagina was thought to be increased by intrauterine exposure to diethylstilboestrol (Herbst et al 1971). With the accrual of more information the risks now seem to be very low and to lie between 0.1 and 1.0 per 1000 (Coppleson 1984, Herbst 1984). Whereas vaginal adenosis and minor anatomical abnormalities of no significance (e.g. cervical cockscomb) are common following intrauterine diethylstilboestrol exposure, the only lesion of any significance that is seen more commonly is CIN (Robboy et al 1984). Uterine malformations may be more common and may result in impaired fecundity in a small minority of cases.

Anatomy

The anatomy of the vagina is described in Chapters 2 and 36.

Pathology

The great majority (92%) of primary vaginal cancers are squamous. Clear cell adenocarcinomas, malignant melanomas, embryonal rhabdomyosarcomas and endodermal sinus tumours are the commonest of the small number of other tumours seen very rarely in the vagina. These are discussed separately.

Natural history

Although the upper vagina is the commonest site for invasive disease, about 25–30% is confined to the lower vagina, usually the anterior wall (Gallup et al 1987, Monaghan 1985b, Pride et al 1979). Squamous vaginal cancer spreads by local invasion initially. Lymphatic spread occurs by tumour embolization to the pelvic nodes from the upper vagina and to both pelvic and inguinal nodes from the lower vagina (Monaghan 1985b). Haematogenous spread is unusual.

Clinical staging

The FIGO clinical staging is shown in Table 41.8.

Table 41.8 FIGO staging for vaginal cancer (Pettersson 1995)

Stage	Definition
Stage 0	Intraepithelial neoplasia
Stage I	Invasive carcinoma confined to vaginal mucosa
Stage II	Subvaginal infiltration not extending to pelvic wall
Stage III	Extends to pelvic wall
Stage IVa	Involves mucosa of bladder or rectum
Stage IVb	Spread beyond the pelvis

Diagnosis and assessment

Before making a diagnosis of primary vaginal cancer, the following criteria must be satisfied: the primary site of growth must be in the vagina; the uterine cervix must not be involved; and there must be no clinical evidence that the vaginal tumour is metastatic disease (Beller et al 2001). To this list, Murad and colleagues (1975) would add that the patient should not have had any antecedent genital cancer. Choo & Anderson (1982) dissent from this view, which they regard as too restrictive. In their series, 11 of the 14 invasive vaginal cancers following radiation therapy for cervical cancer occurred after an interval of more than 10 years and three were of a different histological type.

The most common presenting symptom is vaginal bleeding (53–65%), with vaginal discharge (11–16%) and pelvic pain (4–11%) being less common (Gallup et al 1987, Pride et al 1979). The rate of detection of asymptomatic cancer with vaginal cytology varies greatly (10–42%), depending on the patient population studied, and most of the disease thus detected is at an early stage (Choo & Anderson 1982, Gallup et al 1987, Pride et al 1979).

The most important part of the pretreatment assessment of invasive cancer of the vagina is a careful examination under anaesthesia. Colposcopy will identify co-existing VAIN and help to define the location of the lesion. A combined vaginal and rectal examination will help to detect extravaginal spread. Cystoscopy and proctosigmoidoscopy are indicated if anterior or posterior spread is suspected. A generous, full-thickness biopsy is essential for adequate histological evaluation. A chest X-ray and an intravenous pyelogram are the only radiological investigations required routinely, but lymphangiography can help occasionally in stage II cases to determine the need for teletherapy (external beam therapy). Transrectal ultrasound and magnetic resonance imaging can be used to define the size and extent of the lesion.

Treatment and complications

Radiotherapy

Invasive vaginal cancer is usually treated with radiotherapy. Early cases, stage I–IIa, may be treated entirely with interstitial therapy with iridium-192. In the Hammersmith Hospital this is afterloaded into three concentric rings of stainless steel guide needles located by a specially designed template (Branson et al 1985). The two outer rings of needles are located in the paravaginal space by being inserted through the perineum under general anaesthesia. The inner ring is located in grooves on a vaginal obturator. The objective is to achieve a tumour dose of 70–80 Gy in two fractions, each over 72 hours, 2 weeks apart. Cases with parametrial involvement receive teletherapy to the pelvis as for carcinoma of the cervix, with a tumour dose of 45 Gy followed by interstitial or intracavitary therapy to a total dose of 70–75 Gy. The field may be extended to include the groins if the tumour involves the lower half of the vagina.

Complications of radiotherapy   As with the treatment of vulva carcinoma, the severe complications of radiation have become much less common as a result of modern treatment methods and more sophisticated linear accelerators. Vaginal stenosis may occur and is more likely when advanced tumours are treated (Puthawala et al 1983). There has been a reduction in the instance of vaginal stenosis from 25–32% to 10–15% although it is obviously a problem for sexually active patients. Mucosal ulceration, either immediate or delayed, can be a distressing complication but conservative therapy, sometimes aided by grafts, is usually effective. Approximately 10% of patients develop a fistula or other serious complication (Gallup et al 1987, Pride et al 1979, Puthawala et al 1983) and these are almost invariably associated with teletherapy for advanced disease (Pride et al 1979). Vesicovaginal and rectovaginal fistulae and small bowel complications are especially frequent if previously irradiated patients are treated with radiotherapy (Choo & Anderson 1982).

Surgery

A stage I lesion in the upper vagina can be adequately treated by radical hysterectomy (if the uterus is still present), radical vaginectomy and pelvic lymphadenectomy (Ball & Berman 1982, Johnston et al 1983) (Fig. 41.6). Exenteration is required for more advanced lesions and carries the problems of stomata. However, surgery may be the treatment of choice for women who have had prior pelvic radiotherapy (Choo & Anderson 1982).

Results

Probably as a result of the small numbers of cases in the reported series, the 5-year survival figures described for stage I range widely from 64% to 90% and for stage II from 29% to 66% (Monaghan 1985b). The results of therapy in more advanced disease are less satisfactory, with 5-year figures for stage III of 17–49% (Monaghan 1985b). Some of the best results in a reasonably sized series are quoted by Perez & Camel (1982) and the largest series reported is by Kucera and colleagues (1985) (Table 41.9).

Conclusions

Invasive vaginal cancer is a rare tumour more often seen in association with an antecedent cervical malignancy. Radiotherapy is the main treatment method. Interstitial therapy offers good cure rates in stages I–IIa, with only a small risk of seriously impairing vaginal function. Teletherapy is added for more advanced cases. Previous pelvic radiotherapy greatly increases the risk of serious complications and individualization of treatment regimens is essential for the best results.

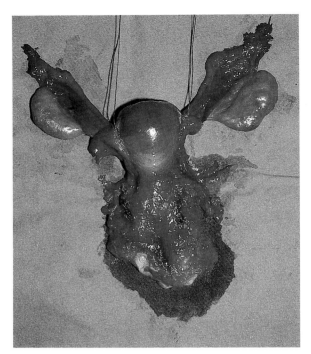

Fig. 41.6   Radical hysterectomy and total vaginectomy for stage I carcinoma extending into the middle third of the vagina.

Table 41.9   Five-year survival rates for vaginal cancer

Stage	Perez & Camel (1982)		Kucera et al (1985)	
	No. of cases	% Alive	No. of cases	% Alive
0	15	90		
I	39	90	67	75
IIa	39	58		
IIb	21	32		
II			120	46
III	12	40	191	29
IV	8	0	83	19

Uncommon vaginal tumours

Clear cell adenocarcinoma

The relation of this rare tumour to intrauterine exposure to diethylstilboestrol is discussed under aetiology. The histology is characterized by vacuolated or clear areas in the cytoplasm and a hobnail appearance of the nuclei of cells displaying a solid, tubulocystic or papillary pattern. Radical surgery or radical radiotherapy is required for invasive lesions. As most are situated in the upper vagina they may be treated as cervical lesions. Lymph node metastases and 5-year survival figures are equivalent to those for cervical cancer (Herbst & Scully 1983).

Malignant melanoma

Melanoma accounts for less than 3% of malignant tumours of vagina. Because the vagina does not have a papillary dermis and reticular dermis the depth of invasion should be measured as a prognostic indication. Vaginal melanoma has a 5-year survival rate of only 7% (Lee et al 1984). Vaginal bleeding and discharge are the most common presenting symptoms. The prognosis depends upon the depth of epithelial invasion. Radical surgery and radiotherapy are of little value if the lesion is deeply invasive because of its propensity to metastasize early via the bloodstream. There is at present no effective chemotherapy.

Rhabdomyosarcoma (sarcoma botryoides)

Some 90% of these rare tumours occur in children less than 5 years old. They present with vaginal bleeding and a grape-like mass in the vagina. The appearance of cross-striations in the rhabdomyoblasts is characteristic of this tumour. The results of radical surgery are poor (Huffman 1968), but chemotherapy alone with VAC (vincristine, actinomycin D and cyclophosphamide) now gives 'cure' in 82% of cases (Raney et al 1983). Indeed, Dewhurst (1985) reported seven alive and well out of a small personal series of nine children followed for 4–19 years. Recent reports confirm the results of these older studies (Crist et al 2001). The results of chemotherapy in postpubertal women are not nearly as good and multimodality treatment is required more often (Hahlin et al 1998).

Endodermal sinus tumour

These very rare tumours may resemble rhabdomyosarcomas but histology shows a primitive adenocarcinoma. Most occur in infants under the age of 2. Although surgery used to be the mainstay of treatment, with an occasional long-term survivor (Dewhurst & Ferreira 1981), chemotherapy with regimens used for this tumour in other sites may offer a hope for more long-term cures (Wiltshaw 1985).

KEY POINTS

1. The prognosis for vulval cancer is good if the lesion is treated adequately at an early stage.
2. Even elderly and relatively unfit women should be treated surgically.
3. There is no place for superficial inguinal lymphadenectomy in the treatment of vulval carcinoma and sentinel node biopsy remains an experimental approach.
4. Inguinofemoral lymphadenectomy should be carried out in all but a small minority of cases which usually present as VIN rather than clinical invasion.
5. Local radical excision must remove the tumour with wide lateral and deep margins.
6. Radiotherapy should be used to treat the pelvis and groins of women with two or more positive groin nodes.
7. Radiotherapy with or without chemotherapy may have a role in treating large tumours prior to surgery but this remains an experimental approach associated with considerable morbidity.
8. Radiotherapy rarely, if ever, causes a vaginal carcinoma.
9. The risks of vaginal cancer in diethylstilboestrol-exposed women now appear to be very low indeed.
10. Early vaginal cancer may be treated with surgery or interstitial brachytherapy but more advanced cases are better treated with radiotherapy.

REFERENCES

Acosta AA, Given FT, Frazier AB, Cordoba RB, Luminari A 1978 Preoperative radiation therapy in the management of squamous cell carcinoma of the vulva: preliminary report. American Journal of Obstetrics and Gynecology 132:198–206

Al-Kurdi M, Monaghan JM 1981 Thirty-two years experience in management of primary tumours of the vagina. British Journal of Obstetrics and Gynaecology 88:1145–1150

Andersen BL, Hacker NF 1983 Psychosexual adjustment after vulvar surgery. Obstetrics and Gynecology 62:457–462

Ansink A, Sie-Go DMDS, Simons EA et al 1999 Sentinel node detection in vulvar cancer patients: a multicentre study. British Journal of Obstetrics and Gynaecology 106:380

Ball HG, Berman ML 1982 Management of primary vaginal carcinoma. Gynecologic Oncology 14:154–163

Ballon SC, Lamb EJ 1975 Separate incisions in the treatment of carcinoma of the vulva. Surgery, Gynecology and Obstetrics 140:81–84

Barrie JR, Brunschwig A 1970 Late second cancers of the cervix after apparent successful initial radiation therapy. American Journal of Roentgenology and Therapeutic Nuclear Medicine 109:109–112

Beller U, Sidei M, Maisonneuve P 2001 Carcinoma of the vagina. 24th Annual Report of the Results of Treatment in Gynaecological cancer. Journal of Epidemiology and Biostatistics 6:141–152

Benedet JL, Murphy KJ, Fairey RN, Boyes DA 1983 Primary invasive carcinoma of the vagina. Obstetrics and Gynecology 62:715–719

Bergeron C, Ferenczy A, Shah K, Naghashfar Z 1987 Multicentric human papillomavirus infections of the female genital tract: correlation of viral types with abnormal mitotic figures, colposcopic presentation and location. Obstetrics and Gynecology 69:736–742

Berman ML, Soper JT, Creasman WT, Olt GT, DiSaia PJ 1989 Conservative surgical management of superficially invasive Stage I vulvar carcinoma. Gynecologic Oncology 35:352–357

Boehm F, Morris JM 1971 Paget's disease and apocrine gland carcinoma of the vulva. Obstetrics and Gynecology 38:185–192

Boice JD, Day NE, Andersen A et al 1985 Second cancers following treatment for cervical cancer. An international collaboration among cancer registries. Journal of the National Cancer Institute 74:955–975

Borgno G, Micheletti L, Barbero M et al 1990 Topographic distribution of groin lymph nodes. Journal of Reproductive Medicine 35:1127–1129

Boronow RC, Hickman BT, Reagan MT et al 1987 Combined therapy as an alternative to exenteration for locally advanced vulvovaginal cancer. American Journal of Clinical Oncology 10:171–181

Branson AN, Dunn P, Kam KC, Lambert HE 1985 A device for interstitial therapy of low pelvic tumours – the Hammersmith Perineal Hedgehog. British Journal of Radiology 58:537–542

Brinton LA, Nasca PC, Mallin K, Baptiste MS, Willbanks GD, Richart RM 1990 Case control study of cancer of the vulva. Obstetrics and Gynecology 75:859–866

Bryson SC, Dembo AJ, Colgan TJ, Thomas GM, DeBoer G, Lickrish GM 1991 Invasive squamous cell carcinoma of the vulva: defining low and high risk groups for recurrence. International Journal of Gynecological Cancer 1:25–31

Burke TW, Stringer CA, Gershenson DM, Edwards CL, Morris M, Wharton JT 1990 Radical wide excision and selective inguinal node dissection for squamous cell carcinoma of the vulva. Gynecologic Oncology 38:328–332

Burrell MO, Franklin EW, Campion MJ, Crozier MA, Stacy PW 1988 The modified radical vulvectomy with groin dissection: an eight year experience. American Journal of Obstetrics and Gynecology 159:715–722

Byron RL, Lamb EJ, Yonemoto RH, Kase S 1962 Radical inguinal node dissection in the treatment of cancer. Surgery, Gynecology and Obstetrics 114:401–408

Carson LF, Twiggs LB, Fukushima M, Ostrow RS, Faras AJ, Okagaki T 1986 Human genital papilloma infections: an evaluation of immunologic competence in the genital neoplasia-papilloma syndrome. American Journal of Obstetrics and Gynecology 155:784–789

Cavanagh D, Ruffolo EH, Marsden DE 1985 Cancer of the vulva. In: Cavanagh D, Ruffolo EH, Marsden DE (eds) Gynecologic cancer – a clinicopathological approach. Appleton-Century-Crofts, Connecticut, pp 1–40

Cavanagh D, Fiorica JV, Hoffman MS et al 1990 Invasive carcinoma of the vulva – changing trends in surgical management. American Journal of Obstetrics and Gynecology 163:1007–1015

Choo YC, Anderson DG 1982 Neoplasms of the vagina following cervical carcinoma. Gynecologic Oncology 14:125–132

Coppleson M 1984 The DES story. Medical Journal of Australia 141:487–489

Cote R, Peterson H, Chaiwan B, for the International Breast Cancer Study Group 1999 Role of immunohistochemical detection of lymph node metastases in management of breast cancer. Lancet 354:896–900

Creasman WT, Gallacher HS, Rutledge F 1975 Paget's disease of the vulva. Gynecologic Oncology 3:133–148

Crist WM, Anderson JR, Meza JL et al 2001 Intergroup rhabdomyosarcoma study-IV: results for patients with nonmetastatic disease. Journal of Clinical Oncology 19:3091–3102

Davidson T, Kissin M, Westbury G 1987 Vulvo-vaginal melanoma: should radical surgery be abandoned? British Journal of Obstetrics and Gynaecology 94:473–476

Deppe G, Cohen CJ, Bruckner HW 1979 Chemotherapy of squamous cell carcinoma of the vulva: a review. Gynecologic Oncology 7:345–348

Dewhurst J 1985 Malignant disease of the genital organs in childhood. In: Shepherd JH, Monaghan JM (eds) Clinical gynaecological oncology. Blackwell, London, pp 270–285

Dewhurst J, Ferreira HP 1981 An endodermal sinus tumour of the vagina in an infant with 7-year survival. British Journal of Obstetrics and Gynaecology 88:859–862

DiSaia PJ, Rutledge F, Smith JP 1971 Sarcoma of the vulva. Obstetrics and Gynecology 38:180–184

DiSaia PJ, Creasman WT, Rich WM 1979 An alternative approach to early cancer of the vulva. American Journal of Obstetrics and Gynecology 133:825–832

Durrant KR, Mangioni C, Lacave AJ et al 1990 Bleomycin, methotrexate, and CCNU in advanced inoperable squamous cell carcinoma of the vulva: a phase II study of the EORTC Gynaecological Cancer Cooperative Group (GCCG). Gynecologic Oncology 37:359–362

Friedrich EG, Wilkinson EJ 1982 The vulva. In: Blaustein A (ed) Pathology of the female genital tract, 2nd edn. Springer-Verlag, New York, pp 13–58

Futoran RJ, Nolan JF 1976 Stage I carcinoma of the uterine cervix in patients under 40 years of age. American Journal of Obstetrics and Gynecology 125:790–797

Gallousis S 1972 Verrucous carcinoma – report of three vulvar cases and review of the literature. Obstetrics and Gynecology 40:502–507

Gallup DG, Talledo OE, Shah KJ, Hayes C 1987 Invasive squamous cell carcinoma of the vagina: a 14-year study. Obstetrics and Gynecology 69:782–785

Green MS, Wendel Naumann R, Elliot M et al 2000 Sexual dysfunction following vulvectomy. Gynecological Oncology 77:73–77

Grimshaw RN, Murdoch JB, Monaghan JM 1993 Radical vulvectomy and bilateral inguinal-femoral lymphadenectomy through separate incisions – experience with 100 cases. International Journal of Gynecological Cancer 3:18–23

Hacker NF, Leuchter RS, Berek JS, Castaldo TW, Lagasse LD 1981 Radical vulvectomy and bilateral inguinal lymphadenectomy through separate groin incisions. Obstetrics and Gynecology 59:574–579

Hacker NF, Berek JS, Lagasse LD, Neiberg RK, Leuchter RS 1984a Individualisation of treatment for Stage I squamous cell vulvar carcinoma. Obstetrics and Gynecology 63:155–162

Hacker NF, Berek JS, Juillard GJF, Lagasse LD 1984b Preoperative radiation therapy for locally advanced vulvar cancer. Cancer 54:2056–2061

Hahlin M, Jaworski RC, Wain GV, Harnett PR, Neesham D, Bull C 1998 Integrated multimodality therapy for embryonal rhabdomyosarcoma of the lower genital tract in postpubertal females. Gynecologic Oncology 70:141–146

Hammond IG, Monaghan JM 1983 Multicentric carcinoma of the female genital tract. British Journal of Obstetrics and Gynaecology 90:557–561

Han SC, Kim DH, Higgins SA, Carcangiu M-L, Kacinski BM 2000 Chemoradiation as primary or adjuvant treatment for locally advanced carcinoma of the vulva. International Journal of Radiation Oncology, Biology and Physics 47:1235–1244

Heaps JM, Fu YS, Montz FJ, Hacker NF, Berek JS 1990 Surgical pathological variables predictive of local recurrence in squamous cell carcinoma of the vulva. Gynecologic Oncology 38:309–314

Helm CW, Hatch K, Austin JM et al 1992 A matched comparison of single and triple incision techniques for the surgical treatment of carcinoma of the vulva. Gynecologic Oncology 46:150–156

Herbst AL 1984 Diethylstilboestrol exposure – 1984. New England Journal of Medicine 22:1433–1435

Herbst AL, Scully RE 1983 Newsletter – Registry for research on hormonal transplacental carcinogenesis.

Herbst AL, Ulfelder H, Poskanzer DC 1971 Adenocarcinoma of the vagina; association of maternal stilbestrol therapy with tumour appearance in young women. New England Journal of Medicine 284:878–881

Hernandez-Linares W, Puthawala A, Nolan JF, Jernstrom PH, Morrow CP 1980 Carcinoma in situ of the vagina: past and present management. Obstetrics and Gynecology 56:356–360

Hildesheim A, Han CL, Brinton LA, Kurman RJ, Schiller JT 1997 Human papillomavirus type 16 and risk of preinvasive and invasive vulvar cancer: results from a seroepidemiological case-control study. Obstetrics and Gynecology 90:748–754

Hoffman JS, Kumar NB, Morley GW 1983 Microinvasive squamous carcinoma of the vulva: search for a definition. Obstetrics and Gynecology 61:615–618

Hoffman M, Greenberg S, Greenberg H et al 1990 Interstitial radiotherapy for the treatment of advanced or recurrent vulvar and distal vaginal malignancy. American Journal of Obstetrics and Gynecology 162:1278–1282

Hoffman MS, Roberts WS, Finan MA et al 1991 A comparative study of radical vulvectomy and modified radical vulvectomy for the treatment of invasive squamous cell carcinoma of the vulva. Gynecologic Oncology 45:192–197

Homesley HD, Bundy BN, Sedlis A, Adcock L 1986 Radiation therapy versus pelvic node resection for carcinoma of the vulva with positive groin nodes. Obstetrics and Gynecology 68:733–740

Homesley HD, Bundy BN, Sedlis A et al 1991 Assessment of current International Federation of Gynaecology and Obstetrics staging of vulvar carcinoma relative to prognostic factors for survival (a Gynecological Oncology Group Study). American Journal of Obstetrics and Gynecology 164:997–1004

Homesley HD, Bundy BN, Sedlis A et al 1993 Prognostic factors for groin node metastasis in squamous cell carcinoma of the vulva (a Gynecologic Oncology Group Study). Gynecologic Oncology 49:279–283

Huffman JW 1968 The gynecology of childhood and adolescence. WB Saunders, Philadelphia

Isaacs JH 1976 Verrucous carcinoma of the female genital tract. Gynecologic Oncology 4:259–269

Iversen T, Aas M 1983 Lymph drainage from the vulva. Gynecologic Oncology 16:179–189

Iversen T, Abeler V, Aalders J 1981 Individualised treatment of Stage I carcinoma of the vulva. Obstetrics and Gynecology 57:85–89

Johnston GA, Klotz J, Boutselis JG 1983 Primary invasive carcinoma of the vagina. Surgery, Gynecology and Obstetrics 156:34–40

Kapteijn BA, Nieweg OE, Liem I et al 1997 Localizing the sentinel node in cutaneous melanoma: gamma probe detection versus blue dye. Annals of Surgical Oncology 4:156–160

Karlen JR, Piver MS, Barlow JJ 1975 Melanoma of the vulva. Obstetrics and Gynecology 45:181–185

Kelly JL III, Burke TW, Tornos C et al 1992 Minimally invasive vulvar carcinoma: an indication for conservative surgical therapy. Gynecologic Oncology 44:240–244

Krag D, Weaver D, Ashikaga T et al 1998 The sentinel node in breast cancer – a multicenter validation study. New England Journal of Medicine 339:941–946

Kraus FT, Perez-Mesa C 1966 Verrucous carcinoma: clinical and pathological study of 105 cases involving oral cavity, larynx and genitalia. Cancer 19:26–38

Kucera H, Langer M, Smekal G, Weghaupt K 1985 Radiotherapy of primary carcinoma of the vagina: management and results of different therapy schemes. Gynecologic Oncology 21:87–93

Lee RB, Buttoni L, Dhru K, Tamimi II 1984 Malignant melanoma of the vagina: a case report of progression from preexisting melanosis. Gynecologic Oncology 19:238–245

Levenback C, Coleman RL, Burke TW, Bodurka-Bevers D, Wolf JK, Gershenon DM 2001 Intraoperative lymphatic mapping and sentinel node identification with blue dye in patients with vulvar cancer. Gynecological Oncology 83:276–281

Lingard D, Free K, Wright RG, Battistutta D 1992 Invasive squamous cell carcinoma of the vulva: behaviour and results in the light of changing management regimens. Australian and New Zealand Journal of Obstetrics and Gynaecology 32:137–145

Magrina JF, Webb MJ, Gaffey TA, Symmonds RE 1979 Stage I squamous cell cancer of the vulva. American Journal of Obstetrics and Gynecology 134:453–459

Micheletti L, Borgno G, Barbero M et al 1990 Deep femoral lymphadenectomy with preservation of the fascia lata – preliminary report on 42 invasive vulvar carcinomas. Journal of Reproductive Medicine 35:1130–1133

Monaghan JM 1985a Management of vulvar carcinoma. In: Shepherd JH, Monaghan JM (eds) Clinical gynaecological oncology. Blackwell, London, pp 133–153

Monaghan JM 1985b Management of vaginal carcinoma. In: Shepherd JH, Monaghan JM (eds) Clinical gynaecological oncology. Blackwell, London, pp 154–166

Monaghan JM 1986 Bonney's gynaecological surgery, 9th edn. Baillière Tindall, Eastbourne, pp 121–128

Monaghan JM, Hammond IG 1984 Pelvic node dissection in the treatment of vulvar carcinoma – is it necessary? British Journal of Obstetrics and Gynaecology 91:270–274

Montana GS, Thomas GM, Moore DH et al 2000 Preoperative chemoradiation for carcinoma of the vulva with N2–3 nodes: a Gynecologic Oncology Group study. International Journal of Radiation Oncology, Biology and Physics 48:1007–1013

Moore DH, Thomas GM, Montana GS, Saxer A, Gallup DG, Olt G 1998 Preoperative chemoradiation for advanced vulvar cancer: a phase II study of the Gynecologic Oncology Group. International Journal of Radiation Oncology, Biology and Physics 42:79–85

Morrow CP, DiSaia PJ 1976 Malignant melanoma of the female genitalia: a clinical analysis. Obstetrical and Gynecologic Survey 31:233–271

Moskovic EC, Shepherd JH, Barton DP, Trott PA, Nasiri N, Thomas JM 1999 The role of high resolution ultrasound with guided cytology of groin lymph nodes in the management of squamous cell carcinoma of the vulva: a pilot study. British Journal of Obstetrics and Gynaecology 106:863–867

Murad TM, Durant JR, Maddox WA et al 1975 The pathologic behaviour of primary vaginal carcinoma and its relationship to cervical cancer. Cancer 35:787–794

Nielsen GP, Rosenberg AE, Koerner FC, Young RH, Scully RE 1996 Smooth-muscle tumors of the vulva. A clinicopathological study of 25 cases and review of the literature. American Journal of Surgical Pathology 20:779–793

OPCS 2001 Cancer statistics registrations in 1995–7. HMSO, London

OPCS 1994 Cancer statistics registrations in 1989. HMSO, London

Parker RT, Duncan I, Rampone J, Creasman W 1975 Operative management of early invasive epidermoid carcinoma of the vulva. American Journal of Obstetrics and Gynecology 123:349–355

Parry-Jones E 1960 Lymphatics of the vulva. Journal of Obstetrics and Gynaecology of the British Commonwealth 67:919–928

Perez CA, Camel HM 1982 Long term follow-up in radiation therapy of carcinoma of the vagina. Cancer 49:1308–1315

Perez CA, Grigsby PW, Galakatos A et al 1993 Radiation therapy in management of carcinoma of the vulva with emphasis on conservative therapy. Cancer 71:3707–3716

Piura B, Masotina A, Murdoch J, Lopes A, Morgan P, Monaghan J 1993 Recurrent squamous cell carcinoma of the vulva: a study of 73 cases. Gynecologic Oncology 48:189–195

Podratz KC, Gaffey TA, Symmonds RE, Johansen KL, O'Brien PC 1983 Melanoma of the vulva: an update. Gynecological Oncology 16:153–168

Pride GL, Schultz AE, Chuprevich TW, Buchler DA 1979 Primary invasive squamous carcinoma of the vagina. Obstetrics and Gynecology 53:218–225

Puthawala A, Syed AMN, Nalick R, McNamara C, DiSaia PJ 1983 Integrated external and interstitial radiation therapy for primary carcinoma of the vagina. Obstetrics and Gynecology 62:367–372

Querci della Rovere G, Bird PA 1998 Sentinel-lymph-node biopsy in breast cancer. Lancet 352:421–422

Ragnarsson-Olding BK, Kanter-Lewensohn LR, Lagerlof B, Nilsson BR, Ringborg UK 1999 Malignant melanoma of the vulva in a nationwide, 25-year study of 219 Swedish females: clinical observations and histopathologic features. Cancer 86:1273–1284

Raney RB, Crist WM, Maurer HM, Foulkes MA 1983 Prognosis of children with soft tissue sarcoma who relapse after achieving a complete response. Cancer 52:44–50

Robboy SJ, Noller KL, O'Brien P et al 1984 Increased incidence of cervical and vaginal dysplasia in 3980 diethylstilbestrol-exposed young women. Journal of the American Medical Association 252:2979–2983

Rotmensch J, Rubin SJ, Sutton HG et al 1990 Preoperative radiotherapy followed by radical vulvectomy with inguinal lymphadenectomy for advanced vulvar carcinomas. Gynecologic Oncology 36:181–184

Rozenberg S, Liebens F, Ham H 1999 The sentinel node in breast cancer: acceptable false-negative rate. Lancet 353:1937–1938

Rutledge FN, Smith JP, Franklin EW 1970 Carcinoma of the vulva. American Journal of Obstetrics and Gynecology 106:1117–1130

Rutledge FN, Mitchell MF, Munsell MF et al 1991 Prognostic indicators for invasive carcinoma of the vulva. Gynecologic Oncology 42:239–244

Schulz MJ, Penalver M 1989 Recurrent vulvar carcinoma in the intervening tissue bridge in early invasive stage disease treated by radical vulvectomy and bilateral groin node dissection through separate incisions. Gynecologic Oncology 35:383–386

Sedlis A, Homesley H, Bundy BN et al 1987 Positive groin nodes in superficial squamous cell vulvar cancer. American Journal of Obstetrics and Gynecology 156:1159–1164

Seeger J, Richman SP, Allegra JC 1986 Systemic therapy of malignant melanoma. Medical Clinics of North America 70:89–94

Shimm DS, Fuller AF, Orlow EL, Dosorctz DE, Aristizabal SA 1986 Prognostic variables in the treatment of squamous cell carcinoma of the vulva. Gynecologic Oncology 24:343–358

Stehman FB, Bundy BN, Dvoretsky PM, Creasman WT 1992a Early Stage I carcinoma of the vulva treated with ipsilateral superficial inguinal lymphadenectomy and modified radical hemivulvectomy: a prospective study of the Gynecologic Oncology Group. Obstetrics and Gynecology 79:490–497

Stehman FB, Bundy BN, Thomas G et al 1992b Groin dissection versus radiation in carcinoma of the vulva: a Gynaecological Oncology Group Study. International Journal of Radiation Oncology, Biology and Physics 24:389–396

Sutton GP, Miser MR, Stehman FB, Look KY, Ehrlich CE 1991 Trends in the operative management of invasive squamous carcinoma of the vulva at Indiana University, 1974 to 1988. American Journal of Obstetrics and Gynecology 164:1472–1481

Taussig FJ 1940 Cancer of the vulva – an analysis of 155 cases (1911–1940). American Journal of Obstetrics and Gynecology 40:764–779

Thigpen JT, Blessing JA, Homesley HD, Lewis GC 1986 Phase II trials of cisplatin and piperazinedione in advanced or recurrent squamous cell carcinoma of the vulva: a Gynecologic Oncology Group study. Gynecologic Oncology 23:358–363

Thomas G, Dembo AJ, Bryson SCP et al 1991 Changing concepts in the management of vulvar cancer. Gynecologic Oncology 42:9–21

Tilmans AS, Sutton GP, Look KY, Stehman FB, Ehrlich CE, Hornback NB 1992 Recurrent squamous carcinoma of the vulva. American Journal of Obstetrics and Gynecology 167:1383–1389

Turner RR, Ollila DW, Krasne DL, Giuliano AE 1997 Histopathological validation of the sentinel lymph node hypothesis for breast carcinoma. Annals of Surgery 226:271–276

van der Velden J, Kooyman CD, Van Lindert ACM, Heintz APM 1992 A Stage Ia vulvar carcinoma with an inguinal lymph node recurrence after local excision. A case report and literature review. International Journal of Gynecological Cancer 2:157–159

Veronesi U, Paganelli G, Galimberti V et al 1997 Sentinel-node biopsy to avoid axillary dissection in breast cancer with clinically negative nodes. Lancet 349:1864–1867

Way S 1948 The anatomy of the lymphatic drainage of the vulva and its influence on the radical operation for carcinoma. Annals of the Royal College of Surgeons of England 3:187–209

Way S 1960 Carcinoma of the vulva. American Journal of Obstetrics and Gynecology 79:692–698

Webb JB, Isoti M, O'Sullivan JC, Azzopardi JG 1984 Combined adenoid cystic and squamous carcinoma of Bartholin's gland. British Journal of Obstetrics and Gynaecology 91:291–295

Weed JC, Lozier C, Daniel SJ 1983 Human papilloma virus in multifocal, invasive female genital tract malignancy. Obstetrics and Gynecology 62:83S–87S

Wharton JT, Gallagher S, Rutledge FN 1974 Microinvasive carcinoma of the vulva. American Journal of Obstetrics and Gynecology 118:159–162

White MJ, Polk HC 1986 Therapy of primary cutaneous melanoma. Medical Clinics of North America 70:71–87

Wilkinson EJ 1991 Superficially invasive carcinoma of the vulva. Clinical Obstetrics and Gynecology 34:651–666

Wiltshaw E 1985 Chemotherapy of ovarian carcinoma and other gynaecological malignancies. In: Shepherd JH, Monaghan JM (eds) Clinical gynaecological oncology. Blackwell, London, pp 215–238

Woodman CBJ, Mould JJ, Jordan JA 1988 Radiotherapy in the management of vaginal intraepithelial neoplasia after hysterectomy. British Journal of Obstetrics and Gynaecology 95:976–979

Yabushita H, Shimazu M, Yamada H et al 2001 Occult lymph node metastases detected by cytokeratin immunohistochemistry predict recurrence in node-negative endometrial cancer. Gynecologic Oncology 80:139–144

42

Malignant disease of the uterus

Michael Quinn   Bleddyn Jones   Roberto Dina
Pat Soutter

INTRODUCTION

Carcinoma of the endometrium continues to be the most common gynaecological malignancy affecting Western women (Creasman et al 1998). It is responsible for 6% of all incident cancers in the United States, with more than 37 000 cases being diagnosed in 1999, and more than 6000 deaths. However, the SEER data show a steady fall in the population death rate from 4.6/100 000 in 1973 to 3.3/100 000 in 1998. The corrected 5-year survival in England and Wales has improved steadily from 61% in 1971–75 to just over 70% in 1991–93 (Quinn et al 2001) but these are still not as good as the results in Norway.

It is reasonable to suggest that endometrial cancer, like ovarian cancer (Junor et al 1994, Kehoe et al 1994), is best managed according to standard treatment protocols involving gynaecological oncologists and that such an approach may impact favourably on survival figures (Tilling et al 1998). There seems little place for the 'occasional' surgeon in the management of endometrial cancer and the myth that this is a 'benign' disease still needs to be dispelled.

A number of controversies still exist as to the optimal investigation and management of the condition. This chapter will examine current information about the aetiology and natural history of the disease and will explore various treatment options.

631

EPIDEMIOLOGY

In Western populations, endometrial cancer is relatively rare in the premenopausal woman, particularly before the age of 40, with more than 90% of patients being postmenopausal at the time of diagnosis (Fig. 42.1). The incidence increases steeply after the age of 44 years but then remains more or less static from 55 years of age onwards (Fig. 42.2).

Geographical and racial variations in incidence

There is a remarkable variety in the incidence of this disease, with rates being highest in North American whites and lowest in women from Asia. This is particularly true of Japanese women, whose incidence of the disease is about five times less than that of North American white women. Asian women who migrate to the United States very quickly develop incidence rates similar to the local population.

Mortality rates for the disease are higher in black women in the US compared to white or Asian women, probably reflecting a later stage of presentation and higher likelihood of poor prognostic histological subtypes. There seems to be little effect of socio-economic status on incidence (Quinn et al 2001).

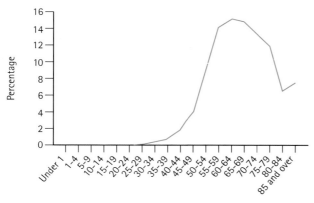

Fig. 42.1 The frequency distribution of new cases of endometrial cancer by age in England and Wales, 1997 (Quinn et al 2001).

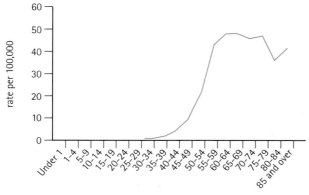

Fig. 42.2 The incidence of endometrial cancer by age in England and Wales, 1997 (Quinn et al 2001).

AETIOLOGY

The precise aetiology is unknown but several factors are known to influence the development of endometrial cancer (Box 42.1). Most relate to the development of the disease in postmenopausal women. Women under the age of 40 who develop this cancer either have polycystic ovarian syndrome or are carriers of a mismatch repair gene defect. There is a strong association with large body mass in premenopausal women (Swanson et al 1993a).

Menstrual and reproductive factors

Early menarche (Brinton et al 1992, La Vecchia et al 1994) and delayed menopause (Kalandidi et al 1996) are associated with a substantial increase in the risk of this disease. Women who menstruated for more than 39 years had four times the risk of endometrial cancer of those who menstruated for less than 25 years (Petterson et al 1986). Nulliparity is associated with a 2–3-fold increased risk in the development of endometrial cancer. The risk falls with increasing number of children (Henderson et al 1983, McPherson et al 1996, Parazzini et al 1991).

Endogenous oestrogen

The strong link with obesity may be because endogenous oestrogen levels in postmenopausal women are directly related to body size, largely due to the conversion of androstenedione to estrone in fat cells and muscle. There is also an association between obesity and reduced levels of sex hormone-binding globulin, thereby leading to an increase in free oestrogen available for uptake in target tissues (Davidson et al 1981). Postmenopausal women with diabetes mellitus have increased oestrogen and reduced gonadotrophin levels independent of body weight, which may explain why they have an increased risk of endometrial cancer (Quinn et al 1981). Rarely, endometrial cancer is associated with an oestrogen-secreting tumour of the ovarian stroma.

Box 42.1 Factors known to alter the risk of developing endometrial cancer

Increase	Decrease
Obesity	Late age at last birth
Diabetes mellitus	Combined oral contraceptive
High-fat/low complex	Smoking
carbo-hydrate diet	Diet with high intake of fruit and
Sedentary lifestyle	vegetables
Early menarche	Physical exercise
Late menopause	
Prolonged/irregular bleeding	
Nulliparity	
Polycystic ovarian syndrome	
Functioning ovarian tumours	
Unopposed oestrogen therapy	
Personal history of breast and colon cancer	
Family history of breast, colon, endometrial cancer	
Tamoxifen use	

43

Gestational trophoblastic tumours

Michael J. Seckl   Edward S. Newlands

INTRODUCTION

The World Health Organization has classified gestational trophoblastic disease (GTD) into two premalignant diseases, termed complete and partial hydatidiform mole (CM and PM), and three malignant disorders, invasive mole, gestational choriocarcinoma and placental site trophoblastic tumour (WHO 1983). These malignant disorders are also frequently referred to as gestational trophoblastic tumours (GTTs) or persistent GTD. GTTs are important to recognize, because they are nearly always curable and in most cases fertility can be preserved. This is mainly because:

- GTTs are exquisitely chemosensitive
- they all produce human chorionic gonadotrophin (hCG), a serum tumour marker with a sensitivity and accuracy in screening, monitoring, management and follow-up of patients which is unparalleled in cancer medicine
- detailed prognostic scoring has permitted 'fine-tuning' of treatment intensity so that each patient receives only the minimum therapy required to eliminate her disease.

GENETICS AND PATHOLOGY

Complete hydatidiform mole (CM)

CMs nearly always contain only paternal DNA and are therefore androgenetic. This occurs in most cases because a single sperm bearing a 23X set of chromosomes fertilizes an ovum lacking maternal genes and then duplicates to form the homozygote, 46XX (Fig. 43.1a). However, in up to 25% of CMs fertilization can take place with two spermatozoa, resulting in the heterozygous 46XY or 46XX configuration (Fig. 43.1b). A 46YY conceptus has not yet been described and is presumably non-viable. Very rarely, a CM can arise from a fertilized ovum which has retained its maternal nuclear DNA and is therefore biparental in origin (Fisher & Newlands 1998).

Macroscopically, the classic CM resembles a bunch of grapes due to generalized (complete) swelling of chorionic villi. However, this appearance is only seen in the second trimester and the diagnosis is today usually made earlier when the villi are much less hydropic. Indeed, in the first trimester the villi microscopically contain little fluid, are branching and consist

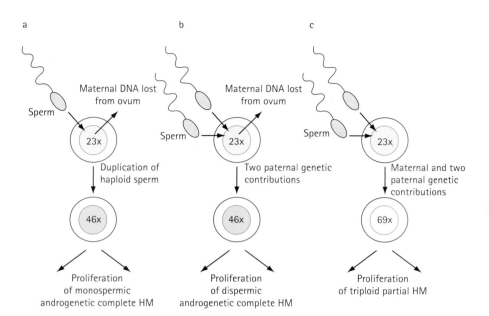

Fig. 43.1 Schematic diagram showing that the androgenetic diploid complete HM is formed either by duplication of the chromosomes from a single sperm **a** or by two sperm fertilizing the ovum **b** which in both cases has lost its own genetic component. The triploid genetic origin of a partial HM is demonstrated in **c**.

of hyperplastic syncytio- and cytotrophoblast with many vessels. Although it was previously thought that CM produced no fetal tissue, histology from 6–8 week abortions reveals evidence of embryonic elements, including fetal red cells (Paradinas 1998). This has resulted in pathologists incorrectly labelling CMs as PMs. The presence of embryonic tissue from a twin pregnancy comprising a fetus and a CM is another source of error which can lead to the incorrect diagnosis of PM.

Partial hydatidiform mole (PM)

PMs are genetically nearly all triploid with two paternal and one maternal chromosome sets (Fig. 43.1c). Although triploidy occurs in 1–3% of all recognized conceptions and in about 20% of spontaneous abortions with abnormal karyotype, triploids due to two sets of maternal chromosome do not become PMs (Lawler et al 1982). Flow cytometry, which can be done in formalin-fixed, paraffin-embedded tissues (Seckl et al 2000), can therefore help in differentiating CM from PM and PM from diploid non-molar hydropic abortions.

In PMs villous swelling is less intense and affects only some villi. Both swollen and non-swollen villi can have trophoblastic hyperplasia which is mild and focal. The villi have characteristic indented outlines and round inclusions. An embryo is usually present and can be recognized macroscopically or inferred from the presence of nucleated red cells in villous vasculature. It may survive into the second trimester but in most cases it dies at about 8–9 weeks gestation and this is followed by loss of vessels and stromal fibrosis. In PMs evacuated early, villous swelling and trophoblastic excess can be so mild and focal that the diagnosis of PM may be missed (Paradinas 1998). Indeed, at uterine evacuation for a 'miscarriage', it is likely that many PMs are misclassified as products of conception. Fortunately, we only see about one patient per year with persistent GTD related to a previously unrecognized PM. Of the increasing number of PMs which are correctly diagnosed very few go on to develop persistent GTD. Indeed, in approximately 3000 PMs

reviewed and followed at Charing Cross between 1973 and 1997, only 15 (0.5%) have required chemotherapy.

Other pregnancies mistaken for PM

Over half of first trimester non-molar abortions are due to trisomy, monosomy, maternally derived triploidy and translocations. These often develop hydrops, but this is small (<3 mm) and PM can be excluded if they are diploid on flow cytometry. Syndromes such as Turner's, Edward's and Beckwith–Wiedemann's can also cause histological confusion with PMs (Paradinas 1998).

Invasive hydatidiform mole

Invasive mole is common and is clinically identified by the combination of an abnormal uterine ultrasound (US) and a persistent or rising hCG level following uterine evacuation of a CM or PM. Pathological confirmation of this condition is rarely required. Moreover, repeat D&C is often contraindicated because of the risks of uterine perforation, infection, life-threatening haemorrhage and subsequent hysterectomy. In occasional cases where histology is available, invasive mole can be distinguished from choriocarcinoma by the presence of chorionic villi.

Choriocarcinoma

Most choriocarcinomas have been shown to have grossly abnormal karyotypes with diverse ploidies and several chromosome rearrangements none of which are specific for the disease (Arima et al 1994). Studies of the origin of GTTs have confirmed that choriocarcinoma may arise from any type of pregnancy including a normal term pregnancy from a homozygous CM or from a heterozygous CM. Until recently, it has been thought that PMs cannot give rise to choriocarcinoma. However, we have now provided incontrovertible genetic evidence that PMs can indeed transform into choriocarcinomas. This is important as there are some centres who wrongly believe it is safe to discontinue hCG follow-up following the diagnosis of PMs.

Choriocarcinoma is highly malignant in behaviour, appearing as a soft, purple, largely haemorrhagic mass. Microscopically it mimics an early implanting blastocyst with central cores of mononuclear cytotrophoblast surrounded by a rim of multinucleated syncytiotrophoblast and a distinct absence of chorionic villi. There are extensive areas of necrosis and haemorrhage and frequent evidence of tumour within venous sinuses. Interestingly, the disease fails to stimulate the connective tissue support normally associated with tumours and induces hypervascularity of the surrounding maternal tissues. This probably accounts for its highly metastatic and haemorrhagic behaviour.

Placental-site trophoblastic tumour (PSTT)

PSTT have been shown to follow term delivery, non-molar abortion or CM. It is conceivable although unproven that PSTT might develop after a PM. Like choriocarcinoma, the causative pregnancy may not be the immediate antecedent pregnancy (Fisher et al 1995). Genetic analysis of some PSTT has demonstrated that they are mostly diploid, originating from either a normal conceptus and therefore biparental or androgenetic from a CM (Newlands et al 1998a).

In the normal placenta, placental-site trophoblast is distinct from villous trophoblast and infiltrates the decidua, myometrium and spiral arteries of the uterine wall. PSTT are rare, slow-growing malignant tumours composed mainly of intermediate trophoblast derived from cytotrophoblast and so produce little hCG. However, they often stain strongly for human placental lactogen (hPL) and β1-glycoprotein. Elevated Ki-67 levels may help in distinguishing PSTT from a regressing placental nodule (Shih & Kurman 1998). In contrast to other forms of GTT, spread tends to occur late by local infiltration and via the lymphatics although distant metastases can occur. More than five mitoses per 10 high power fields may predict tumours with metastasizing potential (Newlands et al 1998a).

EPIDEMIOLOGY AND AETIOLOGICAL FACTORS

Hydatidiform mole

Incidence and ethnic origin
The incidence of CM in Western countries is approximately 1/1000 pregnancies. Recent results indicate that the previously documented higher rates in the Far East have fallen towards the stable levels found in Europe and North America (Hando et al 1998), possibly because of dietary change.

The incidence of PM has been underestimated in the past and is currently 3/1000 pregnancies (Newlands et al 1998b).

Age
CMs are more frequent at the extremes of reproductive age. In one study the relative increased risk compared to the lowest rate between 25–29 years was six-fold in girls under 15 years, three-fold between 40 and 45 years, 26-fold between 45 and 49 years and more than 400-fold over 50 years of age (Bagshawe et al 1983, Newlands et al 1998b). PMs are also more frequent at the extremity of reproductive age although the effect is less pronounced.

Previous pregnancies
Increasing gravidity does not increase the risk of CM. However, following one CM the risk of a subsequent pregnancy being a CM rises from 1 in 1000 to 1 in 76 and to 1 in 6.5 with two previous CMs (Bagshawe et al 1983). Therefore patients with a previous CM must be followed up after each subsequent pregnancy to confirm that their hCG levels return to normal. Although similar data for PMs are not yet available we currently also follow up these patients in the same way.

Choriocarcinoma
The incidence of choriocarcinoma following term delivery without a history of CM is approximately 1:50 000. However, CM is probably the most common antecedent to choriocarcinoma, comprising 29–83% in various studies across the world (WHO 1983). Consequently, the overall incidence of choriocarcinoma after a CM is much higher. Proof of this is frequently difficult to obtain, but when histology was available these tumours were identified as choriocarcinoma in 3% and invasive mole in 16% of previous CMs (rarely as PSTT). Rarely, PMs can give rise to choriocarcinoma.

Unlike HM, choriocarcinoma does not exhibit any clear geographical trends in incidence but the effect of age remains important.

Placental-site trophoblastic tumours

There are currently approximately 150 recorded cases of this tumour in the literature and so estimates of its true incidence may be quite inaccurate (Newlands et al 1998a). Nevertheless, PSTT is thought to constitute about 1% of all trophoblastic tumours (choriocarcinoma, invasive mole and PSTT).

GENETIC FACTORS: THE ROLE OF IMPRINTING

All autosomal genes consist of two alleles (paternal and maternal). However, some alleles are expressed only from one parent and not the other, a phenomenon called genomic imprinting. Interestingly, three closely related genes which are imprinted may be involved in GTT development and in other overgrowth syndromes. These are H19, a putative tumour suppressor gene (Hao et al 1993), p57[kip2], a cyclin-dependent kinase inhibitor (Matsuoka et al 1996), which are both normally expressed by the maternal allele, and the paternally expressed IGF-2, a growth factor commonly implicated in tumour proliferation (Ogawa et al 1993). While p57[kip2] showed the expected pattern of expression in CM and choriocarcinoma (Chilosi et al 1998), CM and post-mole tumours were unexpectedly found to express H19 (Walsh et al 1995), and some post-term tumours showed biallelic expression of both H19 and IGF-2 (Hashimoto et al 1995). This suggests that loss of the normal imprinting patterns of these genes may be an important factor in the development of GTT.

The recent identification of rare families in which several sisters have repeat CMs which are biparental in origin (Fisher & Newlands 1998) is likely to shed further light on the genes involved in CM formation. Indeed, linkage and homozygosity analysis suggested that in two families there is a defective gene located on chromosome 19q13.3–13.4 where at least one imprinted gene is located (Moglabey et al 1999).

RISK OF GTT FOLLOWING CM OR PM

Following evacuation of a CM or PM, the risk of developing a GTT is less than 16% and 0.5%, respectively (Bagshawe et al 1990, Seckl et al 2000). Since it is not yet possible to predict in advance which patients with a CM or PM will develop persistent GTD, all of them must be registered for hCG monitoring. Following this strict protocol enables the identification of individuals with persistent trophoblastic growth who could benefit from lifesaving chemotherapy.

HUMAN CHORIONIC GONADOTROPHIN

β-hCG assays

The family of pituitary/placental glycoprotein hormones includes hCG, follicle-stimulating hormone (FSH), luteinizing hormone (LH) and thyroid-stimulating hormone (TSH). Each hormone comprises an α-subunit which is common between the family members and a distinct β-subunit. Consequently, assays to measure hCG are directed against the β-subunit. Many different β-hCG assays are available. Some detect intact β-HCG and others are either selective for individual fragments or detect various combinations of fragments (Cole 1998). The mechanism of detection is also variable and includes enzyme-linked sandwich assays and radio-immunoassay (RIA). As a result of these differences, great care is required in the interpretation of results obtained. Thus pregnancy tests employing haemagglutination inhibition or complement fixation methods have a lower limit of sensitivity of only 2000 iu/l and may give false-negative results when values for hCG are very high. In contrast, some assays can give false-positive readings leading to unnecessary medical interventions including hysterectomy and chemotherapy (Cole et al 2001). Often these false positives are due to human anti-mouse antibodies (HAMA) crossreacting with the mouse monoclonal antibodies used to detect hCG. As HAMA does not pass into the urine, a simple test for hCG in the urine eliminates this cause of false positives.

Currently, the RIA using a polyclonal antibody recognizing all forms of β-hCG remains the gold standard assay for use in the management of this disease. They are sensitive to 1 iu/l in serum and 20 iu/l in urine.

Use as a tumour marker

hCG has a half-life of 24–36 hours and is the most sensitive and specific marker for trophoblastic tissue. However, hCG production is not confined to pregnancy and GTD. Indeed, hCG is produced by any trophoblastic tissue found, for example, in germ cell tumours and in up to 15% of epithelial malignancies (Vaitukaitis 1979). The hCG levels in such cases can be just as high as those seen in GTD or in pregnancy. Therefore, measurements of hCG do not reliably discriminate between pregnancy, GTD or non-gestational trophoblastic tumours.

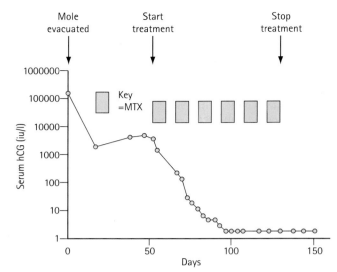

Fig. 43.2 Graph demonstrating the use of monitoring the serum hCG concentration following evacuation of a hydatidiform mole (HM). In this case, after an initial fall the hCG started to rise, indicating the development of invasive HM or choriocarcinoma and so the patient was called up for staging. The prognostic score was low risk (see Table 43.4) and the patient was successfully treated with methotrexate (MTX) and folinic acid (see Box 43.2).

However, serial measurements of hCG have revolutionized the management of GTD for several reasons. The amount of hCG produced correlates with tumour volume so that a serum hCG of 5 iu/l corresponds to approximately 10^4–10^5 viable tumour cells. Consequently, these assays are several orders of magnitude more sensitive than the best imaging modalities available today. In addition, hCG levels can be used to determine prognosis (Bagshawe 1976). Serial measurements allow progress of the disease or response to therapy to be monitored (Fig. 43.2). Development of drug resistance can be detected at an early stage which facilitates appropriate changes in management. Estimates may be made of the time for which chemotherapy should be continued after hCG levels are undetectable in serum in order to reduce the tumour volume to zero. For these reasons hCG is the best tumour marker known.

CLINICAL FEATURES

Complete and partial moles

These most commonly present in the first trimester as a threatened abortion with vaginal bleeding. If the diagnosis is delayed then patients may notice the passing of grape-like structures (vesicles) and occasionally the entire mole may be evacuated spontaneously. The uterus may be any size but is commonly large for gestational age. Patients with marked trophoblastic growth and high hCG levels are particularly prone to hyperemesis, toxaemia and the development of theca lutein cysts which may sometimes be palpable above the pelvis. Toxaemia was diagnosed in 27% of patients with CM (Berkowitz & Goldstein 1981) but is seen less frequently today because of early US diagnosis. Convulsions are rare. The high hCG levels may also produce hyperthyroidism because of cross-reactivity between hCG and TSH at the TSH receptor. Although pulmonary, vaginal and cervical metastases can occur they may disappear spontaneously following removal of the mole. Thus the presence of metastases does not necessarily imply that invasive mole or choriocarcinoma has developed. Patients may rarely present with acute respiratory distress not only because of pulmonary metastases or anaemia but occasionally as a result of tumour embolization. The risk of embolization is reduced by avoiding agents which induce uterine contraction before the cervix has been dilated to enable evacuation of the CM.

Patients with PM usually do not exhibit the dramatic clinical features characteristic of CM (Goldstein & Berkowitz 1994). The uterus is often not enlarged for gestational age and vaginal bleeding tends to occur later so that patients most often present in the late first or early second trimester with a missed or incomplete abortion. In fact the diagnosis is often only suspected when the histology of curettings is available. The pre-evacuation hCG is <100 000 iu/l at diagnosis in over 90% of cases.

Twin pregnancies

Twin pregnancies comprising a normal fetus and a hydatidiform mole occur in between 1:20 000 and 100 000 pregnancies. Some probably abort in the first trimester and so go undiagnosed. However, some are discovered on US examination either routinely or because of complications such as bleeding, excessive uterine size or problems related to a high hCG.

Invasive moles

This is usually diagnosed because serial urine or serum hCG measurements reveal a stable or rising hCG level in the weeks after molar evacuation. Patients may complain of persistent vaginal bleeding or lower abdominal pains and/or swelling. This may occur as a result of haemorrhage from leaking tumour-induced vasculature as the trophoblast invades through the myometrium or because of vulval, vaginal or intra-abdominal metastases. The tumour may also involve other pelvic structures, including the bladder or rectum producing haematuria or rectal bleeding, respectively. Enlarging pulmonary metastases or tumour emboli growing in the pulmonary arteries can contribute to life-threatening respiratory complications (Seckl et al 1991). The risk of these complications is clearly higher in patients where the initial diagnosis of a molar pregnancy was missed and so are not on hCG follow-up.

Choriocarcinoma

Choriocarcinoma can present after any form of pregnancy but most commonly occurs after CM. Histological proof of choriocarcinoma is usually not obtained after a CM because of the risk of fatal haemorrhage caused by biopsy and so it is impossible to distinguish from invasive mole. Choriocarcinoma following a normal pregnancy or non-molar abortion usually presents within a year of delivery but can occur 17 years later (Tidy et al 1995). The presenting features may be similar to HM with vaginal bleeding, abdominal pain and a pelvic mass.

However, one-third of all choriocarcinomas present without pelvic symptoms but have symptoms from distant metastases. In these cases lives can be saved by remembering to include choriocarcinoma in the differential diagnosis of metastatic malignancy (particularly in lungs, brain or liver) presenting in a woman of child-bearing age. Any site may be involved, including skin producing a purple lesion, cauda equina and the heart. Pulmonary disease may be parenchymal, pleural or may result from tumour embolism and subsequent growth in the pulmonary arteries (Savage et al 1998). Thus respiratory symptoms and signs can include dyspnoea, haemoptysis and pulmonary artery hypertension. Cerebral metastases may produce focal neurological signs, convulsions, evidence of raised intracranial pressure and intracerebral or subarachnoid haemorrhage. Hepatic metastases may cause local pain or referred pain in the right shoulder. Although none of these presentations are specific to choriocarcinoma, performing a simple pregnancy test or quantitative hCG assay can provide a vital clue to the diagnosis.

Infantile choriocarcinoma

Choriocarcinoma in the fetus or newborn is exceptionally rare, with approximately 18 reported cases (Kishkuno et al 1997). While a primary choriocarcinoma within the infant is possible, in 11 cases the mother also had the tumour. Interestingly, the diagnosis was often made in the neonate before the mother. In all cases, the infant was anaemic and had a raised hCG but the site of metastasis was variable, including brain, liver, lung and skin. Only two cases have been treated successfully, the rest dying within weeks of initial diagnosis which may have been delayed. Consequently, serum or urine hCG levels should be measured in all babies of mothers with choriocarcinoma. As the disease can present up to 6 months after delivery, an argument could be made for serial monitoring of hCG in these infants.

Placental-site trophoblastic tumour

PSTT grows slowly and can present years after term delivery, non-molar abortion or complete HM. Unlike choriocarcinoma, it tends to metastasize late in its natural history and so patients frequently present with gynaecological symptoms alone. In addition to vaginal bleeding, the production of hPL by the cytotrophoblastic cells may cause hyperprolactinaemia which can result in amenorrhoea and galactorrhoea. Rarely, patients can develop nephrotic syndrome or haematuria and DIC. Metastases may occur in the vagina, extrauterine pelvic tissues, retroperitoneum, lymph nodes, lungs and brain (Newlands et al 1998a).

INVESTIGATION

hCG, chest X-ray, pelvic Doppler ultrasound

All patients who are suspected of having gestational trophoblastic tumours should have an hCG, a chest radiograph and pelvic Doppler ultrasound. The most common metastatic appearance on chest X-ray is of multiple, discrete, rounded lesions but large solitary lesions, a miliary pattern or pleural effusions can occur (Bagshawe & Noble 1965). Furthermore, tumour emboli to the pulmonary arteries can produce an identical picture to venous thromboembolism with wedge-shaped infarcts and areas of decreased vascular markings.

Pulmonary artery hypertension can cause dilatation of the pulmonary arteries. Routine CT scanning of the chest does not add anything to the management of these cases.

US and colour Doppler imaging are not diagnostic but highly suggestive of persistent GTD when there is a combination of a raised hCG, no pregnancy and a vascular mass within the uterus (Fig. 43.3). The last is seen in more than 75% of patients at our centre. The uterine volume and uterine artery blood flow correlate with the amount of disease and the degree of abnormal tumour vasculature respectively. Moreover, both independently predict outcome to therapy. Interestingly, the vascular abnormalities within the pelvis and uterus can persist long after the disease has been eradicated with chemotherapy. Indeed, patients with repeated vaginal haemorrhage from these vascular malformations may require selective arterial embolization. This is usually successful and does not appear to affect fertility (Boultbee & Newlands 1995).

Pelvic US can also demonstrate ovarian theca lutein cysts and other ovarian masses. Metastatic spread outside the pelvis, for example to the liver or kidneys, can also be identified and shown to have an abnormal Doppler signal.

Investigation of drug-resistant disease

When patients develop drug-resistant disease, further investigation is required to more accurately define where the residual tumour is located as resection can be curative. Computed tomography (CT) of the chest and abdomen together with magnetic resonance imaging (MRI) of the brain and pelvis are often helpful and can detect deposits not previously seen. If the CT and MRI are normal then a lumbar puncture to measure the hCG level in cerebrospinal fluid can be useful to detect disease in the central nervous system. An hCG greater than

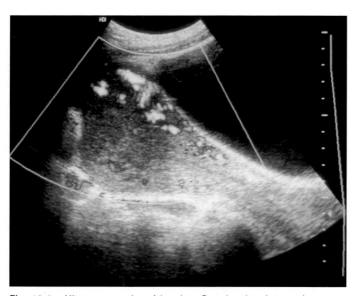

Fig. 43.3 Ultrasonography with colour Doppler showing persistent gestational trophoblastic disease following a CM within the body and wall of the uterus. A typical vesicular or 'snow storm' appearance of residual molar tissue can be seen within the uterus together with a rich blood supply through the endometrium and myometrium. There is no evidence of a fetus.

1:60 of that found in the serum is highly indicative of the presence of trophoblastic disease.

Experimental imaging techniques

Radiolabelled anti-hCG antibodies given intravenously can localize tumours producing hCG when the serum hCG is >100 iu/l (Begent et al 1987). However, both false-positive and -negative results occur and so anti-hCG scanning should be regarded as complementary to other imaging investigations. More recently, positron emission tomography (PET) has provided a novel approach to image many types of tumours using a variety of labels. Whole-body PET has already been reported to distinguish GTT emboli from blood clot in two patients with choriocarcinoma (Hebart et al 1996). Different PET compounds, such as ^{18}fluorodeoxyglucose-PET which can identify tumours missed by other techniques (Beets et al 1994), have yet to be shown to aid in the location of drug-resistant GTTs.

Genetic analysis

On some occasions it can be helpful to perform a comparative genetic analysis of the patient's trophoblastic tumour with their normal tissue and, if available, that of their partner. Thus, if the tumour is suspected of being of non-gestational origin this can be confirmed by the presence of only maternal and the complete absence of paternal DNA. Genetic studies can also determine which of several antecedent pregnancies is the causal pregnancy of the current GTT. This can have an impact on determining appropriate therapy and prognosis (Fisher & Newlands 1998).

MANAGEMENT

Molar evacuation

Evacuation of the uterine cavity using suction gives the lowest incidence of sequelae. When the molar trophoblast invades the myometrium, it is relatively easy to perforate the uterus if a metal curette is used. Medical induction involving repeated contraction of the uterus induced by oxytocin or prostaglandin or other surgical approaches including hysterectomy or hysterotomy increase the risk of requiring chemotherapy 2–3 times compared with suction evacuation. This is thought to be because tumour is more likely to be disseminated by uterine contraction and manipulation. For similar reasons, the use of prostanoids to ripen a nulliparous cervix is not recommended even in nulliparous women (RCOG 1999). If bleeding is severe immediately after suction evacuation, a single dose of ergometrine to produce one uterine contraction may stem the haemorrhage and does not appear to increase the chance of requiring chemotherapy.

In the past it has been common practice for gynaecologists to perform a second and sometimes a third evacuation of the uterine cavity in patients with a molar pregnancy. However, the chance of requiring chemotherapy after one evacuation is only 2.4% but rises markedly to 18% after two evacuations and 81% after four evacuations (Table 43.1). Consequently, a second evacuation may be reasonable and should be discussed

Table 43.1 Correlation between the number of evacuations performed following an HM and the subsequent requirement for chemotherapy at Charing Cross Hospital (1973–86)

Number of evacuations	Patients not treated	Patients treated	% Patients treated
1	4481	109	2.4
2	1495	267	18
3	106	106	50
4	5	22	81

with the local GTD centre if there is vaginal bleeding in the presence of persisting molar trophoblast within the uterine cavity. The use of US control during this procedure may help to reduce the risk of uterine perforation. Further evacuations are not recommended because of the risk of complications and the high chance that the patient will require chemotherapy anyway.

Twin pregnancies

At Charing Cross Hospital in London, we have seen 77 confirmed cases of CM with a separate normal conceptus; 25% of these resulted in a live birth while the remainder had non-viable pregnancies which ended mostly in spontaneous abortions or suction D&Cs. Interestingly, in both the viable and non-viable pregnancies only 20% of women subsequently needed chemotherapy to eliminate persistent GTD and none of these died of resistant disease. Furthermore, although the incidence of pre-eclampsia was 5–10% in those continuing their pregnancies, there were no maternal deaths. Thus, it appears reasonably safe to allow patients with twin pregnancies in which one of the conceptions is a CM to continue to term provided there are no other complications.

Registration and follow-up after uterine evacuation

The majority of patients require no more treatment after evacuation but 16% of patients with CM and <0.5% with PM develop persistent GTD. It is vital that patients with persistent GTD are identified as virtually all of them can be cured with appropriate therapy.

In 1973, under the auspices of the Royal College of Obstetricians and Gynaecologists, a national follow-up service was instituted in the United Kingdom whereby patients with GTD are registered with one of three laboratories located in Dundee, Sheffield and London. Approximately 1400 women are registered per annum and 110–120 require subsequent chemotherapy. After registration the patient's details and pathology together with two weekly blood and urine samples are sent through the post to one of the reference laboratories for confirmation of diagnosis and serial hCG estimations. Following the success of this scheme, other countries have now established or are attempting to establish a similar registration programme to reduce their GTT mortality rates.

In the majority of cases the molar tissue dies out spontaneously, the hCG concentration returns to normal (≤4 iu/l) and the patient can start a new pregnancy after a further

6 months. If the hCG has fallen to normal within 8 weeks of evacuation then marker follow-up can be safely reduced to 6 months as none of these patients have required chemotherapy. However, in patients whose hCG levels are still elevated beyond 8 weeks from the date of evacuation, follow-up should continue for 2 years. Since patients who have had a previous mole or GTT are more at risk of having a second, all patients should have a further estimation of hCG at 6 and 10 weeks following the completion of each subsequent pregnancy.

Indications for chemotherapy

Factors associated with an increased risk of requiring chemotherapy are summarized in Table 43.2. The hormones in the oral contraceptive pill are probably growth factors for trophoblastic tumours and for this reason patients are advised not to use the pill until the hCG levels have returned to normal.

The indications for intervention with chemotherapy in patients who have had a CM or PM are shown in Box 43.1. hCG values ≥20 000 iu/l 4 weeks after evacuation of a mole or rising values in this range at an earlier stage indicate the patient is at increased risk of severe haemorrhage or uterine perforation with intraperitoneal bleeding. These complications can be life-threatening and their risk can be reduced by starting chemotherapy. Withholding chemotherapy from women with metastases in the lung, vulva and vagina is safe only if the hCG levels are falling. However, chemotherapy is required if the hCG levels are not dropping or if the patient has metastases at another site, which can indicate the development of choriocarcinoma.

Table 43.2 Factors increasing the risk of requiring chemotherapy following evacuation of an HM

Factor	Reference
Uterine size > gestational age	Curry et al (1975)
Pre-evacuation serum hCG level >100 000 iu/l	Berkowitz & Goldstein (1981)
Oral contraceptives given before hCG falls to normal	Stone et al (1976)
Bilateral cystic ovarian enlargement	Berkowitz & Goldstein (1981)

Box 43.1 Indications for chemotherapy

- Evidence of metastases in brain, liver or gastrointestinal tract, or radiological opacities >2 cm on chest X-ray
- Histological evidence of choriocarcinoma
- Heavy vaginal bleeding or evidence of gastrointestinal or intraperitoneal haemorrhage
- Pulmonary, vulval or vaginal metastases unless hCG falling
- Rising hCG after evacuation
- Serum hCG @ 20 000 iu/l more than 4 weeks after evacuation, because of the risk of uterine perforation
- Raised hCG 6 months after evacuation even if still falling

Any of the above are indications to treat following the diagnosis of GTD.

Table 43.3 Scoring system for gestational trophoblastic tumours

Prognostic factor	Score*			
	0	1	2	6
Age (years)	<39	>39		
Antecedent pregnancy (AP)	Mole	Abortion or unknown	Term	
Interval (end of AP to chemo at CXH in months)	<4	4–7	7–12	>12
hCG iu/l	10^3–10^4	<10^3	10^4–10^5	>10^5
ABO blood group (female × male)		A × O O × A O or A × unknown	B × A or O AB × A or O	
No. of metastases	Nil	1–4	4–8	>8
Site of metastases	Not detected Lungs Vagina	Spleen Kidney	GI tract	Brain Liver
Largest tumour mass		3–5 cm	>5 cm	
Prior chemotherapy			Single drug	2 or more drugs

* The total score for a patient is obtained by adding the individual scores for each prognostic factor. Low risk, 0–5; medium risk, 6–8; high risk, ≥9. Patients scoring 0–8 currently receive single-agent therapy with methotrexate and folinic acid while patients scoring ≥9 receive combination drug therapy with EMA/CO.

Prognostic factors: scoring versus FIGO staging

The principal prognostic variables for GTTs, which were originally identified by Bagshawe (1976) and since modified by the WHO and our own experience, are summarized in Table 43.3 This has recently been combined with the FIGO staging system to give a unified scoring system, shown in Table 43.4. Each variable carries a score which, when added together for an individual patient, correlates with the risk of the tumour becoming resistant to single-agent therapy. Thus, the most important prognostic variables carry the highest score and include:

- the duration of the disease because drug resistance of GTTs varies inversely with time from the original antecedent pregnancy
- the serum hCG concentration which correlates with volume of viable tumour in the body
- the presence of liver or brain metastases.

ABO blood groups (Table 43.3) contribute little to the overall scoring and therefore have been removed from the current system (Table 43.4).

Chemotherapy

At Charing Cross Hospital, we have used the prognostic scoring system in Table 43.3 to subdivide the patients into three groups termed low, medium and high risk depending on their overall score. Formerly, each risk group corresponded with a separate treatment regimen and so there were three

Table 43.4 Proposed changes to WHO scoring system based on prognostic factors 1998

Prognostic factors[a]	Score[b]			
	0	1	2	4
Age in years	<39	>39		
Antecedent pregnancy	Mole	Abortion	Term	
Interval[c]	<4	4–6	7–12	>12
hCG (iu/litre)	<10^3	10^3–10^4	10^4–10^5	>10^5
Largest tumour (cm)	3–5	>5		
Site of metastases		Spleen, kidney	GI tract	Brain, liver
Number of metastases identified		1–4	5–8	>8[d]
Prior chemotherapy failed			Single	>2

[a] Placental-site trophoblastic tumours are excluded from this table.
[b] The total score for a patient is obtained by adding the individual scores for each prognostic factor. Total score ≤6, low risk; ≥7, high risk.
[c] 'Interval' is the time (in months) between the end of the antecedent pregnancy and the start of chemotherapy.
[d] If all the metastases are in the lung, two or more of these should measure >2 cm on a chest X-ray or CT scan to score 4.

types of therapy termed low, medium and high risk. Several years ago, we discontinued the medium-risk treatment for three reasons:

- the short- and long-term toxicity of this treatment are probably not significantly different from high-risk therapy
- some patients treated with medium-risk have developed drug resistance and subsequently required high-risk therapy anyway
- about 30% of medium-risk patients can still be cured on low-risk chemotherapy which is less toxic than either medium or high-risk chemotherapy (Rustin et al 1996). Moreover, there is no evidence that prior treatment failure with methotrexate is an adverse prognostic variable (Bower et al 1997). Accordingly, patients who score between 5 and 8 now receive low-risk chemotherapy which was previously only given to those with a score ≤5. Patients scoring ≥9 are given high-risk treatment. The details of both low- and high-risk treatment are discussed below. Patients are admitted for the first 3 weeks of either therapy principally because the tumours are often highly vascular and may bleed vigorously in this early period of treatment.

Low- and medium-risk patients

The regimen used since 1964 at Charing Cross Hospital and widely followed in other centres is shown in Box 43.2. This schedule is well tolerated with no alopecia and since the folinic acid dose has been increased from 7.5 mg to 15 mg the incidence of mucosal ulceration has been reduced from 20% to just 2%. Methotrexate can induce serositis, resulting in pleuritic chest pain or abdominal pain. Myelosuppression is rare, but a full blood count should be obtained before each course of treatment. Liver and renal function should also be monitored

Box 43.2   Chemotherapy regimen for low-risk and intermediate-risk patients

Methotrexate (MTX) – 50 mg by IM injection repeated every 48 h × 4
Calcium folinate – 15 mg orally 30 h after each injection of MTX (folinic acid)

Courses repeated every 2 weeks, i.e. days 1, 15, 29, etc.

regularly. All patients are advised to avoid sun exposure or use complete sun block for 1 year after chemotherapy because the drugs can induce photosensitivity.

About 25% of low-risk patients and 69% of medium-risk patients will need to change therapy, most commonly because of drug resistance (Bagshawe et al 1989). However, in our experience all such patients are cured and the only deaths in this group of patients over the last 30 years were one from concurrent but not therapy-induced non-Hodgkin's lymphoma and one from hepatitis (Bagshawe et al 1989). Moreover, a more recent analysis has shown no evidence that methotrexate alone increases the risk of developing a second cancer (Rustin et al 1996).

High-risk patients

These patients are at high risk of developing drug resistance and since 1979 have been treated with an intensive regimen consisting of etoposide, methotrexate and actinomycin D (EMA) alternating weekly with cyclophosphamide and vincristine, otherwise known as Oncovin (CO; see Box 43.3). The regimen requires one overnight stay every 2 weeks and causes alopecia and myelosuppression which are reversible.

The cumulative 5-year survival of patients treated with this schedule is 86% with no deaths from GTT beyond 2 years after the initiation of chemotherapy (Bower et al 1997). While these results are good, the presence of liver or brain metastases correlated with only a 30% or 70% long-term survival, respectively. Early deaths accounted for a significant proportion

Box 43.3   Chemotherapy regimen for high-risk patients

EMA		
Day 1	Etoposide	100 mg/m² by IV infusion over 30 min
	Actinomycin D	0.5 mg IV bolus
	Methotrexate	300 mg/m² by IV infusion over 12 h
Day 2	Etoposide	100 mg/m² by IV infusion over 30 min
	Actinomycin D	0.5 mg IV bolus
	Folinic acid rescue starting 24 h after commencing the methotrexate infusion	15 mg IM or orally every 12 h × 4 doses

CO		
Day 8	Vincristine	1 mg/m² IV bolus
	Cyclophosphamide	600 mg/m² IV infusion over 30 min

EMA alternates with CO every week. To avoid extended intervals between courses caused by myelosuppression, it may occasionally be necessary to reduce the EMA by omitting the day 2 doses of etoposide and actinomycin D.

of the overall mortality, the causes being: respiratory failure, cerebral metastases, hepatic failure and pulmonary embolism. These women did not have preceding moles, were not registered for follow-up and therefore presented with extensive disease. Clearly, it will be difficult to improve the survival of this particular subgroup. However, any woman of child-bearing age presenting with widespread malignancy should have an hCG measurement as very high levels of this hormone are highly suggestive of choriocarcinoma.

The long-term risk of chemotherapy-induced second tumours in patients treated for GTTs in our centre has recently been reviewed (Rustin et al 1996) and is discussed under the section on long-term complications of therapy.

Management of drug-resistant disease

Low-risk disease

Frequent measurement of the serum hCG is a simple way to detect drug resistance at an early stage as the hormone levels will stop falling and may start to rise long before there are other clinical changes. Decisions to alter treatment are not made on the basis of a single hCG result but on a progressive trend over 2–3 values. In patients receiving methotrexate for low-risk disease, if the hCG is ≤100 iu/l when drug resistance occurs the disease can often be cured simply by substituting actinomycin D (0.5 mg IV total dose daily for 5 days every 2 weeks). This drug is more toxic than methotrexate, inducing some hair thinning (occasional complete alopecia), myelo-suppression and more oral ulceration.

Both low-risk and medium-risk patients failing methotrexate whose serum hCG is >100 iu/l are now all treated with EMA/CO.

High-risk disease

Most patients who have failed EMA/CO for high-risk disease can still be salvaged by further chemotherapy and/or surgery (Bower et al 1997). Indeed, the combination of surgical removal of the main site of drug resistance (usually uterus, lung or brain) together with chemotherapy is particularly effective. Preoperative investigations include those outlined above. Following surgery or when surgery is not appropriate, we use the cisplatin-containing regimen, EP (etoposide 150 mg/m² and cisplatin 75 mg/m² with hydration) alternating weekly with EMA (omitting day 2 except the folinic acid). Although this regimen is toxic, the outcome has been impressive with survival rates in excess of 80% (Newlands et al 2000).

Other options include use of some of the new anticancer agents such as the taxanes, topotecan, gemcitabine and high-dose chemotherapy with autologous bone marrow or peripheral stem cell transplantation.

Management of acute disease-induced complications

Haemorrhage

Heavy vaginal or intraperitoneal bleeding is the most frequent immediate threat to life in patients with GTT. The bleeding mostly settles with bedrest and appropriate chemotherapy.

However, occasionally the bleeding can be torrential, requiring massive transfusion. In this situation, if the bleeding is coming from the uterus it may be necessary to consider a uterine pack or emergency embolization of the tumour vasculature. Fortunately, hysterectomy is rarely required. If the bleeding is intraperitoneal and does not settle with transfusion and chemotherapy, laparotomy may be required. Indeed, patients occasionally present this way.

Respiratory failure

Occasionally patients present with respiratory failure due to multiple pulmonary metastases or, more rarely, as a result of massive tumour embolism to the pulmonary circulation (Savage et al 1998). However, in our experience, with appropriate management these patients can be cured. Oxygen support may be required, including masked continuous positive airway pressure ventilation, but mechanical ventilation is usually contraindicated as it results in trauma to the tumour vasculature, leading to massive intrapulmonary haemorrhage and death.

Management of cerebral metastases

Involvement of the central nervous system by GTT may either be overt and require intensive therapy or occult and need prophylaxis. Any patient with a GTT who has lung metastases or who has high-risk disease is at risk of either having or developing central nervous system (CNS) disease (Athanassion et al 1983). Overt CNS disease is treated with modified chemotherapy designed to penetrate the blood–brain barrier and may benefit from early surgery to remove metastases as this may lessen the risk of haemorrhage and raised intracranial pressure. Stereotactic radiotherapy may also be helpful for deep-seated lesions not amenable to resection.

Management of PSTT

PSTT differ from the other forms of GTD in that they produce little hCG, grow slowly, metastasize late and are relatively resistant to combination chemotherapy regimens. Therefore, hysterectomy remains the treatment of choice provided the disease is localized to the uterus. When metastatic disease is present, individual patients can respond to and be apparently cured by chemotherapy (EP/EMA) either alone or in combination with surgery (Newlands et al 1998a). The most important prognostic variable in these patients is the interval from the last pregnancy: where this is <2 years the prognosis is good but thereafter the outlook is poor (Newlands et al 2000). Radiotherapy has produced mixed results and has not yet been proven to cure the disease. Because PSTT is so rare it is unlikely that its treatment will ever be optimized.

PATIENT FOLLOW-UP AFTER CHEMOTHERAPY

On completion of their chemotherapy, patients are followed up regularly with hCG estimations (Box 43.4) to confirm that their disease is in remission. The risk of relapse is about 3% and is most likely in the first year of follow-up. However, we

Box 43.4 Follow-up of patients with gestational trophoblastic tumours who have been treated with chemotherapy

Low/medium/high-risk post chemotherapy patients hCG concentration sampling		
	Urine	Blood
Weekly for the first 6 weeks (outpatient follow-up consultation at 6 weeks post chemotherapy)	✓	✓
Then every 2 weeks until 6 months	✓	✓
Then fortnightly until one year	✓	✗
Then monthly × 12	✓	✗
Then 2 monthly × 6	✓	✗
Then 3 monthly × 4	✓	✗
Then 4 monthly × 3	✓	✗
Then 6 monthly for life	✓	✗

currently continue follow-up for life until a full set of data is available to more accurately guide us as to when it may be safe to stop.

TIMING OF PREGNANCY AFTER TREATMENT

Patients are advised not to become pregnant until 12 months after completing their chemotherapy. This minimizes the potential teratogenicity of treatment and avoids confusion between a new pregnancy or relapsed disease as the cause of a rising hCG. Despite this advice, 230 women on follow-up at our centre between 1973 and 1997 have become pregnant during the first year. Fortunately, this did not appear to be associated with an increased risk of relapse, fetal morbidity and there were no maternal deaths. Indeed, 75% of women continued their pregnancy to term. Consequently, although we continue to advise women to avoid pregnancy for 1 year after completing chemotherapy, those that become pregnant can be reassured of a likely favourable outcome. When a patient becomes pregnant it is important to confirm by US and other appropriate means that the pregnancy is normal. Follow-up is then discontinued until 3 weeks after the end of pregnancy when the hCG due to the pregnancy should have returned to normal.

CONTRACEPTIVE ADVICE

Oral contraceptive use before the hCG is normal following evacuation of an HM increases the risk of developing persistent GTD (Stone et al 1976). For this reason patients are advised to avoid the oral contraceptive pill until the hCG has returned to normal after removal of an HM. Patients who have had chemotherapy for their GTT are advised not to use the oral contraceptive pill until their hCG is normal and chemotherapy is completed.

LONG-TERM COMPLICATIONS OF THERAPY

Most patients, including those who have received intensive chemotherapy, return to normal activity within a few months and the majority of the side-effects are reversible, including alopecia. Late sequelae from chemotherapy have been remarkably rare. In 15 279 patient-years of follow-up, there was no significant increase in the incidence of second tumours (Rustin et al 1996) following methotrexate therapy. In contrast, 26 patients receiving combination chemotherapy for GTT developed another cancer when the expected rate was only 16.45, a significant difference (Rustin et al 1996).

Fertility is an important issue in the management of patients with GTTs. Although combination chemotherapy induces a menopause 3 years earlier than expected (Bower et al 1998), fertility does not otherwise appear to be affected (Woolas et al 1998) and there is no increase in the incidence of congenital malformations compared to the general population (Rustin et al 1984, Woolas et al 1998).

PROGNOSIS

All patients in the low-risk groups can be expected to be cured of their GTTs (Bagshawe et al 1983, Newlands et al 1986). For high-risk patients, survival has progressively improved and is currently 86% (Bower et al 1997). The diagnosis of choriocarcinoma is often not suspected until the disease is advanced. As a result, some deaths occur before chemotherapy has a chance to be effective. The number of such patients can be diminished by a greater awareness of the possibility that multiple metastases in a woman of child-bearing age may be due to choriocarcinoma. The simple measurement of the hCG level in such individuals is a very strong indicator of choriocarcinoma and could help to hasten referrals for life-saving chemotherapy.

CONCLUSION

In the past, many women have died from GTD. However, during the last 50 years we have learnt much about the biology, pathology and natural history of this group of disorders. Furthermore, accurate diagnostic and monitoring methods have been developed together with effective treatment regimens. As a result, the management of GTD today represents one of the modern success stories in oncology, with few women dying from their trophoblastic tumours.

KEY POINTS

1. CM and PM are the commonest forms of GTD.
2. First-trimester bleeding is the commonest presentation.
3. Prostanoids are contraindicated prior to evacuation even in nulliparous women.
4. Second evacuation should be discussed with a GTD centre and >2 evacuations are contraindicated.
5. All confirmed cases should be registered for hCG follow-up.
6. If in doubt get histology reviewed by GTD centre.
7. RIA remains the gold standard for hCG testing in GTD.

KEY POINTS (CONTINUED)

8. Sixteen per cent of CM and 0.5% of PM will require chemotherapy and all can expect to be cured.
9. Deaths from GTT are usually due to late recognition of a post-term choriocarcinoma or from metastatic PSTT which is less chemosensitive.
10. Chemotherapy does not significantly affect fertility but EMA/CO increases the risk of second tumours.
11. Further information can be found at http//www.hmole-chorio.org.uk

REFERENCES

Athanassiou A, Begent RHJ, Newlands ES et al 1983 Central nervous system metastases of choriocarcinoma: 23 years' experience at Charing Cross Hospital. Cancer 52:1728–1735
Arima T, Imamura T, Amada S et al 1994 Genetic origin of malignant trophoblastic neoplasms. Cancer Genetics and Cytogenetics 73:95–102
Bagshawe KD, Dent J, Newlands ES et al 1989 The role of low dose methotrexate and folinic acid in gestational trophoblastic tumours (GTT). British Journal of Obstetrics and Gynaecology 96:795–802
Bagshawe KD, Dent J, Webb J 1986 Hydatidiform mole in the United Kingdom 1973–1983. Lancet ii:673
Bagshawe KD, Lawler SD, Paradinas FJ et al 1990 Gestational trophoblastic tumours following initial diagnosis of partial hydatidiform mole. Lancet 334:1074–1076
Bagshawe KD 1976 Risk and prognostic factors in trophoblastic neoplasia. Cancer 38:1373–1385
Bagshawe KD, Noble MIM 1965 Cardiorespiratory effects of trophoblastic tumours. Quarterly Journal of Medicine 137:39–54
Beets G, Penninckx F, Schiepers C et al 1994 Clinical value of whole body positron emission tomography with [18F]fluorodeoxyglucose in recurrent colorectal cancer. British Journal of Surgery 81:1666–1670
Begent RHJ, Bagshawe KD, Green AJ et al 1987 The clinical value of imaging with antibody to human chorionic gonadotrophin in the detection of residual choriocarcinoma. British Journal of Cancer 55:657–660
Berkowitz RS, Goldstein DP 1981 Pathogenesis of gestational trophoblastic neoplasms. Pathology Annual 11:391
Boultbee JE, Newlands ES 1995 New diagnostic and therapeutic approaches to gestational trophoblastic tumours. In: Bourne TH, Jauniaux E, Jurkovic D (eds) Transvaginal colour doppler. The scientific basis and practical application of colour doppler in gynaecology. Springer, New York
Bower M, Newlands ES, Holden L et al 1997 EMA/CO for high-risk gestational trophoblastic tumours: results from a cohort of 272 patients. Journal of Clinical Oncology 15:2636–2643
Bower M, Rustin GJS, Newlands ES et al 1998 Chemotherapy for gestational trophoblastic tumours hastens menopause by 3 years. European Journal of Cancer 34:1204–1207
Chilosi M, Piazzola E, Lestani M et al 1998 Differential expression of p57kip2, a maternally imprinted cdk inhibitor, in normal human placenta and gestational trophoblastic disease. Laboratory Investigations 78:269–276
Cole LA 1998 hCG, its free subunits and its metabolites. Roles in pregnancy and trophoblastic disease. Journal of Reproductive Medicine 43:3–10
Cole LA, Shahabi S, Butler SA et al 2001 Utility of commonly used commercial human chorionic gonadotropin immunoassays in the diagnosis and management of trophoblastic diseases. Clinical Chemistry 47:308–315
Curry S, Hammond C, Tyrey L, Creasman W, Parker R 1975 Hydatidiform mole: diagnosis, management and long-term follow-up of 347 patients. Obstetrics and Gynecology 45(1):1–8

Fisher RA, Newlands ES 1998 Gestational trophoblastic disease: molecular and genetic studies. Journal of Reproductive Medicine 43:81–97

Fisher RA, Soteriou BA, Meredith L et al 1995 Previous hydatidiform mole identified as the causative pregnancy of choriocarcinoma following birth of normal twins. International Journal of Cancer 5:64–70

Goldstein DP, Berkowitz RS 1994 Current management of complete and partial molar pregnancy. Journal of Reproductive Medicine 39:139–146

Hando T, Masaguki O, Kurose T 1998 Recent aspects of gestational trophoblastic disease in Japan. International Journal of Gynaecology and Oncology 60:S71–76

Hao Y, Crenshaw T, Moulton T et al 1993 Tumor suppressor activity of H19 RNA. Nature 365:764–767

Hashimoto K, Azuma C, Koyama M et al 1995 Loss of imprinting in choriocarcinoma. Nature Genetics 9:109–110

Hebart H, Erley C, Kaskas B et al 1996 Positron emission tomography helps to diagnose tumor emboli and residual disease in choriocarcinoma. Annals of Oncology 7:416–418

Kishkuno S, Ishida A, Takahashi Y et al 1997 A case of neonatal choriocarcinoma. American Journal of Perineonatology 14:79–82

Lawler SD, Fisher RA, Pickthall VG et al 1982 Genetic studies on hydatidiform moles I: the origin of partial moles. Cancer Genetics and Cytogenetics 4:309–320

Matsuoka S, Thompson JS, Edwards MC et al 1996 Imprinting of the gene encoding a human cyclin-dependent kinase inhibitor, p57kip2, on chromosome 11p15. Proceedings of the National Academy of Science USA 93:3026–3030

Moglabey YB, Kircheisen R, Seoud M et al 1999 Genetic mapping of a maternal locus responsible for familial hydatidiform moles. Human Molecular Genetics 8:667–671

Newlands ES, Bagshawe KD, Begent RHJ et al 1986 Development of chemotherapy for medium- and high-risk patients with gestational trophoblastic tumours (1979–1984). British Journal of Obstetrics and Gynaecology 93:63–69

Newlands ES, Bower M, Fisher RA et al 1998a Management of placental site trophoblastic tumours. Journal of Reproductive Medicine 43:53–59

Newlands ES, Mulholland PJ, Holden L et al 2000 EP (etoposide, cisplatin)/EMA (etoposide, methotrexate, actinomycin-D) chemotherapy for patients with high risk gestational trophoblastic tumours (GTT) refractory to EMA/CO chemotherapy and patients presenting with metastatic placental site trophoblastic tumours (PSTT). Journal of Clinical Oncology 18:854–859

Newlands ES, Paradinas FJ, Fisher RA 1998b Recent advances in gestational trophoblastic disease. Hematology and Oncology Clinics of North America 13:225–244

Ogawa O, Eccles MR, Szeto J et al 1993 Relaxation in insulin-like growth factor II gene imprinting implicated in Wilms' tumour. Nature 362:749–751

Paradinas FJ 1998 The diagnosis and prognosis of molar pregnancy. The experience of the National Referral Centre in London. International Journal of Gynaecology and Obstetrics 60:S57–64

Royal College of Obstetricians and Gynaecologists 1999 The management of gestational trophoblastic disease. Guideline no. 18. RCOG, London

Rustin GJS, Booth M, Dent J et al 1984 Pregnancy after cytotoxic chemotherapy for gestational trophoblastic tumours. British Medical Journal 288:103–106

Rustin GJS, Newlands ES, Lutz JM et al 1996 Combination but not single agent methotrexate chemotherapy for gestational trophoblastic tumours (GTT) increases the incidence of second tumours. Journal of Clinical Oncology 14:2769–2773

Savage P, Roddie M, Seckl MJ 1998 A 28 year-old woman with a pulmonary embolus. Lancet 352:30

Seckl MJ, Fisher RA, Salerno GA et al 2000 Choriocarcinoma and partial hydatidiform moles. Lancet 356:36–39

Seckl MJ, Rustin GJS, Newlands ES et al 1991 Pulmonary embolism, pulmonary hypertension, and choriocarcinoma. Lancet 338:1313–1315

Shih IM, Kurman RJ 1998 Ki-67 labelling index in the differential diagnosis of exaggerated placental site, placental site trophoblastic tumour, and choriocarcinoma: a double staining technique using Ki-67 and Mel-CAM antibodies. Human Pathology 29:27–33

Stone M, Dent J, Kardana A et al 1976 Relationship of oral contraceptive to development of trophoblastic tumour after evacuation of hydatidiform mole. British Journal of Obstetrics and Gynaecology 86:913–916

Stone M, Dent J, Kardana A, Bagshawe K 1976 Relationship of oral contraceptive to development of trophoblastic tumour after evacuation of hydatidiform mole. British Journal of Obstetrics and Gynaecology 86:913–916

Tidy JH, Rustin GJS, Newlands ES et al 1995 Presentation and management of choriocarcinoma after nonmolar pregnancy. British Journal of Obstetrics and Gynaecology 102:715–719

Vaitukaitis JL 1979 Human chorionic gonadotrophina – a hormone secreted for many reasons. New England Journal of Medicine 301:324–326

Walsh C, Miller SJ, Flam F et al 1995 Paternally derived H19 is differentially expressed in malignant and non-malignant trophoblast. Cancer Research 55:1111–1116

WHO 1983 Gestational trophoblastic diseases. Technical report series 692. WHO, Geneva

Woolas RP, Bower M, Newlands ES et al 1998 Influence of chemotherapy for gestational trophoblastic disease on subsequent pregnancy outcome. British Journal of Obstetrics and Gynaecology 105(9):1032–1035

44

Benign tumours of the ovary

Pat Soutter   Joanna Girling   Dimitrios Haidopoulos

Benign ovarian cysts are common, frequently asymptomatic and often resolve spontaneously. They are the fourth most prevalent gynaecological cause of hospital admission. By the age of 65 years, 4% of all women in England and Wales will have been admitted to hospital for this reason.

Ninety per cent of all ovarian tumours are benign, although this varies with age. Amongst surgically managed cases the frequency of malignant tumours is 13% in premenopausal women and 45% in postmenopausal women. Thus the major concerns are to exclude malignancy and to avoid cyst accidents, without causing undue morbidity or impairing future fertility in younger women.

Ovarian tumours may be physiological or pathological and may arise from any tissue in the ovary. Most benign ovarian tumours are cystic and the finding of solid elements makes malignancy more likely. However, fibromata, thecomata, dermoids and Brenner tumours usually have solid elements.

PATHOLOGY (Box 44.1)

Physiological cysts

Physiological cysts are simply large versions of the cysts which form in the ovary during the normal ovarian cycle. Most are asymptomatic, being found incidentally as a result of pelvic examination or ultrasound scanning. Although they may occur in any premenopausal woman, they are most common

Box 44.1   Pathology of benign ovarian tumours

Physiological cysts
Follicular cysts
Luteal cysts

Benign germ cell tumours
Dermoid cyst
Mature teratoma

Benign epithelial tumours
Serous cystadenoma
Mucinous cystadenoma
Endometrioid cystadenoma
Brenner

Benign sex cord stromal tumours
Theca cell tumour
Fibroma
Sertoli–Leydig cell tumour

in young women. They are an occasional complication of ovulation induction when they are commonly multiple. They may also occur in premature female infants and in women with trophoblastic disease.

Follicular cyst

Lined by granulosa cells, this is the most common benign ovarian tumour and is most often found incidentally. It results from the non-rupture of a dominant follicle or the failure of normal atresia in a non-dominant follicle. A follicular cyst can persist for several menstrual cycles and may achieve a diameter of up to 10 cm. Smaller cysts are more likely to resolve but may require intervention if symptoms develop or if they do not resolve after 8–12 weeks. Occasionally, oestrogen production may persist, causing menstrual disturbances and endometrial hyperplasia.

Luteal cyst

Less common than follicular cysts, these are more likely to present as a result of intraperitoneal bleeding and this is more commonly on the right side, possibly as a result of increased intraluminal pressure secondary to ovarian vein anatomy. They may also rupture, characteristically on day 20–26 of the cycle. Corpora lutea are not considered to be luteal cysts unless they are greater than 3 cm in diameter.

Benign germ cell tumours

Germ cell tumours are among the most common ovarian tumours seen in women less than 30 years of age. Overall, only 2–3% are malignant but in the under-20s this proportion may rise to a third. Malignant tumours are usually solid, although benign forms also commonly have a solid element. Thus the traditional classification into solid or cystic germ cell tumours, signifying malignant or benign respectively, may be misleading. As the name suggests, they arise from totipotential germ cells and may therefore contain elements of all three germ layers (embryonic differentiation). Differentiation into extraembryonic tissues results in ovarian choriocarcinoma or endodermal sinus tumour. When neither embryonic nor extraembryonic differentiation occurs, a dysgerminoma results.

Dermoid cyst (mature cystic teratoma)

The benign dermoid cyst is the only benign germ cell tumour which is common. It results from differentiation into embryonic tissues and accounts for around 40% of all ovarian neoplasms. It is most common in young women, with a median age at presentation of 30 years (Comerci et al 1994). It is bilateral in about 11% of cases. However, if the contralateral ovary is macroscopically normal, the chance of a concealed second dermoid is very low (1–2%), particularly if preoperative ultrasound has failed to demonstrate typical features (see Chapter 6).

They are usually unilocular cysts less than 15 cm in diameter, in which ectodermal structures are predominant. Thus they are often lined with epithelium like the epidermis and contain skin appendages, teeth, sebaceous material, hair and nervous tissue. Endodermal derivatives include thyroid, bronchus and intestine, and the mesoderm may be represented by bone and smooth muscle.

Occasionally only a single tissue may be present, in which case the term 'monodermal teratoma' is used. The classic examples are carcinoid and struma ovarii, which contains hormonally active thyroid tissue. Primary carcinoid tumours of the ovary rarely metastasize but 30% may give rise to typical carcinoid symptoms (Saunders & Hertzmar 1960). Thyroid tissue is found in 5–20% of cystic teratomas. The term 'struma ovarii' should be reserved for tumours composed predominantly of thyroid tissue and as such comprise only 1.4% of cystic teratomas. Only 5–6% of struma ovarii produce sufficient thyroid hormone to cause hyperthyroidism. Some 5–10% of struma ovarii develop carcinoma. The majority (60%) of dermoid cysts are asymptomatic. However, 3.5–10% may undergo torsion. Less commonly (1–4%), they may rupture spontaneously: either suddenly, causing an acute abdomen and a chemical peritonitis, or slowly, causing chronic granulomatous peritonitis. As the latter may also arise following intraoperative spillage, great care should be taken to avoid this event and thorough peritoneal lavage must be performed if it does occur. During pregnancy, rupture is more common due to external pressure from the expanding gravid uterus or to trauma during delivery.

About 2% are said to contain a malignant component, usually a squamous carcinoma in women over 40 years old. Poor prognosis is indicated by non-squamous histology and capsular rupture. Amongst women aged under 20 years, up to 80% ovarian malignancies are due to germ cell tumours (see Chapter 40).

Mature solid teratoma

These rare tumours contain mature tissues just like the dermoid cyst, but there are few cystic areas. They must be differentiated from immature teratomas which are malignant (see Chapter 40).

Benign epithelial tumours

The majority of ovarian neoplasia, both benign and malignant, arise from the ovarian surface epithelium. They are therefore essentially mesothelial in nature, deriving from the coelomic epithelium overlying the embryonic gonadal ridge, from which develop müllerian and wolffian structures. Therefore, this may result in development along endocervical (mucinous cystadenomata), endometrial (endometrioid) or tubal (serous) pathways or uroepithelial (Brenner) lines respectively. Although benign epithelial tumours tend to occur at a slightly younger age than their malignant counterparts, they are most common in women over 40 years.

Serous cystadenoma

This is the most common benign epithelial tumour and is bilateral in about 10%. It is usually a unilocular cyst with papilliferous processes on the inner surface and occasionally on the outer surface. The epithelium on the inner surface is cuboidal or columnar and may be ciliated. Psammoma bodies are concentric calcified bodies which occur occasionally in these cysts but more frequently in their malignant counterparts. The cyst fluid is thin and serous. They are seldom as large as mucinous tumours.

Mucinous cystadenoma

These constitute 15–25% of all ovarian tumours and are the second most common epithelial tumour. They are typically large, unilateral, multilocular cysts with a smooth inner surface. A recent specimen at Hammersmith Hospital weighed over 14 kg! The lining epithelium consists of columnar mucus-secreting cells. The cyst fluid is generally thick and glutinous.

A rare complication is pseudomyxoma peritonei which is more often present before the cyst is removed rather than following intraoperative rupture. Pseudomyxoma peritonei is most commonly associated with mucinous tumours of the ovary or appendix. Synchronous tumours of the ovary and appendix are common. These are usually well-differentiated carcinomas or borderline tumours (Wertheim et al 1994) which result in seedling growths which continue to secrete mucin, causing matting together and consequent obstruction of bowel loops. The 5-year survival rate is approximately 50% but by 10 years as few as 18% are alive.

Endometrioid cystadenoma

Most of these tumours are malignant as benign endometrioid cysts are difficult to differentiate from endometriosis.

Brenner

These account for only 1–2% of all ovarian tumours and are bilateral in 10–15% of cases. They probably arise from wolffian metaplasia of the surface epithelium. The tumour consists of islands of transitional epithelium (Walthard nests) in a dense fibrotic stroma, giving a largely solid appearance. The vast majority are benign but borderline or malignant specimens have been reported. Almost three-quarters occur in women over the age of 40 and about half are incidental findings, being recognized only by the pathologist. Although some can be large the majority are less than 2 cm in diameter. Some secrete oestrogens and abnormal vaginal bleeding is a common presentation.

Clear cell (mesonephroid) tumours

These arise from serosal cells, showing little differentiation, and are only rarely benign. The typical histological appearance is of clear or 'hobnail' cells arranged in mixed patterns.

Benign sex cord stromal tumours

Sex cord stromal tumours represent only 4% of benign ovarian tumours. They occur at any age from prepubertal children to elderly, postmenopausal women. Many of these tumours secrete hormones and present with the results of inappropriate hormone effects.

Granulosa cell tumours

These are all malignant tumours but are mentioned here because they are generally confined to the ovary when they present and so have a good prognosis. However, they do grow very slowly and recurrences may not be seen until 10–20 years later. They are largely solid in most cases. Call-Exner bodies are pathognomonic but are seen in less than half of granulosa cell tumours. Some produce oestrogens and most appear to secrete inhibin.

Theca cell tumours

Almost all are benign, solid and unilateral, typically presenting in the sixth decade. Many produce oestrogens in sufficient quantity to have systemic effects such as precocious puberty, postmenopausal bleeding, endometrial hyperplasia and endometrial cancer. They rarely cause ascites or Meig's syndrome.

Fibroma

These unusual tumours are most frequent around 50 years of age. Most are derived from stromal cells and are similar to thecomas. They are hard, mobile and lobulated with a glistening white surface. Less than 10% are bilateral. While ascites occurs with many of the larger fibromas, Meig's syndrome – ascites and pleural effusion in association with a fibroma of the ovary – is seen in only 1% of cases.

Sertoli-Leydig cell tumours

These are usually of low-grade malignancy. Most are found around 30 years of age. They are rare, comprising less than 0.2% of ovarian tumours. They are often difficult to distinguish from other ovarian tumours because of the variety of cells and architecture seen. Many produce androgens and signs of virilization are seen in three-quarters of patients. Some secrete oestrogens. They are usually small and unilateral.

AGE DISTRIBUTION OF OVARIAN TUMOURS

In younger women, the most common benign ovarian neoplasm is the germ cell tumour and amongst older women, the epithelial cell tumour. The percentage of ovarian neoplasms which are benign also changes with the age of the woman (Table 44.1).

PRESENTATION

Presentation of benign ovarian tumours is as follows:

- Asymptomatic
- Pain

Table 44.1 Histological distribution of benign ovarian neoplasms treated surgically by age (as %) and percentage of all neoplasms which are benign (n = 650)(modified from Koonings et al 1989)

Histology	Age in years							All ages	
	≤19	20–29	30–39	40–49	50–59	60–69	≥70	% of all benign tumours in each histology group	% of each histology group which is benign
Epithelial	30	27	30	51	63	73	88	38	57
Germ cell	70	72	66	46	21	16	0	58	97
Sex cord	0	1	4	3	17	11	12	4	66
% Benign	92	94	81	59	50	47	71	100	75

- Abdominal swelling
- Pressure effects
- Menstrual disturbances
- Hormonal effects
- Abnormal cervical smear.

Asymptomatic

Many benign ovarian tumours are found incidentally in the course of investigating another unrelated problem or during a routine examination while performing a cervical smear or at an antenatal clinic. As pelvic ultrasound, and particularly transvaginal scanning, is now used more frequently, physiological cysts are detected more often. Where ultrasound was used in trials of screening for ovarian cancer, the majority of tumours detected were benign. Most simple cysts will resolve spontaneously if observed over a period of 6 months (Sasaki et al 1999, Zanetta et al 1996). Use of an oral contraceptive pill does not encourage the resolution of physiological cysts.

Pain

Acute pain from an ovarian tumour may result from torsion, rupture, haemorrhage or infection. Torsion usually gives rise to a sharp, constant pain caused by ischaemia of the cyst. Areas may become infarcted. Haemorrhage may occur into the cyst and cause pain as the capsule is stretched. If the cyst is large, the bleeding may be sufficient to give rise to a haemolytic jaundice, so leading the unwary to diagnose malignancy wrongly. Intraperitoneal bleeding mimicking ectopic pregnancy may result from rupture of the tumour. This happens most frequently with a luteal cyst. Chronic lower abdominal pain sometimes results from the pressure of a benign ovarian tumour but is more common if endometriosis or infection is present.

Abdominal swelling

Patients seldom note abdominal swelling until the tumour is very large. A benign mucinous cyst may occasionally fill the entire abdominal cavity. The bloating of which women complain so often is rarely due to an ovarian tumour.

Hormonal effects

Occasionally the patient will complain of menstrual disturbances but this may be coincidence rather than due to the tumour. Rarely, ovarian tumours present with oestrogen effects such as precocious puberty, menorrhagia and glandular hyperplasia, breast enlargement and postmenopausal bleeding. Secretion of androgens may cause hirsutism and acne initially, progressing to frank virilism with deepening of the voice or clitoral hypertrophy. Very rarely indeed, thyrotoxicosis may occur. Some of these tumours are malignant but are mentioned here because of their ability to produce hormones in some cases.

Predominantly oestrogen-secreting tumours
Granulosa cell tumours These slowly growing malignant tumours are the most common sex cord stromal tumours occurring in the ovary. While the great majority occur in postmenopausal women, 5% present in girls of the prepubertal or pubertal years.

About 70% of these tumours secrete oestrogens or, very rarely, androgens. Among postmenopausal women, 60% will present with vaginal bleeding due to oestrogen secretion from the tumour (Evans et al 1980). Endometrial hyperplasia will develop in 25–50% of these women and 5–10% will develop adenocarcinoma of the endometrium (Malstrom et al 1994). About 50% of women in the reproductive years will complain of menstrual abnormalities and 16% will have secondary amenorrhoea. In the rare cases when the tumour is secreting androgens, hirsutism may be the presenting feature. Precocious puberty is the usual presentation in young girls. The typical signs of abdominal swelling and pain seen in advanced epithelial ovarian cancer appear only when the granulosa cell tumour is larger than 10 cm.

Thecoma Thecomas account for less than 1% of all ovarian tumours. They occur in women of the postmenopausal age group and only a few cases have been reported in women less than 30 years old.

About 70% of thecomas secrete oestrogens but they are less often associated with postmenopausal bleeding than granulosa cell tumours. On the other hand, they are more often associated with endometrial cancer (7% v 2%) (Cronje et al 1999). Endometrial hyperplasia is found in a further 19.8%. Postmenopausal bleeding and abdominal pain are the main presenting features. In the presence of luteinized cells, these tumours can secrete androgens and result in hirsutism.

Pure Sertoli cell tumours (sex cord tumour with annular tubules) These resemble well-differentiated Sertoli–Leydig tumours but contain no Leydig cells. They are benign. The sex cord tumour with annular tubules is a specific variety which resembles gonadoblastomas histologically. Although first described in association with Peutz–Jeghers syndrome, they have also been described in women without this syndrome.

About half of these tumours produce oestrogens and very few secrete androgens. Those secreting oestrogen may cause endometrial hyperplasia, amenorrhoea, menorrhagia or sexual pseudoprecosity. Those associated with Peutz–Jeghers syndrome are usually small, benign, bilateral and partly calcified. In women unaffected by this syndrome, they tend to be larger, unilateral and may be associated with granulosa or Sertoli–Leydig cell tumours. Some are malignant.

Predominantly androgen-secreting tumours
Sertoli–Leydig tumours (androblastomas) Sertoli–Leydig cell tumour, also called androblastoma, is another, rare, malignant, sex cord stromal tumour. Like the normal Leydig cell in males, these tumour cells in female ovaries may produce androgens, resulting in virilization. These tumours should be suspected in women in their second or third decades with an adnexal mass and virilization. However, some Sertoli–Leydig tumours can secrete oestrogen and about 80% are inactive. These usually present as unilateral stage I disease when the prognosis is good, even after fertility-conserving surgery, unless the tumour is poorly differentiated.

Adrenal-like tumours of the ovary   The nomenclature of these tumours is a source of great confusion. The current term, adrenal-like tumours, is now preferred but many others remain in wide use. The alternative names include hilar cell tumours, lipoid cell tumours, luteomas and adrenal rest tumours. These are often very small tumours less than 5 mm in diameter. Most are unilateral and benign. Surgical removal will result in reversal of the symptoms of virilization.

Gonadoblastoma   Gonadoblastoma is the most common neoplasm arising in dysgenetic gonads and arises almost exclusively in them. Although gonadoblastomas are benign, more than half are accompanied by malignant germ cell tumours, usually dysgerminomas, which have probably arisen from premalignant cells within the gonadoblastoma. Metastasis of the dysgerminoma component is uncommon but the other combinations can be highly malignant.

They vary in size from a few millimetres to large masses when other germ cell tumours are present. Most are only a few centimetres in diameter. They are often calcified and can be recognized on plain X-ray. More than half are bilateral.

The great majority occur in phenotypic females who are usually virilized. The age range of reported cases is 1–40 years. The clinical presentation may be abnormal genitalia in phenotypic male infants or primary amenorrhoea with or without hirsutism in phenotypic females. Most have high levels of gonadotrophins due to ovarian virilization failure.

Bilateral gonadectomy is indicated in all these patients because of the risk of malignancy in these non-functioning gonads. This is usually curative for those associated with dysgerminoma, even when large, but chemotherapy will be required for those with other germ cell tumours. The prognosis for such individuals is now good, with modern chemotherapy regimens offering 90% survival.

Miscellaneous

Pressure effects

Gastrointestinal or urinary symptoms may result from pressure effects. In extreme cases, oedema of the legs, varicose veins and haemorrhoids may result. Sometimes, uterine prolapse is the presenting complaint in a woman with an ovarian cyst.

Infrequently, a patient with an abnormal cervical smear will be found to have an ovarian tumour and removal is followed by resolution of the cytological abnormality. Surprisingly, these are often benign tumours.

DIFFERENTIAL DIAGNOSIS

The differential diagnosis of benign ovarian tumours is broad, reflecting the wide range of presenting symptoms.

Pain
- Ectopic pregnancy
- Spontaneous abortion
- Pelvic inflammatory disease
- Appendicitis
- Meckel's diverticulum
- Diverticulitis

Abdominal swelling
- Pregnant uterus
- Fibroid uterus
- Full bladder
- Distended bowel
- Ovarian malignancy
- Colorectal carcinoma

Pressure effects
- Urinary tract infection
- Constipation

Hormonal effects
- All other causes of menstrual irregularities, precocious puberty and postmenopausal bleeding

A full bladder should be considered in the differential diagnosis of any pelvic mass. In premenopausal women, a gravid uterus must always be considered. Fibroids can be impossible to distinguish from ovarian tumours. Rarely, a fimbrial cyst may grow sufficiently to cause anxiety.

Ectopic pregnancy may present as a pelvic mass and lower abdominal pain, especially if there has been chronic intraperitoneal bleeding. Often a ruptured, bleeding corpus luteum will be mistaken for an ectopic gestation. It may be difficult to differentiate between appendicitis and an ovarian cyst. Cooperation between gynaecologist and surgeon is essential to avoid unnecessary surgery on simple ovarian cysts in young women and the effects this may have upon subsequent fertility. Pelvic inflammatory disease may give rise to a mass of adherent bowel, a hydrosalpinx or pyosalpinx.

If the tumour is ovarian, malignancy must be excluded. In many cases this can only be done by a laparotomy. Even then, careful histological examination may be necessary to exclude invasion. Frozen section will only rarely be of value. A pelvic mass may also be caused by a rectal tumour or diverticulitis. Hodgkin's disease may present as a pelvic mass with enlarged pelvic lymph nodes.

INVESTIGATION

The investigations required will depend upon the circumstances of the presentation. The patient presenting with acute symptoms will usually require emergency surgery whereas the asymptomatic patient or the woman with chronic problems may benefit from more detailed preliminary assessment.

Gynaecological history

Details of the presenting symptoms and a full gynaecological history should be obtained with particular reference to the date of the last menstrual period, the regularity of the menstrual cycle, any previous pregnancies, contraception, medication and family history (particularly of ovarian or breast cancer).

General history and examination

Indigestion or dysphagia might indicate a primary gastric cancer metastasizing to the pelvis. Similarly, a history of altered bowel habit or rectal bleeding should be sought as evidence of diverticulitis or rectal carcinoma. However, ovarian carcinoma may also present with these features.

If the patient has presented as an acute emergency, evidence of hypovolaemia should be sought. Hypotension is a relatively late sign of blood loss, as the blood pressure will be maintained for some time by peripheral and central venous vasoconstriction. When decompensation of this mechanism occurs, it often does so very rapidly. It is vital to recognize the early signs – tachycardia and cold peripheries.

The breasts should be palpated and evidence of lymphadenopathy sought in the neck, the axillae and the groins. The chest should be examined for signs of a pleural effusion. Some patients may have ankle oedema. Very occasionally foot drop may be noted as a result of compression of pelvic nerve roots. This would not occur with a benign tumour but suggests a malignancy with lymphatic involvement.

Abdominal examination

The abdomen should be inspected for signs of distension by fluid or by the tumour itself. Dilated veins may be seen on the lower abdomen. Gentle palpation will reveal areas of tenderness and peritonism may be elicited by asking the patient to cough or alternately suck in and blow out her abdominal wall. Male hair distribution may suggest a rare androgen-producing tumour.

The best way of detecting a mass that arises from the pelvis is to palpate gently with the radial border of the left hand, starting in the upper abdomen and working caudally. This is the reverse of the process taught to every medical student for feeling the liver edge. Use of the right hand alone is the most common reason for failing to detect pelviabdominal masses.

Shifting dullness is probably the easiest way of demonstrating ascites but it remains a very insensitive technique. It is always worth listening for bowel sounds in any patient with an acute abdomen. Their complete absence in the presence of peritonism is an ominous sign.

Bimanual examination

This is an essential component of the assessment because, even in expert hands, ultrasound examination is not infallible. By palpating the mass between both the vaginal and abdominal hands, its mobility, texture and consistency, the presence of nodules in the pouch of Douglas and the degree of tenderness can all be determined (Fig. 44.1). While it is impossible to make a firm diagnosis with bimanual examination, a hard, irregular, fixed mass is likely to be invasive.

Ultrasound

The techniques of transabdominal and transvaginal ultrasound are discussed in detail in Chapter 6. Ultrasound can demonstrate the presence of an ovarian mass with reasonable sensitivity and fair specificity and although it cannot distinguish reliably between benign and malignant tumours, solid ovarian masses are more likely to be malignant than their cystic counterparts. CT scanning has no significant advantages over ultrasound in this situation and is more expensive. MRI is sometimes useful in the management.

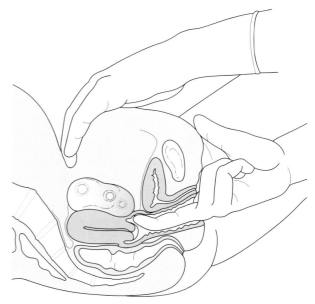

Fig. 44.1 Bimanual examination involves palpating the pelvic organs between both hands.

Ultrasound-guided diagnostic ovarian cyst aspiration

This investigation has been introduced gradually into gynaecological practice from the subspecialty of assisted reproduction where ultrasound-guided egg collection is now commonplace. This has happened without the benefit of appropriate trials to indicate its potential efficacy.

Unfortunately, this technique has up to a 71% false-negative rate and a 2% false-positive rate for the cytological diagnosis of malignancy (Diernaes et al 1987). The degree of risk of dissemination of malignant cells along the needle track or into the peritoneal cavity is not established.

The second potential role of a diagnostic cyst aspiration is to distinguish between functional and benign cysts and in the latter case to determine the type. This is not reliably achieved, even when apparently simple cysts are selected. The inability to inspect the ovarian capsular surface and the peritoneal cavity and the lack of knowledge concerning the long-term behaviour of cysts following aspiration are also important limitations. Overall, ultrasound-guided aspiration of ovarian cysts cannot be recommended as a diagnostic tool.

Radiological investigations

A chest X-ray is essential to detect metastatic disease in the lungs or a pleural effusion which may be too small to detect on auscultation. Occasionally an abdominal X-ray may show calcification, suggesting the possibility of a benign teratoma. An intravenous urogram is often performed but is seldom useful. A barium enema is indicated only if the mass is irregular or fixed or if there are bowel symptoms. A CT scan is seldom indicated.

Blood test and serum markers

It is always sensible to measure the haemoglobin and an elevated white cell count would suggest infection. Platelet count and clotting screen may be useful in the rare case of a large intra-abdominal bleed. Blood may be crossmatched if necessary.

Serum CA125 measurement is used in various risk of malignancy indices (see Chapter 45). However, the predictive value of these tests is rather unsatisfactory. Women with extensive endometriosis may also have elevated levels but the concentration is usually not as high as is seen with malignant disease. The β-hCG concentration might be measured to exclude an ectopic pregnancy but trophoblastic tumours and some germ cell tumours secrete this marker. Oestradiol levels may be elevated in some physiological follicular cysts and sex cord stromal tumours. Androgen concentrations may be increased in Sertoli–Leydig tumours. Raised α-fetoprotein levels suggest a yolk sac tumour.

MANAGEMENT

The management will depend upon the severity of the symptoms; the size and ultrasound characteristics of the cyst; the CA125 results; the age of the patient and therefore the risk of malignancy; and her desire for further children.

The asymptomatic patient

This includes women whose cysts were diagnosed incidentally during investigation of another problem or during investigation of lower abdominal symptoms that may or may not be related to the cyst.

Simple cysts less than 8 cm in diameter with normal CA125

Ovarian cysts are best identified and characterized by transvaginal ultrasound. Larger cysts may also need to be examined by abdominal ultrasound. There is no uniform definition of a simple cyst; the definition used in this chapter has been taken from a study of 1304 women (Ekerhovd et al 2001). A simple cyst is unilocular, echo free without solid parts or papillary formations. These authors also described unilocular cysts with small solid areas or papillary formations on the internal side of the cyst wall or echogenic cyst content; these were defined as complex cysts. They excluded cysts with internal septae, whether bilocular or mutilocular.

Premenopausal women   Young women less than 40 years are both more likely to want the option of further children and less likely to have a malignant epithelial tumour. Only three (0.73%) of 413 premenopausal women who underwent surgery for simple echo-free cysts without solid parts or papillary formations had borderline (2) or malignant (1) tumours (Ekerhovd et al 2001). The malignant tumour was 99 mm in diameter and the borderline lesions were 75 and 82 mm in diameter.

A normal follicular cyst up to 3 cm in diameter requires no further investigation. An echo-free, unilocular cyst of 3–8 cm identified by ultrasound should be re-examined 3–6 months later for evidence of diminution in size. The use of a combined oral contraceptive is unlikely to accelerate the resolution of a functional cyst (Steinkampf & Hammond 1990) and hormonal treatment of endometriosis does not usually benefit an endometrioma. If the cyst does not change in size, observation

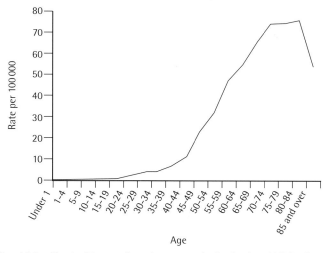

Fig. 44.2   The incidence of ovarian cancer in England and Wales in 1997 (Quinn et al 2001). Note how uncommon ovarian cancer is before the age of 35 years.

Table 44.2   Distribution of malignant ovarian tumours treated surgically, by cell type at different ages, as percentages (n=180)(modified from Koonings et al 1989)

Histology	≤19	20–29	30–39	40–49	50–59	60–69	≥70	All ages
Epithelial	0	33	69	94	96	100	100	86
Germ cell	80	33	8	2	2	0	0	7
Sex cord	20	33	21	4	2	0	0	7

may be continued but laparoscopy or laparotomy will be indicated if there has been a significant increase in size.

The older woman   Women over 50 years of age are far more likely to have a malignancy (Fig. 44.2, Table 44.2) and have less to gain from the conservative management of a pelvic mass. However, the capacity of the postmenopausal ovary to generate benign cysts is greater than previously thought, occurring in up to 17% of asymptomatic women (Levine et al 1992). Over 50% of simple cysts will resolve spontaneously and almost 30% will remain static (Bailey et al 1998, Levine et al 1992, Sasaki et al 1999).

Considerable efforts have been made to safely avoid unnecessary surgery in this older age group. However, one group found malignant tumours in 8.9% of 112 post-menopausal women with monolocular simple cysts studied between 1987 and 1993 with transvaginal ultrasound (Osmers et al 1998). They did not find internal echoes helpful in identifying malignancies. They found malignancies in 4.6% of cysts less than 40 mm in diameter, 10.8% of cysts 40–69 mm in diameter and in 18.2% of cysts more than 69 mm in diameter. Their view was that only cysts less than 3 cm could be managed conservatively. The results of other studies are more reassuring. In particular, a more recent study running from 1992 to 1997 found that only 1.6% of 247 echo-free cysts in postmenopausal women were malignant and that all of these were more than 7.9 cm in diameter (Ekerhovd et al

Box 44.2 The criteria for observation of an asymptomatic ovarian tumour. All these criteria must be met

- Unilateral tumour
- Unilocular cyst without solid elements
- Cyst less than 8 cm in diameter. Premenopausal women with cysts less than 3 cm do not usually require further follow-up
- Normal CA125
- No free fluid or masses suggesting omental cake or matted loops of bowel

2001). It was only cysts with small solid areas or papillary formations on the internal side of the cyst wall or echogenic cyst content that carried a 10% risk of malignancy in the 130 studied. Of the nine invasive cancers detected in this group, five were in cysts less than 8 cm in diameter.

This suggests that simple, echo-free, unilateral cysts without solid parts or papillary formations and less than 8 cm in diameter are very likely to be benign and may safely be managed conservatively with 3–6-monthly ultrasound and CA125 estimation (Ekerhovd et al 2001, Goldstein 1993) (Box 44.2).

All other cysts

Echo-free ovarian cysts more than 7.9 cm in diameter are unlikely to be physiological or to resolve spontaneously and will be malignant in about 5% of premenopausal women and in about 15% of postmenopausal women (Ekerhovd et al 2001). These are probably better removed or at very least re-scanned 3 months later if the woman is unwilling to undergo surgery.

If the cyst is not echo free, unilocular or unilateral or if the CA125 is raised, surgical removal must be advised to all postmenopausal women regardless of the size of the lesion. In premenopausal women, a corpus luteum or an endometrioma will have a complex appearance on ultrasound and the CA125 is often slightly raised. When these are suspected, a repeat scan in 3 months is reasonable with surgery advised if the tumour persists. Otherwise, surgical removal should be advised.

The patient with symptoms

If the patient presents with severe, acute pain or signs of intraperitoneal bleeding, an emergency laparoscopy or laparotomy will be required. More chronic symptoms of pain or pressure may justify pelvic ultrasound if no mass can be felt, but ultrasound is unlikely to contribute to the investigation of a woman in whom both ovaries can be clearly felt to be of a normal size.

The pregnant patient

An ovarian cyst in a pregnant woman may undergo torsion or may bleed. There is said to be an increased incidence of these complications in pregnancy, although the evidence for this is poor. Very occasionally, it can prevent the presenting fetal part from engaging. A dermoid cyst may rupture or leak slowly, causing peritonitis. However, an ovarian cyst is usually discovered incidentally at the antenatal clinic or on ultrasound and occasionally at caesarean section.

The pregnant woman with an ovarian cyst is a special case because of the dangers of surgery to the fetus. These have probably been exaggerated in the past and no urgent operation should be postponed solely because of a pregnancy. Thus, if the patient presents with acute pain due to torsion or haemorrhage into an ovarian tumour or if appendicitis is a possibility, the correct course is to undertake a laparotomy regardless of the stage of the pregnancy. The likelihood of labour ensuing is small. However, the operation should be covered by tocolytic drugs and performed in a centre with intensive neonatal care when possible.

If an asymptomatic cyst is discovered, it is prudent to wait until after 14 weeks' gestation before removing it. This avoids the risk of removing a corpus luteum cyst upon which the pregnancy might still be dependent. In the second and third trimester, the management of an asymptomatic ovarian cyst may be either conservative or surgical. The risks to the mother and fetus of an elective procedure need to be balanced against the chances of a cyst accident, an unexpected malignancy and spontaneous resolution. Cysts less than 10 cm in diameter which have a simple appearance on ultrasound are unlikely to be malignant or to result in a cyst accident, and may therefore be followed ultrasonographically: many will resolve spontaneously (Thornton & Wells 1987). If the cyst is unresolved 6 weeks postpartum, surgery may be undertaken then. The role for cyst aspiration in pregnancy, either diagnostically or therapeutically, is very small. Ovarian cancer is uncommon in pregnancy, occurring in less than 3% of cysts. However, a cyst with features suggestive of malignancy on ultrasound, or one that is growing, should be removed surgically. The tumour marker CA125 is not useful in the pregnant woman, since elevated levels occur frequently as an apparently physiological change. Management may need to include a caesarean hysterectomy, bilateral salpingo-oophorectomy and omentectomy.

The female fetus

Fetal ovarian androgen synthesis commences at 12 weeks' and estradiol and progesterone at 20 weeks' gestation. Thus small follicular cysts up to 7 mm in diameter may occur in up to a third of newborn girls. However, larger cysts are rare and, usually, isolated findings. Most are follicular cysts although luteal cysts, cystic teratomata and granulosa cell tumours also occur. They may undergo torsion or haemorrhage and occasionally necrosis of the pedicle may result in the 'disappearance' of the ovary. Rarely, small bowel compression may cause polyhydramnios but diaphragmatic splinting and consequent pulmonary hypoplasia do not seem to occur. Most resolve spontaneously, either antenatally or, more commonly, postnatally. Consideration may need to be given to the antenatal aspiration of a very large cyst if it is felt that it may obstruct labour or be ruptured during vaginal delivery, although this is reported rarely. Therefore, delivery by caesarean section is not indicated. Cysts which have not resolved by 6 months of age should be explored surgically.

The prepubertal girl

Ovarian cysts are uncommon and often benign. Teratomata and follicular cysts are the most common. Theca and granulosa cell tumours may secrete hormones. Presentation may be with abdominal pain or distension or precocious puberty, either isosexual or heterosexual. Management depends upon relief of symptoms, exclusion of malignancy and conservation of maximum ovarian tissue without jeopardizing fertility.

SURGERY

When treatment is required, it is surgical. Cyst aspiration and oral contraceptives are ineffective.

Therapeutic ultrasound-guided cyst aspiration

The theoretical advantages of this technique are that surgery is avoided and cyst accidents are reduced. However, it assumes that the cyst fluid is unable to reaccumulate and that both physiological (likely to resolve spontaneously) and malignant cysts can be reliably excluded beforehand. Cytological assessment of the aspirated fluid is routinely performed but cannot be relied upon to confirm a benign diagnosis (see above).

A randomized trial of therapeutic cyst aspiration in 278 women with simple cysts diagnosed by ultrasound showed no advantage for aspiration (Zanetta et al 1996). This suggests that there is no place for aspiration of ovarian cysts.

Examination under anaesthesia

Prior to any laparoscopy or laparotomy for a suspected ovarian tumour, it is prudent to perform a bimanual examination under anaesthesia to confirm the presence of the mass. If benign disease seems likely, unilateral salpingo-oophorectomy would be the usual surgical treatment for women under 40 years of age, especially if their family is incomplete, unless probable evidence of malignancy was visible at the time of surgery.

Laparotomy

A clinical diagnosis may not be possible without a laparotomy and even then histological examination is essential for a confident conclusion. Frozen section is seldom of value in this situation as a thorough examination of a tumour is required to exclude invasive disease.

If there is a possibility of invasive disease, a longitudinal skin incision should be used to allow adequate exposure in the upper abdomen. If wider exposure is required after making a transverse incision, the ends of the wound can be extended cranially to fashion a flap from the upper edge of the wound (Fig. 44.3). A sample of ascitic fluid or peritoneal washings should be sent for cytological examination at the beginning of the operation. It is essential to explore the whole abdomen thoroughly and to inspect *both* ovaries.

Women under 35 years of age

In a young woman less than 35 years of age, an ovarian tumour is very unlikely to be malignant. Even if the mass is a primary ovarian malignancy, it is likely to be a germ cell

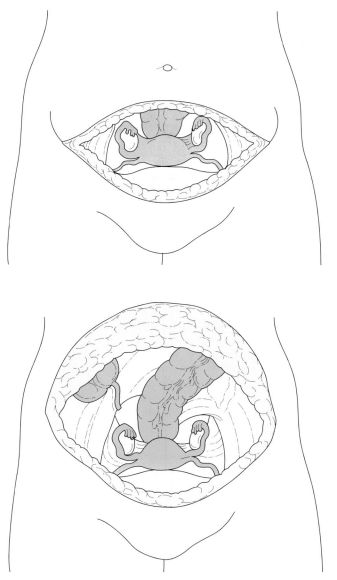

Fig. 44.3 A transverse wound may be enlarged by extending the ends cranially to create a flap from the upper edge.

tumour which is responsive to chemotherapy (see Tables 44.1, 44.2). Thus, ovarian cystectomy or unilateral oophorectomy are sensible and safe treatments for unilateral ovarian masses in this age group (Bianchi et al 1989). It is often said that the contralateral ovary should be bisected and a sample sent for histology in case the tumour is malignant. In practice, most gynaecologists would be unwilling to biopsy an apparently healthy ovary lest this result in infertility from periovarian adhesions. This would be especially true if the tumour was thin-walled and cystic but even apparently solid tumours may be benign. Bilateral dysgerminomas are not common, even allowing for microscopic disease in an apparently normal ovary. Even when the lesion is bilateral, every effort should be made to conserve ovarian tissue. This policy is made possible by the effectiveness of modern chemotherapy for germ cell tumours and is discussed further in Chapter 45.

If malignancy seems likely or if there is a suspicion of malignancy at the time of laparotomy in a young, nulliparous woman with a unilateral tumour and no ascites, unilateral salpingo-oophorectomy may be justifiable after peritoneal washings for cytology and careful exploration to exclude metastatic disease. Curettage of the uterine cavity should be performed to exclude a synchronous endometrial tumour. If the tumour is subsequently found to be poorly differentiated or if the washings are positive, a second operation to clear the pelvis will be necessary. Recurrence rates of 5–9% have been reported after conservative surgery for stage I invasive tumours (Marchetti et al 1998, Zanetta et al 1997).

Women over 34 years of age

It would seem reasonable to individualize treatment of women 35–44 years of age where there are greater benefits to the patient from a conservative approach and where the risks may well be less. If conservative surgery is planned, preliminary hysteroscopy and curettage of the uterus are essential to exclude a concomitant endometrial tumour, a thorough laparotomy is especially important and an appropriate plan of action must be decided in advance with the patient in case more widespread disease is found.

Since epithelial cancer is so much more likely in a woman over the age of 44 years with a unilateral ovarian mass more than 10 cm in diameter, she is probably best advised to have a full staging procedure. This includes peritoneal washings for cytology, a full exploration of the abdomen, removal of the infracolic omentum and total abdominal hysterectomy and bilateral salpingo-oophorectomy. Some also recommend lymph node sampling but the benefit of this remains unproven.

Laparoscopy

The advantages of laparoscopy over laparotomy are largely short term and economic. Hospital stay and time to resumption of normal life are both shortened. In the opinion of an expert group with many years of experience, although these advantages are very attractive, they cannot justify a possible dissemination of tumour and reduction in survival (Canis et al 1999). Even extraction in a bag does not protect against dissemination of malignant disease. This group advises bilateral adnexectomy in postmenopausal women but does not remove the uterus because of the added operating time and morbidity. Instead, they undertake routine cervical smears and hysteroscopy.

They also report that the cosmetic effect is probably similar when comparing a laparotomy tailored to the size of the tumour and a laparoscopic adnexectomy followed by an incision large enough to allow easy extraction without morcellation of the tumour. In premenopausal women with benign-looking cysts, they puncture the cyst and aspirate the cyst fluid which is then sent for routine cytology. The cyst is opened with scissors and the internal cyst wall is inspected for signs of malignancy. In postmenopausal women or premenopausal women with highly suspicious masses, adnexectomy is performed and the cyst opened after removal.

Another group with a large experience in the field treated 493 women laparoscopically in 2 years (Mettler et al 2001).

The mean size of these tumours was 4.5 cm, with a range of 1.1–11 cm. The predominance of functional cysts and corpus luteum cysts suggests that many of these would have resolved spontaneously without intervention.

Laparoscopic procedures

Diagnostic laparoscopy may be of value if there is uncertainty about the nature of the pelvic mass. Thus it may be possible to avoid a laparotomy when there is no pathology. However, it can be difficult to exclude ovarian disease in the presence of marked pelvic inflammatory disease and pelvic adhesions.

The second indication for laparoscopy is if the patient has a cyst suitable for laparoscopic surgery (Nezhat et al 1989). This decision should be made after a full history and careful bimanual examination, ultrasound assessment and a thorough laparoscopic appraisal of the whole abdominal cavity, particularly the contralateral ovary. The patient should be consented for a laparotomy in case malignancy is found or unexpected laparoscopic complications encountered.

These operations require considerable expertise in laparoscopic manipulation and should not be attempted without appropriate training. The following laparoscopic procedures have been used in the management of ovarian cysts:

- aspiration and fenestration
- cystectomy – intraperitoneal, with or without cyst puncture, or extra-abdominal
- oophorectomy or salpingo-oophorectomy.

Aspiration and fenestration (removal of a window of the cyst wall, for histological analysis) has several disadvantages and cannot be recommended. Recurrence, spillage of cyst contents and failure to diagnose a malignant tumour are all possible, even if the inner surface of the cyst is carefully inspected (ovarian cystoscopy), the fluid sent for cytological assessment and careful peritoneal lavage performed. Frozen section is also unreliable and cannot be recommended routinely. It has been suggested that aspiration is reserved for physiological cysts but in general their benign course means that they should not be subjected to surgery unless they fail to resolve spontaneously. Aspiration may be combined with cystectomy.

Cystectomy may be performed using two or three 5 mm puncture trocars, one inserted suprapubically in the midline and the others lateral to the inferior epigastric vessels. The ovarian capsule is incised with either scissors, diathermy or CO_2 laser and either blunt or hydrodissection used to separate the cyst. The CO_2 laser may be particularly useful to vaporize the inner wall of endometriomas. The cyst is then removed, either through a large portal or in a laparoscopic bag to reduce the risk of dissemination of the cyst contents.

Alternatively, following laparoscopic assessment of the cyst, a small suprapubic transverse skin incision allows the ovary to be grasped under laparoscopic view and pulled onto the skin. The parietal peritoneum under the skin incision is only incised once the ovary has been grasped. This extra-abdominal approach is particularly appropriate for the management of larger cysts and seems to combine the best aspects of laparoscopic and 'traditional' surgery.

Prior to oophorectomy, the course of the ureter must be established. The broad ligament and round ligament are coagulated and cut. Endoloops, extracorporeal knots or the Endo-GIA stapler may be used to ligate the infundibulopelvic ligament and ovarian vessels.

KEY POINTS

1. Asymptomatic, benign ovarian cysts in young women often resolve spontaneously.
2. Ovarian cysts with a simple appearance on ultrasound and less than 10 cm in diameter are very rarely malignant.
3. Solid ovarian tumours are often malignant; in young women these are usually germ cell or sex cord stromal tumours.
4. There is no place for ultrasound-directed aspiration of cysts.
5. Laparoscopic removal of ovarian cysts should be confined to those with no features of malignancy.
6. Women over 44 years of age with a unilocular ovarian cyst greater than 10 cm or with any other type of ovarian tumour should usually be advised to have a total abdominal hysterectomy and bilateral salpingo-oophorectomy.
7. A bimanual examination under anaesthesia should be performed prior to any surgery for ovarian tumours to confirm that a mass is still palpable.

In memoriam

In the spring of 2002, Gerardo Zanetta died. The authors express their admiration for the immense contribution that he made to improving the care of women with benign and borderline ovarian tumours and early ovarian carcinoma.

REFERENCES

Bailey CL, Ueland FR, Land GL et al 1998 The malignant potential of small cystic ovarian tumors in women over 50 years of age. Gynecological Oncology 69:3–7

Bianchi UA, Favalli G, Sartori E et al 1989 Limited surgery in non-epithelial ovarian cancer. In: Conte PF, Ragni N, Rosso R, Vermorken JB (eds) Multimodal treatment of ovarian cancer. Raven Press, New York, pp 119–126

Canis M, Mage G, Pomel C et al 1999 Laparoscopic diagnosis of adnexal tumours. In: Querleu D, Childers JM, Dargent D (eds) Laparoscopic surgery in gynaecological oncology. Blackwell Science, Oxford, pp 9–16

Comerci JT, Licciardi F, Bergh PA, Gregori C, Breen JL 1994 Mature cystic teratoma: a clinicopathological evaluation of 517 cases and review of the literature. Obstetrics and Gynecology 84:22–28

Cronje HS, Niemand I, Bam RH, Woodruff JD 1999 Review of the granulosa-theca cell tumours from the Emil Novak Ovarian Tumor Registry. American Journal of Obstetrics & Gynecology 180:323–327

Diernaes E, Rasmussen J, Soersen T, Hasche E 1987 Ovarian cysts: management by puncture? Lancet i:1084

Ekerhovd E, Wienerroith H, Staudach A, Granberg S 2001 Preoperative assessment of unilocular adnexal cysts by transvaginal ultrasonography: a comparison between ultrasonographic morphologic imaging and histopathologic diagnosis. American Journal of Obstetrics and Gynecology 184:48–54

Evans AT, Gaffey TA, Malkasian GD, Annegers JF 1980 Clinicopathological review of 118 granulosa and 83 theca cell tumours. Obstetrics and Gynecology 55:231–237

Goldstein SR 1993 Conservative management of small postmenopausal cystic masses. Clinical Obstetrics and Gynaecology 36 (2):395–401

Koonings PP, Campbell K, Mishell DR, Grimes DA 1989 Relative frequency of primary ovarian neoplasms: a 10 year review. Obstetrics and Gynecology 74:921–926

Levine D, Gosink B, Wolf SI, Feldesman MR, Pretorius DH 1992 Simple adnexal cysts: the natural history in postmenopausal women. Radiology 184:653–659

Malstrom H, Hogberg T, Risberg B, Simonsen E 1994 Granulosa cell tumours of the ovary: prognostic factors and outcome. Gynecological Oncology 52:50–55

Marchetti M, Padoran P, Fracas M 1998 Malignant ovarian tumors: conservative surgery and quality of life in young patients. European Journal of Gynaecological Oncology 19:297–301

Mettler L, Jacobs V, Brandenburg K, Jonat W, Semm K 2001 Laparoscopic management of 641 adnexal tumours in Keil, Germany. Journal of the American Association of Gynaecological Laparoscopists 8:74–82

Nezhat C, Winer WK, Nezhat F 1989 Laparoscopic removal of dermoid cysts. Obstetrics and Gynecology 73:278–281

Osmers RGW, Osmers M, von Maydell B, Wagner B, Kuhn W 1998 Evaluation of ovarian tumors in postmenopausal women by transvaginal sonography. European Journal of Obstetrics Gynecology and Reproductive Biology 77:81–88

Quinn M, Babb P, Brock A, Kirby L, Jones J 2001 Cancer trends in England and Wales 1950–1999. Studies on medical and population subjects no. 66. Stationery Office, London

Sasaki H, Oda M, Ohmura M et al 1999 Follow up of women with simple ovarian cysts detected by transvaginal sonography in the Tokyo metropolitan area. British Journal of Obstetrics and Gynaecology 106:415–420

Saunders AM, Hertzman VO 1960 Malignant carcinoid teratoma of the ovary. Canadian Medical Association Journal 83:602–605

Steinkampf MP, Hammond KR 1990 Hormonal treatment of functional ovarian cysts: a randomised, prospective study. Fertility and Sterility 54:775–777

Thornton JG, Wells M 1987 Ovarian cysts in pregnancy: does ultrasound make traditional management inappropriate? Obstetrics and Gynecology 69:717–720

Wertheim I, Fleischhacker D, McLachlin CM, Rice LW, Berkowitz RS, Goff BA 1994 Pseudomyxoma peritonei: a review of 23 cases. Obstetrics and Gynecology 84:17–21

Zanetta G, Lissoni A, Torri V et al 1996 Role of puncture and aspiration in expectant management of simple ovarian cysts: a randomised study. British Medical Journal 313:1110–1113

Zanetta G, Chiari S, Rota S et al 1997 Conservative surgery for stage l ovarian carcinoma in women of childbearing age. British Journal of Obstetrics and Gynaecology 104:1030–1035

45

Carcinoma of the ovary and fallopian tube

Roberto Dina   Gordon J.S. Rustin   Pat Soutter

CARCINOMA OF THE OVARY

EPIDEMIOLOGY

Carcinoma of the ovary is commoner in developed areas, such as Europe and the USA. In England and Wales, there were just over 6100 new registrations of ovarian cancer in 1997, making it the fourth most common site in women after breast, colorectal and lung (Quinn et al 2001). The overall age-standardized incidence rate rose steadily from the early 1970s to reach 19 per 100 000 in 1997. There are now about 30% more cases than uterine cancer and almost double the number of cervical cancer cases. Because of its much poorer survival, it accounts for 6% of all cancer deaths in women, far more than all the other gynaecological cancers combined.

Most ovarian tumours are of epithelial origin. These are rare before the age of 35 years but the incidence increases with age to a peak in the 50–70-year-old age group. Just under half occur in women aged 45–65 years (Fig. 45.1). Most epithelial tumours are advanced at diagnosis so only 29% of women

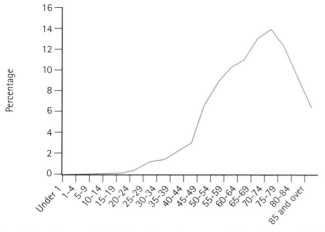

Fig. 45.1 The age distribution of ovarian cancer in England and Wales in 1997 (Quin et al 2001).

with ovarian cancer are alive at 5 years. Eventually 75–80% of women with ovarian cancer will die from their disease. Only 3% of ovarian cancers are seen in women younger than 35 years and the vast majority of these are non-epithelial cancers such as germ cell tumours.

AETIOLOGY

'Incessant ovulation' theory

The factors which lead to the development of ovarian carcinoma are not known. Epithelial tumours are most frequently associated with nulliparity, an early menarche, a late age at menopause and a long estimated number of years of ovulation (Hildreth et al 1981). The infrequent occurrence of carcinoma of the ovary in women of high parity is thought to be due to the suppression of continuous ovulation and there is now good evidence that oral contraceptives play a protective role (Ness et al 2001, Vessey et al 1987). This applies equally to carriers of a mutated BRCA1 gene (Narod et al 2001). However, a very large case control study which confirmed the protective effect of parity also showed that the risk fell with increasing age at first birth in a population in which use of oral contraceptives was very limited (Adami et al 1994). This and the protection associated with tubal ligation and other methods of contraception in multigravid but not nulligravid women (Narod et al 2001, Ness et al 2001) cast doubt upon the 'incessant ovulation' theory.

Infertility treatment

There is an association between infertility and both ovarian and endometrial cancer. This link appears to be strongest in women with unexplained infertility (Venn et al 1995) and in women who have not been able to become pregnant at all (Rodriguez et al 1998). However, a pooled analysis of several case control studies showed a small increased risk for ovarian cancer in infertile women treated with 'fertility drugs' (odds ratio 2.8, 95% CI 1.3–6.1) (Whittemore et al 1992) and 12 cases of granulosa cell tumours were reported after ovarian

stimulation (Willemsen et al 1993). A later paper showed that use of clomiphene for more than a year was associated with an increased risk of borderline or invasive ovarian tumours (relative risk 11.1, 95% CI 1.5–82.3) (Rossing et al 1994). Subsequently, a large study of women who underwent IVF showed no increased risk in up to 15 years after ovarian stimulation (Venn et al 1995). However, these women would not have been treated more than five or six times at most.

Overall, these various studies do suggest the possibility of a link with ovulation induction but only after prolonged treatment. However the situation remains unclear (Shelly et al 1999).

GENETIC FACTORS

These are described in more detail in Chapter 32.

Familial cancer

Inheritance plays a significant role in about 5% of epithelial ovarian cancers. These tumours are usually serous adenocarcinomas. The lifetime risk for a woman with one affected close relative is dependent upon her own age and the relationship with the affected relative (Stratton et al 1998). For a woman aged 45 years or less with one affected relative, the lifetime risk is about 4%. If the one affected relative was her mother, the risk rises to about 7%. With more than one affected relative the risk is about 14%. After the age of 45, the risk falls steadily. It is unusual to find families with multiple cases of only ovarian cancer. More commonly, there are cases of breast or colorectal cancer in the family. The Lynch syndrome consists of families with colorectal cancer, endometrial cancer and ovarian cancer (Watson & Lynch 1992).

The genes involved with ovarian cancer are described in Chapter 36. A woman who has inherited the BRCA1 gene in a well-documented family has a 60% risk of breast cancer by 50 years of age and an 80% lifetime risk. The risk of ovarian cancer is in the region of 40–50%. Although the BRCA2 penetrance for breast cancer is approximately 80% the penetrance for ovarian cancer seems to be lower than for BRCA1 mutations and is approximately 25%. While BRCA1 mutations do occur in sporadic disease, they are relatively uncommon. The management of women with a family history of ovarian cancer is described in Chapter 36.

MOLECULAR BIOLOGY

Much effort has been invested in studying the biology of ovarian cancer in the hope that improved understanding would lead to better treatment or prevention. In recent years, the search has focused on the overexpression of potential oncogenes and on the role of cytokines. Her-2/neu (c-erbB-2) is an oncogene that codes for an epidermal growth factor (EGF) receptor-like molecule. It is overexpressed in about 30% of ovarian carcinomas and may indicate a poor prognosis (Berchuck et al 1990). Inactivating antibodies to the extracellular portion of the HER-2/neu gene product can inhibit the growth of cells that overexpress the gene (Bast et al 1992).

Mutations in the tumour suppressor gene p53 are observed in up to half of women with advanced disease (Marks et al 1991). The lower incidence of mutations in early-stage disease may suggest that p53 mutations are a late event in the development of ovarian cancer. Alternatively, such mutations may result in rapid progression of disease. Another tumour suppressor gene recently discovered by Dr Gabra and his team in Edinburgh is called OBCAM. This encodes a GPI-anchored cell adhesion molecule of the IgLON family. This is strongly expressed in normal ovarian epithelium but only weakly expressed in cancer cell lines.

Most ovarian and endometrial tumours overexpress CSF-1 (M-CSF) and its receptor encoded by the proto-oncogene *c-fms*. CSF-1 can stimulate the growth of tumour cell lines and transfection of the cells with a dominant negative mutant *c-fms* gene inhibits cell growth. This suggests that CSF-1 and *c-fms* can cause an autocrine stimulation of tumour growth. There is also evidence of persistent autocrine stimulation by transforming growth factor alpha (TGF-α) and epidermal growth factor (EGF), both acting through the EGF receptor (EGFR) (Rodriguez et al 1991). Paracrine stimulation by cytokines produced by macrophages may also influence both the growth and invasiveness of tumour cells. Tumour necrosis factor alpha (TNF-α) appears to be particularly potent in this regard (Naylor et al 1995).

CLASSIFICATION OF OVARIAN TUMOURS

Ovarian tumours can be solid or cystic. They may be benign or malignant and in addition there are those which, while having some of the features of malignancy, lack any evidence of stromal invasion. These are called borderline tumours.

The most commonly used classification of ovarian tumours was defined by the World Health Organization (Scully 1999). This is a morphological classification that attempts to relate the cell types and patterns of the tumour to tissues normally present in the ovary. The primary tumours are thus divided into those that are of epithelial type (implying an origin from surface epithelium and the adjacent ovarian stroma), those that are of sex cord gonadal type (also known as sex cord stromal type or sex cord mesenchymal type, and originating from sex cord mesenchymal elements) and those that are of germ cell type (originating from germ cells). A simplified version of the WHO classification is given in Box 45.1.

PATHOLOGY OF EPITHELIAL TUMOURS

These are derived from the ovarian surface epithelium, which is a modified mesothelium with a similar origin and behaviour to the müllerian duct epithelium, and from the adjacent distinctive ovarian stroma. They are subclassified according to epithelial cell type (serous, mucinous, endometrioid, clear, transitional, squamous); the relative amount of epithelial and stromal component (when the stromal is larger than the cystic epithelial component the suffix fibroma is added); and the macroscopic appearance (solid or cystic or papillary). They account for 50–55% of all ovarian tumours but their malignant forms represent approximately 90% of all ovarian cancers in the Western world (Koonings et al 1989). Well-differentiated

Box 45.1   Histological classification of ovarian tumours

I   Common epithelial tumours (benign, borderline or malignant)
   A   Serous tumour
   B   Mucinous tumour
   C   Endometrioid tumour
   D   Clear cell (mesonephroid) tumour
   E   Brenner tumour
   F   Mixed epithelial tumour
   G   Undifferentiated carcinomas
   H   Unclassified tumour
II   Sex cord stromal tumours
   A   Granulosa stroma cell tumour
   B   Androblastoma: Sertoli–Leydig cell tumour
   C   Gynandroblastoma
   D   Unclassified tumour
III   Lipid cell tumours
IV   Germ cell tumours
   A   Dysgerminoma
   B   Endodermal sinus tumour (yolk sac tumour)
   C   Embryonal cell tumour
   D   Polyembryoma
   E   Choriocarcinoma
   F   Teratoma
   G   Mixed tumours
V   Gonadoblastoma
VI   Soft tissue tumours not specific to ovary
VII   Unclassified tumours
VIII   Metastatic tumours

epithelial carcinomas tend to be more often associated with early-stage disease, but the degree of differentiation does correlate with survival, except in the most advanced stages. Diploid tumours tend to be associated with earlier stage disease and a better prognosis. Histological cell type is not of itself prognostically significant.

Comparing patients stage for stage and grade for grade, there is no difference in survival in different epithelial types. However, mucinous and endometrioid lesions are likely to be associated with earlier stage and lower grade than serous cystadenocarcinomas.

Serous carcinoma

Gross features
The majority of serous carcinomas show a mixture of solid and cystic elements, although a significant minority are predominantly cystic. Serous carcinomas have a propensity to bilaterality, ranging from 50% to 90% but in only 25–30% of stage I cases.

Microscopical features
The better differentiated tumours have an obviously papillary pattern with unequivocal stromal invasion and psammoma bodies (calcospherules) are often present (Fig. 45.2). A highly differentiated form of serous papillary carcinoma called psammocarcinoma contains large numbers of psammoma bodies surrounded by no more than 15 well to moderately differentiated serous cells and has a favourable prognosis, even

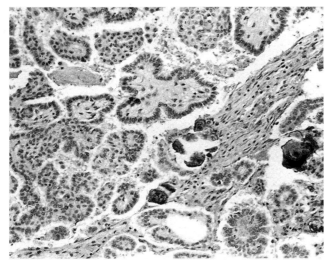

Fig. 45.2 Serous papillary cystadenocarcinoma. A well-differentiated (grade 1) serous carcinoma. The papillary pattern is obvious and a group of psammoma bodies is present at the lower right. Haematoxylin and eosin ×180.

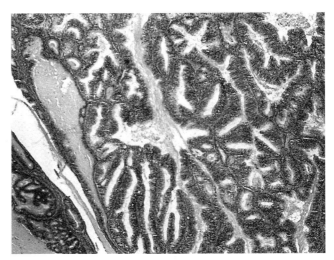

Fig. 45.3 Mucinous adenocarcinoma of the ovary. Haematoxylin and eosin ×180.

if most lesions are found in stage III. None of these features is diagnostic of serous tumours alone. Endometrioid and clear cell carcinomas and, to a lesser extent, mucinous carcinomas may all form papillary structures. The term 'papillary carcinoma of the ovary' therefore should not be used as a diagnosis.

At the other end of the spectrum is the anaplastic tumour composed of sheets of undifferentiated neoplastic cells in masses within a fibrous stroma. Occasional glandular structures may be present to enable a diagnosis of adenocarcinoma to be made. All gradations between these two are seen, sometimes in the same tumour.

Mucinous carcinoma

Gross features
Malignant mucinous tumours comprise about 12% of malignant tumours of the ovary. They are typically multilocular, thin-walled cysts with a smooth external surface, containing mucinous fluid. The locules vary in size and often the tumour may be composed of one major cavity with many smaller daughter cysts apparently within its wall. Mucinous tumours are amongst the largest tumours of the ovary and may reach enormous dimensions; a cyst diameter of 25 cm is quite commonplace.

A mucinous cystadenocarcinoma may look the same as a benign tumour. Some malignant tumours may exhibit obvious solid areas, perhaps with necrosis and haemorrhage. The more advanced carcinomas will show the stigmata of ovarian malignancy, with adhesions to adjacent viscera and malignant ascites.

Microscopical features
Mucinous adenocarcinomas present a variety of histological appearances (Fig. 45.3). They may contain only endocervical-like cells, intestinal-type cells or a combination of the two but are more often composed of mucinous cells without

distinguishing features. The better differentiated examples are composed of cells that retain a resemblance to the tall, picket-fence cells of the benign tumour, although stromal invasion is present. As differentiation is lost, the cells become less easily recognizable as of mucinous type and their mucin content diminishes.

Endometrioid carcinoma

These are ovarian tumours that resemble the malignant neoplasia of epithelial, stromal and mixed origin that are found in the endometrium (Czernobilsky et al 1970). They account for 2–4% of all ovarian tumours. They are accompanied by ovarian or pelvic endometriosis in 11–42% of cases and in up to 30% of cases a transition to endometriotic epithelium can be seen. The pathologist must distinguish metaplastic and reactive changes in endometriosis from true neoplastic changes.

Gross features
There is little to characterize an ovarian tumour as being of endometrioid type by naked-eye examination. Most are cystic, often unilocular and contain turbid brown fluid. The internal surface of the cyst is usually rough with rounded, polypoid projections and solid areas the appearances of which are usually distinct from those of the papillary excrescences seen in serous tumours.

Microscopical features
Endometrioid carcinomas resemble the endometrioid carcinomas of the endometrium (Fig. 45.4). The pattern is predominantly tubular and may resemble proliferative endometrium. The epithelium is tall and columnar, with a high nuclear:cytoplasmic ratio. Endometrioid carcinomas of the ovary are more likely to be papillary than are primary endometrial carcinomas. Five to 10% of cases are seen in continuity with recognizable endometriosis. Ovarian adeno-acanthoma, with benign-appearing squamous elements,

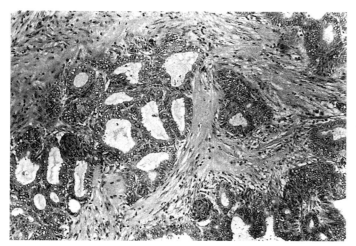

Fig. 45.4 Endometrioid carcinoma of the ovary. Haematoxylin and eosin ×180.

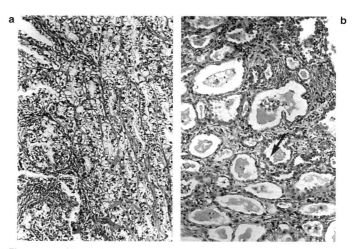

Fig. 45.5 Clear cell carcinoma of the ovary. **a** A moderately differentiated glandular pattern composed entirely of clear cells. Haematoxylin and eosin ×170. **b** A tubulocystic area showing prominent 'hob-nail' cells (arrow). Haematoxylin and eosin ×230.

account for almost 50% in some series of endometrioid tumours.

Associated endometrial carcinoma

It is important to note that 15% of endometrioid carcinoma of the ovary are associated with endometrial carcinoma in the body of the uterus. Although this is sometimes due to a primary in one site and a secondary at the other, in most cases these are two separate primary tumours.

Clear cell carcinoma (mesonephroid)

These are the least common of the malignant epithelial tumours of the ovary, accounting for 5–10% of ovarian carcinomas (Anderson & Langley 1970).

Gross features

There is nothing characteristic about the gross appearances of the clear cell tumour to distinguish it from the other cystadenocarcinomas of the ovary. Most are thick-walled, unilocular cysts containing turbid brown or bloodstained fluid, with solid, polypoid projections arising from the internal surface. About 10% are bilateral.

Microscopical features

Clear cell carcinomas of the ovary are characterized by the variety of their architectural patterns, which may be found alone or in combination in any individual tumour (Fig. 45.5). The appearance from which the tumours derive their name is the clear cell pattern but, in addition, some areas show a tubulocystic pattern with the characteristic 'hob-nail' appearance of the lining epithelium. The third major pattern is papillary.

Association with endometriosis and endometrioid tumours

Because there is a very strong association between clear cell tumours of the ovary and ovarian endometriosis and because clear cell and endometrioid tumours frequently co-exist, it has been suggested that the clear cell tumour may be a variant of endometrioid tumour.

Transitional cell tumours

These represent 1–2% of all ovarian tumours and most are benign. The epithelial component resembles urothelium which may undergo cystic, mucinous or serous metaplasia, the stromal component resembles that of fibromas in the benign or borderline lesions while the malignant counterpart resembles a transitional cell carcinoma.

Borderline epithelial tumours

Approximately 10% of all epithelial tumours of the ovary are borderline tumours, of which 30% are of the mucinous type, followed by the serous type. Other borderline tumours are rare. The histological diagnosis of borderline malignancy can be difficult, particularly in mucinous tumours (Fig. 45.6). These show varying degrees of nuclear atypia and an increase in mitotic activity, multilayering of neoplastic cells and formation of cellular buds, but no invasion of the stroma. Most borderline tumours remain confined to the ovaries and this may account for their much better prognosis.

Peritoneal lesions are present in some cases and although a few are true metastases, many do not grow and even regress after removal of the primary. Surgical pathological stage and subclassification of extraovarian disease into invasive and non-invasive implants are the most important prognostic indicators for serous borderline tumours, the survival for advanced-stage serous tumours with non-invasive implants being 95.3% as opposed to 66% for tumours with invasive implants (Seidman & Kurman 2000).

NATURAL HISTORY

Approximately two-thirds of patients present with disease spread beyond the pelvis. This is probably due to the insidious

681

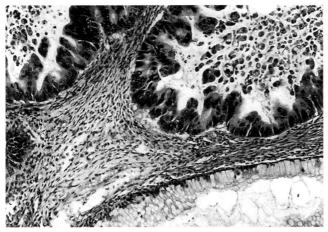

Fig. 45.6 A borderline mucinous tumour with multilayering of the epithelium but no evidence of stromal invasion.

nature of the signs and symptoms of carcinoma of the ovary but may sometimes be due to a rapidly growing tumour. Due to the non-specific nature of most of these symptoms, a diagnosis of ovarian cancer is seldom considered until the disease is in an advanced stage.

Metastatic spread

The pelvic peritoneum and other pelvic organs become involved by direct spread. The peritoneal fluid, flowing to lymphatic channels on the undersurface of the diaphragm, carries malignant cells to the omentum, to the peritoneal surfaces of the small and large bowel and liver and to the parietal peritoneal surface throughout the abdominal cavity and on the surface of the diaphragm. Metastases on the undersurface of the diaphragm may be found in up to 44% of of what otherwise seems to be stage I–II disease. Intraperitoneal metastases are superficial and seldom involve the substance of the organ beneath. Even when the surface of the bowel is extensively involved, the muscularis layer is seldom infiltrated.

Lymphatic spread is generally thought to be mainly along the lymphatics that run with the ovarian vessels to the para-aortic region at the level of the renal vessels. These nodes may be involved in 19% of stages I–II and in 65% of stages III–IV. However, pelvic lymph node involvement occurs more often than previously reported (Table 45.1; Burghardt et al 1991). Spread may also occur to nodes in the neck or inguinal region.

Haematogenous spread usually occurs late in the course of the disease. The main areas involved are the liver and the lung, although metastases to bone and brain are sometimes seen.

Table 45.1 Pelvic and para-aortic node metastases (Burghardt et al 1991)

	Nodes involved	
	Pelvic nodes	Para-aortic nodes
Stage I–II	30%	19%
Stage III–IV	67%	65%

Box 45.2 FIGO staging for primary ovarian carcinoma

I Growth limited to ovaries
   Ia   Growth limited to one ovary
       no ascites; no tumour on external surface; capsule intact
   Ib   Growth limited to both ovaries
       no ascites; no tumour on external surfaces; capsule intact
   Ic   Tumour either stage Ia or Ib but tumour on surface of one or both ovaries; or with capsule ruptured; or with ascites present containing malignant cells; or with positive peritoneal washings

II Growth involving one or both ovaries with pelvic extension
   IIa Extension and/or metastases to the uterus or tubes
   IIb Extension to other pelvic tissues
   IIc Tumour either stage IIa or IIb but tumour on surface of one or both ovaries; or with capsule ruptured; or with ascites present containing malignant cells; or with positive peritoneal washings

III Growth involving one or both ovaries with peritoneal implants outside the pelvis or positive retroperitoneal or inguinal nodes. Superficial liver metastases equals stage III
   IIIa Tumour grossly limited to the true pelvis with negative nodes but with histologically confirmed microscopic seeding of abdominal peritoneal surfaces
   IIIb Tumour with histologically confirmed implants on abdominal peritoneal surfaces, none exceeding 2 cm in diameter. Nodes are negative
   IIIc Abdominal implants greater than 2 cm in diameter or positive retroperitoneal or inguinal nodes

IV Growth involving one or both ovaries with distant metastases. If pleural effusion is present there must be positive cytology to allot a case to stage IV. Parenchymal liver metastasis equals stage IV

CLINICAL STAGING

The staging of ovarian cancer as defined by FIGO is shown in Box 45.2. Peritoneal deposits on the surface of the liver do not make the patient stage IV; the parenchyma must be involved. Similarly, the presence of a pleural effusion is insufficient to put the patient in stage IV unless malignant cells are found on cytological examination of the pleural fluid.

DIAGNOSIS

Abdominal pain or discomfort are the most common presenting complaints and distension or feeling a lump the next most frequent. Patients may complain of indigestion, urinary frequency, weight loss or, rarely, abnormal menses or post-menopausal bleeding. A hard abdominal mass arising from the pelvis is highly suggestive, especially in the presence of ascites. A fixed, hard, irregular pelvic mass is usually felt best by combined vaginal and rectal examination (Fig. 45.7). The neck and groin should also be examined for enlarged nodes.

Haematological investigations include a full blood count, urea, electrolytes and liver function tests. A chest X-ray is essential. It is sometimes advisable to carry out a barium enema to differentiate between an ovarian and a colonic tumour and to assess bowel involvement from the ovarian tumour itself. An IVP is sometimes useful.

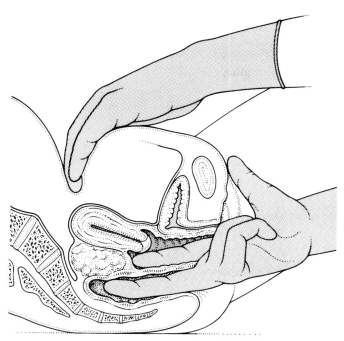

Fig. 45.7 A combined vaginal and rectal examination allows more accurate assessment of the pouch of Douglas.

Imaging techniques

Ultrasonography may help to confirm the presence of a pelvic mass and detect ascites before it is clinically apparent. It is also a relatively reliable tool for examining the liver parenchyma and may detect enlarged pelvic or para-aortic lymph nodes.

Computed axial tomography of the abdomen and pelvis is used as an alternative to ultrasonography but is more expensive and less accurate in the pelvis. Magnetic resonance imaging (MRI) is particularly useful for examining the pelvis in difficult cases but its use is not justifiable in routine management. Radio-immunoscintigraphy is still a research tool but it has some value in detecting spread of ovarian tumour within the abdomen. None of these techniques will detect small peritoneal metastases.

The most accurate method for assessing lymph node involvement is biopsy at the time of surgery. Lymphangiography is accurate only to a degree as it cannot detect micrometastases and false-positive results are frequent.

Markers for epithelial tumours

None of the markers available at the present time is sufficiently accurate or specific to detect ovarian cancer at an early stage. The most useful marker, CA125, derived from a human cancer line, is usually raised in advanced ovarian cancer but it can also be raised in benign conditions such as endometriosis. Using CA125 estimations to monitor women receiving chemotherapy is a useful method for assessing response and can reduce the need for scans. A persistent rise in CA125 may precede clinical evidence of recurrent disease by several months in some cases. However, the values can be normal in the presence of small tumour deposits.

Carcinoembryonic antigen (CEA) is abnormal most often in mucinous cystadenocarcinoma. Concentrations in excess of 20 ng/ml are suggestive of ovarian tumour. The tumour-associated antigens OCCA and OCA are raised in both serous and mucinous cystadenocarcinoma (van Nagell 1983).

Cytology

In patients with pleural effusion or ascites, specimens of fluid may be examined cytologically for the presence of malignant cells. Regardless of FIGO stage, positive peritoneal washing cytology predicts a poor prognosis. It is seldom justifiable to perform a paracentesis for cytology; that can be deferred until the laparotomy. Fine needle aspiration of clinically suspicious lymph nodes in the groin or neck can be very valuable.

Differentiating malignant from benign pelvic masses

It is important to differentiate a malignant from a benign pelvic mass in order to ensure that the woman undergoes surgery in an appropriately staffed department with a gynaecological oncology team of surgeons, oncologists and nurses. Much work has gone into the development of 'risk of malignancy indices' using ultrasound, CA125 and age or menopausal status. However, none of the published methods performs as well when tested on a second population (Aslam et al 2000, Mol et al 2001, Morgante et al 1999). Typically, to obtain a sensitivity of 90% the cut-off value must be set at a level that gives a specificity of only 46–61% and a positive predictive value of only 33%. This means that half of the population would have a positive result, only one-third of these would have cancer and 10% of the women with cancer would be wrongly labelled benign. The sensitivity needs to be reduced to an unacceptable 55% to achieve a specificity of 95%.

It is clear that none of these methods performs terribly well even when most of the malignant tumours were advanced stage. The cut-off value used will depend upon local circumstances and upon whether it is thought to be more important to refer most women with cancer or to reduce the number needing referral to the minimum.

Screening

Because carcinoma of the ovary tends to be asymptomatic in the early stages and most patients present with advanced disease, efforts have been made to define a tumour marker which could be used for screening purposes. So far, none has become available which is truly specific and suitable for the early detection of epithelial carcinoma (MacDonald et al 1998, Oram & Jeyarajah 1994, Urban 1999).

Tumour markers

The only marker assessed in a prospective trial of screening is CA125 (Jacobs et al 1999). Ultrasound was used for all women with abnormal values. In this study of 21 000 women, six cancers were detected by screening and 10 further women in the screened group developed cancer in the subsequent 8 years' follow-up. In the control group, 20 women developed cancer.

The women with ovarian cancer in the screening group had a longer survival than those in the unscreened control group. A greater improvement in median survival from 20 months to 100 months was reported by the Stockholm Screening Study (Einhorn et al 2000).

New markers with promise for the future include macrophage colony-stimulating factor (MCSF) (Suzuki et al 1993); inhibin, a marker for mucinous cancers (Burger 1993) and granulosa cell tumours; and OVX1 (Xu et al 1993). A combination of CA125, MCSF and OVX1 gave 98% sensitivity in patients with stage I disease but 11% false-positive results (Woolas et al 1993).

Ultrasound for screening

After very disappointing results with conventional ultrasound methods, colour flow transvaginal ultrasound was assessed in 1601 women with a family history of ovarian cancer (Bourne at al 1993). A laparotomy or laparoscopy was performed in 61 of these women as a result of an abnormal scan. Six of these had ovarian cancer, five were stage Ia and three of these were borderline tumours.

A more recent report has described somewhat more encouraging results (van Nagell et al 2000). Annual trans-vaginal scans performed on 14 469 asymptomatic women from 1987 to 1999 detected 17 ovarian cancers in 180 women with persistent abnormalities. Two-thirds were detected at stage I and 88% of the women found to have invasive ovarian cancer survived 5 years. The sensitivity, specificity and negative predictive value were 81%, 98.9% and 99.97% respectively but the positive predictive value was only 9.4% and this resulted in surgery for benign and probably harmless disease. Ultrasound is good at detecting early disease but it is labour intensive and operator dependent and there are many false-positive results.

Conclusion

In our present state of knowledge and with the available technology, screening the general population is neither useful nor safe. High-risk patients may take part in trials to assess new screening techniques but should not be led to believe that these have proven value. This subject is well reviewed by Oram & Jeyarajah (1994).

SURGERY

The exploration

Surgery is the mainstay of both the diagnosis and the treatment of ovarian cancer. A vertical incision is required for an adequate exploration of the upper abdomen. A sample of ascitic fluid or peritoneal washings with normal saline, which must be taken for cytology, should be obtained before any manipulation of the tumour to avoid contamination.

The pelvis and upper abdomen are explored carefully, including the omentum, sub-diaphragmatic areas, the paracolic gutters, large and small bowel and small bowel mesentery. Such an exploration is not possible with a low transverse incision. In the absence of gross upper abdominal disease, suspicious areas should be biopsied. A sample for cytology may be taken from the diaphragm with an Ayre's spatula (Griffiths 1987).

The therapeutic objective

The therapeutic objective of surgery for ovarian cancer is the removal of all tumour. While this is achieved in the majority of stage I cases and in some stage II, it is probably impossible in more advanced disease. Because of the diffuse spread of tumour throughout the peritoneal cavity and the retroperitoneal nodes, microscopic deposits will persist in almost all cases even when all macroscopic tumour appears to have been excised. Thus, while surgery alone may be curative in many stage I cases, additional therapy is essential for most of the remainder.

BORDERLINE TUMOURS

Prognosis

Women with borderline ovarian tumours have an excellent prognosis if the tumour is confined to the ovary, as it usually is. DNA ploidy is said by some to be the most important prognostic factor. In one study, patients with diploid stage I tumours had a very good prognosis but those with aneuploid tumours had a 19-fold increased risk of dying (Kaern et al 1993). Patients with aneuploid tumours were more likely to be older, to have mucinous tumours or severe atypia. However, others have not found ploidy to be of prognostic value (Kuoppala et al 1996). The 5-year survival for serous borderline epithelial tumours of all stages is 90–95% and at 15 years is 72–86%. For mucinous tumours the survival rates are 81–91% at 5 years and 60–85% at 15 years. Subclassification of extraovarian disease into invasive and non-invasive implants is the most important prognostic indicator for serous borderline tumours, survival for advanced-stage tumours with non-invasive implants being 95.3% as opposed to 66% for tumours with invasive implants (Seidman & Kurman 2000).

Surgery in borderline tumours

The role of conservative surgery in young women whose families are not complete has been the subject of considerable interest in recent years. In nearly all cases, the diagnosis is not made until the pathology report on the surgical specimen after surgery for an apparently benign ovarian cyst. It is not safe to rely upon a frozen section diagnosis.

It would be normal practice to advise hysterectomy, bilateral salpingo-oophorectomy and omentectomy for a woman with a clinical or ultrasound diagnosis of an ovarian cyst 10 cm or more in diameter who is 40 years old or more and whose family is complete. Younger women or those whose families are not complete usually prefer conservative surgery unless there is a suspicion of invasive malignancy (see Chapter 44). In all these women, the laparotomy should include peritoneal washings for cytology and careful examination of the peritoneal surfaces. Suspicious areas should be biopsied if accessible.

No further treatment is required for women with stage I borderline tumours who have undergone pelvic clearance. Even if a full staging laparotomy with omentectomy has not been performed, there is no indication for further surgery because the likelihood of significant metastatic disease is low. Very few such women will develop recurrent disease. Only three (2.5%) women recurred in an Italian study and all appear to have been treated successfully with further surgery (Zanetta et al 2001a).

If fertility-sparing surgery has been performed, the risk of recurrence is around 15.2% in stage I and 40% in stage II–III (Zanetta et al 2001a). The risk is greater after ovarian cystectomy (36.3%) than after oophorectomy or salpingo-oophorectomy (15.1%) (Morice et al 2001). However, invasive recurrences are rare (2%) and almost all borderline recurrences are treated successfully. The disease-free survival for stage I treated conservatively was 99.3% and treated radically was 100% (Zanetta et al 2001a). In this series in which 56% of the patients were treated conservatively, the overall disease-free survival after a median follow-up of 70 months was 99.6% for stage I, 95.8% for stage II and 89% for stage III.

Decisions about the need for further surgery should be taken in the light of these data and the woman's personal circumstances. In many cases it will be appropriate to do nothing further, particularly if the affected ovary has been removed. However, if only cystectomy has been performed, it may be appropriate to remove the rest of the affected ovary.

Follow-up

It may not be necessary to follow up all these women. Clearly those who have undergone conservative surgery should be followed carefully. Follow-up will have to be prolonged beyond 5 years because so many of those who recur do so late. For the remainder, the risk of recurrence is very small and regular follow-up visits are likely to be normal. However, it is prudent to arrange 4–6-monthly follow-up visits for the first 1–2 years in case there has been a diagnostic error in the initial assessment. Most women will find this reassuring. Thereafter, annual assessment should be sufficient to detect any recurrences in these slow-growing tumours. Some women will prefer not to have the inconvenience of these visits and the investigations associated with them.

Transvaginal ultrasound is the most reliable follow-up test and is better than both clinical examination and CA125 estimation, neither of which adds to the diagnostic accuracy (Zanetta et al 2001b).

There is no place for chemotherapy or radiotherapy in the primary management of these women.

EARLY-STAGE INVASIVE TUMOURS

Most authors consider ovarian carcinoma to be early stage if the tumour is confined to the ovaries and possibly fallopian tubes and/or uterus (FIGO stages I–IIa). It is necessary to ascertain the extent of residual disease and any adverse prognostic factors before deciding if adjuvant therapy should be even considered. The extent of residual disease is partly dependent on the intensity of surgical staging. If no disease is found in biopsies of pelvic peritoneum, the abdominal gutters, the diaphragm and para-aortic nodes and all cytology samples are clear, residual disease is less likely to be missed. However, there is debate as to whether more aggressive staging, including lymphadenectomy, influences survival.

There is a need to define those cases of stage I carcinoma of the ovary where adjuvant therapy is indicated to prevent recurrent disease. While FIGO stage Ic includes cases with capsular penetration by tumour, rupture of the capsule and ascites or positive peritoneal washings, there is little evidence that each of these has the same prognostic value.

Prognostic factors in early-stage ovarian cancer

In a recent study of 1545 patients with FIGO stage I disease, multivariate analysis identified degree of differentiation as the most powerful prognostic indicator of disease-free survival (Vergote et al 2001a). Women with moderately differentiated tumours were three times more likely to die than women with well-differentiated tumours and those with poorly differentiated tumours had nine times greater risk than those with well-differentiated malignancies. The 5-year disease-free survival was 93.7% for patients with well-differentiated tumours. Other significant variables were rupture before surgery (hazard ratio 2.65), rupture during surgery (hazard ratio 1.64) and age. Histological type, dense adhesions, extracapsular growth, ascites, FIGO 1988 stage or size of tumour were no longer of prognostic value.

Many other factors have been investigated as prognostic factors but it will be difficult to confirm their relative value until all the best ones are measured in a large enough sample of patients so they can be subjected to multivariate analysis. DNA ploidy was shown in a prospective study of 162 Scandinavian stage I patients to be the most powerful prognostic factor with a hazard ratio of 6 comparing aneuploid with diploid tumours (Trope et al 2000). Quantitative pathological features such as mitotic activity index, mean nuclear area (MNA) and mean nuclear volume have been investigated as an alternative to ploidy studies. Using a scoring system based on FIGO stage and MNA, Brugghe and colleagues (1998) demonstrated a 6-year survival of 97% among 102 stage I patients in those with a low score compared with 54% in those with a high score.

In an Italian study of 201 stage I patients, the preoperative level of CA125 was found to be the most powerful prognostic factor for survival (Nagele et al 1995). The risk of dying from disease was 6.37 times higher for those with a CA125 level higher than 65 u/ml. There is increasing interest in tumour suppressor genes, oncogenes, angiogenesis markers, drug resistance proteins and proliferation markers (Green et al 1999).

Low-risk patients

Conservative surgery

The resection of all visible tumour usually requires a total hysterectomy and bilateral salpingo-oophorectomy but in a young, nulliparous woman with a unilateral tumour and no ascites, unilateral salpingo-oophorectomy may be justifiable after careful exploration to exclude metastatic disease. Curettage of the uterine cavity should be performed to exclude a synchronous endometrial tumour. Some recommend that the normal-looking ovary is biopsied but the risk of occult spread to that ovary is small and biopsy may impair fertility, negating the purpose of the conservative operation. If the tumour is subsequently found to be poorly differentiated or if the washings are positive, a second operation to clear the pelvis will be necessary. Recurrence rates have been found to be

5–9% after conservative surgery (Marchetti et al 1998, Zanetta et al 1997).

Adjuvant therapy

Patients with stage Ia or Ib well-differentiated tumours do not require adjuvant therapy following surgery. A trial of 81 patients randomized between melphalan chemotherapy or observation showed no significant difference with respect to either 5-year disease-free survival (91% vs 98%) or overall survival (94% vs 98%) (Young et al 1990). The survival after a median follow-up of 48 months was 98% among 45 stage Ia patients given no adjuvant therapy at the Royal Marsden Hospital (Brugghe et al 1998). The excellent survival in this group of patients suggests that adjuvant therapy is not required for these women. Indeed, conservative surgery should be considered if a young patient wishes to maintain fertility and has a stage Ia well-differentiated tumour (see above).

High-risk patients

These patients should undergo radical surgery as described for advanced disease.

There has been great uncertainty as to the value of adjuvant therapy in patients with poor prognosis early-stage disease. Adjuvant therapy has been advocated in the USA ever since it was recommended in the publication of the results of a trial in 141 patients with resected stage II or poorly differentiated stage I disease (Young et al 1990). However, this trial, which compared melphalan with a single intraperitoneal dose of ^{32}P, had no control arm and the 5-year disease-free survival was only 80% in both groups. ^{32}P has since been compared with cisplatin $100 \, \text{mg/m}^2$ plus cyclophosphamide $1000 \, \text{mg/m}^2$ (CP) in a trial of 251 patients by the Gynecologic Oncology Group (GOG). With a median follow-up of 6 years, the investigators reported an estimated 31% reduction in risk of recurrence with the use of CP ($p = 0.075$). Survival at 5 years was 84% with CP and 76% with ^{32}P (Young et al 1999). They concluded that platinum-based therapy should be the standard for patients requiring adjuvant therapy. They are currently comparing three versus six cycles of a combination of carboplatin plus paclitaxel.

The apparent superiority of platinum-based therapy over ^{32}P has also led most doctors to abandon pelvic (P) plus abdominopelvic (AB) irradiation. This had been previously recommended following studies in Toronto which showed an apparent survival advantage of P+AB over P alone in 101 patients most of whom had stage Ib or II disease (Dembo et al 1990).

In European centres, there has been far more uncertainty about the value of adjuvant therapy (Table 45.2). A trial of cisplatin $50 \, \text{mg/m}^2$ versus ^{32}P in a rather heterogeneous group of 347 patients failed to show any difference in survival (Vergote et al 1992). A similar trial in 152 patients with just stage Ic disease showed a 61% reduction in relapse rate but no difference in survival (Bolis et al 1995). The same Italian group also compared cisplatin $50 \, \text{mg/m}^2$ with observation in 83 grade 2 or 3 stage Ia or b patients and found a 65% reduction in relapse rate with cisplatin but no difference in 5-year survival. A trial comparing carboplatin with observation in 162 high-risk stage I patients showed no difference in disease-free survival or survival (Trope et al 2000).

Two groups reported results of trials comparing platinum-based chemotherapy versus observation in a total of 925 high-risk stage I patients at the American Society of Clinical Oncology meeting in 2001. The first International Collaborative Ovarian Neoplasm (ICON) trial included patients with fully resected disease where it was uncertain whether they should receive chemotherapy. The Adjuvant Clinical Trial in Ovarian Neoplasm (ACTION) was organized by the Gynecological Cancer Co-operative Group of the European Organization for Research and Treatment of Cancer (EORTC). Both trials produced similar results showing that adjuvant therapy improves recurrence-free survival by 11% at 5 years and overall survival by 7% (from 75% to 82%) at 5 years.

These data provide a more secure basis upon which to advise patients about chemotherapy when they have high-risk stage I disease. Many women will feel that it is worth enduring the side-effects of chemotherapy for this small but distinct improvement.

ADVANCED INVASIVE DISEASE

Maximal cytoreductive surgery in advanced disease

Maximum cytoreductive surgery aims to remove all macroscopic tumour and to remove tissue like the omentum to which micro-

Table 45.2   Randomized trials of chemotherapy in early-stage ovarian cancer with untreated controls

Study group	Reference	Treatment	No. patients	5-year DFS %	5-year survival %
GICOG	Bolis et al 1995	P50q 4 wk × 6	41	83	88
		Control	42	65	82
NOCOVA	Trope et al 2000	AUC 7q 4 wk × 6	81	70	86
		Control	81	71	85
ICON	Vergote et al 2001b	Pt based × 6	470	Not yet	reported
		Control			
EORTC	Vergote et al 2001b	Pt based ≥ × 4	448	Not yet	reported
		Control			

GICOG, Gruppo Italiano Collaborativo Oncologica Ginecologia
NOCOVA, Nordic Ovarian Cancer Study Group
P, cisplatin; C, carboplatin, Pt, platinum, AUC, area under the curve

scopic spread is common. The minimum operation consists of a total abdominal hysterectomy and bilateral salpingo-oophorectomy and infracolic omentectomy. Some surgeons also include pelvic and para-aortic lymphadenectomy either as a sampling procedure or as a radical removal of retroperitoneal nodes.

Even if no disease is apparent in the upper abdomen, infracolic omentectomy is advisable because microscopic spread can be present when the omentum looks normal. When the omentum is extensively infiltrated it is usually possible to free it from adherent loops of small bowel and to separate it from the transverse colon and stomach. If a limited area of the small bowel or its mesentery is involved it can be resected. However, multiple or extensive resections of small bowel are limited by the need to preserve a functional length of intestine and such patients will still have a poor prognosis.

If the pelvic tumour is large or densely adherent to the pelvic side wall and the colon, it is usually easier to enter the retroperitoneal space at the pelvic brim in order to ligate the ovarian vessels, dissect the ureter from the pelvic peritoneum and mobilize the tumour. The mass can often be freed from the bladder and rectum by peeling the tumour-bearing visceral peritoneum off the underlying organ. The uterine vessels may be ligated at the pelvic side wall and a hysterectomy performed. Sometimes resection of part of the bladder or removal of the sigmoid colon and rectum is necessary. Primary reanastomosis is often possible. Resection of the pelvic colon is indicated if obstruction is imminent but in most other circumstances the prognosis is unlikely to be greatly improved.

Observing a high incidence of pelvic and para-aortic node metastases in their patients, Burghardt and his colleagues (1991) attempted a complete clearance initially of only the pelvic nodes and more recently of pelvic and para-aortic nodes to the level of the renal vessels. It remains to be seen whether radical lymphadenectomy will make a major impact upon the survival of women with this dreadful disease.

Feasibility and morbidity of cytoreductive surgery

The proportion of patients optimally cytoreduced depends on the attitudes and experience of the surgical team. Gynaecological oncologists who are fully trained in this type of surgery with experienced anaesthetists and nurses will successfully cytoreduce patients with advanced disease more often than those with less experience or enthusiasm. Approximately 75% of women with advanced ovarian cancer are amenable to optimal surgery. The postoperative morbidity is surprisingly low for a poor-risk group and seems to relate more to the experience of the team looking after the patient than to the amount of surgery performed.

The value of maximal cytoreductive surgery in advanced disease

For the past 15–20 years, gynaecological oncologists have been advocating maximal cytoreductive surgery in advanced ovarian cancer in the belief that this would improve the prospects for survival and make tumours more amenable to chemotherapy. This view is undergoing revision in the light of more recent data.

Many studies show that women with minimal or no residual disease after surgery have a better prognosis than those in whom more disease remained after surgery. However, it is likely that the latter group includes the more aggressive tumours with an intrinsically worse prognosis. Griffiths and his co-workers (1979) showed that women with no or minimal residual disease (<1.5 cm) after primary surgery survived longer than those with larger residual masses and that patients with residual masses <1.5 cm following surgery did as well as those whose metastases were small from the outset. These data suggested that surgical intervention could indeed influence the prognosis. Unfortunately, an analysis of more modern data has failed to confirm these findings (Hoskins et al 1992).

It has become clear that the prognosis is adversely affected by the volume of metastatic disease at the outset, even when maximum cytoreduction has been successfully performed (Hacker et al 1983). Similarly, women who have undergone bowel surgery as part of successful cytoreduction have a worse prognosis than those without bowel surgery even if cytoreduction was unsuccessful (Potter et al 1991).

No prospective, controlled trials of primary cytoreductive surgery have been reported. However, a study of two different chemotherapy regimens showed no survival advantage for those women operated upon in units with higher rates of successful cytoreduction (Bertelsen 1990). A subsequent meta-analysis of over 6000 cases was based on the principle that groups of women with higher rates of successful cytoreduction should have better survival rates if the surgery was contributing to the outcome (Hunter et al 1992). In this study, maximal cytoreductive surgery had no significant effect on median survival once the effects of chemotherapy had been taken into account.

While it seems likely that primary cytoreductive surgery can improve the quality of life for women with advanced ovarian cancer (Blyth & Wahl 1982) and increase their ability to tolerate chemotherapy, any effect on survival will probably be small. Removal of the majority of the tumour volume should always be attempted and is likely to be successful in some 75% of cases. However, resection of bowel should not be performed except when obstruction is imminent. The meticulous removal of all tiny tumour nodules is unlikely to be helpful. Similarly, radical lymphadenectomy cannot be recommended.

Intervention debulking surgery

An alternative approach when initial surgery has left bulky disease is a planned second laparotomy after 2–4 courses of cytoreductive chemotherapy in those women who respond. The chemotherapy is then resumed as soon as possible after the second operation. A relatively small British study did not show any benefit from this approach (Redman et al 1994). The results of a larger EORTC study are more encouraging (van der Burg et al 1995). These suggest that the median survival in this poor prognosis group may be increased by 6 months and that the survival at 3 years may be improved from 10% to 20%. A more recent retrospective case series study suggested that interval debulking in selected patients did not worsen their prognosis but allowed less aggressive surgery and improved their quality of life (Kayikcioglu et al 2001).

Second-look surgery

Second-look surgery is defined as a planned laparotomy at the end of chemotherapy. The objectives are firstly, to determine the response to previous therapy in order to document accurately its efficacy and to plan subsequent management and secondly, to excise any residual disease. While there is no doubt that second-look surgery gives the most accurate indication of the disease status, laparotomy being more accurate in this respect than laparoscopy, the balance of evidence suggests that neither the surgical resection of residual tumour nor the opportunity to change the treatment has any effect whatever on the patient's survival. Second-look procedures therefore have no place outside clinical trials at the present time.

Postoperative management of advanced invasive disease

First-line chemotherapy

The great majority of patients with FIGO stage IIb disease or higher will have residual tumour following surgery and would relapse rapidly without adjuvant therapy. There is general consensus that cisplatin or carboplatin are the most effective agents for the management of ovarian cancer. Two meta-analyses of individual patient data from nearly 10 000 patients in 45 randomized trials have shown that platinum-based therapy is better than non-platinum-based therapy and that platinum in combination is better than single-agent platinum when used at the same dose (Advanced Ovarian Cancer Trialists Group 1991, 1998). The fact that most patients in the non-cisplatin arm received this drug on relapse explains why only a 5% improvement in survival was seen.

The suggestion of these two meta-analyses that combination therapy was better than single-agent therapy and the result of two other meta-analyses indicating a benefit from adding doxorubicin (A'Hern & Gore, 1995, Ovarian Cancer Meta-Analyses Project 1991) lead to the ICON 2 trial which tested the combination of cyclophosphamide, doxorubicin and cisplatin (CAP) against single-agent carboplatin. Carboplatin was chosen for the single-agent group because at optimal dose, it is less toxic than single-agent cisplatin and the meta-analysis showed no difference in efficacy between the two drugs. The dose of carboplatin was calculated using the area under the curve (AUC) method using the glomerular filtration rate determined by either the radio-isotope method or the Cockroft formula (Calvert et al 1989). The ICON 2 trial on 1526 patients showed no difference in survival between CAP and carboplatin with a median survival of 33 months for both groups (ICON Collaborators 1998).

Carboplatin is now preferred to cisplatin as, in addition to the meta-analysis showing equivalent efficacy between cisplatin and carboplatin, three randomized trials comparing paclitaxel plus cisplatin versus paclitaxel plus carboplatin showed no difference in response rates or progression-free survival (Vermorken 2000a). Carboplatin is also better tolerated than CAP and so became the recommended chemotherapy for advanced ovarian cancer.

Many opinion leaders changed their views when two trials comparing cyclophosphamide and cisplatin versus paclitaxel

Table 45.3 Trials comparing paclitaxel/platinum combinations with a platinum-based control treatment

Trial	Treatment	No. patients	Median PFS months	Median survival months
GOG 111	CP (750/75)	202	13.0	24
	TP (135-24h/75)	184	18.0	38
OV10	CP (750-75)	338	11.5	25.8
	TP (175-200-3h/75)	342	15.5	35.6
GOG-132	P (100)		16.4	30.2
	T (200-24h)		11.4	26.0
	TP (135-24h/75)		14.1	26.6
ICON-3	Control CAP or Cb	1364	16.1	36.1
	TCb (175-3h/AUC ≥5)	710	17.1	37.6

Trials groups see text.
C, cyclophosphamide; P, cisplatin; T, paclitaxel; A, adriamycin; Cb, carboplatin; numbers in parenthesis, dose in mg and duration of infusion in hours – h.

and cisplatin showed an advantage for the paclitaxel arm (Table 45.3). The first study, GOG protocol 111, showed an improvement in median survival from 24 to 38 months in the group receiving paclitaxel 135 mg/m^2 as a 24-hour infusion (McGuire et al 1996). The second trial, OV10, by European and Canadian investigators also showed an improvement in median survival from 25.8 to 35.6 months in the group receiving paclitaxel given at a dose of 175 mg/m^2 over 3 hours (Piccart et al 2000). A combination of carboplatin at a minimum dose of AUC 5 plus paclitaxel 175 mg/m^2 over 3 hours is considered by many to be the standard treatment (Berek et al 1999).

However, two trials have created uncertainty over the value of adding paclitaxel to platinum. GOG protocol 132 compared single-agent cisplatin 100 mg/m^2 with single-agent 24-hour paclitaxel 200 mg/m^2 and with a combination of both as used in GOG 111. The response rates of cisplatin alone or in combination with paclitaxel were identical at 67% whilst the response rate to paclitaxel was only 46% and the median survival of all three arms was the same (Muggia et al 2000). The discrepancy between this trial and GOG 111 and OV 10 has been blamed by some on the large proportion of patients on the single-agents arms of GOG 132 changing to the other arm prior to clinical progression.

This criticism could not be made of the next trial whose results brought into question the value of adding paclitaxel to platinum. Very little crossover occurred prior to progression in the ICON 3 trial in which paclitaxel 175 mg/m^2 plus carboplatin was compared with either of two control arms, carboplatin alone or CAP. These control arms produced survival curves identical to those in ICON 2. The ICON 3 trial is by far the largest ever trial in ovarian cancer with 2074 patients randomized, of whom 1363 had progressed or died at the time of latest analysis (ICON collaborators 2002). There was a non-significant difference in 2-year survival of 1%

from 63% to 64% in favour of the paclitaxel arm. There was a similar non-significant difference in 1-year progression-free survival of 2% from 60% to 62% in favour of the paclitaxel arm.

The results of these trials suggest that giving cisplatin or carboplatin at the optimal dose as single agents is as good as giving a lower platinum dose with paclitaxel.

Intraperitoneal chemotherapy

There is a theoretical attraction of giving certain drugs intraperitoneally as they can attain local concentrations far higher than when given intravenously. However, the penetration of drugs into tumour nodules of more than 1 cm is poor. This fact and the poor results of intraperitoneal therapy in patients with bulky or relapsed disease has lead to its use being confined to patients with minimal or no macroscopic residual disease after primary surgery. No randomized trials have accrued sufficient patients to assess the value of intraperitoneal therapy as consolidation after initial therapy. There are four randomized trials which have investigated intraperitoneal therapy as part of first-line treatment (Vermorken 2000b). The two largest studies showed a significant survival advantage of giving 100 mg/m^2 cisplatin intraperitoneally (Alberts et al 1996, Markman et al 1998). Despite this positive result there remains little enthusiasm for intraperitoneal chemotherapy which mirrors the very slow accrual to these clinical trials.

Radiotherapy

Postoperative abdominopelvic radiotherapy for early ovarian carcinoma no longer has a role in the management of ovarian cancer. Chemotherapy has replaced radiotherapy in the management of early ovarian cancer and has always been used for advanced disease for which radiotherapy is ineffective. Intraperitoneal, colloid-bound, radio-active phosphorus has not been proven to have any advantage over chemotherapy for early-stage disease and can cause serious late bowel problems. Intraperitoneal radio-active antibody therapy is still a research tool.

Summary of postoperative therapy

The overall 5-year survival for women with ovarian cancer in England and Wales has improved from 21% for women treated in 1971–75 to 29% for those treated in 1991–93 (Quinn et al 2001). This may be due in part to increasing registration of women with borderline tumours but at least some of the improvement is likely to be due to the introduction of platinum chemotherapy.

The 5-year survival rate for women with stage I disease is 75–80%. These data suggest that women with stage Ia or Ib disease and well-differentiated tumours may not require further treatment. Adjuvant therapy for a high-risk group with grade 2 or 3 tumours or stage Ic–IIa seems to improve the recurrence-free 5-year survival by 11%. There is no evidence that adjuvant therapy affects the outcome in women with borderline tumours.

All other patients with advanced invasive ovarian carcinoma have a much worse prognosis, with 5-year survival rates that remain in the region of 20–25% in spite of improvements in shorter term and median survival rates. All these women require adjuvant therapy if their physical condition allows. Giving cisplatin or carboplatin at the optimal dose as single agents is probably as good as giving a lower platinum dose with paclitaxel.

TREATMENT FOR PERSISTENT OR RELAPSED EPITHELIAL OVARIAN CANCER

Clinical, scan or CA125 evidence of residual disease will be found at completion of initial chemotherapy in about 30% of patients. There is unfortunately no consolidation therapy that has been shown in randomized trials to prolong survival of these patients. Despite a desire to do something active, we should wait to see if randomized trials show any benefit for agents such as weekly paclitaxel before routinely starting such therapy. The current trials of sequential therapy of different agents will show whether such approaches reduce the proportion of patients with residual disease.

Despite a high response rate to initial therapy, over 80% of patients will relapse. Further remissions can be achieved in a high proportion of patients, with many having repeat remissions with subsequent courses of chemotherapy. It must be remembered that therapy for relapsed disease is palliative so all possible approaches to symptom control should be considered. Although a response to chemotherapy is usually the best way of providing symptom control, a balance must be struck between the toxicity of the therapy and its potential benefit. The role of debulking surgery in recurrent disease is uncertain and is being addressed in an EORTC trial. Patients troubled by recurrent ascites rather than solid masses not responding to chemotherapy may benefit from insertion of a shunt between the peritoneal cavity and subclavian vein. Radiotherapy can be useful for painful or bleeding pelvic disease.

The patients most likely to benefit from further chemotherapy were originally shown to be those with the longest interval from last treatment (Blackledge et al 1989). A multivariate analysis of 704 patients treated by a variety of drugs for relapse has shown serous histology, ≤2 sites of disease and ≤5 cm maximum tumour diameter to be the best predictors of response (Eisenhauer et al 1997). Patients are frequently stratified as platinum resistant if progressing during initial platinum-based therapy or within 6 months, and platinum sensitive if relapsing beyond 6 months. Retreatment with single-agent carboplatin is often considered the best option for those with a long treatment-free interval. It is unclear whether adding other drugs improves the response rate or duration of response, but it invariably increases the toxicity.

Paclitaxel was the first agent to demonstrate a response rate around 20% in patients with cisplatin-refractory disease (Trimble et al 1993). A higher response rate but no improvement in survival was seen when it was given in combination with epidoxorubicin (Bolis et al 1999). An even higher response rate has been reported with weekly cisplatin and paclitaxel (van der Burg et al 1998). Docetaxel might produce a higher response rate than paclitaxel; it causes greater myelosuppression at the standard dose but less neurotoxicity. Unlike carboplatin, they both cause alopecia.

Topotecan given as a 5-day schedule every 3 weeks has been shown to have similar activity to paclitaxel (Bokkel Huinink et al 1997). It is usually well tolerated but neutropenia and thrombocytopenia are common side-effects. Gemcitabine, altretamine, oral etoposide, ifosfamide and liposomal doxorubicin are other agents that have shown response rates in the range of 15–40% in phase II trials. The difference in proportion of platinum-refractory patients between studies makes it difficult to compare response rates unless trials are randomized.

Many new agents are being investigated in women with relapsed ovarian cancer. Inhibitors of matrix metalloproteinases have so far failed to show any benefit. There is an expectation that anti-angiogenic agents or inhibitors of cell-signalling pathways such as epidermal growth factor receptor tyrosine kinase inhibitors may be more successful. Trials of intraperitoneal genetic therapy are under way. Of particular interest is an attenuated adenovirus, Onyx-015, which selectively replicates in cells with absent or non-functional p53.

OTHER TREATMENTS

Hormonal therapy

Hormonal therapy is used fairly widely in ovarian cancer, chiefly because it is devoid of side-effects in comparison to chemotherapy. Cytoplasmic oestrogen and progesterone receptors have been detected in malignant ovarian tumours (Soutter & Leake 1987) but the efficacy of hormone therapy is modest. Response rates of 8–14% are seen with a number of agents. These include tamoxifen, progestational agents, gonadotrophin-releasing hormone analogues and combined oestrogen/progestin preparations (Schwartz et al 1998). Responses are more commonly seen in well or moderately differentiated tumours and might be expected to be higher in patients with endometrioid histology. Hormonal replacement therapy (HRT) is used increasingly in premenopausal women treated for ovarian cancer. A retrospective study which assessed 373 patients given HRT showed no detrimental effect on the prognosis (Eeles et al 1991).

Biological or antibody-based therapy

The propensity of ovarian cancer to remain within the peritoneal cavity for much of its natural history has stimulated evaluation of various forms of targeted biological therapy, using the intraperitoneal route. Trials of immunotherapy using interferon alpha, interleukin-2 (IL-2) and lymphokine-activated killer cells with IL-2 have produced responses. A randomized trial of consolidation intraperitoneal interferon-alpha therapy has failed to demonstrate any survival benefit.

The most promising trial of targeting using antibody localization has used a conjugate of ^{90}Y with the monoclonal antibody HMFG1. Fifty-two patients received this after chemotherapy and it appeared to benefit those patients who were already in complete remission. The 5-year survival of the 21 complete responders who received radio-immunotherapy

was 80% compared to 55% in a matched control group (Nicholson et al 1998). Multinational phase III trials are now under way to define accurately the value of intraperitoneal immunotherapy in ovarian cancer.

NON-EPITHELIAL TUMOURS

Non-epithelial tumours constitute approximately 10% of all ovarian cancers. Because of their rarity and their sensitivity to intensive chemotherapy, it is especially appropriate to refer these patients for specialist care.

Sex cord stromal tumours

Granulosa and theca cell tumours

The most common sex cord stromal tumours are the granulosa and theca cell tumours. They often produce steroid hormones, in particular oestrogens, which can cause postmenopausal bleeding in older women and sexual precocity in prepubertal girls. The hormones may cause cystic glandular hyperplasia or occasionally carcinoma of the endometrium (Fox & Langley 1976). Theca cell tumours are usually benign. The majority of those that are malignant contain both granulosa and theca cells, the malignant element originating in the granulosa cell. Granulosa cell tumours occur at all ages, but are found predominantly in postmenopausal women. The staging system for these tumours is the same as for epithelial tumours and most present as stage I. Bilateral tumours are present in only 5% of cases.

Pathology Granulosa cell tumours are normally solid although, when they become large, cystic spaces may develop and some tumours are predominantly cystic. Like most tumours of the sex cord stromal tumour group, the cut surface is often yellow, reflecting the presence of neutral lipid which is related to sex steroid hormone production. Areas of haemorrhage are also common. The stromal component may be fibromatous or resemble theca externa, theca interna cells or lutein cells. Granulosa cells express α-inhibin. The juvenile form differs in that the granulose cells usually lack the typical nuclear grooves of the adult form and the cytoplasm is luteinized.

Treatment Theca cell tumours, being usually benign, may be treated surgically like any other benign ovarian tumour.

Radical surgery should always be considered as the first option for treating granulosa cell tumours. Unilateral oophorectomy cannot be recommended readily to young women with stage Ia disease because of the probability of a high recurrence rate associated with conservative therapy (Lauszus et al 2001). This study of 37 women with stage I disease reported survival rates of 94%, 82% and 62% after 5, 10 and 20 years. The 10- and 20-year survival rates for women treated with total abdominal hysterectomy and bilateral salpingo-oophorectomy were over 90% compared with 60% and none for those treated conservatively. There are no trials showing any benefit from adjuvant therapy which cannot therefore be recommended.

Recurrence should be treated surgically if possible. These tumours are frequently indolent and lengthy remissions can be obtained following surgical removal of recurrent tumour. A variety of chemotherapy regimens have been used, but should

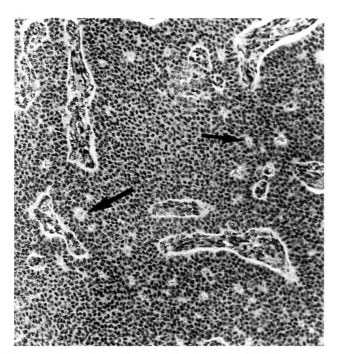

Fig. 45.8 A granulosa cell tumour showing a microfollicular pattern. Call-Exner bodies are shown with the arrows. Haematoxylin and eosin ×170.

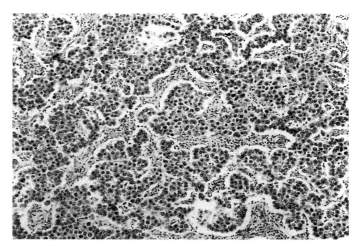

Fig. 45.9 A dysgerminoma with the typical large, pale round cells separated by fibrous septae in which a lymphocytic infiltrate is prominent. Haematoxylin and eosin ×200.

be considered palliative rather than curative. Cisplatin-based regimens, most commonly with etoposide, bleomycin, doxorubicin or cyclophosphamide, produce an overall response rate of 60–80%, but responses are not durable. Many centres use the same regimen as used for germ cell tumours (Gershenson et al 1996). There have been anecdotal reports of response to antioestrogenic therapy.

Sertoli–Leydig cell tumours

Half of these rare neoplasia produce male hormones which can cause virilization. Rarely, oestrogens are secreted. The prognosis for the majority who have localized disease is good and surgery as for granulosa cell tumours is the treatment of choice. Chemotherapy may be used for metastatic or recurrent disease.

Germ cell tumours

Dysgerminomas

Dysgerminomas are uncommon ovarian tumours accounting for 2–5% of all primary malignant ovarian tumours. Originating in the germ cells, 90% occur in young women less than 30 years old. They behave in a similar way to seminoma in men, spreading mainly by lymphatics to para-aortic, mediastinal and supraclavicular glands. All cases need to be investigated by chest X-ray, CT scanning and lymphangiogram. Serum AFP and β-hCG must be assayed to exclude the ominous presence of elements of choriocarcinoma, endodermal sinus tumour or teratoma. Occasionally some cases of pure dysgerminoma have raised levels of β-hCG and, in metastatic disease, placental alkaline phosphatase and lactate dehydrogenase are usually elevated. Pure dysgerminomas have a good prognosis as about 70% are stage I tumours, most being stage Ia (Bjorkholm et al 1990).

Pathology (Gordon et al 1981) Dysgerminomas are solid tumours which have a smooth or nodular, bosselated external surface. They are soft or rubbery in consistency, depending upon the proportion of fibrous tissue contained in them. They may reach a considerable size; the mean diameter is 15 cm. Approximately 10% are bilateral; they are alone among malignant germ cell tumours in having a significant incidence of bilaterality.

Dysgerminoma is composed of groups of large, round tumour cells separated by fibrous tissue septae infiltrated by lymphocytes (Fig. 45.9). The tumour cells possess abundant, pale, slightly eosinophilic cytoplasm which contains glycogen, lipid and alkaline phosphatase, the last being situated predominantly in the periphery of the cell. A minimal lymphocytic response, a high mitotic count, capsular penetration, intraovarian lymphatic or vascular invasion are all associated with a decreased survival.

Immature teratoma, yolk sac tumour or choriocarcinoma are found in 6.7–13.8% of dysgerminomas. Very thorough sampling of all dysgerminomas must be undertaken by the histopathologist to exclude the presence of these more malignant germ cell elements as their presence alters therapy. Approximately 3% of tumours contain syncytiotrophoblastic giant cells which are immunoreactive for hCG. The neoplastic cells are typically reactive for placental-like alkaline phosphatase and vimentin.

Other germ cell tumours

Germ cell tumours other than dysgerminoma also occur in young women under 30 years old. Their very poor prognosis has been greatly improved by combination chemotherapy. Their derivation from germ cells is shown in Figure 45.10 (Teilum 1965). Mature teratomas are benign, the most common being the cystic teratoma or dermoid cyst found at all ages but particularly in the third and fourth decades.

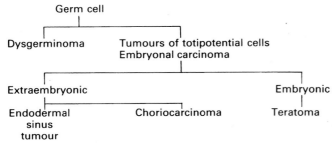

Fig. 45.10 The derivation of germ cell tumours.

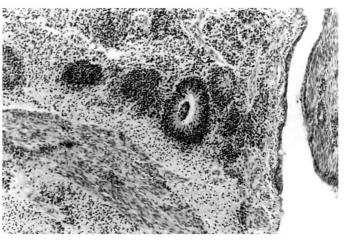

Fig. 45.11 An immature teratoma with prominent neuroectodermal tissue and a well-formed rosette. Haematoxylin and eosin ×170.

Tumour markers are of value in diagnosis, monitoring therapy and in early detection of recurrence. The two main markers are AFP, produced by yolk sac cells, and β-hCG from the syncytiotrophoblast.

Yolk sac (endodermal sinus) tumours Yolk sac tumour is the second most common malignant germ cell tumour of the ovary, making up 10–15% overall and reaching a higher proportion in children. It may present as an acute abdomen due to rupture of the tumour following necrosis and haemorrhage.

The tumour is usually well encapsulated and solid. Areas of necrosis and haemorrhage are often seen, as are small cystic spaces. Its consistency varies from soft to firm and rubbery and its cut surface is slippery and mucoid.

The yolk sac tumour is characterized by the presence of a variety of patterns. The background of the tumour is a loose vacuolated network of microcysts lined by flat cells of mesothelial appearance. The most characteristic feature is the endodermal sinus (Schiller–Duval body). A constant finding is PAS-positive, hyaline globules containing AFP and other metabolic products of the normal yolk sac.

Immature teratomas These tumours are solid and often malignant. It should be noted that solid teratomas are not all of immature type. Immature teratomas are composed of a wide variety of tissues and comprise about 1% of all ovarian teratomas.

The tumours are unilateral in almost all cases and appear as solid masses that have smooth and bosselated surfaces. The cut surface shows mainly solid tissue, although small cystic spaces are visible. The tumour is very heterogeneous and areas of bone and cartilage may be apparent and hair may be seen. Both the gross appearance and the histology may resemble a benign teratoma due to the presence of these mature elements. At a microscopic level, the amount of immature tissue may be quite variable, most of it being represented by neuroectodermal tissue in which rosettes of tightly packed neuroectodermal cells with dark nuclei neuroepithelial rosettes (Fig. 45.11) and glial structures may predominate. Rarely, peritoneal implants of mature or immature neural tissue may be associated with the main lesion. Both immature embryonal epithelial structures and immature mesenchymal elements, such as cartilage, bone or muscle, may be present. The amount of embryonal tissue, its degree of atypia and mitotic activity correlate with the prognosis.

A careful search must be made for elements of yolk sac tumour and choriocarcinoma; the presence of these may have a bearing on prognosis and treatment, particularly if the teratoma is of low grade. Blood levels of β-hCG and AFP should be estimated to exclude their presence even when the tumour appears to be a straightforward immature teratoma.

Treatment of germ cell tumours

With the exception of dysgerminoma, which are bilateral in 10–15% of cases, most malignant ovarian germ cells tumours involve only one ovary even when there is metastatic disease at other sites. Fertility-sparing surgery should be the rule even in the presence of metastatic disease and biopsy of a normal-looking contralateral ovary should be avoided because it very rarely detects disease and it may impair fertility (Zanetta et al 2001c). These patients should be rapidly referred to a centre experienced in managing these curable patients. The only other role for surgery is a second-look procedure with appropriate cytoreduction. This is only recommended for those patients with a teratoma component in the primary, persistent radiological abnormalities and normal serum tumour markers at the end of chemotherapy (Williams et al 1994).

Patients who, after adequate surgical exploration, have stage Ia disease should be considered for adjuvant therapy unless they can have obsessional surveillance from an experienced centre. The 5-year survival of stage I dysgerminoma patients following just unilateral adnexectomy was >90% even before the advent of modern chemotherapy (Bridgewater & Rustin 1999). Virtually all patients on surveillance for stage I endodermal sinus and immature teratoma patients should be cured, providing relapses are detected early and rising tumour markers are not masked by these young patients becoming pregnant (Dark et al 1997). In practice, two-thirds of women receive adjuvant chemotherapy. Radiotherapy is effective for dysgerminomas if future fertility is not desirable but is now seldom used.

Bleomycin, etoposide and cisplatin (BEP) or a combination of cisplatin, vincristine, methotrexate and bleomycin (POMB) alternating with actinomycin-D, cyclophosphamide and etoposide (ACE) are the most commonly used regimens for treating patients with metastatic disease (Bower et al 1996, Gershenson et al 1990). Over 95% of early-stage patients are cured with cure rates in excess of 75% even in those presenting with very advanced disease (Low et al 2000). Most patients recover their fertility, providing they had conservative surgery (Low et al 2000, Zanetta et al 2001c).

OVARIAN CARCINOMA: CONCLUSIONS

Epithelial ovarian carcinoma is still a difficult tumour to treat, partly because of its late presentation and partly because no truly effective therapy has yet been developed. Surgery remains an important part of the management. Prolonged survival is only possible when the surgeon is able to excise the tumour virtually completely. Chemotherapy has had a major impact on the rare, germ cell tumours. Although less effective in the common epithelial malignancies, chemotherapy does extend substantially the life expectancy of many patients.

CANCER OF THE FALLOPIAN TUBE

Cancers of the fallopian tube can be either primary or secondary. Most tumours involving the fallopian tube are metastatic from ovarian cancer but secondary spread from the breast and gastrointestinal tract also occurs. Primary carcinoma is usually unilateral. It is thought to be extremely rare, comprising only 0.3% of gynaecological malignancies. However, only early fallopian tube carcinomas can be distinguished with certainty from ovarian disease. A study of the use of CA125 in screening for ovarian carcinoma detected three cases of early fallopian tube carcinoma and 19 ovarian tumours (Woolas et al 1994). This prevalence of fallopian tube lesions is 25-fold greater than expected. This may be due to a greater sensitivity of CA125 for these tumours or, more probably, they are more common than is realized. The finding that women with fallopian tube cancers have a 15.9% prevalence of BRCA1 or BRCA2 mutations or family histories of early-onset breast or ovarian cancer (Aziz et al 2001) also suggests that some advanced 'ovarian' cancers may actually have originated from the fallopian tubes.

Most present after the menopause, the mean age being 56 years. Many of the patients are nulliparous (45%) and infertility is reported in up to 71% of these women. Tumour spread is identical to that of ovarian cancer and metastases to pelvic and para-aortic nodes are common.

PATHOLOGY

Because of the histological similarity between serous ovarian carcinoma and primary tubal carcinoma, strict criteria must be applied before the diagnosis of tubal carcinoma can be made. Carcinoma of the fallopian tube usually distends the lumen with tumour. The tumour may protrude through the fimbrial end and the tube may be retort shaped, resembling a hydrosalpinx. It is typically very similar to the serous adenocarcinoma of the ovary histologically (Fig. 45.12). The predominant pattern is papillary, with a gradation through alveolar to solid as the degree of differentiation decreases.

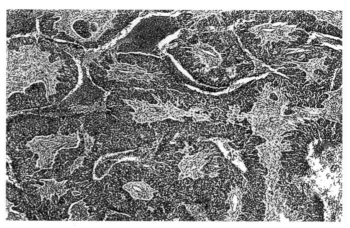

Fig. 45.12 A rather poorly differentiated serous adenocarcinoma of the fallopian tube in which the papillary pattern is still recognizable. Haematoxylin and eosin ×100.

Box 45.3 FIGO staging for fallopian tube carcinoma

 0 Carcinoma *in situ* – limited to the tubal mucosa
 I Growth limited to the fallopian tubes
  Ia One tube involved with extension into the submucosa or muscularis. Not penetrating the serosal surface. No ascites
  Ib Both tubes involved but otherwise as for Ia
  Ic One or both tubes with extension through or onto the tubal serosa; or ascites with malignant cells; or positive peritoneal washings
 II Growth involving one or both fallopian tubes with pelvic extension
  IIa Extension or metastases to the uterus or ovaries
  IIb Extension to other pelvic organs
  IIc Stage IIa or IIb plus ascites with malignant cells; or positive peritoneal washings
 III Tumour involves one or both fallopian tubes with peritoneal implants outside the pelvis or positive retroperitoneal or inguinal nodes. Superficial liver metastases equals stage III. Tumour appears limited to the true pelvis but with histologically proven malignant extension to the small bowel or omentum
  IIIa Tumour is grossly limited to the true pelvis with negative lymph nodes but with histologically confirmed microscopic seeding of abdominal peritoneal surfaces
  IIIb Tumour involving one or both tubes with histologically confirmed implants of abdominal peritoneal surfaces, none exceeding 2 cm in diameter. Lymph nodes are negative
  IIIc Abdominal implants greater than 2 cm in diameter or positive retroperitoneal or inguinal nodes
 IV Growth involving one or both fallopian tubes with distant metastases. If pleural effusion is present, there must be positive cytology. Parenchymal liver metastases equals stage IV

Note: Staging for fallopian tube is by the surgical pathological system. Operative findings designating stage are determined prior to tumour debulking

STAGING

The FIGO clinical staging is similar to that used for ovarian cancer (Box 45.3). Probably because of the difficulty in distinguishing between advanced ovarian and advanced fallopian tube carcinoma, 74% of fallopian tube carcinomas are diagnosed at stage I–IIa while the remaining 26% are stage IIb–IV (Hellström et al 1994).

CLINICAL PRESENTATION AND MANAGEMENT

Most cases of cancer of the fallopian tube are diagnosed at laparotomy. The diagnosis is seldom considered preoperatively. The usual presenting symptom is postmenopausal bleeding and the diagnosis should be considered particularly if the patient also complains of a watery discharge and lower abdominal pain. Unexplained postmenopausal bleeding or abnormal cervical cytology without obvious cause demands a careful bimanual examination and pelvic ultrasound. Laparoscopy may be required in doubtful cases.

The management of cancer of the fallopian tube is as for cancer of the ovary, with surgery to remove gross tumour. This will almost always involve a total abdominal hysterectomy and bilateral salpingo-oophorectomy. Omentectomy should be performed. Postoperative chemotherapy will be required with platinum analogues for all but the earliest cases. The treatment of carcinoma metastatic to the fallopian tube is determined by the management of the primary tumour.

RESULTS

The overall 5-year survival rate is around 35%. The prognosis is improved if the tumour is detected early. The 5-year survival for stage I is in the region of 70%, as is that for stage Ia cases but in stages Ib–IIIc survival falls to 25–30% (Hellström et al 1994). Chemotherapy with platinum agents improves the survival.

KEY POINTS

1. Epithelial ovarian cancer most often occurs between the ages of 45 and 65 years. The disease is usually advanced at presentation and except when the disease is confined to the ovaries and is well or moderately well differentiated, it has a poor prognosis.
2. Oral contraceptive use protects against the development of ovarian cancer.
3. Inheritance plays a significant role in approximately 5% of epithelial ovarian cancers. The BRCA1 gene is associated with 80% of families with both breast and ovarian cancer but the risk of ovarian cancer alone is variable. BRCA1 does not appear to be responsible for many sporadic cases of ovarian cancers.
4. Population screening for ovarian cancer is not yet justified with the techniques evaluated so far.
5. Standard treatment at the present time is surgery followed by a platinum drug-based chemotherapy regimen. This approach allows many women to lead a relatively symptom-free life for periods of up to 2–3 years.

KEY POINTS (CONTINUED)

6. Chemotherapy of epithelial ovarian tumours with platinum agents, either alone or in coombination, will prolong the patient's life but is unlikely to result in an improved long-term survival. Combinations of platinum drugs with paclitaxel may not offer as great an advantage as first appeared to be the case.
7. At present, the biological factors inherent in each tumour, rather than treatment, determine survival.
8. Germ cell tumours occur in young women. They have a much better prognosis than the epithelial tumours. Chemotherapy for germ cell tumours is effective even in advanced and recurrent cases and fertility can be preserved. A young woman with a solid ovarian tumour should be referred to a gynaecological oncologist. If the diagnosis is made postoperatively she should always be referred to a specialist team.
9. Primary carcinoma of the fallopian tube is treated like ovarian carcinoma.

REFERENCES

Adami H-O, Hsieh C-C, Lambe M et al 1994 Parity, age at first childbirth, and risk of ovarian cancer. Lancet 344:1250–1254

Advanced Ovarian Cancer Trialists Group 1991 Chemotherapy in advanced ovarian cancer: an overview of randomised clinical trials. British Medical Journal 303:884–893

Advanced Ovarian Cancer Trialists' Group 1998 Chemotherapy in advanced ovarian cancer: four systematic meta-analyses of individual patient data from 37 randomized trals. British Journal of Cancer 78:1479–1487

A'Hern RP, Gore ME 1995 Impact of doxorubicin on survival in advanced ovarian cancer. Journal of Clinical Oncology 13:726–732

Alberts DS, Liu PY, Hannigan EV et al 1996 Intraperitoneal cisplatin plus intravenous cyclophosphamide versus intravenous cisplatin plus intravenous cyclophosphamide for stage III ovarian cancer. New England Journal of Medicine 335:1950–1955

Anderson MC, Langley FA 1970 Mesonephroid tumours of the ovary. Journal of Clinical Pathology 23:210–218

Aslam N, Banerjee S, Carr JV, Savvas M, Hooper R, Jurkovic D 2000 Prospective evaluation of logistic regression models for the diagnosis of ovarian cancer. Obstetrics and Gynecology 96:75–80

Aziz S, Kuperstein G, Rosen B et al 2001 A genetic epidemiological study of carcinoma of the fallopian tube. Gynecologic Oncology 80:341–345

Bast RC, Xu FJ, Rodriguez GC et al 1992 Inhibition of breast and ovarian tumour cell growth by antibodies and immunotoxins reactive with distinct epitopes on the extracellular domain of HER-2/neu (c-erbB2). In: Sharp F, Mason WP, Creasman W (eds) Ovarian cancer 2: biology, diagnosis and management. Chapman and Hall London, pp 67–71

Berchuck A, Kamel A, Whitaker R et al 1990 Overexpression of HER-2/neu is associated with poor survival in advanced ovarian cancer. Cancer Research 50:4087–4091

Berek JS, Bertelsen K, du Bois A et al 1999 Advanced epithelial ovarian cancer: 1998 consensus statements. Annals of Oncology 10:S87–S92

Bertelsen K 1990 Tumour reduction surgery and long term survival in advanced ovarian cancer: a DACOVA study. Gynecological Oncology 38:203–209

Bjorkholm E, Lundell M, Gyftodimos A, Silfversward C 1990 Dysgerminoma. The Radiumhemmet series 1927–1984. Cancer 65:38–44

Blackledge G, Lawton F, Redman C, Kelly K 1989 Response of patients in phase II studies of chemotherapy in ovarian cancer: Implications for patient treatment and the design of phase II trials. British Journal of Cancer 59:650–653

Blyth JG, Wahl TP 1982 Debulking surgery: does it increase the quality of survival? Gynecological Oncology 14:396–406

Bokkel Huinink T, Bolis G, Gore M, Carmichael JC et al 1997 Topotecan versus paclitaxel for the treatment of recurrent epithelial ovarian cancer. Journal of Clinical Oncology 15:2183–2193

Bolis G, Colombo N, Pecorelli S et al 1995 Adjuvant treatment for early epithelial ovarian cancer: results of two randomised clinical trials comparing cisplatin to no further treatment or chromic phosphate (32P). Annals of Oncology 6:887–893

Bolis G, Parazzini F, Scarfone G et al 1999 Paclitaxel vs epidoxorubicin plus paclitaxel as second-line therapy for platinum-refractory and resistant ovarian cancer. Gynecological Oncology 72:60–64

Bourne TH, Campbell S, Reynolds KM et al 1993 Screening for early familial ovarian cancer with transvaginal ultrasonography and colour blood flow imaging. British Medical Journal 306:1025–1029

Bower M, Fife K, Holden L, Paradinas FJ, Rustin GJ, Newlands ES 1996 Chemotherapy for ovarian germ cell tumours [see comments]. European Journal of Cancer 32A:593–597

Bridgewater JA, Rustin GJS 1999 Managment of non-epithelial ovarian tumours. Oncology, 57:89–98

Brugghe J, Baak JPA, Wiltshaw E, Brinkhuis M, Meijer, GA, Fisher C 1998 Quantitative prognostic features in FIGO I ovarian cancer patients without postoperative treatment. Gynecologic Oncology 68:47–53

Burger HG 1993 Clinical utility of inhibin measurements. Journal of Clinical Endocrinology and Metabolism 76:1391–1396

Burghardt E, Girardi F, Lahousen M, Tamussino K, Stettner H 1991 Patterns of pelvic and paraaortic lymph node involvement in ovarian cancer. Gynecologic Oncology 40:103–106

Calvert AH, Newell DR, Gumbrell S et al 1989 Carboplatin dosage: prospective evaluation of a simple formula based on renal function. Journal of Clinical Oncology 7:1748–1756

Czernobilsky B, Silverman BB, Mikuta JJ 1970 Endometrioid carcinoma of the ovary. A clinicopathologic study of 75 cases. Cancer 26:1141–1152

Dark G, Bower M, Newlands E, Paradinas F, Rustin G 1997 Surveillance policy for stage I ovarian germ cell tumours. Journal of Clinical Oncology 15:620–624

Dembo AJ, Davy M, Stenwig AE et al 1990 Prognostic factors in patients with Stage I epithelial ovarian cancer. Obstetrics and Gynecology 75:263–273

Eeles RA, Tan S, Wiltshaw E et al 1991 Hormone replacement therapy and survival after surgery for ovarian cancer. British Medical Journal 302:259–262

Einhorn N, Bast R, Knapp R, Nilsson B, Zurawski V Jr, Sjovall K 2000 Long term follow-up of the Stockholm screening study on ovarian cancer. Gynecological Oncology 79:466–470

Eisenhauer EA, Vermorken JB, van Glabekke M 1997 Predictors of response to subsequent chemotherapy in platinum pretreated ovarian cancer: a multivariate analysis of 704 patients. Annals of Oncology 8:963–968

Fox H, Lang FA 1976 Tumours of the ovary. Heinemann, London, pp 119–137

Gershenson DM, Morris M, Burke TW, Levenback C, Matthews, CM, Wharton JT 1996 Treatment of poor-prognosis sex cord-stromal tumors of the ovary with the combination of bleomycin, etoposide, and cisplatin. Obstetrics and Gynecology 87:527–531

Gershenson DM, Morris M, Cangir A et al 1990 Treatment of malignant germ cell tumors of the ovary with bleomycin, etoposide, and cisplatin. Journal of Clinical Oncology 8:715–720

Gordon A, Lipton D, Woodruff JD 1981 Dysgerminoma: a review of 158 cases from the Emil Novak ovarian tumor registry. Obstetrics and Gynecology 58:497–504

Green JA, Berns E, Hensen-Logmans S et al 1999 Biological markers in ovarian cancer – implications for clinical practice. CME Journal of Gynecological Oncology 4:13–21

Griffiths CT 1987 Carcinoma of the ovary: surgical objectives. In: Sharp F, Soutter WP (eds) Ovarian cancer–the way ahead. Royal College of Obstetricians and Gynaecologists, London, pp 235–244

Griffiths CT, Parker LM, Fuller AFJ 1979 Role of cystoreductive surgical treatment in the management of advanced ovarian cancer. Cancer Treatment Reports 63:235–240

Hacker NF, Berek JS, Lagasse LD et al 1983 Primary cytoreductive surgery for epithelial ovarian cancer. Obstetrics and Gynecology 61:413–420

Hellström A-C, Silfverswärd C, Nilsson B, Pettersson F 1994 Carcinoma of the fallopian tube. A clinical and histopathological review. The Radiumhemmet series. International Journal of Gynecological Cancer 4:395–400

Hildreth NG, Kelsey JL, LiVolsi VA et al 1981 An epidemiological study of epithelial carcinoma of the ovary. American Journal of Epidemiology 114:389–405

Hoskins WJ, Bundy BN, Thigpen JT, Omura GA 1992 The influence of cytoreductive surgery on recurrence-free interval and survival in small-volume stage III epithelial ovarian cancer: a Gynecologic Oncology Group study. Gynecological Oncology 47:159–166

Hunter RW, Alexander NDE, Soutter WP 1992 Meta-analysis of surgery in advanced ovarian carcinoma: is maximum cytoreductive surgery an independent determinant of prognosis? American Journal of Obstetrics and Gynecology 166:504–511

ICON Collaborators 1998 ICON2: randomised trial of single-agent carboplatin against three-drug combination of CAP (cyclophosphamide, doxorubicin, and cisplatin) in women with ovarian cancer. Lancet 352:1571–1576

ICON Collaborators 2002 ICON3: randomised trial comparing paclitaxel plus carboplatin against standard chemotherapy of either single agent carboplatin or CAP (cyclophosphamide, doxorubicin, cisplatin) in women with ovarian cancer. Lancet 2002 in press

Jacobs IJ, Skates SJ, MacDonald N et al 1999 Screening for ovarian cancer: a pilot randomised controlled trial. Lancet 353:1207–1210

Kaern J, Tropé CG, Kristensen VM et al 1993 DNA ploidy: the most important prognostic factor in patients with borderline tumors of the ovary. International Journal of Gynecological Cancer 3:349–358

Kayikcioglu F, Kose MF, Boran N, Caliskan E, Tulunay G 2001 Neoadjuvant chemotherapy or primary surgery in advanced epithelial ovarian cancer. International Journal of Gynecological Cancer 11:466–470

Koonings PP, Campbell K, Mishell DR, Grimes DA 1989 Relative frequency of primary ovarian neoplasms: a 10 year review. Obstetrics and Gynecology 74:921–926

Kuoppala T, Heinola M, Isola J, Heinonen PK 1996 Serous and mucinous borderline tumours of the ovary: a clinicopathologic and DNA-ploidy study of 102 cases. International Journal of Gynecological Cancer 6:302–308

Lauszus FF, Petersen AC, Greisen J, Jakobsen A 2001 Granulosa cell tumor of the ovary: a population-based study of 37 women with stage I disease. Gynecologic Oncology 81:456–460

Low JJH, Perrin LC, Crandon AJ, Hacker NF 2000 Conservative surgery to preserve ovarian function in patients with malignant ovarian germ cell tumors. Cancer 89:391–398

MacDonald ND, Rosenthal AN, Jacobs IJ 1998 Screening for ovarian cancer. Annals of the Academy of Medicine of Singapore 27:676–682

Marchetti M, Padovan P, Fracas M 1998 Malignant ovarian tumours: conservative surgery and quality of life in young patients. European Journal of Gynaecological Oncology 19:297–301

Markman M, Bundy B, Benda J et al 1998 Randomised phase 3 study of intravenous (iv) cisplatin/paclitaxel versus moderately high dose iv carboplatin followed by iv paclitaxel and intraperitoneal cisplatin in optimal residual ovarian cancer. Proceedings of the American Society of Clinical Oncology 361a

Marks JR, Davidoff AM, Kerns BJM et al 1991 Overexpression and mutation of p53 in epithelial ovarian cancer. Cancer Research 51:2979–2984

McGuire WP, Hoskins WJ, Brady MF et al 1996 Cyclophosphamide and cisplatin compared with paclitaxel and cisplatin in patients with stage III and stage IV ovarian cancer. New England Journal of Medicine 334:1–6

Mol BWJ, Boll D, de Kanter M et al 2001 Distinguishing the benign and malignant adnexal mass: an external validation of prognostic models. Gynecologic Oncology 80:162–167

Morgante G, la Marca A, Ditto A, de Leo V 1999 Comparison of two malignancy risk indices based on serum CA125, ultrasound score and menopausal status in the diagnosis of ovarian masses. British Journal of Obstetrics and Gynaecology 106:524–527

Morice P, Camatte S, El Hassan J, Pautier P, Duvillard P, Castaigne D 2001 Clinical outcomes and fertility after conservative treatment of ovarian borderline tuours. Fertility and Sterility 75:92–96

Narod SA, Sun P, Ghadirian P et al 2001 Tubal ligation and risk of ovarian cancer in carriers of BRCA1 or BRCA2 mutations: a case-control study. Lancet 357:1467–1470

Muggia FM, Braly PS, Brady MF et al 2000 Phase III randomized study of cisplatin versus paclitaxel versus cisplatin and paclitaxel in patients with suboptimal stage III or IV ovarian cancer: a Gynecologic Oncology Group study. Journal of Clinical Oncology 18:106–115

Nagele F, Petru E, Medl M, Kainz C, Graf AH, Sevelda P 1995 Preoperative CA 125: an independent prognostic factor in patients with stage I epithelial ovarian cancer. Obstetrics and Gynecology 86:259–264

Naylor MS, Burke F, Balkwill FR 1995 Cytokines and ovarian cancer. In: Sharp F et al (Eds) Ovarian cancer 3. Chapman and Hall, London, pp 89–97

Ness RB, Grisso JA, Vergona R, Klapper J, Morgan M, Wheeler JE, Study of Health and Reproduction (SHARE) Study Group 2001 Oral contraceptives, other methods of contraception, and risk reduction for ovarian cancer. Epidemiology 12:307–312

Nicholson S, Gooden CSR, Hird V et al 1998 Radioimmunotherapy after chemotherapy compared to chemotherapy alone in the treatment of advanced ovarian cancer: a matched analysis. Oncology Reports 5:223–226

Oram DH, Jeyarajah AR 1994 The role of ultrasound and tumour markers in the early detection of ovarian cancer. British Journal of Obstetrics and Gynaecology 101:939–945

Ovarian Cancer Meta-Analyses Project 1991 CP vs CAP chemotherapy of ovarian carcinoma: a meta-analysis. Journal of Clinical Oncology 9:1668–1674

Piccart MJ, Bertelsen K, James K 2000 Randomized intergroup trial of cisplatin-paclitaxel vs cisplatin-cyclophosphamide in women with advanced epithelial ovarian cancer. Three year results. Journal of the National Cancer Institute 92:699–708

Potter ME, Partridge EE, Hatch KD, Soong S-J, Austin JM, Shingleton HM 1991 Primary surgical therapy of ovarian cancer: how much and when? Gynaecological Oncology 40:195–200

Quinn M, Babb P, Brock A, Kirby L, Jones J 2001 Cancer trends in England and Wales 1950–1999. Studies on medical and population subjects no. 66. Stationery Office, London

Redman CWE, Warwick J, Luesley DM, Varma R, Lawton FG, Blackledge GPR 1994 Intervention debulking surgery in advanced epithelial ovarian cancer. British Journal of Obstetrics and Gynaecology 101:142–146

Rodriguez GC, Berchuck A, Whitaker RS et al 1991 Epidermal growth factor expression in normal ovarian epithelium and ovarian cancer. II Relationship between receptor expression and response to epidermal growth factor. American Journal of Obstetrics and Gynecology 164:745–750

Rodriguez C, Taham LM, Calle EE, Thun MJ, Jacobs EJ, Heath CW Jr 1998 Infertility and risk of fatal ovarian cancer in a prospective cohort of US women. Cancer Causes and Control 9:645–651

Rossing MA, Daling JR, Weiss NS, Moore DE, Self SG 1994 Ovarian tumours in a cohort of infertile women. New England Journal of Medicine 331:771–776

Schwartz P, Kavanagh J, Kudellea A, Vershraegen C 1998 The role of hormonal therapy in the management of ovarian cancer. In: Ovarian cancer: controversies in management. Churchill Livingstone, Edinburgh

Scully RE 1999 WHO international histological classification of tumor. Histologic typing of ovarian tumours. Springer, Heidelberg

Seidman JD, Kurman RJ 2000 Ovarian serous borderline tumors:a critical review of the literature with emphasis on prognostic indicators. Human Pathology 31:539–556

Shelly J, Venn A, Lumley J 1999. Long-term effects on women of assisted reproduction. International Journal of Technology Assessment in Health Care 15:36–51

Soutter WP, Leake RE 1987 Steroid hormone receptors in gynaecological cancers. In: Bonnar J (ed) Recent advances in obstetrics and gynaecology. Churchill Livingstone, Edinburgh, pp 175–194

Stratton J, Pharaoh P, Smith S, Easton D, Ponder B 1998 A systematic review and meta-analysis of family history and risk of ovarian cancer. British Journal of Obstetrics and Gynaecology 105:493–499

Suzuki M, Ohwada M, Aida I et al 1993 Macrophage colony-stimulating factor as a tumour marker for epithelial ovarian cancer. Obstetrics and Gynecology 82:946–950

Teilum G 1965 Classification of endodermal sinus tumours (mesoblastoma vitellinum) and so called 'embryonal carcinoma' of the ovary. Acta Pathologica et Microbiologica 64:407

Trimble EL, Adams JD, Vena D et al 1993 Paclitaxel for platinum-refractory ovarian cancer: results from the first 1,000 patients registered to National Cancer Institute Treatment Referral Centre 9103. Journal of Clinical Oncology 11:2405–2410

Trope C, Kaern J, Hogberg T et al 2000 Randomized study on adjuvant chemotherapy in stage I high-risk ovarian cancer with evaluation of DNA-ploidy as prognostic instrument. Annals of Oncology 11:281–288

Urban N 1999 Screening for ovarian cancer: we now need a definitive randomised trial. British Medical Journal 319:1317–1318

van der Burg M, de Wit R, Stoter GF et al 1998 Phase I study of weekly cisplatin (P) and weekly or 4-weekly taxol (T): a highly active regimen in advanced epithelial ovarian cancer (OC). Proceedings of the American Society of Clinical Oncology 355

Van der Burg ME, van Lent M, Buyse M et al 1995 The effect of dubulking surgery after induction chemotherapy on the prognosis in advanced epithelial ovarian cancer. New England Journal of Medicine 332:629–634

van Nagell JR 1983 Tumour markers in gynaecologic malignancies. In: Griffiths CT, Fuller AF (eds) Gynecologic Oncology. Martinus Nijhoff, Boston, pp 63–79

van Nagell JR Jr, DePriest PD, Reedy MB et al 2000 The efficacy of transvaginal sonographic screening in asymptomatic women at risk for ovarian cancer. Gynecological Oncology 77:350–356

Venn A, Watson L, Lumley J, Giles G, King C, Healy D 1995 Breast and ovarian cancer incidence after infertility and in vitro fertilisation. Lancet 336:995–1000

Vergote I, de Brabanter J, Fyles A et al 2001a Prognostic importance of degree of differentiation and cyst rupture in stage I invasive epithelial ovarian carcinoma. Lancet 357:176–182

Vergote I, Trimbos B, Guthrie D et al 2001b Results of a randomized trial in 923 patients with high-risk early ovarian cancer, comparing chemotherapy with no further treatment following surgery. Proceedings of the American Society of Clinical Oncology 20:201

Vergote IB, de Vos LN, Abeler VM et al 1992 Randomized trial comparing cisplatin with radioactive phosphorus or whole abdominal irradiation as adjuvant treatment of ovarian cancer. Cancer 69:741–749

Vermorken JB 2000a Optimal treatment for ovarian cancer: taxoids and beyond. Annals Oncology 11:131–139

Vermorken JB 2000b The role of intraperitoneal chemotherapy in epithelial ovarian cancer. International Journal of Gynecological Cancer 10:26–32

Vessey M, Metcalfe A, Wells C, McPherson K, Westhoff C, Yeates D 1987 Ovarian neoplasms, functional cysts and oral contraceptives. British Medical Journal 294:1518–1520

Watson P, Lynch HT 1992 Hereditary ovarian cancer In: Sharp F, Mason WP, Creasman W (eds) Ovarian cancer 2. Biology, diagnosis and management. Chapman and Hall, London, pp 9–15

Whittemore A, Harris R, Intyre J, the Collaborative Ovarian Cancer Group 1992 Characteristics related to ovarian cancer risk: collaborative analysis of twelve US case-control studies. II Invasive epithelial cancer in white women. American Journal of Epidemiology 136:1184–1203

Willemsen W, Kruitwagen R, Bastiaans B, Hanselaar T, Rolland R 1993 Ovarian stimulation and granulosa-cell tumour. Lancet 341:986–988

Williams S, Blessing J, DiSaia P, Major F, Ball H, Liao S 1994 Second-look laparotomy in ovarian germ cell tumors: the Gynecologic Oncology Group experience. Gynecological Oncology 52/3:287–291

Woolas RP, Xu FJ, Jacobs IJ et al 1993 Elevation of multiple serum markers in patients with Stage I ovarian cancer. Journal of the National Cancer Institutes 85:1748–1751

Woolas R, Jacobs I, Prys Davies A et al 1994 What is the true incidence of primary fallopian tube carcinoma? International Journal of Gynecological Cancer 4:384–388

Xu FJ, Yu YH, Daly L et al 1993 The OVX1 radioimmunoassay

complements CA 125 for prdicting the presence of residual ovarian carcinoma at second look surgical surveillance procedures. Journal of Clinical Oncology 11:1506–1510

Young RC, Brady MF, Nieberg RM et al 1999 Randomized clinical trial of adjuvant treatment of women with early (FIGO I-IIA high risk) ovarian cancer – GOG #95. Clinical Oncology 18:357

Young RC, Walton LA, Ellenberg SS et al 1990 Adjuvant therapy in stage I and stage II epithelial ovarian cancer: results of two prospective randomized trials. New England Journal of Medicine 322:1021–1027

Zanetta G, Chiari S, Rota S et al 1997 Conservative surgery for stage I ovarian carcinoma in women of childbearing age. British Journal of Obstetrics and Gynaecology 104:1030–1035

Zanetta G, Rota S, Chiari S, Bonazzi C, Bratina G, Mangioni C 2001a Behaviour of borderline ovarian tumours with particular interest to persistence, recurrence, and progression to invasive carcinoma: a prospective study. Journal of Clinical Oncology 19:2658–2664

Zanetta G, Rota S, Lissoni A, Meni A, Brancatelli G, Buda A 2001b Ultrasound, physical examination, and CA 125 measurement for the detection of recurrence after conservative surgery for early borderline ovarian tumours. Gynecological Oncology 81:63–66

Zanetta G, Bonazzi C, Cantu MG et al 2001c Survival and reproductive function after treatment of malignant germ cell ovarian tumours. Journal of Clinical Oncology 19:1015–1020

46

Benign disease of the breast

Poramaporn Prasarttong-Osoth   William Svensson
John Lynn

INTRODUCTION

Breast cancer is such an emotive disease that on discovering a breast-related symptom, many women fear the worst. In fact, around 90% of these women will have benign pathology. A prompt and accurate diagnosis and a plan of treatment are required to alleviate their anxiety. Many breast units have instituted the 'one-stop' clinic, where the patient comes to see a surgeon and have further imaging and cytological investigations on the same visit. Most patients will leave the clinic with a diagnosis, if possible, and the plan of treatment.

Triple assessment is now standard practice for diagnosis of any breast lesion. It is based on the three complementary aspects of clinical examination, imaging and cytology or core biopsy.

HISTORY

These are the common presenting symptoms of the patient in breast clinic and the following questions should be asked.

1. Lump or thickening
   - How long has it been present?
   - Is it changed or affected by the menstrual cycle?
   - Is it painful?
2. Pain or tenderness
   - Is it cyclical or non-cyclical?
   - Does it affect both breasts?
   - Is it generalized or only at the specific point?
3. Nipple discharge
   - Is it from single or multiple ducts?

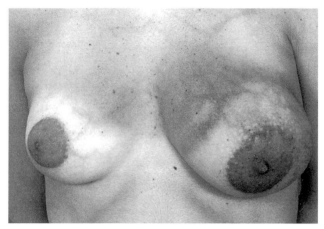

Fig. 46.1   The left breast is clearly larger, more dependent and has visible distended veins. The cause was a giant fibroadenoma.

- What is the colour of the discharge? Has it ever been bloodstained?

Information about previous history of breast disease and biopsies, menstrual history, menopausal status, use of oral contraceptive pill or HRT and family history of breast cancer should also be obtained.

EXAMINATION

The examination should take place in a warm, well-lit and comfortable environment where the patient's privacy is maintained at all times. Examination begins with inspection while the patient is sitting upright, with arms by her sides. The patient is asked to lift her arms above her head and then press her hands on her hips. All through these procedures the examiner looks for asymmetry of the breast contour, differences in the level of the nipples, changes in the skin and nipples and scars (Fig. 46.1).

Palpation of the breasts is performed with the patient lying flat with her arms above the head. All four quadrants should be examined in turn, including the axillary tail and areolar area. Feeling the asymptomatic breast first will give you an idea of the normal breast consistency. If a lump is found, its size, position, consistency, fixity and any overlying skin change should be noted. The patient who complains of a nipple discharge, if not obvious, should be asked to demonstrate where and how to produce the symptom herself. This is less unpleasant for the patient than if it is performed by the physician. Single or multiple duct discharge may give the clue to the causes of the symptoms. The discharge itself can be analysed for haemoglobin, cytology and culture.

Examination of the breast cannot be completed without palpation for enlarged axillary and supraclavicular nodes. Palpable lymphadenopathy increases the suspicion of a breast carcinoma, but can also occur with an inflammatory process.

INVESTIGATIONS

Ultrasonography and mammography are the most frequently used methods of imaging (Box 46.1). Palpable masses within

Box 46.1   Indications for imaging and the advantages of the different techniques

Indication for mammography	Indications for breast ultrasonography
Over 50 years old Breast screening	**Under 35 years old** Clinically benign mass and no significant risk factors for breast cancer
Over 35 years old No recent mammography and a palpable mass and clinical suspicion of carcinoma	**Over 35 years old** • *Benign or equivocal solitary mass* Can be biopsied under direct vision if indicated
Under 35 years old Very strong clinical suspicion of malignancy and normal breast ultrasound and cytology	• *Cysts* Can be diagnosed reliably and needling avoided • *Multiple masses* Solid lesions can be differentiated from cysts and suspicious areas can be biopsied or needled • *Abscess cavities* Can be identified and drained by needle aspiration • *Augmented breast* Not obscured by a prosthesis so silicone granulomas and leakage are more easily diagnosed than by mammography • *Pregnant woman* Because mammography is contraindicated by slight radiation risk

the breast are best imaged with ultrasonography in patients under the age of 35. Over the age of 35, mammography and/or ultrasonography should be performed. If there has been recent mammography, ultrasonography may be the investigation of choice, particularly if there is a previous history of cysts or the palpable lump is thought to be a cyst.

Wherever possible, imaging should precede fine needle aspiration or core biopsy, as these can cause changes within the breast tissue which can be indistinguishable from the mammographic and ultrasound appearance of carcinoma. Tissue diagnosis should be obtained in all breast lesions either by fine needle aspiration cytology (FNA) or core biopsy.

Ultrasonography

Ultrasonography should be performed by an experienced radiologist or ultrasonographer using a high-resolution linear array probe (7–10 MHz) on an ultrasound machine with colour Doppler designed for high-resolution small parts soft tissue imaging. Under the age of 35 ultrasound is the imaging modality of choice for a palpable mass. Over 35 it may also be the most useful, though the indications for mammography are stronger. It also has a place in the imaging of pregnant patients and patients with breast implants. Ultrasound is less helpful than mammography in screening for impalpable lesions. It is rarely, if ever, helpful in identifying microcalcification demonstrated mammographically.

Ultrasound-guided FNA or core biopsy is the new trend in investigation of the breast lesions. Ultrasound-guided interventions are preferable to mammographic guidance, both for the experienced operator and the patient, as the patient lies in a comfortable supine position rather than sitting up for mammographic procedures. Ultrasonography allows real-time imaging and optimum placement of the needle tip under direct vision. It has a significant advantage when differentiating between solid and cystic breast lesions, mastitis and small breast abscesses.

Mammography

Mammography currently has three main applications: in routine screening, investigation of symptomatic breast disease and image-guided FNA, biopsy or excision. Interpretation of mammography should be performed by experienced radiologists with suitable breast imaging training. Oblique and craniocaudal views are usually obtained. Mammography is normally not advised for the patient under age of 35 due to the dense fibroglandular tissue that leads to poor image quality. The sensitivity of mammography alone is over 80% but is considerably less in younger patients.

A mammogram offers the opportunity for early detection of breast cancer, especially in impalpable lesions. It shows mass lesions, areas of parenchymal distortion and microcalcifications. The risks of mammography causing breast cancer are greater in young or large breasts than in old or small breasts. It has been estimated that one cancer is likely to be caused for every three detected in women aged 30–34 years if two views are taken for each breast. At age 40–44 years, the ratio falls to one for every 30 detected, whereas at 50–54 years it decreases to one for every 90 detected. Because of the cumulative effect of radiation, mammographic screening is certainly not indicated below the age of 40 years. It is of benefit in women more than 45 years and clearly beneficial for these over 50.

Ductography

Ductography is the imaging of a duct by injection of X-ray contrast after cannulation of the duct. Indications are continuing discharge after previous surgery and suspicion of a duct abnormality despite a normal ultrasound examination. Most intraductal lesions of any size, such as intraductal papilloma, are demonstrated on ultrasound (Fig. 46.2)

Magnetic resonance imaging

Magnetic resonance imaging (MRI) is the most sensitive technique for diagnosis of breast cancer. Its superior image quality is particularly useful for the implanted breast and the breast after conservative surgery. At present its wider use is limited by cost and availability of the equipment but in the future MRI will be used as the main screening method as it becomes more readily available and less expensive.

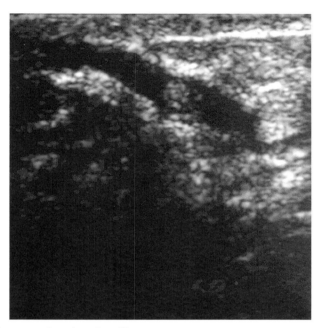
Fig. 46.2 Intraductal papilloma.

Fine needle aspiration cytology (FNAC)

FNAC and core biopsy have resulted in a major change in the management of breast symptoms over the past decade, with a substantial reduction in the need for open biopsy. For optimal results, FNAC requires a consistent sampling technique in conjunction with reporting by a skilled cytopathologist. Results can be generated within minutes. This allows planning of treatment and, for those with benign disorders, has the potential to allay patient fears.

FNAC should be performed with a 21G needle and 10 ml syringe. Local anaesthesia is rarely required, but for the particularly anxious patient EMLA cream can be used topically. The lump is 'fixed' between the thumb and index finger of the surgeon's non-dominant hand. Once the needle has entered the lump, suction is applied to the syringe and maintained during several passes through the lump. The suction is then released and the needle withdrawn. The contents of the syringe are spread over a couple of slides. These are then air-dried or sprayed with fixative and later stained, depending on the cytopathologist's preference.

The breast cytology will be reported as a numerical score:

C1 Inadequate specimen
C2 Benign
C3 Atypia, probably benign
C4 Suspicious of malignancy
C5 Malignant

The majority of patients reported as C3 will have a benign diagnosis.

Complications of FNAC of the breast are rare but pneumothorax, haematoma and acute mastitis have been reported.

Histological biopsy

Core biopsy can be performed under local anaesthesia. It is

now used alongside FNAC or when FNAC has been unhelpful. Core biopsy has the advantage of providing a histological diagnosis. When used to biopsy an impalpable lesion with abnormal calcification, it is important to X-ray the biopsy specimen to prove the presence of microcalcification in the specimen as a means of confirming the accuracy of the biopsy.

Diagnosis of most breast lesions is usually reached by a combination of clinical and radiological assessment with either FNAC or core biopsy results. Open biopsy is rarely performed because of diagnostic uncertainty. Specific indications for biopsy in cases of clinically benign breast disease include cytological or radiological suspicion, heightened patient anxiety and a breast cyst that either recurs or persists after two attempts at aspiration. Recommendations for open biopsy based on age are contentious, with arbitrary limits set at either 35 or 40 years.

SCREEN-DETECTED IMPALPABLE LESIONS

This category has been generated by the growth of breast-screening programmes. As with palpable lesions, a diagnosis must be achieved by a combination of physical examination, radiological imaging and cytological/histological pathology. Further mammography or ultrasound images may be required to allow directed aspiration of the lesion. Where uncertainty still exists, open targeted biopsy should be performed. Guidewire localization is the most commonly used technique. The specimen should always be X-rayed to confirm that the relevant area has been excised.

ABNORMALITIES OF DEVELOPMENT AND INVOLUTION

In the past a variety of names has been given to the condition of painful, often lumpy breasts, including benign mammary dysplasia, fibroadenosis and chronic mastitis. Histological analysis of breast tissue from these women has often shown similar features to those with apparently normal asymptomatic breasts. To resolve this dilemma, the concept of abnormalities of development and involution (ANDI) has been established by the Cardiff Breast Clinic as a framework for benign breast disorders. This proposes that there is a gradation from normal through mild to more pronounced abnormality which presents as frank disease. The scheme encompasses not merely painful nodularity but also other conditions, such as fibroadenomas, adolescent hypertrophy and cystic disease.

Breast pain and/or nodularity

Lumpiness of the breast with or without pain and the pain symptom alone account for more than 50% of the presenting problems in a breast clinic. From the outset, anxiety can be alleviated by the knowledge that most patients with breast pain do not have cancer. Patients with breast pain and a palpable mass should be investigated as dictated by the mass.

The nature of the pain can help to pinpoint the exact cause of the pain. It is important to establish whether the pain originates in the breast itself, whether it is cyclical or non-cyclical, bilateral or unilateral. Cervical spondylosis, cardiac pain, pleurisy, oesophageal lesions and Tietze's disease may mimic breast pain. This last condition is a painful costochondritis deep to the breast. Non-steroidal analgesics are commonly of benefit.

Non-cyclical mastalgia

Non-cyclical breast pain is most commonly seen in the perimenopausal age group. The most likely underlying causes, such as mammary duct ectasia, fat necrosis and sclerosing adenosis, are discussed later in the chapter.

Cyclical mastalgia

Many patients are relieved to hear that cyclical breast pain affects the majority of women to varying degrees at some point in their reproductive life. The condition is usually considered an aberration of the normal cyclical changes, quite possibly hormonal in origin. Major hormonal events, such as pregnancy and the menopause, frequently relieve the pain and spontaneous remission is common. Characteristically, pain occurs in the few days leading up to the onset of menstruation, when the breast feels swollen and

BREAST PAIN CHART

Patient name:

Month	1	2	3	4	5	6	7	8	9	10	11	12	13	14	15	16	17	18	19	20	21	22	23	24	25	26	27	28	29	30	31

Note the degree of breast pain you experience on each day by filling in the relevant square

■ severe pain

◢ mild pain

• no pain

Note when your period starts with the letter "P" for each day

Fig. 46.3 Breast pain chart.

areas of nodularity may be evident. However, the relationship between nodularity and the pain is not constant. Usually both breasts are affected, particularly in the upper outer quadrant. A pain chart kept by the patient over 2–3 months may help to demonstrate the cyclic nature of the pain (Fig. 46.3).

Investigation

Careful history taking, clinical examination and sympathetic explanation of the condition will satisfy around 85% of patients. The remainder require medical treatment. Mammography often has a therapeutic effect, although in the absence of a dominant nodule this should be reserved for those over the age of 35. If no mass is identified and the imaging is negative, no further investigation is indicated and the patient should be reassured.

Areas of focal nodularity are extremely common and should be investigated as any other lump in the breast. In patients over the age of 35 mammography is the first line of investigation. FNAC can be performed but may have a lower diagnostic yield than in other breast conditions. Core biopsy is more accurate than FNAC in this case and an open biopsy is rarely needed. Features of normal breast involution, i.e. fibrosis, adenosis, apocrine change and microcyst formation, will be evident on histological examination.

Treatment

After assessment and reassurance only a small group of patients will require medical treatment. Randomized controlled trials have confirmed the efficacy of drugs in the treatment of mastalgia; the results are generally better in cyclical mastalgia. The role of dietary factors such as caffeine in the aetiology of mastalgia is unclear. Wearing a supportive bra often improves true non-cyclical pain.

Gamolenic acid (γ-linolenic acid)

Evening primrose is a plant rich in γ-linolenic acid, an essential fatty acid. Empirical treatment with oil of evening primrose was noted to produce a reduction in breast pain. It was subsequently demonstrated that women with mastalgia have abnormal fatty acid profiles, which tend to correct after several months with gamolenic acid. Essential fatty acids are intimately related to lipid metabolism and consequently affect such diverse functions as cellular membrane flexibility, hormone receptor affinity and cholesterol transport. Gamolenic acid is now the first-line drug for treatment of cyclical mastalgia. It is almost free of side-effects but response to therapy can be slow. A reduction in pain response is seen in approximately 60% of patients. The recommended dose is 80 mg, 3–4 times a day. The treatment should originally be continued for 3 months and can be extended if effective.

Hormonal agents

Danazol. Danazol is a synthetic steroid which combines androgenic activity with anti-oestrogenic and antiprogestogenic activity. A prospective randomized double-blind trial using danazol in a dose of 200 mg bd showed a significant improve-ment in breast pain, tenderness and nodularity. In cyclical mastalgia a response rate approaching 80% can be anticipated. Unfortunately side-effects, most notably virilization, reduce patient compliance. Use of this drug should therefore be reserved for those unresponsive to gamolenic acid.

Bromocriptine. This drug stimulates dopamine receptors and inhibits prolactin release. Mastalgia is relieved in approximately 60% of patients. Again, the side-effects, especially nausea, vomiting and dizziness, preclude widespread use of the drug. A gradual increase in dose may reduce the frequency of complications.

Tamoxifen. Tamoxifen is an oestrogen receptor antagonist which is of benefit in the treatment of cyclical mastalgia.

EPITHELIAL HYPERPLASIA

A suspicious aspirate (C3 and C4) may indicate a diagnosis of epithelial hyperplasia. This results from exaggerated proliferation of the ductal epithelium. Severe hyperplasia doubles the risk of breast carcinoma, which is further increased in the presence of cellular atypia or a positive family history. Diagnosis is confirmed by open biopsy. Those with cellular atypia warrant close surveillance.

SCLEROSIS

These benign lesions, such as sclerosing adenosis and radial scar, are of clinical significance because they can mimic the presentation of cancer or recurrence at the site of previous excision of carcinoma. Sclerosis may occur during the process of involution and may give rise to diagnostic confusion. Distortion of the terminal duct lobular unit is seen, perhaps provoked by an adjacent scar.

Clinical presentation is either with a breast lump or an abnormality detected on screening mammogram. Unfortunately, these lesions may often be indistinguishable in appearance from carcinoma, both mammographically and ultrasonically. FNAC may help the diagnosis but if there is any doubt, excision biopsy is recommended.

CYSTIC BREAST DISEASE

This is a condition which affects over 5% of women. It most commonly occurs in the decade before the menopause. In contrast with ANDI, in which cysts are also an integral component, in cystic breast disease the cysts are usually larger. Macroscopically the cysts may have a bluish appearance and are known eponymously as the 'blue-domed cyst of Bloodgood'.

Cysts probably arise as an aberration of senile involution associated with active secretion of apocrine epithelium. There may be underlying hormonal imbalance. One theory suggests that altered central regulation of prolactin may be involved and levels of essential fatty acids are lower than in the general population.

Characteristically, breast cysts are discrete, smooth and rounded. The upper outer quadrant is most commonly affected. If tensely filled with fluid, the cyst may cause pain.

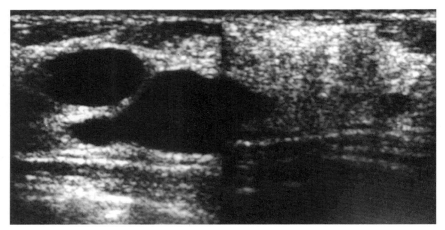

Fig. 46.4 Breast cyst.

Multiple cysts occur in 50% of affected women, with a small percentage reporting over 20 cysts (Fig. 46.4).

Investigation

Ultrasound gives a definite diagnosis of cyst in most cases, with the confirmed by aspiration of the fluid. Mammorgraphically, cysts may classically show a localized opacity with a surrounding halo. Unless the aspirated fluid is bloodstained, cytological analysis is not required.

Treatment

Approximately 2% of patient with breast cysts may have a co-existent carcinoma. Patients who have their cysts aspirated have to be re-examined to exclude an underlying or residual breast lump. If this is discovered, the patient needs to be fully assessed with further imaging and repeated FNAC of the lump.

A further examination should take place 4 weeks later to confirm that the cyst has not reaccumulated. Excision biopsy is required for cytological uncertainty or if the cyst repeatedly refills.

It has been suggested that there is a slightly increased risk of breast carcinoma in patients with breast cysts and the tendency is most marked in those with multiple cysts. This risk is otherwise not considered of clinical significance. This group of patients may undergo regular mammography. Danazol may be effective at reducing the numbers of cysts and the associated discomfort.

FIBROADENOMA

The contemporary view is that these lesions are also aberrations of normal breast development. Clonal analysis has shown that both epithelial and stromal cells are polyclonal, confirming that fibroadenomas, which develop from a whole lobule, are hyperplastic. Furthermore, hyperplastic lobules, histologically indistinguishable from fibroadenomata, are commonly present in the breasts of normal young women.

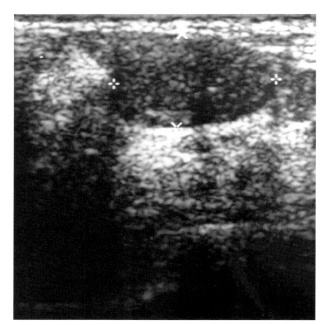

Fig. 46.5 Fibroadenoma.

Fibroadenoma are most commonly found in early adult life and are particularly prevalent in negroid races. Up to the mid-30s fibroadenomas are a more common cause of breast lumps than carcinoma. Juvenile fibroadenomas are occasionally seen in adolescent girls.

The usual presentation is a discrete, firm breast lump, mostly situated in the upper outer quadrant of the breast. Because of their mobility, these lumps are popularly known as breast mice. Fibroadenoma may be multiple in up to 20% of cases. Most lumps are 1–2 cm in diameter; those over 5 cm are defined as giant fibroadenomas (Figs 46.5, 46.6).

Investigation

Although the vast majority of clinically diagnosed fibroadenomas are benign, up to 5% will subsequently be shown to

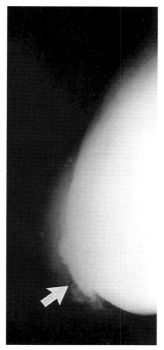

Fig. 46.11 Mammogram showing leaking silicone breast prosthesis (arrowed) which caused pain, lumpiness and local inflammation.

subsequent mammographic interpretation difficult. Modified views may improve visualization of breast parenchyma. Ultrasound is much more helpful in the evaluation of palpable abnormalities. Even after removal of silicone prostheses, residual speculated silicone granulomas may simulate carcinoma on mammography.

MISCELLANEOUS CONDITIONS

Fat necrosis

This condition is most prevalent in plump, middle-aged women. A history of trauma, most commonly seatbelt injury, is reported in about 50% of affected patients. The major significance of fat necrosis is that it mimics many of the features of breast carcinoma, e.g. skin tethering, dimpling, with a poorly defined painless lump. Less commonly the patient may complain of non-cyclical mastalgia.

Investigation is by mammography in conjunction with FNAC or core biopsy. Calcification and fibrosis may be seen mammographically, again leading to confusion with carcinoma. Open biopsy is indicated if the results of these investigations are inconclusive.

Haematoma

These are clearly seen as a fluid-filled low echogenic area within the breast. If the blood has clotted within the haematoma, it is often seen as heterogeneous echogenicity within the low-echogenic area. It is often possible to differentiate haematoma from abscess using colour Doppler, as there is no significant increase in the blood flow around haematomas,

compared with the markedly increased blood flow around infected areas such as abscesses within the breast. Ultrasound allows localization of both haematomas and abscesses for aspiration with a large-bore needle under ultrasound control.

Galactocoele

This cystic lesion always dates from lactation. It presents in a subareolar position and contains milk, either liquid or inspissated. Treatment by aspiration is usually successful. Ultrasound diagnosis is usually definitive.

Mondor's disease

Thrombophlebitis of the superficial veins of the breast and anterior chest wall is known as Mondor's disease. The inflamed vein is palpable as a subcutaneous cord and elevation of the arms throws the adjacent skin into a furrow. Mondor's disease is a self-limiting complaint but symptomatic relief may be required in the early stages when the area is painful.

Enlarged Montgomery's tubercles

Montgomery's tubercles are sebum-producing glands which open on to the areola. Blockage of the drainage duct will produce an areolar lump, which can become secondarily infected. Excision may be necessary for troublesome symptoms.

KEY POINTS

1. If possible, imaging of the breast should precede FNAC or core biopsy to avoid difficulties in interpretation due to the changes caused by these procedures.
2. Ultrasound can now diagnose many benign lesions with a high degree of certainty and is the imaging method of choice for the women under 35.
3. Mammography is not recommended for women less than 35 years old except if required to evaluate a known carcinoma.
4. Cyclical breast pain is very common and 85% of patients are satisfied with explanation alone. The remainder may be treated with gamolenic acid, danazol, bromocriptine or tamoxifen.
5. Women with multiple breast cysts have an increased risk of breast cancer.
6. About 5% of what are thought clinically to be fibroadenomas are in fact malignant. Investigation with ultrasound and fine-needle aspiration or core biopsy is required.
7. Breast abscesses can usually be treated with repeated needle aspiration.

SUGGESTED READING

Asch RH, Greenblatt RB 1977 The use of an impeded androgen – danazol – in the management of benign breast disorders. American Journal of Obstetrics and Gynaecology 127:130–134

Clarke D, Sudhakaran N, Gateley CA 2001 Replace fine needle aspiration cytology with automated core biopsy in the triple assessment of breast cancer. Annals of Royal College of Surgeons of England 83:110–112

Davies EL, Gateley CA, Miers M, Mansel RE 1998 The long-term course of mastalgia. Journal of the Royal Society of Medicine 91:462–464

Goldberg RP, Hall FM, Simon M 1983 Preoperative localization of non-palpable breast lesions using a wire marker and a perforated mammographic grid. Radiology 146:833–835

Klein DL, Sickles EA 1982 Effects of needle aspiration on the mammographic appearance of the breast: a guide to the proper timing of the mammography examination. Radiology 145:44

Law J 1993 Variations in individual radiation dose in a breast screening programme and consequence for the balance between associated risk and the benefit. British Journal of Radiology 66:394–397

Malur S, Wurdinger S, Moritz A, Michels W, Schneider A 2001 Comparison of written reports of mammography, sonography and magnetic resonance mammography for preoperative evaluation of breast lesions, with special emphasis on magnetic resonance mammography. Breast Cancer Research 3:55–60

Mansel RE 1983 Classification of mastalgia – the Cardiff system. In: Benign breast disease. Royal Society of Medicine, London, pp 33–41

Mansel RE, Wisbey JR, Hughes LE 1982 Controlled trial of the antigonadotrophin danazol in painful nodular benign breast disease. Lancet i:928–930

Moskowitz M, Russell P, Fidler J, Sutorius DJ, Law EJ Holle 1975 Breast cancer screening. Preliminary report of 207 biopsies performed in 4128 volunteer screenees. Cancer 36:2245–2250

Preece PE, Hughes LE, Mansel RE, Baum M, Bolton PM, Gravelle IH 1976 Clinical syndromes of mastalgia. Lancet ii:670–673

Sackier JM, Wood CB 1988 The treatment of fibrodenoma and Phylloides tumours. In: Ioannidou-Mouzaka L, Philippakis M, Angelakis P (eds) Mastology. Elsevier, Amsterdam, pp 151–156

Snyder RE 1980 Specimen radiography and pre-operative localization of non-palpable breast cancer. Cancer 46:950–956

Svensson WE, Tohno E, Cosgrove DO, Powles TJ, Al Murrani B, Jones A 1992 Effects of fine needle aspiration on the ultrasound appearance of the breast. Radiology 185:709–711

Tokunaga M, Land CE, Yamamoto T 1984 Breast cancer among atomic bomb survivors. In: Boice JD Jr, Fraumani JF (eds) Radiation carcinogenesis: epidemiology and biological significance. Raven Press, New York, p 45

Westened PJ, Sever AR, Beekman-de Volder HJ, Liem SJ 2001 A comparison of aspiration cytology and core biopsy in the evaluation of breast lesions. Cancer 93:146–150

47

Malignant disease of the breast

Abigail A. Evans   Anthony I. Skene

INTRODUCTION

Breast cancer represents a significant cause of morbidity and mortality worldwide with in excess of 1 million new cases diagnosed each year. In the United Kingdom, where the age-standardized incidence and mortality rates are high, breast cancer causes 14 000 deaths a year and is the leading cause of death in women aged 40–50 years. A woman's lifetime risk of developing breast cancer is approximately 1 in 12 and half of these women will die of their disease. The incidence is increasing, but recent evidence suggests a decline in mortality (Peto et al 2000). This is likely to be a result of earlier detection and improvements in therapy.

RISK FACTORS

The cause of breast cancer is unknown. There are many interrelated factors associated with an increased risk of developing breast cancer but few are clinically relevant and 66% of women with the disease have no identifiable risk factors.

Age

The incidence of breast cancer increases with age to the menopause, levels off and rises again at a reduced rate through the postmenopausal years.

Geographical variation

Incidence rates for breast cancer are six times greater in Western than underdeveloped countries and are greater in women of higher socioeconomic class. The role of environmental factors such as diet (particularly fat consumption) is supported by an increased incidence in immigrants to developed countries within three generations.

Hormones

Although lifetime exposure to endogenous oestrogens is related to breast cancer risk, there is no definitive evidence that the administration of exogenous oestrogens promotes the growth or dissemination of breast cancer.

Oral contraceptive pill

Use of the oral contraceptive pill, particularly from an early age, is associated with a small but independent increased risk of developing breast cancer (relative risk 1.3) (Collaborative

Group on Hormonal Factors in Breast Cancer 1996). This risk diminishes steadily after discontinuing use and returns to normal after 10 years.

Hormone replacement therapy (HRT)

The risk of HRT with regard to breast cancer is controversial. There is evidence that women currently or recently taking HRT are more likely to be diagnosed with breast cancer (Dupont & Page 1991). The relative risk is small, increases with duration of use (2.3% per year of use) and returns to normal 5 years after cessation of use. Between the ages of 50 and 70 years it is estimated that 45/1000 women will be diagnosed with breast cancer. In women using HRT for 5 years from the age of 50 years, this increases to 47/1000 and in those using HRT for 10 years to 51/1000. These increased rates are similar to those associated with a natural delay of the menopause of similar duration (Collaborative Group on Hormonal Factors in Breast Cancer 1997), suggesting that the risk is related to duration of hormone exposure regardless of source.

Breast cancers diagnosed in women on HRT tend to be smaller, of lower grade and are less often associated with metastatic disease. As such, although the incidence may be increased, there may not be any associated increased mortality from breast cancer in HRT users.

When advising patients regarding the use of the OCP and HRT, any increased risk of breast cancer diagnosis needs to be balanced against the benefits of preventing unwanted pregnancy, in the case of the contraceptive pill, and osteoporosis, and disabling menopausal symptoms, in the case of hormone replacement therapy.

Radiation

There is an increased risk of developing breast cancer following exposure to ionizing radiation, particularly at a young age (<30 years). However, exposure to clinically important levels is rare and is usually due to therapeutic irradiation such as mantle irradiation for lymphoma.

Benign breast disease

Women with palpable breast cysts, intraduct papillomas, sclerosing adenosis and florid epithelial hyperplasia have a marginally increased risk of developing breast cancer, but this is not of an order which is clinically significant. The only benign condition associated with a significant risk is atypical hyperplasia (relative risk 4).

Family history

Breast cancer is common and many women have a relative who has been affected by the disease. These women are understandably concerned about the implications for their own and their family's risk. In fact, only 5% of breast cancers are familial, resulting from an inherited germline mutation. Several breast cancer-related genes have been identified, most recently BRCA1 (long arm of chromosome 17) and BRCA2 (long arm of chromosome 13), the mutation of which may

account for as many 40% of inherited breast cancers (Eeles 1996). Other genes whose mutation predisposes to the development of breast cancer are p53 and the ataxia telangiectasia gene, but these probably account for very few breast cancers and there are undoubtedly other important genes yet to be identified. The estimated risk of developing breast cancer for a carrier of a BRCA1 mutation is 51% by the age of 50 years and 85% by the age of 70 years. There is an associated increased risk of ovarian cancer of the order of 44–63%. Mutation of the BRCA2 gene is associated with male breast cancer and carcinoma of the prostate but a lower risk of developing ovarian cancer than that associated with BRCA1 mutation. Inherited breast cancers tend to present at an early age, be of high grade and oestrogen receptor negative.

In assessing the risk of familial breast cancer for an individual, the number of affected relatives, their genetic closeness and the age at which they were diagnosed enables a lifetime risk to be calculated (Table 47.1). Patients with a risk in excess of 1 in 8 may be offered early mammographic screening and regular clinical examination although there is no evidence that this is of any benefit in terms of survival. It is particularly important that women understand that screening does not equate with prevention.

Specific genetic testing is available for affected relatives for whom blood samples are available. If a mutation is identified, both affected and unaffected relatives can be tested for that specific mutation. Pre-test counselling is extremely important as a negative test does not exclude a mutation in an as yet

Table 47.1 Maximum lifetime risk of developing breast cancer according to family history together with recommendations for screening

Family history	Lifetime risk (max)	Risk category	Early mammography	Genetic clinic
1 relative:				
>40 yrs	1 in 8	Low	No	No
<40 yrs	1 in 6	Low/Mod	Yes	No
<30 yrs or male at any age	1 in 6	Low/Mod	Yes	No
2 relatives:				
50–60 yrs	1 in 8	Low	No	No
40–49 yrs	1 in 4	Moderate	Yes	No
30–39 yrs	1 in 3	High	Yes	Yes
3 relatives:				
average 50–60 yrs	1 in 4	Moderate	Yes	Yes
average 40–50 yrs	1 in 3	High	Yes	Yes
Breast & other cancers:				
≥1 <50 yrs + ≥1 ovarian cancer at any age	>1 in 6	Moderate/High	Yes	Yes
1 relative breast & ovarian cancer	>1 in 6	Moderate/High	Yes	Yes
1 breast cancer & 1 childhood malignancy		High	Avoid mammos prior to genetic review	Yes

unidentified gene and in the presence of a mutation, the limitations of prevention and screening must be understood. Certain ethnic groups are at higher risk of specific mutations; for example, Ashkenazi Jews have a high incidence of BRCA1 mutations. In such groups genetic testing may be worthwhile with a weaker pedigree.

PREVENTION

There are considerable medical and ethical dilemmas regarding the management of women identified as high risk. In the absence of any clear causative factors for the majority of breast cancers, the options for effective prevention are limited. Any preventive agent must have a low-risk profile.

Medical prevention

The observation that women receiving tamoxifen as adjuvant treatment for breast cancer developed fewer contralateral breast cancers than expected suggested that this drug may be effective in reducing the incidence of breast cancer in other women at higher than normal risk. Such medical prevention is currently available only within the context of national and international trials, of which there are several still recruiting. Most of these are double-blind placebo trials involving the use of tamoxifen and/or other anti-oestrogens. Currently there are no clear results from these trials but it is likely that there is some protective benefit from tamoxifen.

Surgical prevention

Prophylactic mastectomy is becoming more common with the advent of genetic testing. Women at high risk, in particular those with a proven gene mutation, may be offered bilateral prophylactic mastectomies with or without immediate reconstruction. The risk of developing breast cancer after bilateral mastectomies is reduced by at least 90%, but not to zero because it is unlikely that all breast cells will be removed (Hartmann et al 1999). Recent evidence suggests that prophylactic mastectomy with reconstruction reduces psychological morbidity and anxiety in women identified as high risk and does not have a detrimental effect on their body image or sexual functioning (Hatcher et al 2001).

PATHOLOGY

The most important distinction in the pathology of breast cancer is between invasive and in situ disease.

Invasive carcinoma

Eighty per cent of invasive carcinomas are ductal, 5% are lobular and the remainder are classified as special types, which include tubular, medullary, mucinous and papillary. The distinction between types has few implications for management. Lobular carcinomas are more likely to be multifocal and bilateral and tumours of special type tend to have a more favourable prognosis. The most important histological information for invasive tumours is the size, grade, presence of vascular or lymphatic invasion, oestrogen receptor status and lymph node status as all these factors have implications for prognosis and treatment.

In situ disease

Carcinoma cells which are contained within the duct/lobular unit and have not invaded through basement membrane into the adjacent stroma of the breast are termed carcinoma in situ.

Lobular carcinoma in situ

LCIS is usually an incidental finding in a breast biopsy and is a marker for increased risk of developing invasive disease, often elsewhere in the same breast or even in the contralateral breast. Management of LCIS is controversial but in view of the increased risk of invasive disease (30% at 20 years), these women should be offered regular follow-up and additional screening. Some advocate prophylactic mastectomies.

Ductal carcinoma in situ

DCIS is more common than LCIS and may present symptomatically with a palpable mass or bloodstained nipple discharge. More commonly, it is detected as an area of pleomorphic calcification on a mammogram performed for an unrelated symptom or as part of the breast-screening programme. Prior to the introduction of routine breast screening, DCIS accounted for 5% of all breast cancers but this has now increased to 20%. DCIS is classified pathologically according to grade. If untreated, it is believed that some DCIS, especially of high grade, will progress to invasive disease, but the timescale for this is unknown.

Treatment is surgical excision which, if complete, should be curative. If local recurrence occurs it does so in the form of invasive disease in 50% of cases. The value of adjuvant therapies in the treatment of DCIS is uncertain and is the subject of several ongoing trials involving the use of radiotherapy and/or tamoxifen. There is some evidence that local recurrence, particularly of high-grade disease, can be significantly reduced by adjuvant radiotherapy (Fisher 1998).

PRESENTATION

Breast cancer may present as symptomatic or screen-detected disease.

Screen-detected disease

The UK NHS breast-screening programme was introduced in 1988 following recommendations of the Forrest Report (1986), the principal finding of which was that the introduction of mass screening by mammography would lead to a reduction of breast cancer deaths by 25%. Women between the ages of 50 and 64 years (to be extended to 70 years from 2003) are invited for 3-yearly mammography. The success of the programme depends upon screening of at least 70% of the invited population. The benefit of screening mammography below the age of 50 years has not been established although screening in this age group is routinely offered in some countries. After the

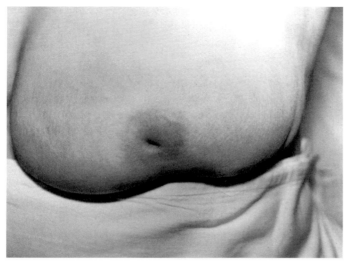

Fig. 47.1 Carcinoma of the left breast causing skin and nipple retraction.

age of 64 years women can self-refer for screening. Women with an abnormality are recalled for further assessment, which may include further mammographic views, ultrasound scan, clinical assessment and biopsies. After assessment women may be returned to routine screening, put onto early recall or referred for surgical intervention. The aim of the assessment clinics is to make a diagnosis of any abnormality detected so that definitive treatment can be undertaken, but sometimes a diagnostic surgical biopsy is required.

Considerable debate exists over the value of breast screening, particularly with regard to lead-time bias and the anxiety caused by false-positive results. However, the programme is well established and likely to remain despite these reservations.

Symptomatic disease

The majority of breast cancers present symptomatically with a discrete lump, skin changes (distortion or ulceration), nipple changes (Fig. 47.1) and, rarely, pain. In the UK, symptomatic guidelines have been issued to all general practitioners by the Department of Health informing them of those symptoms that are deemed sufficiently suspicious of breast cancer to warrant urgent referral to a breast clinic (Box 47.1). These patients must be referred within 24 hours of being seen by their GP and must be seen by a breast specialist within 2 weeks of the referral date.

DIAGNOSIS

The management of women with breast disease should be undertaken in a specialist multidisciplinary unit with close co-operation between an appropriately trained surgeon, radiologist, cytologist, histopathologist and clinical oncologist.

Triple assessment

Patients undergo a full clinical assessment, appropriate radiological imaging and cytological +/− histological investigation.

Box 47.1 Breast symptoms/signs warranting urgent referral to a breast clinic

Discrete lump >30 years
Nipple changes – eczema, inversion, ulceration, distortion
Skin changes – dimpling, ulceration, peau d'orange

This is known as triple assessment. The positive predictive value of triple assessment is high, with a low false-positive rate. The aim of triple assessment is to make a diagnosis so that the patient can be fully counselled before proceeding to definitive treatment.

Mammography

Mammography is the commonest imaging tool over the age of 35 years. Malignant lesions present as asymmetrical densities, which tend to be irregular or spiculated (Fig. 47.2), or show architectural distortion or pleomorphic microcalcifications. Up to 10% of breast cancers are not visible on mammography and 55% of screen-detected cancers are impalpable. In addition to its use in screening, mammography can be used to detect the presence of multifocal or contralateral disease and recurrent cancer. Impalpable but mammographically

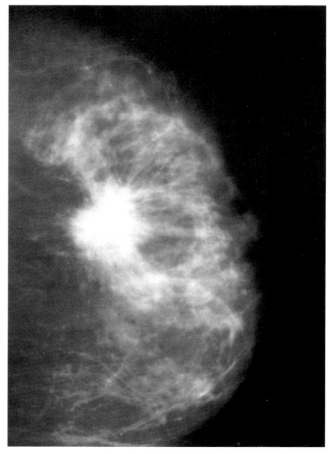

Fig. 47.2 Mammogram showing a central, large, spiculated carcinoma.

Box 47.2   Reporting grades of fine needle aspiration cytology

C0 = no cells
C1 = insufficient cells to make a diagnosis
C2 = benign epithelial cells
C3 = atypical cells
C4 = suspicious of carcinoma
C5 = carcinoma

Box 47.3   The UICC TNM staging system for breast cancer

T Tumour size
T0   Impalpable
T1a/b   2 cm
T2a/b   2–5 cm
T3a/b   >5 cm
T4a   Direct chest extension
T4b   Skin infiltration or oedema or peau d'orange or satellite
        nodules in same breast
T4c   T4a + T4b
(a = no deep fixation; b = with deep fixation)

N Nodal status
N0   No palpable nodes
N1a   Palpable homolateral axillary nodes
        Clinically non-malignant
N1b   Palpable homolateral axillary nodes
        Clinically malignant
N2   Palpable fixed malignant nodes
N3   Clinically malignant homolateral clavicular nodes or oedema
        of arm

M Metastases
M0   No clinically apparent distant metastases
M1   Distant metastases apparent

suspicious lesions may be localized prior to surgical excision by placing a percutaneous hook needle alongside the lesion under mammographic guidance. Limited excision based on palpation of the needle tip is then carried out and excision of the lesion can be confirmed by specimen radiology.

Ultrasound

Ultrasound scanning is usually used as an adjunct to mammography for indeterminate lesions and to differentiate between solid and cystic masses. Malignant lesions are usually solid, irregular, of mixed echogenicity and are highly vascular.

Fine needle aspiration cytology (FNAC)

FNAC is a safe and reliable outpatient procedure, which can be performed on clinically palpable abnormalities or on impalpable lesions under radiological guidance. FNAC has a high sensitivity, specificity and positive predictive value but accurate results are dependent on the expertise of both the aspirator and cytologist. Results are reported as shown in Box 47.2 (Trott 1991).

The commonest complication of FNAC is haematoma formation. Infection and pneumothorax are extremely rare. The main limitation of cytological analysis is that it cannot differentiate between in situ and invasive disease. This requires either a core biopsy or a formal excision biopsy.

Core biopsy

Core biopsy is also a safe outpatient procedure, which is performed under local anaesthetic on suspicious or indeterminate lesions. It allows differentiation between in situ and invasive disease and may also enable tumour grade and oestrogen receptor status to be determined. This information is important for assessment of systemic risk and decisions regarding the sequence of treatment modalities.

Staging Investigations

In the absence of specific symptoms, staging investigations are not routinely performed on patients with a diagnosis of breast cancer. Currently available tests are not sufficiently sensitive or specific, yielding both high false-positive and false-negative results.

STAGING

Breast cancer is staged by the TNM system based on UICC criteria (Box 47.3). This has been promoted to enhance the

comparison of results of trials worldwide and provide information that can be used to choose treatment regimes. It is, however, observer biased, dependent on the extent of axillary surgery, the completeness of excision and the staging investigations that are carried out.

LOCAL TREATMENT

The management of breast cancer within the context of a multidisciplinary team of specialists facilitates rapid and accurate diagnosis as well as selection of appropriate treatment for all stages of disease. Breast cancer is an emotive subject and the specialist team must include breast care nurses who have a vital supporting and counselling role.

One of the most difficult roles of an oncologist is that of breaking bad news. It requires time, patience, sensitivity and compassion. There are significant differences in an individual woman's requirements for information, choice and support at the time of breast cancer diagnosis. These differences are best achieved by creating an environment in which an individual can secure the information, autonomy and support that suits her needs.

In common with other cancers, the treatment of breast cancer has two main objectives, namely to cure the disease and to maintain or improve quality of life. The achievement of one objective often impinges on the chances of achieving the other and these treatment dilemmas should be fully discussed. When contemplating treatment options, women and their doctors must appreciate that the initial management of breast cancer offers the best hope of cure and this opportunity should be grasped.

There are two aspects to the treatment of breast cancer, that of local disease and systemic disease. The majority of women dying of breast cancer do so as a result of the failure to control systemic disease. Many of these women will have initially presented with clinically localized disease (confined to the breast and axilla) which has been adequately controlled by a combination of surgery and radiotherapy. Despite this, about 50% of these women ultimately develop systemic disease, suggesting that occult micrometastases are present at the time of diagnosis, a concept which has important implications for primary treatment. Women at risk of metastases need to be identified at presentation and offered systemic treatment if cure is to be a realistic objective.

Surgery

Breast

The aim of surgical treatment is complete removal of the primary tumour. The benefits of local disease control have established surgery as the initial treatment modality in the majority of breast cancers, but surgery may follow down-staging by other treatment modalities. Surgical treatment of the primary tumour has essentially evolved into two basic procedures: complete local excision and total mastectomy. In deciding which of these options is suitable for an individual patient, the clinical and radiological size of the tumour relative to the overall size of the breast must be considered. If complete excision cannot be achieved with an acceptable cosmetic result, mastectomy should be advised. A conservative approach requires patients to be aware that if the margins of excision are not clear, re-excision or mastectomy will be necessary to avoid a high risk of local recurrence. Women undergoing mastectomy should be offered the option of a breast reconstruction.

Axilla

Surgical treatment of the axilla is designed to achieve two simultaneous aims: disease control and staging. There is a continuing debate on the optimal extent of axillary surgery required to achieve these aims, ranging from no surgery to full axillary clearance. Axillary surgery is not required for in situ disease.

Non-operative techniques rely either on clinical examination alone, which has a very poor correlation with histological node status, or non-invasive imaging methods, which are still the subject of research.

Axillary sampling aims to excise a minimum of four nodes on the assumption that these will predict the overall axillary nodal status. Formal axillary block dissection is both diagnostic and therapeutic with a very low, local recurrence rate (<1.5% at 5 years). However, complications are more common with this extent of surgery, including breast and arm lymphoedema (7%), intercostobrachial nerve syndrome, infection, seroma and shoulder discomfort.

Sentinel node biopsy is a relatively new technique utilizing radio-isotope and/or dye to localize key node(s) that drain directly from the tumour bed, in the hope that they will predict the status of the whole axilla. Initial results are encouraging, with 97.5% accuracy reported (Veronesi et al 1997).

Radiotherapy

Radiotherapy is usually used in the adjuvant setting for the local control of breast cancer, but on occasions can be utilized as a primary treatment for locally advanced disease.

Radiotherapy to the breast

Radiotherapy to the breast is standard following conservative surgery for invasive cancer, consistently showing a highly significant reduction in local recurrence from 25–35% to 4–5% at 5 years (Early Breast Cancer Trialists Collaborative Group 1995). Radiotherapy is not routinely given after mastectomy but tends to be reserved for those with bulky, high-grade tumours and extensive node involvement who are at high risk of local recurrence. Chest wall recurrences may be difficult to control and it is preferable to prevent them.

Radiotherapy to the axilla

Axillary radiotherapy is usually advocated only in the presence of positive nodes that have not been treated surgically (axillary sampling) or in the presence of extensive node-positive disease with extranodal extension of tumour.

Radiotherapy services are often provided on a regional basis and patients may have to travel long distances daily for treatment. This in itself may influence a patient's choice regarding therapy. In women who are at high risk of systemic disease, adjuvant radiotherapy can safely be deferred until adjuvant chemotherapy is completed.

SYSTEMIC TREATMENT

Hormone manipulation

Oestrogens and progestogens are involved in the growth regulation of both normal and malignant breast tissue. Expression of oestrogen receptors (ER) can be demonstrated in 60% of tumours (McGuire et al 1975). In premenopausal women, the ovary is the major source of oestrogens. In postmenopausal women levels of oestrogen are much lower and the principal site of origin is the peripheral fat where adrenal androgens are converted to oestrogens by aromatase enzymes. The aim of hormone manipulation is to prevent oestrogenic stimulation of tumour cells. This can be achieved by removing the main source of oestrogen or by blocking its actions on tumour cells.

Ovarian ablation

In premenopausal women ovarian ablation can be achieved surgically, medically or by radiotherapy. Gonadotrophin-releasing hormone agonists can achieve hormone levels similar to surgical ablation but with the advantage of reversibility on stopping treatment. Any method of ovarian ablation can produce a similar reduction in mortality in ER-positive women to systemic chemotherapy (Pritchard 2000). In postmenopausal women levels of circulating oestrogens can be decreased by the use of aromatase inhibitors, such as anastrozole.

Tamoxifen

Tamoxifen is a synthetic partial oestrogen agonist that acts primarily through binding to the oestrogen receptor. It is the most commonly used hormone in the management of breast cancer with proven value in both the adjuvant and metastatic setting (Early Breast Cancer Trialists' Collaborative Group 1992). It may also have a role in chemoprevention. Tamoxifen has primarily antagonistic actions on breast cancer cells but oestrogenic activity in other tissues such as bone and the endometrium. Additional mechanisms of action include effects on apoptosis, angiogenesis and growth factors.

Use of tamoxifen is associated with a highly significant improvement in disease-free and overall survival (Early Breast Cancer Trialists' Collaborative Group 1992). There is also a 35–40% reduction in the risk of contralateral disease (Early Breast Cancer Trialists' Collaborative Group 1998). The effects of tamoxifen are greater in women with ER-positive tumours and in women over the age of 50 years. The standard dose of tamoxifen is 20 mg daily and there is no evidence to suggest a higher dose is any more effective. The optimal duration of therapy is still uncertain but 5 years of treatment gives greater protection than 2 years.

The side-effects of tamoxifen can be explained largely by its anti-oestrogenic activity. The most common is hot flushes. In premenopausal women tamoxifen can produce vaginal atrophy, dryness and loss of libido. However, the drug is generally well tolerated and only 3% of patients stop taking it because of side-effects. Long-term use of tamoxifen is associated with endometrial hyperplasia and an increased risk of carcinoma of the endometrium. However, the magnitude of this risk is small and outweighed by the reduction in the number of contralateral breast cancers (Early Breast Cancer Trialists' Collaborative Group 1998). There is no evidence that endometrial screening with transvaginal ultrasound is of benefit in women on tamoxifen but any abnormal vaginal bleeding should be investigated appropriately. Beneficial oestrogenic effects of tamoxifen include preservation of bone density, decrease in plasma cholesterol levels and an associated reduction in cardiovascular morbidity.

More selective oestrogen receptor modifiers have been designed, but are currently available only within the context of clinical trials. One of these, raloxifene, is licensed for use in the prevention of osteoporosis.

Aromatase inhibitors

This group of drugs is currently indicated as second-line hormone therapy in postmenopausal women in whom first-line treatment with tamoxifen has failed. The third-generation aromatase inhibitors have high oral specificity for the aromatase enzyme. Their role as first-line agents in metastatic disease and use as adjuvant therapy is currently the subject of ongoing clinical trials.

Biological therapy

With the development of increasingly sophisticated biological techniques, understanding of the molecular mechanisms involved in the pathogenesis of breast cancer is providing opportunities for the identification of better prognostic factors and the development of new biological treatment modalities that can be targeted more specifically at tumour cells.

C-erbB2 is an epidermal growth factor receptor (EGF-R) related transmembrane protein. Overexpression of c-erbB2 occurs in about 20% of primary breast cancers and is believed to be associated with a poor prognosis (Perren et al 1991). A chimeric monoclonal antibody has been developed against the extracellular component of c-erbB2 and the first to be licensed for clinical use has recently become available for the treatment of metastatic breast cancer. Clearly this antibody is only suitable for use in a small proportion of patients, but early results show response rates of up to 40%, which may translate to an overall survival benefit.

Chemotherapy

There are many chemotherapeutic agents available for the treatment of breast cancer and numerous regimes have been developed. Combination therapy has a more prolonged benefit than single agents and is usually given in 4–6 cycles over a period of 3–6 months.

Recommendations for the use of chemotherapy should be made within a multidisciplinary setting supervised by a medical or clinical oncologist and are based on the potential oncological gains balanced against the side-effect profiles of the agents used.

Chemotherapy is used mainly in the adjuvant setting for women deemed to be at high risk of systemic disease. However, it is increasingly being considered as a primary treatment for patients with large, locally advanced or inflammatory carcinomas, which are unsuitable for surgery.

The aim of primary medical therapy is to downstage disease prior to definitive surgical treatment. Overall response rates are of the order of 70% with a complete response rate of 10% (Fisher et al 1997). In complete responders, surgery may be deferred and patients proceed directly to adjuvant radiotherapy and close follow-up.

Assessment of risk and adjuvant systemic treatment

Adjuvant systemic therapy is a fundamental component of breast cancer treatment which aims to eradicate micro-metastatic disease. Prevention of the development of clinically evident metastatic disease will extend disease-free survival and should improve overall survival. When considering which patients are suitable for treatment, an assessment of systemic risk is made based on a number of prognostic factors. Numerous factors have been identified but few are of independent significance and suitable for routine clinical use. The most powerful prognostic factor is axillary lymph node status, hence the importance of axillary surgery as part of primary surgical treatment. Other prognostic factors in routine clinical use are: tumour size; tumour grade; presence of lymphovascular invasion; and oestrogen receptor status.

Patients deemed to be at significant risk of systemic relapse based on assessment of these factors are offered adjuvant systemic therapy. There is strong evidence from meta-analysis of breast cancer trials that there is a significant reduction in annual risk of recurrence and death after systemic treatment for both node-positive and node-negative patients with breast cancer (Early Breast Cancer Trialists' Collaborative Group 1992). The average magnitude of this effect is a 30% reduction in risk of relapse and a 20% reduction in the risk of death at 10 years. The absolute reduction in risk is obviously smaller.

ADVANCED DISEASE

Advanced disease includes inoperable local disease and metastatic disease. Locally advanced disease is clinically determined by the presence of tumour infiltrating the skin or chest wall or by the presence of fixed lymph nodes. Treatment is aimed at achieving local disease control. The modalities available are the same as for early breast cancer, but surgery is often not appropriate as first-line treatment. Systemic treatment or radiotherapy may be used to control or to downstage disease prior to surgery. In the absence of metastatic disease, radical surgical techniques involving chest wall reconstruction may be indicated.

Metastatic breast cancer is currently incurable so palliation with maintenance of quality of life is the aim of treatment. Surgery is rarely indicated. Radiotherapy is useful for the treatment of symptomatic bone metastases and for cerebral disease. Hormonal manipulation or chemotherapy may be suitable for women with soft tissue disease (liver and lung).

BREAST CANCER AND PREGNANCY

Breast cancer and its relationship to pregnancy can be considered in several different contexts: premenopausal women who have the potential to become pregnant; women who are pregnant at diagnosis; and women who wish to become pregnant after treatment is completed.

Treatment of women who may become pregnant

Potentially fertile women undergoing treatment for breast cancer are advised to take precautions to avoid pregnancy. Some treatments, in particular chemotherapy, may be directly harmful to the fetus and there is a theoretical risk that the hormone levels associated with pregnancy may act as growth factors for the cancer. A more sensitive issue when counselling a fertile woman is the issue of morbidity and mortality – she may not survive to bring up her child or may be too unwell to care for it.

Treatment of breast cancer during pregnancy

Breast cancer during pregnancy is uncommon, with a prevalence of 1:4000 pregnancies. However, in the under-35 age group where breast cancer is itself rare, 25% of breast cancers are diagnosed during or within 1 year of pregnancy. There is no consistent evidence that breast cancer during pregnancy is more aggressive than at other times, but the diagnosis may be delayed due to the physiological changes in the breast, which can make a discrete mass difficult to distinguish both clinically and radiologically. Women tend to present at a more advanced stage with nodal involvement in 70% of cases. Decisions in the early stages of pregnancy involve the dilemma of continuing pregnancy through treatment or of terminating the pregnancy. Therapeutic abortion has not been shown to improve survival of the mother, but there may be significant treatment-associated risks to the fetus.

Surgery remains the primary treatment of choice and can be performed safely throughout pregnancy with only a small anaesthetic risk of spontaneous abortion in the first trimester. Radiotherapy should not be delivered during pregnancy because of detrimental effects on the fetus. Chemotherapy can be given, but is associated with a small risk of congenital abnormalities in the first trimester and low birth weight at term. Diagnosis in the third trimester can be managed surgically with early delivery at 32 weeks to allow prompt administration of adjuvant treatments. Early delivery also allows patients with locally advanced or inflammatory tumours to have primary chemotherapy in an attempt to downstage disease prior to surgery. Hormone manipulation is clearly not appropriate during pregnancy. Tamoxifen is known to be teratogenic and should be avoided.

Pregnancy after treatment for breast cancer

Adjuvant treatments for breast cancer may have an adverse affect on fertility, either directly as in the case of hormone manipulation or indirectly through toxic effects on the ovaries. Pregnancy after breast cancer is uncommon, experience is limited and the implications for recurrence are unknown. There are theoretical risks from circulating hormones, but studies have not demonstrated an adverse effect. It is usual to recommend a post-treatment delay of at least 2 years before planning a pregnancy. This is based on survival data and the fact that 80% of recurrences will have occurred during this time. Lactation is often impaired from a breast treated with radiotherapy.

BREAST CANCER IN THE ELDERLY

Almost 40% of breast cancers occur in women over the age of 70 years. Historically these women have been treated by hormone manipulation alone, but local control was frequently unsatisfactory, necessitating surgical intervention or radiotherapy at a later stage. Since the biology of cancers in this age group is similar to that in younger women, the majority of elderly patients presenting with breast cancer should be managed in the standard way. Primary hormonal treatment should be reserved for those women who decline surgical intervention or in whom co-morbidity is such that their disease is unlikely to progress significantly within their natural lifetime. In practice, very few patients are unfit for surgery. Elderly women presenting with bulky ER-positive disease may benefit from primary endocrine therapy to downstage their disease.

FOLLOW-UP

Most follow-up protocols are not evidence based and have evolved over time. In practice, the majority of recurrences are detected by patients themselves or by mammography. The aims of follow-up are:

- early detection of local recurrence
- early detection of metastatic disease
- screening for new primary breast cancer
- detection of treatment-related toxicities
- provision of psycho-oncological support.

Most local recurrences after mastectomy occur in the first 2 years, but after breast-conserving surgery there is a steady relapse rate. Women with a history of invasive breast cancer have a fivefold increased risk of developing a second primary with an annual risk of contralateral breast cancer of 0.6%.

Mammography is therefore an important component of follow-up and should be performed annually for at least the first 5 years. After breast-conserving surgery and radiotherapy, mammography may be difficult to interpret, in which case magnetic resonance imaging (MRI) or scintimammography may be useful.

HRT AFTER TREATMENT FOR BREAST CANCER

Menopausal symptoms are common after treatment for breast cancer. This is because the majority of women diagnosed with breast cancer are postmenopausal and most are advised to stop taking HRT because of the risk of stimulating tumour growth. In addition, most women undergoing hormone manipulation develop variable symptoms of oestrogen blockade.

The commonest symptom is hot flushes, which can sometimes be controlled with clonidine or low-dose megestrol acetate (20 mg bd). Topical oestrogens can be used sparingly for vaginal symptoms. For women in whom menopausal symptoms severely compromise quality of life, HRT has been used alone or in combination with tamoxifen with no apparent risk of worsening prognosis.

BREAST RECONSTRUCTION

Despite a move away from radical surgery for the treatment of breast cancer, there are still several indications for removal of the entire breast. Mastectomy may be associated with considerable psychological morbidity and although disease control is of primary importance, quality of life issues must be considered in making treatment decisions. Women undergoing mastectomy should be offered breast reconstruction as either an immediate or delayed procedure.

To be acceptable, a reconstructed breast must have appropriate shape, symmetry, projection and comfort with minimal scarring. Following a standard mastectomy both skin and volume need to be replaced. The simplest way to achieve this is with an expandable implant placed beneath the muscle of the chest wall. More complex methods of reconstruction involve importing autologous tissue from elsewhere in the form of myocutaneous flaps.

Tissue expanders

These implants have a shell of silicone surrounding a central saline-filled chamber, which is inflatable by means of an integral or remote injection port. Following insertion as either an immediate or delayed procedure, the implant is inflated over a period of weeks to the required volume, gradually stretching the skin to accommodate it. Correct positioning at the time of insertion and a period of overinflation of the implant allow a degree of ptosis to be achieved in the reconstructed breast. This type of reconstruction is only suitable for women with small breasts and minimal ptosis (Fig. 47.3).

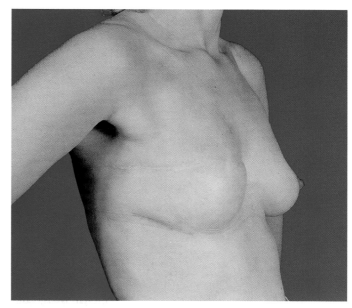

Fig. 47.3 Right breast reconstruction with subpectoral tissue expander.

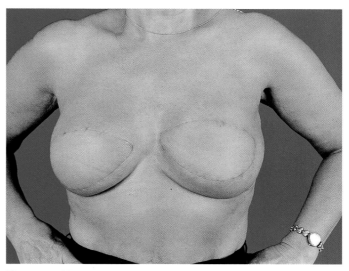

Fig. 47.4 Bilateral latissimus dorsi flap breast reconstructions – immediate on the right, delayed on the left.

Myocutaneous flaps

Two myocutaneous flaps are commonly used for breast reconstruction, the latissimus dorsi flap and the transverse rectus abdominis flap. These are usually used as pedicle flaps but are also suitable for free flaps.

Latissimus dorsi flap (LDF)

The latissimus dorsi muscle and a paddle of overlying skin from the ipsilateral side of the back, are mobilized on the thoracodorsal pedicle and tunnelled beneath the skin and subcutaneous tissue of the lateral chest wall to sit in the defect following mastectomy (Fig. 47.4). Although these flaps can be

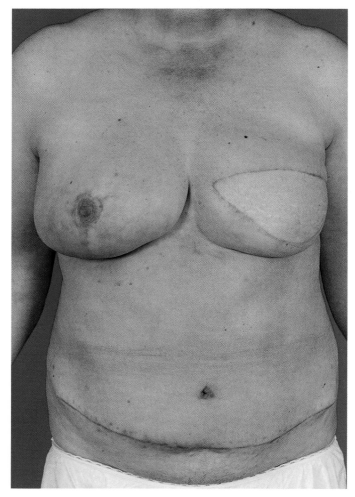

Fig. 47.5 Immediate left TRAM flap breast reconstruction and contralateral mastopexy (6 weeks postoperatively).

quite bulky, it is usually necessary to supplement them with an implant to achieve the required volume in the reconstructed breast. LDFs are safe, reliable, associated with minimal long-term morbidity and are suitable for most patients undergoing breast reconstruction.

Transverse rectus abdominis (TRAM) flap

The contralateral rectus muscle with an ellipse of skin from the lower abdomen is mobilized on the superior epigastric vessels and tunnelled beneath the skin and subcutaneous tissue of the abdominal wall to fill the defect on the anterior chest wall (Fig. 47.5). TRAM flaps are particularly suitable for women with a thick layer of abdominal fat. The flaps are usually of sufficient bulk that an implant is rarely required to augment them, even in large-breasted women. The defect in the abdominal wall muscle is closed either primarily or with a synthetic mesh, but there is a significant risk of postoperative hernia formation and there have been reports of long-term back problems following this procedure.

Nipple-areola reconstruction and adjustments to the contralateral breast to maximize symmetry are usually performed as a delayed procedure. Overall, the cosmetic results

are good and there is evidence that the psychological morbidity associated with mastectomy is decreased in women undergoing breast reconstruction.

KEY POINTS

1. Breast cancer is common and is the cause of significant morbidity and mortality worldwide.
2. The incidence of breast cancer is increasing, but the mortality is decreasing.
3. The incidence of breast cancer increases with age.
4. There is a small increased risk of breast cancer diagnosis in women taking hormone replacement therapy, but this needs to be balanced against the benefits of treatment.
5. Familial breast cancer accounts for only 5% of cases and nearly half of these are due to mutations in BRCA1 and BRCA2.
6. Breast cancer may present as symptomatic or screen-detected disease.
7. The diagnosis and management of breast cancer should be undertaken by a multidisciplinary team of specialists.
8. Diagnosis is based on triple assessment – clinical examination, radiological imaging and cytology/histology.
9. The aim of primary surgical treatment is complete removal and hence control of local disease.
10. DCIS is treated by complete surgical excision. Axillary surgery is not required. The role of adjuvant treatments is uncertain.
11. Women undergoing mastectomy should be offered breast reconstruction.
12. Radiotherapy to the breast is standard after breast-conserving surgery for invasive disease to minimize the risk of local recurrence.
13. Patients with axillary node disease should have axillary clearance or radiotherapy.
14. All oestrogen receptor-positive patients should receive adjuvant tamoxifen for 5 years.
15. Adjuvant chemotherapy is offered to patients deemed to be at high risk of systemic relapse.
16. Metastatic disease is incurable and treatment is palliative.
17. Breast cancer in pregnancy usually presents at a more advanced stage, but the prognosis stage for stage is the same.
18. New hormonal and biological therapies for breast cancer are becoming available.

REFERENCES

Collaborative Group on Hormonal Factors in Breast Cancer 1996 Breast cancer and hormonal contraceptives: collaborative reanalysis of individual data on 53 297 women with breast cancer and 100 239 women without breast cancer from 54 epidemiological studies. Lancet 347:1713–1727

Collaborative Group on Hormonal Factors in Breast Cancer 1997 Breast cancer and hormone replacement therapy: collaborative reanalysis of data from 51 epidemiological studies of 52 705 women with breast cancer and 108 411 women without breast cancer. Lancet 350:1047–1059

Dupont WD, Page DL 1991 Menopausal oestrogen replacement therapy and breast cancer. Archives of Internal Medicine 151:67–72

Early Breast Cancer Trialists' Collaborative Group 1992 Systemic treatment of early breast cancer by hormonal, cytotoxic, or immune therapy: 133 randomised trials involving 31 000 recurrences and 4 000 deaths among 75 000 women. Lancet 339:1–15, 71–85

Early Breast Cancer Trialists' Collaborative Group 1995 Effects of radiotherapy and surgery in early breast cancer: an overview of the randomised trials. New England Journal of Medicine 333:1444–1455

Early Breast Cancer Trialists' Collaborative Group 1998 Tamoxifen for early breast cancer: an overview of the randomised trials. Lancet 351:1451–1467

Eeles R 1996 Testing for the breast cancer predisposition gene, BRCA1. British Medical Journal 313:572–573

Fisher B 1998 Lumpectomy and radiation therapy for the treatment of intraductal breast cancer: findings from National Surgical Adjuvant Breast and Bowel Project B-17. Journal of Clinical Oncology 16:441–452

Fisher B, Brown A, Mamounas E et al 1997 Effects of preoperative chemotherapy on loco-regional disease in women with operable breast cancer: findings from National Surgical Adjuvant Breast and Bowel Project B-18. Journal of Clinical Oncology 15:2483–2493

Forrest P 1986 Breast cancer screening report to the health ministers of England, Wales, Scotland and Northern Ireland by working group chaired by Professor Sir Patrick Forrest. Her Majesty's Stationery Office, London

Hartmann LC, Schaid DJ, Woods JE et al 1999 Efficacy of bilateral prophylactic mastectomy in women with a family history of breast cancer. New England Journal of Medicine 340:77–84

Hatcher MB, Fallowfield L, A'Hern R 2001 The psychological impact of bilateral prophylactic mastectomy: prospective study using questionnaires and semistructured interviews. British Medical Journal 322:76–81

McGuire WL, Carbonne PP, Sears ME, Escher GC 1975 Estrogen receptors in human breast cancer: an overview. In: McGuire WL, Carbonne PP, Vollmer EP (eds) Estrogen receptors in human breast cancer. Raven Press, New York, pp 1–7

Perren TJ 1991 c-erbB2 oncogene as a prognostic marker in breast cancer. British Journal of Cancer 63:328–332

Peto R, Boreham J, Clarke M, Davies C, Beral V 2000 UK and USA breast cancer deaths down 25% in year 2000 at 20–69 years. Lancet 355:1822

Pritchard KI 2000 Current and future directions in medical therapy for breast carcinoma: endocrine treatment. Cancer 88:3065–3072

Trott PA 1991 Aspiration cytodiagnosis of the breast. Diagnostic Oncology 1:79–87

Veronesi U, Paganelli G, Galimberti V et al 1997 Sentinel-node biopsy to avoid axillary dissection in breast cancer with clinically negative lymph nodes. Lancet 349:1864–1867

48

Supportive care for gynaecological cancer patients: psychological and emotional aspects

Karen Summerville

INTRODUCTION

The patient

The aim of this chapter is to identify and discuss the psychological, psychosocial, psychosexual, emotional and practical needs of women affected by a gynaecological cancer. It considers ways in which we can provide care and support to meet the needs of patients and their families throughout their cancer journey. The role of the professional carer and the knowledge and skills required to assess the individual needs of these women will be explored and recommendations for practical interventions aimed at providing support will be discussed. These issues affect both cancer survivors and those in the palliative stage of their disease process.

When a woman is diagnosed with gynaecological cancer, it affects her life in many ways. At the time of diagnosis it may feel like an emotional onslaught and the effects can be both abrupt and long lasting. Sometimes issues and feelings remain long after the cancer has gone. The challenge is how best to help the woman to cope with the knowledge of her disease and its implications for herself and her family. Support may be required for an extended period of time, in a variety of forms and from a number of different people. This should not be seen as a task that is the sole responsibility of one individual, but will inevitably involve 'the team'. This is best managed by a multidisciplinary team approach, within a designated gynaecological oncology centre, where all members of the specialist support team are available (COG 1999) and with strong links to both hospital and community palliative care services.

The carers

The needs of the carers will also be addressed. In order to deal effectively and sensitively with the emotional and practical challenges with which they are confronted through caring for these women, healthcare professionals must understand their own feelings, develop insight into their reactions and coping mechanisms. They themselves may need to explore strategies in order to improve their ability to cope more effectively with the emotional onslaught to which they too are exposed through their own personal experience of care giving.

SPIRITUAL AND EMOTIONAL PAIN

Spiritual well-being has several components: a sense of purpose and meaning in life; a sense of relationship with self, others and a supreme being; and a feeling of hope (Clark et al 1991, Miller 1985, Moberg 1982). Both Clinebell (1966) and Ellison (1983) have identified four categories of basic spiritual needs: meaning, challenge in life; a reason for being; continuing on in the face of adversity. A person's spiritual outlook makes a tremendous difference to the process of both living and dying (Moberg 1982). Spirituality functions as a resource during multiple losses and change (Reed 1987).

The diagnosis of cancer changes the patient's life forever, causing her to confront her own mortality. The doctor or nurse who cares for these women confronts his or her own mortality an equal number of times (Pace 2000).

If we are able to understand and learn to accept that mental pain is inevitable for both the patient and the carer, we may be freed from feelings of inadequacy and futility, which inhibit important discussion of the woman's hopes and fears.

In order to be effective in these painful situations, doctors and nurses must understand their own feelings and be aware of the natural devices they might use to avoid what may often be a difficult situation and one for which they have received no formal training. Saunders & Baines (1989) use the concept of 'staff pain'. They emphasize the need for staff to grieve the loss of a patient and the importance of group support for staff and 'debriefing' sessions to allow opportunities to express these feelings in a safe and supportive environment.

Recognition of our own feelings of pain, and acceptance of help from others within the team and/or from a trained external facilitator is the only way to retain the resilience, sense of oneself and the humanity required in order to continue to 'care'.

Times of crisis can usually be turned into opportunities and the intimacy of such moments between the woman and the doctor or nurse can produce deep feelings, sometimes tears. At times it is appropriate to sit in silence and just the sense of being there can be recognition enough (Pace 2000). The most important point of all, at the core of every nursing or medical care situation, is the woman's need for someone who is genuine. The need the honest truth, not evasion or empty reassurances. If the healthcare professional has not questioned and analysed his or her own beliefs for the reassurance, doubts and answers they provide, there may be little of value to offer the patient who is forced to confront the ultimate truths and uncertainties of all that comes thereafter.

Box 48.1 Three steps in the spiritual growth of both doctors and nurses (Lane 1987)

- Developing a 'greater awareness of the spirit within self' in order to be a better listener for the patient.
- Opening the 'self' by being totally present with the patient.
- Allowing the patient to share her feelings and emotions without reserve on the health professional's part.

Care that integrates the spiritual dimensions creates a nurse or doctor who is actually involved in a human relationship. Qualities that demonstrate the ability to provide better spiritual care include a supportive approach to the patient; what has been termed a sense of benevolence to the patient; awareness of the patient, self and the impact of family and significant others; empathy; and non-judgemental understanding (Dickenson 1975).

It takes more than just education for a nurse or doctor to feel comfortable with spiritual issues. Introspection and an awareness of their own personal spiritual journey are required to integrate the spiritual domain into patient care (Pace 2000).

It is emphasized that healthcare professionals need to take care of their own spiritual needs. Failure to do so will lead to emotional exhaustion (Lane 1987).

QUALITY OF LIFE

What is quality of life?

Quality of life was broadly defined as early as 1947, when the World Health Organization described it as: 'a state of complete physical, mental and social well-being, and not merely absence of disease and infirmity' (King et al 1997).

Quality of life is a complex phenomenon that affects an individual's personality and lifestyle. It is developed over time with physical, psychological, sociocultural, sexual and spiritual effects (Woods 1975). It is affected by change in appearance, mental states and personal and social factors and, in the case of cancer, the effects of disease process and treatments. It is tied closely to the concept of body image, self-esteem and self-concept and is affected by attitudes, beliefs and behaviours (Penson et al 2000).

Poor body image can result in the patient feeling worthless as a person, physically unattractive or even repulsive and unable to feel valued, loved or able to express themselves sexually (Box 48.2) (Dudas 1992). For some women, quality of life means feeling alive. It is personal and individual and what is considered normal or acceptable to one person or couple may be unacceptable to another.

Box 48.2 The changes in sexuality and their effects

- Reduced physical contact
- Loss of intimacy
- Loss of sex drive and desire disorders
- Early menopause
- Infertility
- Reduced human warmth

Effects of gynaecological cancer

The patient

Both the diagnosis and management of gynaecological cancer can have a major impact on every aspect of a woman's quality of life (Donovan et al 1989). It can be an overwhelming experience for a woman and her family, Then, before the woman has had time to work through her feelings of shock and grief relating to the diagnosis, she must begin treatment. There is no doubt that a diagnosis of gynaecological cancer can potentially compromise the key elements described for quality of life: body image, sexual health and relationships (Auchinloss 1989, Colyer H. 1996). Women of childbearing age experience sadness and anger at the loss of fertility and women of all ages may view the loss of female organs as a loss of femininity (Steginga & Dunn 1997).

The short- and long-term side-effects of treatment may also affect a woman's self-worth, self-esteem and confidence and have potential or actual psychosocial and psychosexual implications (Box 48.3) (Anderson 1985, Sacco Ezzell 1999). For example, a premature menopause, hair loss, lymphoedema, a stoma or a surgical scar may impact further on the reaction to the actual cancer (Anderson 1993).

However, it is also important to remember that body image may be altered and affect sexual health and quality of life without any change in appearance, function or control (Price 1990). Being told the diagnosis of cancer may alter body image, as this new knowledge of change may affect the woman's perception of herself and her health. This perception of change can lead to a distortion of body image; the woman may sense that something in herself or in her way of relating to others has changed, even before cancer or treatment have any physical effect. Smithman (1981) points out: 'Some changes in function can be purely psychological, and yet the potential for disturbed self-concept is great'. It is therefore widely accepted that body image, sexual health and overall quality of life are affected by physical factors, physical sensations, emotional and social reactions.

The partner

It is also important to assess the partner's understanding and needs, as the effect of the cancer is on the relationship as a result of change to either individual. A needs assessment among cancer patients and their partners showed that 63% of the participants would have liked to receive more information about sexual functioning after treatment and that 64% would

participate in a specific counselling programme on the quality of life changes, if this was offered (Bullard et al 1980).

Model's article (1990) examines reactions to body image change following surgery in some depth and links these to concepts of grief and loss. It is useful as it considers how nurses support both patients and their partners psychologically. Modd suggests that we are far from doing this successfully and that it is important to create an atmosphere in which patients and their partners feel accepted and understood if they experience anxiety, anger or grief and to provide a medium through which they can express, share and clarify their feelings. She recommends that the whole healthcare team work together to do this, which does indeed seem vital, given that many patients and their partners express feelings of isolation following discharge from treatment and for some time thereafter (Colyer 1996).

A high proportion of women are anxious (31%) and depressed (41%) after surgery for gynaecological cancer (Corney et al 1992). The majority have chronic sexual problems and a high proportion would like further information on after-effects – physical, sexual and emotional. Fifty per cent of young women would have liked their partners to be involved and 25% of the 40 partners who were involved would have preferred further information.

Ten years on from the publication of these studies, there remains a lack of consistency within both nursing and the medical professions in the ongoing assessment process used to identify change and impact on quality of life for both women and their partners.

What we must try to achieve

The specialist multidisciplinary gynaecological oncology support team has an important role in patient education and management of side-effects, aimed at maintaining or improving quality of life.

Faced with multiple adjustment demands relating to the cancer, the treatments, survivorship issues or palliation of disease and its symptoms, it is important that the couple are encouraged to prioritize what is important to them and have ownership over agreed interventions. It is essential that this assessment not only covers the cancer diagnosis and treatment, but takes into account what life was like for the woman and her partner/family before the cancer (Box 48.4).

It is important that we view the woman as much more than a 'cancer diagnosis' and consider her uniqueness by asking ourselves 'who is this woman we are trying to the help?'. In this way we can establish how actual or potential change may impact on her current measures for her quality of life. Roles, identity and relationships such as being a wife/partner, lover, mother, daughter, sister, employee or employer, friend and carer may be challenged, threatened and even altered either temporarily or permanently. Issues such as housing, transport, finances, insurance and ongoing responsibilities for paying the bills and childcare, along with the challenge of a cancer diagnosis and treatment, may affect her ability to cope. Her usual resources and coping mechanisms and strategies may be challenged to the limit and all this will impact on quality of life.

Box 48.3 Physical effects of gynaecological cancer and its treatment

- Pain
- Fatigue and lethargy
- Weight loss and anorexia
- Weight gain (steroids, ascites, lymphoedema)
- Skin irration
- Odour, fistula, stomas
- Discharge, bleeding
- Vaginal change – stenosis, scarring, dryness
- Abdominal distension (bowel obstruction, ascites)

Box 48.4 Aspects of quality of life that may change

- Altered body image
- Low self-confidence
- Low self-esteem
- Unable to deal with losses, i.e. fertility/premature menopause
- Loss of self-concept
- Loss of self-perception
- Loss of femininity
- Loss of control

Emotional impact (grieving scenario)
- Anxiety
- Fear
- Powerlessness
- Anger
- Depression
- Guilt
- Feelings of isolation

Social impact
- Feeling of isolation from:
  - partner/children
  - family
  - friends
  - work colleagues
- Changes in roles/relationships:
  - partner
  - family/mother
  - work
  - socio/cultural
- Impact on resources/finances:
  - unable to work – reduces income
  - unable to afford to socialize
  - transport – reduced mobility/isolation
  - unable to afford new clothes/extra laundry bills
  - equipment issues/extra bedding

Box 48.5 The assessment process

- Listening to how patients talk about their body, in positive or negative terms.
- Observation of how patients behave towards damaged body parts.
- Listening to relatives' visitors' reports about the woman and her methods of coping – is this typical coping behaviour?
- Observing for social withdrawal.
- Identify social network/support.
- Listening to patients' verbal accounts about how they anticipate life will be beyond the stay in hospital, e.g. how they anticipate others may react to their appearance or body function.

Box 48.6 Evaluating adaptation to the cancer and treatment effects

- Has resumed former lifestyle.
- Can verbalize concerns over body image change.
- Demonstrates healthy coping abilities.
- Can touch and look at body and accept change due to any scars, stomas, body shape.
- Can incorporate necessary change to allow enjoyable activity.
- Has incorporated altered body image as part of 'self'.
- Shows evidence of high self-esteem.
- Is willing to resume sexual relations/intimacy.
- Can discuss and consider reconstruction of lifestyle.

Assessing the needs

The effects of both the cancer and treatments have the potential to be both abrupt and long lasting, even when the goal is cure. The impact of altered body image resulting from treatments and/or surgical procedures for chronic illness extends beyond the immediate patient (Wilson & Williams, 1988). Therefore, the need for individualized assessment on how this will impact on quality of life both before and following cancer treatment is fundamental (Box 48.5). Assessment must be as specific as possible (Box 48.6) and address the woman's concerns by self-assessment techniques.

The changing focus of need

Typically, the focus both before and following cancer treatment is on a physical need. However, issues such as being unable to continue to work and the consequent reduced income or transport issues due to reduced mobility preventing use of public transport may be paramount and need to be given priority for the woman and her family. In the initial stages of diagnosis and treatment for a gynaecological cancer, quality of life issues may not seem so important and the focus of concern may be on the tremendous physiological demands that occur as a result of coping with the disease process and treatments.

However, as the illness trajectory lengthens, previously held notions may change as a woman adjusts to a new identity as a person with cancer.

Quality of life assessment and issues relating to the impact of actual or potential change require reassessment during treatment, at follow-up and as part of the long-term rehabilitation process. In women where the cancer progresses or recurs, the goals may change from cure to prolongation of life with the best possible quality for the woman and her family. Criteria for futility must be established to guide the transition from active to palliative management.

Rehabilitation and palliation both begin at *diagnosis* and continue throughout treatment and follow-up. They address the specific desires of each person and it is recommended that they incorporate the contribution of every member of the multidisciplinary healthcare team (van Eschenback & Schover 2000).

The challenge facing all healthcare professionals is to achieve improvement in the quality of the patient's life, by reducing dysfunction and disruption and providing support with physical, psychological, social and spiritual aspects. In order to achieve this it is important to identify information needs and individual coping strategies, to explore issues identified as important to the patients themselves and set realistic and achievable goals.

Whilst families are often the primary source of ongoing support to female cancer patients, women also derive considerable support from other patients and from healthcare professionals. The medical team should aim to develop psychological and psychosexual skills to cope with this important area of care. Further research is also needed into how support groups may best meet patient's needs (Veronesi et al 1999) and those of the care providers.

What we must learn

The following are essential in empowering both nurses and doctors to undertake their role: a comprehensive understanding of the aetiology of the gynaecological cancer and of the effects of both the disease and treatment; and knowledge of the ways of minimizing adverse problems and of assisting the woman and her partner in managing their needs.

Healthcare professionals must develop an appreciation of the wider issues and literature surrounding sexual health, altered body image, gender identity, role identity, cultural issues, religious beliefs and how all the factors can influence self-esteem and body image and impact on quality of life in either a positive or negative way (Masters et al 1995).

Concern is often expressed in clinical practice that healthcare professionals lack the time and skills to deal with psychological and quality of life issues, although the literature suggests that giving patients the opportunity to express such concerns can be preventive of problems as well as therapeutic (Auchinloss 1989).

Despite its importance, quality of life is rarely a reported outcome in randomized clinical trials in cancer patients. Gynaecology oncology nurses, clinicians, educators and researchers must continue to work collaboratively to enhance the knowledge base regarding quality of life issues and to improve care provided to women with gynaecological cancer (King et al 1997). The impact of a gynaecological cancer on a woman's quality of life is an important outcome parameter that may be measured as survival without significant morbidity (Anderson & Lutgendorf 1997).

PSYCHOSOCIAL ISSUES AND RETURNING TO NORMALITY

The woman may have undertaken several different roles and responsibilities prior to the cancer diagnosis and treatments. She may have been the central supporting figure in a household of some complexity and may have provided the economic support, as well as the responsibility of motherhood, a partner, a lover and a homemaker. The very act of returning to any or all of these roles is often a significant milestone in recovery.

Apart from the obvious anxieties about her prognosis and family relationships, financial worries and change in role can both be an immense source of stress for the patient and partner. The potential for this needs to be assessed prior to treatment and at subsequent follow-up.

Often practical help can be offered, such as a letter to the employer or facilitating the intervention of social services and giving information on benefit entitlements and grants (e.g. Macmillan), where patients are unaware of possible financial assistance, and help in dealing with transport problems.

For patients living with severe ongoing disability due to the cancer or its treatment, or those with progressive disease where the aim is no longer cure but palliation, additional grants such as disability living allowance, attendance allowance and 'special rules' or palliative care funding may be applied for and the benefits helpline should be contacted to clarify eligibility.

The issues that must be addressed (Box 48.7) may be ongoing and follow-up appointments provide an opportunity

to assess how the woman and her family are readjusting to life following cancer.

SEXUALITY AND PSYCHOSEXUAL ISSUES RELATING TO GYNAECOLOGICAL CANCER

In 1986 the World Health Organization stated that key elements of sexual health were:

- a capacity to enjoy and control sexual and reproductive behaviour in accordance with a social and personal ethic.
- Freedom from fear, shame, guilt, false beliefs and other psychological factors inhibiting sexual response and impairing sexual relationships.
- Freedom from organic disorders, diseases and deficiencies that interfere with sexual and reproductive function

A gynaecological cancer diagnosis and treatment may threaten or actually change the key elements described for sexual health and are associated with considerable sexual dysfunction (COG 1999).

The background

A woman's physical genital development, her attitudes and security about being a woman and her view of herself in relation to others, especially in intimate relationships, are all part of her uniqueness. Sexual functioning and concerns vary throughout one's lifespan and cannot be assumed for any age group or extent of disease. A woman's genital region may be perceived as psychologically very special, being both exquisitely sensitive and primal in sexual arousal. A malignancy in this area may be especially disturbing and significantly different in its emotional effects from cancer in other parts of the body. Reactions may vary according to feelings of the individual woman about her genitalia prior to developing a gynaecological cancer. However, there is no doubt that cancer of the vulva, which necessitates very evident vulval mutilation as a consequence of surgical treatment, can produce severe problems with psychosexual function (COG 1999).

The quality of a woman's life needs to be considered and assessed in relation to what it was before she became ill. An unsatisfactory relationship prior to a cancer diagnosis may be improved by a couple having to cope and coming closer together. Alternatively, poor relationships may continue to be devoid of intimacy and affection. How the effects of the cancer and its treatment impact on either of these scenarios needs ongoing assessment.

Effects of gynaecological cancer

A study by Cull et al (1993) included 83 women with early-stage cervical cancer, half of whom had received surgery and half radiotherapy. They were studied by standard self-report questionnaires and semi-structured interview. Over half reported deterioration in sexual function and the irradiated women suffered more with loss of sexual pleasure. Many women felt their psychological needs were not being met adequately.

A similar UK study included 105 women who had undergone radical pelvic surgery, of whom 65% had been treated for primary cervical cancer (Corney et al 1993). The mean time since treatment was 2 years. Of 73 women in whom the vagina had been preserved and who were in a sexual relationship, 16% never resumed intercourse. Two-thirds were experiencing sexual difficulties and around half reported a deterioration in their sexual relationship. However, this study highlights the need to never 'assume' as, interestingly, around one-third of these couples felt their marital relationship had actually improved.

The need to provide information

The inadequate information about the effects of disease and its therapeutic interventions on people's sexual function and alterations in their quality of life is also reflected in the scarce amount of empirical research available on these issues. All oncology professionals should be aware of the importance of recognizing and addressing issues of sexual function as an integral aspect of quality of life for people with cancer and their partners (Gallo-Silver 2000) and both nurses and doctors need to develop skills in talking to patients and partners about sexual concerns and in taking a sexual history (Green 1999, Smith 1989).

Sexual function is an essential and fundamental area of the assessment process and should be discussed in a continuous rather than a haphazard or one-off fashion. A woman diagnosed with a gynaecological cancer and needing to undergo any form of treatment may have concerns relating to potential change in her sexuality or sexual function. However, she may be too embarrassed to ask and may worry or fear that it may be perceived as inappropriate to ask or discuss.

in a society that has moved rapidly towards an awareness of sexuality of all ages, these patients will demand, not without justification, that medical science passes both appreciation and expertise concerning this dimension of their disease.
They will require and expect therapeutic interventions which will assist them in becoming psychosexually as well as physically rehabilitated (Derogatis 1980)

The goal of intervention

The goal of sexual rehabilitation is to restore the patient's ability to engage in intimate interpersonal relationships and incorporates the restoration of self-esteem and bodily function or adaption to change (Bancroft 1989). When appropriate and desired, sexual rehabilitation includes restoring physical ability to engage in sexual activity. Sexuality is an important aspect of quality of life and has a tremendous impact on an individual, their partner and families (Rutter 2000).

Listening and asking

Loss of sex drive may arise from an altered body image or there may be unresolved feelings such as guilt or fear of an association between sexual intercourse and cancer. Full assessment, discussion and information given about the facts, in order to remove any misconceptions, are essential. The effect of the diagnosis on the partner is often overlooked but it cannot be emphasized too strongly that preparation for the couple is the key to preventing avoidance or silence. The partner may fear that he could hurt or harm the woman and other misconceptions that he can 'catch' cancer himself through being intimate may cause a barrier between them. Simple explanations and reassurance both before and following treatment, involving both partners if possible, can prevent problems arising or minimize problems by recognizing the important issues early.

Sexual functioning should be enquired into at the early follow-up visits and continually assessed, so that if any changes or difficulties occur they can be recognized and support offered and appropriate interventions or specialist psychosexual referrals made as appropriate.

Sexuality may be expressed in a multitude of ways so it is imperative that healthcare professionals do not make assumptions about sexual behaviour and understand that information assists women in regaining a sense of control over their behaviour and destiny (Burke 1996). This applies just as much to the late stages of the disease as to the early phases of the journey.

When physical love and intimacy have been important and suddenly are withdrawn, their loss is felt. Even when they have not been important, their need may now be recognized. We cannot assume. However, loving touch in the palliative stage of the disease process may be avoided for fear that it may lead to more sexual intimacy. This may be overcome if both partners are able to discuss their anxieties, either with each other or facilitated by a healthcare professional.

The woman may not touch her partner or avoid closeness for fear that it might lead to physical sex. The man may be just as fearful that coitus would damage or hurt his partner and consequently keeps his distance. Both should be reassured that sexual intercourse is 'acceptable' at any stage of the disease process if there is sexual desire and drive on both sides and if it is physically possible. However, when coitus is not physically possible, methods of mutual masturbation can be explored and sexual expression using sensate focus techniques can be explained (see below).

Communicating a willingness to assist women to ways to express their sexuality in spite of the cancer and consequences of treatment can be a challenge (MacElveen-Hoehn & McCorkle 1985). Basic counselling skills such as listening, a non-judgemental approach and an open and accepting attitude with clear boundaries help legitimize concerns as normal and valid (Lamb 1985, Laurent 1994).

Intervention

Both cognitive and behavioural sexual rehabilitation interventions have been suggested to assist women and their partners to adjust to the physical, psychological and psychosexual change due to cancer and the impact on their relationship (Gallo-Silver 2000). The interventions described are aimed at increasing understanding and gradual adjustment, allowing the woman and her partner to have 'ownership' over the interventions chosen and take back control.

Understanding and familiarity of appropriate use of the following interventions can prepare healthcare professionals to assist patients and their partners with sexual needs and concerns.

- Educating patients about the phases of sexual functioning and the impact of treatment.
- Giving permission to explore their ability to respond to sexual stimulation by using self-pleasuring exercises.
- Teaching sensate focus exercises that structure non-coital foreplay and suggesting changes in coital positions to increase both access and comfort.

The P-LI-SS-IT model (Box 48.8) (RCN 2000) is a framework for assessment of sexual need and can be useful as part of the multidisciplinary team approach to assessment of sexuality in women with cancer.

All patients need permission and limited information, frequently dispelling myths and eliminating ignorance about the disease and treatment effects on their sexuality. This is often enough to enable patients to resume sexual expression and intimacy. Specific suggestions can help patients whose radical surgery or radiotherapy treatment has resulted in physiological or anatomical alterations, such as a stoma formation or vaginal stenosis, or when the mechanisms of sexual response have been affected.

Despite careful assessment and interventions, problems may still arise and expectations may not be met. The need for the skills and expertise to provide in-depth assessment of need and intensive structured therapy in the form of marital or sexual counselling is recognized in the P-LI-SS-IT-model (Bancroft 1989, Persan et al 2000). Doctors and nurses need to be secure in the knowledge that it is appropriate to refer to a sexual therapist as the need is identified with the patient or couple.

Behavioural therapy

Direct behavioural approaches for treating sexual dysfunction due to performance anxiety are advocated (Masters & Johnson 1970). Sensate focus may be useful as it is aimed at regaining intimacy within the relationship through mutual touching and physical sexual sensation and stimulation of each other's body parts, while not necessarily needing to involve the genitals or the act of intercourse. It is essentially about being able to communicate and relax with their partner and developing a sense of trust and closeness which may have been lost (Leiblum & Rosen 1989). The sensate focus method restructures and reorientates how couples may ordinarily approach sexual interactions, allowing them to move away from old familiar habits and reinvent the physical side of their

Box 48.8 Outline of P-LI-SS-IT model (RCN 2000)

Level 1: Permission (P)
The challenge for all healthcare professionals at level 1 is to create a comfortable environment that gives patients permission to discuss concerns and problems related to their sexuality and sexual health by:

- ensuring the physical environment is comfortable and private
- communicating to the patient using acceptable counselling skills such as openness, reflection and paraphrasing
- using cue questions to give the patient the opportunity to raise any sexuality and sexual health concerns
- giving reassurance, where required, that the patient's current sexual practices are appropriate and healthy or that experimentation is appropriate
- having a range of information available that is educational and non-personal
- knowing where to get further information from and routes of referral for the patient
- acknowledging the needs of sexual partners
- acknowledging the sexuality and sexual health needs of patients in relation to their cultural background.

Level 2: Limited Information (LI)
This is where healthcare professionals provide non-expert or limited information relating to sexuality and sexual health. For example, a woman receiving pelvic radiotherapy will need to know about vaginal dryness and possible implications for her future fertility.

Level 3: Specific Suggestions (SS)
To provide specific suggestions to help patients with sexuality and sexual health needs, healthcare professionals complete training at specialist practitioner level.

Level 4: Intensive Therapy (IT)
The most advanced level of addressing sexuality and sexual healthcare involves complex interpersonal and psychological issues and is used with patients who have specific sexual problems such as dyspareunia or vaginismus. Relationship counselling falls into this category. Further training is needed in psychosexual medicine and relationship therapy to undertake this stage.

relationship. It is about touching and being touched. However, at the heart of the programme is an initial ban on sexual intercourse, particularly genital contact and penetration, until performance anxiety and fear of failure have subsided and trust within the relationship has been re-established.

Finally

For a woman to be sexually complete she must feel secure and this is a fundamental need for a woman facing the future especially when she is terminally ill. Respect, trust and love are needed in order to establish security. Fear, distrust and anger need to be dispelled. Respect includes self-respect and this may have been absent even before the occurrence of cancer. Altered body image may exacerbate already fragile and vulnerable emotions around oneself. To acknowledge the hurt and pain of emaciation, hair loss, discharge, bleeding, abdominal distension, colostomy or urostomy is difficult and it can help to share this difficulty by not avoiding the important issues for the woman. Love of the person rather than the body must be constantly reinforced. There is an opportunity to engender new self-respect and trust, in discussing openly and honestly the issues that may be painful but most important to the woman at that time.

BREAKING 'BAD NEWS'

'Bad news' can be defined as any information that dramatically alters a patients' view of her future for the worse (Kay 1996). The way bad news is delivered affects both the patient's and the family's ability to cope and should therefore be done in a sensitive and, where possible, planned and supportive way.

It is in the nature of gynaecological malignancies that the possibility of cancer is uppermost in the patient's mind even before the investigations that confirm her worst fear. Most studies in which patients with cancer have been asked how much information they want report that over 90% want all the information available, good or bad (National Cancer Guidance Group 1998).

Bad news may be broken in the following circumstances:

- at the point of diagnosis
- at the point of recurrence
- when entering the terminal phase of illness

The manner in which this responsibility is undertaken determines the subsequent relationship between the patient and the healthcare professional. Trust and respect established at this time will ease future care and the relationship between them.

Breaking bad news well is important for the following reasons:

- To maintain trust which enables the relationship between the patient and healthcare professional to be based on openness and honesty.
- Truthfulness about the disease allows open communication with the patient and fosters discussion about the disease process and its management.
- Uncertainty may be reduced.
- To prevent the demoralization caused by unrealistic hope.
- To allow appropriate adjustment of the patient and her family, empowering them to make informed decisions about their future care.
- To prevent collusion with family members which destroys family communication and prevents mutual support.
- Information/bad news given to the patient and her family must be communicated to the patient's primary, secondary or tertiary care team to allow open and sensitive communication between care settings.

Standards of care suggested for breaking bad news

The specialist in charge must ensure that members of the multidisciplinary team have appropriate training and skills in breaking bad news. The patient's autonomy must be respected when making management plans. In this way the patient will be given the option of involving a family member or carer to support her at the time of breaking of bad news. The doctor or specialist should plan, whenever possible, how this will be done, the setting and with a specialist nurse or appropriate member of the team present. It is the responsibility of the specialist team to ensure swift communication and liaison between the hospital-based team and the primary care services when bad news is broken.

The actual process of breaking bad news

Preparation

- Ensure all information is available, e.g. diagnostic information, knowledge of all the facts.
- Have a defined treatment plan/options available prior to the interview.
- Give the woman notice of the interview to enable her to invite a family member or friend.
- Invite a specialist nurse/support nurse to be with you whilst breaking bad news.
- Ensure privacy is maintained with no interruptions, no phones, bleeps or pagers and an 'engaged' or 'do not disturb' sign on the door.
- Set time aside, indicate how long and indicate that arrangements can be made to meet again if needed.
- Book an interpreter if needed. Do not use a family member to break bad news.

The doctor's role in the breaking of bad news

- Give time, do not appear to hurry. Sit down facing the patient and her family (if present).
- Make any necessary introductions, including the family members and specialist/support nurse.
- Make eye contact.
- Find out the patient's perception of the situation.
- Ask if the patient wants more information, e.g. 'I have the results of your tests, would you like me to explain them to you now?'
- Avoid the use of medical jargon, use the patient's language. Be honest and clear.
- Give a warning shot, e.g. 'I'm afraid it looks rather serious'. Simple sensitive explanation, avoiding too much detail at this stage, unless the patient asks, as she will not remember everything that is said because of the shock process.
- Be optimistic and maintain realistic hope, e.g. 'There are things we can do to help you'.
- Use the word cancer and avoid the use of euphemisms.
- Stop at this point. Allow the patient time for expressions of feelings or stunned silence.
- At this point check the patient's understanding of her situation now.
- Continue at the patient's pace with information giving.
- Expect expression of feelings and sometimes angry questions.
- Be prepared to repeat yourself as details will not be remembered.
- Discuss treatment plan, time scales and other written information.
- Ensure the interview is closed sensitively and inform the woman when she will see you next or how to contact you if necessary.
- Offer to meet other members of family separately.

- Bad news will always be bad and always be remembered, as will empathy and simple, clear, well-planned, sensitive and honest explanation.

The nurse's role in the breaking of bad news

- Be prepared to co-ordinate the process.
- Ensure a quiet room is available or screen off the bedside – no interruptions, bleeps or pagers or phones.
- Make sure the patient and family are comfortable and all seated.
- Ensure the doctor is able to sit down comfortably to enable him/her to maintain eye contact throughout.
- The nurse's role is to support the patient, the family and the doctor.
- Ensure the patient's dignity is maintained at all times, e.g. dressed/covered before the consultation begins.
- If the woman is an out patient, ensure that if she is alone, there are transport arrangements home and someone to collect her if in shock.
- It is necessary to ask the patient's permission to contact her GP and any community support service, i.e. Macmillan.
- Stay with the patient and family following the interview. Allow time for them to compose themselves and the opportunity to ask questions.
- Offer relevant written information and contact numbers for the patient and family to access further information or advice, e.g. Macmillan nurse/support groups.

After the consultation

- The nurse should be available to the patient and family for as long as necessary.
- Ensure the next appointment is made for further investigations, treatment, symptom review and follow-up.
- Offer nurse-led follow-up in the form of personal or phone contact.
- Ensure the GP is informed and local community support as appropriate, i.e. Macmillan team/district nurses, as soon as possible by either phone or fax regarding the bad news given, treatment plan and how the patient and family received the news. Indicate the name and contact number of the support/specialist nurse involved.

Dealing with collusion and the conspiracy of silence

Family distress at anticipated bad news can lead to collusion which in turn leads to poor communication between the family, patient and the healthcare team. Some patients may not wish to have detailed information and elect to permit their information to be discussed with the family or a carer.

To prevent collusion occurring the following should be addressed.

- Deal with the patient's main concerns first.
- Ask the patient's permission to see the family/carer.
- Talk to the family/carer. Gain their trust to enable them to give 'permission' to talk openly and honestly.
  - Acknowledge they know the patient best.
  - Check the family's understanding of the illness.
  - Check why the family do not want information given to the patient.
  - Indicate potential difficulties the family may experience if the patient is not told the information if she asks.
  - Ask permission to talk to the patient alone to elicit what she would like to know.
- Talk with the patient.
- Talk with the patient and family together.
- Document the outcome of discussions.

Relatives often ask that the patient should not be told the diagnosis. This wish can sometimes be very strongly stated and may be driven by a strong desire to protect the patient. It is important to discover whether this is because their own fears are too great to face.

If the opportunity is given to discuss the woman's illness, with care and support for the whole family to cope, a very positive outcome can result. The alternative is that the strain of pretence will undermine patient and family alike, with both sides usually being unaware of the reality of the situation, even if this is not admitted (Twycross & Lack 1983).

Modern cancer treatment, often involving radical complex surgery, chemotherapy and radiotherapy, can hardly be carried out without the patient realizing she has cancer. Even if the medical and nursing staff collude with relatives to conceal the diagnosis, day-to-day discussion and comparison of treatments with other patients will usually result in her guessing the truth.

If an open, honest approach is not adopted from the onset of the relationship with the healthcare team it imposes an almost intolerable burden on the person who is fully informed. There is a tragic irony in the situation where the nearest relative has been told the diagnosis but tries to preserve a façade, while the patient who has guessed the truth attempts to maintain a brave face for the benefit of her relatives. They are each left to face alone the prospect of uncertainty around the diagnosis of cancer and the relatives are separated from the woman by this conspiracy of silence. It is far more constructive to be able to discuss their fears with each other and to provide the close emotional support that they both need and deserve.

Giving the patient opportunities to ask and replying honestly

Simple questions such as 'Have I made myself clear?' or 'Is there anything I have not yet explained that you wish to know?' will give the woman a cue to discuss concerns. It is important to be aware of body language, both our own and the patient's as this can speak volumes. Try to sit at the same level as the patient and maintain eye contact. Avoid any obstacles to open communication such as lack of privacy, constant interruptions, phone calls or even interposing large desks. If an authoritarian posture is avoided, patients will be more likely to express their fears and feelings around what is always going to be a difficult subject.

Letting the news sink in

Patients' frequent dissatisfaction with the explanations given to them may not be due solely to a failure of communication or lack of time. They may not retain the information or may even suppress it when the content of the conversation is emotionally distressing and too painful to absorb.

Women often report that they 'shut off' and 'could no longer bear to listen'. Hogbin & Fallowfield (1989) and the National Cancer Guidance Group (1998) have suggested that tape recording 'bad news' consultations and giving the tape to the patient to take away with them may help them understand the problem, overcome failures of recall and explain the diagnosis and any treatment plan to their relatives.

However, this approach may not suit every patient and may create further obstacles to communication by preventing the interview from achieving the degree of privacy and intimacy which is necessary for two-way open interaction.

Another suggestion is to write down the facts from the information given verbally following the consultation in which bad news is broken and allow the patient an opportunity to absorb the information at her own pace over time and once the shock process has started to shift. Once the reality of her new situation has sunk in, the need for more factual information and exploration of the options in order to take back some control often takes over from initial fear, shock and stunned silence (COG 1999). Written information following the breaking of bad news can then be extremely useful in helping the patient and family to formulate their questions prior to their next consultation with the specialist team.

Many areas also have local cancer support groups and there are national cancer helplines which may also be useful in helping patients come to terms with the 'bad news' given (see Sources of support below).

Being realistic

It is important always to be realistic and avoid giving false reassurance. At the same time, it is important not to deny the patient all hope. Encouraging a positive but realistic attitude will help. The importance of this stage cannot be emphasized too strongly. If the multidisciplinary care team forms an open and honest relationship when there is hope for cure, this will be far easier for the woman to accept if disease recurs or her condition does not respond to treatment and she enters the palliative stage of her journey. Some women will choose to cope with the news by denial. They should not be assaulted with the truth but allowed to come to terms with the situation in their own time. No response is needed other than gentle reiteration of the truth, relating to the known facts when requested. Denial may, in part, be responsible for a woman's apparent lack of understanding after the initial interview. In this case it should be carefully noted for use in further meetings, in order to manage her care in a professional, sensitive and individualized manner.

TALKING TO CHILDREN ABOUT CANCER

What makes cancer especially difficult are the many unknowns. Living with uncertainty is part of having cancer. There are some questions that cannot be answered. Helping the patient and her partner accept that fact and to find out all they can to make the unknown more familiar to them is the first step in allowing them to be able to talk to their children and help them to accept the fact too.

Children need to be given information about their mother's condition, to a degree dependent on their maturity, in order to understand and cope with what is happening. Honesty is very important when communicating with children. The best person to give children information is the parent or another close family member. If they feel unable to do this, they can enlist the help of a professional, for example a member of the multidisciplinary specialist cancer care team, a counsellor or social worker. However, it is important that the parent is present when the child is told bad news so that they know exactly what has been said and can comfort them with their immediate reaction to it.

Everyone who has a relationship with the patient will be affected by the cancer diagnosis, even if they don't show their feelings. If their mother is frequently absent or not well enough to care for and play with them as she did prior to her illness, children may feel inexplicably rejected. Without reassurance, a child may feel responsible for his or her mother's illness or subsequent death.

A child's understanding of illness and death, although not the same as an adult's, is often underestimated. Children can often accept the inevitable more easily than their elders. Sometimes all that is needed is time to adjust and the maintenance of some routine and stability. However, there are things that parents can say or do to help their children to cope with change and uncertainty.

Children need to be given information in a way they can understand. It is important that jargon and excessive medical details are avoided. Tell children what has happened; explain what will happen next and be prepared to repeat the information and to ask children questions to check whether they have understood what they have been told. The use of drawings or story books can help younger children to understand. Children need accurate information about cancer, not fears and assumptions gleaned from other sources.

It is important to ask children whether they have any questions and to let them know it is all right to ask anything they want. Children often take a long time to process information and may need to come back much later and ask more. As well as telling them about changes, it is important for them to know what will stay the same. Reassurance that they will always be looked after and loved in spite of the illness will help maintain feelings of security. However, false promises must be avoided, as cancer involves great uncertainty.

It is important to listen to children, as they will let us know what they can cope with. Honesty about what adults don't know is as important as sharing what we do, if children are to continue to trust. A child has a right to know anything that affects the family, as cancer does. Not telling them may feel like a breach of trust and children usually know when something is wrong. If parents try to protect them by saying nothing, they may actually develop fears which are worse than the real situation. Children can be left feeling isolated if they are not told the truth. Attempts to protect them may enhance their anxiety. Children have an amazing ability and capacity to deal with truth. Even sad truths can relieve the anxiety of too much uncertainty. Through sharing their feelings and being prepared to acknowledge and express sadness, the parents can offer support for their children.

Coping with cancer in the family can be an opportunity for children to learn about the body, cancer, treatment and

- feel angry with the deceased, medical profession or God
- be relieved that the deceased's suffering is over
- feel anxious, lonely, exhausted, depressed or despairing
- search for reasons why they have lost their loved one
- feel that they are 'going mad' because of the strength of their feelings
- feel disappointed and/or cheated about plans and expectations that will never be fulfilled
- have difficulties eating, concentrating and sleeping (due to persistent thoughts of the deceased or nightmares)
- feel unwell or generally run down
- find everyday situations and relationships hard to deal with
- feel that no one understands how they feel
- find it impossible to think about the future or believe that they could ever be happy again
- find that they have changes in sexual drive and desire.

There are some suggested 'Dos' and Don'ts' that may help the bereaved person and their family in their grief.

Do
- remember that grief is a normal process
- talk about your feelings
- resume a normal routine 2–3 weeks after the death
- allow children to go back to school and keep their normal activities such as hobbies or playing sport
- allow children to share the grief by expressing their feelings and asking questions. Allow them to attend the funeral if they want to
- accept support, both practical and emotional, from family and friends
- take care of yourself – eat a balanced diet and take plenty of rest. Illness and accidents are more common when people are going through a traumatic time
- allow yourself time to grieve. When you are feeling low, take one day at a time grief cannot be hurried or avoided

Do not
- cut yourself off from sources of support
- bottle up feelings and emotions
- dispose of the deceased's belongings until you are ready
- make major life decisions or changes in the first year of a bereavement, if it can be avoided
- turn to drugs, alcohol or heavy smoking.

SOURCES OF SUPPORT

The bereaved person may feel they have enough support from family, friends, the church or other organizations. However, feelings may sometimes seem too intense to cope with or the bereaved may feel that they have no one to talk to who understands. They may find it helpful to talk about their feelings to someone outside their family and friends or to meet people in a similar situation. This will not take away the pain of their loss, but may help them to cope better.

There are national support organizations who help and support bereaved individuals.

- CRUSE – bereavement care. Tel: 020 8940 4818
- National Association of Bereavement Services. Tel: 020 7709 9090
- Samaritans. Tel: 020 7734 2800 or 0345 909090
- London Bereavement Network. Tel: 020 7700 8134

Other useful organizations involved in the support and provision of information for women and families affected by a gynaecological cancer include the following.

- Ovacome – ovarian cancer information and support organisation. Tel: 07071 781861
- Jo's Trust – cervical cancer information service.
- Radical Vulvectomy Support Group for women with vulval cancer. Tel: 01977 640234
- Cancer Bacup – cancer information and helpline. Tel: 0808 8001 2734
- Cancer Link – cancer information and helpline. Tel: 0207 696 9000
- Macmillan Cancer Relief. Tel: 0845 601 6161
- Benefits Enquiry Line. Freephone 0800 882200
- Amarant Trust – advice line for women undergoing the menopause. Tel: 01293 413000
- National Society of Gynaecological Oncology Nurses – specialist gynae/oncology nurses information and support group for all healthcare professionals. Tel: 0208 383 3317

KEY POINTS

1. Most patients prefer to be told the truth about their condition.
2. Supportive care is not the sole responsibility of one person but the onus lies with her doctor.
3. Staff need to be aware of their own feelings and attitudes to illness and death.
4. Staff must watch and listen carefully and respond to what they observe, rather than have any preconceived ideas about the woman's feelings and needs.
5. Time with the patient must be protected from interruption and adequate time allocated.
6. Accepting the inevitability of mental pain in the patient frees the physician from feelings of inadequacy.
7. There must be no conspiracy of silence in the family and children need to be included.
8. Many sexual problems can be avoided by simple discussion and encouragement.
9. Analgesia should usually be given orally in regular doses.
10. Intravenous fluids should be avoided in obstruction unless it is clear that surgical correction is a feasible option.
11. Cyclizine and haloperidol are very useful for controlling nausea in obstruction.
12. The general practitioner can play a central role in mobilizing local help.
13. Bereavement affects both family and staff. Both need to mourn.

REFERENCES

Anderson BL 1985 Sexual functioning and morbidity among cancer survivors: patient status and future research directions. Cancer 55(8):1835–1842

Anderson BL 1993 Predicting sexual and psychological morbidity and improving the quality of life for women with gynaecology cancer. Cancer 71(4):1678–1690

Anderson B & Lutgendorf S 1997 Quality of life in gynaecologic cancer survivors. Cancer: A Journal for Clinicians 47:218–225

Auchinloss C 1989 Sexual dysfunction in cancer patients: issues in evaluation and treatment. In: Holland J, Rowland J (eds) Handbook of psych-oncology. Oxford University Press, New York

Bancroft J 1989 Human sexuality and its problems, 2nd edn. Churchill Livingstone, Edinburgh

Bullard D, Causey G, Newman A 1980 Sexual health care and cancer: A needs assessment. In: Vaeth J (ed) Frontiers of radiation therapy in oncology. Basel Karger, Basel

Burke LM 1996 Sexual dysfunction following radiotherapy for cervical cancer. British Journal of Nursing 4:239–244

Clark C, Cross J, Deane D, Lowry L 1991 Spirituality: integral to quality care. Holistic Nursing Practice 5(3):67–76

Clinebell HJJ 1966 Basic types of pastoral counselling. Abington Press, Nashville, Tennessee

COG 1999 Guidelines on Commissioning Cancer Services. Improving Outcomes in Gynaecological Cancers: The Research Evidence and NHS Executive. Good Practice.

Colyer H 1996 Women's experiences of living with cancer (body image and sexuality in gynaecological cancer patients, focusing on three patient histories). Journal of Advanced Nursing 23(3):496–501

Corless I 1992 Hospice and hope: an incompatible duo. American journal of Hospice and Palliative Care 9(3):10–12

Corney R, Everett H, Howells A, Crowther M 1992 The care of patients undergoing surgery for gynaecological cancer, the need for information, emotional support and counselling. Journal of Advanced Nursing 17(6):667–671

Corney RH, Crowther ME, Everett H et al 1993 Psychosexual dysfunction in women with gynaecological cancer following radical pelvic surgery. British Journal of Obstetric and Gynaecology 100:73–78

Cull A, Cowie VJ, Farquharson D et al 1993. Early stage cervical Cancer: psychosocial and sexual Outcomes of treatment. British Journal of Cancer 68:1216–1220

Derogatis L 1980 Breast and gynaecological cancers: their unique impact on body image and sexual identity in women. In: Vaeth J (ed.) Frontiers of radiation therapy and oncology. Karger, Basel

Dickenson C 1975 The search for spiritual meaning. American Journal of Nursing 75(10):1789–1793

Donovan K, Sanson-Fisher RW, Redman S 1989 Measuring quality of life in cancer patients. Journal of Clinical Oncology 7(7):959–968

Dudas S 1992 Manifestations of cancer treatment. In: Groenwold S, Hanson-Frogge M, Goodman M, Henke-Yarbo C (eds) Cancer Symptom Management. Jones and Bartlett, Boston

Ellison E 1983 spiritual well-being: conceptualization and measurement. Journal of Psychology and Theology 11(4):330–340

Faulkner A, Maguire P 1994 Talking to cancer patients and their relatives. Oxford Medical Publications, Oxford

Frankl VE 1987 Man's search for meaning, 50th edn. Hodder and Stroughton, London

Gallo-Silver L 2000 The sexual rehabilitation of persons with cancer. Cancer Practice 8(1):10–15

Green J 1999 Taking a sexual history. Trends in Urology/Gynaecology and Sexual Health Sept/Oct:31–33

Hogbin B, & Fallowfield L 1989 Getting it taped: the 'bad news'. Consultation with cancer patients. British Journal of Hospital Medicine 41:330–333

Kay P 1994 A–Z pocket book of symptom control. EPL Publications, London

Kay P 1996 Breaking bad news, EPL Publications, London

King CR, Harman M, Berry DL et al 1997 Quality of life and the cancer experience: the state of the knowledge. Oncology Nursing Forum 24(1):27–41

Lamb M 1985 Sexual dysfunction in gynaecology oncology patients. Seminars in Oncology Nursing 1(1):9–17

Lane J 1987 The care of the human spirit. Journal of Professional Nursing 3(6):332–337

Laurent, M 1994 Talking treatment: nursing counsellor's role in helping patients deal with the psychosocial and sexual problems of treatment for cervical cancer. Nursing Times 10:14–15

Leiblum SR Rosen RC (Eds) 1989 Principles and practice of sex therapy. Guilford Press, New York

Lichter I 1987 Communication in cancer care. Churchill Livingstone, Edinburgh.

Lichter I, Hunt M 1990 Hospice patients. Journal of Palliative Care 6:7–15

MacElveen-Hoehn P, McCorkle R 1985 Understanding sexuality in progressive disease. Seminars in Oncology Nursing 1(1):56–62

Maguire P 1993 Handling the withdrawn patients – a flow diagram. Palliative Medicine 7:333–338

Massie MJ, Holland JC 1989 Overview of normal reactions and prevalence of psychiatric disorders. In: Holland JC, Rowlands JH (eds) Handbook of psycho-oncology. Oxford Medical Press, Oxford

Masters WH, Johnson VE 1970 Human sexual inadequacy. Churchill, London

Masters W, Johnson V, Kolodny R 1995 Human sexuality. Harper Collins, New York

Miller J 1985 Assessment of loneliness and spiritual well-being in Chronically ill and healthy adults. Journal of Professional Nursing 1(2):79–85

Moberg D 1982 Spiritual well-being of the dying. In: Lesnoff-Caravaglia G (ed) Aging and the human condition. Human Sciences Press, Springfield, Illinois

Model G 1990 A new image to accept: psychological aspects of stoma care. Professional Nurse 3:10–16

Pace JC 2000 Spirituality issues. In: Women and Cancer: A Gynaecological Oncology Nursing Perspective 15:579–598.

Persan RT, Gallagher J, Giorella M et al 2000 Sexuality and cancer: conversation comfort zone. Oncologist 5(4):336–344

Price B 1990 Body image: nursing concepts and care. Prentice Hall, London

RCN 2000 P-LI-SS-IT model. In: Sexuality and Sexual Health in Nursing Practice. RCN, London

Reed P 1987 Spirituality and well-being in terminally ill hospitalized adults. Research in Nursing and Health 10:335–344

Rutter M 2000 The impact of illness on sexuality. In: Wells D (ed) Caring for sexuality in health and illness. Churchill Livingstone, Edinburgh

Sacco Ezzell P 1999 Managing the effects of gynaecological cancer treatment on quality of life and sexuality. Society of Gynaecological Nursing Oncologists 8(3):23–26

Saunders C, Baines M, 1989 Living with dying. Oxford Medical Publications, Oxford

Smith DB 1989 Sexual rehabilitation of the cancer patient. Cancer Nursing 12(1):10–15

Smithman C 1981 Nursing actions for health care promotion. FA Davis, Philadelphia

Steginga K, Dunn J 1997 Women's experiences following treatment for gynaecological cancer, Oncology Nurses Forum 24(8):1403–1407

Twycross R 1997 a Symptom management in advanced cancer, 2nd edn. Radcliffe Medical Press, Oxford

Twycross R 1997b Introductory palliative care, 2nd edn. Radcliffe Medical Press, Oxford

Twycross R, Lack S 1983 Symptom control in far advanced cancer: pain relief. Pitman Medical, Tunbridge Wells

Veronesi U, ven Kleist S, Redmond K et al 1999 Caring About Woman and Cancer (CAWAC): a European survey of the perspectives and experiences of women with female cancers. European Journal of Cancer 35(12):1667–1675

Wilson E, Williams H 1988 Oncology nurses' attitudes and behaviours related to sexuality of patients with cancer. Oncology Nursing Forum 15(1):49–53

Woods N 1975 Human sexuality in health and illness. CV Mosby, St Louis

World Health Organization 1986 concepts for sexual health. Regional Office for Europe, Copenhagen

FURTHER READING

Hammersmith Hospital Trust 2001 Breaking bad news: guidelines for staff. HHT Palliative Care Team, London

Hammersmith Hospital Trust 2001 Talking to children about cancer: guidelines. HHT Palliative Care Team, London

Section 4
UROGYNAECOLOGY

49

Classification of urogynaecological disorders

Stuart L. Stanton

INTRODUCTION

If the body were divided into specialties by physiological rather than anatomical boundaries, there would be no need for an explanation of urogynaecology. As it is, this specialty represents an interface between gynaecologist and urologist. Physiological events or disease affecting gynaecological organs invariably affect the urinary tract, as they will also sometimes affect the adjacent alimentary system.

It is increasingly recognized that colorectal surgeons have an important role in the management of pelvic floor disorders. The studies of Snooks et al (1984a, b) and Sultan et al (1993) show the traumatic effects of vaginal delivery on the pelvic floor and anal sphincters. Wall & de Lancey (1991) have succinctly summarized the need for a holistic approach involving gynaecologists, urologists and colorectal surgeons in the management of pelvic floor disorders.

Following the introduction of subspecialization by the American College of Obstetricians and Gynecologists, the Royal College of Obstetricians and Gynaecologists considered and then recommended subspecialization in 1982. Four subspecialties were created, among them urogynaecology. This comprised the following disorders: congenital anomalies, incontinence, voiding difficulties, urinary fistulae, bladder neuropathy, genital prolapse, urgency and frequency, and urinary tract infection. By common consent, all 'supravesical' conditions and neoplasia arising anywhere in the urinary tract belong to the realm of urology.

To these might now be added disordered bowel motility, descending perineum and rectal prolapse, anal sphincter injuries, rectovaginal fistula, perineal hernia and faecal and flatal incontinence.

TERMINOLOGY

As in any developing branch of medicine and science, old terms and definitions have become inadequate. To provide a common language for both clinician and researcher, the International Continence Society's (ICS 1973) standardization committee drew up standards of terminology of lower urinary tract function.

Nine reports have now appeared, four since the last edition of *Gynaecology* (1997), and these are:

1. the standardization of terminology of lower urinary tract dysfunction (Abrams et al 1988)
2. lower urinary tract rehabilitation techniques: seventh report on the standardization of terminology of lower urinary tract function (Anderson et al 1992)
3. standardization of terminology of female pelvic organ prolapse and pelvic floor dysfunction (Bump et al 1996)
4. standardization of terminology and assessment of functional characteristics of intestinal urinary reservoirs (Thuroff et al 1996)
5. the standardization of terminology of lower urinary tract function: pressure-flow studies of voiding, urethral resistance and urethral obstruction (Griffiths et al 1997)
6. standardization of outcome studies in patients with lower urinary tract dysfunction: a report on general principles from the Standardization Committee of the International Continence Society (Mattiasson et al 1998)
7. outcome measures for research in adult women with symptoms of lower urinary tract dysfunction (Lose et al 1998)
8. outcome measures for research of lower urinary tract dysfunction in frail older people (Fonda et al 1998)
9. the standardization of terminology in neurogenic lower urinary tract dysfunction (Stöhrer et al 1999).

The term 'stress incontinence' was coined by Sir Eardley Holland in 1928 and meant the loss of urine during physical effort. It came to be used not only as a symptom and sign, but also as a diagnostic term. As the pathophysiology of urinary incontinence became more clearly understood, it was apparent that the term 'stress incontinence' was ambiguous as it could be applied to a symptom, a sign and a diagnosis – indeed, the symptoms and sign of stress incontinence can be found in most types of incontinence.

Nowadays the term 'stress incontinence' is retained for the symptom of involuntary loss of urine on physical exertion and the sign of urine loss from the urethra immediately on increase in abdominal pressure. The term 'genuine stress incontinence' was proposed by the ICS in 1976 (Bates et al 1976) to mean the condition of involuntary loss of urine when 'the intravesical pressure exceeds the maximum urethral pressure in the absence of a detrusor contraction'. This condition has a number of synonyms: urethral sphincter incompetence, stress urinary incontinence and anatomical stress incontinence. I prefer the term 'urethral sphincter incompetence' because this accurately describes the pathophysiology of this condition.

In a similar way, the term 'dyssynergic detrusor dysfunction' was introduced by Hodgkinson et al in 1963 and other synonyms followed: urge incontinence, uninhibited bladder, bladder instability/unstable bladder and more recently, the overactive bladder (OAB). In 1979, the ICS defined an unstable bladder as one 'shown objectively to contract, spontaneously or on provocation during the filling phase, while the patient is attempting to inhibit micturition. Unstable contractions may be asymptomatic and do not necessarily imply a neurological disorder'. The contractions are phasic. Another term, 'low compliance', is used to mean a gradual increase in detrusor pressure without a subsequent decrease during bladder filling. The term 'neurogenic detrusor overactivity' is used for phasic uninhibited contractions when there is objective evidence of a relevant neurological disorder. Terms to be avoided include 'hypertonic', 'spastic', 'automatic' and 'automatic'.

CLASSIFICATION

Congenital anomalies (see Ch. 1)

The subject of congenital anomalies reaffirms the principle that a lesion affects multiple systems. Often these present to the urologist as a primary urological problem (e.g. bladder exstrophy, horseshoe kidney). The gynaecologist's expertise lies in the area of diagnosis and management of dubious sexuality or later, when reconstructive surgery may be required for epispadias or haematocolpos.

Incontinence

Urinary incontinence forms the major proportion of urogynaecology. It is defined by the ICS as 'an involuntary loss of urine which is objectively demonstrable and a social or hygienic problem'.

Incontinence is considered to be involuntary; for two categories of patients further explanation is needed. In a child under 3 years of age control of continence has not yet developed; however, careful observation shows that the normal child is dry between involuntary voids, whereas the incontinent child is wet the whole time. On the other hand, the mentally frail or elderly demented patient may be incontinent because she has lost her social consciousness and appreciation of the need to be dry.

The social isolation caused by incontinence is demonstrated by 25% of patients delaying for more than 5 years before seeking advice, owing to embarrassment (Norton et al 1988). Ostracism and rejection by relatives may lead to an elderly patient being institutionalized solely because of incontinence; paradoxically, some allegedly 'caring' institutions will not accept an elderly patient if she is incontinent.

It is now accepted that incontinence should be objectively demonstrable using urodynamic studies which will define the cause and detect other conditions such as voiding disorders and the OAB.

The hygienic aspect of incontinence occupies some 25% of nursing time in hospitals, and unless managed, urinary odour is offensive to both patient and relatives alike.

Incontinence may be divided into urethral and extraurethral conditions (Fig.49.1).

Urethral conditions

1. The commonest form is urethral sphincter incompetence (urodynamic stress incontinence), which can present from childhood (see Ch. 52). This condition has several causes. The original classification of type 1, 2 and 3 is facile. It is realistic to acknowledge that whilst only some patients have 'urethral hypermobility', all will have some degree of sphincter incompetence, otherwise they would not leak.

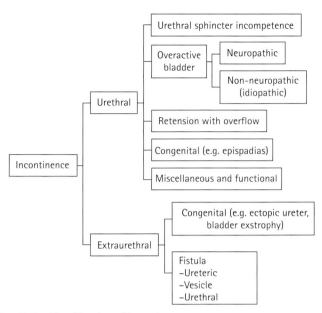

Fig. 49.1 Classification of incontinence.

Type 3 is gross incontinence with a maximum urethral closure pressure below $20 \, cm \, H_2O$ (and more usefully termed 'intrinsic sphincter defect') and for them, conventional bladder neck elevating surgery or even mid-urethral support surgery is unlikely to succeed and what is required is something to restore urethral pressure, such as an artificial urinary sphincter. For the vast majority (i.e. old type 1 and 2) either a bladder neck elevating procedure such as a colposuspension or sling or a mid-urethral support procedure such as a TVT will likely suffice. The latter has shown that lack of mid-urethral support is a significant cause of sphincter incompetence.

2. *Overactive bladder* (see Ch. 53). Depending on its cause, this may be subdivided into neuropathic or idiopathic. Some patients with overactive bladder and a competent sphincter mechanism may remain dry. If, however, there is coexistent sphincteric incompetence ('mixed incontinence'), the patient may complain of stress incontinence and urge incontinence.

3. *Urinary retention and overflow* (see Ch. 54). This may be acute or chronic; the former is usually sudden in onset and painful. There may be an obvious cause, such as an impacted pelvic mass. Chronic retention, on the other hand, is often painless and insidious and frequently undetected, so errors in diagnosis are often made. It occurs more commonly in the elderly as a result of neuropathy, e.g. peripheral diabetic neuropathy or stenosis of the lumbar spinal canal.

4. *Congenital disorders.* Epispadias is usually detected during childhood, but occasionally it is not diagnosed until adult life.

5. *Miscellaneous.* These causes include urethral diverticulum, urinary tract infection (temporary and commonest in the elderly), faecal impaction, drugs (such as α-adrenergic blocking agents) and functional disorders. These are rare and the patient should be fully investigated and all the above causes excluded before this diagnosis is made. The loss of social awareness of the need to be continent is usually associated with dementia or a space-occupying lesion of the frontal cortex.

Extraurethral conditions

These may be divided into congenital and acquired. Extraurethral conditions may be distinguished from urethral conditions by the symptom of continuous incontinence. The congenital disorders include ectopic ureter and bladder exstrophy. Acquired conditions include urinary fistulae, which in the Western world are largely iatrogenic, the majority occurring after abdominal hysterectomy for benign conditions (see Ch. 57). Other causes include pelvic carcinoma and its attendant surgery or radiotherapy. In the developing world, obstetrical causes such as obstructed labour with an impacted vertex are more common. If the fistula is small, skill and patience are required to detect it.

Voiding difficulties (see Ch. 54)

These are uncommon in the female and are frequently undiagnosed. If untreated they can lead to recurrent urinary tract infection or acute or chronic retention following otherwise successful bladder neck surgery for incontinence.

Urinary fistulae

These have already been referred to and are dealt with at length in Chapter 57.

Bladder neuropathy

This is rightfully dealt with by the urologist, but it is important for the gynaecologist to be aware of and recognize these disorders.

Genital prolapse

Prolapse should not be considered in isolation as it is sometimes associated with urethral sphincter incompetence or with perineal descent and faecal incontinence (see Ch.55). The latter conditions represent an important interface with the colorectal surgeon.

Urgency and frequency

These symptoms can of course be part of a urinary disease process, such as urinary tract infection or overactive bladder, but can often present as single or combined symptoms in the absence of an obvious pathology (see Ch. 56).

Urinary tract infection (see Ch. 58)

This is of common interest to the obstetrician/gynaecologist, urologist and nephrologist and the experience of all three may be required for difficult cases. However, the majority of patients are treated by the general practitioner without referral to hospital, although urinary tract infection is frequently unproven. Inadequate treatment during pregnancy can lead to acute pyelonephritis and abortion and, if neglected in later life, can lead to chronic pyelonephritis, hypertension and later renal failure.

CONCLUSION

This classification is an introduction to urogynaecology and the ensuing chapters will cover more depth. For more specialized reading a list of selected books is given after the references.

KEY POINTS

1. Trauma, denervation and the menopause affect the whole of the pelvic floor.
2. Urogynaecology needs to include rectal prolapse, anal sphincter injury and rectovaginal fistula.
3. Standardized terminology and methodology, as suggested by the International Continence Society, should be used.
4. Incontinence has a variety of causes which need urodynamic studies for their accurate diagnosis.
5. Stress incontinence is a symptom and a sign and *not* a diagnosis.

REFERENCES

Abrams P, Blaivas J, Stanton SL, Andersen J 1988 Standardization of terminology of lower urinary tract function. International Continence Society. Scandinavian Journal of Urology and Nephrology 114(suppl):5–19

Anderson JT, Blaivas JG, Cardozo L, Thüroff J 1992 Lower urinary tract rehabilitation techniques: seventh report on the standardisation of terminology of lower urinary tract function.

Bates P, Bradley W, Glen E et al 1976 First report on standardization of terminology of lower urinary tract function. International Continence Society. British Journal of Urology 48:39–42

Bump R, Mattiasson A, Bo K et al 1996 Standardization of terminology of female pelvic organ prolapse and pelvic floor dysfunction. ICS Committee on Standardization of Terminology. American Journal Obstetrics and Gynecology 175:10–17

Fonda D, Resnick NM, Colling J, Burgio K et al 1998. Outcome measures for research of lower urinary tract dysfunction in frail older people. Neurourology and Urodynamics 17:173–281

Griffiths D, Hofner K, van Mastrigt R et al 1997 Standardization of terminology of lower urinary tract function: pressure flow studies of voiding, urethral resistance and urethral obstruction. Neurourology and Urodynamics 16:1–18

Hodgkinson CP, Ayers M, Drukker B 1963 Dyssynergic detrusor dysfunction in the apparently normal female. American Journal of Obstetrics and Gynecology 87:717–730

Lose G, Fantl JA, Victor A, Walter S et al 1998 Outcome measures for research in adult women with symptoms of lower urinary tract dysfunction. Neurourology and Urodynamics 17:255–262

Mattiasson A, Djurhuus JC, Fonda D et al 1998 Standardization of outcome studies in patients with lower urinary tract dysfunction: a report on general principles from the Standardisation Committee of the International Continence Society: Neurourology and Urodynamics 17:249–253

Norton P, MacDonald L, Sedgwick P, Stanton SL 1988 Distress and delay associated with urinary incontinence, frequency and urgency in women. British Medical Journal 297:1187–1189

Snooks S, Barnes P, Swash M 1984a Damage to innervation of the voluntary anal and periurethral sphincter musculature in incontinence: an electrophysiological study. Journal of Neurology, Neurosurgery and Psychiatry 47:1269–1273

Snooks S, Swash M, Henry M, Setchell M 1984b Injury to innervation of pelvic floor sphincter musculature in childbirth. Lancet ii:546–550

Stöhrer M, Goepel M, Kondo A et al 1999 The standardisation of terminology in neurogenic lower urinary tract dysfunction. Neurourology and Urodynamics 18:139–158

Sultan A, Kamm M, Hudson C, Thomas J, Bartram C 1993 Anal sphincter disruption during vaginal delivery. New England Journal of Medicine 329:1905–1911

Thuroff J, Mattiasson A, Anderson JT, Hedlund H et al 1996 Standardization of terminology and assessment of functional characteristics of intestinal urinary reservoirs. Neurourology and Urodynamics 15:499–511

Wall LL, de Lancey J 1991 The politics of prolapse: a revisionist approach to disorders of the pelvic floor in women. Perspectives in Biology and Medicine 34:486–496

SUGGESTED READING

Cardozo L, Staskind D 2001 Textbook of female urology and urogynaecology. Martin Dunitz, London

Lentz G 2000 Urogynecology. Arnold, London

Mundy A, Stephenson T, Wein A 1994 Urodynamics: principles, practice and application, 2nd edn. Churchill Livingstone, Edinburgh

Ostergard D, Bent A 1996 Urogynecology and urodynamics: theory and practice, 4th edn. Williams and Wilkins, Baltimore

Sand P, Ostergard D 1995 Urodynamics and evaluation of female incontinence. Springer-Verlag, London

Stanton SL, Tanagho E 1986 Surgery of female incontinence, 2nd edn. Springer-Verlag, Heidelberg

Stanton SL, Owyer PL 2000 Urinary tract infection in the female. Martin Dunitz, London

Stanton SL, Monga A 2000 Clinical urogynaecology, 2nd edn. Churchill Livingstone, London.

Stanton SL, Zimmern P 2002 Female pelvic reconstructive surgery. Springer-Verlag, London

Wall L, Norton P, de Lancey J 1993 Practical urogynaecology. Williams and Wilkins, Baltimore

Walters M, Karram M 1999 Urogynecology and reconstructive surgery, 2nd edn. Mosby, St Louis

Zacharin RF 1988 Obstetric fistula. Springer-Verlag, Vienna

50

The mechanism of continence

Ash Monga   Abdul Sultan

URINARY INCONTINENCE

Introduction

Urinary incontinence may be defined as a condition in which an involuntary loss of urine is a social or hygienic problem and is objectively demonstrable. Therefore continence is the ability to retain urine within the bladder between voluntary acts of micturition. In order to comprehend fully the pathological processes which lead to the development of urinary incontinence, a clear understanding of normal mechanisms for the maintenance of continence is fundamental.

Anatomy of the lower urinary tract

The bladder

The bladder consists of three layers of smooth muscle, known collectively as the detrusor, which functions as one syncytial mass with the exception of the trigone. The outer smooth muscle layer is oriented longitudinally, the middle circularly and the inner longitudinally.

Histochemically, the detrusor muscle has been shown to be rich in acetylcholinesterase by virtue of its rich cholinergic parasympathetic nerve supply. In contrast, the trigone comprises only two layers of smooth muscle. The inner layer is similar to the rest of the detrusor but the outer layer consists of smooth muscle bundles with a sparse parasympathetic nerve supply. The outer layer extends to, and is continuous with, the proximal urethra and the distal portion of the ureter, where it may have a role in preventing ureteric reflux. The smooth muscle that forms the bladder neck is separate from the detrusor, with little or no sphincteric effect. Two or three layers of transitional epithelia cover the detrusor and secrete a protein on to their luminal surface that forms a watertight blood–bladder barrier.

When empty, the urothelium relaxes into numerous folds or rugae.

The urethra

The normal female urethra is 30–50 mm in length. It comprises smooth and striated muscle. The smooth muscle is continuous with that of the detrusor but has minimal parasympathetic innervation and little sphincteric effect in contrast to the profusion of acetylcholinesterase within the detrusor cells. The external urethral sphincter (rhabdosphincter) is one of two striated muscle components surrounding the urethra. Its fibres are bulked anteriorly at the midurethral level, are slow twitch in nature and are involved in maintaining continence at rest. The second striated muscle component is the peri-urethral portion of the levator ani, which is separated from the external urethral sphincter by a connective tissue septum. The fibres are bulked anterolaterally at a lower level than the external urethral sphincter, are fast twitch in nature and are involved in maintaining continence under stress.

The mucosa of the urethra is lined by pseudostratified transitional epithelia proximally, changing to non-keratinized stratified squamous epithelia distally. The junction between the two cell types alters with age and oestrogenic status, which may affect urinary symptoms. In young females, the submucosa has a rich venous supply which engorges the tissues, helping to close the urethra. This ceases after the menopause and may be involved in the development of stress incontinence later in life due to poor urethral closure.

The pelvic floor

For the context of this chapter the pelvic floor structures that will be described are the levator ani muscles, the endopelvic fascia and condensations of this fascia which form the ligaments. The levator ani muscles are often described as funnel-shaped structures but in vivo imaging has revealed that in fact they are more horizontal. The fibres of each side pass downwards and inwards. The two muscles, one on each side, constitute the pelvic diaphragm. Defects in the levator ani allow the urethra, vagina and rectum to pass. It is subdivided into the pubococcygeus, iliococcygeus and coccygeus. The pubococcygeus arises anteriorly from the posterior aspect of the pubic bone and from the anterior portion of the arcus tendineus (white line) which is a condensation of the obturator internus fascia. The medial fibres of the pubococcygeus merge with the fibres of the vagina and perineal body and have been given various names, such as puborectalis, pubourethralis and pubovaginalis. The iliococcygeus arises from the remainder of the arcus tendineus, partly overlapping the pubococcygeus on its perineal surface and extending to the medial surface of the ischial spine. The coccygeus or ischiococcygeus is a rudimentary muscle arising from the tip of the ischial spine and quite often constitutes only a few muscle fibres on the sacrospinous ligament. Posteriorly, the muscles of the levator ani or pelvic diaphragm insert into the sides of the coccyx and the anococcygeal raphe, which is formed by the interdigitation of muscle fibres from either side. The most medial fibres of the pubococcygeus that pass round the rectum at the anorectal junction form the puborectalis muscle (Fig. 50.1).

The endopelvic fascia invests all the structures that lie within the pelvis and is composed mainly of loose areolar tissue although smooth muscle cells have been identified. The layer between the bladder, urethra and vagina is termed the vesicovaginal fascia and the layer between the vagina and rectum is known as the rectovaginal fascia, rectovaginal septum or Denonvillier's fascia. Laterally both these layers attach to a condensation of fascia known as the arcus tendineus fasciae pelvis. This is a condensation of the endopelvic fascia which runs from the posterior part of the pubic ramus to the ischial spine and attaches to the stronger underlying obturator internus muscle fascia. The urethra has an intimate attachment to the lower one-third of the vagina and therefore the supports for these structures are identical. The urethra has a further condensation of endopelvic fascia which attaches to the symphysis pubis. These are known as the pubourethral ligaments and lie at the midportion of the urethra. They are fairly loose attachments and allow movement of the bladder neck during straining and also by voluntary contraction of the levator ani muscles.

The uterus, cervix and upper third of the vagina are attached to the pelvic side wall by broad condensations of endopelvic fascia with a high content of smooth muscle cells known as the cardinal and uterosacral ligaments. These ligaments originate from the region of the greater sciatic foramen and the lateral aspects of the sacrum. In the erect position these ligaments run almost vertically and suspend their attached structures.

The levator ani muscles, ligaments and endopelvic fascia work in synergy. If any of these structures is not intact then the mechanisms of support and continence may be affected.

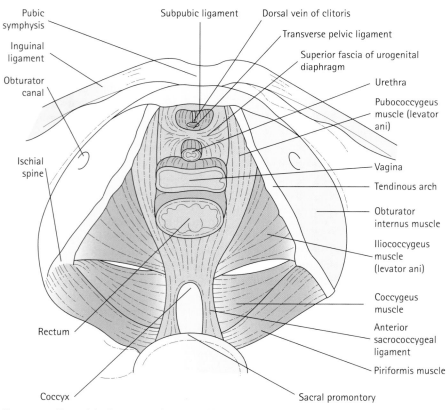

Fig. 50.1 The pelvic floor musculature and ligaments.

THE MECHANISM OF CONTINENCE

Innervation of the bladder and urethra

The bladder has a rich parasympathetic nerve supply (Fig. 50.2). The postganglionic cell bodies lie either in the bladder wall or pelvic plexuses, innervated by preganglionic fibres that originate from cell bodies in the grey columns of S2–4. There is little sympathetic innervation of the bladder, although greater quantities of noradrenergic terminals can be detected in the bladder neck or trigone. Noradrenergic affects can be either inhibitory or excitatory, depending on the receptor type present.

- α-Receptors, located predominantly in the bladder base, cause detrusor contraction.
- They can be manipulated with limited success with α-adrenergic agonists to treat mild stress incontinence.
- β-Receptors which cause detrusor relaxation are found in the dome of the bladder.

The cell bodies of the sympathetic nerves originate in the grey matter of T10–L2, pass through the sympathetic chain via the lumbar splanchnic nerve and left and right hypogastric nerves to the pelvic plexus. It is thought the sympathetic nervous system exerts its effects by inhibiting the parasympathetic nervous system rather than direct action. The visceral nerve afferents pass along the sacral and thoracolumbar visceral efferents, relaying sensations of touch, pain and distension: however, transection has little or no effect on micturition. The urethra possesses similar autonomic innervation. Parasympathetic efferents cause contraction but the functional significance of this remains in doubt. There is no obvious sphincteric function but contraction produces shortening and widening of the urethra along with detrusor contraction during micturition. Sympathetic efferents innervate the predominantly α-adrenoreceptors.

Innervation of striated muscle

The rhabdosphincter muscle is supplied via the pelvic splanchnic nerves travelling with the parasympathetic fibres to the intrinsic smooth muscle of the urethra. This is analogous to the puborectalis muscle.

The extrinsic periurethral muscle of the levator ani is innervated by motor fibres of the perineal branch of the pudendal nerve. This is in common with the external anal sphincter. The pudendal nerve also supplies the striated elements of the levator ani on both sides and there are associated somatic afferent fibres which travel with the pudendal nerves and they ascend via the dorsal columns to convey proprioception from the pelvic floor.

Central nervous control of continence

The connections of the lower urinary tract within the central nervous system are complex (Fig. 50.3). There are many discrete areas which influence micturition and these have been identified within the cerebral cortex, in the superior frontal and anterior cingulate gyri of the frontal lobe and the paracentral lobule: within the cerebellum, in the anterior vermis and fastigial nucleus; and in subcortical areas including the

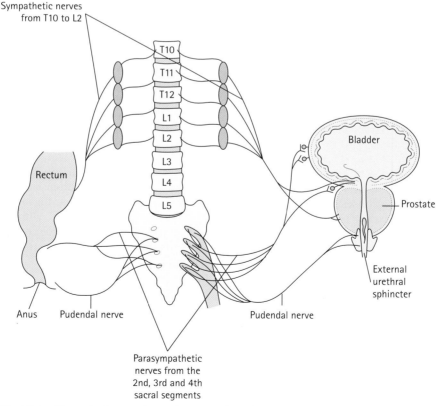

Fig. 50.2 The major innervation pathways at the pelvic level that are basic to control of micturition and continence.

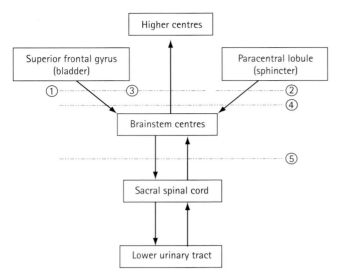

Fig. 50.3 The interaction of the nervous system in micturition. Locations of possible nervous lesions are denoted by numbers.
1. Lesions isolating superior frontal gyrus prevent voluntary postponement of voiding. 2. Lesions ilosating paracentral louble, often with hemiparesis, will cause spasticity of urethral sphincter and retention. 3. Pathways of sensation are not known accurately. In theory, isolated lesion of sensation above brainstem would lead to unconscious incontinence. Defective conduction of sensory information would explain enuresis. 4. Lesions above brainstem centres lead to involuntary voiding that is coordinated with sphincter relaxation. 5. Leisons below brainstem centres but above the sacral spinal cord lead, after a period of bladder paralysis, to involuntary 'reflex' voiding that is not coordinated with sphincter relaxation.

thalamus, the basal ganglia, the limbic system, the hypothalamus and discrete areas of the mesencephalic pontine medullary reticular formation. The full function and interactions of these various areas are incompletely understood, although the effects of ablation and tumour growth in humans and stimulation studies in animals have given some insights.

The centres within the cerebral cortex are important in the perception of sensation in the lower urinary tract and the inhibition and subsequent initiation of voiding. Lesions in the superior frontal gyrus and the adjacent anterior cingulate gyrus reduce or abolish both the conscious and unconscious inhibition of the micturition reflex. The bladder tends to empty at low functional capacity. Sometimes the patient is aware of the sensation of urgency and sometimes micturition may be entirely unconscious. These areas, which now have been localized by functional magnetic resonance imaging, are supplied by the anterior cerebral and pericallosal arteries, spasm or occlusion of which produces incontinence.

Localized lesions more posteriorly in the paracentral lobule may produce retention rather than incontinence because of the combination of impaired sensation and spasticity of the pelvic floor.

The thalamus is the principal relay centre for pathways projecting to the cerebral cortex and ascending pathways activated by bladder and urethral receptors synapse on neurones in specific thalamic nuclei which have reciprocal connections with the cortex. Electrical stimulation of the basal ganglia in animals leads to suppression of the detrusor reflex, whereas ablation has resulted in detrusor hyperreflexia; patients with parkinsonism commonly are shown to have detrusor instability on cystometric examination.

Within the pontine reticular formation are two closely related areas with inhibitory and excitatory affects on the sacral micturition centre in the conus medullaris. Lesions of the cord below this always lead to inco-ordinate voiding with a failure of urethral relaxation during detrusor contraction; lesions above this level may be associated with normal though involuntary micturition.

The mechanism of urinary continence

The mechanism of urinary continence is a complex dynamic process which relies on intact fascia, ligaments and muscles with their accompanying nerve and vascular supply. It relies on maximum urethral pressure being higher than maximum detrusor pressure. There are special features of physiology and anatomy that contribute to the maintenance of a low detrusor pressure and adequate urethral closure and positioning. These features are now discussed.

Bladder
An intravesical pressure that exceeds urethral pressure will lead to incontinence. There are a number of factors which maintain a low intravesical pressure.

The hydrostatic pressure at the bladder neck. Any fluid within the bladder will itself have a pressure. This is due to a vertical gravitational pressure gradient. For clinical purposes, the intravesical pressure defines the pressure in the bladder with respect to atmospheric pressure measured at the level of the upper border of the symphysis pubis. This pressure works against the mechanisms that produce urethral closure and very rarely amounts to more than $10\,cmH_2O$.

Transmission of intra-abdominal pressure. The bladder is normally an intra-abdominal organ and is subject to the pressures of adjacent organs and abdominal pressure. The pressures are normally equally transmitted to the bladder and the bladder neck and proximal areas of the urethra and this helps to maintain continence.

Tension in the bladder wall. Due to higher control of the basic visceral reflexes, the bladder does not contract in response to stretch receptors within the bladder wall. This and the actual ability of the bladder to be compliant, i.e. allow for a large rise in volume and a little rise in pressure, make it an ideal storage organ.

Urethra
There are several components of urethral function that are necessary to maintain good urethral closure.

The hermetic seal. We have already mentioned the vascularity in the submucosal urethral plexuses and there are also secretions that allow this seal to be maintained. This may fail after the menopause.

The intrinsic smooth and striated and the extrinsic striated muscles. The intrinsic smooth and striated muscles exert a constant pressure from their constant tone and the

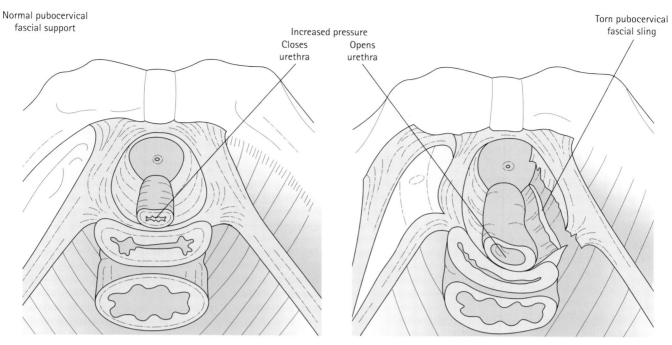

Normal pubocervical
fascial support

Increased pressure
Closes
urethra

Opens
urethra

Torn pubocervical
fascial sling

Fig. 50.4   Fascial breaks.

extrinsic striated muscle contracts during moments of stress to maintain urethral closure. It has been estimated from urethral pressure studies that resting urethral pressure is one-third due to external striated muscle effects, one-third due to smooth muscle effects and one-third due to its vascular supply. The hightest pressure is found in the mid-urethral point.

Urethral support.   From cadaveric studies and ultrasound and MRI imaging, it is postulated that the urethra is supported by a hammock (Fig. 50.4). This hammock is contributed to by its immediate intimate relationship with the vagina, the pubocervical fascia that lies between them and attaches laterally to the arcus tendineus fascia pelvis which attaches to muscle fascia and which are in connection with the levator ani muscles themselves. During any rise in abdominal pressure these may cause a comprsssion of the urethra against the anterior vaginal wall. In this model it is the stability of the supporting structures rather than the height of the urethra that determines stress continence. In an individual with a firm supportive layer, the urethral compression can be compared to the way you can stop the flow of water through a garden hose by stepping on it and compressing it against concrete. The pubourethral ligaments also contribute to mid-urethral support.

Normal micturition cycle

Filling and storage phase

The bladder normally fills with urine by a series of peristaltic contractions at a rate of between 0.5 and 5 ml/min. Under these conditions the bladder pressure increases only minimally. Urethral closure is maintained by the three mechanisms already mentioned. During the early stages of bladder filling, proprioceptive afferent impulses from the stretch receptors within the bladder wall pass via the pelvic nerves to sacral dorsal roots S2–4. These impulses ascend in the cord via the lateral spinothalamic tracts and any detrusor motor response is inhibited by descending impulses from higher centres. As bladder filling continues further afferent impulses ascend to the cerebral cortex and eventually a first sensation to desire is appreciated. This is usually at approximate half of functional bladder capacity. The impulses increase as volume increases and reinforce conscious inhibition and micturition occurs when a suitable site and posture for micturition is found. At this time, in addition to the cortical suppression of detrusor activity, there may also be a voluntary pelvic floor contraction in an attempt to improve urethral closure.

Initiation phase

When a suitable time, site and posture for micturition have been selected the process of voiding commences. Relaxation of the pelvic floor occurs early in the process of initiation and micturition. This can be observed radiologically and also by performing electromyography where an electrical silence is recorded. It is likely that a simultaneous relaxation of the intrinsic striated muscle also occurs since a marked fall in intraurethral pressure is seen before the intravesical pressure rises. A few seconds later the descending inhibitory influences are suppressed, allowing rapid discharge of efferent para-sympathetic impulses via the pelvic nerves to cause detrusor contraction at the bladder neck. There is probably also efferent sympathetic discharge encouraging urethral relaxation.

Voiding phase

When the falling urethral and increasing intravesical pressures equate, urine flow will commence. As bladder emptying occurs the radius of the bladder falls. However, the pressure remains constant during voiding and therefore it is likely that the tension of the wall falls as voiding continues. If micturition is voluntarily interrupted midstream by contraction of the periurethral striated muscle, the urethral pressure rises rapidly and therefore urine flow stops. The detrusor is much slower to relax and therefore goes on contracting against the sphincter and isometric contraction occurs. At the end of micturition the intravesical pressure gradually falls as urine flow diminishes. The pelvic floor and intrinsic striated muscle are contracted and flow is interrupted in the mid urethra and a process of milkback occurs where a few drops of urine are forced back into the bladder as urethral closure occurs in a cephalad direction.

Pathophysiology of urinary incontinence

The pathophysiology of major causes of incontinence is discussed in some detail in the following chapters. A few general principles are considered here.

If the lower urinary tract is intact then urine flow can only occur when the intravesical pressure exceeds the maximum urethral pressure or when the maximum urethral pressure becomes negative. Causes of this are discussed in later chapters but may be largely due to childbirth, with direct mechanical injury to the supports including muscle and connective tissue and following denervation injury to those muscles. Ageing also plays a part as does pelvic floor surgery and radiotherapy. Incontinence therefore may occur as a result of:

- a fall in urethral pressure associated with an increase in intravesical pressure. This can occur during normal voiding or in cases of detrusor instability (Fig. 50.5a)
- an increase in intravesical pressure associated with an increase in urethral pressure where the latter rise is insufficient to maintain a positive closure pressure. This may be the case in detrusor instability with associated detrusor – sphincter dyssynergia (Fig. 50.5b)
- an abnormally steep rise in detrusor pressure during bladder filling, suggesting impaired bladder compliance. This can occur after pelvic irradiation or with conditions that cause chronic inflammation such as tuberculosis or interstitial cystitis (Fig. 50.5c)
- loss of urethral pressure alone. This can occur in urethral instability and also in women who have urethral insufficiency or, as it is otherwise termed, intrinsic sphincter deficiency. This can commonly occur in the menopause or after radiotherapy or surgery (Fig. 50.5d)
- during periods of stress the intravesical pressure rises to a greater extent than the intraurethral pressure. this is usually due to a lack of urethral support or an abnormally positioned bladder neck and proximal urethra where equal pressure transmission does not occur (Fig. 50.5e).

Effect of continence surgery on mechanisms of continence

There are many operations for stress incontinence and the mechanism of their actions is debated. Operations such as the Burch colposuspension and Marshall–Marchetti–Krantz

elevate the bladder neck and this is assumed to restore it to its zone of equal pressure transmission. This has been shown using pressure transmission ratios where there is increased pressure transmitted to the proximal quartile of the urethra but there are obviously obstructive components that also contribute. Bladder neck injectables have been used to again increase urethral length, allowing better transmission to the proximal urethra. Finally, more recently, tension-free vaginal tape has caused great interest and this is thought to work by increasing the support of the urethra in the midurethral zone rather than influencing bladder neck position.

ANAL CONTINENCE

Definition

Faecal incontinence is defined as 'the involuntary or inappropriate passage of faeces' (RCP 1995). This definition, however, is incomplete as it may not include incontinence to flatus and therefore many adopt the term 'anal incontinence' to include flatus. Furthermore, this definition includes transient episodes of incontinence that may be experienced following a bout of gastrointestinal upset and therefore a definition similar to that proposed by the International Continence Society for urinary incontinence may be more appropriate: namely, anal incontinence is the involuntary loss of flatus or faeces that is a social or hygienic problem.

Prevalence of anal incontinence

The estimated community prevalence of faecal incontinence is 4.2 per 1000 in men aged 15–64 years, 10.9 in men aged 65 or over, 1.7 per 1000 in women aged 15–64 and 13.3 per 1000 in women aged 65 or over. In residential homes for the elderly the incidence was found to be 10.3% but may approach 60% in the elderly. Although the incidence of faecal incontinence in 45-year-old women is eight times higher than in men of the same age, its prevalence has not been accurately assessed in the younger age groups. Even a minor degree of faecal incontinence can be very distressing and is a cause of great embarrassment and therefore very few admit to it and seek medical assistance. In one study half the patients referred to a gastrointestinal clinic complaining of diarrhoea were incontinent but less than half of them volunteered this information. Moreover, clinicians may also not enquire or document this symptom and therefore the true prevalence of faecal incontinence can be grossly underestimated. A validated scoring system would therefore be more representative for epidemiological and research purposes. The Wexner scoring system is very popular and includes the need to wear a pad and alteration in lifestyle (Table 50.1). A modified version of the Wexner score has also been introduced to include faecal urgency, the ability to defer defaecation and the use of antidiarrhoeal medications.

The anal sphincter mechanism

The puborectalis and the external anal sphincter (EAS)

Proximally the external anal sphincter lies in contiguity with the posterior half of the puborectalis; distally it merges with

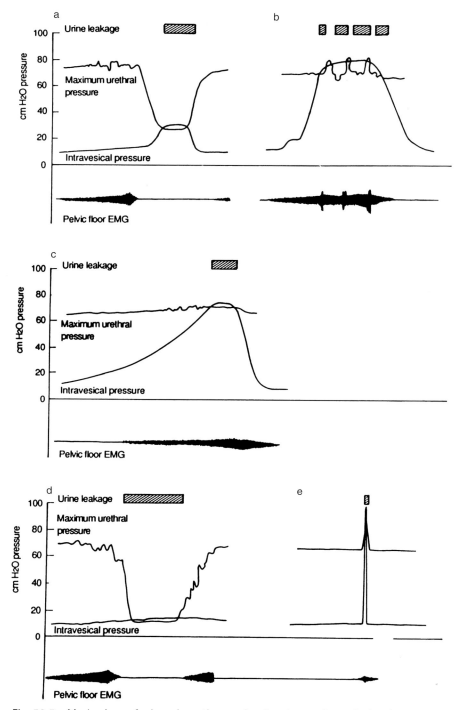

Fig. 50.5 Mechanisms of urinary incontinence showing changes in urethral and intravesical pressure and pelvic floor electromyogram (EMG) at various stages of bladder filling, in different types of incontinence. **a** Normal voiding or detrusor instability; **b** detrusor instability with detrusor–sphincter dyssynergia; **c** impaired bladder compliance; **d** urethral instability; **e** genuine stress incontinence.

the perianal skin. Like the levator ani it is primarily composed of striated muscle. There is lack of consistency in the literature with regard to the structural subdivisions of the EAS. Some authors describe it as one structure while others have subdivided it into two or even three components, the subcutaneous and

deep EAS as annular muscles not attached to the coccyx and the superficial EAS (middle layer) as being elliptical with fibres running anteroposteriorly from the perineal body to the coccyx and the anococcygeal raphe (Fig. 50.6). The deep EAS has anterior fibres which cross over to the opposite side and

Table 50.1 The Wexner score

Type of incontinence	Never	Rarely	Sometimes	Usually	Always
			Frequency		
Solid	0	1	2	3	4
Liquid	0	1	2	3	4
Gas	0	1	2	3	4
Wears pad	0	1	2	3	4
Lifestyle alteration	0	1	2	3	4

Never: 0
Rarely: <1/month
Sometimes: <1/week, ≥1/month
Usually: <1/day, ≥1/week
Always: ≥1/day
0 = perfect continence
20 = complete incontinence

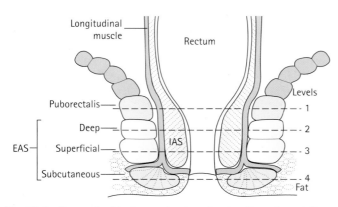

Fig. 50.6 The anal sphincter mechanism showing the puborectalis and external anal sphincter (EAS), the longitudinal muscle, and the internal anal sphincter (IAS).

combine with the superficial transverse perinei attaching to the ascending ramus of the ischium. Electrophysiological techniques have shown that the motor supply of the puborectalis is via direct branches of the sacral nerves (S3 and S4) and that of the EAS is via the pudendal nerve (S2, S3, S4). This supports the contention that the puborectalis is part of the levator ani and separate from the anal sphincter. Nevertheless, close cohesion between these muscles would seem to be essential because without it, peristalsis would pull the rectum upwards and over its contents without expelling them through the anus. Frustration in attempts to identify these subdivisions of the EAS led some authors to propose that the EAS is in fact a single structure with no real subdivision. As these subdivisions are not identified during surgery, they do not appear to be clinically relevant. However, a clear understanding of normal anatomy and variants is important during imaging (ultrasound and MRI) of the anal sphincter in order to avoid misinterpretation.

The longitudinal muscle (LM)

The LM of the anal canal is a direct continuation of the smooth LM of the rectum. Between the lower border of the IAS

and the upper border of the subcutaneous EAS, it attaches to the anal skin to form the anal intermuscular septum. Many of the fibres then pass outwards, traversing the subcutaneous EAS to insert into the perianal skin to form the 'corrugator cutis ani'. The functional significance of this muscle is unknown.

The internal anal sphincter (IAS)

The IAS is continuous with the inner circular smooth muscle of the rectum and terminates in a sharply defined, thickened, rounded lower margin, separated from the subcutaneous EAS by the anal intermuscular septum. The IAS measures about 3 mm in length and 5 mm in thickness. It is tonically active and under autonomic control, namely excitatory (sympathetic L1–2) and inhibitory (parasympathetic S2–4).

The defaecation cycle

The main reservoir for faeces is the transverse colon and the rectum is usually empty. Although the rectum has a poor supply of intraepithelial receptors, it is sensitive to distension and the first sensation of rectal filling occurs at a volume of 50 ml with a maximum tolerated volume of 200 ml. Depending on various factors such as gut motility and stool consistency, colonic contents are delivered at a variable rate to the rectum.

Following rectal distension with either faeces or flatus, the internal sphincter relaxes to allow sampling of rectal contents to take place by the specialized sensory epithelium of the anal canal (Fig. 50.7). This relaxation is mediated via myenteric connections modulated by the autonomic nervous system and is known as the rectoanal inhibitory reflex. If it is socially convenient, the puborectalis and external sphincter relax and evacuation occurs. If the time for evacuation is inappropriate, EAS contraction extends the period of continence to allow the compliance mechanisms within the colon to make adjustments in order to accommodate the increased rectal volume. Thereafter the stretch receptors are no longer activated and afferent stimuli are abolished together with the sensation of faecal urgency.

The factors contributing to the mechanism of incontinence will now be discussed in detail.

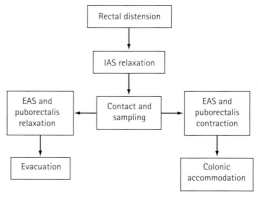

Fig. 50.7 The mechanism of defaecation.

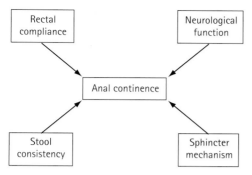

Fig. 50.8   The mechanism of anal continence.

Anal continence mechanisms

The mechanism that maintains continence is complex and affected by various factors such as mental function, lack of a compliant rectal reservoir, changes in stool consistency and volume, diminished anorectal sensation and enhanced colonic transit (Fig. 50.8). However, analogous to urinary continence, anal continence can be maintained provided that the anal pressure exceeds the rectal pressure. As shown in Figure 50.6, the ultimate barrier to rectal contents is provided by the puborectalis sling and anal sphincters. An increased volume of liquid stool coupled with rapid colonic transit may overwhelm the compliant rectal reservoir. Therefore if the rectum is able to function effectively as a rectal reservoir and in the presence of normal stool consistency, faecal incontinence can usually be attributed to defective function of the anal sphincter complex.

The physiological role of various components of this complex in maintaining continence will be considered separately.

The puborectalis muscle and the anorectal angle

The anorectal angle is formed by the anteriorly directed pull of the puborectalis. The angle varies from 60° to 105° at rest and during defaecation the angle straightens, allowing the rectum to empty. Two theories have been proposed to explain how the anatomical angulation at the anorectal junction may contribute to maintain continence. The first is the 'flutter' valve which is created as the rectum passes through the slit-like aperture in the pelvic floor caused by the forward pull of the puborectalis; a rise in intra-abdominal pressure would create a high-pressure zone and result in apposition of the rectal walls at the anorectal junction. The second is the flap valve theory: contraction of the puborectalis creates an acute anorectal angle and intra-abdominal forces compress the anterior rectal wall against the upper anal canal. However, both these theories have lost credibility; for a flutter valve to produce such a high-pressure zone, intra-abdominal forces would have to be applied below the pelvic floor. Moreover, both theories would account for rectal pressures in excess of anal canal pressures without evacuation of rectal contents. As rectal pressures have been shown to be consistently lower than anal pressures in healthy subjects, continence must be sphincteric and not valvular.

The puborectalis is considered by some to be the most important muscle in maintaining continence. In children with congenital anomalies and absence of the anal sphincter, a high degree of continence can be maintained with the puborectalis. However, posterior division of the puborectalis in the treatment of chronic constipation made no difference to the anorectal angle and was not associated with incontinence of solid stool. Furthermore, following successful postanal repair for faecal incontinence, no significant change was observed in the anorectal angle. The role of the anorectal angle in maintaining continence therefore remains controversial.

The puborectalis muscle functions in concert with the external anal sphincter and it is probable that if damage occurs to one muscle, the other may compensate functionally. Faecal incontinence may ensue if, in addition, other factors in the continence mechanism (see below) are compromised or if the remaining muscle cannot compensate adequately.

Internal anal sphincter

There are conflicting opinions on the role of the IAS in maintaining continence. As 70% of the resting tone is contributed by the IAS, it is a major factor in keeping the anal canal closed at rest. This is supported by the finding that symptoms of incontinence can develop in up to 40% following lateral internal anal sphincterotomy. Faecal incontinence has also been reported following anal dilatation with sonographic evidence of internal sphincter disruption and a reduced resting pressure.

Ultrastructural changes have been identified in the morphology of the internal sphincter of patients suffering from neurogenic faecal incontinence. Although these changes are probably not the primary cause of faecal incontinence, they may have some relevance to IAS function. In addition, abnormalities of adrenergic innervation with a diminished sensitivity of the IAS to α-adrenergic agents in vitro have been demonstrated in patients with idiopathic faecal incontinence. These changes could be attributed to an intrinsic degeneration of the muscle and its receptors or to simultaneous direct injury to the striated muscle of the pelvic floor.

The rectoanal inhibitory reflex (RAIR)

The RAIR or rectosphincteric reflex is a transient relaxation of the IAS when the rectum is distended. This response has been shown to persist in patients with cauda equina lesions and after complete transection of the spinal cord, indicating that it occurs independently of central control. It appears that the RAIR is mediated by intramural myenteric neurones because topical anaesthesia of the rectal mucosa blocks the reflex and it is absent in patients with Hirschsprung's disease.

The RAIR causes equalization of rectal and upper canal resting pressures and allows rectal contents to enter the anal canal. The contents are then analysed by the specialized sensory epithelium in the anal canal (sampling reflex). This is accompanied by a reflex contraction of the external sphincter and puborectalis (inflation reflex) which temporarily maintains the high-pressure zone in the anal canal until either evacuation occurs or the anal contents are pushed back into the rectum. The sampling reflex occurs as a normal physiological process about seven times per hour. The absence of the reflex in patients with faecal incontinence would indicate a weakness of the IAS whereas in Hirschsprung's disease (segmental aganglionosis) it would be associated with obstructive defaecation rather than faecal incontinence. However, the value of this test is limited as the RAIR may be difficult to elicit consistently even in healthy subjects.

The external anal sphincter (EAS)

The EAS is inseparable from the puborectalis posteriorly and both muscles appear to function as a single unit electrophysiologically. It has been shown that while contraction of the puborectalis accentuates the anorectal angle, it does not increase the intraluminal pressure of the anal canal.

The EAS, similar to the IAS, is in a state of tonic contraction even at rest and the activity is reflexly raised when intra-abdominal pressure is increased, e.g. when coughing, laughing or lifting. Activity is maximally raised when the EAS is contracted voluntarily but contraction can only be maintained for 1–2 minutes. Stimulation of the perianal skin also results in a reflex EAS contraction via the pudendal nerve, called the cutaneo-anal reflex. Electrical activity usually decreases during straining and when defaecation is attempted, although this is described as a variable response in some subjects.

The EAS contributes up to 30% of the resting pressure and the increment of the squeeze pressure above the resting pressure reflects predominantly EAS function. The maintenance of tone is, however, also dependent on a sensory input as it is lost if the sensory roots are destroyed, e.g. tabes dorsalis.

The response to changes in intra-abdominal pressure suggests that the EAS is actively involved in the preservation of continence. Further support for this hypothesis is that division of the internal sphincter alone can be associated with minor degrees of incontinence to flatus and liquid stool but not usually to solid stool. These properties of the EAS may be diminished either by denervation, mechanical trauma or a combination of factors.

The anal cushions

The anal cushions, consisting of epithelium, subepithelium and the underlying haemorrhoidal plexuses, can contribute up to 15% of resting pressure. The anal sphincters cannot obliterate the lumen completely without the sealing effect of the anal cushions. The thickened cushions may account for the increased resting pressures seen in patients with haemorrhoids. The fall in resting pressure following haemorrhoidectomy may explain the development of minor anal incontinence although inadvertent damage to the sphincter, particularly the internal sphincter, has been observed using anal endosonography.

Rectal compliance

A compliant rectal reservoir that can accommodate large volumes of stool without significant increases in pressure is an important prerequisite for the effective function of barrier mechanisms of continence. Patients who have a reduction in rectal capacity, as occurs in colitis and radiation proctitis, often suffer from faecal urgency and incontinence.

Anorectal sensation

The epithelium of the anal canal is richly supplied with sensory nerve endings exquisitely sensitive to pain, heat and cold. The afferent nerve pathways for anal canal sensation is via the posterior inferior haemorrhoidal branches of the pudendal nerve and anterior haemorrhoidal branches of the perineal nerve to the sacral roots of S2, S3 and S4 but in addition, direct anal and urethral branches arise from S4 and S5. Sampling has been shown to occur less frequently in incontinent patients compared to controls.

Central control of anal continence

The upper motor neurones for the voluntary sphincter muscles lie close to those of the lower limb musculature in the parasagittal motor cortex. They communicate by a fast conducting oligosymptomatic pathway with the Onuf nucleus situated in the sacral ventral grey matter, mainly S2 and S3. The frontal cortex is important for the conscious awareness of the need to defaecate and appropriate social behaviour. Disease affecting the upper neurone motor pathway usually results in urgency and urge incontinence and provided the lower motor pathway is still intact, reflex defaecation will still be possible. Neurological diseases such as multiple sclerosis, Parkinson's disease and disorders of the spinal cord or cauda equina can be accompanied by incontinence because the central pathways which control sphincter function are located in the vicinity of the corticospinal tracts. Patients suffering with diabetes mellitus can have an autonomic neuropathy and this can also lead to faecal incontinence.

The lower motor neurones innervating the striated pelvic floor and urethral and anal sphincters arise from the Onuf nucleus. The commonest cause of a lower motor neurone lesion in the adult is chronic stretching of the pudendal nerve, usually as a result of chronic straining at stool and/or childbirth. Damage to the pudendal nerve results in progressive denervation and reinnervation of the pelvic floor–anal sphincter complex causing weakness and atrophy of these muscles.

Pathophysiology

The development of anal incontinence may be due to either mechanical disruption or neuropathy but sometimes both may co-exist. Obstetric trauma is a major cause of such injury although the peak incidence appears to be in the perimenopausal years. The development of anal endosonography has revolutionized our understanding of anal incontinence and it has now been demonstrated that about one-third of primiparous women develop anal sphincter injury that is not recognized during vaginal delivery. However, even when it is recognized and repaired, the outcome is suboptimal as one-third continue to suffer impaired continence. Attention is now being focused on improved training in anatomy and repair techniques. However, there are other factors such as the effect of ageing, collagen weakness, progression of pelvic neuropathy, oestrogen deficiency, concurrent irritable bowel syndrome, primary degeneration of the internal anal sphincter, severe constipation and uterovaginal/rectal prolapse that may contribute to a deterioration in anorectal function.

Effects of continence surgery on mechanisms of continence

The commonest operation for faecal incontinence is an overlap anterior sphincteroplasty which serves to re-establish the continuity of the anal sphincter muscle ring in patients with a sphincter defect. In addition, some surgeons perform a levatoroplasty while others imbricate the internal sphincter. This operation has a success rate of 70–80% although this can deteriorate to nearer 50% by 5 years. Anal pressures, particularly the voluntary squeeze pressure, increase. Pelvic neuropathy can cause atrophy of the sphincter muscles and hence have an adverse outcome. Some studies have suggested that a prolonged pudendal nerve latency prognosticates a poor outcome but other studies have failed to identify a correlation. An abnormally prolonged latency of >2.4 ms in isolation correlates poorly with anal squeeze pressures and therefore some neurophysiologists believe that this is not a good test of neuropathy as it is only a measure of conduction in the fastest conducting motor fibres of the pudendal nerve.

The postanal repair is performed when faecal incontinence is due to a neurogenic cause leading to pelvic floor atrophy. The intention is to recreate the anorectal angle by placating the levators at the back of the rectum. However, current evidence indicates that this operation does not have a significant effect on the anorectal angle but appears to increase the functional length of the anal canal and may improve anal canal sensation.

COMPARISON BETWEEN BLADDER AND BOWEL

Reflex adaptation of the rectum and bladder in response to filling are fairly analogous. There is an inverse relationship between distension and compliance. The 'irritable bladder' is more often found in patients with irritable bowel syndrome. The aetiology of faecal and urinary incontinence may also be comparable and Table 50.2 compares bladder and bowel conditions.

CONCLUSION

An understanding of the mechanism of urinary and anal continence is essential before one can discuss incontinence. Furthermore, if treatment is to be appropriately targeted then one must understand the anatomical deficiencies as repair of these often results in correction of function without causing new dysfunction. In the light of this kind of knowledge meaningful investigations can be carried out and treatment modalities selected on an individual basis.

Table 50.2 Comparison of bladder and bowel conditions

Bladder	Bowel
Detrusor instability	Irritable bowel syndrome
Genuine stress incontinence	Faecal incontinence
Detrusor sphincter dyssynergia	Anismus
Urgency	Urgency
Hypotonic bladder	Constipation

KEY POINTS

1. The muscular, connective tissue and nerve components of the urethral and anal sphincter continence mechanisms are very similar. The levator ani and their contribution by means of the pubourethralis and puborectalis muscles play an important extrinsic striated muscle role for continence. Both mechanisms have smooth muscle components and a nerve supply largely from the pudendal nerves.

2. The bladder and urethra and the rectum and anal sphincter have complex autonomic innervation in addition to the somatic innervation that allows reflex interplay with the spinal cord and higher centres that provide us with proprioreceptive information from either bowel or rectum. Closure of the urethra and the anal canal is vital in maintaining continence and our ability to choose the time to relax these mechanisms is essential for normal control of both continence mechanisms.

3. Mechanical damage to both the fascia and muscles is thought to be the most important factor in the aetiology of both urinary and faecal incontinence and anal sphincter defects certainly have been shown to correlate with anal incontinence.

4. Successful repair for both urinary and faecal incontinence is aimed at restoring anatomy and function and methods of imaging are useful to help us to identify defects that can then be appropriately repaired.

FURTHER READING

Urinary continence

Abrams P, Blaivas J, Stanton SL. Anderson J 1990 The standardisation of terminology of lower urinary tract function. British Journal of Obstetrics and Gynaecology 97 (suppl 6)

Asmussen M, Ulmsten U 1983 On the physiology of continence and pathophysiology of stress incontinence in the female. In: Umsten U (ed) Contributions to gynaecology and obstetrics, vol 10, female stress incontinence. Karger, Basel, pp 32–50

Bradley WE, Timm TW, Scott FB 1974 Innervation of the detrusor muscle and urethra. Urological Clinics of North America 1:3–27

Constantinou CE 1985 Resting and stress urethral pressures as a clinical guide to the mechanism of continence. Clinics in Obstetrics and Gynaecology 12:343–356

Coolsaet B 1984 Cystometry. In: Stanton SL (ed) Clinical gynaecological urology. CV Mosby, St Louis, pp 59–81

DeLancey JO 1988 Structural aspects of the extrinsic continence mechanism. American Journal of Obstetrics and Gynecology 72:296–301

Gosling JA, Dixon J, Critchley HOD, Thompson SA 1981 A comparative study of human external sphincter and periurethral levator ani muscle. British Journal of Urology 53:35–41

Griffiths DJ 1980 Urodynamics. Adam Hilger, Bristol

Hilton P 2000 Mechanism of continence. In: Stanton SL, Monga AK (eds) Clinical Urogynaecology. Churchill Livingstone pp 31-40

Monga AK, Phillips C 1999 Structural urogynaecology. In: Thomas E, Stones RW (eds) Gynaecology Highlights. Health Press Oxford. pp 43-52

Wein A 1986 Physiology of micturition. Clinics in Geriatric Medicine 2(4):689–699

Zacharin RF 1963 The suspension mechanism of the female urethra. Journal of Anatomy 97:423–427

Anal continence

Henry MM, Swash M (eds) 1992 Coloproctology and the pelvic floor. Butterworth-Heinemann, London, pp 196–206

Spence-Jones C, Kamm MA, Henry MM, Hudson CN 1994 Bowel dysfunction: a pathogenic factor in uterovaginal prolapse and urinary stress incontinence. British Journal of Obstetrics and Gynaecology 101:147–152

Sultan AH, Kamm MA, Hudson CN, Thomas JM, Bartram CI 1993 Anal sphincter disruption during vaginal delivery. New England Journal of Medicine 329:1905–1911

Sultan AH, Monga AK, Stanton SL 1996 The pelvic floor sequelae of childbirth. British Journal of Hospital Medicine 55(9):575–579

Sultan AH 1997 Anal incontinence after childbirth. Current Opinion in Obstetrics and Gynecology 9:320–324

51

Urodynamic investigations

Vikram Khullar   Con J. Kelleher

INTRODUCTION

Evaluation of lower urinary tract dysfunction

Symptoms of lower urinary tract dysfunction are common amongst women of all ages and are the cause of significant quality of life impairment. A thorough assessment of the symptoms, their impact and cause is the key to their successful treatment.

Urinary symptoms are normally assessed as part of clinical history taking using structured questioning or standardized symptom questionnaires. The bother that symptoms cause can be assessed using symptom bother scores, and quality of life questionnaires, and these are increasingly used for the assessment of patients with urinary tract dysfunction in both clinical practice and clinical trials. Urodynamic investigations are both simple and complex tests performed to objectively determine the cause and quantify urinary symptom severity.

Urinary symptoms

The relationship between urinary symptoms, urodynamic investigations and quality of life impairment is complex. Weak relationships have been found between the presence of lower urinary tract symptoms (including incontinence) and clinical measures such as urodynamics. Although urodynamic investigations determine the cause of urinary symptoms they do not quantify their impact on women's quality of life.

Urinary symptoms alone have been found to inaccurately reflect the cause of lower urinary tract dysfunction and hence the need for urodynamic investigations (Cundiff et al 1997). Jarvis et al (1980) compared the results of clinical and urodynamic diagnosis for 100 women referred for investigation of lower urinary tract disorders. There was agreement in 68% of cases of genuine stress incontinence but only 51% of cases of overactive bladder. Although nearly all the women with genuine stress incontinence complained of symptoms of stress incontinence, 46% also complained of urgency. Of the women with overactive bladder, 26% also had symptoms of stress incontinence.

Versi et al (1991), using an analysis of symptoms for the prediction of genuine stress incontinence in 252 patients, found that they achieved a correct classification of 81% with a false-positive rate of 16%. Lagro-Jansson et al (1991) showed that symptoms of stress incontinence in the absence of symptoms of urge incontinence had a sensitivity of 78%, specificity of 84% and a positive predictive value of 87%. Where stress incontinence is the only symptom reported, then genuine stress incontinence is likely to be present in over 90% of cases (Farrer et al 1975, Hastie & Moisey 1989). Even when women who complain only of stress incontinence and have a normal frequency/volume chart are investigated, 65% have genuine stress incontinence and 8% have overactive bladder (James et al 1997).

The severity of urinary symptoms is often used as a measure of the impact of lower urinary tract dysfunction in both clinical practice and clinical trials. At its simplest, severity may reflect symptom frequency, for example the number of incontinent episodes, the number of daily voids or the number of episodes of nocturia. Measuring symptom frequency is relatively easy but offers little insight into their impact.

Quality of life assessment

Incontinence research requires that morbidity is measured by endpoints that assess different aspects and are not always independent, such as the number of micturitions and volume voided. The relationship of these endpoints to the lives of women is not well understood. For example, do fewer incontinent episodes or reduced volume of an incontinent episode improve quality of life most? Incontinent women find that many aspects of their lives are affected by the condition, including social, psychological, occupational, domestic, physical and sexual aspects.

Symptoms alone do not adequately assess the impact of urinary incontinence on an individual's life – this requires the use of symptom bother or generic/condition-specific quality of life (QoL) questionnaires. Several authors have found weak relationships between the perceived impact of incontinence and clinical measures of urine loss (Aslaksen et al 1990, Uebersax et al 1995, Wyman et al 1987). Hunskaar & Vinsnes 1991 used the Sickness Impact Profile (a generic QoL questionnaire) to evaluate incontinent women with stress or urge incontinence. Mean scores on the SIP were low for both groups, but the study concluded that the impact of incontinence on quality of life was both age and symptom dependent. Grimby et al (1993) compared the Nottingham Health Profile scores for women divided into three groups according to pad tests, a urinary diary, a cough provocation test and clinical history of urge incontinence, stress incontinence or both. A significantly higher level of emotional impairment and social isolation was found amongst those with urge and mixed incontinence than those with stress incontinence.

Wyman et al (1987), using the Incontinence Impact Questionnaire (IIQ), showed that women with overactive bladder experienced greater psychosocial dysfunction as a result of their urinary symptoms than women with genuine stress incontinence, although no relationship was found between the questionnaire score and urinary diary or pad test results. More recently, Kobelt et al (1999) have shown that the severity of symptoms of incontinence as expressed as frequency of voids and leakage correlates well with the patient's quality of life and health status, as well as the amount they are willing to pay for a given percentage reduction in their symptoms.

Severity may also be measured as the impact of symptoms on patients' lives, namely how much bother individual symptoms cause. The bother caused by symptoms is probably the most important assessment from the patient's perspective and forms an important part of many disease-specific QoL questionnaires for the assessment of incontinent patients.

Although it is of value to measure the bother caused by individual symptoms, it is important to appreciate that the majority of patients present with a multitude of different symptoms. These may change as a result of time and adaptive change or as a result of treatment. It is accepted that patients with stress incontinence may develop frequency in order to limit stress leakage and that these symptoms may be more problematic than the stress urinary leakage itself. Irritative symptoms and voiding dysfunction can follow surgery for genuine stress incontinence and voiding dysfunction in addition to distressing antimuscarinic side-effects can follow drug treatment of the overactive bladder. Such changes can negatively impact on the overall QoL of patients.

The King's Health Questionnaire is a good example of a disease-specific QoL questionnaire which incorporates both symptom bother and QoL questions (Kelleher et al 1997). It was specifically designed for the assessment of women with urinary symptoms and has been shown to have good sensitivity to clinically relevant improvement in urinary symptoms in clinical practice and clinical trials (Kobelt et al 1999). In one study the KHQ was used to assess the outcome of surgery (colposuspension) for the treatment of genuine stress incontinence. There was a broad general agreement between objective urodynamic changes demonstrating continence as a result of surgery and symptom and QoL score improvements (Bidmead et al 2001).

URODYNAMIC INVESTIGATIONS

Measuring the presence of symptoms, their severity and impact does not determine their cause; this requires urodynamic investigation. This entails both simple and complex investigations which measure lower urinary tract function and provide a diagnosis and explanation of dysfunction.

Midstream urine specimen

A midstream urine specimen must be taken from all women presenting with urinary symptoms. Urinary symptoms can be caused by a urinary tract infection and once the infection is treated the symptoms may resolve. A significant bacteriuria is growth of 10^5 organisms per millilitre of urine and is usually associated with pyuria. The presence of epithelial cells, erythrocytes and casts is also noted. Urine can be screened for infection using Multistix strips which test for nitrites, blood and leucocytes. This has been shown to pick up 95% of urinary tract infection.

Urodynamic studies produce a 1% risk of urinary tract infection (Coptcoat et al 1988) so there is no need for these women to have prophylactic antibiotics. However, if a woman has risk factors for urinary tract infection such as diabetes or voiding difficulties, she may benefit from prophylactic antibiotics.

Urinary diary

A urinary diary is a simple paper record of when and how much fluid a woman drinks and voids (Fig. 51.1). The diary should be completed for 5 days. Leakage episodes are also recorded and ideally the precipitating event is also noted. This information helps to determine when the urinary problem is worst and link this with other activities. The documented record is more accurate than memory alone, having reasonable test–retest reliability particularly for incontinence episodes (Wyman et al 1991). The functional capacity of the bladder is also obtained and overdrinking (<2 l) as a cause of incontinence can be excluded. Unfortunately the diary does not differentiate between the different urodynamic diagnoses (Larsson & Victor 1992; Larsson et al 1991). The urinary diary can also be used as a baseline for monitoring of women undergoing bladder retraining.

Pad test

Pad tests differ according to the length of the test and volume of fluid within the bladder. A 1-hour pad test with a 500 ml oral fluid load has been defined by the International Continence Society (Abrams et al 1990). The woman wears a weighed sanitary towel, drinks 500 ml of water and rests for

BLADDER RECORD CHART (FREQUENCY AND VOLUME)

Name.. Date...........................

Approx. time	Day 1			Day 2			Day 3			Day 4			Instructions	
	IN	OUT	WET	IN	OUT	WET	IN	OUT	WET	IN	OUT	WET	In	When you have a drink, write the amount (in mls) in this column opposite the appropriate time
6:00 AM														
7:00 AM														
8:00 AM														
9:00 AM														
10:00 AM													Out	Measure the amount of urine passed in a jug, and record the amount (in mls) in this column opposite the appropriate time.
11:00 AM														
12:00 PM														
1:00 PM														
2:00 PM														
3:00 PM														If you are unable to measure place a tick in the column
4:00 PM														
5:00 PM														
6:00 PM													Wet	Place an X in this column each time you wet yourself. This includes one drop or enough to wet your clothes.
7:00 PM														
8:00 PM														
9:00 PM														
10:00 PM														
11:00 PM														EXAMPLE

	IN	OUT	WET
6:00 AM	100		
7:00 AM		350	X
8:00 AM			
9:00 AM	200	50	
10:00 AM			X

Approx. time	Day 1			Day 2			Day 3			Day 4		
12:00 AM												
1:00 AM												
2:00 AM												
3:00 AM												
4:00 AM												
5:00 AM												
TOTAL												

Fig. 51.1   Urinary diary showing the input and output for each day. The woman records the timing and amount of leakage and precipitating events.

15 minutes. She then performs half an hour of gentle exercise, such as walking and climbing stairs, followed by 15 minutes of more provocative exercise, including bending, standing and sitting, coughing, hand washing and running if possible. The sanitary towel is removed and re-weighed. An increase in weight of greater than 1 g is considered significant. The problem with a 1-hour pad test and an oral fluid load is that it is not reliable unless a fixed bladder volume is used (Lose et al 1988).

A 24-hour pad test correlates well with symptoms of incontinence, has good reproducibility and is positive if the weight gain is over 4 g (Lose et al 1989).

A simple pad test can be performed on all women presenting with incontinence and also is an easy follow-up measure after continence surgery.

The extended pad test is a more lengthy and objective measurement of leakage and can be used to confirm or refute

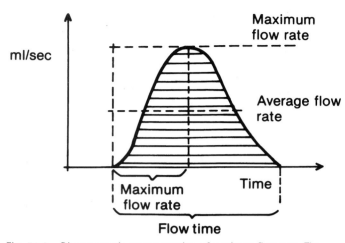

Fig. 51.2 Diagrammatic representation of a urinary flow rate. The shaded area represents voided volume.

leakage in those women complaining of stress incontinence, which has not been demonstrated on cystometry.

Uroflowmetry

Uroflowmetry is a simple non-invasive investigation and can be easily performed as an outpatient. Flowmeters are relatively inexpensive and give a permanent graphic record.

Indications

Measurement of the flow rate is indicated in women with complaints of difficulty in voiding, with neuropathy, with a past history of urinary retention and prior to continence surgery. It is advisable for any incontinent woman to exclude voiding difficulties.

Measurements

The flow rate is defined as the volume of urine (in ml) expelled from the bladder each second (Fig. 51.2). The flow time is the total duration of the void and includes interruptions in a non-continuous flow. The maximum flow rate is the maximum measured rate of flow and the average flow is the volume voided divided by the flow time. The total volume voided can be calculated from the area under the flow curve. The two most useful parameters are the maximum flow rate and the voided volume, which should be greater than 150 ml. In women with intermittent flow the same parameters can be used but time intervals between flow episodes must be discounted.

Equipment

There are three main types of flow meter. The gravimetric transducer measures the weight of urine voided over time and this is converted to a flow rate (Fig. 51.3). The rotating disc flow meter has a disc spinning at a constant speed. The voided urine slows the rotating disc. The flow rate is calculated from the amount of power needed to maintain the disc spinning at a constant speed. This is a simple and relatively inexpensive system but is more fragile and more liable to mechanical failure. The capacitance flow meter has a metal strip capacitor attached to a plastic dipstick inserted vertically into the jug

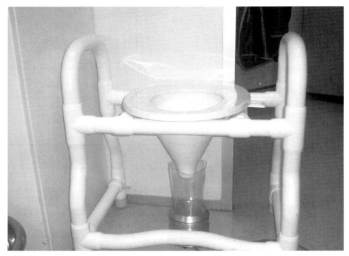

Fig. 51.3 Gravimetric urinary flowmeter.

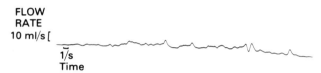

Fig. 51.4 Urinary flow rate showing a prolonged flow with a low maximum peak flow rate suggestive of a voiding disorder.

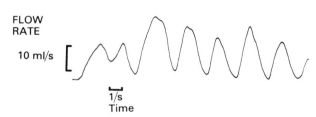

Fig. 51.5. A straining flow rate also suggestive of a voiding disorder.

containing the voided urine. The rate and volume changes are measured by a change in electrical conductance across the capacitor. This is the most expensive type of flow meter but is robust and very reliable.

Abnormal flow rates

Nomograms for peak and average urine flow rates in women have been constructed from flow rates of 249 normal women (Haylen et al 1989). These allow comparison of a single value with a standard flow rate. A flow rate below 15 ml/s on more than one occasion is taken as abnormal in women. The voided volume should be above 150 ml, as flow rates on smaller volumes than this are not reliable.

A low peak flow rate and a prolonged voiding time suggest a voiding disorder (Fig. 51.4). Straining can give abnormal flow patterns with interrupted flow (Fig. 51.5). The cause of voiding dysfunction is better determined by simultaneously measuring intravesical pressure.

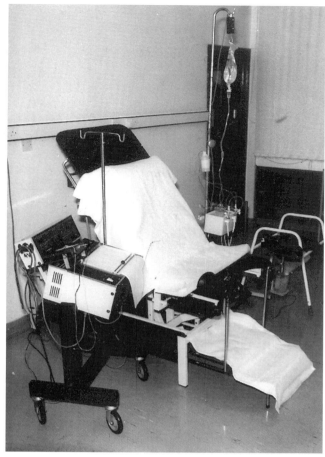

Fig. 51.6 Urodynamic equipment showing the computerized cystometry unit.

Cystometry

Cystometry involves the measurement of the pressure/volume relationship of the bladder during filling and voiding and is the most useful test of bladder function. It is a simple and accurate investigation and is easy to perform, taking between 15 and 20 minutes.

Indications
Cystometry is indicated in the investigation of the following bladder disorders.

- Multiple urinary symptoms, i.e. urge incontinence, stress incontinence and frequency.
- Voiding disorder.
- Prior to any bladder neck surgery.
- Previous unsuccessful continence surgery.
- Neuropathic bladder disorders.

Equipment
Modern twin-channel cystometry requires two transducers, a recorder and an amplifying unit (Fig. 51.6). Bladder pressure is measured using a fluid-filled line attached to an external pressure transducer or a solid-state microtip pressure catheter. To measure abdominal pressure, a rectal catheter is required, a

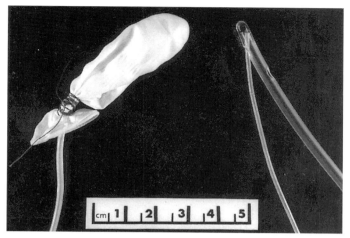

Fig. 51.7 Pressure lines for cystometry. From left to right: bladder and rectal filling lines.

fluid-filled 2 mm diameter catheter covered with a rubber finger cot to prevent blockage with faeces when the catheter is inserted into the rectum (Fig. 51.7). The upper edge of the pubic symphysis is the zero reference for all measurements, which are made in centimetres of water (cmH_2O).

External transducers are cheaper and less fragile but the microtip transducer does not suffer from movement artefact.

The bladder is filled using a 12 F catheter with a continuous infusion of normal saline at room temperature. The standard filling rate is between 10 and 100 ml/min and is provocative for overactive bladder. Slow-fill cystometry at a rate below 10 ml/min is indicated in women with neuropathic bladders. Rapid filling at over 100 ml/min is rarely used, but can be a further provocative test for overactive bladder.

Measurements
The parameters measured are the intravesical pressure (P_{ves}, measured with the bladder transducer) and the intra-abdominal pressure (P_{abd}, measured with the rectal line). The detrusor pressure (P_{det}) is obtained by subtracting the abdominal pressure from the intravesical pressure and if twin-channel cystometry is used this subtracted value is displayed simultaneously. The flow rate, filling and voided volumes are also displayed.

Method
Prior to performing cystometry, the woman voids on the flow meter. On catheterization the residual volume is noted. During filling the woman is asked to indicate her first desire to void and the maximal desire to void and the volumes of these events are noted. Systolic detrusor contractions are noted and their association with urgency. Precipitating factors, such as coughing or running water, are also noted. Any symptomatic detrusor pressure rise on standing is again recorded.

At the end of filling, the filling line is removed and the woman stands. She is asked to cough and leakage is noted. Provocative tests for overactive bladder, such as listening to running water and handwashing, are performed at this stage. The woman then transfers to the commode and voids with the pressure lines still in place.

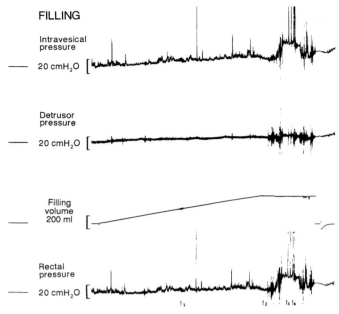

Fig. 51.8 Cystometric trace showing genuine stress incontinence. The detrusor line remains flat. Each arrow (1–4) indicates a cough, when leakage occurred.

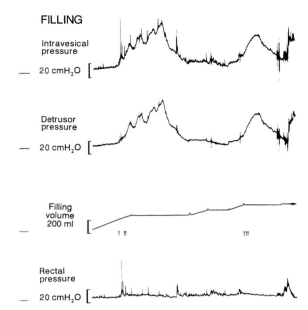

Fig. 51.9 Cystometric trace showing detrusor instability. The arrows indicate where the woman complained of urgency and leakage occurred.

Normal cystometry

The following are parameters of normal bladder function.

- Residual urine of less than 50 ml.
- First desire to void between 150 and 200 ml.
- Capacity (taken as strong desire to void) of greater than 400 ml.
- No detrusor pressure rise on filling.
- Absence of systolic detrusor contractions.
- No leakage on coughing.
- A detrusor pressure rise on voiding (maximum voiding pressure) of less than $50\,cmH_2O$, with a peak flow rate of greater than 15 ml/s for a voided volume over 150 ml.

Abnormal cystometry

If leakage on coughing occurs in the absence of a rise in detrusor pressure, genuine stress incontinence is diagnosed (Fig. 51.8). It is therefore a diagnosis of exclusion, as cystometry by itself cannot determine bladder neck or urethral function; radiographic imaging or the addition of urethral function tests is required. Detrusor instability is diagnosed during the filling phase, if spontaneous or provoked detrusor contractions occur while the woman is attempting to inhibit micturition (Fig. 51.9). Systolic overactive bladder is shown by phasic contractions, whereas low compliance is diagnosed where the pressure rise is greater than $15\,cmH_2O$ on filling the bladder with 500 ml of fluid and does not settle after filling is stopped.

Ambulatory monitoring

Laboratory urodynamics does not provide a diagnosis in 15–25% of symptomatic women consistent with the woman's symptoms. This has been thought to be due to the test occurring in an artificial environment, the test period being short and the filling rate not being physiological. The test also renders the woman immobile and bladder abnormalities produced by movement may be missed. Ambulatory urodynamic monitoring (AUM) was introduced to avoid these problems using portable digital data storage units attached to the women for periods of several hours (Anders et al 1997, van Waalwijk et al 1991, Webb et al 1991).

Technique

The woman wears her normal outdoor clothing and has the digital recording system which is the size of a Walkman (Fig. 51.10). Intravesical and rectal pressures are recorded using microtip pressure transducers at a rate of 1 Hz. The ambulatory recording device also has an electronic leakage detection system and when the woman wishes to void she connects the recorder to a flow meter and then voids. The test can last up to 6 hours in clinical practice. The women are encouraged to mobilize and continue normal daily activities, including gentle exercise. In our practice, fluids are encouraged and a minimum intake of 180 ml every 30 minutes is requested (Salvatore et al 1999). Antibiotic cover is not given as infection rates are less than 1%. At the end of the test the woman is requested to attend with a full bladder and various provocative manoeuvres are carried out.

This investigation is available in specialist units and tends to be reserved for women in whom routine cystometry gives conflicting or unexpectedly negative results. This technique has been found to increase the detection of abnormal overactive bladder in symptomatic women who had previously not been found to have an abnormality on laboratory urodynamics (van Waalwijk et al 1996, Webb et al 1991). More recently, high rates of overactive bladder have been reported in investigating asymptomatic controls (Heslington & Hilton 1996, Robertson et al 1994, van Waalwijk et al 1992). However, using a strict

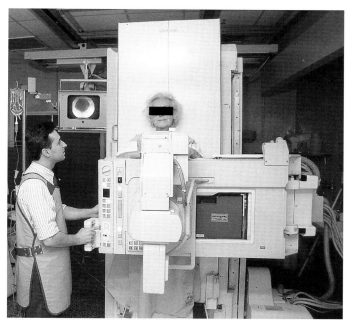

Fig. 51.10 Woman undergoing a videocystourethrogram. The woman lies on an X-ray table which is then tilted vertically for the voiding phase.

protocol for investigation and reporting, the high false-positive detection of overactive bladder in asymptomatic women is corrected (Salvatore et al 1996). There is some evidence that overactive bladder which develops after colposuspension can be detected preoperatively using ambulatory urodynamics (Khullar et al 1995). Ambulatory monitoring is time consuming and sometimes technically difficult. The equipment is expensive and fragile, which is important when women are being discharged home with equipment in situ. Discomfort is a problem but is usually mild and more common in male than female patients.

Radiology

General radiology

A plain abdominal X-ray is useful when symptoms suggest bladder calculi. Osteitis pubis is a rare complication of the Marshall–Marchetti–Krantz procedure, presenting with suprapubic pain, and is diagnosed on an anteroposterior pelvic X-ray. Sacral and lumbar spine X-rays are indicated if a congenital abnormality is suspected, e.g. spina bifida and meningomyelocoele, which are important causes of neuropathic bladder disorders in children. Spinal cord trauma and tumours can also cause disturbances of micturition. Disc prolapse is common and is demonstrated on a myelogram.

Intravenous urography

Intravenous urography is not indicated in most women with lower urinary tract symptoms unless for neuropathic bladder, suspected ureterovaginal fistula or haematuria.

Videocystourethrography

Videocystourethrography (VCU) is radiological screening of the bladder synchronized with pressure studies of the bladder recorded with a sound commentary on video (Fig. 51.11).

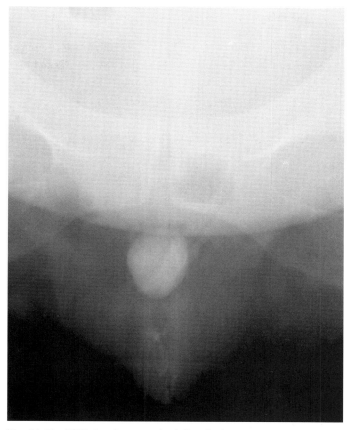

Fig. 51.11 VCU showing a urethral diverticulum.

Stanton (1988) reviewed 200 cases of urinary incontinence following failed surgery and concluded that VCU had an advantage over a cystometrogram in only a few selected groups of women. VCU was indicated in women complaining of postmicturition dribble, which may be due to diverticula (Fig. 51.12), where incontinence occurred on standing up, where ureteric reflux may be a cause of urinary symptoms associated with pain or in the investigation of the neuropathic bladder. It was not necessary in the routine evaluation of female incontinence.

Technique. The procedure is the same as cystometry except the filling medium is Urografin 35% and the test is performed in a X-ray screening room. The main differences from cystometry are that the woman is tilted upright and positioned in the erect lateral oblique position. She is asked to cough and strain. Leakage, bladder neck opening and bladder base descent are all noted with X-ray screening. Any ureteric reflux and detrusor contractions are also noted. The woman then commences voiding and is screened simultaneously; once the flow is established, she is asked to interrupt it. The ability of the urethra to milk contrast back into the bladder is noted.

All data are recorded and displayed at the same time as the bladder image. A sound commentary can also be recorded simultaneously.

Micturating cystogram

This investigation also involves radiological screening of the bladder but without pressure or flow measurements and is

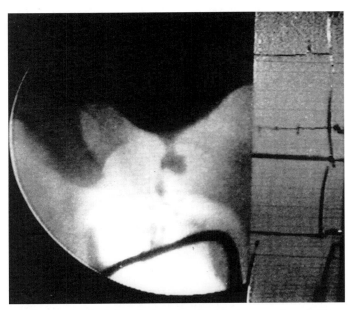

Fig. 51.12   Urethral diverticulum visualized during a session of VCU.

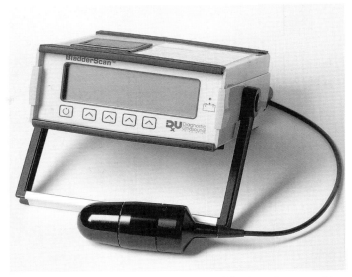

Fig. 51.13   Portable ultrasound scanner used for detecting postvoid urinary residuals.

therefore less useful in the investigation of incontinence. Its main value is to demonstrate vesicoureteric reflux, abnormalities of bladder and urethral anatomy, e.g. diverticula, and bladder and urethral fistulae. It is not useful for the assessment of incontinence.

Lateral chain X-rays

A lateral pelvic X-ray with a metallic bead chain can be used to outline the urethra and bladder neck. Downward and backward displacement of the bladder neck during coughing and straining can be demonstrated (Hodgkinson et al 1998). Lateral chain X-rays have been advocated in the assessment of women with failed continence surgery, based on the premise that if the bladder neck has not been moved upwards and forwards compared with the preoperative position, the operation is a technical failure. Wall and colleagues (1994) examined lateral chain X-rays on 98 women undergoing one of four different bladder procedures and confirmed that no useful information was obtained about diagnosis or surgical cure. Radiographic evaluation of the posterior urethral angle is neither reliable nor consistent in clinical practice.

Ultrasound

Ultrasound is becoming more widely used in urogynaecology. Its most simple use is in the estimation of postmicturition residual urine volume and to assess the bladder neck and surrounding area.

Postmicturition urine estimation

This useful technique obviates the need for urethral catheterization with its risk of introducing infection. It is indicated in the investigation of women with voiding difficulties, either idiopathic or preoperative, and also occasionally following postoperative catheter removal. The bladder is scanned in two planes and three diameters are measured. As the bladder only

approaches a spherical shape when it is full, a correction factor has to be applied. Several different formulae have been devised: the most common is to multiply the product of three diameters (height × width × depth) by a figure of 0.625 (Hakenberg et al 1983). This has an error rate of 21%, which is acceptable. Ultrasound machines are expensive and not always available in the community setting, in clinic or on the postoperative ward where residual volumes often need to be measured. The bladder scan is a portable ultrasound device designed for the measurement of bladder volume (Fig. 51.13). The machine calculates the urine volume using preconfigured settings without the operator needing to perform any mathematical calculations and results are similar to those obtained with complex ultrasound technology for the assessment of residual urine assessment.

Bladder neck position

Ultrasound scanning of the bladder neck has been used as an alternative to radiological screening and has been reported to give equivalent information to the clinician (Brown et al 1985, Richmond et al 1986). Ultrasound does not need X-ray contrast or catheterization and avoids irradiation while providing good visualization of the structures around the bladder neck.

Ultrasound of the bladder neck has been performed using the transabdominal (White et al 1980), rectal (Shapeero et al 1983), vaginal (Hol et al 1995) and transperineal (Khullar et al 1994a) routes. The transabdominal view of the bladder neck is difficult in obese women and there is no fixed reference point when assessing bladder neck movement. Transperineal measurement of bladder neck excursion with a specific Valsalva pressure antenatally appears to predict the development of stress incontinence postnatally (King & Freeman 1998).

Vaginal, rectal and perineal probes use the lower border of the public symphysis as a fixed reference. The rectal probe is less acceptable to women and difficulties arise with rotation of the probe, causing loss of the image.

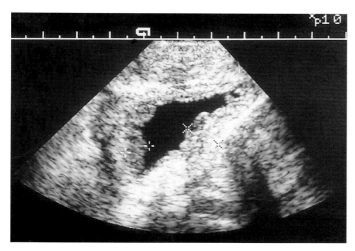

Fig. 51.14 Transvaginal ultrasound picture showing measurement of bladder wall thickness in a woman with a diagnosis of detrusor instability.

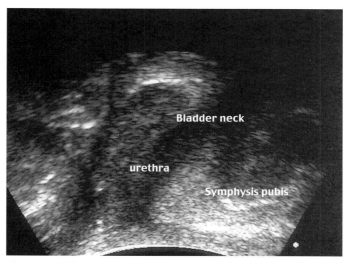

Fig. 51.15 Transperineal 2-D ultrasound scan of the bladder neck.

Transvaginal ultrasound

The vaginal probe has been used successfully to image the bladder neck. Descent of the bladder base, together with bladder neck opening, has been demonstrated in a majority of women with stress incontinence but not in controls (Quinn 1990). However, bladder neck opening also occurs with overactive bladder and this may be difficult to distinguish from stress incontinence unless there is a concomitant bladder pressure recording. The bladder neck can be compressed by the transvaginal ultrasound probe, preventing urinary leakage (Wise et al 1992). The potential for distortion of the bladder neck by the probe has not been fully assessed. Transvaginal ultrasonography has been used to measure bladder wall thickness (Khullar et al 1994b, 1996a) (Fig. 51.14). Women with urodynamically diagnosed overactive bladder were found to have significantly thicker bladder walls than those with genuine stress incontinence and this has been proposed as a screening and diagnostic test.

Perineal ultrasound

Perineal scanning is the most readily available and least expensive technique. It is less likely to cause pelvic distortion, is more acceptable to the woman and is feasible in the obese woman (Fig. 51.15). The technique has been shown to be as accurate as lateral chain urethrocystography in the assessment of women with failed continence surgery. The equipment is accurate, portable and available in most gynaecology departments (Gordon et al 1989). It may be of use in the determianation of causes of failed continence surgery (Creighton et al 1994).

Urethral ultrasound

Urethral cysts and diverticula can be examined using ultrasound. The disadvantage of this method is that unless the opening of the diverticulum is seen directly, the two cannot be differentiated. Intraurethral ultrasonography of the urethral sphincter has been described (Schaer et al 1998) and shows an association between decreased sphincter cross-sectional area

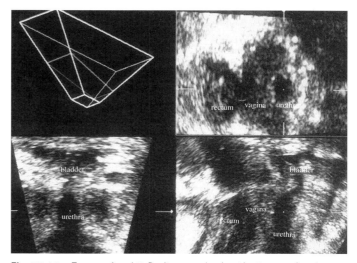

Fig. 51.16 Transperineal 3-D ultrasound using the transperineal approach.

and genuine stress incontinence. There is no clinical use of this at present.

Three-dimensional ultrasound of the urethra and urethral sphincter has been described (Khullar et al 1994c). This uses a perineal probe which records 150 ultrasound 'slices' as the probe scans 90° on its axis. A three-dimensional image is reconstructed, giving views of the urethra and rhabdosphincter (Fig. 51.16). The volume of the urethral sphincter is larger in continent women compared with those diagnosed with genuine stress incontinence (Athanasiou et al 1995, Khullar et al 1996b). Evidence of damage to the rhabdosphincter is present in some women with severe genuine stress incontinence.

Investigations of urethral function

Urethral pressure measurement

Continence is achieved if the urethral pressure is higher than the intravesical pressure. Many methods of measuring urethral pressure have been used. It is usually measured with a

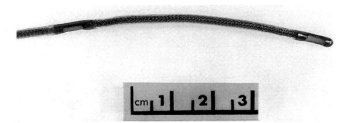

Fig. 51.17 Gaeltec urethral pressure catheter.

catheter-tip dual-sensor microtransducer, although in the past infusion catheters using fluid or gas and intraluminal balloons have been tried. The microtransducer system has two transducers which are 6 cm apart and each is 12 mm long and 1.6–2.3 mm in diameter, mounted on a 7 F catheter (Fig. 51.17). These catheters are easy to use but fragile and expensive.

Technique The bladder is filled with 250 ml of physiological saline and the catheter passed so that both sensors are within the bladder. The catheter is then connected to a catheter withdrawal mechanism set at a standard speed of 5 cm/min and a chart recorder. The static urethral pressure is the urethral intraluminal pressure along its length with the bladder at rest. The dynamic urethral pressure (the urethral closure pressure) is the difference between the maximal urethral pressure and the intravesical pressure while the woman gives a series of coughs. Women with stress incontinence have a lower urethral closure pressure than continent women and this is directly proportional to the severity of their incontinence (Hilton & Starton 1983).

Clinical value. Urethral pressure measurements are useful in defining the physical properties; however, their value in clinical practice is not certain. The static urethral pressure profile is useful to detect a low-pressure urethra where the urethral pressure is less than $20\,cmH_2O$ as these women have a 50% failure rate with conventional continence surgery. It has been suggested that they would benefit from a more obstructive procedure (Sand et al 1987). A static profile is also of value in the detection of the ostium of a urethral diverticulum, aiding preoperative counselling.

The dynamic urethral pressure profile more closely approximates to the clinical problem, but there is a large overlap for both the functional urethral length and the urethral closure pressure between normal and stress-incontinent women and it is not possible to separate the two groups on urethral pressure profile alone. Versi (1990) compared the urethral pressure profile with VCU as the 'gold standard' investigation and found that accurate diagnosis was not possible with the urethral pressure profile alone.

Urethral pressure measurements may be of value for the assessment of women following failed surgery and for the study of urethral diverticula or strictures.

Leak point pressure

Leak point pressures can be detrusor or abdominal. The detrusor leak point pressure is indicated in women who have incontinence and a neuropathic condition or those who are unable to empty their bladders (McGuire & Brady 1979).

Abdominal leak point pressure is the pressure at which leakage occurs during either a cough or Valsalva manoeuvre.

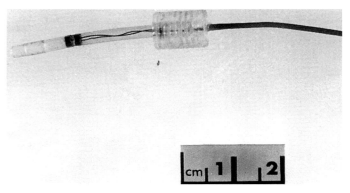

Fig. 51.18 DUEC catheter. The two gold-plated brass electrodes can be seen mounted towards the tip of the catheter.

The pressure can be measured using pressure catheters in the bladder, vagina or rectum. It has been proposed as a measure of urethral resistance of the urethral sphincter to increased intra-abdominal pressure (Robinson & Brocklehurst 1983). It is highly reproducible with a strong correlation with maximum urethral closure pressure. It is not clear whether this test is useful in the evaluation of urinary incontinence and long-term results are awaited.

Urethral electrical conductance

This technique uses changes in electrical conductance to detect movement of urine along the urethra (Janez et al 1993). Two gold-plated electrodes are mounted on a 7 F catheter. A non-stimulatory voltage of 20 mV is applied and the electrode connected to a meter calibrated in mA. The current measured between the two electrodes is proportional to whatever substance is between them. The conductance of urine is much higher than that of urothelium and causes a deflection on the meter. Therefore, entry of urine into the urethra can be sensitively detected. The catheter is either short and positioned in the distal urethra (distal urethral electrical conductance, DUEC; Fig. 51.18) or long and lies at the bladder neck (bladder neck electrical conductance, BNEC). Urethral electrical conductance profiles can be measured by withdrawing the BNEC catheter at a fixed speed from the bladder to the external meatus. DUEC measurement is used during cystometry following removal of the filling line, to detect stress incontinence more accurately than just by observation. Three different patterns of DUEC have been shown. Types 1 and 2 patterns (deflections of greater than 8 mA, with a quick return to the baseline; Fig. 51.19a) are associated with a cystometric diagnosis of stress incontinence and type 3 (deflections of greater than 8 mA lasting longer than 3 s; Fig. 51.19b) is associated with a cystometric diagnosis of overactive bladder (Peattie et al 1988a). Any reduction in urethral pressure is invariably associated with an increase in urethral electrical conductance if the two parameters are measured simultaneously in women with genuine stress incontinence (Hilton 1988). DUEC has been suggested as an alternative screening test to cystometry for the detection of incontinence (Creighton 1991).

BNEC is performed in the investigation and treatment of women with overactive bladder and sensory urgency. Both of these conditions can demonstrate bladder neck opening

Conductivity

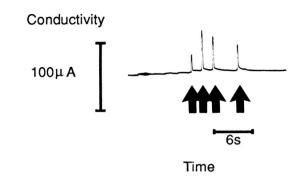

a

Time

Conductivity

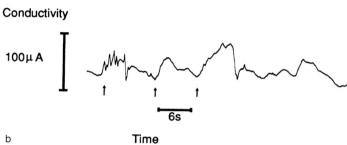

b

Time

Fig. 51.19 **a** Type 1 DUEC pattern. At each cough a spike of increase in conductance demonstrates leakage. **b** Type 3 DUEC pattern. In this pattern the coughs provoke a more sustained rise in urethral electrical conductance.

associated with urgency and if this occurs, it can be used for biofeedback (Peattie et al 1988b).

Cystourethroscopy

Cystoscopy allows the urethra and bladder to be visualized optically. It is indicated in a small group of women with incontinence but is not a part of the routine investigation of incontinence as it gives little information about function.

Indications

- A reduced bladder capacity at cystometry.
- Recent (<2 years) history of urinary symptoms, e.g. frequency and urgency.
- A suspected urethrovaginal or vesicovaginal fistula.
- Suspicion of interstitial cystitis.
- Haematuria unrelated to urinary tract infection.
- A need to exclude neoplasm in the presence of persistent urinary infection.

Cystoscopy comprises part of the operative technique in continence operations, such as the tension-free vaginal tape (TVT) procedure, to ensure that the TVT introducer needle has not passed through the bladder or in assisting in the placement of injectables such as GAX collagen (Bard) or Macroplastique (Uroplasty).

Technique

Cystoscopy is a sterile technique performed under general or local anaesthetic. If it is used to assess reduced bladder capacity during urodynamic studies, it must be performed under a general anaesthetic. The urethra is difficult to examine in women and is best done by withdrawing the cystoscope and using a urethroscope sheath. Residual urine should be noted, although it is not always accurate if the woman has not recently voided.

Bladder capacity is the volume at which filling usually stops, using a 1 litre bag of fluid under gravity feed. Using a 70° scope, the mucosa should be inspected for abnormalities, such as signs of infection or tumour. A note is made on the state of the bladder and urethral mucosa and the presence of normally situated ureteric orifices. Interstitial cystitis may be suggested by the presence of splits which bleed on decompression and a reduced capacity. If diverticula are present an attempt must be made to see inside to exclude carcinoma and calculi. Bladder calculi may be present, particularly in women with neuropathic bladder and/or indwelling catheters. Abnormal areas must be biopsied.

Most makes of cystoscope are similar and, as they are often not interchangeable, it is preferable to stick to one kind. A standard set should include a cystoscope, urethroscope sheath, 0°, 30° and 70° telescopes, a catheterizing bridge and a fibre-optic light. A biopsy forceps is essential, as is a method for dilating the urethra, such as a set of Hegar dilators or an Otis urethrotome. Flexible cystoscopes are more suitable for cystoscopy under local anaesthetic, but have the disadvantage that the image is less clear, particularly if irrigation is required, and discomfort may limit the ability to carry out a thorough examination. If flexible cystoscopy has proven suboptimal a formal rigid cystoscopy should be performed.

Electrophysiological tests

Electromyography

Electromyography is the study of bioelectrical potentials generated by smooth and striated muscles and can be used to evaluate pelvic floor damage in women with urinary or faecal incontinence and prolapse. A motor unit comprises a motor nerve and the fibres it innervates. The electrical potential generated during a contraction is called the motor nerve unit action potential and this can be measured using electromyography. If denervation occurs the remaining nerves sprout collaterals to reinnervate the muscle fibres, thus increasing the dispersion of the motor unit so that more fibres of a particular unit will fire together at one time. This is seen on electromyography as an increase in the amplitude, duration and number of phases of the action potential. If reinnervation is present, polyphasic potentials are seen.

Partial denervation has been proposed as the mechanism by which childbirth contributes to the aetiology of stress incontinence. Allen et al (1990) performed transvaginal electromyography on primiparous women before and after delivery and detected a highly significant increase in mean motor unit potential duration which was positively associated with birthweight and length of second stage of labour. Smith et al (1989) studied anal sphincter fibre density in women with stress incontinence and/or prolapse and found an increased fibre density in all groups compared to normal controls.

Electromyography can be performed using surface electrodes such as anal or vaginal plugs and ring electrodes

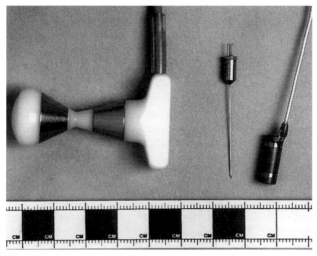

Fig. 51.20 Electrodes for electromyography. From left to right: anal plug electrode, concentric needle electrode and urethral ring electrode.

mounted on a urethral catheter or it can be performed using needle electrodes inserted into the external anal sphincter or periurethral muscles (Fig. 51.20). Single-fibre needles give more selective recordings and allow measurement of motor unit fibre density. A single-fibre reading is more difficult to obtain than concentric needle signals as the sampling area of the needle is less (Kreiger et al 1988) but it can be improved using ultrasound (Fischer et al 2000).

Sacral reflexes

Sacral reflexes indicate the integrity of the sacral reflex arc by measuring the conduction time between a stimulus and an evoked muscle contraction. Electrical stimuli can be applied to the skin over the clitoris while recording from the pelvic floor muscle using an electromyography needle, a ring electrode on a Foley catheter or an anal plug electrode. This technique has been used in the investigation of neurogenic bladder disorders, although its usefulness in the detection of 'lower motor neurone' bladder disorders is not clear.

Pudendal terminal motor latencies

Terminal motor latency of the pudendal nerve has been used extensively to investigate neurogenic disorders of the pelvic floor. Motor latency only reflects the conduction velocity of the fastest conducting muscle fibres, whereas terminal motor latency will be prolonged if there is demyelination of the nerve between the site of stimulation and the muscle. The pudendal nerve is difficult to access and must be stimulated using a fingerstall-mounted electrode applied to the ischial spine via a rectal examination. Weak responses with an increased latency have been observed in women with urethral sphincter incompetence. Snooks et al (1984) found an increased pudendal nerve latency to the anal sphincter in women following a vaginal delivery, compared to women who had had caesarean section. Smith and colleagues (1989) found that terminal motor latency to the urethral sphincter (perineal terminal latency) was prolonged in women with stress incontinence. These techniques have been invaluable in the study of pelvic floor damage sustained during childbirth and its contribution to the later development of incontinence.

CONCLUSION

Urinary symptoms cause significant morbidity. Evaluation requires detailed symptom, quality of life and urodynamic assessment. Whilst understanding the nature of urinary symptoms and their impact on patients' lives is important, determining their cause requires simple and sometimes complex urodynamic investigations. Only by fully understanding the cause of lower urinary tract pathology can we hope to improve our understanding of lower urinary tract dysfunction and provide appropriate treatment.

KEY POINTS

1. Urinary infection must be excluded before any urodynamic investigation takes place.
2. Clinical history is often not a good predictor of urodynamic findings.
3. Peak urinary flow rate measurement is indicated in all women with voiding difficulty, particularly prior to continence surgery, which may aggravate this.
4. Stress incontinence diagnosed on cystometry is a diagnosis of exclusion; it is assessed by leakage in the absence of detrusor contractions.
5. Cough-induced detrusor instability may clinically mimic genuine stress incontinence.
6. All women undergoing repeat continence surgery must have urodynamic studies (VCU) performed.
7. Intravenous urography is not indicated in the routine investigation of incontinent women.
8. Ultrasound is becoming more widely used in the assessment of the incontinent woman, with the advantage that radiological screening can be avoided.
9. Cystoscopy must be performed in the case of recurrent urinary tract infections to exclude malignancy.
10. Partial denervation of the pelvic floor following childbirth contributes to the development of both incontinence and vaginal prolapse.

REFERENCES

Abrams P, Blaivas JG, Stanton SL, Andersen JT 1990 The standardisation of terminology of lower urinary tract function. British Journal of Obstetrics and Gynaecology suppl 6:1–16

Allen RE, Hosker GL, Smith AR, Warrell DW 1990 Pelvic floor damage and childbirth: a neurophysiological study. British Journal of Obstetrics and Gynaecology 97:770–779

Anders K, Khullar V, Cardozo LD et al 1997 Ambulatory urodynamic monitoring in clinical urogynaecological practice. Neurourologic and Urodynamic 16:510–512

Aslaksen A, Baerheim A, Hunskaar S, Gothlin JH 1990 Intravenous urography versus ultrasonography in evaluation of women with recurrent urinary tract infection. Scandinavian Journal of Primary Health Care 8:85–89

Athanasiou S, Hill S, Cardozo LD et al 1995 Three dimensional ultrasound of the urethra, periurethral tissues and pelvic floor. International Urogynaecology Journal 6:239

Bidmead J, Cardozo L, McLellan A, Khullar V, Kelleher CJ 2001 A comparison of the objective and subjective outcomes of colposuspension for stress incontinence in women. British Journal of Obstetrics and Gynaecology 108:408–413

Brown MC, Suthurst JR, Murray A, Richmond DH 1985 Potential use of ultrasound in place of X-ray fluoroscopy in urodynamics. British Journal of Urology 57:88–90

Coptcoat MJ, Reed C, Cumming J, Shah PJR, Worth PHL 1988 Is antibiotic prophylaxis necessary for routine urodynamics? British Journal of Urology 61:302–303

Creighton SM 1991 Innovative techniques in the investigation and management of female urinary incontinence. MD Thesis, University of London

Creighton SM, Clark A, Pearce JM, Stanton SL 1994 Perineal bladder neck ultrasound: appearances before and after continence surgery. Ultrasound in Obstetrics and Gynecology 14:428–433

Cundiff GW, Harris RL, Coates KW, Bump RC 1997 Clinical predictors of urinary incontinence in women. American Journal of Obstetrics and Gynecology 177:262–266

Farrar DJ, Whiteside CG, Osborne JL, Turner-Warwick RT 1975 A urodynamic analysis of micturition symptoms in the female. Surgery in Gynecology and Obstetrics 141:875–881

Fischer JR, Heit MH, Clark MH, Benson JT 2000 Correlation of intraurethral ultrasonography and needle electromyography of the urethra. Obstetrics and Gynecology 95:156–159

Gordon D, Pearce M, Norton P, Stanton SL 1989 Comparison of ultrasound and lateral chain urethrocystography in the determination of bladder neck descent. American Journal of Obstetrics and Gynecology 160:182–185

Grimby A, Milsom I, Molander U, Wiklund I, Ekelund P 1993 The influence of urinary incontinence on the quality of life of elderly women. Age and Ageing 22:82–89

Hakenberg OW, Ryall RL, Langlois SL, Marshal VR 1983 The estimation of bladder volume by sonocystography. Journal of Urology 130:249–251

Hastie KJ, Moisey CU 1989 Are urodynamics necessary in female patients presenting with stress incontinence? British Journal of Urology 63:155–156

Haylen BT, Ashby D, Sutherst JR, Frazer MI, West CR 1989 Maximum and average flow rates in normal male and female populations–the Liverpool nomograms. British Journal of Urology 64:30–38

Heslington K, Hilton P 1996 Ambulatory monitoring and conventional cystometry in asymptomatic female volunteers. British Journal of Obstetrics and Gynaecology 103:434–441

Hilton 1988 Urethral pressure variations: the correlation between pressure measurement and electrical conductance in genuine stress incontinence. Neurourology and Urodynamics 7:175–176

Hilton P, Stanton SL 1983 Urethral pressure measurement by microtransducer: the results in symptom-free women and in those with genuine stress incontinence. British Journal of Obstetrics and Gynaecology 90:919–933

Hodgkinson CP, Dank HP, Kelly WT 1958 Urethrocystogram: metallic bead chain technique. Clinical Obstetrics and Gynecology 1:668–677

Hol M, van Bolhuis C, Vierhout ME 1995 Vaginal ultrasound studies of bladder neck mobility. British Journal of Obstetrics and Gynaecology 102:47–53

Hunskaar S, Vinsnes A 1991 The quality of life in women with urinary incontinence as measured by the sickness impact profile. Journal of the American Geriatrics Society 39:378–382 [erratum appears in Journal of American Geriatrics Scociety 1992;40:976–7].

James MC, Jackson SL, Shepherd AM et al 1997 Can overactive bladder really be discounted with a history of pure stress urinary incontinence? International Urogynecology Journal 8:S53

Janez J, Rodi Z, Mihelic M, Vrtacnik P, Vodusek DB, Plevnik S 1993 Ambulatory distal urethral electric conductance testing coupled to a modified pad test. Neurourology and Urodynamics 2:324–326

Jarvis GJ, Hall S, Stamp S, Millar DR, Johnson A 1980 An assessment of urodynamic examination in incontinent women. British Journal of Obstetrics and Gynaecology 87:893–896

Kelleher CJ, Cardozo LD, Khullar V, Salvatore S 1997 A new questionnaire to assess the quality of life of urinary incontinent women. British Journal of Obstetrics and Gynaecology 104:1374–1379

Khullar V, Abbott D, Cardozo LD et al 1994 a Perineal ultrasound measurement of the urethral sphincter in women with urinary incontinence: an aid to diagnosis? British Journal of Radiology 54:134–135

Khullar V, Athanasiou S, Cardozo L, Salvatore S, Kelleher CJ 1996b Urinary sphincter volume and urodynamic diagnosis. Neurourology and Urodynamics 15:334–336

Khullar V, Salvatore S, Cardozo LD, Kelleher CJ, Bourne TH 1994 A novel technique for measuring bladder wall thickness in women using transvaginal ultrasound. Ultrasound in Obstetrics and Gynecology 14:220–223

Khullar V, Cardozo L, Salvatore S, Hill S 1996a Ultrasound: a noninvasive screening test for overactive bladder. British Journal of Obstetrics and Gynaecology 103:904–908

Khullar V, Salvatore S, Cardozo L, Yip A, Kelleher CJ, Hill S 1995 Prediction of the development of overactive bladder after colposuspension. Neurourology and Urodynamics 14:486

Khullar V, Salvatore S, Cardozo LD et al 1994c Three dimensional ultrasound of the urethra and urethral pressure profiles. International Urogynaecology Journal 5:319

King JK, Freeman RM 1998 Is antenatal bladder neck mobility a risk factor for postpartum stress incontinence? British Journal of Obstetrics and Gynaecology 105:1300–1307

Kobelt G, Kirchberger I, Malone-Lee J 1999 Review. Quality-of-life aspects of the overactive bladder and the effect of treatment with tolterodine. British Journal of Urology 83:583–90.

Krieger MS, Gordon, Stanton SL 1988 Single fibre EMG – a sensitive tool for evaluation of the urethral sphincter. Neurourology and Urodynamics 7:239–240

Lagro-Jansson AL, Debruyne FM, van Weel C 1991 Value of patient's case history in diagnosing urinary incontinence in general practice. British Journal of Urology 67:569–572

Larsson G, Abrams P, Victor A 1991 The frequency/volume chart in overactive bladder. Neurourologic and Urodynamics 10:533–543

Larsson G, Victor A 1992 The frequency/ volume chart in genuine stress incontinent women. Neurourologic and Urodynamics 11:23–31

Lose G, Jorgensen L, Thunedborg P 1989 24 hour home pad weighing test versus 1 hour ward test in the assessment of mild stress incontinence. Acta Obstetrica Gynecologica Scandinavica 68:211–215

Lose G, Rosenkilde P, Gammelgaard J, Schroeder T 1988 Pad-weighing test performed with standardized bladder volume. Urology 32:78–80

McGuire EJ, Brady S 1979 Detrusor sphincter dyssynergia. Journal of Urology 21:774–777

Peattie AB, Plevnik S, Stanton S 1988a The use of bladder neck electrical conductance (BNEC) in the investigation and management of sensory urge incontinence in the female. Journal of the Royal Society of Medicine 81:442–444

Peattie AB, Plevnik S, Stanton SL 1988b Distal urethral electric conductance (DUEC) test: a screening test for female urinary incontinence? Neurourology and Urodynamics 7:173–174

Quinn MJ 1990 Vaginal ultrasound and urinary stress incontinence. Contemporary Reviews in Obstetrics and Gynaecology 2:104–110

Richmond DH, Sutherst JR, Brown MC 1986 Screening of the bladder base and urethra using linear array transrectal ultrasound scanning. Journal of Clinical Ultrasound 14:647–651

Robertson AS, Griffiths CJ, Ramsden PD, Neal DE 1994 Bladder function in healthy volunteers: ambulatory monitoring and conventional urodynamic studies. British Journal of Urology 73:242–249

Robinson JM, Brocklehurst JC 1983 Emepronium bromide and flavoxate hydrochloride in the treatment of urinary incontinence associated with overactive bladder in elderly women. British Journal of Urology 55:371

Salvatore S, Khullar V, Cardozo L et al 1996 Controlling for artefacts on ambulatory urodynamics. Neurourologic and Urodynamic 15:272–2731

Salvatore S, Khullar V, Cardozo LD et al 1999 Ambulatory urodynamics: do we need it? Neurourology and Urodynamics 18:257–258

Sand PK, Bowen LW, Panganiban R, Ostergard DR 1987 The low pressure urethra as a factor in failed retropubic urethropexy. Obstetrics and Gynecology 69:399–402

Schaer GN, Schmid T, Peschers U, Delancey JO 1998 Intraurethral ultrasound correlated with urethral histology. Obstetrics and Gynecology 91:60–64

Shapeero LG, Friedland GW, Perkash I 1983 Transrectal sonographic voiding cystourethrography: studies in neuromuscular bladder dysfunction. American Journal of Roentgenology 141:83–90

Smith AR, Hosker GL, Warrell DW 1989 The role of partial denervation of the pelvic floor in the aetiology of genitourinary prolapse and stress incontinence of urine. A neurophysiological study. British Journal of Obstetrics and Gynaecology 96:24–28

Snooks SJ, Setchell M, Swash M, Henry MM 1984 Injury to innervation of pelvic floor sphincter musculature in childbirth. Lancet 2:546–550

Stanton 1988 Videocystourethrography: its role in the assessment of incontinence in the female. Neurourology and Urodynamics 7:172–173

Uebersax JS, Wyman JF, Shumaker SA, McClish DK, Fantl JA 1995 Short forms to assess life quality and symptom distress for urinary incontinence in women: the Incontinence Impact Questionnaire and the Urogenital Distress Inventory. Continence Program for Women Research Group. Neurourology and Urodynamics 14:131–139

van Waalwijk van Doorn ES, Meier AH, Ambergen AW, Janknegt RA 1996 Ambulatory urodynamics: extramural testing of the lower and upper urinary tract by Holter monitoring of cystometrogram, uroflowmetry, and renal pelvic pressures. Urologic Clinics of North America 23:345–371

van Waalwijk van Doorn ES, Remmers A, Janknegt RA 1991 Extramural ambulatory urodynamic monitoring during natural filling and normal daily activities: evaluation of 100 patients. Journal of Urology 146:124–131

van Waalwijk van Doorn ES, Remmers A, Janknegt RA 1992 Conventional and extramural ambulatory urodynamic testing of the lower urinary tract in female volunteers. Journal of Urology 47:1319–1326

Versi E 1990 Discriminant analysis of urethral pressure profilometry data for the diagnosis of genuine stress incontinence. British Journal of Obstetrics and Gynaecolology 97:251–259

Versi E, Cardozo L, Anand D, Cooper D 1991 Symptoms analysis for the diagnosis of genuine stress incontinence. British Journal of Obstetrics and Gynaecology 98:815–819

Wall LL, Helms M, Peattie AB, Pearce M, Stanton SL, 1994 Bladder neck mobility and the outcome of surgery for genuine stress urinary incontinence, A logistic regression analysis of lateral bead-chain cystourethrograms. Journal of Reproductive Medicine 39:429–435

Webb RJ, Ramsden PD, Neal DE 1991 Ambulatory monitoring and electronic measurement of urinary leakage in the diagnosis of overactive bladder and incontinence. British Journal of Urology 68:148–152

White RD, McQuown D, McCarthy TA, Ostergard DR, 1980 Real-time ultrasonography in the evaluation of urinary stress incontinence. American Journal of Obstetris and Gynecology 138:235–237

Wise BG, Burton G, Cutner A, Cardozo LD 1992 Effect of vaginal ultrasound probe on lower urinary tract function. British Journal of Urology 70:12–16

Wyman JF, Harkins SW, Choi SC, Taylor JR, Fantl JA 1987 Psychosocial impact of urinary incontinence in women. Obstetrics and Gynecology 70:378–381

Wyman JF, Elswick RK, Wilson MS, Fantl JA 1991 Relationship of fluid intake to voluntary micturitions and urinary incontinence in women. Neurourology and Urodynamics 10:132–143

misdiagnosing or missing detrusor instability with simple cystometry, although there is no consensus to this point (Fonda et al 1993, Scotti & Myers 1993, Sutherst & Brown 1984, Wall et al 1994b)

Urethral pressure profilometry and Valsalva leak point pressure

This study involves measurement of urethral pressure. As continence depends on the urethral pressure exceeding vesical pressure at all times except during voiding, this parameter has been an attractive means by which many have attempted to explain GSI. Sand et al (1987) defined the low-pressure urethra as having closure pressure $<20 \, cmH_2O$ and found this entity to represent a significant risk factor for failure of Burch colposuspension. These findings have also been reported by others (Koonings et al 1990). Comparisons of pre-and post-operative profilometry findings in continent controls and incontinent patients, however, have failed to support urethral pressure as a culprit in the aetiology of GSI (Faysal et al 1981, Versi et al 1986). The Valsalva leak point pressure (VLPP) is generally determined during cystometry. It provides a dynamic assessment of the patient's urethral closure pressure and is determined by having the patient strain while the urethra is observed for loss of urine. The vesical pressure at which urine loss is documented is considered the VLPP. It represents the true detrusor pressure plus the subject-generated abdominal pressure that overcomes urethral closure pressure, permitting loss of urine. VLLP less than $60 \, cmH_2O$ is considered abnormally low and evidence for sphincteric incompetence. The primary drawback to the VLLP test is its lack of reproducibility.

Uroflowmetry and pressure voiding studies

Uroflowmetry is an assessment of a subject's urine flow. It may identify patients with abnormal voiding mechanisms, but is not particularly helpful with diagnosis of urinary incontinence. Nor has it played a particularly useful role in predicting poor outcome after incontinence surgery.

Imaging

Radiology

We generally reserve radiological studies for evaluation of potential operative complications and to assess the upper urinary tract in patients in whom we suspect that congenital or iatrogenic ureteral abnormalities might contribute to their symptoms. Plain abdominal films can screen for upper tract stones and soft tissue and bony abnormalities. An intravenous pyelogram may detect duplicated or ectopic ureters and ureterovaginal fistulae.

Fluoroscopy

These techniques permit real-time assessment of the lower urinary tract. A voiding cystourethrogram permits evaluation of the bladder and urethra. Bladder and pelvic floor relaxation can be assessed when the patient is asked to empty her bladder of the radio-opaque dye during fluoroscopy. This may assist in identification of vesicovaginal fistula and urethral diverticula. It may also detect vesicoureteral reflux.

Ultrasound

Ultrasound can be used as a non-invasive means to measure postvoid residual volume. It has been used to measure bladder neck mobility and can detect bladder and urethral diverticula. It is also an excellent tool for detecting hydronephrosis and hydroureter. Transrectal ultrasound has also evolved into an invaluable means of assessing the anal sphincter.

CONSERVATIVE TREATMENT

Every subject with GSI should be offered a trial of conservative therapy prior to committing to surgical intervention. Conservative therapies are not only less expensive but generally involve less risk to the patient as well. Furthermore, as has been discussed above, it is sometimes difficult to distinguish between incontinence secondary to detrusor instability and GSI. A small percentage of the time, all the patient's subjective complaints will be resolved due to treatment of her bladder instability. One must also keep in mind that incontinence is for the most part a quality of life problem. Even partial improvement due to conservative therapy may be more than acceptable to the patient.

Behavioural therapies

Two important interventions are patient education and pelvic floor muscle exercises. Subjects who are unable to generate an adequate pelvic floor muscle response may benefit from biofeedback, electrical stimulation or evaluation by a pelvic floor physical therapist. Consideration of habitual behaviours is also important. Smoking and caffeine cessation should be discussed as well as weight loss, fluid intake and the fibre component of the subject's diet.

Pelvic floor muscle exercises (PFE) were introduced by Kegel in the 1950s to address urinary incontinence in women (Kegel 1951). Subjective cure rates have been reported in up to 36% of patients (Elia & Bergman 1993). Rate of improvement is anywhere from 17% to 75% (Mouritsen et al 1991, Urinary Incontinence Guideline Panel 1992). In general one can expect better results in patients who have mild incontinence or who have a weak pelvic floor response. Older women may respond more slowly to exercises and achieve less improvement. There is one study that reported objective findings in the treatment of GSI with PFEs at two different centres. Cure was determined by pad test before and after treatment and occurred at rates of 35% and 50% (Henalla et al 1988).

Patient education is a vital component to PFEs. The strength of pelvic floor muscle contraction must be assessed at the time of pelvic exam. On simple verbal command to squeeze their pelvic floor muscles around the examiner's fingers, many women are unable to do so or they inadvertently contract their abdominal or gluteal muscles. The pelvic exam provides an opportunity to teach the patient which muscles she needs to strengthen. Bump et al (1991) underscored the importance of education in a study in which women were given only verbal or simple written instructions to perform PFEs; 25% of the subjects were doing the exercises incorrectly, despite their perception that they were performing PFEs.

Biofeedback can maximize rehabilitation in patients who have difficulty in performing PFEs after brief instruction.

Biofeedback is any signal, auditory or visual, which tells the patient that she is contracting the correct muscles. Simple verbal affirmation of a good pelvic floor muscle contraction at the time of pelvic exam is a form of biofeedback. More sophisticated forms include perineometers that consist of a rectal or vaginal probe, a visual or auditory analogue signal and abdominal electromyography electrodes. When the patient correctly contracts her pelvic floor an analogue signal through the probe tells her she is utilizing the proper muscles. Similarly, an auditory signal via the EMG tells her to what degree, if any, she is recruiting her abdominal muscles. Biofeedback in addition to PFEs has been shown to yield a better result than PFE alone (Burns et al 1990).

Weighted vaginal cones represent another form of bio-feedback (Fig. 52.1). The patient places the lightest cone in the vagina for 15 minutes twice daily and goes about her normal activities. She is forced to contract her pelvic floor muscles to keep the cone from falling out of her vagina. When this weight becomes easy to manage she exchanges this cone for the next heaviest. Objective assessment of this intervention has shown improvement or cure in 70% (Peattie et al 1988).

Patients who are unable to perform PFEs despite biofeedback may be candidates for functional electrical stimulation. Direct mechanical stimulation of the pudendal nerve is delivered by either vaginal or rectal probe, causing contraction of the pelvic floor musculature. Eriksen & Eik-Nes (1989) and Meyer et al (1992) utilized this technique followed by biofeedback and reported success rates of 56–95% in patients with mild to moderate GSI. Recently this intervention has been adapted to a specially designed chair that stimulates the pelvic floor. The chair, produced by Neotonus Incorporated, produces what the company calls Extracorporeal Magnetic Innervation (ExMI™) which non-invasively builds pelvic floor muscle strength and endurance. Treatment involves subjects sitting fully clothed in the chair for 20 minutes twice weekly for 2 months. This device has won praise due to the significant improvement in patient comfort.

Devices

An assortment of vaginal and urethral devices have been marketed to treat GSI. The urethral devices function to occlude the urethra and are placed either within the urethra or over the external meatus. The primary drawbacks to these devices are the risk of infection and patient discomfort. There are also several vaginal devices: pessaries, tampons and bladder neck support prostheses. The vaginal devices all function in primarily the same way: to provide preferential support to the bladder neck. As long as the subject does not object or find it uncomfortable to keep a device in the vagina they may be quite beneficial. Of course, the device must be removed periodically and cleaned and the patient must have regular follow-up to check for irritation or erosion of the vaginal wall.

Pharmacotherapy

As noted above, GSI is generally not very amenable to pharmacologic therapy. In some cases of mild urinary incontinence, however, the patient may gain significant benefit with use of a medication. Medicines to treat GSI all act to increase urethral resistance. We generally give patients desirous of non-surgical treatment a trial of anticholinergic therapy to treat as well as to rule out any component of detrusor instability.

The sympathetic nervous system acts at the detrusor via β-adrenergic receptors to inhibit contraction and at the bladder neck and proximal urethra via α-adrenergic receptors to stimulate contraction. The net result is prevention of micturition. Pseudoephedrine, ephedrine, norephedrine and phenylpropanolamine are all α-agonists. They can be given, when not medically contraindicated, in an attempt to increase urethral tone. They may aggravate or cause hypertension, hyperthyroidism, cardiac arrhythmias and angina and must be used cautiously in patients at risk for these disorders. Phenylpropanolamine has also been known to rarely cause seizure, stroke and death. Various trials of these medications report reduction of urinary leakage in 55–70% of subjects (Diokno & Taub 1975, EK et al 1978). Appropriate dosages are listed in Table 52.2.

Imipramine (Tofranil) is a tricyclic antidepressant that has both α-agonist and anticholinergic effects. It increases urethral tone and causes relaxation of the detrusor. It therefore is the first-line pharmacologic agent in the treatment of mixed urinary incontinence. Patients taking MAO inhibitors and subjects with narrow-angle glaucoma, hypertension, angina, hyperthyroidism, cardiac arrhythmia or other contraindication to tricyclic therapy should not be offered this medication. One study of 21 patients with GSI on imipramine found a 71% cure rate and improvements in functional urethral length and maximal urethral closure pressure (Gilja et al 1984).

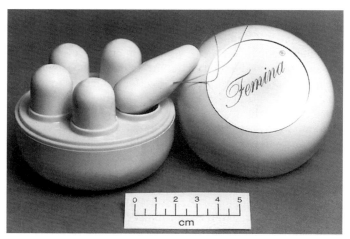

Fig. 52.1   Vaginal cones (Colgate Medical).

Table 52.2   Pharmacologic therapy for genuine stress incontinence

Drug	Dose
Ephedrine	15–30 mg po tid/qid
Pseudoephedrine	30–60 mg po tid/qid
Norephedrine	100 mg po bid
Phenylpropanolamine	25–75 mg po bid/tid
Imipramine	10–25 mg po qd/tid
Oestrogen	0.3–1.25 mg po qd
	2–4 g vaginally 3–7 times/week

Because of oestrogen's beneficial effects in the vagina and urethra it is an attractive therapeutic entity to apply to the treatment of GSI. While several non-randomized studies initially showed improvement in both stress and urge incontinence, randomized trials have had very mixed results (Fantl et al 1994, 1996, Walter et al 1990). When giving oestrogen, orally or vaginally, patients must be made aware of the risks and benefits of this medication including risk of breast/uterine cancer, venous thrombosis, liver disease and gallstones. When giving oestrogen vaginally to a woman with a uterus, concomitant progesterone therapy must also be administered.

SURGICAL TREATMENT

Aims

The aim of any surgical procedure for urinary incontinence should be to correct whatever anatomic defect is responsible for the loss of urine. Primarily, this comes down to three of the theories described above: descent of the bladder neck outside the sphere of intra-abdominal pressure, intrinsic sphincteric weakness or loss of urethral support. One must also be mindful not to be too aggressive lest the unfortunate outcomes of voiding dysfunction or urinary retention occur. Of course, the surgeon must also be cognizant of the unique challenges provided by each individual patient: medical/surgical history, age, severity of symptoms and concurrence of prolapse or other related conditions.

Choice of surgery

Taking the above concerns into account, one must decide whether an abdominal or vaginal approach is best. The untoward side-effects of each operation must also be considered. As has been alluded to above, clinical opinion continues to play a large role in choice of operation. While transvaginal needle suspension and Kelly plication have fallen out of favour due to their inability to provide lasting cure, they still may play an important role in certain carefully selected patients.

The primary approach to stress incontinence today usually involves a choice between bladder neck suspension procedures and sling operations. Gynaecologists have traditionally reserved sling operations for cases of recurrent incontinence or in patients with evidence of obvious ISD, while many urologists employ the sling procedure as a primary treatment of GSI. From a theoretical standpoint, the major drawback of sling procedures has been concern for voiding dysfunction caused by the obstructive nature of the sling operation. In comparison, patients undergoing retropubic suspension are not immune to voiding dysfunction and may be at risk for development of pelvic organ prolapse due to the preferential support given to the anterior vaginal compartment.

In general, with concomitant prolapse, we favour a vaginal route, which means a type of sling procedure. If the patient is undergoing an abdominal procedure for any reason we typically perform a Burch urethropexy, an operation of which the long-term complications and cure rates are known. This procedure can also be performed laparoscopically if appropriate.

The advantages and disadvantages of several operations for GSI are reviewed below.

Useful operations for incontinence

There are several prospective randomized controlled trials that have been performed that have shaped the current surgical approach to GSI. In 1979, Stanton and Cardozo compared the Burch colposuspension procedure to anterior colporrhaphy and found the Burch to be superior, with cure rates at 6 months of 84% and 36% respectively. A similar study by Kammerer-Doak et al in 1999 had equivalent findings. Bergman & Elia (1995) compared the Burch, anterior colporrhaphy and Stamey needle suspension with 5-year follow-up and again found the Burch to be superior. The Burch and Marshall–Marchetti–Krantz (MMK) operations were compared prospectively in randomized fashion by Colombo et al (1994). Although the success rate in the Burch group was higher the difference did not reach statistical significance. Currently, we feel the retropubic urethropexy remains the gold standard operation for GSI, in large part because of the results of such randomized trials and the existence of long-term data on cure and complication rates.

Retropubic urethropexy

The Burch procedure was developed as a modification of the MMK procedure in 1961. These are two of the most commonly performed surgeries for urinary incontinence. Their purpose is to return the bladder neck to an intra-abdominal location so that it encounters the same transmural pressure as the bladder. As noted above, low urethral closure pressure (<20 cmH$_2$O) has been shown to be a risk factor for failure of these operations, but pre- and post-operative urethral pressure studies have failed to support this concept (Faysal et al 1981, Koonings et al 1990, Sand et al 1987, Versi et al 1986).

In 1949, Marshall et al reported the empirical observation that suturing the periurethral tissues to the pubic bone alleviated stress urinary incontinence (Fig. 52.2). The original description of the operation reported using number 1 chromic suture, but the procedure is now usually performed with a permanent suture. The patient is placed into the dorsal lithotomy position to permit access to the vagina. A Pfannenstiel incision is made and the rectus abdominis is divided along its midline raphe. The surgeon's hand is then passed beneath the rectus muscles above the peritoneum in the direction of the pubic symphysis; blunt dissection in this fashion opens the retropubic space. The operation can be performed with the peritoneum opened or closed. Once the retropubic space is exposed, the bladder neck is identified with the operator's non-dominant hand in the vagina using the Foley balloon as a guide. A Kitner or sponge stick is then used to sweep the fatty and vascular tissue off the periurethral fascia while the vaginal fingers elevate the anterior vagina (Fig. 52.3a). Keeping the vaginal fingers elevated, the surgeon is then able to take a full-thickness figure-of-eight bite of tissue (excluding the vaginal mucosa if possible) just lateral to the urethrovesical junction (Fig. 52.3b inset). This suture is then passed through the periosteum or fibrocartilage of the pubic bone and tied in such fashion that the bladder neck is barely brought in contact with

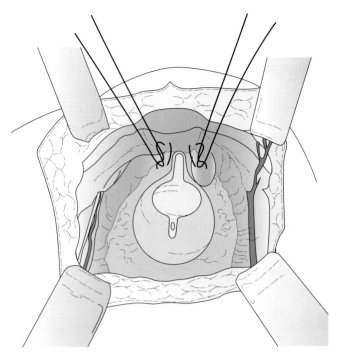

Fig. 52.2   Marshall–Marchetti–Krantz procedure. One suture is placed bilaterally at the level of the bladder neck and then into the periosteum of the pubic symphysis (reproduced with permission from Karram MM, Baggish MS (eds) 2001 Atlas of pelvic anatomy and gynecologic surgery. Harcourt. New York.

the symphysis. A similar suture is then placed on the opposite side.

The Burch procedure is performed in much the same fashion as the MMK. The retropubic space is developed and exposed and permanent suture is placed on both sides of the bladder neck. In this case two sutures are placed on both sides of the bladder neck, one 2 cm lateral to the urethrovesical junction and the other 2 cm lateral to the proximal urethra. Each suture is then passed through the ipsilateral iliopectineal ligament on the posterolateral surface of the pubic bone (Fig. 52.3B). When the sutures are tied the surgeon should be able to pass two fingers between the pubic bone and the urethra.

Cure rates of the retropubic procedures are 65–90% at 1–10 years (Alcalay et al 1995, Colombo et al 1994). Alcalay et al (1995) reported on Burch patients followed for 10–20 years and found that the cure rate for this procedure is approximately 90% at 1 year, but then declines to approximately 70% at 10 years where the cure rate appears to remain thereafter. Complications of both procedures include post operative voiding dysfunction (5–27%), infection, haemorrhage, injury to bladder/urethra/ureter and pelvic organ prolapse (Alcalay et al 1995, Corneua 1997). The MMK also has a 2.5% incidence of osteitis pubis. Because of the risk of injury to the bladder and adjoining structures it is recommended that cystoscopy be performed after both of these procedures.

In 1991 Vancaillie and Schuessler described a laparoscopic approach for Burch colposuspension. Proposed advantages ascribed to this operation over the open technique are minimal invasiveness and lower cost. Cure rates and complication rates

are reported to be 60–91% and 0–25% respectively (Paraiso et al 1999). A single randomized prospective study found the open technique to be superior, but the author had only performed 10 laparoscopic Burch procedures prior to starting the study and it has been reported that the learning curve for this operation is about 35 cases (Burton 1997, Lose 1998). While studies have shown the hospital stay to be shorter, costs, presumably due to laparoscopic equipment and operative time, have not been lower than the open technique (Kohli et al 1997).

Sling operations

Sling operations were initially described more than 100 years ago. They have evolved over the decades as surgeons have attempted to support the urethra and augment urethral sphincter tone. Recent studies, however, have not shown urethral closure pressure to increase significantly after sling procedures (Enzelsberger et al 1996, Rottenberg et al 1985). It is more likely that these operations succeed in maintaining continence by occluding the urethra during increases in intra-abdominal pressure. There is a single prospective randomized trial comparing the sling procedures to MMK, in which both were shown to have similarly excellent results (Henriksson & Ulmsten 1978). Because of their occlusive nature, sling procedures are generally performed in more severe or recurrent cases of GSI. Typically, patients selected to undergo a sling have a low pressure urethra.

Slings are performed with the patient in the dorsolithotomy position. A small horizontal incision is made approximately 2 cm above the pubic symphysis. The subcutaneous fat is dissected, providing visualization of the rectus fascia. If rectus fascia is to be harvested from the patient the incision may need to be longer. An alternative source of sling material is fascia lata that is obtained from the patient's thigh by excision or the use of a fascial stripper (Fig. 52.4). Once a 4 × 4 cm piece (for a patch-type sling) or two 2 × 8 cm portions (which are sewn end to end to create a long enough graft for a full-length sling) of fascia have been excised, the defect is closed with delayed absorbable suture. If the patient permits, cadaveric donor fascia can be used. It saves time, is abundant and risk is minimal. The fascia is kept in saline until it is required.

Attention is then turned to the perineum where a midline anterior vaginal incision is made. The vaginal wall is dissected off the underlying bladder and urethra. This dissection is continued laterally to both sides of the bladder neck until the underside of the pubic symphysis is encountered. At this point a curved instrument such as a Kelly clamp or Stamey needle is passed from the abdominal incision, through the rectus fascia just above the symphysis. It traverses uneventfully through the retropubic space by keeping the instrument in constant contact with the back of the pubic bone, finally emerging into the vagina where the vaginal dissection was carried to the underside of the pubic bone. The entry of the instrument into the vaginal dissection is assisted by placing a vaginal finger lateral to the bladder neck along the underside of the symphysis. The instrument is aimed at this finger and guided into the vagina. The same procedure is repeated on the other side. Cystoscopy should be performed after each passage of the instrument to ensure that no injury to the bladder has occurred.

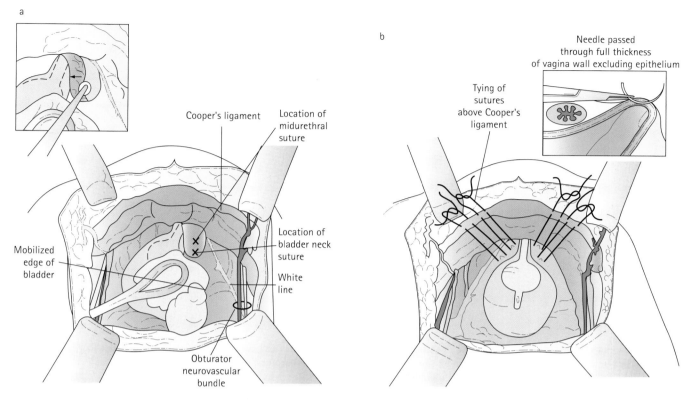

Fig. 52.3 **a** Burch colposuspension. The bladder is gently mobilized to the opposite side utilizing sponge sticks. The anterior vaginal wall is elevated by the middle finger of the surgeon's non-dominant hand. The position of the sutures should be at least 2 cm lateral to the proximal urethra and bladder neck. Xs mark the ideal placement of the Burch colposuspension sutures. Inset: The anterior vaginal wall on the right side is being elevated by a vaginal finger. A Kitner is passed on top of the finger mobilizing the fat medially. **b** Sutures have been appropriately placed on each side of the proximal urethra and bladder neck. Note figure-of-eight bites are taken through the vagina. Double-armed sutures are utilized so the end of each suture can be brought up through the ipsilateral Cooper's ligament, thus allowing the sutures to be tied above the ligament. Inset: Detail of the suture being placed over the surgeon's vaginal finger. Note suture should include full-thickness vaginal wall excluding the epithelium (reproduced with permission from Karram MM, Baggish MS (eds) 2001 Atlas of pelvic anatomy and gynecologic surgery: Harcourt, New York.

When placing a full-length sling the centre portion of the graft is sewn in place at the level of the bladder neck with an absorbable suture. Each end of the sling is then pulled up through the retropubic space using the previously passed instruments (Fig. 52.5). Once the end of the graft is above the level of the abdominal rectus fascia it is either sewn to the fascia on either side or in the midline to the other end of the graft. For patch slings, the tissue is folded or trimmed to the correct size then sewn in place at the bladder neck (Fig. 52.6). A permanent suture is then fixed to either side of the patch and the ends are pulled up through the retropubic space to the abdominal incision as described for the full-length sling. Similarly, the ends of the permanent suture can be tied to one another across the midline. Alternatively, the Stamey needle can be passed through the rectus fascia in two different locations on both sides (a total of four passes) and each end of the permanent suture can be brought up through its own tract. The two left ends are tied to one another on the left side and the two right ends tied on the right.

The most challenging part of a sling procedure is determining the correct amount of tension to apply. The balance one tries to obtain is continence without creating postoperative voiding dysfunction. In general, the sling should be tied under as little tension as possible. This can be accomplished by placing a right angle clamp between the sling and the bladder neck at the time when the abdominal portion of the graft is being tied. Some advocate using a Q-tip to assist in tightening the sling until an angle of 0° to + 10° is achieved. Others perform this portion of the procedure with a cystoscope in place and still others simply fill the bladder and adjust the sling until there is no leakage. Unfortunately, there is no substitute for experience when it comes to performing this part of the procedure.

Cure rates with slings are reported to be 70–95% (Iosif 1983, Morgan et al 1985). It should be noted that it is difficult to assess results of sling procedures because there is so much variation in technique and materials used. Complications are similar to retropubic procedures, including postoperative voiding dysfunction/retention (up to 30%), detrusor instability/urgency/frequency (up to 50%), haemorrhage, infection, injury to the bladder and adjoining structures, fistula formation and nerve entrapment. If synthetic mesh is used for the sling material there is also a risk of mesh erosion (Jarvis 1994, Kohli & Karram 1994).

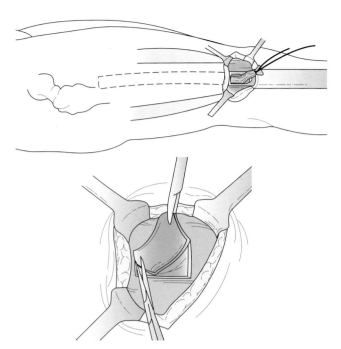

Fig. 52.4 Techniques for obtaining fascia for sling operations. **a** Obtaining fascia lata with a vein stripper. **b** Excising a small piece of fascia lata from just above the knee for a patch sling (reproduced with permission from Karram MM, Walters MD (eds) 1999 Urogynecology and reconstructive pelvic surgery, 2nd edn. Mosby, St Louis.

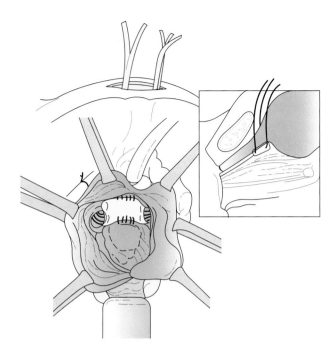

Fig. 52.6 Patch sling. Permanent suture, which is fixed to both sides of the suburethral patch, is passed from the vagina, through the space of Retzius on both sides of the bladder neck and fixed to the anterior rectus fascia (reproduced with permission from Karram MM, Walters MD (eds) 1999 Urogynecology and reconstructive pelvic surgery, 2nd edn. Mosby, St Louis.

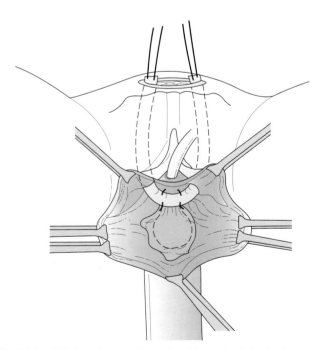

Fig. 52.5 Full-length suburethral sling. The ends of the fascia are fixed to the anterior rectus fascia (reproduced with permission from Karram MM, Walters MD (eds) 1999 Urogynecology and reconstructive pelvic surgery, 2nd edn. Mosby, St Louis.

In 1998 Nilsson published some of his initial results with an operation called tension-free vaginal tape (TVT) (Fig. 52.7). This procedure is a type of suburethral sling. A Prolene tape is passed vaginally to either side of the midurethra with specially designed needles. Minimal dissection is required and the tape is not sutured to any structure and is not under tension – hence the name. The mechanism by which this operation is believed to achieve continence is improved midurethral support. Success rates are reported to be 85–90% at 3 years (Nilsson 1998, Ulmsten et al 1998). There have been isolated cases of erosion of the Prolene tape. The minimal invasiveness, short operative time and high cure rate of this operation make it an attractive surgical option for GSI. Many surgeons are currently using the TVT as a primary operation for incontinence. More long-term and comparative data are needed.

Non-primary operations for incontinence

The success of retropubic suspensions and sling procedures makes these operations the clear choices for the first-line surgical approach to GSI. There are several other operations, however, which still merit mention.

Periurethral injection is a simple technique that may be performed in the office. It can be used in cases of recurrent GSI and is a good option for patients with contraindications to surgery. A bulking agent (collagen, Macroplastique or a newer agent called Durasphere™) is injected transurethrally via an operative cystourethroscope into the urethral submucosa at the bladder neck (Fig. 52.8). Alternatively a periurethral approach

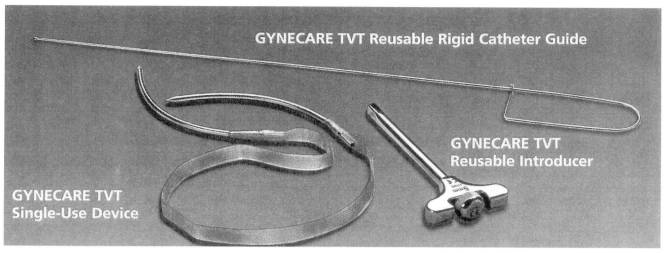

Fig. 52.7 Tension-free vaginal tape. The needles are passed to either side of the midurethra with the help of the removable handle. Also shown is the catheter guide that is used during passing of the tape to divert the bladder neck away from the path of the needle (courtesy of Ethicon Inc.).

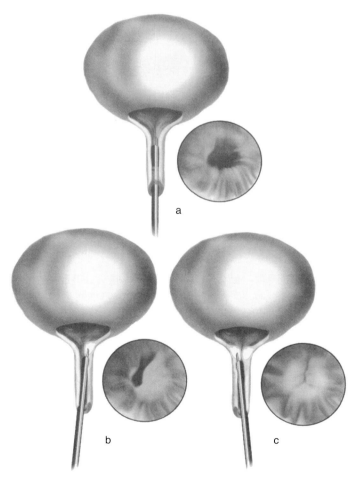

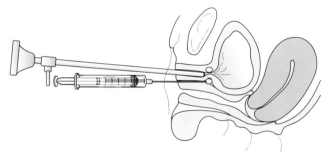

Fig. 52.9 Technique for periurethral injection of urethral bulking agents (reproduced with permission from Karram MM, Walters MD (eds) 1999 Urogynecology and reconstructive pelvic surgery, 2nd edn. Mosby, St Louis).

Fig. 52.8 Technique for transurethral injection of urethral bulking agents. **a** Bladder neck open prior to injection. **b** Submucosal placement of needle at one site partially closes bladder neck. **c** Complete closure of bladder neck at completion of the procedure (reproduced with permission from Karram MM, Walters MD (eds) 1999 Urogynecology and reconstructive pelvic surgery, 2nd edn. Mosby, St Louis).

may be utilized in which the needle is passed alongside the urethra and injection is aided with the use of a separate urethroscope (Fig. 52.9). Small amounts are injected in such a fashion that a wheal is formed just beneath the mucosa. Usually several wheals are made until the mucosa on one side of the bladder neck just touches the mucosa on the opposite side. Success rates are reported to be 63–90% with both methods (Flora 1997). Retrospective study has shown that co-existing urethral hypermobility does not decrease cure rates (Steele et al 2000). Less than 5% of patients will exhibit a hypersensitivity response to collagen, therefore skin testing is indicated 30 days prior to injection. Skin testing is not required with Macroplastique or Durasphere™. Other complications include retention requiring temporary self-catheterization, bleeding and infection. Collagen unfortunately begins to degrade after about 3 months, thus patients will typically require subsequent injections. Macroplastique and Durasphere™ are not reabsorbed, but long-term studies to evaluate cure rate have not been done.

Anterior colporrhaphy has been described as an anti-incontinence procedure for decades. It is believed to achieve

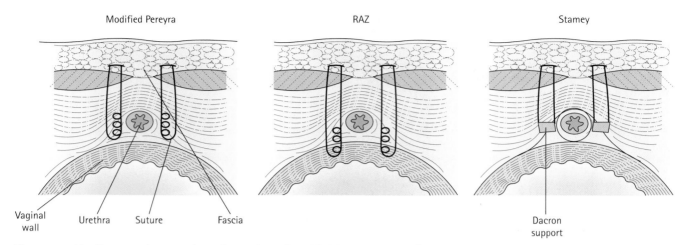

Fig. 52.10   Needle suspension procedures. Comparison of modified Pereyra, Raz and Stamey operations: coronal section of the bladder neck and surrounding tissues. VW, vaginal wall; U, urethra; S, suture; DS, Dacron support; F, fascia.

continence by preferentially supporting the bladder neck. Unfortunately, long-term cure rates are only 30–35% (Bergman & Elia 1995, Kammerer–Doak et al 1999, Stanton & Cardozo 1979). The operation does have the advantage of little risk for postoperative voiding dysfunction and can be performed under local anaesthesia if needed.

Needle suspension procedures (Pereyra, Stamey and Raz) were at one time very popular (Fig. 52.10). Randomized controlled trials have shown them to be less effective than either the retropubic suspensions or slings (Bergman & Elia 1995, Hilton 1989). They can be done quite quickly under local anaesthesia, however, and therefore may be viable choices in the case of poor operative candidates.

The paravaginal repair is a surgery designed to repair a specific lateral support defect resulting in a cystocoele. In this operation the endopelvic fascia, which normally supports the bladder and has been found to be torn away from the arcus tendineus fascia pelvis (white line of the pelvis), is reattached to the pelvic side wall. It was noted to make some women continent, presumably by elevation of the bladder neck. Unfortunately, the results are not lasting. In a randomized trial versus the Burch procedure, the paravaginal repair was clearly inferior in treating GSI (Colombo et al 1996). In patients with paravaginal defects and GSI, the defect should be repaired and Burch colposuspension sutures should be placed (Fig. 52.11).

The artificial sphincter is an implantable device that occludes the urethra, but which can be voluntarily opened by the patient when she desires to empty her bladder (Fig. 52.12). The procedure is more complex than other incontinence operations and patients must have good manual dexterity to be candidates. While success rates are high (80–100%), device malfunction (21%), infection and erosion are significant concerns (Kohli & Karram 1999, Valaitis & Stanton 1995).

EVALUATION OF TREATMENT: QUALITY OF LIFE

In our zeal to report findings objectively, it is easy to forget that the physician's and patient's definitions of cure might not be the same and that it is really the patient's desires that need to

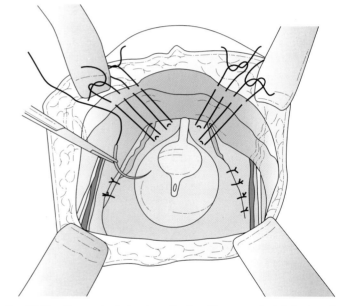

Fig. 52.11   Paravaginal plus. In patients with paravaginal defects and stress urinary incontinence the paravaginal defects are repaired and then Burch colposuspension sutures are placed (reproduced with permission from Karram MM, Baggish MS (eds) 2001 Atlas of pelvic anatomy and gynecologic surgery. Harcourt, New York).

be satisfied. The postoperative subject who presents to the office stating that she had daily loss of large amounts of urine prior to her anti-incontinence procedure, but now only leaks a few drops when she sneezes or coughs might not be considered cured by objective standards. In her mind, however, she may be cured. When one considers the possible untoward effects of a more aggressive repair, one realizes that this patient has likely struck the perfect balance.

Complete evaluation of treatment techniques for incontinence clearly requires some subjective considerations, yet there still must be some way of standardizing these tools (Filbeck et al 1999). One such approach is quality of life assessment. There are several tools that have been designed, applied to clinical

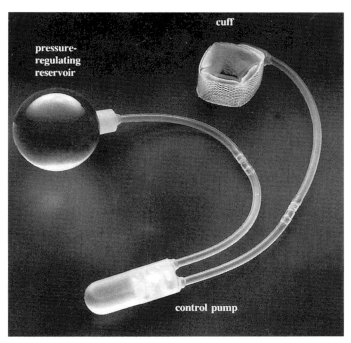

Fig. 52.12 AMS 800 artificial urinary sphincter. Note small button on control pump for activation and deactivation of device (American Medical Systems).

use and tested for reproducibility. We use the Incontinence Impact Questionnaire (IIQ-7) and the Urogenital Distress Inventory (UDI-6) in our practice (see Table 52.1). These are 7- and 6-question surveys respectively, which can be filled out by the patient in less than 5 minutes. Studies have shown these tools to be valid and strongly correlated with longer questionnaires which otherwise would be impractical for clinical use (Uebersax et al 1995). We have the patients complete these surveys before and after treatment. Each patient is then her own control and we get a much clearer sense of the life impact that the treatment has afforded her.

MANAGEMENT OF RECURRENT INCONTINENCE

Patients who present postoperatively with persistent troublesome urinary incontinence will typically have one of the following aetiologies: cystitis, de novo urge incontinence, fistula or simple operative failure. We evaluate such patients with urine culture and empiric anticholinergic medication to address the first two causes. Subjects whose symptoms persist beyond 6–8 weeks, when any inflammation present should be resolved, undergo a complete evaluation as described above, including urodynamics and cystourethroscopy. These latter studies will identify detrusor instability and will help determine if the aetiology is loss of anatomic support or an intrinsic problem with the urethral sphincter. Such studies will also rule out fistula or iatrogenic injury to the lower urinary tract. If the urethra is well supported, we would then consider injection with a urethral bulking agent. Classically these patients will have a fixed, scarred, low-pressure urethra. Some form of sling operation would be the procedure of choice if recurrent urethral hypermobility is noted.

CONCLUSION

It is apparent that the exact aetiology of GSI cannot be determined in every case, thus making the selection of operation less straightforward. For this reason, and because every surgical intervention has its own undesired effects, conservative therapies should be attempted first. If this approach fails surgery should be offered based on the best evidence-based data available. In most cases this will be a retropubic suspension or sling procedure. However, one must still further tailor the treatment to each individual case, taking into consideration urodynamic findings, age and medical history. Assessment by objective methods must be enhanced by subjective quality of life measurements.

KEY POINTS

1. Urethral sphincter incompetence (genuine stress incontinence) has multiple aetiologies including loss of support of the bladder neck, loss of urethral support and inadequate urethral pressure.
2. It is possible that other mechanisms, yet to be elucidated, may exist to explain some cases of urethral sphincter incompetence.
3. There are multiple risk factors to the development of this disorder including parturition, advanced age, oestrogen deficiency, obesity and loss of pelvic tissue support.
4. Stress incontinence is not limited to the elderly, occuring in up to 50% of women aged 17–25 years.
5. Approximately 30% of women with urinary incontinence will have a mixed aetiology for their urine loss.
6. The diagnosis of stress urinary incontinence requires careful consideration, often involving several diagnostic tests, as relying on symptoms alone will lead to misdiagnosis and improper treatment in up to 25% of subjects.
7. All patients should be given a trial of conservative measures. These interventions may improve symptoms in up to 75% of patients. Such measures require significant and concerted efforts on the part of the subject and the caregiver.
8. Patients who are not cured by conservative treatments or whose quality of life is not adequately improved should be offered surgical treatment for their stress urinary incontinence based on urodynamic data, concomitant pathology, age and medical history.
9. The risks and untoward effects of the surgical options must be discussed in detail with the patient.
10. Patients with persistent recurrent stress urinary incontinence must be thoroughly evaluated to rule out complications of their prior incontinence operation. Choice of operation in these cases is based on degree of urethral support.

REFERENCES

Abrams P, Blaivas JG, Stanton SL et al 1988 The standardization of terminology of lower tract function. Scandinavian Journal of Urology and Nephrology 114(suppl):5

Alcalay M, Monga A, Stanton SL 1995 Burch colposuspension: a 10–20 year follow up. British Journal of Obstetrics and Gynaecology 102:740–745

Bailey KV 1956 Clinical investigation into uterine prolapse with stress incontinence. Journal of Obstetrics and Gynaecology of the British Empire 63:663–676

Bergman A, Elia G 1995 Three surgical procedures for genuine stress incontinence: five-year follow-up of a prospective randomized study. American Journal of Obstetrics and Gynecology 173:66–71

Bergman A, Koonings PP, Ballard CA 1989 Negative Q-tip test as a risk factor for failed incontinence surgery in women. Journal of Reproductive Medicine 34:193–197

Bowen LW, Sand PK, Ostergard DR, Franti CE 1989 Unsuccessful Burch retropubic urethropexy: a case-controlled urodynamic study. American Journal of Obstetrics and Gynecology 160:452–458

Bump RC, Hurt WG, Fantl JA, Wyman JF 1991 Assessment of Kegel pelvic floor muscle exercise performance after brief verbal instruction. American Journal of Obstetrics and Gynecology 165:322

Bump RC, Sugerman HJ, Fantl JA et al 1992 Obesity and lower urinary tract function in women: effect of surgically induced weight loss. American Journal of Obstetrics and Gynecology 167:392

Burns PA, Pranikoff K, Nochajski T et al 1990 Treatment of stress incontinence with pelvic floor exercises and biofeedback. Journal of the American Geriatric Society 38:341

Burton G 1997 A randomized comparison of laparoscopic and open colposuspension Neurourology and Urodynamics 16:497–498

Colombo M, Milani R, Vitobello D, Maggioni A 1996 A randomized comparison of Burch colposuspension and abdominal paravaginal defect repair for female stress urinary incontinence. American Journal of Obstetrics and Gynecology 175:78–84

Colombo M, Scalambrino S, Maggioni A, Milani R 1994 Burch colposuspension versus modified Marshall–Marchetti–Krantz urethropexy for primary genuine stress urinary incontinence: a prospective, randomized clinical trial. American Journal of Obstetrics and Gynecology 171:1573–1579

Cornella JL 1997 Long-term complications of retropubic urethropexy: a review and clinical opinion. Association of Urogenital Surgeons Quarterly Report 15:1

DeLancey JOL 1997 The pathophysiology of stress urinary incontinence in women and its implications for surgical treatment. World Journal of Urology 15:268–274

Diokno A, Taub M 1975 Ephedrine in treatment of urinary incontinence. Urology 5:624

Diokno AC, Brown MB, Brock BM et al 1989 Prevalence and outcome of surgery for female incontinence. Urology 33:285–290

Ek A, Andersson KE, Gullberg B et al 1978 The effects of long-term treatment with norephedrine on stress incontinence and urethral closure pressure profile. Scandinavian Journal of Urology and Nephrology 12:105

Elia G, Bergman A 1993 Pelvic muscle exercises: when do they work? Obstetrics and Gynecology 81:283–286

Enhorning G 1961 Simultaneous recording of intraurethral and intravesical pressure: a study of urethral closure and stress incontinent women. Acta Chirurgica Scandinavica 276(Suppl):1–68

Enzelsberger H, Helmer H, Schatten C 1996 Comparison of Burch and lyodura sling procedures for repair of unsuccessful incontinence surgery. Obstetrics and Gynecology 88:252–265

Eriksen BC, Eik-Nes SH 1989 Long-term electrostimulation of pelvic floor: primary therapy in female stress incontinence? Urology International 49:90

Fantl JA, Bump RC, Robinson D et al 1996 Efficacy of estrogen supplementation in the treatment of urinary incontinence. The Continence Program for Women Research Group. Obstetrics and Gynecology 88:745

Fantl JA, Cardozo L, McClish DK 1994 Estrogen therapy in the management of urinary incontinence in postmenopausal women: a meta-analysis. First report of the Hormones and Urogenital Therapy Committee. Obstetrics and Gynecology 83:12

Faysal MH, Constantinou CE, Rother LF, Govan DE 1981 The impact of bladder neck suspension on the resting and stress urethral pressure profile: a prospective study comparing controls with incontinent patients preoperatively and postoperatively. Urology 125:55–60

Fedorkow DM, Sand PK, Retzky SS, Johnson DC 1995 The cotton swab test, receiver-operating characteristic curves. Journal of Reproductive Medicine 40:42–46

Filbeck T, Ullrich T, Pichlmeier U et al 1999 Correlation of persistent stress urinary incontinence with quality of life after suspension procedures: is continence the only decisive postoperative criterion of success? Urology 54:247–251

Flora R 1997 Urethral bulking agents: periurethral versus transurethral approach. Issues in Incontinence 4:3–8

Fonda D, Brimage PJ, d'Astoli M 1993 Simple screening for urinary incontinence in the elderly: comparison of simple and multichannel cystometry. Urology 42:536–540

Frewen WK 1971 Foley catheter urethrography in stress incontinence. Journal of Obstetrics and Gynaecology of the British Commonwealth 78:660–663

Gilja I, Radej M, Kovacic M et al 1984 Conservative treatment of female stress incontinence with imipramine. Journal of Urology 132:909

Green TH 1962 Development of a plan for the diagnosis and treatment of urinary stress incontinence. American Journal of Obstetrics and Gynecology 83:632–648

Henalla SM, Kirwan P, Castleden CM et al 1988 The effect of pelvic floor exercises in the treatment of genuine urinary stress incontinence in women at two hospitals. British Journal Obstetrics and Gynaecology 95:602–606

Henriksson L, Ulmsten U 1978 A urodynamic evaluation of the effects of abdominal urethrocystopexy and vaginal sling urethroplasty in women with stress incontinence. American Journal of Obstetrics and Gynecology 131:77–82

Hilton P 1989 A clinical and urodynamic study comparing the Stamey bladder neck suspension and suburethral sling procedures in the treatment of genuine stress incontinence. British Journal of Obstetrics and Gynaecology 96:213–220

Hutch JA 1967 A new theory of the anatomy of the internal urinary sphincter and the physiology of micturition. Obstetrics and Gynecology 30:309–317

Iosif CF, Batra S, EK A 1981 Estrogen receptors in the human female lower urinary tract. American Journal of Obstetrics and Gynecology 141:817

Iosif CS 1983 Results of various operations for urinary stress incontinence. Archives of Gynecology 233:93–100

James MJ, Jackson S, Shepard A, Abrams P 1999 Pure stress leakage symptomatology: is it safe to discount detrusor instability? British Journal of Obstetrics and Gynaecology 106:1255–1258

Jarvis GJ 1994 Surgery for genuine stress incontinence. British Journal of Obstetrics and Gynaecology 101:371–374

Jensen JK, Nielson R, Ostergard DR 1994 The role of patient history in the diagnosis of urinary incontinence. Obstetrics and Gynecology 83:904–909

Kammerer-Doak DN, Dorin MH, Rogers RG, Cousin MO 1999 A randomized trial of Burch retropubic urethropexy and anterior colporrhaphy for stress urinary incontinence. Obstetrics and Gynecology 93:75–78

Karram MM, Bhatia NN 1988 The Q-tip test: standardization of the technique and its interpretation in women with urinary incontinence. Obstetrics and Gynecology 71:807–811

Karram MM, Bhatia NN 1989 Management of coexistent stress and urge urinary incontinence. Obstetrics and Gynecology 73:4–7

Kegel AM 1951 Physiologic therapy for urinary stress incontinence. JAMA 146:915

Kohli N, Jacobs PA, Sze EHM et al 1997 Open compared with laparoscopic approach to Burch colposuspension: a cost analysis. Obstetrics and Gynecology 90:411–415

Kohli N, Karram MM 1999 Surgery for geniune stress incontinence. In: Karram MM, Walters MD (eds) Urogynecology and reconstructive pelvic surgery 2nd edn. Mosby, St Louis

Koonings PP, Bergman A, Ballard CA 1990 Low urethral pressure and stress urinary incontinence in women: risk factor for failed retropubic surgical procedure. Urology 36:245–248

Kromann-Anderson B, Jakobson H, Thorup Anderson J 1989 Pad-weighing tests: a literature survey on test accuracy and reproductibility. Neurourology and Urodynamics 8:237–242

Lose G 1998 Laparoscopic Burch colposuspension. Acta Obstetrica and Gynecologia Scandinavica 77 (suppl) 29–33

Marshall VF, Marchetti AA, Krantz KE 1949 The correction of stress incontinence by simple vesicourethral suspension. Surgery, Gynecology and Obstetrics 509–518

Meyer S, Dhenin T, Schmidt N, DeGrandi P 1992 Subjective and objective effects of intravaginal electrical myostimulation and biofeedback in patients with genuine stress urinary incontinence. British Journal of Urology 69:584–588

Mommsen S, Foldspang A 1994 Body mass index and adult female urinary incontinence. World Journal of Urology 12:319

Montz FJ, Stanton SL 1986 Q-tip test in female urinary incontinence. Obstetrics and Gynecology 67:258–260

Morgan JE, Farrow GA, Stewart FE 1985 The Marlex sling operation for the treatment of recurrent stress urinary incontinence: a 16-year review. American Journal of Obstetrics and Gynecology 151:224–226

Mouritsen L, Berild G, Hertz J 1989 Comparison of different methods for quantification of urinary leakage in incontinent women. Neurourology and Urodynamics 8:579–587

Mouritsen L, Frimodt-Moller C, Moller M 1991 Long-term effect of pelvic floor exercises on female urinary incontinence. British Journal of Urology 68:32–37

Nemir A, Middleton RP 1954 Stress incontinence in young nulliparous women. American Journal of Obstetrics and Gynecology 68:1166–1168

Nilsson CG 1998 The tension free vaginal tape procedure (TVT) for treatment of female urinary incontinence. Acta Obstetrica Gynecologica Scandinavica 77 (suppl) 34–37

Norton PA, MacDonald ID, Sedgwick PM, Stanton SL 1988 Distress and delay associated with urinary incontinence-frequency, and urgency in women. British Medical Journal 397:1187–1189

Olsen AL, Smith VJ, Bergstrom JO et al 1997 Epidemiology of surgically managed pelvic organ prolapse and urinary incontinence. Obstetrics and Gynecology 89:501–506

Paraiso MFR, Falcone T, Walters M 1999 Laparoscopic surgery for genuine stress incontinence. International Urogynecology Journal 10:237–247

Peattie AB, Plevnik S, Stanton SL 1988 Vaginal cones: a conservative method of treating genuine stress incontinence. British Journal of Obstetrics and Gynaecology 95:1049–1053

Raz R, Stamm WE 1993 A controlled trial of intravaginal estriol in postmenopausal women with recurrent urinary tract infections. New England Journal of Medicine 329:753

Rottenberg RD, Weil A, Brioschi PA, Bischof P, Krauer F 1985 Urodynamic and clinical assessment of the lyodura sling operation for urinary stress incontinence. British Journal of Obstetrics and Gynaecology 92:829–834

Rud T 1980 Urethral pressure profile in continent women from childhood to old age. Acta Obstetrica et Gynecologica Scandinavica 59:335

Sand PK, Bowen LW, Panganiban R, Ostergard DR 1987 The low pressure urethra as a factor in failed retropubic urethropexy. Obstetrics and Gynecology 69:399–402

Scott JC 1969 Stress incontinence in nulliparous women. Journal of Reproductive Medicine II(2):96–97

Scotti RJ, Myers DL 1993 A comparison of the cough stress test and single-channel cystometry with multichannel urodynamic evaluation in genuine stress incontinence. Obstetrics and Gynecology 81:430–433

Stanton SL, Cardozo LD 1979 A comparison of vaginal and suprapubic surgery in the correction of incontinence due to urethral sphincter incompetence. British Journal of Urology 51:497–499

Steele AC, Kohli N, Karram MM 2000 Periurethral collagen injection for stress incontinence with and without urethral hypermobility. Obstetrics and Gynecology 95:327–331

Sultan AH, Kamm MA, Hudson CN 1994 Pudendal nerve injury during labor: prospective study before and after childbirth. British Journal of Obstetrics and Gynaecology 101:22

Summitt RL, Bent AE, Ostergard DR, Harris TA 1990 Stress incontinence and low urethral closure pressure. Journal of Reproductive Medicine 35:877–880

Sutherst JR, Brown MC 1984 Comparison of single and multichannel cystometry in diagnosing bladder instability. British Medical Journal 9:1720–1722

Uebersax JS, Wyman JF, Shumaker SA et al 1995 Short forms to assess life quality and symptom distress for urinary incontinence in women: the incontinence impact questionnaire and the urogenital distress inventory. Neurourology and Urodynamics 14:131–139

Ulmsten U, Falconer C, Johnson P et al 1998 A multicenter study of tension-free vaginal tape (TVT) for surgical treatment of stress urinary incontinence. International Urogynecology Journal 9:210–213

Urinary Incontinence Guideline Panel 1992 Urinary incontinence in adults: clinical practice guideline. Agency for Healthcare Policy and Research, Public Health and Human Services Rockville, Maryland

Valaitis SR, Stanton SL 1995 Surgery for genuine stress incontinence. Contemporary Obstetrics and Gynaecology 40:65–80

Vancaillie TG, Schuessler W 1991 Laparoscopic bladderneck suspension. Journal of Laparoendoscopic Surgery 1: 169–173

Versi E, Cardozo L, Studd J, Cooper D 1986 Evaluation of urethral pressure profilometry for diagnosis of genuine stress incontinence. World Journal of Urology 4:6–9

Wall LL, Helms M, Peattie AB, Pearce M, Stanton SL 1994a Bladder neck mobility and the outcome of surgery for genuine stress urinary incontinence. Journal of Reproductive Medicine 39:429–435

Wall LL, Wiskind AK, Taylor PA 1994b Simple bladder filling with a cough stress test compared with subtracted cystometry for the diagnosis of urinary incontinence. American Journal of Obstetrics and Gynecology 171: 1472–1479

Walter S, Kjaergaard B, Lose G et al 1990 Stress urinary incontinence in postmenopausal women treated with oral estrogen (estriol) and alpha-adrenoreceptor-stimulating agent (phenylpropanolamine): a randomized double-blind placebo-controlled study. International Urogynecology Journal 1:74

Wein AJ 1998 Pathophysiology and categorization of voiding dysfunction. In: Walsh PC, Retik AB, Vaughan ED et al (eds) Campbell's Urology 7th edn. WB Saunders, Philadelphia

Wilson PD, Herbison RM, Herbison GP 1996 Obstetric practice and the prevalence of urinary incontinence three months after delivery. British Journal of Obstetrics and Gynaecology 103:154

Wilson PD, Mason MV, Herbison GP, Sutherst JR 1989 Evaluation of the home pad test for quantifying incontinence. British Journal of Urology 64:155–157

Wolin LH 1969 Stress incontinence in young, healthy nulliparous female subjects. Journal of Urology 101:545–549

53
Overactive bladder

Linda Cardozo   Dudley Robinson

INTRODUCTION

The normal adult human bladder is stable, is under voluntary control and does not contract except during micturition. Conversely, an unstable bladder is one which contracts involuntarily or can be provoked to do so. Raised bladder pressure was first reported in certain neurological conditions over 60 years ago (Langworthy et al 1936, Rose 1931) but its clinical significance was not appreciated until 1963, when Hodgkinson et al demonstrated urinary incontinence as a result of detrusor contractions in 64 neurologically normal women. They called this condition 'dyssynergic detrusor dysfunction'. Various other names have been used, including uninhibited detrusor, detrusor reflex instability, overactive bladder and detrusor hyperreflexia – the latter is now reserved for abnormal detrusor activity secondary to a neuropathy. The term 'overactive bladder' (or the unstable bladder) was coined by Bates et al (1970) to describe 'the objectively measured loss of ability to inhibit detrusor contraction even when it is provoked to contract by filling, change of posture, coughing, etc.'. Detrusor instability has been defined by the International Continence Society (ICS) as a condition in which the bladder is shown to contract, either spontaneously or with provocation, during bladder filling whilst the subject is attempting to inhibit micturition (Abrams et al 1990).

INCIDENCE

Detrusor instability is a common condition and it has been suggested that it may be a variant of normal, occurring in about 10% of the population who have not learnt bladder control at the appropriate age. Versi & Cardozo (1988) have shown that 10% of postmenopausal women complaining of climacteric symptoms, but without urological complaints, have unstable bladders. In the adult female population overactive bladder is the second commonest cause of urinary incontinence after urodynamic stress incontinence, accounting for 30–50% of cases investigated (Torrens & Griffiths 1974). Among the elderly overactive bladder is the commonest cause of urinary incontinence (Castleden & Duffin 1985) and has been shown to exist in as many as 80% of those presenting for urodynamic assessment because of urinary incontinence (Malone-Lee & Wahedena 1993).

AETIOLOGY

No specific underlying cause for overactive bladder has been identified but some probabilities are idiopathic, psychosomatic, neuropathic (hyperreflexia), incontinence surgery and outflow obstruction (men).

During infancy, prior to potty training it is normal for the bladder to contract uninhibitedly at a critical volume and an unstable bladder may be the result of poorly learnt bladder control. Zoubek et al (1990) studied 46 toilet-trained children all of whom developed isolated urinary frequency. In 40% of cases a 'trigger' was identified prior to the onset of symptoms. This often involved problems at school. All cases were self-limiting or resolved following counselling or removal of the 'trigger'. There is a strong association between childhood nocturnal enuresis and overactive bladder presenting in adult life (Whiteside & Arnold 1975).

In the majority of women who suffer from overactive bladder no cause can be found, although some have neurotic personality traits (Freeman et al 1985) and they may respond well to psychotherapy. The psychoneurotic status of women with overactive bladder has been assessed by several authors, with conflicting results. Walters et al (1990) evaluated 63 women with incontinence and 27 continent controls using formal psychometric testing. They reported no difference in the test results between women with urodynamic stress incontinence and those with overactive bladder. Women with overactive bladder scored significantly higher than controls on the hypochondriasis, depression and hysteria scales. They concluded that these abnormalities may be related to incontinence in general and not to the specific diagnosis. Norton et al (1990) psychiatrically assessed 117 women prior to urodynamic investigation. There was no increased psychiatric morbidity in women with overactive bladder compared to women with urodynamic stress incontinence. Interestingly, women in whom no urodynamic abnormality could be detected had the highest scores for anxiety and neuroticism. These levels were comparable to those of psychiatric outpatients.

Moore & Sutherst (1990) have evaluated the response to treatment of overactive bladder, using oxybutynin, in relation to psychoneurotic status. Poor responders had a higher mean psychoneurotic score than responders, although one-third of poor responders were normal. Patients who responded well to therapy had scores similar to normal urban females. Many women with overactive bladder therefore show little evidence of psychoneuroticism. Using validated generic and disease-specific quality of life questionnaires Kelleher and colleagues (1993) have shown that overactive bladder has a more severe adverse effects on quality of life than does urodynamic stress incontinence.

Neurological lesions such as multiple sclerosis and spinal injuries may cause uninhibited bladder contractions, which play an aetiological role in only a small group of women with detrusor hyperreflexia. Following incontinence surgery there is an increased incidence of overactive bladder (Brown & Hilton 1999, Cardozo et al 1979, Steel et al 1985) for which no specific cause has been found, but it may be due to extensive dissection around the bladder neck as it is more commonly seen after multiple previous operations. Alternatively, it may be failure to diagnose the abnormality prior to surgery or relative outflow obstruction caused by the operation itself. Outflow obstruction is rare in women and does not seem to cause overactive bladder in the same way that prostatic hypertrophy does in men. In a large study only one of 3000 women with overactive bladder had bladder neck obstruction on urodynamic testing (Webster 1975). The increased incidence of overactive bladder in the elderly may be due to the onset of occult neuropathy, e.g. senile atherosclerosis or dementia.

PATHOPHYSIOLOGY

A detrusor contraction is initiated in the rostral pons. Efferent pathways emerge from the sacral spinal cord as the pelvic parasympathetic nerves and run forwards to the bladder. Acetylcholine is released at the neuromuscular junction and

results in a co-ordinated contraction. Thus a balance between sympathetic and parasympathetic stimulation is required for normal detrusor function.

The pathophysiology of overactive bladder remains a mystery. In vitro studies have shown that the detrusor muscle in cases of idiopathic overactive bladder contracts more than normal detrusor muscle. These detrusor contractions are not nerve mediated and can be inhibited by the neuropeptide vasoactive intestinal polypeptide (Kinder & Mundy 1987). Other studies have shown that increased α-adrenergic activity causes increased detrusor contractility (Eaton & Bates 1982). There is evidence to suggest that the pathophysiology of idiopathic and obstructive overactive bladder is different. From animal and human studies on obstructive instability, it would seem that the detrusor develops postjunctional supersensitivity, possibly due to partial denervation (Sibley 1997), with reduced sensitivity to electrical stimulation of its nerve supply but a greater sensitivity to stimulation with acetylcholine (Sibley 1985). If outflow obstruction is relieved the detrusor can return to normal behaviour and reinnervation may occur (Speakman et al 1987).

Relaxation of the urethra is known to precede contraction of the detrusor in a proportion of women with overactive bladder (Wise et al 1993a). This may represent primary pathology in the urethra which triggers a detrusor contraction or may merely be part of a complex sequence of events which originate elsewhere. It has been postulated that incompetence of the bladder neck, allowing passage of urine into the proximal urethra, may result in an uninhibited contraction of the detrusor. However, Sutherst & Brown (1978) were unable to provoke a detrusor contraction in 50 women by rapidly infusing saline into the posterior urethra using modified urodynamic equipment.

Brading & Turner (1994) have suggested that the common feature in all cases of overactive bladder is partial denervation of the detrusor which may be responsible for altering the properties of the smooth muscle, leading to increased excitability and increased ability of activity to spread between cells, resulting in co-ordinated myogenic contractions of the whole detrusor (Brading 1997). They dispute the concept of 'hyperreflexia', that is, increased motor activity to the detrusor, as the underlying mechanism in overactive bladder, proposing that there is a fundamental abnormality at the level of the bladder wall with evidence of altered spontaneous contractile activity consistent with increased electrical coupling of cells, a patchy denervation of the detrusor and a supersensitivity to potassium (Mills et al 2000). Charlton et al (1999) suggest that the primary defect in the idiopathic and neuropathic bladders is a loss of nerves accompanied by hypertrophy of the cells and an increased production of elastin and collagen within the muscle fascicles.

CLINICAL PRESENTATION

Symptoms and signs

Detrusor instability usually presents with a multiplicity of symptoms. Those most commonly seen are urgency, frequency (>7 times per day), nocturia (>once per night), urge incon-

Box 53.1 Common causes of frequency and urgency of micturition

Urological
Urinary tract infection
Detrusor instability
Small–capacity bladder
Interstitial cystitis
Chronic urinary retention/chronic urinary residual
Bladder mucosal lesion, e.g. papilloma
Bladder calculus
Urethral syndrome
Urethral diverticulum
Urethral obstruction

Gynaecological
Pregnancy
Genuine stress incontinence
Cystocoele
Pelvic mass, e.g. fibroids
Previous pelvic surgery
Radiation cystitis/fibrosis
Postmenopausal urogenital atrophy

Sexual
Coitus
Sexually transmitted disease
Contraceptive diaphragm

Medical
Diuretic therapy
Upper motor neurone lesion
Impaired renal function
Congestive cardiac failure (nocturia)
Hypokalaemia

Endocrine
Diabetes mellitus
Diabetes insipidus
Hypothyroidism

Psychological
Excessive drinking
Habit
Anxiety

tinence, stress incontinence, nocturnal enuresis and coital incontinence.

The most common symptoms are urgency and frequency of micturition, which occur in about 80% of patients (Cardozo & Stanton 1980a). However, there are numerous other causes of urgency and frequency (Box 53.1).

Frequency and polyuria due to numerous cups of tea or coffee should be detected by means of a frequency/volume chart. Most women who are incontinent develop voluntary frequency, initially in order to try to leak less. Nocturia is also a common symptom in overactive bladder, occurring in almost 70% of cases (Cardozo & Stanton 1980a). However, being woken from sleep for some other reason and voiding because one is awake does not constitute nocturia. There is an increasing incidence of nocturia with increasing age and it is normal over the age of 70 years to void twice and over the age of 80 years to void three times during the night.

Urge incontinence is usually preceded by urgency (a strong and sudden desire to void) and is due to an involuntary detrusor contraction. However, some women are unaware of any sensation associated with their detrusor contractions and just notice that they are wet. There seems to be a strong correlation between nocturnal enuresis, either childhood or current, and idiopathic overactive bladder (Whiteside & Arnold 1975). Some women complain of incontinence during sexual intercourse and they can be broadly divided into two groups: those who leak during penetration and tend to have urodynamic stress incontinence and those who leak at orgasm who tend to have overactive bladder (Hilton 1988).

The most noticeable feature of the symptomatology of overactive bladder is its infinite variability. Some patients may be severely incapacitated when at work but virtually asymptomatic when they go on holiday; others complain of severe urgency and frequency in the mornings but void normally during the rest of the day; and others say that they are incontinent when they do the washing-up or put the door key in the lock (latch-key incontinence).

There are no specific clinical signs in women with overactive bladder but it is always worth looking for vulval excoriation, urogenital atrophy, a residual urine and stress incontinence. Occasionally an underlying neurological lesion such as multiple sclerosis will be discovered by examining the cranial nerves and S2, 3 and 4 outflow.

Quality of life (QoL)

Health as defined by the World Health Organization (WHO) is 'not merely the absence of disease, but complete physical, mental and social well-being' (WHO 1978). The term 'quality of life', however, has no formal definition although it has been accepted to mean a combination of patient-assessed measures such as physical function, role function, social function, emotional or mental state, burden of symptoms and sense of well-being (Slevin et al 1988). Quality of life is assessed by the use of questionnaires completed by the patient alone or as part of the consultation and its measurement allows the quantification of morbidity and the evaluation of treatment efficacy and also acts as a measure of how lives are affected and coping strategies adopted.

There are many validated questionnaires although all have the same structure, consisting of a series of sections (domains) designed to gather information regarding particular aspects of health. Generic questionnaires, such as the Short Form 36 (Jenkinson et al 1993), are general measures of QoL and are therefore applicable to a wide range of populations and clinical conditions whilst disease-specific questionnaires have also been designed to focus on lower urinary tract symptoms.

The King's Health Questionnaire (KHQ) is a reliable, validated disease-specific tool used to assess women with lower urinary tract dysfunction (Kelleher et al 1997). Experience using the KHQ has shown that incontinence impact scores were significantly worse for women with overactive bladder than for those with urodynamic stress incontinence and significantly better in women with normal urodynamics. Interestingly, the perception of severity of urinary incontinence

KINGS COLLEGE HOSPITAL
FREQUENCY VOLUME CHART

Time	Day 1			Day 2			Day 3			Day 4			Day 5		
	In	Out	Wet	In	Out	Wet	In	Out	Wet	In	Out	Wet	In	Out	Wet
6 am		75		180	50		180	125					240	300	✓
7 am	180									125	225	✓			
8 am	180	150	✓	360	125		360	125			50 60		360	125	
9 am		100					180	350	✓	320	100			100	
10 am	360	75		180	250	✓					100 75	✓		125	✓
11 am							180	200	✓	180	50		180	100	✓
12 pm	180	225	✓	180	325	✓		100							
1 pm		100		180			180	75		180	300 75	✓	180	125	✓
2 pm	100	50			100						200				
3 pm		25 75		180	25 75		220	220	✓	360	100	✓	240		
4 pm	240	100	✓				75	90		75			180	320	✓
5 pm				220	200	✓					100			100	
6 pm	180	220	✓	220	50		100	125		120			180	100	
7 pm	180				50			200			100	✓			
8 pm		225					200			240				75	
9 pm				180	100			150	✓				360		
10 pm	180	100		180	75		180	100		180	225	✓		150	
11 pm								75 25		180	150		180	200	✓
12 am	240	100		180	150	✓	240				100		180	225	
1 am								100	✓						
2 am				180	125	✓				180	100			350	✓
3 am	180	300	✓										220		
4 am					300	✓		225	✓	180	100			100	✓
5 am													180		

Fig. 53.1   Frequency volume chart from a woman with overactive bladder.

was greater in women with urodynamic stress incontinence than overactive bladder although this did not reach significance.

INVESTIGATIONS

Urine culture

A midstream specimen of urine should be sent for microscopy, culture and sensitivity in all cases of incontinence. An infection may contribute to the symptomatology and investigations, which are mainly invasive, may exacerbate this. Such investigations are certainly uncomfortable when an infection is present and the results may be inaccurate.

Frequency/volume chart

It is our practice to send all patients a frequency/volume chart with their appointment for urodynamic investigations, so that when they arrive we can evaluate their fluid intake and voiding pattern. They are asked to complete the chart (Fig. 53.1) for 5 days but are told that they need not measure their voided volumes when at work if this proves difficult. Some women find that this is a useful exercise, similar to home bladder drill.

Uroflowmetry

Although voiding difficulties are uncommon in women, a large chronic urinary residual may present with symptoms of urgency and frequency of micturition, so it is relevant to measure the urine flow rate prior to urodynamic assessment. Usually, in uncomplicated idiopathic overactive bladder the flow rate is high and the voiding time short, with only a small volume being passed each time.

Cystometry

The diagnosis of overactive bladder is made when detrusor contractions are seen on a cystometrogram. The recorded detrusor pressure rise may take different forms on the cystometrogram trace. Most commonly, uninhibited systolic contractions occur during bladder filling (Figs 53.2, 53.3). Not all cases of overactive bladder will be diagnosed on supine filling alone (Turner-Warwick 1975). Some show an abnormal detrusor pressure rise on the change of posture and may void precipitately on standing (Fig. 53.4) or there may be detrusor contractions provoked by coughing which manifest as stress incontinence. Sometimes a steep detrusor pressure rise occurs during bladder filling (Fig. 53.5). This usually represents low compliance of the detrusor but may be due to involuntary detrusor activity in some cases. It can be difficult to differentiate between systolic (phasic) overactive bladder and low compliance, which may co-exist. Both conditions usually produce the same symptoms.

During the cystometrogram it is important to ask the patient about her symptoms and relate them to the recorded changes. Most patients will complain of urgency when a detrusor contraction occurs or urge incontinence if the detrusor pressure exceeds the urethral pressure. Thus, in order to diagnose or exclude overactive bladder, subtracted provocative cystometry must be employed. Other common, although not universal, features of the cystometrogram in women with overactive bladder are early first sensation, small bladder capacity and inability/or difficulty in interrupting the urinary stream. The latter may be associated with a high isometric detrusor contraction (Fig. 53.4) or, if videocystourethrography is performed, slow or absent milk-back of contrast medium from the proximal urethra into the bladder.

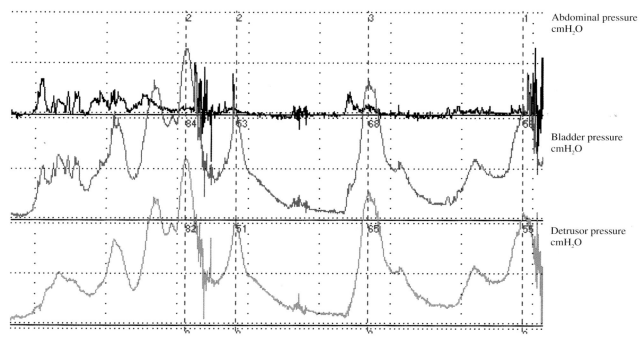

Fig. 53.2 Cystometrogram showing severe systolic detrusor contractions during filling.

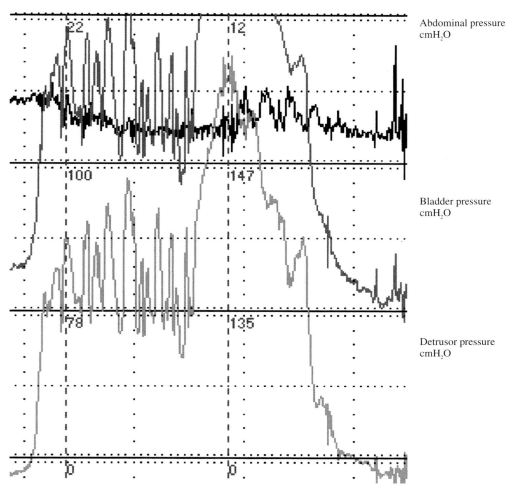

Fig. 53.3 Cystometrogram showing neurogenic detrusor overactivity during filling in a patient with multiple sclerosis.

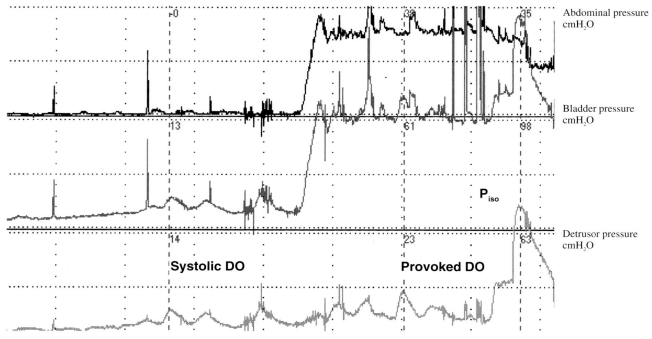

Fig. 53.4 Cystometrogram showing provoked and systolic overactive bladder in addition to a high isometric contraction (P_{iso}).

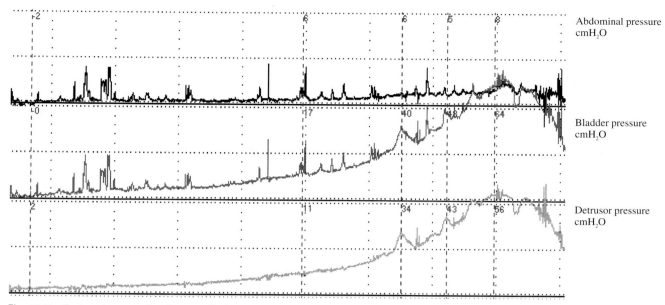

Abdominal pressure cmH$_2$O

Bladder pressure cmH$_2$O

Detrusor pressure cmH$_2$O

Fig. 53.5 Cystometrogram showing systolic detrusor contractions and low compliance during bladder filling.

In the absence of subtracted cystometry single-channel cystometry provides a useful screening test with fairly high levels of sensitivity, although rather poor specificity (Cutner et al 1992, Sutherst & Brown 1984).

Ambulatory urodynamics

Ambulatory monitoring, although still principally a research tool, is becoming more popular and is believed to be more physiological and therefore more accurate in the diagnosis of overactive bladder (Griffiths et al 1989) (Fig. 53.6). In a large study of women with symptoms of urinary incontinence but normal laboratory urodynamic investigation, overactive bladder was detected in 65% of cases on ambulatory testing (Khullar & Cardozo 1994, unpublished data). The presence of uninhibited detrusor contractions has also been detected in asymptomatic 'normal' controls during ambulatory monitoring (van Waalwijk van Doorn et al 1992) and therefore a consensus needs to be reached regarding the definition of 'normal', a standardization document having recently been published (van Waalwijk van Doorn et al 2000). In addition, detailed instructions allowing accurate completion of the patient symptom diary will improve the sensitivity of the study and decrease the number of false-positive findings. The number of spurious pressure rises misclassified as abnormal detrusor activity may be reduced by 64% if such measures are adopted (Salvatore et al 1998, 2001).

Cystourethroscopy

Endoscopy is not helpful in diagnosing overactive bladder but may be used to exclude other causes for the symptoms, such as a bladder tumour or calculus. Coarse trabeculation and diverticulae of the bladder may be noted in long-standing cases of overactive bladder. Bladder diverticulae (Fig. 53.7)

and trabeculation (Fig. 53.8) can also be seen during video-cystourethrography.

Other urodynamic tests are of limited benefit in overactive bladder. Urethral pressure profilometry (Hilton & Stanton 1983) may reveal co-existent urethral instability but its clinical significance is uncertain. A positive bladder neck electric conductance test (Holmes et al 1989) has been found to correlate well with the symptom of urgency, but this test has not gained widespread popularity and requires further evaluation.

Additional information may be acquired by undertaking videocystourethrography with pressure and flow studies, rather than subtracted cystometry, although this will not increase the diagnostic accuracy. However, when severe overactive bladder has caused upper urinary tract damage vesicoureteric reflux may be observed (Fig. 58.8).

TREATMENT

Not all women with overactive bladder require treatment. Once the problem has been explained to them some will be able to control their own symptoms by behaviour modification, such as drinking less and avoiding tea, coffee and alcohol (which are bladder stimulants). However, most women with overactive bladder request treatment and although many different therapies have been tried, none has proved universally satisfactory. The major therapeutic interventions which are currently in use attempt to either improve central control, as in behavioural intervention, or alter detrusor contractility using drugs or surgical denervation techniques. When these measures fail to adequately control the patient's symptoms over a long period of time augmentation cystoplasty may be undertaken. Conventional bladder neck surgery (as is used to treat urodynamic stress incontinence) rarely cures women with overactive bladder and may make the symptoms of urgency and frequency worse.

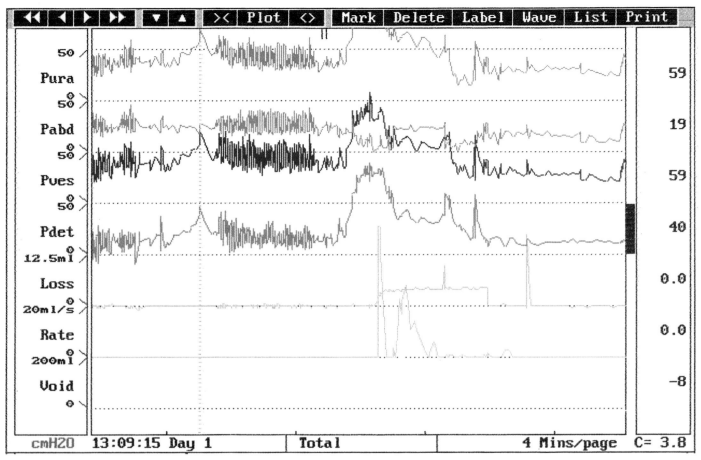

Fig. 53.6 Cystometrographic recording obtained during ambulatory monitoring. A detrusor contraction (P_{det}) is associated with pressure rises in both bladder lines (P_{ves}, P_{ura}) and leakage of urine (loss).

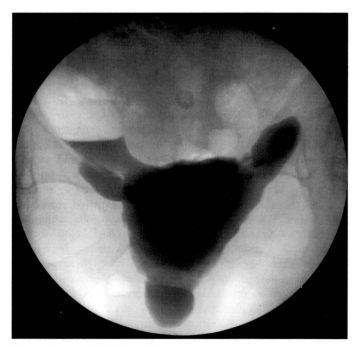

Fig. 53.7 Multiple bladder diverticulae.

Methods of treatment currently employed are drug therapy, behavioural intervention, maximal electrical stimulation, acupuncture, augmentation cystoplasty and urinary diversion. Other types of treatment which have been tried include vaginal denervation (Hodgkinson & Drukker 1977, Ingleman-Sundberg 1978, Warrell 1977), caecocystoplasty, selective sacral neurectomy (Torrens & Griffiths 1974), cystodistension (Higson et al 1978, Pengelly et al 1978, Ramsden et al 1976) and bladder transection (Mundy 1983). All give some short-term benefit in carefully selected cases but may produce significant morbidity and none has stood the test of time.

General management

All incontinent women benefit from advice regarding simple measures which they can take to help alleviate their symptoms. Many patients drink too much and they should be told to limit their fluid intake to between 1 and 1.5 litres per day and to avoid tea, coffee and alcohol if these exacerbate their problem. The use of drugs which affect bladder function, such as diuretics, should be reviewed and if possible stopped. If there is co-existent urodynamic stress incontinence then pelvic floor exercises with or without electrical stimulation may be helpful.

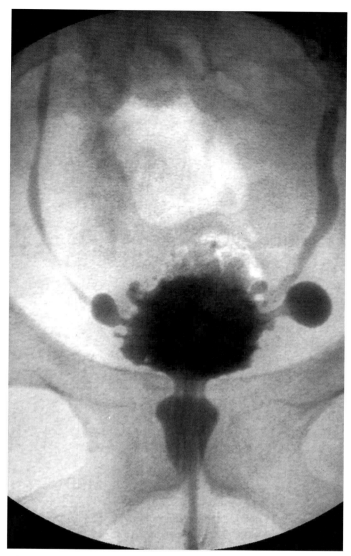

Fig. 53.8 Trabeculated bladder secondary to long-standing overactive bladder, with bladder diverticulae and bilateral vesicoureteric reflux. The bladder neck is open during a detrusor contraction with associated leakage.

It is usually preferable in cases of mixed incontinence to treat overactive bladder prior to resorting to surgery for the urethral sphincter incompetence. Such treatment may obviate the need for surgery (Karram & Bhatia 1989). In addition, there is always the risk that the incontinence operation may exacerbate the symptoms of overactive bladder.

For younger women who leak only when exercising, a tampon in the vagina during sporting activities may be helpful. For a peri- or postmenopausal woman hormone replacement therapy is unlikely to cure the problem but may increase the sensory threshold of the bladder and may also make urinary symptoms easier to cope with. The most degrading aspect of urinary incontinence for many patients is the odour and staining of their clothes and this can be helped by good advice regarding incontinence pads and garments.

Box 53.2 Drugs used in the treatment of overactive bladder

Anticholinergic drugs
Propantheline bromide
Emepronium bromide/carrageenate
Tolterodine
Darifenacin
Trospium

Musculotrophic drugs
Oxybutynin chloride

Anticholinergic/calcium antagonists
Propiverine

Calcium antagonists
Nifedipine
Flunarizine

Potassium channel openers
Cromakalim
Nicorandil
Pinacidil

Tricyclic antidepressants
Imipramine
Doxepin

Prostaglandin synthetase inhibitors
Flurbiprofen
Indomethacin

Neurotoxins (vanilloids)
Capsaicin
Resiniferatoxin

Other drugs
Desmopressin (DDAVP)

Pharmacology

Drug therapy has an important role in the management of women with irritative urinary symptoms caused by overactive bladder although there are none which specifically act on the bladder and urethra which do not have systemic effects. The large number of drugs available is indicative of the fact that none is ideal and it is often their systemic adverse effects which limit their use in terms of efficacy and compliance. Drugs which may be useful in the treatment of overactive bladder (Box 53.2) fall into three main categories:

1. those that inhibit bladder contractility
2. those that increase outlet resistance
3. those that decrease urine production.

In practice only the first group are prescribed regularly. Neurotransmission in the detrusor is muscarinic and so most of the agents used to treat overactive bladder have some antimuscarinic properties. Unfortunately, it is very difficult to assess the clinical benefit of drugs prescribed for this condition because they may act at more than one site, have different effects in vitro and in vivo and may have different short- and long-term effects. Many drugs have been investigated but few have been subjected to placebo-controlled clinical trials and consequently few are in regular clinical use (Wein 1986).

GYNAECOLOGY

Antimuscarinic drugs

The detrusor is innervated by the parasympathetic nervous system (pelvic nerve), the sympathetic nervous system (hypogastric nerve) and by non-cholinergic, non-adrenergic neurones. The motor supply arises from S2, 3 and 4 and is conveyed by the pelvic nerve. The neurotransmitter at the neuromuscular junction is acetylcholine, which acts upon muscarinic receptors. Antimuscarinic drugs should therefore be of use in the treatment of overactive bladder. Atropine is the classic non-selective anticholinergic drug with antimuscarinic activity; however, its non-specific mode of action makes it unacceptable for clinical use because of the high incidence of side-effects. All antimuscarinic agents produce competitive blockade of acetylcholine receptors at postganglionic parasympathetic receptor sites. They all, to a lesser or greater extent, have the typical side-effects of dry mouth, blurred vision, tachycardia, drowsiness and constipation. Unfortunately, virtually all the drugs which are truly beneficial in the management of overactive bladder produce these unwanted systemic side-effects.

Tolterodine Tolterodine is a competitive muscarinic receptor antagonist with relative functional selectivity for bladder muscarinic receptors (Ruscin & Morgenstern 1999). Whilst it shows no specificity for receptor subtypes it does target the bladder muscarinic receptors rather than those in the salivary glands (Nilvebrant et al 1997). Several randomized, double-blind, placebo-controlled trials have demonstrated a significant reduction in incontinent episodes and micturition frequency (Hills et al 1998, Jonas et al 1997, Millard et al 1999) whilst the incidence of adverse effects has been shown to be no different to placebo (Rentzhog et al 1998). When compared to oxybutynin in a randomized double-blind placebo-controlled parallel group study, it was found to be equally efficacious and to have a lower incidence of side-effects, notably dry mouth (Abrams et al 1998). Consequently this has been shown to be associated with improved patient compliance (Appell 1997). In summary, the available evidence would suggest that tolterodine is as effective as oxybutynin although since it has fewer adverse effects patient tolerability and compliance are improved.

Propantheline Propantheline bromide is a related drug with fewer side-effects. It is a quaternary ammonium analogue with both antimuscarinic and antinicotinic properties, which acts at both the ganglionic level and at the neuromuscular junction. Blaivas et al (1980) have shown that intramuscular injection of propantheline abolishes involuntary detrusor contractions in 79% of cases of overactive bladder. However, 50% of patients required short-term intermittent self-catheterization for resulting urinary retention. When given orally in a dose of 15 mg four times daily it is often ineffective due to low bioavailability (5–10%). The dose may therefore be increased as high as 90 mg four times daily, but introduced slowly to minimize side-effects. Gastrointestinal absorption is aided by taking the drug before meals (Gibaldi & Grundhofer 1975). Propantheline is cheap, with few side-effects, and is particularly useful when frequency of micturition is a major problem. Unfortunately, there have been no good recent clinical trials.

Emepronium Emepronium bromide has antimuscarinic activity at both peripheral and ganglionic levels and has to be taken in doses above 200 mg tds. Unfortunately, it is poorly absorbed from the gastrointestinal tract (Ritch et al 1977) and at high doses causes oesophageal ulceration. Emepronium carragenate, which is available in some parts of Europe, does not have this problem and has been shown to improve symptoms when administered in high doses (Massey & Abrams 1986). Unfortunately, emepronium is no longer licensed in the United Kingdom.

Trospium chloride Trospium chloride is a quaternary ammonium compound which is non-selective for muscarinic receptor subtypes and has recently been launched in the UK. A placebo-controlled, randomised, double-blind multicentre trial has shown trospium to increase cystometric capacity and bladder volume at first unstable contraction, leading to significant clinical improvement without an increase in adverse effects over placebo (Cardozo et al 2000). When compared to oxybutynin it has been found to have comparable efficacy although was associated with a lower incidence of dry mouth (4% vs 23%) and patient withdrawal (6% vs 16%) (Madersbacher et al 1995). At present trospium chloride would appear to be equally effective as oxybutynin although it may be associated with fewer adverse effects.

Darifenacin Darifenacin is a highly selective muscarinic receptor antagonist which has a fivefold affinity for the M_3 (bladder) muscarinic receptor than for the M_1 (salivary gland) receptors (Alabaster 1997). Studies have shown darifenacin to be equipotent with atropine in the ileum and bladder and six times less potent at inhibiting muscarinic receptors in the salivary gland. Although currently still under development, early studies (Rosario et al 1995) suggest that it may prove clinically useful.

Musculotropic drugs

Oxybutynin Oxybutynin is a tertiary amine which has local anaesthetic effects and direct muscle relaxant effects in addition to antimuscarinic action and antihistaminic properties. Given in the maximum recommended dose of 5 mg three times daily, many women find the side-effects less tolerable than the symptoms of overactive bladder. The worst problems seem to be a very dry mouth and throat with a lingering bad taste, with 10–23% of women discontinuing medication (Kelleher et al 1994a). However, oxybutynin does cause significant improvement in the symptom of urgency, but this may be at the expense of an increased urinary residual volume (Cardozo et al 1987). In those patients who can tolerate this drug a 70% improvement rate can be expected.

In a large randomized double-blind multicentre study conducted by Thuroff et al (1991) the degree of symptomatic improvement and objective improvement in urodynamic parameters was significantly greater for those treated with oxybutynin than with either propantheline or placebo. However, the dose of propantheline was too low to be considered effective therapy for the majority of women with overactive bladder.

Oxybutynin is contraindicated in patients with glaucoma. It has a half-life of only 5 hours and is therefore rapidly effective following ingestion. A dose may be taken as prophylaxis to control symptoms for short periods, when the individual feels it is necessary (Burton 1994). Alternatively, the side-effects may be reduced by lowering the dose to 3 mg three times daily

(Moore et al 1990) without significantly reducing the efficacy. Intravesical administration of oxybutynin is an effective and useful alternative for patients with neurogenic detrusor overactivity who need to self-catheterize or who suffer from 'bypassing' an indwelling catheter (Madersbacher & Jilg 1991). In addition, the rectal route may also be used (Collas & Malone-Lee 1997).

More recently controlled-release preparations using an osmotic system (OROS) have been developed which have been shown to have comparable efficacy with immediate-release preparations but are associated with fewer adverse effects (Anderson et al 1999). The incidence of dry mouth is also reduced (23%) with only 1.6% of women discontinuing the medication due to adverse effects (Gleason et al 1999).

In summary, the efficacy of oxybutynin is well documented although very often its clinical usefulness is limited by adverse effects. Alternative routes and methods of administration may produce better patient acceptability and compliance.

Propiverine Propiverine has both antimuscarinic and calcium channel-blocking actions (Haruno et al 1989). Open studies have demonstrated a beneficial effect in patients with overactive bladder (Mazur et al 1995) and detrusor hyper-reflexia (Stoher et al 1999). Dry mouth was experienced by 37% in the treatment group as opposed to 8% in those taking placebo, with dropout rates being 7% and 4.5% respectively. Whilst propiverine would appear to be a promising new development at present there is a need for further long-term studies to fully evaluate efficacy and safety.

Flavoxate Flavoxate is a tertiary amine with direct smooth muscle relaxant properties through calcium antagonistic activity, local anaesthetic properties and an ability to inhibit phosphodiesterase. It is still commonly prescribed in a dose of 200 mg three times daily, but is poorly absorbed from the gut and in clinical trials its effect has not been shown to be superior to that of placebo (Briggs et al 1980, Chapple et al 1990). Thus efficacy remains to be established.

Tricyclic antidepressants

These drugs have a complex pharmacological action. Imipramine has antimuscarinic, antihistamine and local anaesthetic properties. It may increase outlet resistance caused by peripheral blockage of noradrenaline uptake and it also acts as a sedative. The side-effects are antimuscarinic, together with tremor and fatigue. Imipramine is particularly useful for the treatment of nocturia and nocturnal enuresis (Castleden et al 1981). Imipramine together with propantheline may be used to treat the combined symptoms of diurnal frequency and nocturia. A dose of up to 150 mg may be given safely but the standard dosage is 50 mg twice daily. Other tricyclic antidepressants such as amitriptyline may be substituted for imipramine if specific side-effects are a problem whilst doxepin has been found to be more potent in its musculotropic relaxant and antimuscarinic activity (Lose et al 1989). A tricyclic given prophylactically before sexual intercourse may be a benefit to patients with coital incontinence at orgasm (Cardozo 1988).

At therapeutic levels tricyclic drugs can cause orthostatic hypotension and ventricular arrhythmias. In addition, allergic rashes, hepatic dysfunction, obstructive jaundice and agranulocytosis may also occur. Consequently women taking

medication should be closely monitored and treatment should be tailed off gradually rather than suddenly.

Other drugs

Calcium channel antagonists The influx of extracellular calcium is important for detrusor muscle contractions and calcium anatagonists such as nifedipine have been shown to be effective at reducing the frequency and amplitude of unstable bladder contractions (Rud et al 1979) although this has not been confirmed by other authorities (Laval & Lutzeyer 1980). At present their use is principally restricted to research although calcium channel antagonists may play an important therapeutic role in the future.

Potassium channel–opening drugs The opening of K^+ ion channels in the membrane of the detrusor muscle cell leads to an increase in K^+ movement out of the cell, resulting in membrane hyperpolarization (Andersson 1997). This reduces the opening probability of ion channels involved in membrane depolarization and hence excitability is reduced (Andersson 1992). These agents act during the filling phase and whilst abolishing spontaneous detrusor contractions, are not thought to affect normal bladder contractions. Their clinical usefulness is limited by significant cardiovascular effects with cromakalin and pinacidil being found to be up to 200 times more potent as inhibitors of vascular preparations than of detrusor muscle (Edwards et al 1991). At present none are commercially available although the development of sub-type selective drugs may lead to a role in the management of overactive bladder (Lawson 1996).

Desmopressin (1-desamino-8-D-arginine vasopressin; DDAVP) Synthetic vasopressin (DDAVP) has been shown to reduce nocturnal urine production by up to 50%. It can be used for children or adults with nocturia or nocturnal enuresis (Norgaard et al 1989), but must be avoided in patients with hypertension, ischaemic heart disease or congestive cardiac failure (Hilton & Stanton 1982). There is good evidence to show that it is safe to use in the long term (Knudsen et al 1989, Rew & Rundle 1989) and it may be given orally or as a nasal spray, the latter giving better bio-availability.

Oestrogens Oestrogen deficiency following the menopause causes changes in all layers of the urethra, which has abundant oestrogen receptors (Tapp & Cardozo 1986), but the bladder itself possesses fewer receptors. There have been few placebo-controlled trials using objective as well as subjective outcome measures, but a meta-analysis of the worldwide literature would suggest that oestrogens may produce some symptomatic improvement in urinary symptoms, including urgency and frequency of micturition (Fantl et al 1994). In addition, sensory urgency, which may be due to generalized urogenital atrophy, does respond to oestrogen replacement therapy (Fantl et al 1988, Wise et al 1993b). Whilst oestrogens would appear to improve irritative symptoms there is no proven benefit in the treatment of overactive bladder.

Capsaicin This is the pungent ingredient found in red chillies and is a neurotoxin of substance P-containing (C) nerve fibres. Patients with neurogenic detrusor overactivity secondary to multiple sclerosis appear to have abnormal C fibre sensory innervation of the detrusor, which leads to premature activation of the holding reflex arc during bladder filling

(Fowler et al 1992). Intravesical application of capsaicin dissolved in 30% alcohol solution appears to be effective for up to 6 months. The effects are variable (Chandiramani et al 1994) and the long-term safety of this treatment has not yet been evaluated.

Resiniferatoxin This is a phorbol-related diterpene isolated from the cactus and is a potent analogue of capsaicin that appears to have a similar efficacy but with fewer side-effects of pain and burning during intravesical instillation (Kim & Chancellor 2000). It is 1000 times more potent than capsaicin at stimulating bladder activity (Ishizuka et al 1995). As with capsaicin, the currently available evidence does not support the routine clinical use of the agents although they may prove to have a role as an intravesical preparation in neurological patients with neurogenic detrusor overactivity.

Prostaglandin synthetase inhibitors Prostaglandins are known to play a role in detrusor contractions in addition to PGE_2 causing urethral smooth muscle relaxation and $PGF_{2\alpha}$ leading to an increase in urethral smooth muscle tone. Sensory afferent nerves may be sensitized by prostaglandins, thereby increasing the afferent input at lower bladder volumes and leading to involuntary detrusor contractions and prostaglandins have been shown to cause detrusor contractions in vitro. Flurbiprofen, a prostaglandin synthetase inhibitor, has been shown to increase the bladder volume at which unstable bladder contractions occur but did not inhibit spontaneous detrusor contractions (Cardozo et al 1980). In addition, indomethacin has been shown to cause symptomatic improvement in women with overactive bladder although it was associated with a high incidence of side-effects (Cardozo & Stanton 1980b). At present these drugs do not have a role in the management of overactive bladder although further development may lead to them being clinically useful.

Behavioural therapy

As continence is normally learned during infancy it is logical to suppose that it can be relearned during adult life. Bladder re-education includes bladder drill, biofeedback and hypnotherapy. Bladder discipline was first described as a method of treating urgency incontinence by Jeffcoate & Francis (1966) in the belief that it was exacerbated or even caused by underlying psychological factors. Since then Frewen (1970) has shown that many women with overactive bladder are able to correlate the onset of their symptoms with some untoward event, which can be identified by taking a careful history. He showed that both inpatient and outpatient bladder drill can be effective forms of treatment for many such women.

The technique for performing inpatient bladder drill has been established by Jarvis (1989) and is shown below. It may be performed either as an inpatient or in an outpatient setting.

Technique for bladder drill
1. Exclude pathology and admit to hospital (if possible).
2. Explain rationale to patient.
3. Instruct the patient to void every one-and-a-half hours during the day (either she waits or is incontinent).
4. When one-and-a-half hours are achieved, increase by half an hour and continue with 2-hourly voiding, etc.
5. Allow a normal fluid intake (1500 ml/24 h).
6. The patient keeps a fluid balance chart.
7. She meets a successful patient.
8. She receives encouragement from patients, nurses and doctors.

Jarvis & Millar (1980) performed a controlled trial of bladder drill in 60 consecutive incontinent women with idiopathic overactive bladder. They showed that following inpatient treatment, 90% of the bladder drill group were continent and 83.3% remained symptom free after 6 months. In the control group 23.2% were continent and symptom free due to the placebo effect. Despite the excellent early results it has been shown that up to 40% of patients relapse within 3 years (Holmes et al 1983).

Biofeedback

Biofeedback is a form of learning or re-education in which the patient is given information about a normally unconscious physiological process in the form of an auditory, visual or tactile signal. The objective effects of biofeedback in the treatment of overactive bladder can be recorded on a polygraph trace, but the subjective changes may be difficult to separate from the placebo effect. This technique was originally described by Cardozo et al (1978a). Thirty women aged between 16 and 65 years of age suffering from idiopathic overactive bladder which was resistant to conventional therapy were treated in two centres (Cardozo et al 1978b). Some 80% of the women were cured or significantly improved subjectively and 60% were cured or improved objectively. Long-term follow-up revealed a relatively high relapse rate (Cardozo & Stanton 1984) consistent with the long-term effects of bladder drill. Other reports suggest that bladder training with or without biofeedback can be effectively used to treat incontinence due to overactive bladder (Burgio et al 1986, Millard & Oldenberg 1983). However, this type of treatment is time consuming and requires trained personnel and currently biofeedback is used almost exclusively to treat children with maladaptive voiding problems.

Hypnotherapy

Hypnotherapy can be used in one of two ways: either symptom removal by suggestion alone or by attempting to help the patient disclose hidden emotions or memories which may be pathogenic. Freeman & Baxby (1982) treated 61 women with idiopathic overactive bladder using 12 sessions of hypnosis over a period of 1 month. They achieved an overall improvement rate of over 80%, but unfortunately at 2-year follow-up only nine of the women remained symptom free (Freeman 1989). This type of treatment is not currently employed in the management of overactive bladder.

Acupuncture

Acupuncture is thought to act by increasing levels of endorphins and encephalins in the cerebrospinal fluid. Encephalins are known to inhibit detrusor contractility in vitro (Klarskov 1987). Naloxone, an opiate antagonist, conversely causes decreased bladder capacity and increased detrusor pressure (Murray & Feneley 1982). Several studies have shown symptomatic improvement (Philp et al 1988) or decreased frequency and urinary leakage (Pigne et al 1985) in patients with overactive bladder treated with acupuncture. Gibson et al (1990) utilized infrared low-power laser on acupuncture points successfully initially, but unfortunately there was a high relapse rate at 6 months. Acupuncture is as effective as oxybutynin in the treatment of symptoms associated with idiopathic low compliance and it is acceptable to patients but time consuming for the operator (Kelleher et al 1994b).

Maximal electrical stimulation

Electrical stimulation, applied either vaginally or anally, may inhibit spontaneous detrusor contractions and thus represents a therapeutic alternative for the management of overactive bladder (Plevnik et al 1986). The neurophysiological basis for the resulting prolonged bladder inhibition remains unclear. The technique is safe and inexpensive and can be performed by specialist nurses. A success rate (cure or significant improvement) of 77% on objective follow-up at 1 year after an average initial treatment regimen of seven sessions has been reported by Eriksen et al (1989).

We have compared maximal electrical stimulation with oxybutynin in women with overactive bladder (Wise et al 1992). Both treatments were associated with a significant reduction in symptoms. Although 20% of the women who received oxybutynin withdrew due to treatment side-effects, maximal electrical stimulation was universally acceptable and should therefore be considered as an alternative to pharmacological agents. More recently, the efficacy of functional electrical stimulation has been reviewed, with rates of improvement being 50–90% (Okada et al 1999).

All forms of bladder retraining in the treatment of overactive bladder are advantageous because there are few unpleasant side-effects and no patient is ever made worse. Mild to moderate overactive bladder can be cured or significantly improved by re-educating the bladder. However, the relapse rate is very high and although this type of treatment avoids the morbidity associated with surgery and the side-effects of drug therapy, it requires skilled personnel and is time consuming for both the patient and the operator. A recent meta-analysis has concluded that bladder retraining is more effective than placebo and medical therapy although there is insufficient evidence to support the effectiveness of electrical stimulation and too few studies to evaluate the effect of pelvic floor exercises and biofeedback in women with urinary urge incontinence (Berghmans et al 2000).

Neuromodulation

Stimulation of the dorsal sacral nerve root using a permanent implantable device in the S3 sacral foramen has been developed for use in patients with overactive bladder and neurogenic detrusor overactivity. The sacral nerves contain nerve fibres of the parasympathetic and sympathetic system providing innervation to the bladder as well as somatic fibres providing innervation to the muscles of the pelvic floor. The latter are larger in diameter and hence have a lower threshold of activation, meaning that the pelvic floor may be stimulated selectively without causing bladder activity. Prior to implantation temporary cutaneous sacral nerve stimulation is performed to check for a response and if successful, a permanent implant is inserted under general anaesthesia. Initial studies in patients with overactive bladder refractory to medical and behavioural therapy have demonstrated that after 3 years, 59% of 41 urinary urge incontinent patients showed greater than 50% reduction in incontinence episodes, with 46% of patients being completely dry (Seigel et al 2000).

Whilst neuromodulation remains an invasive and expensive procedure, in the future it may offer a useful alternative to medical and surgical therapies in patients with severe, intractable overactive bladder.

Transvesical phenol

Originally described for the treatment of neurogenic detrusor overactivity (Ewing et al 1982), this treatment has since been used for women with idiopathic overactive bladder. Using a cystoscope, a semirigid needle is inserted under the bladder epithelium midway between the ureteric orifice and the bladder neck and 10 ml of 6% aqueous phenol is injected on each side. In the largest published series, Blackford et al (1984) reported improvement for at least 1 year in 88 of 116 women treated. They found that the response to treatment was best in those women over the age of 55. A number of side-effects and complications were recorded, of which transient postoperative haematuria was the most common. However, they said that there was no significant morbidity. Other workers in the field have been less enthusiastic about the long-term results of transvesical phenol and more concerned about the incidence of significant complications (Rosenbaum et al 1988). This form of treatment is now only rarely employed.

Surgery

Approximately 10% of women with overactive bladder remain refractory to medical and behavioural therapy and may be considered for surgery. Various different surgical techniques have been developed although currently auto-augmentation is the most commonly performed technique using a clam cystoplasty or detrusor myectomy.

Clam cystoplasty

In the clam cystoplasty (Bramble 1990, Mast et al 1995) the bladder is bisected almost completely and a patch of gut (usually ileum) equal in length to the circumference of the bisected bladder (about 25 cm) is sewn in place. This often cures the symptoms of overactive bladder (McRae et al 1987) by converting a high-pressure system into a low-pressure system although inefficient voiding may result. Patients have to learn to strain to void or may have to resort to clean intermittent self-catheterization, sometimes permanently. In addition, mucus retention in the bladder may be a problem, but this can be partially overcome by ingestion of 200 ml of cranberry juice each day (Rosenbaum et al 1989) in addition to intravesical mucolytics such as acetylcysteine. The chronic exposure of the ileal mucosa to urine may lead to malignant change (Harzmann & Weckerman 1992). There is a 5% risk of adenocarcinoma arising in ureterosigmoidostomies, where colonic mucosa is exposed to N-nitrosamines found in both urine and faeces, and a similar risk may apply to enterocystoplasty. Biopsies of the ileal segment taken from patients with clam cystoplasties show evidence of chronic inflammation of villous atrophy (Nurse & Mundy 1987) and diarrhoea due to disruption of the bile acid cycle is common (Barrington et al 1995). This may be treated using cholestyramine. In addition, metabolic disturbances such as hyperchloraemic acidosis, B_{12} deficiency and occasionally osteoporosis secondary to decreased bone mineralization may occur.

Detrusor myectomy

Detrusor myectomy offers an alternative to clam cystoplasty by increasing functional bladder capacity without the complications of bowel interposition. In this procedure the whole thickness of the detrusor muscle is excised from the dome of the bladder, thereby creating a large bladder diverticulum with no intrinsic contractility (Cartwright & Snow 1989). Whilst there is a reduction in episodes of incontinence there is little improvement in functional capacity and thus frequency remains problematic (Kennelly et al 1994, Snow & Cartwright 1996).

Urinary diversion

As a last resort, for those women with severe overactive bladder or neurogenic detrusor overactivity who cannot manage clean intermittent catheterization, it may be more appropriate to perform a urinary diversion. Usually this will utilize an ileal conduit to create an incontinent abdominal stoma for urinary diversion. An alternative is to form a continent diversion using the appendix (Mitrofanoff) or ileum (Koch pouch) which may then be drained using self-catheterization.

CONCLUSION

Detrusor instability is a common condition affecting people of all ages. It is characterized by multiple symptoms which, although not life-threatening, may cause much embarrassment and a very restricted lifestyle. Our lack of understanding of the underlying pathology of overactive bladder is reflected in the many different methods of treatment which are currently employed, none of them wholly satisfactory. Conventional bladder neck surgery is not useful in the treatment of overactive bladder unless there is concomitant urethral sphincter incompetence and therefore it is important to make an accurate diagnosis before treatment is concerned.

Surgical procedures such as augmentation cystoplasty are reserved for women with severe symptoms in whom other forms of treatment have been tried and failed. Behavioural intervention seems to be the best type of treatment of idiopathic overactive bladder because it may produce a permanent cure without any significant morbidity or side-effects. However, the majority of patients are still treated with drug therapy, which they may need to take indefinitely as symptoms usually return once the tablets are discontinued.

Fortunately, overactive bladder is a disease of spontaneous exacerbations and remissions and therefore short courses of drug therapy, when symptoms are at their worst, may be sufficient for the sufferer to maintain a normal lifestyle. Although it is rare to cure a patient completely with any form of treatment, most can have their symptoms significantly reduced. The elucidation of the patient's main complaints is therefore of great importance. As the pathophysiology of the condition becomes clearer, leading to the development of new drugs offering greater efficacy and improved compliance, we can expect significant advances in the management of overactive bladder.

KEY POINTS

1. Detrusor instability is a disease of spontaneous exacerbations and remissions.
2. Detrusor instability may occur in 10% of the normal population and be asymptomatic.
3. It is the second commonest cause of incontinence in young and middle-aged women but the commonest cause in the elderly.
4. The cause of idiopathic overactive bladder is unknown but many patients have a neurotic personality trait.
5. The diagnosis of overactive bladder can be suggested by symptoms but confirmed only on cystometry.
6. Bladder retraining and behaviour modification are important treatments which can be augmented by antimuscarinic drug therapy.
7. Most antimuscarinic drugs need to be given at a dosage which will produce parasympathetic side-effects.
8. Mild overactivity can be cured or improved by bladder retraining but the relapse rate is high.
9. Where overactivity and genuine stress incontinence co-exist, it is preferable to treat the overactivity first.

REFERENCES

Abrams P, Blavis JG, Stanton SL, Anderson JT 1990 the standardisation of terminology of lower urinary tract function. British Journal of Obstetrics and Gynaecology 97 (suppl 6):1–16

Abrams P, Freeman R, Anderstrom C, Mattiasson A 1998 Tolterodine, a new antimuscarinic agent: as effective but better tolerated than oxybutynin in patients with an overactive bladder. British Journal of Urology 81:801–810

Alabaster VA 1997 Discovery and development of selective M3 antagonists for clinical use. Life Science 60:1053–1060

Anderson RU, Mobley D, Blank B et al 1999 Once daily controlled versus immediate release oxybutynin chloride for urge urinary incontinence. OROS Oxybutynin Study Group. Journal of Urology 161:1809–1812

Andersson KE 1992 Clinical pharmacology of potassium channel openers. Pharmacology and Toxicology 70:244–245

Anderson KE 1997 The overactive bladder: pharmacologic basis of drug treatment. Urology 50:74–89

Appell RA 1997 Clinical efficacy and safety of tolterodine in the treatment of overactive bladder: a pooled analysis. Urology 50:90–96

Barrington JW, Fern Davies H, Adams RJ, Evans WD, Woodcock JP, Stephenson TP 1995 Bile acid dysfunction after clam enterocystoplasty. British Journal of Urology 76:169–171

Bates CP, Whiteside CG, Turner-Warwick RT 1970 Synchronous cine-pressure–flow cystourethrography with special reference to stress and urge incontinence. British Journal of Urology 50:714–723

Berghmans LC, Hendricks HJ, de Bie RA, van Waalwijk van Doorn ES, Bo K, van Kerrebroeck PE 2000 Conservative treatment of urge urinary incontinence in women: a systematic review of randomised clinical trials. British Journal of Urology International 85:254–263

Blackford W, Murray K, Stephenson TP, Mundy AR 1984 Results of transvesical infiltration of the pelvic plexus with phenol in 116 patients. British Journal of Urology 56:647–649

Blaivas JG, Labib KB, Michalik SJ, Zayed AAH 1980 Cystometric response to propantheline in detrusor hyperreflexia. Therapeutic implications. Journal of Urology 124:259–262

Brading AF 1997 A myogenic basis for the overactive bladder. Urology 50:57–67

Brading AF, Turner WH 1994 The unstable bladder: towards a common mechanism. British Journal of Urology 73:3–8

Bramble FJ 1990 The clam cystoplasty. British Journal of Urology 66:337–341

Briggs RS, Castleden CM, Asher MJ 1980 The effect of flavoxate on uninhibited detrusor contractions and urinary incontinence in the elderly. Journal of Urology 123:665–666

Brown K, Hilton P 1999 The incidence of overactive bladder before and after colposuspension: a study using conventional and ambulatory urodynamic monitoring. British Journal of Urology International 84(9):961–965

Burgio KL, Robinson JC, Engel BT 1986 The role of biofeedback in Kegel exercise training for stress incontinence. American Journal of Obstetrics and Gynecology 154:64–88

Burton G 1994 A randomised cross over trial comparing oxybutynin taken three times a day or taken 'when needed'. Neurourology and Urodynamics 13:351–352

Cardozo LD 1988 Sex and the bladder. British Medical Journal 296:587–588

Cardozo LD, Stanton SL 1980a Genuine stress incontinence and overactive bladder: a review of 200 cases. British Journal of Obstetrics and Gynaecology 87:184–190

Cardozo LD, Stanton SL 1980b A comparison between bromocriptine and indomethacin in the treatment of overactive bladder. Journal of Urology 123:399–401

Cardozo LD, Stanton SL 1984 Biofeedback: a five year review. British Journal of Urology 56:220

Cardozo LD, Stanton SL, Robinson H, Hole D 1980 Evaluation on flurbiprofen in overactive bladder. British Medical Journal 280:281–282

Cardozo LD, Stanton SL, Allan V 1978a Biofeedback in the treatment of overactive bladder. British Journal of Urology 50:250–254

Cardozo LD, Abrams PH, Stanton SL, Feneley RCL 1978b Idiopathic overactive bladder treated by biofeedback. British Journal of Urology 50:521–523

Cardozo LD, Stanton SL, Williams JE 1979 Detrusor instability following surgery for urodynamic instability. British Journal of Urology 51:204–207

Cardozo LD, Cooper D, Versi E 1987 Oxybutynin chloride in the management of idiopathic overactive bladder. Neurourology and Urodynamics 6:256–257

Cardozo LD, Chapple CR, Toozs-Hobson P et al 2000. Efficacy of trospium chloride in patients with overactive bladder: a placebo-controlled, randomized, double-blind, multicentre clinical trial. British Journal of Urology International 85:659–664

Cartwright PC, Snow BW 1989 Bladder autoaugmentation: partial detrusor excision to augment the bladder without use of bowel. Journal of Urology 142:1050–1053

Castleden CM, Duffin HM 1985 Factors influencing outcome in elderly patients with urinary incontinence and overactive bladder. Aging 14:303–307

Castleden CM, George CF, Renwick AG, Asher MJ 1981 Imipramine – a possible alternative to current therapy for urinary incontinence in the elderly. Journal of Urology 125:318–320

Chandiramani VA, Peterson T, Beck RO, Fowler CJ 1994 Lessons learnt from 44 intravesical instillations of capsaicin. Neurourology and Urodynamics 13:348–349

Chapple CR, Parkhouse H, Gardener C, Milroy EJG 1990 Double blind placebo-controlled cross over study of flavoxate in the treatment of idiopathic overactive bladder. British Journal of Urology 66:491–494

Charlton RG, Morley AR, Chambers P, Gillespie JI 1999 Focal changes in nerve, muscle and connective tissue in normal and unstable human bladder. British Journal of Urology International 84(9): 953–960

Collas D, Malone-Lee J 1997 The pharmacokinetic properties of rectal oxybutynin – a possible alternative to intravesical administration. Neurourology and Urodynamics 16:346–347

Cutner A, Wise BS, Cardozo LD, Burton G, Abbott D, Kelleher CJ 1992 Single channel cystometry as a screening test for abnormal detrusor activity. Neurourology and Urodynamics 11(4):455–456

Eaton AC, Bates CP 1982 An in vitro physiological, study of normal and unstable human detrusor muscle. British Journal of Urology 54:653–657

Edwards G, Henshaw M, Miller M, Weston WH 1991 Comparison of the effects of several potassium-channel openers on rat bladder and rat portal vein in vitro. British Journal of Pharmacology 102:679–686

Eriksen BC, Bergmann S, Eik-Nes SH 1989 Maximal electro-stimulation of the pelvic floor in female idiopathic overactive bladder and urge incontinence. Neurourology and Urodynamics 8:219–230

Ewing R, Bultitude ME, Shuttleworth KGD 1982 Subtrigonal phenol injection for urge incontinence secondary to overactive bladder in females. British Journal of Urology 54:689–692

Fantl JA, Wyman JF, Anderson RL, Matt DW, Bump RC 1988 Postmenopausal urinary incontinence: a comparison between non-estrogen supplemented and estrogen supplemented women. Obstetrics and Gynecology 71:823–828

Fantl JA, Cardozo LD, McLish D 1994 The Hormones and Urogenital Therapy Committee. Estrogen therapy in the management of urinary incontinence in postmenopausal women: a meta-analysis. Obstetrics and Gynecology 83:12–18

Fowler CJ, Jewkes D, McDonald WI, Lynn B, DeGroat WC 1992 Intravesical capsaicin for neurogenic bladder dysfunction. Lancet 339:1239

Freeman RM 1989 Hypnosis and psychomedical treatment. In: Freeman RM, Malvern J (eds) The unstable bladder. Wright, Bristol, pp 73–80

Freeman RM, Baxby K 1982 Hypnotherapy for incontinence caused by the unstable detrusor. British Medical Journal 284:1831–1834

Freeman RM, McPherson FM, Baxby K 1985 Psychological features of women with idiopathic overactive bladder. Urologia Internationalis 40:247–259

Frewen WK 1970 Urge and stress incontinence: fact and fiction. Journal of Obstetrics and Gynaecology of the British Commonwealth 1977:932–934

Gibaldi M, Grundhofer S 1975 Biopharmaceutic influences on the anticholinergic effect of propantheline. Clinical Pharmacology and Therapeutics 18:457–461

Gibson JS, Pardley J, Neville J 1990 Infra-red low power laser therapy on acupuncture points for treatment of the unstable bladder. Proceedings of the 20th Meeting of the International Continence Society, pp 146–147

Gleason DM, Susset J, White C, Munoz DR, Sand PK 1999 Evaluation of a new once daily formulation of oxybutynin for the treatment of urinary urge incontinence. Ditropan XL Study Group. Urology 54:420–423

Griffiths CJ, Assi M, Styles RA, Ramsden PD, Neal DE 1989 Ambulatory monitoring of bladder and detrusor pressure during natural filling. Journal of Urology 142:780–784

Harzmann R, Weckerman D 1992 Problem of secondary malignancy after urinary diversion and enterocystoplasty. Scandinavian Journal of Urology and Nephrology 142 (suppl):56

Haruno A, Yamasaki Y, Miyoshi K et al 1989 Effects of propiverine hydrochloride and its metabolites on isolated guinea pig urinary bladder. Folia Pharmacologica Japonica 94:145–150

Higson RH, Smith JC, Whelan P 1978 Bladder rupture: an acceptable complication of distension therapy? British Journal of Urology 50:529–534

Hills CJ, Winter SA, Balfour JA 1998. Tolterodine. Drugs 55:813–820

Hilton P 1988 Urinary incontinence during sexual intercourse: a common but rarely volunteered symptom. British Journal of Obstetrics and Gynaecology 95:377–381

Hilton P, Stanton SL 1982 Use of desmopressin (DDAVP) in nocturnal urinary frequency in the female. British Journal of Urology 54:252–255

Hilton P, Stanton SL 1983 Urethral pressure measurement by microtransducer: the results in symptom-free women and those with urodynamic stress incontinence. British Journal of Obstetrics and Gynaecology 90:919–933

Hodgkinson CP, Drukker BH 1977 Infravesical nerve resection for detrusor dyssynergia (the Ingleman-Sundberg operation). Acta Obstetrica et Gynecologica Scandinavica 56:401–408

Hodgkinson CP, Ayers MA, Drukker BH 1963 Dyssynergic detrusor dysfunction in the apparently normal female. American Journal of Obstetrics and Gynecology 87:717–730

Holmes DM, Stone AR, Barry PR, Richards CJ, Stephenson TP 1983 Bladder training – years on. British Journal of Urology 55:660–664

Holmes D, Plevnik S, Stanton SL 1989 Bladder neck electric conductivity in female urinary urgency and urge incontinence. British Journal of Obstetrics and Gynaecology 96:816–820

Ingleman-Sundberg A 1978 Partial bladder denervation for detrusor dyssynergia. Clinical Obstetrics and Gynaecology 21:797–805

Ishizuka O, Mattiasson A, Andersson K-E 1995 Urodynamic effects of intravesical resiniferatoxin and capsaicin in conscious rats wth and without outflow obstruction. Journal of Urology 154:611–616

Jarvis GT 1989 Bladder drill. In: Freeman R, Malvern J (eds) The unstable bladder. Wright, Bristol, pp 55–60

Jarvis GT, Millar DR 1980 Controlled trial of bladder drill for overactive bladder. British Medical Journal 281:1322–1323

Jeffcoate TNA, Francis WJA 1966 Urgency incontinence in the female. American Journal of Obstetrics and Gynecology 94:604–618

Jenkinson C, Coulter A, Wright L 1993 Short Form 36 (SF-36) health survey questionnaire. Normative data for adults of working age. British Medical Journal 306:1437–1440

Jonas U, Hofner K, Madesbacher H, Holmdahl TH 1997 Efficacy and safety of two doses of tolterodine versus placebo in patiets with detrusor overactivity and symptoms of frequency, urge incontinence, and urgency: urodynamic evaluation. World Journal of Urology 15:144–151

Karram MM, Bhatia NW 1989 Management of coexistent stress and urge urinary incontinence. Obstetrics and Gynecology 73:4–7

Kelleher C, Khullar V, Cardozo LD 1993 Psychoneuroticism and quality of life in healthy incontinent women. Neurourology and Urodynamics 12(4):393–394

Kelleher CJ, Cardozo LD, Khullar V, Salvatore S, Hill S 1994a Anticholinergic therapy: the need for continued surveillance. Neurourology and Urodynamics 13:432–433

Kelleher CJ, Filsche J, Burton G, Cardozo LD 1994b Acupuncture and the treatment of irritative bladder symptoms. Acupuncture in Medicine 12(1):9–12

Kelleher CJ, Cardozo LD, Khullar V, Salvatore S 1997 A new questionnaire to assess the quality of life of urinary incontinent women. British Journal of Obstetrics and Gynaecology 104:1374–1379

Kennelly MJ, Gormley EA, McGuire EJ 1994 Early clinical experience with adult bladder autoaugmentation. Journal of Urology 152:303–306

Kim DY, Chancellor MB 2000 Intravesical neuromodulatory drugs: capsaicin and resiniferatoxin to treat the overactive bladder. Journal of Endourology 14:97–103

Kinder RB, Mundy AR 1987 Pathophysiology of idiopathic overactive bladder and detrusor hyperreflexia – an in vitro study of human detrusor muscle. British Journal of Urology 60:509–515

Klarskov P 1987 Gukephaline inhibits presynaptically the contractility of urinary tract smooth muscle. British Journal of Urology 59:31–35

Knudsen UB, Rittig S, Pedersen JP, Norgaard JP, Djurhuus JC 1989 Long-term treatment of nocturnal enuresis with desmopressin – influence on urinary output and haematological parameters. Neurourology and Urodynamics 8:348–349

Langworthy DR, Kolb LG, Dees JE 1936 Behaviour of the human bladder freed from cerebral control. Journal of Urology 36:577–597

Laval KU, Lutzeyer W 1980 Spontaneous phasic activity of the detrusor: a cause of uninhibited contractions in the unstable bladder. Urology International 35:182–187

Lawson K 1996 Is there a therapeutic future for 'potassium channel openers'? Clinical Science 91:651–663

Lose G, Jorgensen L, Thunedborg P 1989 Doxepin in the treatment of female detrusor overactivity: a randomized double-blind cross over study. Journal of Urology 142:1024–1027

Madersbacher H, Jilg S 1991 Control of detrusor hyperreflexia by the intravesical instillation of oxybutynin hydrochloride. Paraplegia 29:84–90

Madersbacher H, Stoher M, Richter R et al 1995 Trospium chloride versus oxybutynin: a randomised, double-blind multicentre trial in the treatment of detrusor hyperrflexia. British Journal of Urology 75:452–456

Malone-Lee J, Wahedena I 1993 Characterisation of detrusor contractile function in relation to old age. British Journal of Urology 72:873–880

Massey JA, Abrams P 1986 Dose titration in clinical trials: an example using empronium carageenate in overactive bladder. British Journal of Urology 58:125–128

Mast P, Hoebeke, Wyndale JJ, Oosterlinck W, Everaert K 1995 Experience with clam cystoplasty. A review. Paraplegia 33:560–564

Mazur D, Wehnert J, Dorschner W, Schubert G, Herfurth G, Alken RG 1995 Clinical and urodynamic effects of propiverine in patients suffering from urgency and urge incontinence. Scandinavian Journal of Urology and Nephrology 29:289–294

McRae P, Murray KH. Nurse DE, Stephenson JP, Mundy AR 1987 Clam entero-cystoplasty in the neuropathic bladder. British Journal of Urology 60:523–525

Millard RJ, Oldenberg BF 1983 The symptomatic, urodynamic and psycho-dynamic results of bladder re-education programmes. Journal of Urology 130:717–719

Millard R, Tuttle J, Moore K et al 1999 Clinical efficacy and safety of tolterodine compared to placebo in detrusor overactivity. Journal of Urology 161:1551–1555

Mills IW, Greenland JE, McMurray G et al 2000 Studies of the pathophysiology of idiopathic overactive bladder: the physiological properties of the detrusor smooth muscle and its pattern of innervation. Journal of Urology 163(2):646–651

Moore KH, Sutherst JR 1990 Response to treatment of overactive bladder in relation to psychoneurotic status. British Journal of Urology 66:486–490

Moore KH, Hay DM, Irvine AE, Watson A, Goldstein M 1990 Oxybutynin hydrochloride (3mg) in the treatment of women with idiopathic overactive bladder. British Journal of Urology 66:479–485

Mundy AR 1983 The long-term results of bladder transection for urge incontinence. British Journal of Urology 55:642–644

Murray KH, Feneley RCL 1982 Endorphins – a role in lower urinary tract function? The effect of opioid blockade on the detrusor and urethral sphincter mechanism. British Journal of Urology 54:638–640

Nilvebrant L, Andersson K-E, Gillberg P-G, Stahl M, Sparf B 1997 Tolterodine – a new bladder selective anti-muscarinic agent. European Journal of Pharmacology 327:195–207

Norgaard JP, Rillig S, Djurhuus JC 1989 Nocturnal enuresis: an approach to treatment based on pathogenesis. Journal of Pediatrics 114:705–709

Norton KRW, Bhat AV, Stanton SL 1990 Psychiatric aspects of urinary incontinence in women attending an outpatient clinic. British Medical Journal 31:271–272

Nurse DE, Mundy AR 1987 Cystoplasty infection and cancer. Neurourology and Urodynamics 6:343–344

Okada N, Igawa Y, Nishizawa O 1999 Functional electrical stimulation for overactive bladder. International Urogynecology Journal and Pelvic Floor Dysfunction 10:329–335

Pengelly AW, Stephenson TP, Milroy EJG, Whiteside CG, Turner-Warwick R 1978 Results of prolonged bladder distension as treatment for overactive bladder. British Journal of Urology 50:243–245

Philp T, Shah PJR, Worth PHL 1988 Acupuncture in the treatment of bladder instability. British Journal of Urology 61:490–493

Pigne A, Degansac C, Nyssen C, Barratt J 1985 Acupuncture and the unstable bladder. In: Proceedings of the 15th International Continence Society Meeting, pp 186–187

Plevnik S, Janez J, Vrtacnik P, Trsinar B, Vodusek DB 1986 Short-term electrical stimulation: home treatment for urinary incontinence. World Journal of Urology 4:24–26

Ramsden PD, Smith JC, Dunn M, Ardran GM 1976 Distension therapy for the unstable bladder: late results including an assessment of repeat distensions. Journal of Urology 48:623–629

Rentzhog L, Stanton SL, Cardozo LD, Nelson E, Fall M, Abrams P 1998

Efficacy and safety of tolterodine in patients with overactive bladder: a dose ranging study. British Journal of Urology 81:42–48

Rew DA, Rundle JSH 1989 Assessment of the safety of regular DDAVP therapy in primary nocturnal enuresis. British Journal of Urology 63:352–353

Ritch AES, George CF, Castleden CM, Hall MRP 1977 A second look at emepromium bromide in urinary incontinence. Lancet 1:504–505

Rosario DJ, Leaker BR, Smith DJ, Chapple CR 1995 A pilot study of the effects of multiple doses of the M3 muscarinic receptor antagonist darifenacin on ambulatory parameters of detrusor activity in patients with overactive bladder. Neurourology and Urodynamics 14:464–465

Rose DK 1931 Clinical application of bladder physiology. Journal of Urology 26:91–105

Rosenbaum TP, Shah PJR, Worth PHL 1988 Transtrigonal phenol – the end of an era? Neurourology and Urodynamics 7:294–295

Rosenbaum TP, Shah PJR, Rose GA, Lloyd-Davies RW 1989 Cranberry juice helps the problem of mucus production in enterouroplasties. Neurourology and Urodynamics 8:344–345

Rud T, Andersson K, Ulmsten U 1979 The effects of nifedipine in women with unstable bladders. Urology International 34:421–429

Ruscin JM, Morgenstern NE 1999 Tolterodine use for symptoms of overactive bladder. Annals of Pharmacotherapy 33(10):1073–1082

Salvatore S, Khullar V, Anders K, Cardozo LD 1998 Reducing artifacts in ambulatory urodynamics. British Journal of Urology 81(2):211–214

Salvatore S, Khullar V, Cardozo L, Anders K, Zocchi G, Soligo M 2001 Evaluating ambulatory urodynamics: a prospective study in asymptomatic women. British Journal of Obstetrics and Gynaecology 108:107–111

Seigel SW, Cantanzaro F, Dijkema He et al 2000 Long term results of a multicentre study on sacral nerve stimulation for treatment of urinary urge incontinence, urgency-frequency and retention. Urology 56:87–91

Sibley GNA 1985 An experimental model of overactive bladder in the obstructed pig. British Journal of Urology 57:292–298

Sibley GN 1997 Developments in our understanding of overactive bladder. British Journal of Urology 80:54–61

Slevin M, Plant H, Lynch D, Drinkwater J, Gregory WM 1988 Who should measure quality of life, the doctor or the patient? British Journal of Cancer 57:109–112

Snow BW, Cartwright PC 1996 Bladder autoaugmentation. Urologic Clinics of North America 23:323–331

Speakman MJ, Brading AF, Gilpin CJ, Dixon JS, Gilpin SA, Gosling JA 1987 Bladder outflow obstruction – cause of denervation supersensitivity. Journal of Urology 183:1461–1466

Steel SA, Cox C, Stanton SL 1985 Long-term follow-up of overactive bladder following the colposuspension operation. British Journal of Urology 58:138–142

Stoher M, Madersbacher H, Richter R, Wehnert J, Dreikorn K 1999 Efficacy and safety of propiverine in SCI-patients suffering from detrusor hyperreflexia: a double-blind, placebo-controlled clinical trial. Spinal Cord 37:196–200

Sutherst JR, Brown M 1978 The effect on the bladder pressure of sudden entry of fluid into the posterior urethra. British Journal of Urology 50:406–409

Sutherst JR, Brown M 1984 Comparison of single and multichannel cystometry in diagnosing bladder instability. British Medical Journal 288:1720–1722

Tapp AJS, Cardozo LD 1986 The postmenopausal bladder. British Journal of Hospital Medicine 35:20–23

Thuroff JW, Burke B, Ebner A et al 1991 Randomised double-blind multicentre trial on treatment of frequency, urgency and incontinence related to detrusor hyper-activity: oxybutynin versus propantheline versus placebo. Journal of Urology 145:813–817

Torrens MJ, Griffiths HB 1974 The control of the uninhibited bladder by selective sacral neurectomy. British Journal of Urology 46:639–644

Turner-Warwick RT 1975 Some clinical aspects of detrusor dysfunction. Journal of Urology 113:539–544

van Waalwijk van Doorn ESC, Remmers A, Janknegt RA 1992 Conventional and extramural ambulatory urodynamic testing of the lower urinary tract in female volunteers. Journal of Urology 47:1319–1326

van Waalwijk van Doorn, Anders K, Khullar V et al 2000 Standardisation of ambulatory urodynamic monitoring: report of the Standardisation Sub-committee of the ICS for Ambulatory Urodynamic Studies. Neurourology and Urodynamics 19(2):113–125

Versi E, Cardozo LD 1988 Oestrogens and lower urinary tract function. In: Studd JWW, Whitehead M (eds) The menopause. Blackwell Scientific Publications, Oxford, pp 76–84

Walters MD, Taylor S, Schoenfeld LS 1990 Psychosexual study of women with overactive bladder. Obstetrics and Gynaecology 75:22–26

Warrell DW 1977 Vaginal denervation of the bladder nerve supply. Urology International 32:114–116

Webster JR 1975 Combined video/pressure/flow cystometry in female patients with voiding disturbances. Urology 5:209–213

Wein AJ 1986 Pharmacology of the bladder and urethra. In: Stanton SL, Tanagho E (eds) Surgery of female incontinence, 2nd edn. Springer-Verlag, Heidelberg, pp 229–250

Whiteside CG, Arnold GP 1975 Persistent primary enuresis: a urodynamic assessment. British Medical Journal 1:364–369

Wise BG, Cardozo LD, Cutner A, Kelleher C, Burton G 1992 Maximal electrical stimulation: an acceptable alternative to anticholinergic therapy. International Urogynecology Journal 3(3):270

Wise BG, Cardozo LD, Cutner A, Benness CJ, Burton G 1993a The prevalence and significance of urethral instability in women with overactive bladder. British Journal of Urology 72:26–29

Wise BG, Benness CJ, Cardozo LD, Cutner A 1993b Vaginal oestradiol for lower urinary tract symptoms in post-menopausal women. A double blind placebo-controlled study. In: Proceedings of the 7th International Congress on the Menopause, Stockholm, p 15

World Health Organization 1978 Definition of health. Constitution of the WHO 28th edn. WHO, Geneva

Zoubek J, Bloom D, Sedman AB 1990 Extraordinary urinary frequency. Pediatrics 85:1112–1114

54
Voiding difficulties
Gary E. Lemack   Philippe E. Zimmern

INTRODUCTION

Voiding disorders in women are frequently difficult to characterize and often even more difficult to treat effectively. While some patients have an obvious source to which the sudden development of voiding disorders can be traced, there is often no clear origin for what can be a slowly developing, yet progressive symptom complex. Knowing when to alter the diagnostic strategy, and in which direction, remain critical aspects of the treating physician's evaluation. That various pathological processes can produce similar symptomatology makes diagnosis and treatment challenging. For example, urinary urgency, frequency and nocturia can all be caused by a urinary tract infection, a bladder tumour, a neurological condition, bladder outlet obstruction (BOO) or other causes. When no cause can be found despite thorough investigation, one is left treating symptoms rather than the pathological entity itself.

In this chapter, we describe the complaints frequently reported by women who enter a clinic that specializes in voiding dysfunction. We explain our approach to evaluation and management of voiding disorders and discuss the more common pathological processes underlying these conditions.

TERMINOLOGY

Lower urinary tract symptoms (LUTS)

A term encompassing a variety of symptoms normally associated with bladder storage or emptying functions. Specific areas used to determine LUTS during history taking typically include:

- frequency of daytime and nighttime voiding
- urgency associated with the need to urinate
- pain associated with (or relieved by) voiding
- need to strain, bend over or otherwise alter positions to void
- force of the urinary stream
- hesitancy in voiding
- the nature of the urinary stream (smooth vs interrupted)
- the sensation of incomplete emptying.

Urine leakage related to urgency (urge incontinence) or activities that increase intra-abdominal pressure (stress urinary incontinence) may also be included as LUTS.

Overactive bladder

A term to convey symptoms normally associated with detrusor activity during the storage phase (bladder filling). Typical symptoms include urinary frequency, urgency and urge-related incontinence.

Urinary retention

Can be acute or chronic. Acute retention is normally associated with severe pelvic discomfort and a precipitating event, such as flaring of a progressive neurological injury (e.g. multiple sclerosis) or other neurological event (e.g. spinal cord injury, epidural anaesthetic). Often, acute retention will be noticed after extensive pelvic surgery, such as abdominoperineal resection or low anterior resection for rectal cancer. It can also be associated with the use of medication(s), particularly narcotics.

Chronic retention, on the other hand, is usually painless. It is often associated with the surreptitious finding of elevated postvoid residuals (greater than the voided volumes) when evaluating vague bladder complaints, recurrent urinary tract infections or postvoid dribbling (when the patient experiences overflow incontinence). Chronic retention is often associated with other chronic conditions (e.g. diabetes, dementia), severe constipation, bladder prolapse, bladder obstruction (congenital or acquired) or sacral spinal cord injuries.

INCIDENCE

A clear linear relationship seems to exist between the development of bladder symptoms and ageing. For example, Schatzl and colleagues (2000) noted that only 3.1% of women younger than 30 experienced nocturia greater than twice per night, whereas 26.7% of those aged 60 and older did. This seems to be true of most irritative symptoms as well as urinary incontinence. In fact, increases in residual volumes and decreases in maximum flow rate, voided volume and bladder capacity have been noted in patients of advancing age of both sexes. Similarly, voiding difficulties, thought to be fairly unusual in women, were found in 9.1% of women over the age of 60. Although surprisingly high, this figure may be even higher, as recent urodynamic studies estimate BOO to be present in as many as 20% of women visiting a centre for voiding disorders.

AETIOLOGY AND PATHOPHYSIOLOGY

Chronic conditions

Several chronic conditions have been linked to bladder dysfunction. Perhaps the most common is diabetes mellitus, which frequently leads to chronic bladder distension and detrusor hypocontractility over time. Microangiopathy is thought to be responsible for the development of the diabetic neuropathy that commonly affects the genitourinary system and overall bladder dysfunction is normally present in 25–50% of diabetics, though overt symptoms are commonly absent during the initial phases. Ultimately, impaired bladder sensation, elevated residuals and recurrent urinary tract infections indicate more significant dysfunction.

Neurogenic

Virtually all neurological conditions can affect the bladder. Cerebrovascular accidents, for example, often lead to urgency and frequency as a result of detrusor hyperreflexia (DH) or unstable bladder contractions during filling. Parkinson's disease can lead to LUTS in both men and women before the neurological disease becomes advanced.

Multiple sclerosis (MS) is also often associated with urgency and urge incontinence, though urodynamic findings can include detrusor areflexia and lack of co-ordination between the detrusor and external sphincter (detrusor sphincter dyssynergia – DSD) in addition to DH. As a result, the clinical presentation can vary and urinary retention is not uncommon in women with MS.

Depending on the level and extent, spinal cord injury often results in bladder dysfunction. Immediately after the injury, the bladder enters a spinal shock phase in which detrusor activity ceases. In cases of suprasacral injuries, after the spinal shock phase passes (usually in 3–6 months), DH and DSD may present as urgency and urge incontinence and there is potential for renal damage if intravesical pressures remain elevated. With sacral lesions, detrusor areflexia persists. Consequently, the patient is unable to void spontaneously. Other lesions of the cord, such as herniated discs, may also be associated with bladder dysfunction.

Obstructive

While BOO is much less common in women than men, it can still cause severe voiding dysfunction.

Congenital

Urethral strictures (intrinsic or luminal lesions), thought to be very uncommon in women, are rarely responsible for BOO and can often be diagnosed during cystoscopy or voiding cysto-urethrography. Ectopic ureterocoeles can similarly obstruct the urethra.

Neoplasm

Rarely, malignant neoplasms can cause urethral obstruction (e.g. urethral squamous cell carcinoma, sarcoma botryoides), as can benign vaginal neoplasms (leiomyoma) or cysts. Large bladder neck neoplasms (most commonly transitional cell) produce BOO, but also do so rarely.

Prolapse

Severe anterior vaginal wall prolapse (cystocoele) may cause significant voiding dysfunction. Both detrusor instability and impaired detrusor contractility can occur as a result, particularly when a severely prolapsed bladder is present in combination with an adequately supported urethra (often after bladder neck suspension or pubovaginal sling). In this case, outlet resistance is enhanced, which leads to elevated postvoid residuals and, often, to recurrent infections.

Iatrogenic

BOO is an unfortunate outcome of some anti-incontinence procedures (1–20% of cases). Regardless of the type of procedure done to improve incontinence, overzealous tightening of the bolstering mechanism used to restore urethral position or to provide suburethral support can increase outlet resistance and create obstructive voiding patterns, elevated postvoid residuals, urinary urgency and recurrent urinary tract infections. Periurethral fibrosis, thought to be a result of scarring related to surgery at the bladder neck and along the urethra, may also be responsible for BOO and is best diagnosed by urethral MRI.

Inflammatory

Chronic inflammatory diseases that affect the bladder, such as eosinophilic cystitis and malacoplakia, can produce storage and voiding abnormalities. Initial strategies seek to confirm the diagnosis, often by biopsy, so as to rule out neoplasm. Typical management strategies include oral steroid or antihistamine use (eosinophilic cystitis) or prolonged antibiotic and anticholinergic therapy (malacoplakia). Interstitial cystitis (IC) is a chronic inflammatory condition of uncertain aetiology that may affect as many as 70 per 100 000 women in the United States (covered in detail in Chapter 56).

Infectious

Acute and chronic bacterial cystitis can result in voiding abnormalities (typically dysuria), sensation of incomplete emptying and occasionally postvoid dribbling. Other infectious aetiologies, such as tuberculous disease, should be considered in certain patient populations (e.g. immunocompromised patients, travel history, presence of sterile pyuria). Fungal infections may also cause bladder dysfunction, most typically in patients with indwelling catheters, those receiving broad-spectrum antibiotics or those who are immunosuppressed. Viral infections, while difficult to diagnose, are thought to result in irritative bladder symptoms and haematuria, particularly in children and immunocompromised adults.

Miscellaneous

Medications containing α-adrenergic agonist agents, such as many over-the-counter decongestants containing pseudoephedrine, may have a contractile effect on the bladder neck and proximal urethra that results in increased outlet resistance and elevated residuals. Psychotropic drugs or anticholinergic medications can also affect detrusor function and provoke various degrees of urinary retention.

It is not uncommon for patients to experience a transient period of retention following major surgery, regardless of the type (abdominal, neurosurgical, etc.). Usually, a short period of clean intermittent catheterization is all that is required and residuals taper off within the first 2 weeks. An even shorter period of retention in the postpartum period has also been reported and has no recognized long-lasting sequelae if appropriately diagnosed and treated.

Rarely, patients with a large cervical myoma will experience difficulty voiding due to a direct compressive effect on the bladder neck. In those cases, hysterectomy may be the only solution, though video-urodynamic evaluation is mandatory to confirm the diagnosis prior to proceeding. Similarly, patients with haematocolpos due to an imperforate hymen may also experience voiding symptoms due to direct compression.

Finally, some young women may suffer from Fowler's syndrome, an inability to relax the external sphincter at the time of voiding. This can lead to elevated bladder pressures and residuals. Pelvic floor retraining and biofeedback are essential in teaching these women how to void successfully.

Idiopathic

Despite a thorough evaluation, the source of voiding dysfunction will not be discovered in many women with LUTS. Age alone correlates with its development, regardless of coexisting risk factors. This may be caused by a number of processes such as occult supratentorial CNS lesions, neurogenic or myogenic dysfunction at the level of the bladder and changes in extracellular matrix composition at the level of the bladder and urethra.

PRESENTATION

Voiding disorders are associated with hesitancy, straining to void, weak flow, intermittent stream and/or the feeling of incomplete emptying. Frequency, urgency and nocturia are also quite common, although less directly suggestive of BOO. The detrusor muscle can become overactive in reaction to an obstructive mechanism. Certainly, a high index of suspicion for BOO should exist when a patient states that her flow has decreased since her most recent operation.

None the less, using question number 5 of the Urogenital Distress Inventory-6 questionnaire in 128 women complaining of LUTS, Lemack et al (1999) found that most patients who answered that incomplete emptying was their most bothersome symptom had urodynamically proven BOO (61%) and most women with a different main complaint were unobstructed (73%, $p <0.002$).

Patients who have developed acute retention may be in pain and require prompt drainage. Chronic retention presents with frequency and then overflow incontinence. All of these may be associated with symptoms of a primary cause. Urinary tract infection, with its usual presenting symptoms, may occur in response to high levels of residual urine.

PHYSICAL EXAMINATION

Patients suspected of having a voiding disorder should undergo a general abdominal examination, a focused neurological examination with inspection of the back for stigmata of an underlying neurological lesion (e.g. spina bifida occulta) and a detailed and combined vaginal/perineal examination. Clinical examination may disclose a palpable bladder (assuming a retention volume over 150 ml in a non-obese patient) and signs of the primary cause may be present. Occasionally, LUTS can be the first manifestation of MS or a herniated disk. During vaginal examination, the entire length of the urethra should be palpated for any tender area or mass. An overcorrected urethra from previous surgery with dense periurethral scarring should be noted. The urethral meatus should be carefully examined for urethral caruncle or luminal narrowing. Urethral calibration, however, is not necessary since the external appearance has not been correlated with openness during

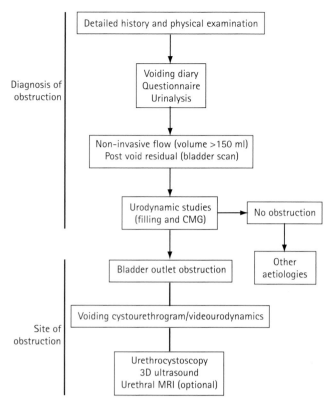

Fig. 54.1   Evaluation of lower urinary tract symptoms in woman.

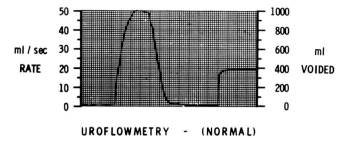

UROFLOWMETRY - (NORMAL)

Fig. 54.2   Normal flow rate.

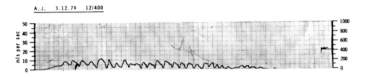

Fig. 54.3   Flow rate showing voiding difficulty with an attenuated flow not exceeding 15 ml/sec.

voiding. Presence of a cystocoele, anterior vaginal wall scar(s) from prior Kelly plication or other vaginal procedures, cervical appearance and position with straining should be assessed and a bimanual examination to determine uterine size should be performed.

INVESTIGATION (Fig. 54.1)

Urine culture and sensitivity

A urine sample (midstream) should be analysed for all patients with voiding difficulty. Urinary infection may occasionally precipitate acute retention and infection is often a sequel of incomplete bladder emptying.

Urinary diary

Accurate record of fluid intake and output is important and most patients can easily maintain a urinary diary. Several variations for collecting a urinary diary have been reported, with time periods ranging from 3 to 14 days. Critical diary parameters include mean voided volume, number of voiding episodes per day and night, maximum and minimum bladder volumes and overall daily fluid intake. When catheterization is carried out for acute retention, it is essential to note the volume of urine drained and the frequency of catheterization. Bladder overdistension (over 500 ml) should be discouraged to avoid permanent damage to the smooth muscle fibres of the detrusor. When catheterized volumes consistently decrease to

100–150 ml, intermittent catheterization can usually be discontinued.

Uroflowmetry

Measuring the rate of free urine flow is a good indicator of voiding function. Despite its ease, wide availability and inexpensive nature, the uroflowmetry should be interpreted with caution. Accurate interpretation in men necessitates a minimal voided volume of 150 ml. Although this guideline has never been replicated in women, it is commonly applied when interpreting uroflow data.

Maximum flow rate (Q_{max}), voiding time and the shape of the uroflow curve must be assessed. Although age-normative values are lacking, flow rates consistently below 15 ml for a volume greater than 150 ml indicate some voiding dysfunction. This may be due to an obstructive process or to abnormal detrusor contractility (hypocontractility or impaired contractility). The shape of the curve is also important. The normal, bell-shaped cone (Fig. 54.2) should be compared with the attenuated and intermittent flow rate of the patient with voiding difficulty (Fig. 54.3). Following uroflowmetry, an estimate of postvoid residual (PVR) by catheterization or ultrasound (bladder scan) is necessary to determine functional bladder capacity.

Filling and voiding cystometrogram (CMG)

Based on the physical principle that obstruction exists in a fluid-transporting system if elevated pressure is required to transport flow through a relative narrowing, the simultaneous measurement of detrusor pressure and urine flow during voiding offers the best objective evidence for diagnosing BOO in women. Both filling and voiding studies help establish whether there is a neurogenic bladder component. Suprapontine and cord lesions above S2, 3 and 4 may show uninhibited detrusor contractions (Fig. 54.4a) and/or changes in bladder compliance.

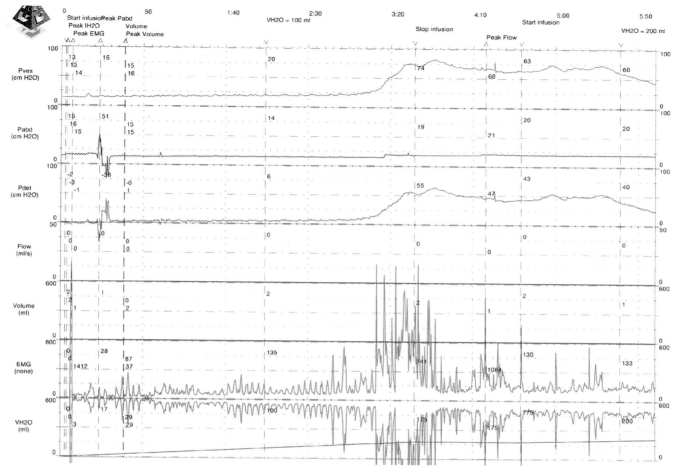

Fig. 54.4 **a** Urodynamics study demonstrating an unstable detrusor contraction at 175 cc (noted on first and third tracings) and sphincter dyssynergia (EMG tracing) simultaneously.

Peripheral lesions of the cord will show late sensation to void, a large-capacity bladder with a normal or low voiding pressure and residual urine (Fig. 54.4b). Both may show impaired detrusor contractility, especially in older patients.

According to the International Continence Society, the filling CMG evaluates time to first bladder filling sensation, presence of uninhibited detrusor contractions (magnitude, bladder volume when it arises), bladder compliance and maximum bladder capacity. Variations in the test include prolapse reduction (pessary or pack), EMG patches to document proper relaxation during voiding (exclude dysfunctional voider) and recording – through a small suprapubic catheter – when urethral pain/pathology is present to avoid urethral instrumentation. Many urodynamic laboratories repeat the filling and voiding cycles to ensure the data are reproducible (two 'fill and void') and compare intubated flow against non-invasive flow pattern to account for the possible obstructive effect of the urethral catheter. The latter effect can be minimized by using a small (6 F or 7 F) double-lumen urethral catheter.

Computerized equipment enhances the interpretation of urodynamic studies (Fig. 54.5). None the less, age-normative data are scant. Therefore, most studies reporting cut-off values for BOO in women use symptomatic control groups (LUTS or stress urinary incontinence).

Our current criteria, based on a large-scale, prospective study using receiver operator characteristics (ROC) curves, suggest that, regardless of the mechanism of obstruction, detrusor pressure at maximum flow ($P_{det}Q_{max}$) above 21 cm H_2O combined to a maximum flow (Q_{max}) less than 11 ml/sec is highly suggestive of BOO. In contrast, control groups generally exhibit $P_{det}Q_{max}$ values at 20–25 cmH$_2$O combined with Q_{max} above 20 ml/sec. These criteria do not apply to dysfunctional voiders, patients in complete retention, patients unable to void during the study and patients with long-standing obstruction in whom detrusor decompensation is suspected.

Videocystourethrography (the combination of CMG, uroflowmetry and radiological screening during bladder filling and voiding) provides a comprehensive study of bladder function, but whether this is necessary in all cases of voiding difficulty is debatable. In addition to the information provided by CMG alone, videocystourethrography will show abnormal bladder morphology, e.g. formation of sacculation and diverticulum, and presence of vesicoureteric reflux.

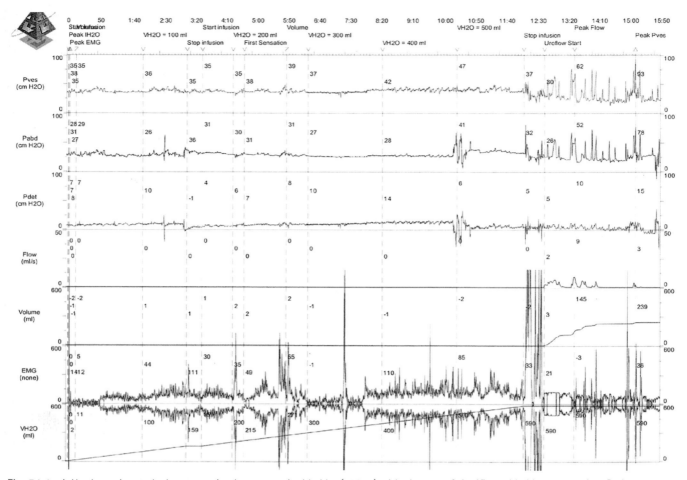

Fig. 54.4 **b** Urodynamics study demonstrating large capacity bladder (590 cc) with absence of significant bladder contraction. Patient urinates by straining (note increase in both intravesical and intra-abdominal pressures on first and second tracings) and voids less than half of instilled volume (239 cc).

Video-urodynamic studies, which are primarily available only in larger medical centres, can certainly help determine the site of BOO. Absence of bladder neck opening or excessive ballooning of the proximal urethra suggest proximal and distal sites (Fig. 54.6) for obstruction, respectively. When overlying bony structures in the oblique or lateral positions render the study doubtful, a voiding cystourethrogram with lateral films can help determine the exact site of obstruction.

Radiology

An abdominal X-ray can disclose a large amount of residual urine. A lumbosacral spine X-ray is important to exclude congenital (e.g. sacral agenesis; spina bifida occulta: Fig. 54.7) or acquired (intervertebral disc) lesions. Both can produce a peripheral neurological disorder. Intravenous urography is less useful than it was because ultrasound now produces comparable information on back-pressure effects (hydronephrosis) on the ureter and kidney. Upper tract studies are recommended when high voiding pressures, changes in compliance and/or a large cystocoele are found.

A voiding cystourethrogram (VCUG) is a simple, safe, easily reproducible study with which to evaluate the lower urinary tract in standing position (Table 54.1). During voiding, bladder neck funnelling, urethral configuration (angulation, distortion) and active reflux can all be observed. Normal urethral angle on a lateral view ranges from 0 to 30°. A patient with LUTS suggestive of BOO who demonstrates a negative angle after a prior anti-incontinence procedure may suffer from over-correction.

Ultrasonography

Abdominal ultrasound scanning provides an estimate of residual urine to within 20%, which is sufficiently accurate. Intravesical lesions such as an ectopic ureterocoele can be demonstrated. Office bladder scanners have become popular for rapid assessment of PVR. Three-dimensional ultrasound has helped screening for urethral or periurethral lesions (diverticulum).

Cystourethroscopy

Cystoscopy can be performed in an office setting with a rigid or flexible cystoscope. Difficulty in instrumenting the urethra

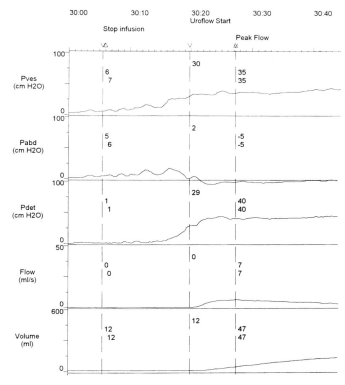

Fig. 54.5. Voiding cystometrogram demonstrating a maximum flow (Q_{max}) at 7 ml/sec with an intravesical pressure around 30 cmH$_2$O ($P_{det}Q_{max}$ 35 – minus 5 cmH$_2$O baseline). Because of relaxation during voiding, the abdominal pressure dropped slightly, thus artificially raising $P_{det}Q_{max}$.

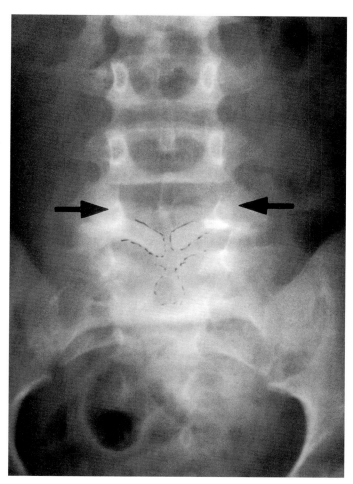

Fig. 54.7 Lumbosacral spine X-ray showing spina bifida occulta (arrows).

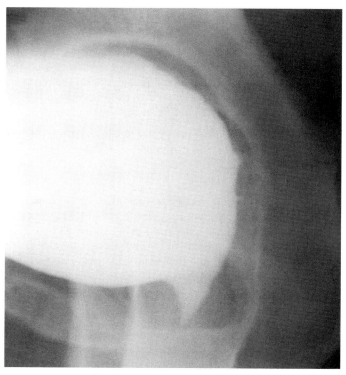

Fig. 54.6. VCUG (voiding study) demonstrating distal urethral beaking and marked distension of middle and proximal urethra in a urodynamically obstructed woman.

Table 54.1 Voiding cystourethrogram checklist

Film	Information
Scout	Calculi (diverticular, urinary tract); bony abnormalities (osteitis pubis, vertebral defect); soft tissue/pelvic mass; foreign body (bone anchors); metal clips from previous surgery
Anteroposterior view	Bladder trabeculation, diverticulum, reflux Tumour/filling defects Bladder neck position in relation to symphysis pubis
Lateral view	Urethral axis (normal, overcorrected, hypermobility)
Rest/Straining	Bladder base descent (severity of cystocoele)
Voiding view	Opening of bladder neck, active reflux, urethral diverticulum, ballooning of the proximal urethra, distal urethral narrowing, overcorrected urethra, vaginal voiding
Post void	Postvoid residual; urethral diverticulum

arises when there is significant urethral narrowing (e.g. urethral stenosis) or other pathologies (e.g. diverticular opening, tumour). Cystoscopy demonstrates whether there is any intravesical pathology and whether trabeculation, sacculation and diverticulum have occurred. These findings suggest long-standing obstruction but do not indicate its cause.

Electrophysiological tests

Concentric or single-fibre needle electromyography of the pelvic floor and urethral sphincter mechanism (with terminal motor latency studies of the perineal branch of the pudendal nerve) indicates whether denervation or nerve damage to these structures has occurred. In evaluating neurological conditions, EMG is important to diagnose detrusor–sphincter dyssynergia.

Urethral MRI

With enhancement of high-resolution images obtained with endorectal coil MRI, this imaging modality has helped diagnose complex cases of BOO involving the urethral wall or periurethral tissues. Our group has reported normative female urethral measurements that then allowed recognition of site and extent of periurethral fibrosis, excessive injection of periurethral material (i.e. fat, collagen) or recurrent scarring periurethrally after extensive urethrolysis.

TREATMENT

Principles of therapy

Both the primary condition and its effects on the bladder may need treatment. In cases of acute retention, these may require simultaneous treatment.

Catheterization can be urethral or suprapubic. Urethral is quickest and simplest but is uncomfortable for some patients and, if maintained for longer than 5–7 days, is associated with a higher incidence of urinary tract infection than a suprapubic catheter (unless prophylactic, low-dose antibiotic therapy is prescribed). Moreover, it is impossible to see whether a patient can resume spontaneous voiding with a urethral catheter in place. However, it is ideal for short-term situations.

Clean intermittent self-catheterization is a non-sterile technique that enables the patient (or her caregiver) to catheterize herself to manage chronic urinary retention. The catheters are disposable and changed periodically. A suprapubic catheter is used mainly to monitor the degree of urinary retention following bladder neck suspension or sling surgery. Despite being placed intraoperatively, the suprapubic catheter must be inserted carefully to avoid bowel injury.

Drugs may be used either to treat symptoms of voiding difficulty or as an adjunct to catheterization, but they are often ineffective. They may relax the sphincter mechanism or stimulate detrusor contraction.

α-Adrenergic blockers (e.g. phenoxybenzamine 10 mg bd) are non-selective α-blocking agents that have the unwanted side effects of tachycardia and fainting due to α_2 stimulation. Terazosin (1–10 mg once daily), doxazosin (2–8 mg once daily) and tamsulosin (0.4 mg once daily) are more selective α_1-blocking agents with unproven efficacy in treating women with lower urinary tract symptoms. Baclofen (5 mg tds to 25 mg qds) is a striated muscle relaxant used to treat spasticity. Diazepam (10–15 mg once daily) acts centrally as a muscle relaxant and has an anxiolytic effect. Both baclofen and diazepam may be used to relax the sphincter.

Muscarinic agents (e.g. bethanechol chloride 20–100 mg qds) should be used with caution among elderly patients, asthmatic patients and patients with cardiovascular disease or parkinsonism. The efficacy of bethanechol in treating women with voiding dysfunction is questionable. Anticholinesterase agents such as distigmine bromide (5 mg/day) have been tried, but they have little proven effect.

Prophylaxis

It is a simple and wise precaution to obtain a non-invasive flow rate and a PVR in any patient scheduled for continence surgery. Many of these procedures (sling especially) are 'obstructive' and any predisposition to voiding difficulty may result in retention or marked changes in voiding pattern (straining, bending over, double voiding).

Asymptomatic voiding difficulty

Patients with asymptomatic voiding difficulty need supervision to help avoid urinary tract infection. Upper tract dilatation rarely occurs in females unless it is associated with a neuropathy.

Symptoms only

Patients with only symptoms of voiding difficulty may be treated with α-adrenergic blocking agents in the dosages detailed above, though experience with this approach is largely anecdotal. The dosage will often be limited by the side-effects of hypotension.

Retention

Acute retention
Where cause is likely to recur (postpartum), simply relieving retention and then removing the catheter is likely to lead to renewed retention. If the amount of urine withdrawn exceeds 1 litre, the bladder is unlikely to recover immediately. In these situations, it is sensible to either insert a suprapubic catheter or to teach the patient or her family to perform intermittent catheterization. Use of a follow-up diary to record voided volumes against residual volumes helps indicate when proper emptying has been re-established.

When there is not an obvious cause and a urine amount less than 1 litre is removed, a Foley catheter can be left in place for 24–48 hours. A voiding trial can then be attempted.

Chronic retention
Chronic retention includes iatrogenic conditions or advanced

processes which result in significant and permanent damage to the detrusor wall (e.g. hypocontractile bladder, impaired contractility).

Clean intermittent self-catheterization is ideal for the manually dextrous patient and should be carried out 4–6 times daily, depending on the amount of fluid intake. Most patients develop urinary colonization and antibiotics are only required for symptoms of urinary tract infection.

For the patient who is not manually dextrous or who is unwilling to perform clean intermittent self-catheterization, a suprapubic catheter can be considered. This catheter should be changed monthly and removed when residuals consistently drop below 100–150 ml.

Some conditions (e.g. distal urethral stenosis) will benefit from dilatation under general anaesthesia (up to 41 F) or an Otis urethrotomy. The latter procedure, once very popular, is seldom performed because of the risk of bleeding, sphincteric damage and secondary periurethral scarring. Technically, the epithelium and submucosa of the urethra is cut in three longitudinal incisions at 4, 7 and 12 o'clock and a large Foley catheter is left in place for 5–7 days. Urethral dilatation is quite painful in the office setting, especially beyond larger diameters (over 30 F). Maximal effectiveness to 'break' the ring of urethral scar may necessitate the use of larger sounds, requiring intravenous sedation. Recurrent urethral stenosis can be corrected by distal urethroplasty.

Although rare, urethral tumours can present with obstructive symptoms and should be managed according to biopsy findings (histology type, grade of cellular differentiation) and local or distant spread (distal urethrectomy, radical cystourethrectomy, radiation therapy).

Patients with chronic retention (due to inefficient or absent reflex micturition, usually after spinal cord injury) who are resistant to conservative therapy may choose electrostimulation using a sacral anterior root stimulator of S2, 3 and 4. If detrusor–sphincter dyssynergia exists, complete sacral rhizotomy of S2 to S5 is offered as well. A three-channel stimulator, for both sides of S2, 3 and 4, is implanted with cables led to three independent receivers to allow separate stimulation of S2, 3 and 4. It is activated by a battery-driven oscillator block that is placed over the three receivers (Brindley 1994). Other surgical interventions, such as augmentation cystoplasty or continent supravesical diversions (with catheterizable cutaneous stoma), can be considered in patients able to perform clean intermittent self-catheterization.

Urethrolysis

Surgical urethrolysis remains the mainstay of treatment in patients with BOO after a previous anti-incontinence procedure. Most cases are amenable to a transvaginal approach. The extent of urethrolysis (lateral, anterior, circumferential) depends on the nature of the previous surgery and intraoperative findings. When the obstruction is due to a fascial or synthetic procedure, the sling material can be incised at the undersurface of the urethra to restore normal voiding function. However, recurrent stress urinary incontinence can ensue. Thus, resuspension is advocated by several authors at the risk of reinducing obstruction. Following urethrolysis, a Martius labial fat pad

graft can be used to wrap the urethra and prevent rescarring. Similar success rates have been reported with transvaginal or retropubic approaches (60–80%), with variable definitions of successful outcome. Preoperative recognition of detrusor instability carries a bad omen in most studies, with persistence of these irritative symptoms in many patients despite relief of BOO.

Other outflow–relieving surgical procedures

Meatoplasty (using vaginal or vestibular flaps) is indicated in established cases of meatal stenosis or distal periurethral fibrosis. This reconstructive procedure is generally considered when urethral dilatation under anaesthesia has led to temporary improvement in symptomatology. Large cystocoeles, which can also cause obstruction by a kinking effect, can be repaired either transvaginally or transabdominally with the goals of restoring bladder base support, improving voiding parameters and maintaining a normal vaginal axis and depth. A pessary may be considered in surgically unfit patients or temporarily to detect SUI. Urethral hypermobility which is often associated with large cystocoeles can be prophylactically corrected by a simple bladder neck suspension at the time of cystocoele repair. Some experts prefer to rely on preoperative urodynamic findings of SUI (following reduction of the cystocoele with pack or pessary) to decide on the concomitant need for providing urethral support. In rare instances a hysterectomy may be indicated (enlarged or retroverted uterus compressing or displacing the bladder neck area). Likewise the occasional patient with crippling BOO and stress or urge incontinence after many failed corrective surgeries may be considered for bladder neck closure and supravesical diversion.

Treatment outcome

There is a dearth of literature on how to assess medical and surgical outcomes for voiding dysfunction. Ideally, combined subjective (questionnaire, diary, examination) and objective (uroflow, residual, VCUG, urodynamic studies) measures should be available to determine success or failure of a given treatment modality. Follow-up intervals should also be specified to ensure durability of results.

CONCLUSION

Voiding difficulties form a spectrum of disorders, which range from symptoms only to established retention. Often these are poorly recognized and inadequately treated. Prevention, early diagnosis and a range of treatment modalities starting with catheterization and possibly involving surgical intervention, where indicated, are key points. Future improvements will derive from the development of disease-specific questionnaires, refinements in urodynamic definition of BOO and comparison with normal age-matched women, surgical innovation into minimally invasive, non-obstructive, anti-incontinence procedures providing durable outcomes and critical use of outcomes tools.

KEY POINTS

1. Voiding disorders may be asymptomatic and occasionally lead to upper tract dilatation.
2. Normal voiding in the female occurs by detrusor contraction, pelvic floor relaxation or abdominal straining. Failure of co-ordination of the first two may lead to voiding difficulty.
3. The epidural in labour is a potent cause of undiagnosed urinary retention and subsequent voiding difficulty.
4. Symptoms of poor or intermittent urinary stream are the best markers of voiding difficulty.
5. Uroflowmetry is the simplest screening test. When combined with cystometrograms, it is sufficient to diagnose most voiding disorders.
6. Treatment is directed towards bladder emptying and management of the primary cause.
7. Drug therapy has little proven clinical effect.
8. Surgical relief of iatrogenic obstruction should be considered when voiding symptoms started following an anti-incontinence procedure.

REFERENCES

Brindley G 1994 Electrical stimulation in vesicourethral dysfunction: practical devices. In: Mundy A, Stephenson T, Wein A (eds) Urodynamics: principles, practice and application, 2nd edn. Churchill Livingstone, London, pp 489–493

Schatzl G, Temml C, Schmidbauer J et al 2000 Cross-sectional study of nocturia in both sexes: analysis of a voluntary health screening project. Urology 56:71–75

Lemack GE, Foster B, Zimmern PE 1999 Urethral dilation in women: a questionnaire-based analysis of practice patterns. Urology 54:37–43

SUGGESTED READING

Abrams P, Wein AJ 1999 The overactive bladder and incontinence: definitions and a plea for discussion. Neurourology and Urodynamics 18:413–416

Curhan GC, Speizer FE, Hunter DJ et al 1999 Epidemiology of interstitial cystitis: a population based study. Journal of Urology 161:549–552

Carlson VK, Rome S, Nitti VW 2000 Dysfunctional voiding in women. Journal of Urology 165:143–148

Carr LK, Webster GD 1996 Bladder outlet obstruction in women. Urologic Clinics of North America 23:385–391

Diokno AC, Brock BM, Brown MB et al 1986 Prevalence of urinary incontinence and other urological symptoms in the noninstitutionalized elderly. Journal of Urology 136:1022–1025

Faerman I, Maler M, Jadzinsky M et al 1971 Asymptomatic neurogenic bladder in juvenile diabetics. Diabetologia 7:168–172

FitzGerald MP, Brubaker L 2001 The etiology of urinary retention after surgery for genuine stress incontinence. Neurourology and Urodynamics 20:13–21

Groutz A, Blaivas JG, Chaikin DC 2000 Bladder outlet obstruction in women: definition and characteristics. Neurourology and Urodynamics 19:213–220

Goldman HB, Rackley RR, Appell RA 1999 The efficacy of urethrolysis without re-suspension for iatrogenic urethral obstruction. Journal of Urology

Hilton P, Laor D 1989 Voiding symptoms in the female: the correlation with urodynamic voiding characteristics. Neurourology and Urodynamics 8:308–310

Hilton P 1990 Bladder drainage. In: Stanton SL (ed) Clinical urogynaecology, 2nd edn. Churchill Livingstone, London

Haylen BT 2000 Editorial – voiding difficulty in woman. International Urogynecology Journal 11:1–3

Kahan M, Goldberg PD, Mandel EE 1970 Neurogenic vesical dysfunction and diabetes mellitus. New York State Journal of Medicine 70:2448–2455

Kumar A, Mandhani A, Gogoi S, Srivastava A 1999 Management of functional bladder neck obstruction in women: use of α-blockers and pediatric resectoscope for bladder neck incision. Journal of Urology 162:2061–2065

Lemack GE, Zimmern PE 2000 Pressure-flow analysis can aid in identifying women with outflow obstruction. Journal of Urology 163:1823–1828

Lemack GE, Dewey RB, Roehrborn CG et al 2000 Questionnaire-based assessment of bladder dysfunction in patients with mild to moderate Parkinson's disease. Urology 56:250–254

Lemack GE, Zimmern PE 1999 Predictability of urodynamic findings based on the urogenital distress inventory-6 questionnaire. Urology 54:461–466

Madersbacher S, Pycha A, Schatzl G et al 1998 The aging lower urinary tract: a comparative urodynamic study of men and women. Urology 51:206–212

Shaw PJR 1992 Voiding difficulties and retention. In: Stanton SL (ed) Clinical urogynaecology, 2nd edn. Churchill Livingstone, Edinburgh

Snooks SJ, Swash M 1984 Abnormalities of the innervation of the urethral striated musculature in incontinence. British Journal of Urology 56:401–405

Stanton SL, Ozsoy C, Hilton P 1983 Voiding difficulties in the female: prevalence, clinical and urodynamic review. Obstetrics and Gynecology 61:144–147

Smith RNJ, Cardozo L 1997 Early voiding difficulty after colposuspension. British Journal of Urology 80:911–914

Worth P 1986 Urethrotomy. In: Stanton SL, Tanagho EA (eds) Surgery of female incontinence, 2nd edn. Springer-Verlag, Heidelberg

Webster GD, Kreder KJ 1990 Voiding dysfunction following cystourethropexy: its evaluation and management. Journal of Urology 144:670–763

Zimmern PE, Hadley HR, Leach GE et al 1987 Female urethral obstruction after Marshall–Marchetti–Krantz operation. Journal of Urology 138:517

55

Vaginal prolapse

Stuart L. Stanton

INTRODUCTION

Prolapse, rather than urinary incontinence, is now the great clinical and academic challenge for urogynaecology. Significant advances in diagnosis, medical and surgical treatments have contributed to a higher cure rate for primary and secondary incontinence than primary and secondary prolapse.

The reasons for this may lie in the incentive, because of the greater impairment of quality of life for incontinence than prolapse and, therefore, the greater challenge in the knowledge that a sharper and more distinct endpoint exists for continence than prolapse. Both gynaecologists and urologists see incontinence as a competitive challenge whereas prolapse has, until recently, been the province solely of the gynaecologist for which there was little glamour in cure. Finally, there are the fundamental and structural difficulties in achieving a cure rather than an improvement and the inherent risks of recurrence of prolapse surgery.

PREVALENCE

About 50% of parous women have prolapse, which is symptomatic in 20%. Symptoms of coital laxity may be reported by 5% of women. Olsen et al (1997), reporting on a population of North American women, noted that by 80 years of age 11.1% had undergone surgery for prolapse or urinary incontinence and that 29% of them required repeat surgery later. Prolapse is frequently accompanied by urinary or faecal incontinence with increasing severity of symptoms in postmenopausal women. Up to 51% may have anterior vaginal wall prolapse while 27% may have posterior wall prolapse and 20% have uterine or vault prolapse. No trend has been noted between prolapse and menopausal age (Versi et al 2001). Vaginal vault prolapse may be found in 1.8% of women who had a hysterectomy for benign disease, but up to 11.6% when hysterectomy had been performed for prolapse (Marchioni et al 1999).

CLASSIFICATION

A prolapse represents protrusion of an organ or structure outside its normal anatomical boundaries. It may be classified according to its anatomical position.

The pelvis can be divided into three compartments.

- Anterior – including the urethra (urethrocoele) and bladder (cystocoele).
- Middle – including the uterus or vault descent and enterocoele (containing small bowel or omentum).
- Posterior – containing the rectum (rectocoele), perineal hernia or rectal prolapse.

As vaginal delivery is the most common aetiological factor, it is sensible to assume that the whole pelvic floor rather than just one compartment will be adversely affected.

There are many grading systems. None is perfect and some are complex and impractical. Some vaginal laxity is normal – prolapse is a matter of degree rather than being absolute. The scoring system which has survived the longest is the Baden & Walker classification (1972) (Fig. 55.1).

Grade I   Descent of any organ to the vaginal midplane
Grade II   Descent to the hymenal ring
Grade III   Descent to halfway through the introitus
Grade IV   Complete eversion

For some, this system has lacked scientific accuracy and in 1996 the International Continence Society (ICS) Committee for

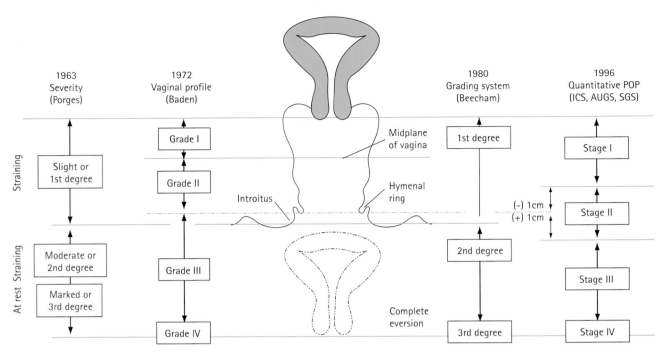

Fig. 55.1 Comparison of the four most commonly used pelvic organ prolapse grading systems (with kind permission of Steven Swift and John Theofrastous).

Standardization published its Pelvic Organ Prolapse (POP) quantitative scoring system which has been adopted by the AUGS and SGS (Bump et al 1996). Its staging is similar to that of Baden & Walker.

0   No descent of pelvic organs during straining
I   Leading surface of the prolapse does not descend below 1 cm above the hymenal ring
II   Leading edge of the prolapse extends from 1 cm above to 1 cm below the hymenal ring
III From 1 cm beyond the hymenal ring but without complete vaginal eversion
IV   The vagina is completely everted

For all measurements, the condition of the examination must be specified, i.e. position of the patient, at risk or straining and whether traction is employed. Figures 55.2 and 55.3 show the representation of points recorded for the ICS POP classification system. A comparison of the four most commonly used POP grading systems is shown in Figure 55.1.

PELVIC ANATOMY

Pelvic floor

The pelvic floor includes the levator ani, internal obturator and piriform muscles and superficial and deep perineal muscles (Fig. 55.4). The levator ani (which is in two parts, pubococcygeus and iliococcygeus) is covered by pelvic fascia and arises from the pelvic surface of the pubic bone (lateral to the symphysis pubis) and posteriorly from the ischial spine. In between, it takes its origin from the internal obturator fascia (tendinous arch). The pubococcygeus fans out and forms two

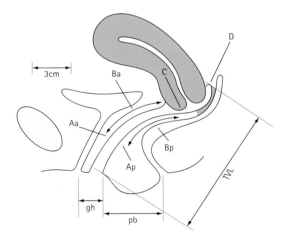

Fig. 55.2 Graphic representation of points used to quantify prolapse. GH, genital hiatus; PB, perineal body; TVL, total vaginal length. Aa is midline point of the anterior vaginal wall 3 cm proximal to the external meatus. Ba is most distal/dependent position of the anterior vaginal wall from the vaginal vault or anterior fornix to Aa. C, most distal/dependent edge of cervix or vault. D, location of the posterior fornix. Bp, most distal/dependent point on posterior vaginal wall from vault or posterior fornix to Ap. Ap, point on midline posterior vaginal wall 3 cm proximal to hymen. (ICS Standardization of terminology of female pelvic organ prolapse and pelvic floor dysfunction, 1996.)

parts, which are inserted differently. The anterior fibres decussate around the vagina and pass to the perineal body and anal canal. Although anteriorly the fibres of the pubococcygeus are in close relation to the urethra, they are not structurally attached to it (Gosling 1981). Posterior fibres join the raphe

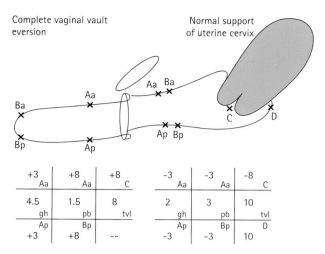

Complete vaginal vault eversion

Normal support of uterine cervix

+3 Aa	+8 Aa	+8 C		-3 Aa	-3 Aa	-8 C
4.5 gh	1.5 pb	8 tvl		2 gh	3 pb	10 tvl
+3 Ap	+8 Bp	--		-3 Ap	-3 Bp	10 D

Fig. 55.3 Contrasting measurement between normal support and post-hysterectomy vaginal eversion. a (right) normal support of uterus and cervix; b (left) complete vaginal vault eversion. (ICS Standardization of terminology of female pelvic organ prolapse and pelvic floor dysfunction, 1996.)

from the tip of the coccyx to the anus. The muscle is supplied by the anterior primary rami of S3 and S4.

The coccygeus is a flat, triangular muscle arising from the ischial spine and in the same place as the iliococcygeus. It is inserted into the lateral margin of the lower two pieces of the sacrum and the upper two pieces of the coccyx. Its nerve supply is the anterior primary rami S3 and S4.

Both of these muscles act as support for the pelvic viscera and as sphincters for the rectum and vagina. Contraction of the pubococcygeus will also arrest the urinary stream.

These muscles are aided by the muscles of the urogenital diaphragm – the superficial and deep perineal muscles that originate from the ischial rami and are inserted into the perineal body (Fig. 55.5). They are supplied by the perineal branch of the pudendal nerve (S2 and S4) and brace the perineum against the downward pressure from the pelvic floor. The muscles are covered superiorly by fascia continuous with that over the levator ani and internal obturator muscles and inferiorly by fascia called the perineal membrane.

Pelvic ligaments

The pelvic ligaments are condensations of pelvic fascia that sling the cervix, uterus and upper part of the vagina from the walls of the pelvis. They include the following.

- The *pubocervical ligament* (pubocervical fascia) extends from the anterior aspect of the cervix to the back of the body of the pubis.

formed by the iliococcygeus. The deeper fibres of each side unite behind the anorectal junction to form the puborectalis muscle, which slings the anorectal junction from the pubic bone. The fibres of the iliococcygeus proceed downwards medially and backwards to be inserted into the last two pieces of the coccyx and into a median fibrous raphe that extends

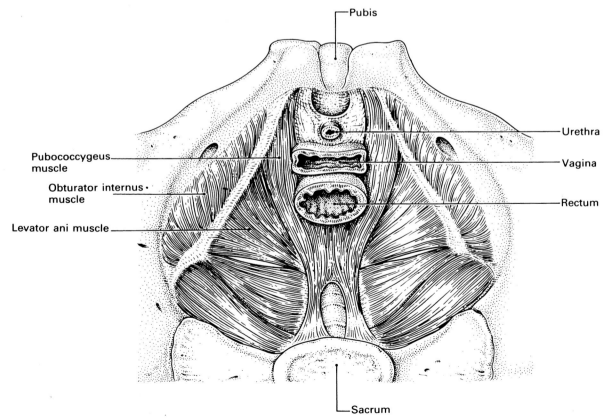

Fig. 55.4 Pelvic floor muscles from above.

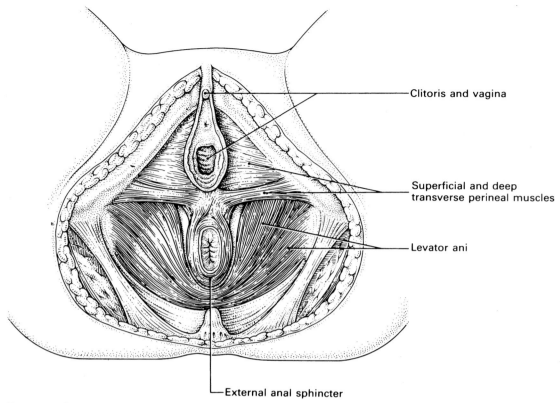

Fig. 55.5 Superficial and deep perineal muscles.

- The *lateral cervical ligament* (transverse cervical, Mackenrodt or cardinal ligaments) extends from the lateral aspect of the cervix and upper vagina to the pelvic side walls. It is the lower part of the broad ligament and nerves and vessels pass through from the pelvic side walls to the uterus. The ureter passes underneath it to the ureterovesical junction. The upper edge of the broad ligament contains the ovarian vessels.
- The *uterosacral ligament* extends from the back of the uterus to the front of the sacrum.
- The *posterior pubourethral ligament* extends from the posterior inferior aspect of the symphysis to the anterior aspect of the middle third of the urethra and on to the bladder (Fig. 55.6). It maintains elevation of the bladder neck and prevents excess posterior displacement of the urethra (Gosling 1981). It may facilitate micturition and is important in maintaining continence.
- The *round ligament*, which is not ligamentous but is formed of smooth muscle, passes from the uterine cornu through the inguinal canal to the labium majus. It is believed to keep the uterus anteflexed but probably plays little part in actually supporting it.

Endopelvic fascia

The endopelvic fascia is a fibromuscular sheet comprised of collagen, elastin and smooth muscle and supported by blood vessels and nerves. It is continuous with the uterus, cervix and vaginal walls and envelops and attaches these to the pelvic side walls. DeLancey (1992) suggested dividing the fascia into three levels to help understand the attachments and supports of the pelvic organs. Level I is the parametrium, comprising uterosacral and cardinal ligaments, and suspends the uterus, cervix and upper vagina to the pelvic side wall and sacrum. Level II attaches the anterior and posterior walls to the pelvic side wall and is attached anteriorly to the fascia overlying the obturator internus and levator ani (arcus tendineus) and posteriorly attached to the superior fascia over the levator ani. At level III the endopelvic fascia fuses anteriorly with the urethra, urogenital diaphragm and pubis, laterally with the levator ani fascia and posteriorly with the perineal body. This concept does not help, however, with the main strategies of surgical treatment.

Discrete fascial breaks in the anterior and posterior pelvic fascia have been identified by Richardson et al (1976) and Richardson (1995) and are said to be responsible for prolapse and their repair will be an adequate correction. This is unlikely to be so for secondary surgery and until appropriate randomized controlled trials exist between fascial repair and mesh-reinforced surgery, little substantive conclusion should be drawn. The role of fascia in surgical correction is disputed by some, including myself, and it does seem doubtful to attempt to repair an already weakened tissue without any additional organic or inorganic material and hope for a lasting cure.

AETIOLOGY

Congenital weakness of pelvic floor ligaments and fascia is found in spina bifida and bladder exstrophy and when there is an abnormality in connective tissue – principally a lesser amount

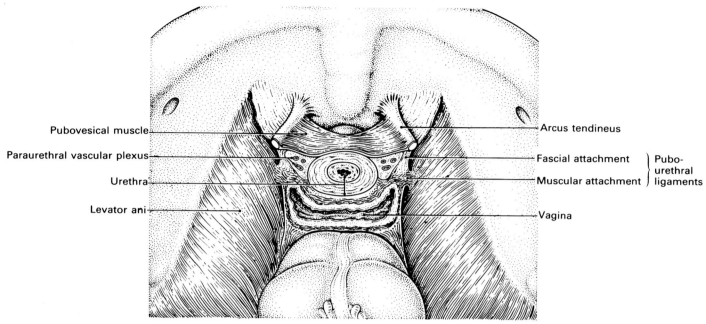

Fig. 55.6 Posterior pubourethral ligaments and arcus tendineus.

of type I collagen (native collagen) and greater amounts of type III collagen, which is more elastic (Norton 1993), and elastin, e.g. type IV Ehlers–Danlos and Marfan's syndrome (Carley & Schaffer 2000). Patients with joint hypermobility have a higher prevalence of genital prolapse than patients with normal joints (Norton et al 1995). A deep uterovesical pouch and a deep pouch of Douglas, the menopause, increasing age and white rather than black genetic make-up, obesity, chronic cough, constipation, occupational physical stress and a prior hysterectomy are all adverse factors.

By far the worst factor is vaginal delivery, with over 90% of patients with prolapse being parous (odds ratio 4.7; Carley et al 1999) and particularly instrumental delivery with a macrosomic infant and a long second stage. Vaginal delivery traumatizes the pelvic floor muscles, ligaments and fascia and causes pudendal nerve damage, resulting also in urinary and faecal incontinence in addition to prolapse.

Electrophysiological studies confirm denervation changes in the pelvic floor and urinary and anal sphincters (Allen et al 1990, Sultan et al 1994, Weidner et al 2000) following vaginal delivery.

PRESENTATION

Symptoms

Prolapse symptoms are very variable both in magnitude and according to the site of the prolapse: a large prolapse can be asymptomatic. Common to all prolapse is a feeling of a lump or dragging below or back ache, aggravated by standing and eased by lying down. It may be difficult to insert a tampon, which is more likely to be extruded. Intercourse may be uncomfortable because of a feeling of a lump below. Finally, when the prolapse extrudes, there may be a feeling of horror on seeing it. Clinical examination shows a lump at the vulva.

Box 55.1   Urinary symptoms

Stress incontinence
Incomplete emptying, voiding difficulty and urinary tract infection
Digitation to initiate voiding
Positional change to initiate voiding
Hesitancy, frequency and urgency

Anterior compartmental prolapse may also present with urinary symptoms (Box 55.1).

Middle compartmental prolapse presents with protrusion of the cervix which may become ulcerated, leading to a blood-stained purulent discharge. Vague symptoms of vaginal discomfort may indicate the presence of an enterocoele or vault descent. Rarely, dehiscence of the vault can occur with acute pain and protrusion of small bowel at the vulva. This can strangulate and is an acute abdominal emergency (Fig. 55.7).

Posterior compartmental prolapse may have bowel symptoms (Box 55.2).

In addition, the following sexual symptoms may be present: inability to have coitus, slackness at coitus or dyspareunia, lack of sensation, satisfaction or orgasm.

Signs

Certain predisposing conditions to prolapse, such as chronic cough, constipation and peritoneal dialysis may be present. The patient should be examined in the lithotomy or left lateral position using a Sims' speculum. Stress incontinence is most likely to be demonstrated if the bladder is full. The patient is asked to cough or bear down and any anterior wall prolapse or uterine descent will be demonstrated by retracting the posterior vaginal wall. To demonstrate uterine descent and after an appropriate explanation, a single tooth vulsellum is applied to the cervix with gentle traction.

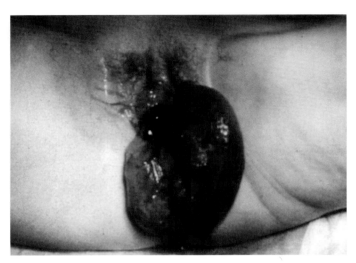

Fig. 55.7 Dehiscence of vault and presentation of small bowel at vulva.

Box 55.2 Bowel symptoms

Difficulty defaecating
Vaginal or anal digitation
Incomplete bowel emptying
Incontinence of flatus or stool
Faecal urgency
Painful lump at the anal margin (rectal prolapse)

A perineal hernia may be diagnosed by observation of the patient's buttocks on straining. A rectal prolapse may require an examination whilst the patient is straining on a toilet or commode.

Enterocoele and rectocoele can be demonstrated by using the speculum to retract the anterior vaginal wall. If the rectocoele protrudes and obscures an enterocoele, it can be reduced by the examining finger, and an enterocoele will be either seen at the tip of the examining finger or felt as an impulse on coughing. Further differentiation can be made by asking the patient to cough while the rectum and vagina are simultaneously examined. If the cervix protrudes outside the vagina, it may be ulcerated and hypertrophied, with thickening of the epithelium and keratinization. Carcinoma of the cervix may be a co-incidental finding – it is not a sequel to long-standing procidentia. A full pelvic examination should always be performed to exclude a pelvic mass that may be the primary cause of the prolapse.

Sometimes the patient may have to stand up and strain to show prolapse or stress incontinence.

Differential diagnosis

A variety of conditions can mimic prolapse of the anterior vaginal wall, such as a congenital anterior vaginal wall cyst (e.g. a remnant of the mesonephric duct system or Gartner's duct), a urethral diverticulum, metastases from a uterine tumour (e.g. choriocarcinoma) and an inclusion dermoid cyst following trauma or surgery. Procidentia can be confused with a large cervical or endometrial polyp or chronic uterine inversion.

INVESTIGATION

When urinary symptoms are present, an MSU should be sent for culture and sensitivity before any investigations or surgery are performed. If there is frequency a urinary diary ought to be completed and, if necessary, three early morning urines sent for acid-fast bacilli culture.

Many clinicians, myself included, now carry out urodynamic studies where:

- the patient complains of incontinence or voiding difficulty
- there is anterior vaginal wall prolapse requiring surgery
- there is grade II or more prolapse of the remaining compartments of the pelvis.

It is known that prolapse can mask incontinence which then presents once prolapse has been corrected. If it is detected preoperatively a continence procedure can be carried out at the same time as any prolapse correction.

If there is thought to be a persistent residual urine, an ultrasound rather than catheterization should be performed to estimate this. When there is doubt about bladder capacity, a cystoscopy under general anaesthesia should be performed.

Renal damage can occur in two situations. A grade III or IV cystourethrocoele can cause ureteric obstruction when the ureters are exteriorized with the cystourethrocoele, leading to ureteric dilatation and hydronephrosis. This may also rarely occur with detrusor overactivity which can produce a persistently high intravesical pressure. The patient needs assessment with a renal ultrasound and, if in doubt, an intravenous urogram.

Confirmation of the clinical assessment of prolapse can be made using the following techniques.

- *Ultrasound.* Perineal and transvesical ultrasound have been used to visualize the pelvic floor simultaneously with bladder pressure measurements (Creighton et al 1992). This technique is straightforward and avoids irradiation.
- *Pelvic floor fluoroscopy.* This technique is particularly useful for the detection of an enterocoele. It involves introduction of a barium contrast into the bladder, small bowel, vagina and rectum. The patient sits on a commode and is encouraged to contract the pelvic floor muscles and then strain down and evacuate bladder and rectum during fluoroscopy (Fig. 55.8). The technique is invasive, involves irradiation and doubt has been cast on its ability to reliably correlate with vaginal examination (Kenton et al 1996).
- *Magnetic resonance imaging* (MRI). Dynamic MRI is regarded as having many advantages, despite costs, over the two previous techniques. It is safer and has superior anatomical imaging and detail (Stoker et al 2001). Healy et al (1997) found that MRI clearly demonstrated prolapse in all compartments and confirmed that pelvic floor damage is often global, affecting all compartments. Both Gufler et al (1999) and Lienemann et al (2000) confirm that MRI is superior to pelvic fluoroscopy in the detection of enterocoele. However, MRI should ideally be performed in the upright position.

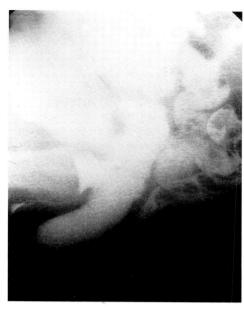

Fig. 55.8   Pelvic fluoroscopy showing a cystourethrocoele, rectocoele and enterocoele during the emptying phase.

- *Isotope defaecography.* This is used to demonstrate a rectocoele and the ability of the rectum and rectocoele to empty. Technetium-99m labelled 'porridge' is introduced into the rectum and a gamma camera image records the descent of the pelvic floor and rectum, together with the mean evacuation times of the rectum and rectocoele and the amounts retained with both (Fig. 55.9) (Hutchinson et al 1993).

TREATMENT

It is important to ensure that symptoms are caused by prolapse and not by other pelvic or spinal conditions. The patient should be told that, provided there is no urinary tract obstruction or infection, prolapse carries no risk to life. It is preferable to have completed child bearing before surgery, because a successful pelvic floor repair can be disrupted by a further vaginal delivery. Coital activity must be taken into account and narrowing of the vagina carefully avoided. Obese patients should be referred to a dietitian for dietary control and chronic cough and constipation should be corrected as far as possible.

Prevention

To date, there is no evidence that prophylactic pelvic exercises are effective, but they may prevent stress incontinence due to urethral sphincter incompetence and as they do no harm, they should be positively encouraged. Sultan et al (1993) and others have shown that multiparity, forceps delivery, macrosomia and a prolonged second stage are harmful. An episiotomy may lead to a decreased incidence of cystocoele and rectocoele. There is a need for a large RCT to demonstrate whether elective caesarean section for selected high-risk women (where there is already evidence of connective tissue disorder) would be protective for prevention of both prolapse and urinary and faecal incon-

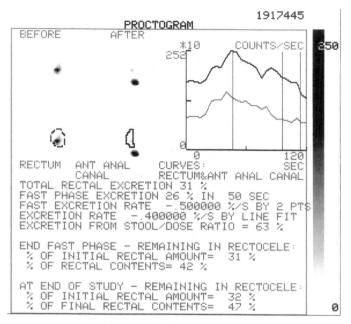

Fig. 55.9   Isotope defaecography (proctogram). Of the three vertical lines on the graph, the one on the left represents the start of defaecation and the one on the extreme right represents the end of defaecation. The upper black line represents total rectal contents, the lower line represents rectocoele contents. This study represents poor rectocoele evacuation with 32% initial rectal amount and 47% of the final rectal content remaining in the rectocoele. Courtesy of Devinder Kumar.

tinence. Similarly, an RCT is needed to establish whether HRT has any protective role in avoiding the development or deterioration of prolapse.

Hysterectomy is a risk factor for prolapse and correct closure of the vault with attention to prevention of an enterocoele by uterosacral ligament apposition is important (Cruikshank & Kovac 1999).

Conservative

Vaginal pessaries have been used for many years to correct prolapse. They are indicated particularly in the patient who is unfit for or refuses or wishes to defer surgery. They come in a variety of sizes and shapes and have to be individually fitted to each patient (Fig. 55.10). The complications include urinary incontinence, vaginal discharge and vaginal ulceration which if neglected can occasionally lead to vesical or rectal fistula. The pessary should fit comfortably, not cause pain and the patient should not be aware of it. It should be changed every 6–12 months and local oestrogen may be helpful in preventing some of the complications.

Surgery

Prolapse surgery is directed towards:

- restoring anatomy
- restoring vaginal function
- correcting urinary and faecal incontinence
- preventing de novo prolapse and incontinence.

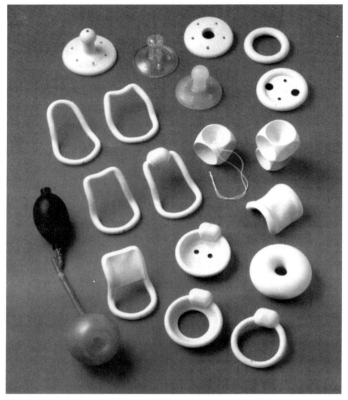

Fig. 55. 10 Variety of pessaries used to control prolapse. Courtesy of Milex Products.

A broad view must be taken of reconstructive surgery and a thorough pelvic examination, with imaging if necessary, performed beforehand to ensure that surgery corrects all the significant defects; birth trauma is global and does not just affect one compartment.

Surgery is the mainstay of prolapse treatment but the following topics have yet to be resolved and in some cases justified.

- Role of mesh
- Fascial defects
- Laparoscopic repairs
- Abdominal versus vaginal route
- Rectocoele surgery
- Role of local anaesthetic repair

Role of mesh
Organic meshes are increasingly used where secondary prolapse requires correction. Amid (1997) has described four categories of mesh according to pore size. The most suitable is type 1 or macroporous, where the pore size exceeds 75 microns. This allows access by leucocytes to infection, so that when this occurs, the mesh can be left in place and treatment with antibiotics may be all that is necessary. Polypropylene examples include Prolene (Gynecare/Johnson & Johnson) and Marlex (Bard). Microporous meshes, e.g. polytetrafluorethylene (Mersilene and Teflon, Ethicon; Teflon, Bard; Goretex, Gore), have to be removed if infection occurs. All meshes have a propensity to contract by up to 20% and, therefore, a mesh should never be

inserted under tension. There is a good review of mesh in gynaecology by Iglesia et al (1997).

Fascial defects
In 1976 Richardson & colleagues described breaks in the endopelvic fascia and ascribed prolapse and stress incontinence to them (Fig. 55.11). It was suggested that these conditions could be corrected by repairing the defects. Whilst this might be so for primary prolapse, I remain sceptical that secondary prolapse correction by these techniques will be long-lasting and evidence from long-term follow-up RCTs is needed to substantiate these claims.

Laparoscopic repairs
I think the role of laparoscopic sacrocolpopexy has been convincingly demonstrated (Mahendren et al 1996, Wattiez et al 2001) but there is as yet insufficient evidence to take claims for repair of enterocoele and rectocoele seriously. Yet again, there need to be RCTs with conventional surgery for a long-term follow-up before laparoscopic prolapse surgery can be recommended.

Abdominal versus vaginal route
These should not necessarily be seen as competitive, but rather as choices to suit the individual patient's characteristics. Benson et al (1996) reported on an RCT with a 29% good outcome for vaginal surgery and a 58% good outcome for abdominal surgery; however, there were too many confounding factors, particularly the multiplicity of additional surgeries for both groups, to make these findings really secure. Roovers et al (2001) compared vaginal hysterectomy and anterior and posterior repair with sacrocolpopexy and preservation of the uterus and found that further prolapse surgery and more micturition symptoms were more common in the abdominal group.

Whilst the abdominal route anecdotally seems to give a more lasting cure with less risk of reducing vaginal length, the vaginal route certainly offers a less painful recovery. Carey & Dwyer (2001) favour the abdominal route for the younger patient who has undergone previous prolapse surgery and the vaginal route for primary surgery in the medically compromised and frail woman. They emphasize that every reconstructive surgeon should be proficient with either route.

Rectocoele surgery
The rectocoele is the meeting ground for the gynaecologist and colorectal surgeon. The former favours the posterior repair, whilst the latter favours a transanal correction. In a randomized controlled trial of these two operations, Kahn et al (1999) found that both operations improved symptoms of impaired evacuation, but only the posterior repair addressed posterior vaginal wall prolapse. The main debate continues as to whether a fascial or conventional levator ani repair is best. Studies by Cundiff et al (1998) and Kenton et al (1999a) indicate that up to a 2-year follow-up, between 77% and 82% of patients were relieved of vaginal prolapse with fewer side-effects by a fascial repair than with conventional levator plication. A longer follow-up with an RCT comparing the two techniques is required.

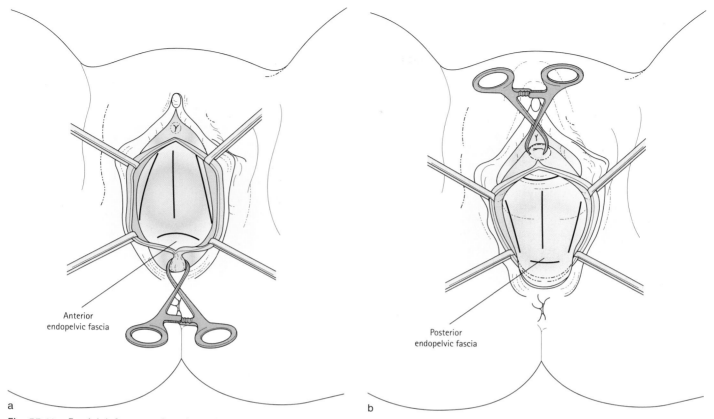

a

b

Fig. 55.11 Fascial defects. **a** = Anterior endopelvic fascia. **b** = Posterior endopelvic fascia. Discrete defects can occur in the endopelvic fascia centrally and inferiorly, superiorly or laterally at its peripheral attachments. Sites of discrete defects in the anterior and posterior endopelvic fascias are shown (reproduced with permission from Stanton S, Monga A 2000 Clinical urogynaecology. Churchill Livingstone).

Role of local anaesthetic repair

Recently, day case repair of prolapse under local anaesthetic has been tried and advocated. The advantages are clear. Dorflinger et al (2001) studied patients with at least a grade II cystocoele, rectocoele or both and repaired these under local anaesthetic with fascial techniques; 75% of patients were cured at a median follow-up of 6 months. A follow-up of at least 2 years is required and a full assessment of the advantages and disadvantages of an early return home is also needed.

Compartmental surgery

Anterior compartment. Traditionally an anterior colporrhaphy (repair) has been used to correct a cystourethrocoele. If there is accompanying stress incontinence, a continence procedure (e.g. tension-free vaginal tape) should be used as well. The essentials of the operation are to reduce the prolapse using interrupted absorbable sutures placed in the pubocervical fascia, cautious excision of surplus vaginal skin and then approximation of the remaining vaginal skin with a continuous locking suture for haemostasis and to avoid shortening the anterior wall. If there is a secondary repair then the inclusion of type I mesh such as Prolene or Vypro (Ethicon, Johnson & Johnson) is recommended.

Alternatively the fascial defects can be displayed by vaginal or abdominal dissection and corrected using either absorbable or permanent (for the abdominal route) sutures. If the fascia is

attenuated, mesh can be used. Using these techniques, up to 97% success has been claimed. Nguyen (2001) reviewed transvaginal and abdominal correction of paravaginal defects and concluded that both offered favourable cure rates.

The best abdominal operation to correct both cystourethrocoele and stress incontinence is the Burch colposuspension; however, it has a legacy of enterocoele and rectocoele formation afterwards (Alcalay et al 1995).

Uterine prolapse. Where a woman wishes to retain her uterus, a sacrohysteropexy is performed. The junction of the cervix and uterus is attached, by a mesh which is peritonealized, to the anterior longitudinal ligament over the first or second sacral vertebra. In a study on 13 women who had at least a 2° uterine prolapse, all were cured at the mean follow-up time of 16 months. There were no significant intra- or postoperative complications (Leron & Stanton 2001).

Where the uterus does not have to be conserved then vaginal hysterectomy rather than Manchester repair is the preference for correction of uterine prolapse. The hysterectomy can be combined with an anterior or posterior colporrhaphy and uterosacral ligaments must be coapted to prevent or correct an enterocoele.

The assessment for vaginal hysterectomy is important. The subpubic arch should be sufficiently wide to accommodate two fingers, which will allow the operator access to the uterus. There should be sufficient vaginal capacity and laxity of the pelvic tissues to allow the surgery to be carried out and clinical experience with the help of an episiotomy will determine this. Unless morcellation is intended, the uterine size should not be larger than 14 weeks. Where there has been previous pelvic surgery, such as a ventral suspension or complicated bowel surgery, a vaginal hysterectomy could be hazardous.

The principles of vaginal hysterectomy include careful upward displacement of the bladder and ureters, ligation of each main pedicle and repair of any enterocoele. The ovaries are inspected and if there is ovarian pathology or the woman has consented and is over 50 years of age, vaginal oophorectomy should be carried out at the same time (Sheth 1991). The pedicles are then approximated to each other in pairs to reform the roof of the vault and the uterosacral ligaments are united and attached to the posterior fornix epithelium and the vault is closed.

Enterocoele or vault repair. Most enterocoeles can be repaired at the time of abdominal surgery, by coaptation of the uterosacral ligaments. The Moschowitz procedure is not recommended because of the risk of including the ureter when inserting purse-string sutures into the pouch of Douglas peritoneum and in any case, there is little inherent strength in the peritoneum. The Halban procedure is safer and better.

The initial decision to use the vaginal suprapubic route will depend on the patient's general state. The sacrospinous operation (Nichols 1982) does not compromise vaginal size, but the surgery is carried out under limited visibility and there is a significant risk of damage to pudendal vessels and nerves. There is also a high risk of cystocoele and stress incontinence following this procedure.

Maher et al (2001) reviewed a series of matched pairs of women who underwent sacrospinous fixation and iliococcygeal fixation for vault prolapse. Whilst the correct of prolapse was very similar (89% versus 86% of patients reported cure), the patients' satisfaction rate for ICF was less and the cystocoele recurrence was more common. Shull et al (2000) are strong enthusiasts for the technique of reattaching the vaginal vault by means of the pubocervical fascia and rectovaginal fascia to the uterosacral ligaments. Because of the proximity of sutures to the ureters, it is important to cystoscope afterwards and check for ureteric patency. The procedure is anatomically convincing but one has to be sure to identify the uterosacral ligament remnants which are not always so visible following hysterectomy and the surgery is technically quite difficult. Long-term follow-up is awaited.

Where there is recurrent prolapse most clinicians prefer the abdominal route and would choose the sacrocolpopexy. The vault is attached by a mesh (Prolene or Vypro) to the anterior longitudinal ligament over the first or second sacral vertebra. Care has to be taken here because the venous plexus is in front of this ligament and the pelvic nerves are lateral. The mesh is peritonealized, to avoid bowel attaching to the mesh or becoming trapped underneath it.

Results indicate that although this is an effective operation for the support of the vault, stress incontinence may occur in up to 33% of patients, presumably due to excess tension on the anterior vaginal wall interfering with the urethral sphincter mechanism.

Carey & Dwyer (2001) reported a 98% cure of vault prolapse,

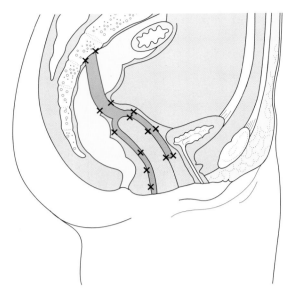

Fig. 55.12 Sacrocolpopexy with mesh insertion anteriorly to correct a high cystocoele and posteriorly down to the perineal body to correct a rectocoele.

but 7% developed a rectocoele and required further surgery and 12% developed de novo stress incontinence. Mesh erosion was found in 2%. In a smaller series of 29 patients, we used a sacrocolpopexy and mesh interposition between the vagina and rectum to correct a secondary vault descent and rectocoele. At 14 months all women had correction of the grade II prolapse: one mesh became infected and had to be removed (Fox & Stanton 2000) (Fig. 55.12). Subsequent follow-up has shown that in up to 20% of patients, there was some migration proximally of the mesh from the perineal body.

Rectocoele Because of complications following posterior colporrhaphy, namely dyspareunia and bowel symptoms, this operation should not be carried out as a routine accompaniment to anterior colporrhaphy, but instead there should be sound indications for its use. Any patient with coincident bowel dysfunction, such as faecal incontinence or constipation, may need anorectal investigation before undergoing surgery (Kahn & Stanton 1997).

The operation commonly used to correct rectocoele is the conventional posterior colporrhaphy, using either levator plication or fascial repair and placement of a mesh between the vagina and rectum if there has been a previous colporrhaphy.

MANAGEMENT OF COMPLEX PROLAPSE

Complex prolapse includes the following.

- Recurrent prolapse
- Prolapse with urinary or faecal incontinence
- Nulliparous prolapse
- Prolapse in a frail patient
- Vaginal and rectal prolapse.

Following on from what has already been stated, complex prolapse needs careful clinical assessment and investigation. Its surgery should only be carried out by clinicians familiar with both abdominal and vaginal approaches and who have had the necessary training and see sufficient cases to be familiar with the relevant techniques of repair. The final decision on surgery will depend on the patient's symptoms, signs and expectations, i.e. a fit and physically and coitally active woman will make more demands on her surgery than a frail patient who is not coitally active.

Recurrent prolapse needs careful assessment and management of pre-disposing factors such as those which raise the intrabdominal pressure (lifestyle – heavy lifting, chronic cough, obesity and constipation), steroid usage and peritoneal dialysis. The use of supportive tissue preferably inorganic Type I mesh rather than fascial replacement or reconstruction is advised, and avoidance of unnecessary heavy lifting after surgery is mandatory.

Where there is co-existent faecal incontinence or rectal prolapse, collaboration with a colorectal surgeon may be necessary.

For the nulliparous patient with prolapse, every effort must be made to retain the uterus. A future pregnancy, if the prolapse remains cured, should be delivered by an elective caesarean section.

Prolapse in the frail patient should usually be managed conservatively, but where this fails, expert anaesthesia and preferably nursing before and after on a medical ward is preferable to a surgical ward, for the insidious slide into respiratory, cardiovascular or neurological failure is better detected in the former than in the latter.

The combination of vaginal and rectal prolapse, rather like the combination of prolapse and incontinence, are conditions which can be repaired at the same sitting by either one surgeon or a combination of surgeons. Using this philosophy for patients at the Combined Pelvic Floor Clinic at St George's Hospital over the past 8 years, we have not had any increase in morbidity and patients have benefited from a single admission and anaesthetic.

CONCLUSION

Pelvic floor weakness may affect all compartments and the correction of prolapse must be thorough and include surgery for any accompanying urinary and faecal incontinence. Ideally, a pelvic reconstructive surgeon should have training in gynaecology, urology and colorectal surgery and collaboration to ensure that the patient has this experience available to her is paramount.

KEY POINTS

1. Prolapse is a common condition with a long-term cure rate which may not exceed 70%.
2. Vaginal delivery is the commonest cause.
3. Prolapse may affect all compartments and both urinary and anal sphincters and therefore examination and investigation must include all of these.
4. Validated outcome measures, rather than terms like 'slight' or 'moderate', should be used.
5. Preventive measures include avoidance of unnecessary lifting, straining at stool and a prolonged second stage of labour.

KEY POINTS (*CONTINUED*)

6. A variety of pessaries are available and should be used when appropriate.
7. Urinary incontinence may be masked by prolapse and urodynamic studies are advised before prolapse surgery.
8. Surgery for recurrent prolapse may need mesh reinforcement.
9. Complex prolapse should only be attempted by those familiar with, and trained in, prolapse surgery.

REFERENCES

Alcalay M, Monga A, Stanton SL 1995 Burch colposuspension: a 10–20 year follow up. British Journal of Obstetrics and Gynaecology 102:740–745

Allen R, Hosker G, Smith A, Warrell D 1990 Pelvic floor damage and childbirth: a neurophysiological study. British Journal of Obstetrics and Gynaecology 97:770–779

Amid P 1997 Classification of biomaterials and their related complications in abdominal wall surgery. Hernia 1:15–21

Baden W, Walker T 1972 Genesis of the vaginal profile: a correlated classification of vaginal relaxation. Clinical Obstetrics and Gynecology 15:1048–1054

Benson T, Lucenti V, McClellan E 1996 Vaginal versus abdominal reconstructive surgery for the treatment of pelvic support defects: a prospective randomised study with long term outcome evaluation. American Journal of Obstetrics and Gynecology 175:1418–1422

Bump R, Mattiasson A, Bo K et al 1996 The standardisation of terminology of female pelvic organ prolapse and pelvic floor dysfunction. American Journal of Obstetrics and Gynecology 175:10–17

Carey M, Dwyer P 2001 Genital prolapse: vaginal versus abdominal route of repair. Current Opinion in Obstetrics and Gynecology 13:499–506

Carley M, Schaffer J 2000 Urinary incontinence and pelvic organ prolapse in women with Marfan or Ehlers Danlos syndrome. American Journal of Obstetrics and Gynecology 182:1021–1023

Carley M, Turner R, Scott D et al 1999 Obstetric history in women with surgically corrected adult urinary incontinence and pelvic organ prolapse. Journal of the American Association of Gynecologic Laparoscopists 6:39–44

Creighton S, Pearce J, Stanton SL 1992 Perineal videoultrasonography in the assessment of vaginal prolapse – early observations. British Journal of Obstetrics and Gynaecology 99:310–313

Cruikshank S, Kovac S 1999 Randomised comparison of 3 surgical methods used at the time of vaginal hysterectomy to prevent posterior enterocele. American Journal of Obstetrics and Gynecology 180:859–865

Cundiff G, Weidner A, Visco A et al 1998 An anatomic and functional assessment of the discrete defect rectocele repair. American Journal of Obstetrics and Gynecology 179:1451–1457

DeLancey J 1992 Anatomic aspects of vaginal eversion after hysterectomy. American Journal of Obstetrics and Gynecology 166:1717–1728

Dorflinger A, Gelman W, O'Sullivan S, Monga A 2001 Surgical outcome and patient's satisfaction after prolapse repair under local anaesthetic. International Urogynecology Journal 12:S88–89

Fox S, Stanton SL 2000 Vault prolapse and rectocele: assessment of repair using sacrocolpopexy with mesh interposition. British Journal of Obstetrics and Gynaecology 107:1371–1375

Gosling J 1981 Why are women continent? Proceedings of symposium on 'The Incontinent Woman'. RCOG, London

Gufler H, Laubenberger J, de Gregorio G et al 1999 Pelvic floor descent: dynamic MR imaging using a $\frac{1}{2}$Fourier RARE sequence. Journal of Magnetic Resonance Imaging 9:378–383

Healy J, Halligan S, Reznek R et al 1997 Patterns of prolapse in women with symptoms of pelvic floor weakness: assessment with magnetic resonance imaging. Radiology 203:77–81

Hutchinson R, Mostafa A, Grant A et al 1993 Scintigraphic defaecography: quantitative and dynamic assessment of ano-rectal function. Diseases of the Colon and Rectum 36:1132–1138

Iglesia C, Fenner D, Brubaker L 1997 Use of mesh in gynecologic surgery. International Urogynecology Journal 8:105–115

Kahn M, Stanton SL 1997 Posterior colporrhaphy: its effects on bowel and sexual function. British Journal of Obstetrics and Gynaecology 104:82–86

Kahn M, Kumar D, Stanton SL, Fox S 1999 Is posterior colporrhaphy superior to the transanal repair for treatment of posterior vaginal vault prolapse? Neurourology and Urodynamics 18:329–330

Kenton K, Shott S, Brubaker L 1999a Outcome after rectovaginal fascia reattachment for rectocele repair. American Journal of Obstetrics and Gynecology. 180:1360–1364

Kenton K, Sadowski D, Shott S, Brubaker L 1999b A comparison of women with primary and recurrent pelvic prolapse. American Journal of Obstetrics and Gynecology 180:1415–1418

Leron E, Stanton SL 2001 Sacrohysteropexy with synthetic mesh for the management of uterovaginal prolapse. British Journal of Obstetrics and Gynaecology 108:629–633

Lienemann A, Anthuber C, Baron A et al 2000 Diagnosing enteroceles using dynamic magnetic resonance imaging. Diseases of the Colon and Rectum 43:205–212

Mahendren D, Prashar S, Smith ARB et al 1996 Laparoscopic sacrocolpopexy in the management of vaginal vault prolapse. Gynaecological Endoscopy 5:217–222

Maher CF, Murray C, Carey M et al 2001 Iliococcygeus or sacrospinous fixation for vault prolapse: prespinous v sacrospinous. Obstetrics and Gynecology 98:40–44

Marchioni M, Bracco G, Checcucci V et al 1999 True incidence of vaginal vault prolapse. Journal of Reproductive Medicine 44:679–684

Nguyen J 2001 Current concepts in the diagnosis and surgical repair of anterior vaginal prolapse due to paravaginal defects. Obstetrics and Gynecological Survey 56:239–246

Nichols DH 1982 Sacrospinous fixation for massive eversion of the vagina. American Journal of Obstetrics and Gynecology 1942:901–904

Norton P 1993 Pelvic floor disorders: the role of fascia and ligaments. Clinical Obstetrics and Gynecology 36:926–938

Norton P, Baker J, Sharp H et al 1995 Genitourinary prolapse and joint hypermobility in women. Obstetrics and Gynecology 85:225–228

Olsen A, Smith V, Bergstrom J et al 1997 Epidemiology of surgically managed pelvic organ prolapse and urinary incontinence. Obstetrics and Gynecology 89:501–506

Richardson AC 1995 The anatomic defects in rectocele and enterocele. Journal of Pelvic Surgery 1:214–221

Richardson AC, Lyon J, Williams N 1976 A new look at pelvic relaxation. American Journal of Obstetrics and Gynecology 1:568–573

Roovers J, van der Vaart C, van der Born J et al 2001 A randomised control trial comparing abdominal and vaginal surgery of patients with Grade II–IV uterine descent. International Urogynecology Journal 12:S109

Sheth S 1991 The place of oophorectomy in vaginal hysterectomy. British Journal of Obstetrics and Gynaecology 98:662–666

Shull B, Bachofen C, Coates K et al 2000 A transvaginal approach to repair of apical and other associated sites of pelvic organ prolapse using uterosacral ligaments. American Journal of Obstetrics and Gynecology 183:1365–1373

Stoker J, Halligan S, Bartram C 2001 Pelvic floor imaging. Radiology 218:621–641

Sultan A, Kamm M, Hudson C et al 1993 Anal sphincter disruption during vaginal delivery. New England Journal of Medicine 329:1905–1911

Sultan A, Kamm M, Hudson C 1994 Pudendal nerve damage during labour: prospective study before and after childbirth. British Journal of Obstetrics and Gynaecology 101:22–28

Versi E, Harvey M, Cardozo L 2001 Urogenital prolapse and atrophy at menopause: a prevalence study. International Urogynecology Journal 12:107–110

Wattiez A, Canis M, Mage G et al 2001 Promontofixation for the treatment of prolapse. Urological Clinics of North America 28:151–157

Weidner A, Barber M, Visco A et al 2000 Pelvic muscle electromyography of levator ani and external anal sphincter in nulliparous women and women with pelvic floor dysfunction. American Journal of Obstetrics and Gynecology 183:1390–1401

56

Frequency, urgency and the painful bladder

Peter Dwyer   Michael Fynes

INTRODUCTION

Urinary frequency, urgency, suprapubic pain and dysuria are symptoms of altered lower urinary tract sensation and may be of recent onset (acute) or long-standing and recurrent (chronic). Accurate diagnosis and appropriate therapy require careful patient evaluation and a sound understanding of the differential causes of these symptoms. Acute irritative urinary symptoms can be caused by intravesical conditions such as urinary tract infection, calculi, drug-induced cystitis, tumour or extravesical pelvic pathology such as a complicated ovarian cyst.

Once the cause is found, treatment is both specific and effective. Women with long-standing or recurrent chronic symptoms are often treated for presumed recurrent urinary tract infection and it is only after a poor response to antibiotics or failure to culture uropathogens that an alternative diagnosis is considered. It is essential that these women have careful and full evaluation (Fig. 56.1) to exclude any serious underlying pathology (e.g. carcinoma) so that effective treatment can be commenced. Women with chronic irritative symptoms frequently have conditions such as interstitial cystitis and urethral syndrome where the pathogenesis is poorly understood and response to current therapy is often unsatisfactory.

PREVALENCE

Bungay et al (1980) reported that approximately 20% of women suffer from urinary frequency and this figure was unaffected by age. Other reports suggest that the prevalence of urinary frequency is increased in the elderly (23%) and in women with neurological disorders (32%) (Diokno et al 1986, McGrother et al 1987). Fifteen per cent of women report urinary urgency (Bungay et al 1980) and this figure also increases after the menopause. The relative role of oestrogen deficiency versus the ageing process alone is controversial. The prevalence of dysuria and suprapubic pain is unknown and frequently women delay presentation for evaluation secondary to embarrassment (Norton et al 1988).

AETIOLOGY

Irritative bladder symptoms can be caused by a number of conditions originating within the lower urinary tract (Box 56.1). Urinary tract infection and functional disorders such as detrusor instability or voiding dysfunction may cause urge symptoms and should be excluded. These conditions should also be differentiated from more generalized systemic disorders (e.g. pregnancy, diabetes mellitus, diabetes insipidus, renal disease). Pelvic inflammation or gynaecological surgery

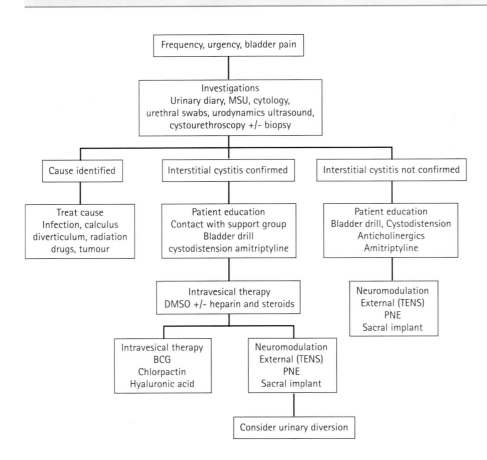

Fig. 56.1 Management strategy for women presenting with irritative lower urinary tract symptom. Adapted from Rosamilia & Dwyer (1998).

Box 56.1 Non-infective sensory disorders of the lower urinary tract

Inflammatory bladder conditions
Interstitial cystitis, drug-induced cystitis, chemical cystitis, eosinophilic cystitis, granulomatous cystitis, radiation cystitis

Non-malignant conditions affecting the lower urinary tract
Proliferative – cystitis cystica, cystitis glandularis
Metaplastic – keratinizing and non-keratinizing squamous metaplasia, intestinal metaplasia
Other – endometriosis, nephrogenic adenomatosis, amyloidosis

Benign and malignant bladder and urethral tumours
Papillomas, polyps, carcinoma in situ, bladder and urethral carcinoma (primary or secondary), benign and malignant non-epithelial tumours

Miscellaneous
Bladder or urethral calculi, urethrovesical foreign bodies (e.g. sutures, mesh erosion), urethral diverticulum, atrophic urethritis, urethral mucosal prolapse, urethral caruncle, acute and chronic urethral syndromes, Reiter's syndrome

may also cause secondary bladder irritation and a pelvic mass may cause symptoms due to bladder compression.

ASSESSMENT

History

A detailed history should be undertaken including specific questions regarding gynaecological and urinary symptoms. The presence of frequency, urgency and nocturia in association with incontinence is likely to reflect underlying detrusor instability. In contrast, chronic severe urgency and bladder pain in the absence of incontinence are likely to be secondary to intravesical pathology such as infective or non-infective cystitis (see Fig. 56.1).

Urinary frequency is defined as voiding more than seven times during waking hours and nocturia is arousal from sleep to micturate more than once at night (Stanton 1984). Nocturia increases with age but is also dependent on fluid/caffeine intake and medications such as diuretics. Urinary urgency is a strong and sudden desire to void which, if not relieved, may lead to incontinence. Bladder pain can be severe and frequently ill defined with radiation to the vagina and rectum. It is often aggravated by bladder distenstion, sexual intercourse, spicy foods, alcohol and caffeine and relieved by voiding. These symptoms can be well documented by a detailed urinary frequency volume diary (Fig. 56.2)

Dysuria is urethral pain during micturition and may be secondary to obvious pathology such as infection or a urethral diverticulum or less clearcut causes (e.g. atrophic urethritis or urethral syndrome). Haematuria is an important symptom, which always requires urgent evaluation to exclude carcinoma. A history of present and past medications (e.g. diuretics, tiaprofenic acid (Surgam) and cyclophosphamide), previous UTI and pelvic surgery should be sought. Possible predisposing factors such as sexual intercourse (e.g. 'honeymoon cystitis'), barrier contraceptive methods (e.g. diaphragm, condoms) and contact irritants (e.g. vaginal douches, spermicidal agents) should be elucidated.

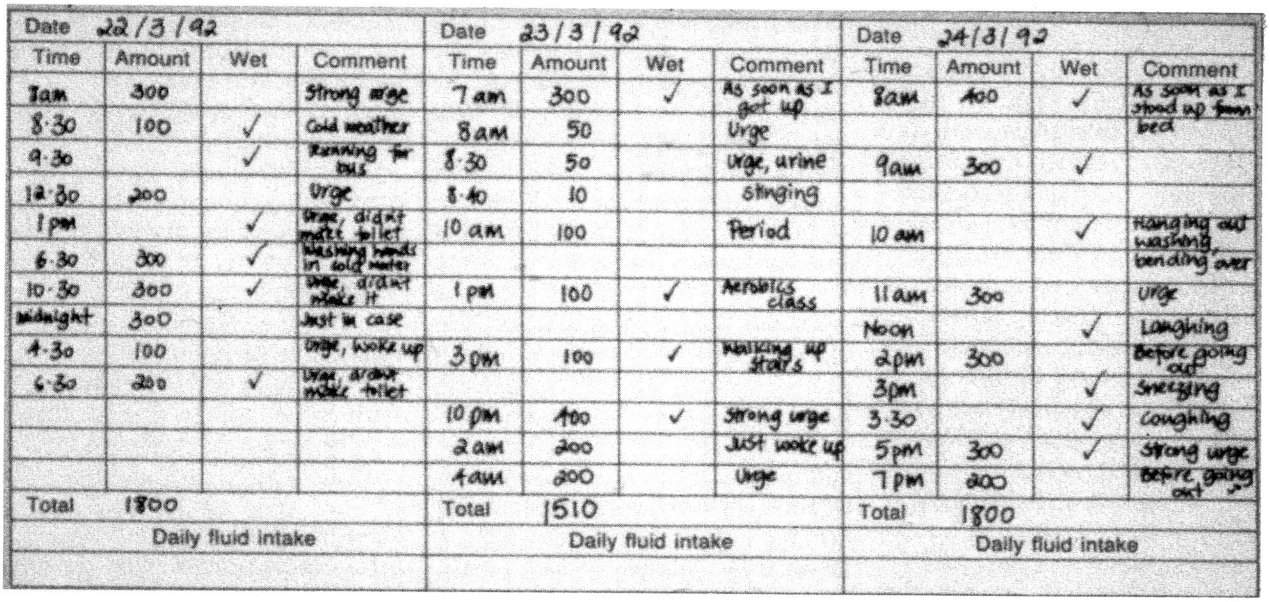

Date 22/3/92				Date 23/3/92				Date 24/3/92			
Time	Amount	Wet	Comment	Time	Amount	Wet	Comment	Time	Amount	Wet	Comment
7am	300		Strong urge	7am	300	✓	As soon as I got up	8am	400	✓	As soon as I stood up from bed
8.30	100	✓	Cold weather	8am	50		Urge				
9.30		✓	Running for bus	8.30	50		Urge, urine stinging	9am	300	✓	
12.30	200		Urge	8.40	10						
1pm		✓	Urge, didn't make toilet	10am	100		Period	10am		✓	Hanging out washing, bending over
6.30	300	✓	Washing hands in cold water								
10.30	300	✓	Urge, didn't make it	1pm	100	✓	Aerobics class	11am	300		Urge
midnight	300		Just in case					Noon		✓	Laughing
4.30	100		Urge, woke up	3pm	100	✓	Walking up stairs	2pm	300		Before going out
6.30	200	✓	Urge, didn't make toilet					3pm		✓	Sneezing
				10pm	400	✓	Strong urge	3.30		✓	Coughing
				2am	200		Just woke up	5pm	300	✓	Strong urge
				4am	200		Urge	7pm	200		Before going out
Total	1800			Total	1510			Total	1800		
Daily fluid intake				Daily fluid intake				Daily fluid intake			

Fig. 56.2   Urinary frequency volume diary.

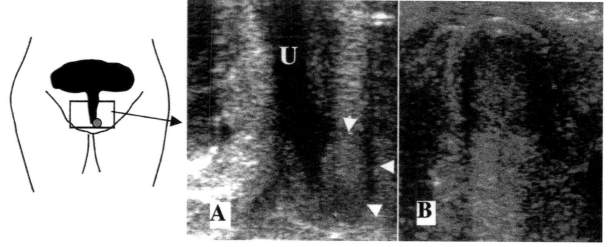

Fig. 56.3   Transperineal high-frequency ultrasound and corresponding line diagram demonstrating a large urethral diverticulum. U, urethra.

Voiding dysfunction may be suspected when symptoms of hesitancy, poor urinary stream with straining and incomplete emptying are present. Impaired bladder emptying secondary to detrusor underactivity or urethral obstruction can be idiopathic or secondary to neurological disease, pelvic surgery or uterovaginal prolapse. In a group of women referred for urodynamic studies (Dwyer & Desmedt 1994) urinary frequency, urgency and urge incontinence were similar in women with normal and impaired voiding, although nocturia was more than twice as common in the voiding dysfunction group.

Examination

Abdominal examination may reveal a palpable bladder secondary to urinary retention, a pelvic mass or bladder tenderness from cystitis. A neurological examination with specific attention to the S2–4 nerve roots, which innervate the bladder, should be performed. Vaginal examination should be performed with a Sims speculum to visualize both the anterior and posterior walls and exclude prolapse, atrophy, inflammation or localized infection. Urethral inspection may reveal a mass (Fig. 56.3), mucosal prolapse or caruncle. Paraurethral masses can also be identified on bimanual examination by compressing the urethra and paraurethral tissues against the back of the symphysis; expression of urethral pus would suggest a urethral diverticulum.

INVESTIGATIONS

Urinary diary

A detailed 3-day urinary frequency and volume diary is an important part of the initial and ongoing assessment. These diaries are more accurate than patient recall and allow rapid and accurate assessment of urinary frequency, nocturia, voided volumes, functional bladder capacity, episodes of urgency, pain, incontinence and their temporal relationship (Fig. 56.2). A urinary diary will also educate the patient regarding voiding habits and is an essential part of bladder retraining.

Urine analysis

A midstream urine (MSU) sent for microscopy, cytology, culture and sensitivity will diagnose any urinary tract infection and confirm or exclude the presence of leucocytes, nitrites, red blood cells and any abnormal tumour cells shed from a bladder cancer. Isolated haematuria with a negative MSU can be caused by inflammatory cystitis or carcinoma and is an indication for cystoscopy.

Microbiology

Urethral swabs are indicated where the MSU is negative and there is urethral tenderness, discharge or the patient is sexually active. In these cases appropriate culture media should also be used for *Chlamydia trachomatis* and *Neisseria gonorrhoeae*. Other organisms commonly identified include coliforms and *Staphylococcus saprophyticus*. Tuberculosis is still prevalent, especially in developing countries, and should be considered in any woman with persistent sterile cystitis and pyuria. Diagnosis is based on a positive Lowernstein-Jensen culture performed on three early morning urine specimens.

Urodynamics

Urodynamic studies should be considered once infection has been excluded and urgency symptoms have not responded to conservative treatment, especially if urinary incontinence is an associated problem. This investigation may identify underlying stress incontinence, detrusor instability or voiding dysfunction. A diagnosis of bladder hypersensitivity is based on the following findings at urodynamics: stable bladder, capacity <350 ml and urgency at <150 ml. Both the urodynamic assessment and a urinary diary will give an indication of functional bladder capacity and severity of bladder hypersensitivity. Women with severe interstitial cystitis frequently are unable to hold more than 50–100 ml.

Imaging

Imaging of the lower and upper urinary tracts can be performed using ultrasound or contrast radiography, either alone or synchronously with urodynamic assessment (videocysto-urethrography). The presence of haematuria in the absence of any identifiable uropathogens, a negative cystoscopy or recurrent UTIs are indications for assessment of the upper urinary tract using contrast intravenous urography (IVU) or renal ultrasound. In women with recurrent UTIs, 5% will have an abnormality identified (e.g. calculus, duplex system, PUJ obstruction, tumour). In women with irritative lower urinary tract symptoms and a paraurethral mass, a micturating cystogram or double balloon contrast urethrogram may identify a communicating tract with a urethral diverticulum. Transperineal ultrasound provides comparable information, is less invasive and allows differentiation between solid (e.g. fibroid, lipoma), cystic lesions (diverticulum, Skene's cyst or abscess, Gartner's duct cyst) and vascular lesions (haemangioma, fibroid). Mixed echogenic contents suggest an infected diverticulum or paraurethral abscess.

A plain abdominal X-ray will demonstrate 90% of calculi present in the kidney, ureters or bladder due to the presence of calcium or cystine (Fig. 56.4). Computed tomography (CT) will occasionally be required to provide a clearer picture of upper and lower urinary tract pathology.

CYSTOURETHROSCOPY

Evaluation of the lower urinary tract by cystourethroscopy is an essential skill for all gynaecological surgeons, not only in

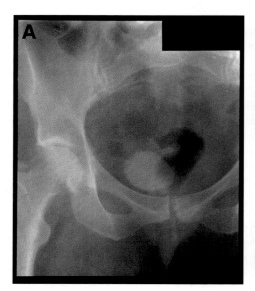
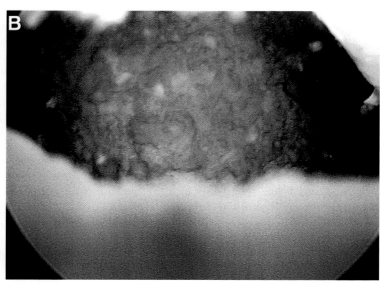

Fig. 56.4 A plain abdominal X-ray **a** and corresponding cystoscopic image **b** demonstrating a large bladder calculus.

the assessment of urinary symptoms and pain but during pelvic surgery for the prevention and early treatment of bladder and ureteral injury (Dwyer et al 1999). Cystoscopy is indicated in the presence of haematuria, abnormal urinary cytology, recurrent UTI or whenever urge symptoms persist despite conservative treatment. At cystourethroscopic evaluation, the lower urinary tract should be carefully visualised using a 70° or 30° scope for the bladder and a 0° scope with Sasche sheath for the urethra. Ideally this should be performed with a video camera and monitor to obtain optimum views and facilitate teaching. Features such as mucosal trabeculation, bladder diverticula, mucosal tumours, squamous metaplasia, bladder calculi and foreign bodies are readily identifiable. Women with misplaced intravesical sutures following stress incontinence surgery frequently present with urgency, bladder pain or urinary tract infection (Dwyer et al 1999). Early diagnosis with cystoscopic removal of the suture is important to avoid medicolegal conseqences. A bladder biopsy should be taken of any suspicious localized lesion to exclude carcinoma.

Miscellaneous

Renal function, endocrine profile, glucose tolerance test, serum calcium or urinary osmolality tests may be indicated in some individuals, especially in the presence of polyuria and polydipsia which is usually detected on a urinary diary. If any of these investigations are positive then referral to an appropriate specialist for further investigation is necessary.

TREATMENT

The management strategy for women presenting with frequency, urgency and bladder pain is outlined in Figure 56.1. Initial evaluation will depend on the presentation, severity and duration of symptoms. An MSU for microscopy and culture and a urinary diary is appropriate in all women with symptoms of frequency and urgency, with or without pain. Simple patient education with reduction of caffeine, fluid or alcohol intake, adjustment of diuretic or other medications and bladder retraining, with or without the use of anticholinergic medication, is frequently effective. The aim of bladder retraining is to normalize voiding habits by encouraging women to increase their voided volumes and time between micturitions. If symptoms are severe or do not respond to conservative treatment then further evaluation, particularly with cystourethroscopy and cystodistension, is warranted to identify any treatable cause. Women with frequency, urgency and bladder pain who have a reduced functional bladder capacity on their urinary diary and urodynamic assessment but no abnormality on cystoscopy may have early interstitial cystitis (IC) or a different condition (idiopathic sensory urgency). The majority of these women will respond to a conservative approach and cystodistension. Cystodistension also provides short-term relief in 30% of patients with IC (Hanno 1994).

Interstitial cystitis

Interstitial cystitis is a disabling condition characterized by frequency, urgency, often severe bladder pain and a significant reduction in quality of life. Guy Hunner first described this condition in 1914 and the mucosal tearing and fissuring, which he described as an ulcer, still carries his name. However, the pathophysiology of this disease process remains poorly understood, the diagnostic criteria are controversial and often ill defined and the treatment frequently unsuccessful.

The prevalence of IC is estimated to be 30–50 per 100 000 of the population (Griffith-Jones et al 1991), more common in women (9:1) and Caucasians. Most women present between 40 and 60 years and there is often a long history of symptoms prior to diagnosis (Parsons 1994). It is estimated that between 5% and 50% of women with symptoms of recurrent cystitis have underlying interstitial cystitis (Hanash & Pool 1970, Hand 1949). The pain of IC is often poorly localized and may be described as pelvic, suprapubic, perineal, vaginal or rectal and may mimic other gynaecological conditions such as pelvic infection or endometriosis. The incidence of hysterectomy is doubled in women with IC.

The diagnostic criteria for the diagnosis of interstitial cystitis are symptoms of frequency (>8 voids per day) associated with urgency and usually pain, a functional bladder capacity of <350 ml diagnosed on urinary diary or urodynamics and the cystoscopic findings of mucosal fissuring or tearing (Hunner's ulcer) seen during bladder distension (Fig. 56.5a) and petechial haemorrhages (glomerulations) usually seen after distension when the bladder is being emptied (Fig. 56.5b). There must be no other pathological (e.g. infection, calculi) or functional (detrusor instability) cause for the patient's symptoms. Urine cytology and bladder biopsy should be performed to exclude other pathology (Ca in situ). There are no specific pathological changes diagnostic of IC. Mucosal denudation, leucocyte and plasma cell infiltration, vascular congestion, haemorrhage and fibrosis are often found in women with IC, but are absent in 50% of cases (Rosamilia et al 1999).

Current theories regarding the pathogenesis of IC are numerous and predominantly conjecture. Proposed aetiologies include an infective agent, allergic or autoimmune conditions, abnormal 'leaky' urothelium secondary to a defective glycosaminoglycan (GAG) layer, urinary toxins, psychological disease, lymphatic or vascular abnormalities and neurogenic inflammation. Any of these pathological changes may be a result rather than the cause of the disease process and there may be more than one aetiological factor operating at any one patient. Therefore treatment efficacy may vary from one patient to the next and often multiple treatment modalities are necessary directed at different disease processes (e.g. bladder retraining, neuromodulation, polypharmacy) if a successful outcome is to be achieved.

Interstitial cystitis is a diagnosis of exclusion so other urogynaecological and systemic pathology should be excluded (see Fig. 56.1). Once the diagnosis is confirmed, an honest and clear explanation of this condition should be given, specifically that it is a non-malignant disorder and usually non-progressive. Although there are many successful treatment options available, cures are rare and relapses are common. Sympathetic support by family, medical staff and IC self-help groups and associations is invaluable. Dietary modification, easy toilet access and stress reduction techniques should be used in

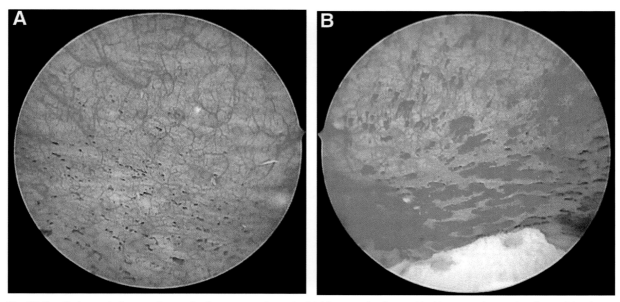

Fig. 56.5 Cystoscopic images demonstrating progressive petechial haemorrhaging on bladder emptying under direct vision in a patient with interstitial cystitis.

conjunction with the standard oral and intravesical therapy outlined in Figure 56.1. Major urological surgery involving ulcer resection, bladder denervation, partial or total cystectomy with urinary diversion should be considered a last resort and may not be curative.

Drug-induced cystitis

A careful history of present and past medications is important as drug-induced cystitis can occur immediately following administration or may manifest many years later. The term 'drug-induced' cystitis is therefore dependent on objective evidence of:

- the onset of irritative symptoms and inflammatory changes at cystoscopy following drug administration
- resolution following withdrawal
- recrudescence with readministration of the drug.

Implicated drugs include cyclophosphamide, tiaprofenic acid (Surgam), sulphasalazine, fenfluramine, fluoxetine, simvastatin, danazol and a number of the NSAIDs.

Radiation cystitis

Radiation cystitis may occur as an early or late complication following radiotherapy. The total single dose, duration of the radiotherapy treatment cycle, preceding surgery, pre-existent infection and previous radiotherapy all influence the risk of radiation cystitis. Acute radiation cystitis presents with mild to severe irritative symptoms with or without haematuria and occasionally may lead to bladder perforation and fistula formation. Chronic radiation cystitis may result in a small fibrotic non-compliant bladder with severe frequency, urgency and incontinence.

Eosinophilic cystitis

This rare condition probably represents a type 1 hypersensitivity reaction to exogenous allergens such as contact irritants, micro-organisms or some drugs. Affected individuals typically have a history of atopy and present with irritative urinary symptoms, haematuria, proteinuria and pyuria. Eosinophiluria occurs in 30% but up to 50% will have a raised serum eosinophil count. The cystoscopic appearance is variable with either diffuse or localized changes which may include the following: bullous oedema, mucosal thickening or trabeculation, petechial haemorrhages, ulceration and well-circumscribed yellow plaques (5–10 mm in diameter). Histology usually identifies a significant inflammatory cell infiltrate within the lamina propria. Oral steroid therapy may provide symptomatic relief although the condition usually resolves spontaneously.

Granulomatous cystitis

This condition may arise following bladder resection, bladder biopsy, bacterial infection or BCG instillation and should be distinguished from tuberculosis. The patient may be asymptomatic or present with haematuria, frequency, urgency and pain. Discrete plaques or nodules may be evident at cystoscopy. At histology diffuse granulomas or histiocytic inflammation is usually identified.

Malakoplakia refers to an uncommon condition in older women with a similar clinical and cystoscopic presentation. Histology identifies aggregates of histiocytes within the lamina propria with a superficial granulomatous reaction.

Proliferative and metaplastic lesions of the bladder

'Brunn's nests', cystitis cystica, cystitis glandularis and squamous metaplasia are common findings at cystoscopy, which are likely to represent normal histological variants. They are usually located on the trigone and anterior wall of the female bladder. Co-existent symptoms of frequency, urgency or bladder pain are more likely to be associated with infection or other inflammatory pathology.

Proliferative cystitis typically starts with 'Brunn's nests' which are clusters of pale yellow cells, 1–5 mm in diameter, within the lamina propria. These lesions are usually confined to the trigone but may be diffuse; differentiation from carcinoma requires biopsy for histological analysis. Cystitis cystica is a result of dilatation of these Brunn's nests within the lamina propria, which are lined by stratified or squamous epithelium and in cystitis glandularis by columnar epithelium.

Squamous metaplasia is a well-delineated 'whitepatch' confined to the trigone and is present in oestrogen-producing women. Keratinizing squamous metaplasia is also known as leucoplakia. It is generally diffuse and associated with recurrent infection and chronic irritation. It often occurs in association with bladder calculi, urethral diverticula or a foreign body. Macroscopically the affected areas of the bladder have a thickened white and shiny appearance interspersed with areas of bladder inflammation. Bladder biopsies typically demonstrate mature keratinized stratified squamous epithelium. This condition may be premalignant and requires surveillance (Benson et al 1984).

Intestinal metaplasia usually occurs in the setting of chronic or recurrent cystitis. It may be isolated or occur in association with proliferative bladder changes such as cystitis cystica or cystitis glandularis. Careful surveillance with cystoscopy and biopsy is required to exclude malignant change.

Nephrogenic adenomatosis

This condition is a variant of urothelial metaplasia and typically presents with microscopic haematuria and irritative bladder symptoms. It arises most commonly in the bladder, usually in the trigone and less often in the urethra. In most cases the stimulus for metaplastic adenomatous change appears to be acute or chronic infective or non-infective cystitis (Gonzales et al 1988). The lesions are usually papillary and multiple although solitary lesions may occur. Histopathology usually demonstrates irregularly branching tubules set in an oedematous stroma, which resemble primitive renal tubule structures, hence the name 'nephrogenic adenomatosis'. The condition is not premalignant and treatment should be aimed at eradication of the primary stimulus and excision of the lesions.

Lower urinary tract tumours

Carcinoma in situ may be asymptomatic or associated with urgency, frequency and dysuria (Utz & Farrow 1984), with a cystoscopic appearance that varies from normal to inflamed and congested. Histology usually demonstrates abnormal pleomorphic transitional cells confined to the urothelium. Urine cytology is positive in 80–90% of cases. Intravesical therapy using BCG vaccine is associated with regression in >50% of cases and is the preferred treatment modality (Coplen et al 1990). Surgical resection or ablation using transvesical laser or diathermy are indicated for persistent disease, but recurrence or progression to muscle invasion will occur in >40% of these women.

The majority of primary invasive lower urinary tract tumours present with painless haematuria, with symptoms of bladder irritation the second most common presentation. Urinary tract infection is a frequent association. The most common histological type of primary bladder carcinoma is transitional cell (>90%). In the developing world, however, schistosomiasis is associated with an increased incidence of squamous carcinoma. Adenocarcinoma is uncommon but may arise in the embryological remnants of the urachus.

Lower urinary tract calculi

Bladder and urethral calculi in women often arise secondary to a foreign body (e.g. suture material, mesh erosion) (see Fig. 56.4) or structural abnormalities such as a bladder or urethral diverticulum. They commonly present with recurrent urinary tract infection or irritative bladder symptoms (Dwyer et al 1999). Treatment is directed at removal of the calculus by cystoscopy or lithotripsy and correction of the underlying abnormality.

Urethral diverticulum

Evidence of asymptomatic paraurethral cystic lesions is found in 2–6% of women at routine ultrasound, many of which may represent urethral diverticula (Fynes et al 2001). Urethral diverticula may be embryonic cystic remnants or acquired and post inflammatory in origin (Boyd & Raz 1983). It has been suggested that infection in the paraurethral glands may lead to abscess formation with spontaneous marsupialization into the urethra. Constant irritation from pooled urine results in epithelialization of the track and formation of a urethral diverticulum (Routh 1980). This theory suggests that there is a prerupture stage with a paraurethral cystic structure and no urethral communication (Davis & Robinson 1970, Fynes et al 2001, Stewart et al 1981).

Urethral diverticula may be asymptomatic or present with dysuria, frequency, stress urinary incontinence or an anterior vaginal wall mass (see Fig. 56.3) (Boyd & Raz 1983). Calculi may form in the base of the diverticulum secondary to chronic infection or stasis; these women often have a history of recurrent urinary tract infection or may complain of pain exacerbated by intercourse. A micturating cystogram or retrograde positive-pressure urethrogram using a Tratner double-balloon catheter will usually identify a urethral diverticulum (Lang & Davis 1959); high-frequency transperineal ultrasound and Doppler may be helpful (Fynes et al 2001). Surgical excision is necessary in symptomatic women. Postoperative complications include urethral stricture or scarring (Fig. 56.6), recurrence, stress incontinence and urethrovaginal fistula.

Urethral syndrome

Urethral syndrome is a non-specific group of lower urinary tract symptoms which include pain (suprapubic or urethral) with urinary frequency and urgency. The pain is typically exacerbated by micturition. The diagnosis can only be made where routine investigations fail to identify any pathology.

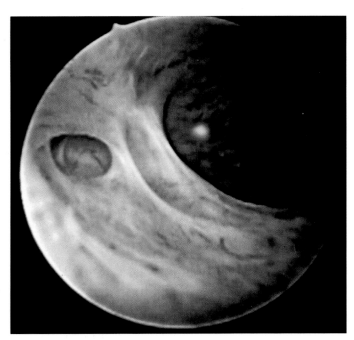

Fig. 56.6 Urethroscopy using a 0° scope and Sashe sheath. This 36-year-old woman had undergone previous excision of a urethral diverticulum and presented with severe type 3 stress incontinence. This image demonstrates extensive urethral scarring.

Such investigations should exclude infectious and non-infectious causes of cystitis, urethral inflammation secondary to trauma, foreign bodies, contact irritation or localized paraurethral lesions (Skene's abscess, urethral stricture, diverticulum, tumour) and urethral manifestations of systemic disorders (Reiter's syndrome, Stevens–Johnson syndrome). Careful cystourethroscopic visualization, particularly of the urethra, using a 0° scope and Sasche sheath is necessary to exclude pathology (see Fig. 56.6). A diagnosis of urethral syndrome is therefore one of exclusion. An MSU and urethral swab should be performed for both microscopy and culture. The latter investigation is only indicated if the woman is sexually active.

In women with recent-onset dysuria and frequency (acute urethral syndrome) and an MSU specimen which demonstrates pyuria with $<10^5$ micro-organisms per ml, an infective cause is often identified (Stamm et al 1980). The most common organisms isolated on culture of urinary specimens or urethral swabs include coliforms, *Chlamydia trachomatis*, *Staphylocoocus saprophyticus* and *Neisseria gonorrhoeae*. If the cultures are negative empirical antibiotic therapy with doxycycline alone or in combination with a sulphonamide should be considered and is frequently associated with symptomatic resolution (Latham & Stamm 1894).

In women with chronic urethral symptoms an infective cause is less likely but should be excluded. In the past urethral dilatation was frequently performed based on the assumption that the condition was due to urethral obstruction, with 80% of women reporting amelioration of their symptoms (Rutherford et al 1988). Comparable symptomatic improvement, however, is also noted following cystoscopy alone and urethral dilatation may be associated with urethral fibrosis or

the development of intrinsic urethral sphincter deficiency and secondary stress urinary incontinence. Pharmacological agents such as the benzodiazepines have also been used; their presumed effect is to reduce spasm of the smooth and striated urethral muscles although there is no objective evidence to support this hypothesis.

This condition may represent an extension of the chronic pain syndromes, which are both complex and poorly understood. There is no current consensus on the appropriate management of this condition. Amitriptyline is used in the treatment of other chronic pain syndromes and is often helpful in women with urethral syndrome. In addition, this agent also has a beneficial anticholinergic effect. Pharmacological therapy, however, should be combined with education and psychological counselling to improve coping strategies for both the patient and their support group.

SUMMARY

Sensory disorders of the lower urinary tract are common and frequently unrecognized. This often leads to many years of suffering before an accurate diagnosis is made. This is distressing for both the affected individual and their family and may occasionally be potentially serious. A sound working knowledge of the clinical presentation, differential diagnoses and diagnostic criteria for these conditions are essential for all practising gynaecologists. While some of these disorders have specific and effective therapeutic options, others remain poorly understood. Interstitial cystitis in particular is an undulating and painful bladder condition, where current therapy is of limited efficacy. Further research is required to evaluate the pathogenesis of these conditions as it is likely that only when the disease process itself is understood will effective therapeutic protocols be developed.

KEY POINTS

1. Urge/frequency syndromes are common and are caused by a wide variety of localized and systemic conditions. A detailed history, examination and sound basic knowledge are required to provide an accurate diagnosis and therapy.
2. Frequency volume diaries are an inexpensive and accurate way to assess symptom severity and response to behavioural therapy.
3. Cystoscopic evaluation of the lower urinary tract is an essential skill for all gynaecological surgeons, not only in the assessment of urinary symptoms and pain but during pelvic surgery for the prevention and early treatment of bladder and urethral injury.
4. Patient education and access to support networks are an important aspect in the management of interstitial cystitis and other chronic pain syndromes.
5. Bladder retraining, oral and intravesical drug therapy, cystodistension and neuromodulation are effective treatment for the management of interstitial cystitis or urge/frequency syndrome.
6. Where urinary cultures are negative, empirical therapy with antibiotics may result in symptom resolution in women with 'urethral syndrome'.

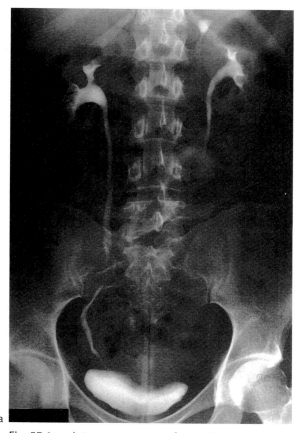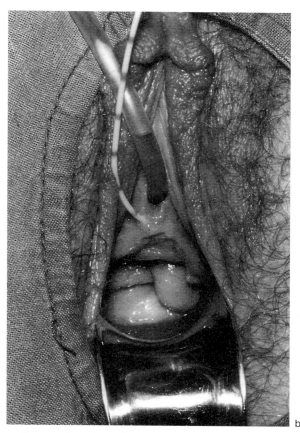

Fig. 57.1 **a** Intravenous urogram from patient presenting with continuous urinary incontinence; a small discrete upper pole element is visible, although the upper pole ureter is not clearly seen. **b** Appearance of vulva with urethral catheter in place and a ureteric catheter placed in the ectopic ureteric opening just below external urethral meatus.

Circumcision has been practised in various forms in much of North Africa and is still practised widely in Sudan and other Moslem cultures. The most extreme form, pharaonic circumcision, involves removal of the labial minora, most of the labia majora, the mons veneris and often the clitoris (Fig. 57.4), the introitus being reduced to pin-hole size. The effect in labour is to produce significant delay in the second stage. This will often necessitate wide episiotomy, often with an anterior incision to allow delivery, and contributes to the development of both vesicovaginal fistulae and rectovaginal fistulae or third-degree tears.

Tahzib (1983, 1985) reported on the epidemiological determinants of vesicovaginal fistulae in northern Nigeria. In 84% of cases obstructed labour was the major aetiological factor; 33% had undergone gishiri and in 15% this was felt to be the main aetiological factor.

In considering obstetric fistulae, however, it is perhaps as much if not more relevant to consider not simply the direct physical injury to the lower urinary tract but the social, cultural and geographical influences. Obstructed labour is most often due to a contracted pelvis. This usually results from stunting of growth by malnutrition and untreated infections in childhood and adolescence. Where women retain a subservient role in society and standards of education are limited, early marriage and the absence of family planning

service result in an early start to child bearing; where first pregnancies occur soon after the menarche, before growth of the pelvis is complete, this also contributes to obstruction in labour.

The influence of these factors is illustrated in the epidemiological studies alluded to earlier. Tahzib (1983) reported that over 50% of the cases of vesicovaginal fistulae seen in northern Nigeria were aged under 20; over 50% were in their first pregnancy and only 1 in 500 had received any formal education. Murphy (1981) from the same area reported that 88% of patients had married at 15 years of age or less and 33% had delivered their first child before the age of 15 years. In different third world societies, however, these factors do seem to have variable influence and, for example, in south-east Nigeria (Hilton & Ward 1998) and the north-west frontier of Pakistan (WHO 1989), fistula patients seem to be somewhat older and of higher parity; they also appear to have a higher literacy rate and to be more likely to remain in a married relationship after the development of their fistula (Hilton & Ward 1998). It is likely that the development of fistulae here reflects other biosocial variations (Table 57.2). It is clear that in these populations, even where skilled maternity care is available, uptake may be poor. Mistrust of hospital is commonplace, antenatal care poorly attended and delivery commonly conducted at home by elderly relatives or unskilled traditional

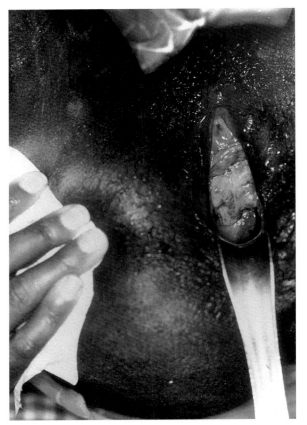

Fig. 57.2   Puerperal patient following prolonged obstructed labour. An area of devitalized tissue is seen on the anterior vaginal wall, about to slough with resultant fistula formation.

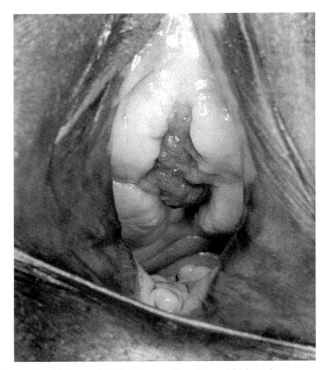

Fig. 57.3   Vesicovaginal fistula resulting from gishiri cut in a young Hausa girl.

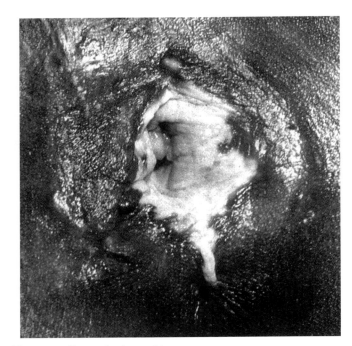

Fig. 57.4   Pharaonic circumcision.

birth attendants. Where labour is prolonged transfer to hospital may only be used as a last resort.

Surgical

Genital fistula may occur following a wide range of surgical procedures within the pelvis (Table 57.1, Fig. 57.5a–f). It is often supposed that this complication results from direct injury to the lower urinary tract at the time of operation. Certainly, on occasions this may be the case; careless, hurried or rough surgical technique makes injury to the lower urinary tract much more likely. However, of 152 fistulae referred to the author in the UK over the last 12 years, 107 have been associated with pelvic surgery and 84 followed hysterectomy; of these, only four presented with leakage of urine on day 1. In other cases compromise to the blood supply may result in tissue necrosis and subsequent leakage or alternatively a small pelvic haematoma may develop in association with the vaginal vault which subsequently becomes infected and discharges with the characteristic puff of haematuria 5–10 days later and incontinence follows shortly thereafter. Recent animal studies suggest that the inadvertent placement of vault sutures into the bladder wall at hysterectomy may not carry as great a risk of fistula formation as previous thought (Meeks et al 1997).

Although it is important to remember that the majority of surgical fistulae follow apparently straightforward hysterectomy in skilled hands, several risk factors may be identified making direct injury more likely (Table 57.3). Obviously anatomical distortion within the pelvis by ovarian tumour or fibroid will increase the difficulty and abnormal adhesions between bladder and uterus or cervix following previous surgery or associated with previous sepsis, endometriosis or malignancy may make fistula formation more likely. Preoperative or early radiotherapy

Table 57.2 Epidemiological aspects of obstetric fistula as illustrated in five studies from Nigeria, Ethiopia and Pakistan

	Northern Nigeria* n = 100	Northern Nigeria ** n = 1443	Ethiopia[†] n = 309	Southeast Nigeria[††] n = 2389	Pakistan[†††] n = 325
Mean age (yrs)	20	21	22	28	32
Mean parity	?	1.6	2.1	3.5	?
% in first pregnancy	65	52	63	31	15
Divorced/deserted (%)	54% divorced/sep'd	?	52% deserted	10% divorced/sep'd	?
Literacy (%)	8	0.2	?	29	?
Delivered at home (%)	?	64	58	27	?

* Murphy 1981; ** Tahzib 1983;[†] Kelly & Kwast 1993;[††] Hilton & Ward 1998;[†††] WHO 1989

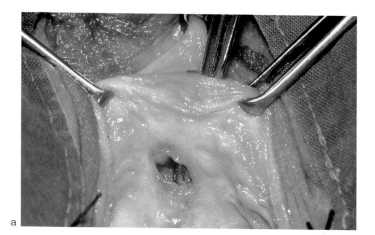
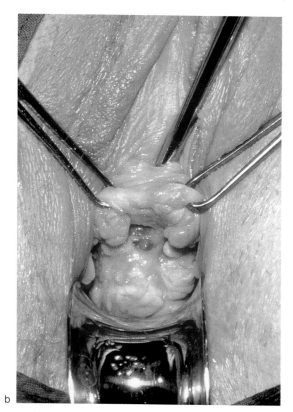
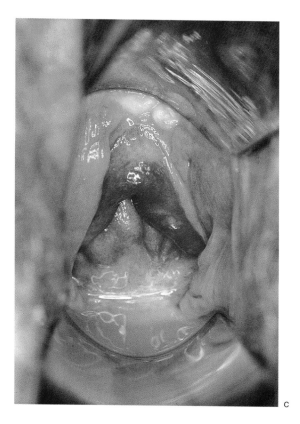
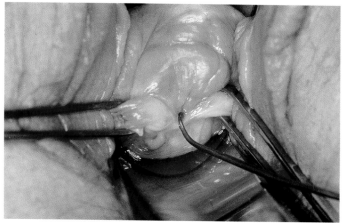

Fig. 57.5 Urogenital fistulae of varying aetiologies. **a** Following anterior colporrhaphy; **b** urethral diverticulectomy; **c** radical hysterectomy; **d** simple abdominal hysterectomy.

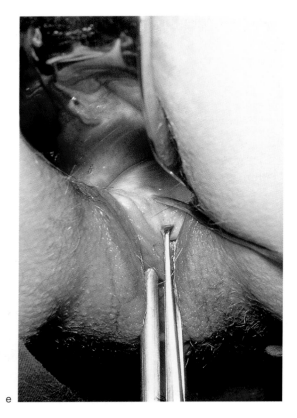

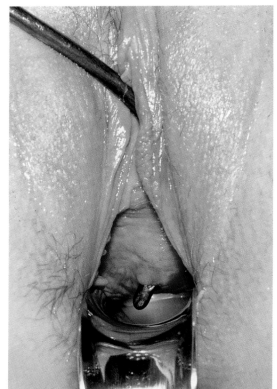

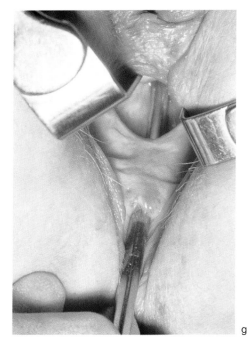

Fig. 57.5 e colposuspension (the fistula in the latter case was fixed retropubically in the midline at the bladder neck and the photograph shows the patient prone, in the reverse lithotomy position); f subtrigonal phenol injection; g radiotherapy for carcinoma of cervix.

may decrease vascularity and make the tissues in general less forgiving of poor technique.

Issues of training and surgical technique are of course also important. The ability to locate and if necessary dissect out the ureter must be part of our routine gynaecological training, as should the first aid management of lower urinary tract injury when it arises. The use of gauze swabs to separate the bladder

from the cervix at caesarean section or hysterectomy should be discouraged; sharp dissection with knife or scissors does less harm, especially where the tissues are abnormally adherent.

It has recently been shown that there is a high incidence of abnormalities of lower urinary tract function in fistula patients (Hilton 1998); whether these abnormalities antedate the surgery or develop with or as a consequence of the fistula

Table 57.3   Risk factors for postoperative fistulae

Risk factor	Pathology	Specific example
Anatomical distortion		Fibroids
		Ovarian mass
Abnormal tissue adhesion	Inflammation	Infection
		Endometriosis
	Previous surgery	Caesarean section
		Cone biopsy
		Colporrhaphy
	Malignancy	
Impaired vascularity	Ionizing radiation	Preoperative
	Metabolic abnormality	radiotherapy
	Radical surgery	Diabetes mellitus
Compromised healing		Anaemia
		Nutritional deficiency
Abnormality of bladder function		Voiding dysfunction

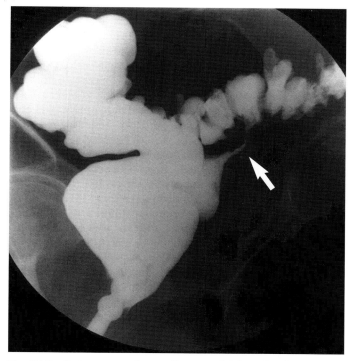

Fig. 57.6   Barium enema from patient complaining of vaginal discharge; demonstrates extensive diverticular disease and obvious colovaginal fistula.

cannot be answered from these data. It is, however, likely that patients with a habit of infrequent voiding or with inefficient detrusor contractility may be at increased risk of postoperative urinary retention; if this is not recognized early and managed appropriately, the risk of fistula formation may be increased.

Radiation

As noted above, preoperative pelvic irradiation increases the risk of postoperative fistula development, but irradiation itself may be a cause of fistula (Fig. 57.5 g). The obliterative endarteritis associated with ionizing radiation in therapeutic dosage proceeds over many years and may be aetiological in fistula formation long after the primary malignancy has been treated. Of the 19 radiation fistulae in the author's series, the fistula has developed at intervals between 1 and 30 years following radiotherapy. Not only does this ischaemia produce the fistulae, it also causes significant damage in the adjacent tissues so that ordinary surgical repair has a high likelihood of failure and modified surgical techniques are required.

Malignancy

The treatment of pelvic malignancy by either surgery or radiotherapy is associated with a risk of fistula development but tissue loss associated with malignant disease itself may result in genital tract fistula. Carcinoma of cervix, vagina and rectum are the most common malignancies to present in this way. It is relatively unusual for urothelial tumours to present with fistula formation, other than following surgery or radiotherapy. The development of a fistula may be a distressing part of the terminal phase of malignant disease; it is nevertheless one deserving not simply compassion but full consideration of the therapeutic or palliative possibilities.

Inflammatory bowel disease

Inflammatory bowel disease is the most significant cause of intestinogenital fistulae in the UK, although these rarely present directly to the gynaecologist. Crohn's disease is by far the most important and appears to be increasing in frequency in the Western world. A total fistula rate approaching 40% has been reported and in females the involvement of the genital tract may be up to 7%.

Ulcerative colitis has a small incidence of low rectovaginal fistulae. Diverticular disease can produce colovaginal fistulae and rarely colouterine fistulae, with surprisingly few symptoms attributable to the intestinal pathology. The possibility should not be overlooked if an elderly woman complains of faeculent discharge or becomes incontinent without concomitant urinary problems (Fig. 57.6).

Miscellaneous

Among other miscellaneous causes of fistulae in the genital tract, the following should be considered.

Infection
- Lymphogranuloma venereum
- Schistosomiasis
- Tuberculosis
- Actinomycosis
- Measles
- Noma vaginae

Other
- Penetrating trauma
- Coital injury
- Neglected pessary
- Other foreign body
- Catheter-related injury

PREVALENCE

The prevalence of genital fistulae obviously varies from country to country and continent to continent as the main causative factors vary. Accurate figures are impossible to obtain since those areas with the highest overall prevalence are also those with the poorest systems of health data collection. Data from the regional health authority information units in England and Wales suggest an average of eight vesicovaginal and urethrovaginal fistula repairs per health region per year and a national incidence of approximately 152 per year (Hilton 1995, 1997). Other estimates range between 135 (Lawson 1990, personal communication) and 350 (Kelly 1983) fistulae per year in the UK, with a post-hysterectomy fistula rate of approximately 1 per 1300 operations (Hilton 1997). Studies from Finland suggest a similar rate of post-hysterectomy fistulae overall, with approximately 1 per 1000 abdominal hysterectomies and 1 per 450 laparoscopic hysterectomies (Harkki-Siren et al 1998). Similarly, ureteric injury may be up to six times as common following laparoscopic as compared to open hysterectomy (Harkki-Siren et al 1998) and 2–10 times as common following radical hysterectomy and exenteration (Averette et al 1993, Bladou et al 1995, Emmert & Kohler 1996). In the studies of Sultan and colleagues (1994) third-degree tears followed 0.6% of vaginal deliveries and in 6% of these (1 in 3000 deliveries overall) a rectovaginal fistula resulted.

In the developing world, many fistula cases are unknown to medical services, being separated from their husbands and ostracized from society. Although the true prevalence in the developing world is unknown, particularly high prevalence rates are reported in Nigeria, Ethiopia, Sudan and Chad. The estimated third world prevalence is 1–2 per 1000 deliveries with perhaps 50 000–100 000 new cases each year. Although several units exist in Nigeria, Ethiopia and Sudan which deal with 100–700 cases per year, these nowhere nearly meet the demand and there are estimated to be perhaps 500 000 untreated cases worldwide (Waaldijk & Armiya'u 1993).

CLASSIFICATION

Many different fistula classifications have been described in the literature on the basis of anatomical site; these are often subclassified into simple cases (where the tissues are healthy and access good) (Fig. 57.7a,b) or complicated (where there is tissue loss, scarring, impaired access, involvement of the ureteric orifices or a co-existent rectovaginal fistula) (Fig. 57.7c). Urogenital fistulae may be classified into urethral, bladder neck, subsymphysial (a complex form involving circumferential loss of the urethra with fixity to bone), midvaginal, juxtacervical or vault fistulae, massive fistulae extending from bladder neck to vault and vesicouterine or vesicocervical fistulae. It is interesting to note that whereas over 60% of fistulae in the third world are midvaginal, juxtacervical or massive (reflecting their obstetric aetiology) (Hilton & Ward 1998), such cases are relatively rare in Western fistula practice; by contrast 50% of the fistulae managed in the UK are situated in the vaginal vault (reflecting their surgical aetiology).

PRESENTATION

Fistulae between the urinary tract and the female genital tract are characteristically said to present with continuous urinary incontinence, both by day and night. In patients with large fistulae the volume of leakage may be such that they rarely feel any sensation of bladder fullness and normal voiding may be infrequent. Where there is extensive tissue loss, as in obstetric fistulae from obstructed labour, or radiation fistulae, this typical history is usually present, the clinical findings gross and the diagnosis rarely in doubt. With postsurgical fistulae, for example, the history may be atypical and the orifice small, elusive or occasionally completely invisible. Under these circumstances the diagnosis can be much more difficult and a high index of clinical suspicion must be maintained.

Occasionally a patient with an obvious fistula may deny incontinence and this is presumed to reflect the ability of the levator ani muscles to occlude the vagina below the level of the fistula. Some patients with vesicocervical or vesicouterine fistula following caesarean section may maintain continence at the level of the uterine isthmus and complain of cyclical haematuria at the time of menstruation or menouria (Falk & Tancer 1956, Youssef 1957). In other cases patients may complain of little more than a watery vaginal discharge or intermittent leakage, which seems posturally related. Leakage may appear to occur specifically on standing or on lying supine, prone or in left or right lateral positions, presumably reflecting the degree of bladder distension and the position of the fistula within the bladder; such a pattern is most unlikely to be found with ureteric fistulae.

Although in the case of direct surgical injury leakage may occur from day 1, in most surgical and obstetric fistulae, symptoms develop between 5 and 14 days after the causative injury; the time of presentation, however, may be quite variable. This will depend to some extent on the severity of symptoms but as far as obstetric fistulae in the third world are concerned, it is determined more by access to healthcare. In a review of cases from Nigeria the average time for presentation was over 5 years' and in some cases over 35 years, after the causative pregnancy (Hilton & Ward 1998).

Urethrovaginal fistulae distal to the sphincter mechanism will often be asymptomatic and require no specific treatment. Some may lead to obstruction and are more likely to present with postmicturition dribbling than other types of incontinence; they can therefore be very difficult to recognize. More proximally situated urethral fistulae are perhaps most likely to present with stress incontinence, since bladder neck competence is frequently impaired.

Ureteric fistulae have similar aetiologies to bladder fistulae and the causative mechanism may be one of direct injury by incision, division or excision or of ischaemia from strangulation by suture, crushing by clamp or stripping by dissection (Yeates 1987). The presentation may therefore be similarly variable. With direct injury leakage is usually apparent from the first postoperative day. Urine output may be physiologically reduced for some hours following surgery and if there is significant operative or postoperative hypotension, oliguria may persist longer. Once renal function is restored, however, leakage will usually be apparent promptly. With other mechanisms

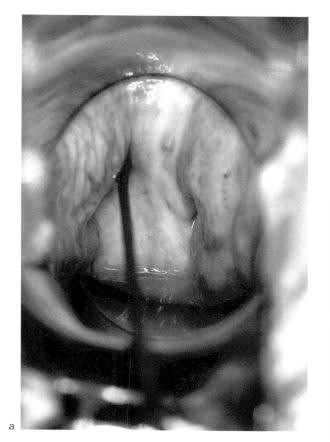
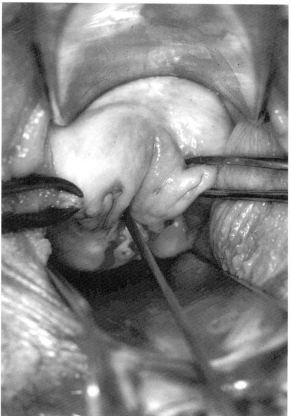
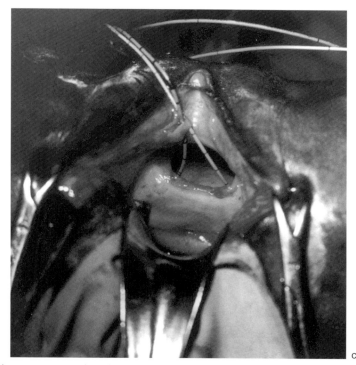

Fig. 57.7   a Simple post-hysterectomy vault vesicovaginal fistula. b Same case as above illustrating tissue mobility and ease of access for repair per vaginam. c Complex obstetric fistula; a massive VVF with involvement of both ureteric orifices and co-existent RVF.

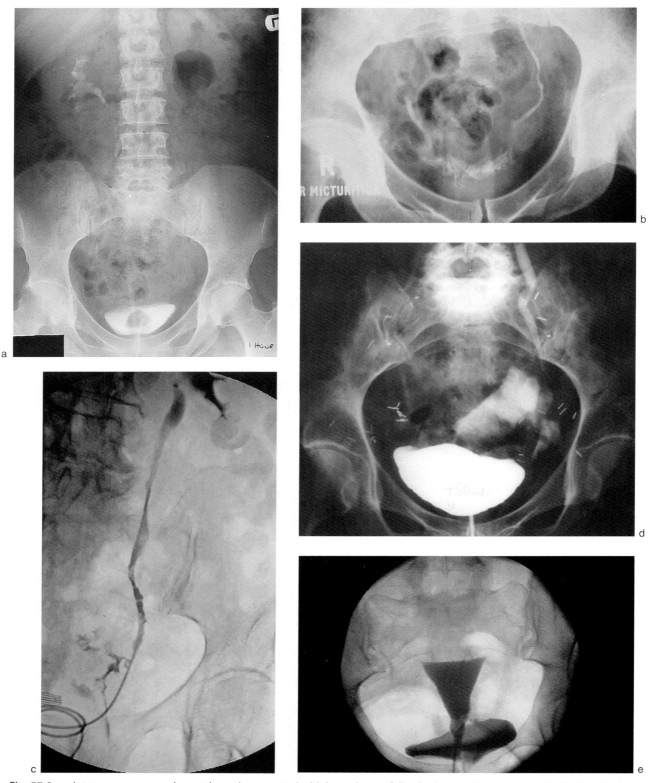

Fig. 57.8 **a** Intravenous urogram in a patient who presented with incontinence following hysterectomy, presumed initially to be due to a vesicovaginal fistula. Apparent resolution of the leakage following catheterization in fact was due to progressive obstruction above the level of a ureterovaginal fistula. **b** Intravenous urogram showing periureteric flare typical of ureterovaginal fistula. **c** Retrograde pyelogram demonstrating ureterovaginal fistula. **d** Intravenous urogram (with simultaneous cystogram) demonstrating a complex surgical fistula occurring after radical hysterectomy. After further investigation including cystourethroscopy, sigmoidoscopy, barium enema and retrograde cannulation of the vaginal vault to perform fistulography, the lesion was defined as an uretero-colo-vesico-vaginal fistula. **e** Hysterosalpingogram in patient with vesicocervical cervical fistula following caesarean section.

obstruction is likely to be present to a greater or lesser degree and the initial symptoms may be of pyrexia or loin pain, with incontinence occurring only after sloughing of the ischaemic tissue, from around 5 days up to 6 weeks later. On occasion the reverse pattern may be seen with apparent relief of leakage resulting from the development of obstruction as scarring in the ureter proceeds (Fig. 57.8a).

With intestinal fistulae the history may be much more misleading. A small communication with the large bowel may cause only an offensive discharge. Even fistulae of obstetric origin may be rendered relatively asymptomatic by the cicatrization of the vagina, which occurs following sloughing. A small high posterior horseshoe-shaped fistula may only become apparent during division of constricting bands for the repair of a vesicovaginal fistula. Most typically, however, patients will complain of incontinence of liquid stool and flatus and whilst they may often be unsure as to whether stool is from the vagina or anus, the sensation of flatus from the vagina is rarely misinterpreted.

INVESTIGATIONS

If there is suspicion of a fistula but its presence is not easily confirmed by clinical examination with a Sims' speculum, further investigation will be necessary to confirm or fully exclude the possibility. Even where the diagnosis is clinically obvious, additional investigation may be appropriate for full evaluation prior to deciding treatment.

Microbiology

Urinary infection is surprisingly uncommon in fistula patients, although especially where there have been previous attempts at surgery urine culture should be undertaken and appropriate antibiotic therapy instituted. Urine culture is not easily obtained when a fistula produces severe incontinence, but a pipette may be used to obtain a small intravesical sample for investigation.

Dye studies

When the diagnosis is in doubt, it is important first to confirm that the discharge is urinary, second that the leakage is extraurethral rather than urethral and third to establish the site of leakage. Although other imaging techniques undoubtedly have a role (see below), carefully conducted dye studies remain the investigation of first choice.

Excessive vaginal discharge or the drainage of serum from a pelvic haematoma postoperatively may simulate a urinary fistula. If the fluid is in sufficient quantity to be collected, biochemical analysis of its urea content in comparison to that of urine and serum will confirm its origin. Phenazopyridine may be used orally (200 mg tds) or indigo carmine intravenously to stain the urine and hence confirm the presence of a fistula. The identification of the site of a fistula is best carried out by the instillation of coloured dye (methylthioninium chloride (methylene blue) or indigo carmine) into the bladder via a catheter with the patient in the lithotomy position. The traditional 'three swab test' has its limitations and is not recommended and the examination is best carried out with direct inspection; multiple fistulae may be located in this way. It is important to be alert for leakage around the catheter, which may spill back into the vagina, creating the impression of a fistula. It is also important to ensure that adequate distension of the bladder occurs as some fistulae do not leak at small volumes; conversely, some fistulae with an oblique track through the bladder wall may leak at small volumes but not at capacity. If leakage of clear fluid continues after dye instillation a ureteric fistula is likely and this is most easily confirmed by a 'two dye test', using phenazopyridine to stain the renal urine and methylthioninium chloride (methylene blue) to stain bladder contents (Raghavaiah 1974).

Dye tests are less useful for intestinal fistulae, although a carmine marker taken orally may confirm their presence. Rectal distension with air via a sigmoidoscope may be of more value; if the patient is kept in a slight head-down position and the vagina filled with saline, the bubbling of any air leaked through a low fistula may be detected.

Imaging

Excretion urography

Although intravenous urography is a particularly insensitive investigation in the diagnosis of vesicovaginal fistula, knowledge of upper urinary tract status may have a significant influence on treatment measures applied and should therefore be looked on as an essential investigation for any suspected or confirmed urinary fistula (Fig. 57.8a,b). Compromise of ureteric function is a particularly common finding when a fistula occurs in relation to malignant disease or its treatment (by radiation or surgery).

Dilatation of the ureter is characteristic in ureteric fistula and its finding in association with a known vesicovaginal fistula should raise suspicion of a complex uretero-vesico-vaginal lesion. Whilst essential for the diagnosis of ureteric fistula, intravenous urography is not completely sensitive, although the presence of a periureteric flare is highly suggestive of extravasation at this site (Fig. 57. 8b).

Retrograde pyelography

Retrograde pyelography is a more reliable way of identifying the exact site of a ureterovaginal fistula and may be undertaken simultaneously with either retrograde or percutaneous catheterization for therapeutic stenting of the ureter (see below) (Fig.57.8c).

Cystography

Cystography is not particularly helpful in the basic diagnosis of vesicovaginal fistulae and a dye test carried out under direct vision is likely to be more sensitive. It may, however, occasionally be useful in achieving a diagnosis in complex fistulae (Fig. 57.8d) or vesicouterine fistulae, where a lateral view may show the cavity of the uterus filled with radio-opaque dye behind the bladder.

Fistulography

This is a special example of the X-ray technique commonly referred to as sinography. For small fistulae a ureteric catheter is suitable, although if the hole is large enough a small Foley catheter may be used to deliver the radio-opaque dye; this is of particular value for fistulae for which there is an intervening abscess cavity. If a catheter will pass through a small vaginal aperture into an adjacent loop of bowel its nature may become apparent from the radiological appearance of the lumen and haustrations, although, further imaging studies are usually required to demonstrate the underlying pathology.

Colpography and hysterosalpingography

If a fistula opening cannot be directly identified colpography or hysterography may occasionally be helpful. If a large Foley catheter with a large balloon is distended in the lower vagina, injection of a non-viscous opaque medium under pressure may outline a fistulous track to an adjacent organ. However, failure to demonstrate a fistula by this means does not exclude its presence. If a patient with a vesicouterine fistula has no history of incontinence but complains of cyclical haematuria, contrast studies carried out through the uterus may be more rewarding than cystography. Again a lateral view is necessary to detect the anterior leak (Fig.57.8e).

Barium enema, barium meal and follow-through

Either or both of these may be required for the evaluation of the intestinal condition when an intestinal fistula is present above the anorectum. Aside from confirming the presence of a fistula, evidence of malignant or inflammatory disease may be identified.

Ultrasound, computerised tomography and magnetic resonance imaging

These may occasionally be appropriate for the complete assessment of complex fistulae. Endoanal ultrasound and MRI are particularly useful in the investigation of anorectal and perineal fistulae.

Examination under anaesthesia

Careful examination, if necessary under anaesthetic, may be required to determine the presence of a fistula and is deemed by several authorities to be an essential preliminary to definitive surgical treatment (Chassar Moir 1967, Jonas & Petri 1984, Lawson 1978, Lawson & Hudson 1987). A malleable silver probe is invaluable for the exploration of the vaginal walls and tissue forceps or plastic surgical skin hooks helpful to put tension on the tissues for the identification of small fistulae. If the probe passes directly into the rectum it may be felt digitally or seen via the proctoscope; in the bladder or urethra it may be identified by a metallic click against a silver catheter or seen by a cystoscope. In either case the diagnosis is then obvious.

It is also important at the time of examination to assess the available access for repair vaginally and the mobility of the tissues (Fig. 57.7a,b). The decision between the vaginal and abdominal approaches to surgery is thus made; when the vaginal route is chosen, it may be appropriate to select between the more conventional supine lithotomy with a head-down tilt and the prone (reverse lithotomy) with head-up tilt (Fig. 57.9). This may be particularly useful in allowing the operator to look down onto bladder neck and subsymphysial fistulae and is also of advantage in some massive fistulae in encouraging the reduction of the prolapsed bladder mucosa (Lawson 1967).

Endoscopy

Cystoscopy

Although some authorities suggest that endoscopy has little role in the evaluation of fistulae, it is the author's practice to perform cystourethroscopy in all but the largest defects. Although in some obstetric and radiation fistulae, the size of the defect and the extent of tissue loss and scarring may make it difficult to distend the bladder, nevertheless much useful information is obtained. The exact level and position of the fistula should be determined and its relationship to the ureteric

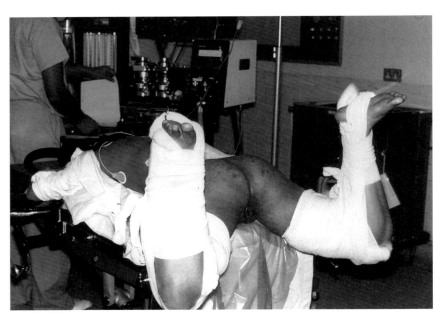

Fig. 57.9 Patient in prone (reverse lithotomy) position with head-up tilt, in preparation for repair of a fixed subsymphysial fistula.

orifices and bladder neck are particularly important. With urethral and bladder neck fistulae the failure to pass a cystoscope or sound may indicate that there has been circumferential loss of the proximal urethra, a circumstance which is of considerable importance in determining the appropriate surgical technique and the likelihood of subsequent urethral incompetence. Similar considerations may apply to investigation of the lower bowel following major obstetric injuries in which segmental circumferential loss of the upper rectum may have occurred.

The condition of the tissues must be carefully assessed. Persistence of slough means that surgery should be deferred and this is particularly important in obstetric and postradiation cases. Biopsy from the edge of a fistula should be taken in radiation fistulae, if persistent or recurrent malignancy is suspected. Malignant change has been reported in a long-standing benign fistula, so where there is any doubt at all about the nature of the tissues biopsy should be undertaken (Hudson 1968). In areas of endemicity evidence of schistosomiasis, tuberculosis and lymphogranuloma may become apparent in biopsy material and again, it is important that specific antimicrobial treatment is instituted prior to definitive surgery. If calculi are identified in the bladder, vaginal vault or diverticulum clinically, radiologically or endoscopically, their removal prior to any attempt at surgical correction is essential.

Sigmoidoscopy and proctoscopy

These examinations are important for the diagnosis of inflammatory bowel disease, which may not have been suspected before the occurrence of a fistula. Biopsies of the fistula edge or any unhealthy-looking area should always be obtained.

MANAGEMENT

Immediate management

Before epithelialization is complete an abnormal communication between viscera will tend to close spontaneously, provided that the natural outflow is unobstructed. Normal continence mechanisms, however, involve the intermittent physiological contraction of urethral and anal sphincters (see Chapter 50). As a result, although spontaneous closure of genital tract fistulae does occur, it is the exception rather than the rule. Bypassing the sphincter mechanisms or diverting flow around the fistula, for example by urinary catheterization or defunctioning colostomy, may, however, encourage closure.

The early management is of critical importance and depends on the aetiology and site of the lesion. If surgical trauma is recognized within the first 24 hours postoperatively, immediate repair may be appropriate, provided that extravasation of urine into the tissues has not been great.

However, the majority of surgical fistulae are recognized between 5 and 14 days postoperatively and these should be treated with continuous bladder drainage. It is worth persisting with this line of management in vesicovaginal or urethrovaginal fistulae for 6–8 weeks, since spontaneous closure may occur within this period (Davits & Miranda 1991).

Obstetric fistulae developing after obstructed labour should also be treated by continuous bladder drainage (Waaldijk 1994a), combined with antibiotics to limit tissue damage from infection. Indeed, if a patient is known to have been in obstructed labour for any significant length of time or is recognized to have areas of slough on the vaginal walls in the puerperium, prophylactic catheterization should be undertaken. If sloughing of the rectal wall has also occurred faecal discharge will adversely affect spontaneous healing and temporary defunctioning colostomy should be performed.

The management of ureterovaginal fistulae is outwith the skill of most gynaecologists and even those with specialist skills in urogynaecology are likely to liaise with urological and radiological colleagues in this situation. Whilst in the past ureteric reimplantation has been the preferred approach in most cases, the use of stents inserted either endoscopically or percutaneously is successful in the majority of cases (Chang et al 1987, Schwartz & Stoller 2000). Where stenting cannot be achieved or does not result in closure of the fistula, definitive surgery should be undertaken at 4–6 weeks, unless progressive calyceal dilatation demands earlier intervention.

The immediate management of obstetric third-degree tears has traditionally been thought to provide good outcome. Recent data suggest that about half of patients sustaining such injuries will have subsequent defaecatory symptoms, as a result of sphincter disruption rather than denervation, and 6% may end up with rectovaginal fistulae (Sultan et al 1994). Whether primary repair by a more experienced surgeon or delayed repair would improve outcome has not been investigated.

It is important to appreciate that some fistulae may be associated with few symptoms and even if persistent, these do not require surgical treatment. Small distal urethrovaginal fistulae, uterovesical fistulae with menouria and some low rectovaginal fistulae may fall into this category.

Palliation and skin care

During the waiting period from diagnosis to repair incontinence pads should be provided in generous quantities so that patients can continue to function socially to some extent. Fistula patients usually leak very much greater quantities of urine than those with urethral incontinence from whatever cause and this needs to be recognized in terms of provision of supplies.

The vulval skin may be at considerable risk from ammoniacal dermatitis and liberal use of silicone barrier cream should be encouraged. Steroid therapy has been advocated in the past as a means of reducing tissue oedema and fibrosis, although these benefits are refuted and there may be a risk of compromise to subsequent healing (Jonas & Petri 1984). Local oestrogen has been recommended by some authors (Jonas & Petri 1984, Kelly 1983) and whilst empirically one might expect benefit in postmenopausal women or those obstetric fistula patients with prolonged amenorrhoea, the evidence for this is lacking.

Nutrition

Because of social ostracism and the effects of prolonged sepsis, patients with obstetric fistulae may also suffer from malnutrition and anaemia. To maximize the prospects for postoperative healing it is essential, therefore, that the general health of the patient should be optimized. Where there is severe inflammatory bowel disease the question of an elemental diet or even total parenteral nutrition may need to be considered in consultation with the gastroenterologist involved.

Physiotherapy

Obstetric fistulae are commonly associated with lower limb weakness, foot drop and limb contracture. In a group of 479 patients studied prospectively 27% had signs of peroneal nerve weakness at presentation and a further 38%, whilst having no current signs, gave a history of relevant symptoms (Waaldijk & Elkins 1994). Early involvement of the physiotherapist in preoperative management and rehabilitation of such patients is essential.

Antimicrobial therapy

In tropical countries the treatment of malaria, typhoid, tuberculosis and parasitic infections should be rigorously undertaken before elective surgery. There is no evidence of benefit from prophylactic antibiotics in the management of obstetric fistulae (Tomlinson & Thornton 1998). Opinions differ on the desirability of prophylactic antibiotic cover for surgery in the developed world, some avoiding their use other than in the treatment of specific infection and some advocating broad-spectrum treatment in all cases. The author's current practice is for single-dose prophylaxis in urinary fistulae and 5 days' cover for intestinal fistulae, in each case using metronidazole and cefuroxime. It advisable to collect urine for culture and sensitivity every 48 hours, although only symptomatic infection need be treated in the catheterized patient.

Bowel preparation

Although surgeons vary in the extent to which they prepare the bowel prior to rectovaginal fistula repair, it is the author's preference to carry out formal preparation in all cases of intestinogenital fistula, whatever the level of the lesion. A low-residue diet should be advised for a week prior to admission, followed by a fluid-only diet for 48 hours preoperatively. Polyethylene glycol 3350 (Kleneprep) four sachets in 4 litres of water over a 4-hour period or alternatively sodium picosulphate (Picolax) 10 mg repeated after 6 hours is given orally on the day before operation. Bowel washout should be carried out on the evening before surgery and if bowel content is not completely clear this should be repeated on the morning of surgery.

Counselling

Surgical fistula patients are usually previously healthy individuals who entered hospital for what was expected to be a routine procedure and they end up with symptoms infinitely worse than their initial complaint. Obstetric fistula patients in the developing world are social outcasts. In both situations, therefore, these women are invariably devastated by their situation It is vital that they understand the nature of the problem, why it has arisen and the plan for management at all stages. Confident but realistic counselling by the surgeon is essential and the involvement of nursing staff or counsellors with experience of fistula patients is also highly desirable. The support given by previously treated sufferers can also be of immense value in maintaining patient morale, especially where a delay prior to definitive treatment is required.

General principles of surgical treatment

Details of individual operations are outside the scope of this chapter and readers wanting further information about this aspect of fistula management are referred to operative surgical texts or more specific texts on the subject. (Chassar Moir 1967, Lawson & Hudson 1987, Mundy 1993, Waaldijk 1994b, Zacharin 1998).

Timing of repair

The timing of surgical repair is perhaps the single most contentious aspect of fistula management. Whilst shortening the waiting period is of both social and psychological benefit to what are always very distressed patients, one must not trade these issues for compromise to surgical success. The benefit of delay is to allow slough to separate and inflammatory change to resolve. In both obstetric and radiation fistulae there is considerable sloughing of tissues and it is imperative that this should have settled before repair is undertaken. In radiation fistulae it may be necessary to wait 12 months or more. In obstetric cases most authorities suggest that a minimum of 3 months should be allowed to elapse, although Waaldijk (1994a) has advocated surgery as soon as slough is separated.

With surgical fistulae the same principles should apply and although the extent of sloughing is limited, extravasation of urine into the pelvic tissues inevitably sets up some inflammatory response. Although early repair is advocated by several authors (Iselin et al 1998), again most would agree that 10–12 weeks postoperatively is the earliest appropriate time for repair.

Pressure from patients to undertake repair at the earliest opportunity is always understandably great but never more so than in the case of previous surgical failure. Such pressure must, however, be resisted and 8 weeks is the minimum time that should be allowed between attempts at closure.

Route of repair

Many urologists advocate an abdominal approach for all fistula repairs, claiming the possibility of earlier intervention and higher success rates in justification. Others suggest that all fistulae can be successfully closed by the vaginal route (Waaldijk 1994b). Such arguments have little merit and both approaches have their place. Surgeons involved in fistula management must be capable of both approaches, and have the versatility to modify their techniques to select that most appropriate to the individual case. Where access is good and the vaginal tissues sufficiently mobile, the vaginal route is usually most appropriate. If access is poor and the fistula cannot be brought down, the abdominal approach should be used. Although such difficulties can sometimes be handled vaginally, where there is concurrent

Table 57.4 Route of primary repair (i.e. 1st repair at referral centre) of urogenital fistulae in two series, from the north of England (Hilton, unpublished), and from southeast Nigeria (Hilton & Ward 1998)

Route of repair	NE England n = 131		SE Nigeria n = 2485	
	%	%	%	%
Abdominal	33.6		17.0	
Transperitoneal		16.1		13.4
Transvesical		7.6		
Ureteric reimplantation/stenting		7.6		3.0
Uretero-sigmoid transplantation		0.0		0.6
Ileal conduit		2.3		0.0
Vaginal lithotomy	64.9		80.0	
Layer dissection		41.2		
Layer dissection + Martius graft		16.8		
Colpocleisis		6.9		
Vaginal reverse lithotomy	1.5		3.0	
Total	100.0		100.0	

involvement of ureter or bowel in a surgical fistula an abdominal procedure may be used to advantage.

Overall, more surgical fistulae are likely to require an abdominal repair than obstetric fistulae, although in the author's series of cases from the UK, and those reviewed from Nigeria, two-thirds of cases were satisfactorily treated by the vaginal route regardless of aetiology (Table 57.4).

Instruments

All operators have their own favoured instruments, although those described by Chassar Moir (1967) and Lawson (1967) are eminently suitable for repair by any route (Fig. 57.10).

Dissection

Great care must be taken over the initial dissection of the fistula and one should probably take as long over this as over the repair itself. Preliminary infiltration with a 1 in 200 000 solution of adrenaline may help separate planes and reduce oozing. The fistula should be circumcized in the most convenient orientation, depending on size and access. All things being equal, a longitudinal incision should be made around urethral or midvaginal fistulae, so that during repair sutures tend to close the bladder neck; conversely vault fistulae are better handled by a transverse elliptical incision, so that during repair sutures do not tend to approximate the ureters (Fig. 57.11a).

The tissue planes are often obliterated by scarring and dissection close to a fistula should therefore be undertaken with a scalpel or scissors (Fig. 57.11b). Sharp dissection is easier with countertraction applied by skin hooks, tissue forceps or retraction sutures. Blunt dissection with small pledgets may be helpful once the planes are established and provided one is away from the fistula edge. Wide mobilization should be performed, so that tension on the repair is minimized (Fig. 57.11c).

There are arguments over the benefits of excision of the fistula track itself. Excision of the bladder walls is probably unwise, as it enlarges the defect and may increase the amount of bleeding into the bladder. Limited excision of the scarred vaginal wall is, however, usually appropriate (Fig. 57.11d).

Bleeding is rarely troublesome with vaginal procedures, except occasionally with proximal urethrovaginal fistulae. Diathermy is best avoided and pressure or underrunning sutures are preferred.

Suture materials

Although a range of suture materials have been advocated over the years and a range of opinion still exists, the author's view is that absorbable sutures should be used throughout all urinary fistula repair procedures. Polyglactin (Vicryl) 2/0 suture on a 25 mm heavy taper-cut needle is preferred for both the

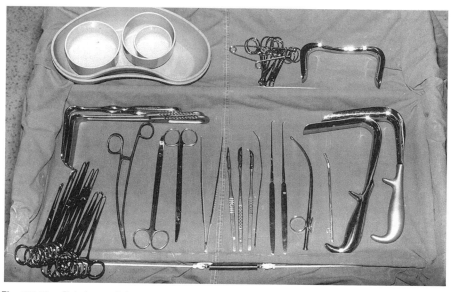

Fig. 57.10 Fistula repair instruments.

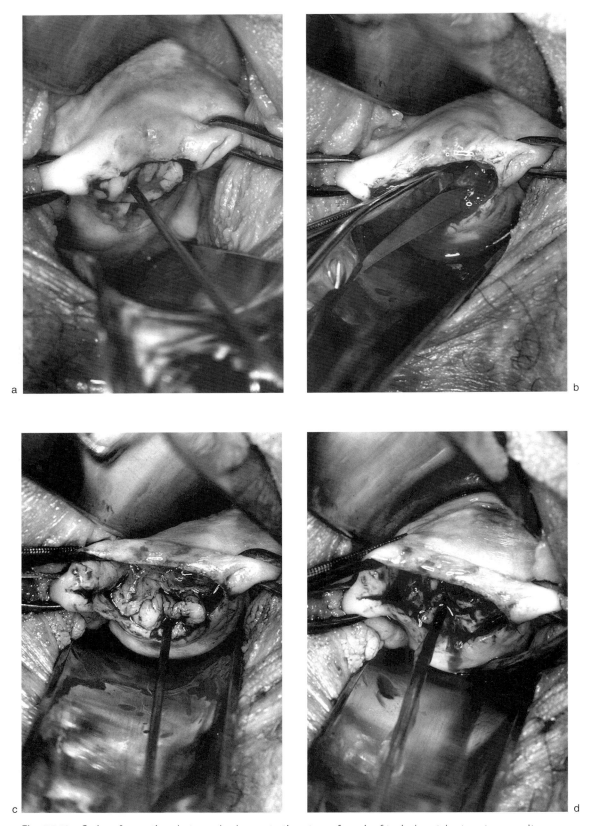

Fig. 57.11 Series of operative photographs demonstrating steps of repair of typical post-hysterectomy vault fistula. **a** Fistula circumcised using no. 12 scalpel; **b** sharp dissection around fistula edge; **c** fistula fully mobilized; **d** vaginal scar edge trimmed.

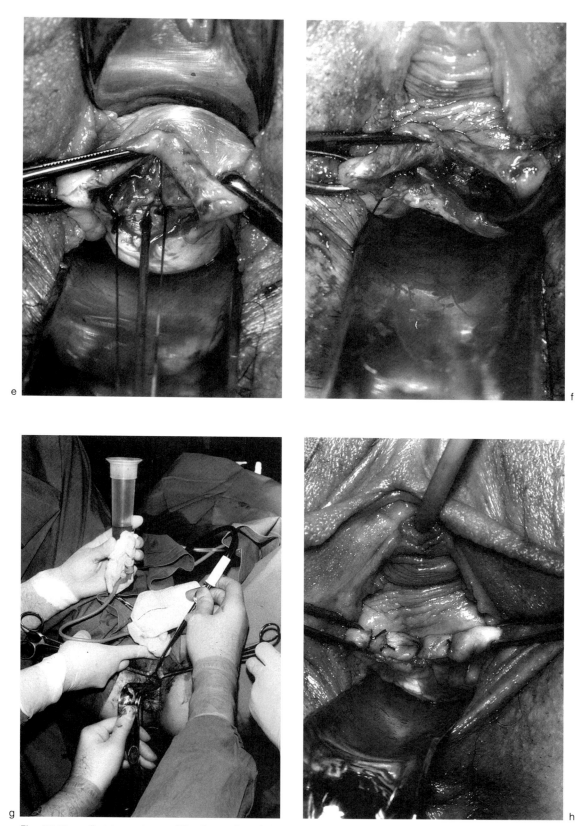

Fig. 57.11 e first two sutures of first layer of repair in place lateral to the angles of the repair;
f second layer completed, sutures catching back of vaginal flaps to close off dead space; g testing the repair with
methylthioninium chloride (methylene blue) dye instillation; h final layer of mattress sutures in the vaginal wall.

bladder and vagina and polydioxanone (PDS) 4/0 on a 13 mm round-bodied needle is used for the ureter. 3/0 sutures on a 30 mm round-bodied needle are used for bowel surgery, polydioxanone (PDS) for the small bowel and either poly-dioxanone (PDS) or braided polyamide (Nurolon) for large bowel reanastomosis.

Testing the repair

The closure must be watertight and so should be tested at the end of vaginal repairs by the instillation of dye into the bladder under minimal pressure; a previously unsuspected second fistula is occasionally identified this way. Testing after abdominal procedures is impractical.

Specific repair techniques

Vaginal procedures

Dissection and repair in layers   There are two main types of closure technique applied to the repair of urinary fistulae: the classic saucerization technique described by Sims (1852) and the much more commonly used dissection and repair in layers. Sutures must be placed with meticulous accuracy in the bladder wall, care being taken not to penetrate the mucosa, which should be inverted as far as possible. The repair should be started at either end, working towards the midline, so that the least accessible aspects are sutured first (Fig. 57.11e). Interrupted sutures are preferred and should be placed approximately 3 mm apart, taking as large a bite of tissue as is feasible. Stitches that are too close together, or the use of continuous or purse-string sutures, tend to impair blood supply and interfere with healing. Knots must be secured with three hitches, so that they can be cut short, leaving the minimum amount of material within the body of the repair.

With dissection and repair in layers, the first layer of sutures in the bladder should invert the edges (Fig. 57.11e); the second adds bulk to the repair by taking a wide bite of bladder wall but also closes off dead space by catching the back of the vaginal flaps (Fig. 57.11f). After testing the repair (Fig. 57.11g) (See above) a third layer of interrupted mattress sutures is used to evert and close the vaginal wall, consolidating the repair by picking up the underlying bladder wall (Fig. 57.11h).

Saucerization   The saucerization technique involves converting the track into a shallow crater, which is closed without dissection of bladder from vagina using a single row of interrupted sutures. The method is only applicable to small fistulae and perhaps residual fistulae after closure of a larger defect; in other situations the technique does not allow secure closure without tension.

Vaginal repair procedures in specific circumstances The conventional dissection and repair in layers as described above is entirely appropriate for the majority of midvaginal fistulae, although modifications may be necessary in specific circumstances. In juxtacervical fistulae in the anterior fornix, vaginal repair may be feasible if the cervix can be drawn down to provide access. Dissection should include mobilization of the bladder from the cervix. The repair must be undertaken transversely to reconstruct the underlying trigone and prevent distortion of the ureteric orifices.

Vault fistulae, particularly those following hysterectomy, can again usually be managed vaginally. The vault is incised transversely and mobilization of the fistula is often aided by deliberate opening of the pouch of Douglas (Lawson 1972). The peritoneal opening does not need to be closed separately but is incorporated into the vaginal closure.

With subsymphysial fistulae involving the bladder neck and proximal urethra as a consequence of obstructed labour, tissue loss may be extensive and fixity to underlying bone a common problem. The lateral aspects of the fistula require careful mobilization to overcome disproportion between the defect in the bladder and the urethral stump. A racquet-shaped extension of the incision facilitates exposure of the proximal urethra. Although transverse repair is often necessary, longitudinal closure gives better prospects for urethral competence.

Where there is substantial urethral loss reconstruction may be undertaken using the method described by Chassar Moir (1967) or Hamlin & Nicholson (1969). A strip of anterior vaginal wall is constructed into a tube over a catheter. Plication behind the bladder neck is probably important if continence is to be achieved. The interposition of a labial fat or muscle graft not only fills up the potential dead space but also provides additional bladder neck support and improves continence by reducing scarring between bladder neck and vagina.

With very large fistulae extending from bladder neck to vault, the extensive dissection required may produce considerable bleeding. The main surgical difficulty is to avoid the ureters. They are usually situated close to the superolateral angles of the fistula and if they can be identified they should be catheterized (See Fig. 57.7c). Straight ureteric catheters passed transurethrally or double pigtail catheters may both be useful in directing the intramural portion of the ureters internally; nevertheless great care must be taken during dissection.

Radiation fistulae present particular problems in that the area of devitalized tissue is usually considerably larger than the fistula itself. Mobilization is often impossible and if repair in layers is attempted, the flaps are likely to slough; closure by colpocleisis is therefore required. Some have advocated total closure of the vagina although it is preferable to avoid dissection in the devitalized tissue entirely and to perform a lower partial colpocleisis converting the upper vagina into a diverticulum of the bladder. It is usually necessary to fill the dead space below this with an interposition graft (See below).

Abdominal procedures

Transvesical repair   Repair by the abdominal route is indicated when high fistulae are fixed in the vault and are therefore inaccessible per vaginam. Transvesical repair has the advantage of being entirely extraperitoneal. It is often helpful to elevate the fistula site by a vaginal pack and the ureters should be catheterized under direct vision. The technique of closure is similar to that of the transvaginal flap-splitting repair except that for haemostasis the bladder mucosa is closed with a continous suture.

Transperitoneal repair   It is often said that there is little place for a simple transperitoneal repair, although a combined transperitoneal and transvesical procedure is favoured by urologists and is particularly useful for vesicouterine fistulae following caesarean section. A midline split is made in the vault of the bladder; this is extended downwards in a racquet shape around the fistula. The fistulous track is excised and the vaginal or cervical defect closed in a single layer. The bladder is then closed in two layers.

For ureteric fistulae not manageable by stenting re-implantation is considered preferable to reanastomosis of the ureter itself, which carries a greater risk of stricture. Several techniques are described for ureteroneocystostomy and the most appropriate will depend on the level of the fistula and the nature of the antecedent pathology. The most widely used techniques are direct reimplantation using a psoas hitch or the creation of a flap of bladder wall – the Boari–Ockerblad technique. There are few lesions which are too high for this approach although where there is significant deficiency it may be necessary to perform an end-to-side anastomosis between the injured ureter and the good contralateral ureter, i.e. a ureteroureterostomy, or to interpose a loop of small bowel.

Interposition grafting

Several techniques have been described to support fistula repair in different sites. In each case the interposed tissue serves to create an additional layer in the repair, to fill dead space and to bring in new blood supply to the area. The tissues used include the following.

- *Martius graft* – labial fat and bulbocavernosus muscle passed subcutaneously to cover a vaginal repair; this is particularly appropriate to provide additional bulk in a colpocleisis and in urethral and bladder neck fistulae may help to maintain competence of closure mechanisms by reducing scarring.
- *Gracilis muscle* passed either via the obturator foramen or subcutaneously (Hamlin & Nicholson 1969) or rectus abdominis muscle (Bruce et al 2000) may also be used as above.
- *Omental pedicle grafts* (Kiricuta & Goldstein 1972, Turner-Warwick 1976) may be dissected from the greater curve of the stomach and rotated down into the pelvis on the right gastroepiploic artery; this may be used at any transperitoneal procedure, but has its greatest advantage in postradiation fistulae.
- *Peritoneal flap graft* (Jonas & Petri 1984) is an easier way of providing an additional layer at transperitoneal repair procedures, by taking a flap of peritoneum from any available surface, most usually the paravesical area.

Postoperative management

Fluid balance

Nursing care of patients who have undergone fistula repair is of critical importance and obsessional postoperative manage-ment may do much to secure success. As a corollary, however, poor nursing may easily undermine what the surgeon has achieved. Strict fluid balance must be kept and a daily fluid intake of at least 3 litres and output of 100 ml per hour should be maintained until the urine is clear of blood. Haematuria is more persistent following abdominal than vaginal procedures and intravenous fluid is therefore likely to be required for longer in this situation.

Bladder drainage

Continuous bladder drainage in the postoperative period is crucial to success and where failure occurs after a straight-forward repair, it is almost always possible to identify a period during which free drainage was interrupted. Nursing staff should check catheters hourly throughout each day, to confirm free drainage and check output. Catheters should of course drain into a sterile closed drainage system with a non-return valve (Hilton 1987). In circumstances where supplies of sterile disposables are limited or where standards of nursing are poor, as in many developing countries, open drainage has been advocated, with good success and low infection rates. Bladder irrigation and suction drainage are no longer recommended.

Views differ as to the ideal type of catheter. The calibre must be sufficient to prevent blockage, although whether the suprapubic or urethral route is used is mainly a matter of individual preference. A urethral Foley catheter should probably be avoided following bladder neck fistulae and either a suprapubic catheter or a non-balloon urethral catheter sutured in place would be preferred. The bladder should not be distended to insert a suprapubic catheter after a vaginal repair, although it could be inserted preoperatively, by the technique of cutting onto a sound. The author's usual practice is to use a belt-and-braces approach of both urethral and suprapubic drainage initially, so that if one becomes blocked free drainage is still maintained. The urethral catheter is removed first and the suprapubic retained and used to assess residual volume, until the patient is voiding normally (Hilton 1987).

The duration of free drainage depends on the fistula type. Following repair of surgical fistulae, 12 days is adequate. With obstetric fistulae up to 21 days' drainage may be appropriate and following repair of radiation fistulae 21–42 days is required. In any of these situations, it is wise to carry out dye testing (See above) prior to catheter removal if there is any doubt about the integrity of the repair. Where a persistent leak is identified free drainage should be maintained for 6 weeks.

Bowel management

If patients are restricted to bed following urogenital fistula repair, a laxative should be administered to prevent excessive straining at stool. Following abdominal repair of intesti-novaginal fistulae patients should either have a nasogastric tube inserted or be kept nil by mouth until they are passing flatus; the majority prefer the latter approach. Once oral intake is allowed or following vaginal repair of rectovaginal fistulae, a low-residue diet should be administered until at least the 5th postoperative day. Enemas and suppositories should be avoided although a mild aperient such as dioctyl sodium (Docusate) is advised to ease initial bowel movements.

Subsequent management

On removal of catheters most patients will feel the desire to void frequently, since the bladder capacity will be functionally reduced, having been relatively empty for so long. In any case it is important that they do not become overdistended and hourly voiding should be encouraged and fluid intake limited. It may also be necessary to wake them once or twice through the night for the same reason. After discharge from hospital patients should be advised to gradually increase the period between voiding, aiming to be back to a normal pattern by 4 weeks postoperatively.

Tampons, pessaries, douching and penetrative sex should be avoided until 3 months postoperatively.

PROGNOSIS

Results

It is difficult to compare the results of treatment in different series, since the lesions involved and the techniques of repair vary so greatly. Cure rates should be considered in terms of closure at first operation and vary from 60% to 98% (Chassar Moir 1973, Elkins et al 1988, Goodwin & Scardino 1979, Hamlin & Nicholson 1969, Hilton 1994, Hilton & Ward 1998, Hudson et al 1975, Lee et al 1988, O'Conor 1980, Patil et al 1980, Turner-Warwick et al 1967, Wein et al 1980, WHO 1989). On average one might anticipate 80% cures, with 10% failures and, in the case of obstetric fistulae at least, 10% suffering from post-fistula stress incontinence (see below).

Of the 152 patients in the author's series managed in the UK (Hilton 1998), 10 (3.6%) healed without operation, nine declined surgery, one (with co-existent detrusor instability) was asymptomatic on medical treatment, three (2.3%) underwent primary urinary diversion and one with a radiotherapy fistula died from recurrent disease during the course of assessment. Of the remaining 128 who have undergone repair surgery, 121 (94.5%) were cured by the first operation; of the 72 fistulae following simple hysterectomy, 71 (98.6%) have been cured at their first operation.

Of the largely obstetric fistulae reviewed from Nigeria by Hilton & Ward (1998), 81.2% were cured by a first operation and 97.7% eventually successfully anatomically repaired, with only 0.6% undergoing urinary diversion.

A law of diminishing returns has previously been reported (Lawson 1978). Although repeat operations are certainly justified, the success rate decreases progressively with increasing numbers of previous unsuccessful procedures. In the series reported from Nigeria, although the cure rate at first operations was 81.7%, the success rate for those patients requiring two or more procedures fell to 65% (Hilton & Ward 1998). It cannot be overemphasized that the best prospect for cure is at the first operation and there is no place for the well-intentioned occasional fistula surgeon, be they gynaecologist or urologist.

Post-fistula stress incontinence

Stress incontinence has long been recognized as a complication of vesicovaginal fistulae (Lawson 1967). It is most likely to occur in obstetric fistula patients when the injury involves the sphincter mechanism, particularly if there is tissue loss (Waaldijk 1989), although it has also been reported in a large proportion of surgical fistulae involving the urethra or bladder neck (Hilton 1998). It affects at least 10% of all fistula patients.

The extent of scarring in the area means that conventional approaches to bladder neck elevation may be technically difficult and of limited success. The use of a labial musculo-fat graft in the initial repair may reduce the likelihood of the complication (Waaldijk 1994b) and a number of other techniques have been attempted (Hudson et al 1975, Waaldijk 1994b). The implantation of an artificial urinary sphincter or neo-urethral reconstruction might from a theoretical point of view be appropriate (Hilton 1990) but the former would be prohibitively expensive and both excessively morbid for use in the developing world. Periurethral injections hold promise as a minimally invasive technique particularly appropriate in the situation of urethral insufficiency with a relatively fixed immobile urethra and have recently been reported with initial success in post-fistula stress incontinent patients (Hilton et al 1998).

Subsequent pregnancy

Although many patients with obstetric vesicovaginal fistula will experience amenorrhoea for 2 years or more after the causative pregnancy (Hilton & Ward 1998), where tissue loss is not great, hypothalamic function often returns to normal immediately after successful repair and fertility may be relatively normal. Most authorities emphasize the need for caesarean section in any subsequent pregnancy (Lawson 1978). Kelly (1979), however, reported on 33 patients who became pregnant within 1 year of fistula repair, 12 of whom were delivered vaginally without damage to the repair. The criteria he used for attempting vaginal delivery were: that the fistula arose from a non-recurring cause (i.e. malpresentation as opposed to pelvic contraction); that an interposition graft had been utilized in the repair; and that the labour was conducted under skilled supervision in hospital (Kelly 1979).

The management of delivery in women who have had a previous third-degree tear has not been prospectively studied, although it has been suggested that there may be benefit in assessing the sphincter prior to delivery by endoanal ultrasound; where minor defects are present potentially traumatic vaginal delivery should be avoided and where more major defects are identified caesarean section might be offered (Sultan et al 1994).

PREVENTION

It is estimated by the World Health Organization (1989) that there are approximately 500 000 maternal deaths per year worldwide and it is clear that the prevalence of obstetric fistulae and maternal mortality rates are closely related. Indeed, one might look on the vesicovaginal fistula patient as being the 'near miss' maternal death. In recognition of this fact WHO established, through their 'Safe Motherhood Initiative', a technical working group to investigate the problems of prevention and management of obstetric fistulae. The recommendations from that working group included the extension of antenatal and intrapartum care; the transfer of women in prolonged labour for delivery by skilled personnel; the identification of areas where fistulae are still prevalent, so that resources could be mobilized to deal with fistulae more effectively; the creation of specialized centres for management, training and research, with a specific aim of treating existing cases within 5 years (WHO 1989).

One thousand years ago Avicenna recognized the problems of early child bearing, saying: 'In cases where women are married too young the physician should instruct the patient in the ways of prevention of pregnancy. In these patients the bulk of the fetus may cause a tear in the bladder which results in incontinence of urine which is incurable and remains until death' (Hilton 1995). Clearly the achievement of the WHO's aims and recommendations is critically dependent on major social change in areas of endemicity. Without improvement in the status of women, an extension of primary education, deferment of marriage and child bearing, improved nutritional status and contraceptive services, and skilled attendants in childbirth throughout the world, the problem of obstetric fistulae will remain with us well into the new millennium.

In the developed world our concern must lie with the prevention and management of fistulae following gynaecological surgery. Primarily we need to be aware of those factors increasing the likelihood of lower urinary tract injury during surgery and must recognize the limits of our own, and perhaps more importantly our trainees', surgical skills. We should not expect staff in training to undertake surgery in cases where risk factors are known to be present without adequate supervision and support. We should be equally aware of the signs of injury in the postoperative period and should have standard regimens for the management of patients with voiding difficulty in the postoperative period if bladder overdistension and risk of late damage are to be avoided. One might perhaps anticipate that with advances in minimally invasive surgery and techniques of endometrial ablation, the need for hysterectomy and the risk of surgical vesicovaginal fistula might reduce considerably. Hysterectomy will, however, always be necessary for fibroids, endometriosis, sepsis and malignancy and these carry the greatest risk of lower urinary tract injury. If these are the only cases on which our trainees can train then there is a danger that surgical skills in general may decline, in the same way that skills in vaginal breech delivery and rotational forceps delivery have declined with increasing use of caesarean section.

KEY POINTS

1. In developing countries over 90% of fistulae are of obstetric origin and are due to pressure necrosis from prolonged obstructed labour.
2. In the UK over 70% of fistulae follow pelvic surgery and half of these cases are associated with simple abdominal hysterectomy.
3. The characteristic presentation with continuous urinary leakage and reduced frequency and bladder sensation is not always present in patients with small fistulae and a high index of suspicion must be maintained if the diagnosis is not to be missed. With intestinal fistulae the history may be similarly misleading.
4. The upper urinary tracts should be assessed by intravenous urogram in all patients with urogenital fistulae.

KEY POINTS (CONTINUED)

5. The best estimate is that vesicovaginal fistula complicates 1 in 1300 hysterectomies; this is rarely due to direct injury and most often results from tissue ischaemia or subclinical haematoma or infection. Although poor surgical technique increases the risk, the mere development of a fistula following hysterectomy does not imply negligence.
6. Where bladder damage is suspected or fistula confirmed following surgery or childbirth, catheterization should be undertaken and continuous drainage maintained; spontaneous healing may occur up to 8 weeks after the initiating event.
7. The possibility of inflammatory bowel disease should always be considered in patients with intestinogenital fistula, even in the absence of specific bowel symptoms. Of the inflammatory causes, Crohn's disease is the most important and surgical treatment should ideally only be undertaken when the bowel pathology is quiescent.
8. Biopsy of the fistula edge or any unhealthy-looking local tissue should be undertaken before embarking on repair of radiation, inflammatory or potentially infective fistulae.
9. Malnutrition, anaemia and infection should be treated before attempting surgical closure; this applies most particularly in patients with obstetric fistulae in the developing world.
10. Surgery for urogenital or intestinogenital fistulae should only be undertaken by surgeons with the appropriate training and experience and with the versatility to undertake the most appropriate operation by the most appropriate route.
11. Layered closure with avoidance of tension on the suture lines, good haemostasis and obliteration of dead space are important technical points for successful closure.
12. Interposition grafting with pedicled fat or muscle may be a useful adjunct in fistula surgery, by providing an additional layer to the repair, filling dead space, bringing new blood supply and encouraging tissue mobility.
13. Successful anatomical closure of a urinary or intestinal fistula is not necessarily associated with restoration of complete functional normality. Incompetence of sphincter mechanisms may occur, with residual urinary stress incontinence, faecal soiling or incontinence of flatus.
14. Diversion of urinary or faecal stream should rarely be required as definitive measures for the management of fistula patients.

REFERENCES

Averette HE, Nguyen HN, Donato DM et al 1993 Radical hysterectomy for invasive cervical cancer. A 25-year prospective experience with the Miami technique. Cancer 71:1422–1437

Bladou F, Houvenaeghel G, Delpero JR, Guerinel G 1995 Incidence and management of major urinary complications after pelvic exenteration for gynecological malignancies. Journal of Surgical Oncology 58:91–96

Bruce RG, El-Galley RES, Galloway NTM 2000 Use of rectus abdominis muscle flap for the treatment of complex and refractory urethrovaginal fistulas. Journal of Urology 63:1212–1215

Chassar Moir J 1967 The vesico-vaginal fistula, 2nd edn. Baillière, London

Chassar Moir J 1973 Vesico-vaginal fistulae as seen in Britain. Journal of Obstetrics and Gynaecology of the British Commonwealth 80:598–602

Chang R, Marshall F, Mitchell S 1987 Percutaneous management of benign ureteral strictures and fistulas. Journal of Urology 137:1126–1131

Davits R, Miranda S 1991 Conservative treatment of vesico-vaginal fistulas by bladder drainage alone. British Journal of Urology 68:155–156

Elkins TE, Drescher C, Martey JO, Fort D 1988 Vesicovaginal fistula revisited. Obstetrics and Gynecology 72:307–312

Emmert C, Köhler U 1996 Management of genital fistulas in patients with cervical cancer. Archives of Gynecology and Obstetrics 259:19–24

Falk F, Tancer M 1956 Management of vesical fistulas after Caesarean section. American Journal of Obstetrics and Gynecology 71:97–106

Goodwin WE, Scardino PT 1979 Vesicovaginal and ureterovaginal fistulas: a summary of 25 years of experience. Transactions of the American Association of Genitourinary Surgeons 71:123–129

Hamlin R, Nicholson E 1969 Reconstruction of urethra totally destroyed in labour. British Medical Journal 2:147–150

Harkki-Siren P, Sjoberg J, Tiitinen A 1998 Urinary tract injuries after hysterectomy. Obstetrics and Gynecology 92:113–118

Hilton P, Ward A 1998 Epidemiological and surgical aspects of urogenital fistulae: a review of 25 years experience in south-east Nigeria. International Urogynecology Journal and Pelvic Floor Dysfunction 9:189–194

Hilton P, Ward A, Molloy M, Umana O 1998 Periurethral injection of autologous fat for the treatment of post-fistula repair stress incontinence: a preliminary report. International Urogynecology Journal and Pelvic Floor Dysfunction 9:118–121

Hilton P 1998 The urodynamic findings in patients with urogenital fistulae. British Journal of Urology 81:539–542

Hilton P 1997 Debate: post-operative urogenital fistulae are best managed by gynaecologists in specialist centres. British Journal of Urology 80 (suppl 1):35–42

Hilton P 1995 Sims to SMIS – an historical perspective on vesico-vaginal fistulae. In: Yearbook of the RCOG, 1994. RCOG, London, pp 7–16

Hilton P 1990 Surgery for genuine stress incontinence: which operation and for which patient? In: Drife J, Hilton P, Stanton S (eds) Micturition. Proceedings of the 21st RCOG Study Group. Springer-Verlag, London, pp 225–246

Hilton P 1987 Catheters and drains. In: Stanton S (ed) Principles of gynaecological surgery. Springer-Verlag, Berlin, pp 257–283

Hudson C, Hendrickse J, Ward A 1975 An operation for restoration of urinary continence following total loss of the urethra. British Journal of Obstetrics and Gynaecology 82:501–504

Hudson C 1968 Malignant change in an obstetric vesico-vaginal fistula. Proceedings of the Royal Society of Medicine 61:121–124

Iselin CE, Aslan P, Webster GD 1998 Transvaginal repair of vesicovaginal fistulas after hysterectomy by vaginal cuff excision. Journal of Urology 160:728–730

Jonas U, Petri E 1984 Genitourinary fistulae. In: Stanton S (ed) Clinical gynecologic urology. CV Mosby, St Louis, pp 238–255

Kelly J 1983 Vesico-vaginal fistulae. In: Studd J (ed) Progress in obstetrics and gynaecology 3rd edn. Churchill-Livingstone, Edinburgh, pp 324–333

Kelly J, Kwast B 1993 Epidemiologic study of vesico-vaginal fistula in Ethiopia. International Urogynecology Journal 4:278–281

Kelly J 1979 Vesicovaginal fistulae. British Journal of Urology 51:208–210

Kiricuta I, Goldstein A 1972 The repair of extensive vesicovaginal fistulas with pedicled omentum: a review of 27 cases. Journal of Urology 108:724–727

Lawson J 1978 The management of genito-urinary fistulae. Clinics in Obstetrics and Gynaecology 6:209–236

Lawson J 1972 Vesical fistulae into the vaginal vault. British Journal of Urology 44:623–631

Lawson L, Hudson C 1987 The management of vesico-vaginal and urethral fistulae. In: Stanton S, Tanagho E (eds) Surgery for female urinary incontinence. Springer-Verlag, Berlin, pp 193–209

Lawson J 1967 Injuries to the urinary tract. In: Lawson J, Stewart D (eds) Obstetrics and gynaecology in the tropics and developing countries. Edward Arnold, London, pp 481–522

Lee R, Symmonds R, Williams T 1988 Current status of genitourinary fistula. Obstetrics and Gynecology 71:313–319

Meeks GR, Sams JO, Field KW, Fulp KS, Margolis MT 1997 Formation of vesicovaginal fistula: the role of suture placement into the bladder during closure of the vaginal cuff after transabdominal hysterectomy. American Journal of Obstetrics and Gynecology 177:1298–1304

Mundy A 1993 Urodynamic and reconstructive surgery of the lower urinary tract. Churchill Livingstone, Edinburgh

Murphy M 1981 Social consequences of vesico-vaginal fistula in Northern Nigeria. Journal of Biosocial Sciences 13:139–150

O'Conor VJ 1980 Review of experience with vesicovaginal fistula repair. Journal of Urology 123:367–369

Patil U, Waterhouse K, Laungani G 1980 Management of 18 difficult vesicovaginal and urethrovaginal fistulas with modified Ingelman–Sundberg and Martius operations. Journal of Urology 123:653–656

Raghavaiah N 1974 Double-dye test to diagnose various types of vaginal fistulas. Journal of Urology 112:811–812

Schwartz BF, Stoller ML 2000 Endourologic management of urinary fistulae. Techniques in Urology 6:193–195

Sims J 1852 On the treatment of vesico-vaginal fistula. American Journal of the Medical Sciences XXIII:59–82

Sultan AH, Kamm MA, Hudson CN, Bartram CI 1994 Third degree obstetric and sphincter tears: risk factors and outcome of primary repair. British Medical Journal 308:887–891

Tahzib F 1985 Vesicovaginal fistula in Nigerian children. Lancet 2:1291–1293

Tahzib F 1983 Epidemiological determinants of vesicovaginal fistulas. British Journal of Obstetrics and Gynaecology 90:387–391

Tomlinson AJ, Thornton JG 1998 A randomised controlled trial of antibiotic prophylaxis for vesico-vaginal fistula repair. British Journal of Obstetrics and Gynaecology 105:397–399

Turner-Warwick R 1976 The use of the omental pedicle graft in urinary tract reconstruction. Journal of Urology 116:341–347

Turner-Warwick RT, Wynne EJ, Handley-Ashken M 1967 The use of the omental pedicle graft in the repair and reconstruction of the urinary tract. British Journal of Surgery 54:849–853

Waaldijk K 1994a The immediate surgical management of fresh obstetric fistulas with catheter and/or early closure. International Journal of Gynaecology and Obstetrics 45:11–16

Waaldijk K 1994b Step-by-step surgery for vesico-vaginal fistulas. Campion, EdinburghWaaldijk K, Elkins T 1994 The obstetric fistula and peroneal nerve injury: an analysis of 947 consecutive patients. International Urogynecological Journal 5:12–14

Waaldijk K, Armiya'u Y 1993 The obstetric fistula: a major public health problem still unsolved. International Urogynecology Journal 4:126–128

Waaldijk K 1989 The surgical management of bladder fistula in 775 women in Northern Nigeria. MD thesis, University of Amsterdam

Wein AJ, Malloy TR, Carpiniello VL, Greenberg SH, Murphy JJ 1980 Repair of vesicovaginal fistula by a suprapubic transvesical approach. Surgery, Gynecology and Obstetrics 150:57–60

World Health Organization 1989 The prevention and treatment of obstetric fistulae: a report of a Technical Working Group. WHO, Geneva

Yeates W 1987 Uretero-vaginal fistulae. In: Stanton S, Tanagho E (eds) Surgery for female urinary incontinence, 2nd edn. Springer-Verlag, Berlin, pp 211–217

Youssef A 1957 "Menouria" following lower segment Caesarean section: a syndrome. American Journal of Obstetrics and Gynecology 73:759–767

Zacharin R 1988 Obstetric fistula. Springer-Verlag, Vienna

58

Urinary tract infections

Charlotte Chaliha   Stuart L. Stanton

INTRODUCTION

Urinary tract infections are a common cause of morbidity in women, affecting 50% of adult women at least once in their lives. In women aged 20–56 years at least 20% will suffer an infection each year. Each year about 5% of women will present to their general practitioners with dysuria and frequency (Hamilton-Miller 1994) and approximately half of these will have a urinary tract infection. It has been estimated that on average a case of uncomplicated acute cystitis results in 6.1 days of symptoms, 2.4 days of restriction of activities and 0.4 days in bed (Foxman & Frerichs 1985a). The incidence of UTIs increases in girls and women with age and with the onset of sexual activity and is highest amongst the elderly. In children under 1 year of age the prevalence is higher in boys than girls, with a male to female ratio of 3:1 to 5:1. Urinary tract infection in the neonate should be considered to be secondary to an underlying anatomical abnormality until proven otherwise (Kunin 1987).

With increasing age the prevalence increases significantly and is higher in women than men. In the elderly the prevalence may be as high as 50% especially if the woman is institutionalized (Boscia & Kaye 1987). This high prevalence in the elderly is thought to be secondary to cerebrovascular accidents, a reduced mental and functional capacity, the use of bladder catheters and diabetes.

TERMINOLOGY

An *uncomplicated UTI* is one that occurs in young healthy women with no functional or anatomical abnormality of the urinary tract whereas a *complicated UTI* is associated with conditions that increase the risk of serious complications or treatment failure. These are usually by causing obstruction or stasis of urinary flow (Box 58.1).

Bacteriuria is defined as the presence of living bacteria in a freshly voided urine sample or a sample taken via suprapubic aspiration. The presence of $>10^5$ colony-forming units (cfu) per ml of urine has been defined as significant bacteriuria (Kass 1956) based on studies of women with acute pyelonephritis and asymptomatic bacteriuria. However, this may be too high a threshold for the diagnosis of infection, as up to one half of cases with acute cystitis have less than 10^5 cfu per ml of urine (Johnson & Stamm 1987). It has been proposed that a more appropriate cut-off for diagnosis of cystitis is $>10^3$ cfu per ml of urine and for pyelonephritis $>10^4$ cfu per ml of urine (Rubin et al 1992). *Asymptomatic bacteriuria* is defined as the presence of $>10^5$ cfu per ml of urine in two samples of urine in the absence of symptoms (Zhanel et al 1990). *Cystitis* is an inflammation of the bladder but the term is often used to describe an acute infection of the bladder although it can occur without the presence of infection. The term *urethral syndrome* is used when there is dysuria and frequency without the presence of bacteriuria.

Acute bacterial pyelonephritis indicates acute infection of the kidneys whereas in *chronic pyelonephritis* there is chronic inflammation of the renal and tubular tissue associated with scarring and a reduction in glomerular and tubular function.

A *recurrent UTI* refers to a UTI that occurs after resolution of a previous UTI. A *relapse* occurs with the same infecting organism within 2 weeks of treatment whereas a *reinfection* is a recurrent UTI from the same organism 2 weeks after treatment or

Box 58.1 Conditions associated with a complicated UTI

Obstruction/structural abnormalities	Presence of stones, catheters, stents or nephrostomy tubes
	Urinary tract malignancy
	Diverticuli
	Fistula
	Ileal conduits/urinary diversions
	Co-existing pelvic malignancy or inflammatory bowel conditions
Functional abnormality	Neurogenic bladder
	Anticholinergic drugs – leading to incomplete bladder emptying
Miscellaneous	Diabetes mellitus
	Pregnancy
	Renal failure
	Immunosuppression
	Hospital-acquired/resistant infections

with infection by a different strain. Reinfection accounts for 80% of recurrent UTIs.

BACTERIOLOGY

The majority of urinary tract infections are caused by bacteria and occasionally by fungi and viruses. These bacteria are usually aerobic Gram-negative rods or Gram-positive cocci derived for the bowel flora. The spectrum of causative organisms differs between community-acquired and hospital-acquired infections and with time and the occurrence of antibiotic resistance. *Escherichia coli* accounts for up to 70% of community-acquired infections (Grüneberg 1994). The rest are caused by *Staphylococcus saprophyticus, Klebsiella pneumoniae, Proteus mirabilis* and enterobacter.

In hospital-acquired infections approximately 50% are secondary to *Escherichia coli,* 15% by *Enterococcus faecalis* and the remainder by klebsiella, enterobacter, citrobacter, serratia, pseudomonas, providencia, enterococcus and *Staphylococcus epidermidis* (Bryan & Reynolds 1984). These complicated urinary infections are those which are often found in association with indwelling catheters, urinary tract instrumentation and urinary tract abnormalities.

AETIOLOGY

There are both host and bacterial factors that may increase the susceptibility to infection.

Bacterial virulence factors

The ability of bacteria to adhere to uroepithelial cells is a prerequisite for infection to occur and reduces the chance of the bacteria being cleared from the urinary tract during voiding. There are various adherence factors, called adhesins; *E. coli* possess surface organelles called pili that act as adhesins. These adhesins attach to complementary structures on the uroepithelial cell wall and act not only to promote infection but also to help promote growth and toxin production (Zafiri et al 1987). Other virulence factors that may facilitate infection are

specific to each pathogen. These include the surface antigens on *E. coli* and haemolysins that are produced to help degrade cells and aerobactins that enhance iron uptake which encourages *E. coli* growth.

Host factors

Regular voiding flushes the urinary tract of pathogens and the acidity of urine inhibits bacterial growth. Lactobacilli and uromucoid in the urine also interfere with bacterial adherence and colonization. The glycosaminoglycan layer of the bladder also serves as a protective layer preventing bacterial adherence.

Factors that increase the risk of infection include the following.

- Impaired bladder emptying which can occur with neurogenic disorders such as diabetes, multiple sclerosis, cerebrovascular events and anatomical abnormalities. Anticholinergic drugs may also impair bladder emptying.
- Instrumentation of the urinary tract which may traumatize the urethra.
- Foreign bodies such as catheters and stones increase the risk of infection as they are a focus for infection.
- Pelvic tumours and inflammatory bowel disorders may directly invade the bladder and also affect bladder emptying.
- Glycosuria that occurs in diabetes mellitus is a potent culture medium for bacterial growth.
- Genetic factors have been postulated to increase the risk of recurrent infection. Women with recurrent infection are more likely to be non-secretors of histo-blood group antigens and *E. coli* is found to adhere better to uroepithelial cells of non-secretors than secretors (Lomberg et al 1986, Sheinfeld et al 1989).
- In menopausal women the lack of oestrogen reduces lactobacillus growth and, with the rise in vaginal pH, leads to a predisposition to growth of enterobacteria (Cardozo 1996).
- Sexual intercourse and contraception are strongly associated with the onset of UTIs (Foxman et al 1997, Hooton et al 1996). Sexual intercourse not only results in trauma and disruption to the uroepithelial cells, but may also introduce rectal and vaginal bacteria into the urethra. In a woman who has had sex in the previous 48 hours, the odds ratio for a UTI is increased 60 times over a woman who has not (Nicolle et al 1982). The use of spermicides with diaphragms alters vaginal flora, increases vaginal pH and decreases lactobacilli concentration, promoting colonization with *E. coli.*

NATURAL HISTORY

In children up to 1 year of age 1.1% of girls and 1.2% of boys may suffer a symptomatic UTI. In school-age children a UTI has been reported in 8% of girls and 2% of boys (Hansson et al 1997). The sequelae of UTI in neonates and young children include pyelonephritis and renal scarring especially if infection has occurred before the age of 5 years. Vesicoureteric reflux is a significant aetiological factor in the occurrence of UTI in the young.

In young women UTI can result as asymptomatic bacteriuria, cystitis and pyelonephritis. These do not usually affect renal function except in the elderly where bacteriuria has been associated with a decrease in the glomerular filtration rate. In pregnancy, UTI have been associated with an increased risk of prematurity, perinatal mortality and perinatal complications (Maclean 2000). The incidence of asymptomatic bacteriuria is similar to non-pregnant women (4–7%) (Patterson & Andriole 1997); however, in pregnancy the risk of developing a symptomatic UTI is much higher and 10–30% of women with asymptomatic bacteriuria (ASB) develop pyelonephritis.

PRESENTATION

A UTI may present either as an asymptomatic bacteriuria, acute cystitis or more seriously as acute pyelonephritis, bacteraemia and renal failure. The classic symptoms of acute cystitis include dysuria, frequency, urgency and suprapubic pain. If the upper urinary tract is involved haematuria, loin pain, renal angle tenderness and fever may also occur. In children and the elderly the classic clinical features of a UTI may not be present. In young children clinical features of a UTI may be failure to thrive or a non-specific abdominal pain. In the elderly UTI often present as confusion and general malaise.

PHYSICAL SIGNS

In cases of acute cystitis or urethritis there is often suprapubic tenderness and occasionally fever. The clinical presentation of acute pyelonephritis is often much more florid, the patient often looking unwell with a pyrexia and tachycardia. There is usually loin tenderness and if severe, features of septicaemia may be present. In young children and the elderly, as with symptoms, clinical signs may be non-specific and atypical in nature.

Other associated physical signs which may point to the aetiology are a sensory neuropathy or evidence of a spinal cord lesion in cases of a UTI secondary to a neuropathic bladder.

MANAGEMENT

History and examination

In many women infection can be diagnosed on the basis of history and clinical examination alone. A history should be taken to identify any predisposing features such as recent urinary tract infection, recent urinary tract operations, recent sexual intercourse and the use of the contraceptive diaphragm and condom. Poor bladder emptying secondary to neurological disorders or the use of anticholinergic therapy, pregnancy, the presence of pelvic tumours and diabetes mellitus may also predispose to infection.

Clinical examination should include a general systemic examination especially if the patient is pyrexial. Examination of the renal angles is required to elicit signs of pyelonephritis. If a neuropathy is suspected a neurological examination of the S2–4 nerve roots should be performed, assessing for sensation around the buttocks. A gynaecological examination should be done to exclude residual urine, a pelvic mass or pregnancy. The differential diagnoses that should be considered include detrusor instability, cystitis, bladder stones or tumours, ovarian torsion or cysts and an ectopic pregnancy or miscarriage.

Investigations

The aim of investigating is not only to select appropriate treatment but to determine if there is an underlying cause which may be corrected to prevent recurrence (Arnold 2000).

Urinalysis

Inspection of urine can often be revealing, infected urine often looking cloudy and smelling offensive. There are also commercial stick tests available for the rapid analysis of urine. These are based on photometry or bioluminescence and test for bacteriuria, pyuria or haematuria. The test most commonly used is the nitrite test which tests for urinary nitrite formed from the conversion of urinary nitrate by bacteria. This test should be performed on the first voided sample of the day, as false-negative results are more likely with later samples as the urine needs to remain within the bladder at least 1 hour for conversion of nitrate to nitrite. The nitrite tests have been shown to correctly identify 89% of urine samples that were subsequently culture positive and 79% of culture-negative samples (Ditchburn & Ditchburn 1990). Combination of the nitrite tests with an esterase test is marginally more sensitive in the diagnosis of infection. The esterase test suggests the presence of pyuria by a substrate colour change caused by the esterase found in leucocytes.

However, though these tests are sensitive in indicating infection they do not detect low count bacteriuria $<10^4$–10^5 organisms/ml and false-negative rates are as high as 40–80% (Stevens 1987). Despite this, they are useful in situations where laboratory culture of urine is not readily available. In women with a positive nitrite test and symptoms and signs of infection, empirical treatment may be commenced in order to reduce delay in treatment. In pregnancy, those with complicated infections and where previous empirical therapy has failed, it is imperative that urine culture is performed.

Urine microscopy and culture

Urine culture has traditionally been the gold standard for the diagnosis of infection. The sample should be a clean-catch sample performed with the labia held apart. Cleaning of the perineum is not required. If a catheter is in place the sample should be taken by syringe aspiration or via a drainage port. The sample should ideally be cultured within 4 hours and if necessary stored only for a few hours at 4°C, preserved in borate or a dip slide used, otherwise bacterial proliferation occurs, which leads to a falsely high count.

Microscopy of a centrifuged urine sample assesses the presence of bacteria, pus and red blood cells with the presence of pus cells being seen in nearly all cases of urinary infection. It has a high specificity of 90% and sensitivity of 80% in predicting infections at colony counts greater than 10^4 organisms/ml (Fihn & Stamm 1983) but is less sensitive at lower colony counts and if the urine is not centrifuged adequately. Urine culture has the advantage of allowing detection of the organism and appropriate antibiotic sensitivities. If there is mixed bacterial growth this may indicate sample contamination or delay in sample transport and ideally a repeat sample should be performed. If tuberculous infection is suspected then at least three early morning urine specimens should be sent for Lowenstein–Jensen culture.

Imaging studies

These should be performed in any woman with recurrent and unexplained infection. A combination of a pelvic ultrasound and plain abdominal X-ray has been shown to be superior to and without the disadvantages of irradiation from an intravenous urogram in the detection of urinary tract abnormalities (Lewis-Jones et al 1989, Spencer et al 1990).

Ultrasound   This has the advantage of being free of radiation and therefore can be used in child-bearing women. It can be used to delineate the contours of the kidneys, assess obstruction and bladder emptying. However, the use of ultrasound is limited in the visualization of the mid-portion of the urethra which is often the site of obstructive lesions or stones. Ultrasound is useful for the detection of parenchymal tumours but it has low specificity for the detection of urothelial tumours of the renal pelvis or urinary tract.

Ultrasound can also measure postvoid residual volume which may be useful if poor bladder emptying is suspected.

Plain abdominal radiograph   This can be used to detect stones or foreign bodies. If stones are present 90% will be visualized as they contain calcium or cystine and so are radio-opaque. Calcification in lymph nodes or renal tumours may also be seen.

Micturating cystogram (MCU)   This is useful in the detection of vesicoureteric reflux, particularly in children, which often results in renal damage. This investigation should also be considered in women with recurrent upper tract infection or evidence of upper tract damage.

Nuclear medicine scanning   Nuclear medicine scans are generally of use only in complicated infections. They can be used to detect obstruction and also to evaluate differential function within each kidney.

The DMSA (dimercaptosuccinate) nucleotide is retained in the renal tubules and therefore this scan delineates renal anatomy and function. In patients with acute pyelonephritis, the affected area or scarring may be seen and any deterioration in proximal function. It should be considered in women with severe or unresolving pyelonephritis. In children under the age of 5 years it is more sensitive than ultrasound and IVU in detecting renal scars (Mansour et al 1987). If obstruction is suspected then a DTPA (diethylenetriamine penta-acetic acid) or MAG3 (mercaptoacetyl triglycerine) scan is useful, as obstruction will result in delayed washout of the isotope from the renal pelvis. It will also allow calculation of the glomerular filtration rate and assessment of the contribution of each kidney to total renal function. MAG3 scans are also useful in delineating areas of reduced uptake and renal scars.

Intravenous urography   This has largely been superseded by ultrasound and isotope studies which do not utilize high-dose radiation and are free of the risk of allergy. It does, however, have the advantage that it delineates the anatomical relationships of the ureter and can detect the level and severity of obstructive lesions. It is particularly indicated in the investigation of unexplained haematuria.

Cystoscopy   This is rarely useful in the diagnosis of uncomplicated infection but it is indicated in all cases of haematuria and may be considered in women with symptoms of recurrent cystitis or infection. It can be used to identify any predisposing factors for infection such as a bladder tumour or stone.

Computed tomography (CT)   In the majority of cases ultrasound and IVU are sufficient to reach a diagnosis; however, CT scanning is a useful adjunctive test where US and IVU fail to make a diagnosis. In acute pyelonephritis it can be used to delineate focal or diffuse changes in the renal architecture and define the extent of hydronephrosis (Talner et al 1994). Spiral CT scan images, which are very much faster, can also detect ureteric stones or abscesses.

Blood tests

If deterioration of renal function is suspected then plasma creatinine and urea estimation should be performed. If diabetes is suspected then a fasting glucose test or glucose toleration test should be performed.

Treatment

There are three principles in the management of infection. General supportive measures relieve symptoms and may help eradicate infection. Antimicrobial therapy should be instituted appropriately and if an underlying cause is found, such as obstruction, this should be treated. Finally prevention of further infections will help reduce recurrence.

General measures

Patients should be advised to maintain a high fluid intake of at least 2 litres per day and to void regularly to ensure adequate bladder emptying. In the majority of cases this can help eradicate uncomplicated UTI. If the patient is septicaemic then more intensive supportive measures and monitoring are required. Intravenous fluids, vasoactive drugs and treatment of the septicaemia should be considered.

Antimicrobial therapy

The aim of antimicrobial therapy is to eradicate pathogenic organisms with minimal local and systemic side-effects. A suitable antimicrobial should have high urinary excretion in the active form, with broad Gram-negative and -positive activity. There should be minimal effect on vaginal and bowel flora, low potential to develop bacterial resistance and a good side-effect profile. Treatment should also account for local resistance patterns, which may vary geographically and are dependent on whether the infection is hospital or community acquired. Side-effects include hypersensitivity reactions and gastrointestinal disturbances as well as vulvovaginal candidiasis.

For effective action the drug must be able to bind to the organism, interfere with growth and remain on the organism for sufficient time to reach and penetrate the cell wall. To avoid rapid serum levels associated with a higher incidence of side-effects, rapid renal excretion is preferable; however, if this is too rapid then this may reduce the serum level below the therapeutic range. The duration and dosage pattern will depend on the serum concentrations.

In uncomplicated infection amoxycillin, nalidixic acid, nitrofurantoin or trimethoprim are often suitable. Alternative therapy for resistant organisms includes co-amoxiclav (amoxycillin with clavulinic acid), an oral cephalosporin or a quinolone. Hexamine should not be used as it is not bactericidal, only bacteriostatic, and has a high incidence of side-effects.

Trimethoprim This is a suitable first-line drug as it is effective for 70% of urinary pathogens at a standard dose of 200 mg twice daily (Winstanley et al 1997) but not against pseudomonas and enterococcus. It is a bacteriostatic, not bactericidal, agent that blocks bacterial folate metabolism. It can be used alone or in combination with sulphamethoxazole and the combination is thought to act synergistically. Higher cure rates are seen with trimethoprim and trimethoprim-sulphamethoxazole combinations compared to the penicillins due to the higher resistance of strains to the latter and the faster clearance of penicillins. The resistance rates of trimethoprim are <10%. Side-effects of trimethoprim include rashes, sore tongue and nausea.

Penicillins Ampicillin and amoxycillin are no longer acceptable as first-line agents for treatment as there is a high proportion (20–50%) of resistance to *E. coli* and a risk of allergic reaction and Stevens–Johnson syndrome (Winstanley et al 1997). The mechanism of resistance is the production of β-lactamase enzymes by various bacterial strains. Allergic reactions are common and include diarrhoea, nausea, vomiting and rashes. Vaginal candidiasis may occur in up to 25% of patients.

In women on oral contraceptives high doses of ampicillin reduce the contraceptive efficacy and they should be recommended to use alternative precautions up to 7 days after therapy is completed.

Nitrofurantoin This is also a suitable first-line drug with 15% of urinary pathogens resistant to nitrofurantoin (Winstanley et al 1997). It is active against most Gram-negative bacteria and enterococci, but not against proteus and pseudomonas. Side-effects include nausea and vomiting which are dose related. Skin rashes, pneumonitis and chronic hepatitis have also been reported. Nitrofurantoin should be used with caution in the elderly and patients with a reduced glomerular filtration rate as it is ineffective and there is a risk of partially reversible peripheral neuropathy.

Cephalosporins The cephalosporins cause less resistance amongst bowel flora than the penicillins and are excreted in a high concentration in the urine. However, they also affect vaginal flora, resulting in vaginal candidiasis in approximately 15% of women. Adverse reactions with cephalosporins are rare but there is a 10–20% cross-reactivity to these antimicrobials in patients with a history of allergic reaction to penicillins.

Quinolones The quinolone class of antibiotics, nalidixic acid derivatives, e.g norfloxacin, ofloxacin and ciprofloxacin, are well tolerated and have a broad spectrum of activity. They are particularly effective against pseudomonas species and multiple antibiotic-resistant organisms. These antimicrobials are effective against Gram-negative organisms and also *Pseudomonas aeruginosa* and Gram-positive bacteria such as staphylococci and enterococci. A 3-day regime can be recommended with fluroquinolones such as ciprofloxacin,

enoxacin, norfloxacin and ofloxacin. A single dose can be used with pefloxacin, fleroxacin and rufloxacin which have a longer half-life. Side-effects include dizziness, headache, visual disturbance, seizures, gastrointestinal disturbances, photosensitivity, abnormal transaminases and allergic reactions.

Quinolones are contraindicated in patients under 13 years as there is a risk of osteochondritis. They should also be avoided in pregnant women, patients with a history of seizures and asthmatics on theophylline. Simultaneous use of antacids, calcium and iron reduces absorption by 50%. Drug resistance has been reported in 5% but this may increase with the wider use of this class of drug. Therefore it is suggested that they are not used as first-line therapy unless there are complicating features.

Duration of therapy

The duration of therapy has come under considerable debate. Traditional 7- and 14-day regimes have been replaced by shorter 1–3-day regimes in the treatment of uncomplicated infections. The advantages of these shorter regimes are that they increase compliance, are less expensive and have less effect on vaginal and faecal flora and probably reduce the risk of the emergence of resistant strains. Single-dose therapy regimes include amoxycillin 3 g, trimethoprim 200–400 mg, trimethoprim-sulphamethoxazole 320 mg plus 1600 mg and various sulphonamides. However, single-dose therapy is more likely to result in recurrent infection, especially in patients with complicated infections or occult renal infection (Johnson & Stamm 1989, Norrby 1990). This recurrence is thought to be secondary to persistent colonization from faecal and vaginal reservoirs from which the organism has not been eradicated.

Three-day regimes have been found to be more effective than single-day regimes and appear as effective as 5- or 7-day regimes (Norrby 1990). Unlike single-dose regimes, they reduce rectal carriage of Gram-negative bacteria. Longer duration of therapy should be considered in pregnant women, those patients with systemic disease such as diabetes, those with a history of pyelonephritis, recurrent infection, a childhood history or known abnormalities of the urinary tract. In patients with acute cystitis whose symptoms persist despite 3 days of empirical therapy, a urine culture should be obtained for culture and sensitivity.

Prevention

For many women with recurrent infections, suggested preventive measures include maintaining a high fluid intake, instructions on perineal hygiene such that the perineum is wiped from front to back after defaecation and micturition, reducing the risk of faecal contamination of the urethra, the avoidance of bubble baths and vaginal deodorants and specific underwear. The benefits of these practices are unclear and they have not been shown to reduce the frequency of infections in case control studies (Foxman & Frerichs 1985b, Remis et al 1987).

There is, however, a strong association of sexual behaviour and contraceptive use (Foxman & Chi 1990) and so if sexual intercourse is a precipitating factor then postcoital treatment and voiding are recommended. In women using spermicides and diaphragms for contraception, alternative methods may be recommended.

The beneficial effects of cranberry juice are receiving increasing attention as a simple remedy that reduces the incidence of recurrent infection. There are two postulated mechanisms of action: competitive inhibition of the *E. coli* fimbrial subunit to the uroepithelial cells or prevention of the expression of the normal fimbrial subunits (Patel & Daniels 2000). In a randomized double-blind trial to determine the effect of cranberry juice on bacteriuria and pyuria in 153 elderly women, there was a reduced frequency of bacteruria with daily ingestion of 300 ml of cranberry juice (Avorn et al 1994).

In postmenopausal women there is an increased susceptibility to infection secondary to the changes in the vaginal flora and uroepithelium secondary to oestrogen deficiency. There are few randomized trials of hormone replacement therapy in the prevention of UTI. Raz & Stamm (1993) found, in a double-blind placebo-controlled trial of estriol cream for the treatment of recurrent infection, that those on HRT had a lower incidence of UTI. In a later study by Cardozo et al (1998) estriol cream (3 mg/day) was found to be superior to placebo in the treatment of recurrent UTI.

Low-dose prophylactic antibiotics can be considered if the frequency of attacks is two or more per 6 months. The aim of treatment is to eradicate urinary bacteria without affecting the healthy flora of the bowel and vagina or causing the development of resistant strains. The usual suppressive dose is one-quarter to one-third of the antimicrobial dose required to treat an acute infection. This is usually prescribed at night to maintain a high antimicrobial concentration for as long as possible. The antibiotics of choice are trimethoprim, trimethoprim and sulphamethoxazole, nitrofurantoin, nalidixic acid and cephalexin (Harding et al 1982). In patients with neuropathic bladders, long-term indwelling catheters or ileal conduits who are at increased risk of recurrent infections, it is not advisable to begin long-term prophylaxis as this increases the risk of resistance and antimicrobial side-effects. In these cases the patient should be advised to seek early treatment when a UTI is suspected.

Future approaches to treatment

There has been much research looking at reducing bacterial colonization of the urinary tract and overcoming bacterial virulence mechanisms. Bacterial adherence is a prerequisite for infection and deficiencies of the glycosaminoglycan (GAG) mucin layer may increase the susceptibility to infection.

The identification of various *E. coli* adhesins, including the type I and P fimbriae, has stimulated the search for vaccines against the development of UTI. Animal studies have shown that vaccination with antibodies to the FimH adhesin, which mediates binding to the bladder mucosa, reduces bacterial binding and bacteriuria and pyuria (Langermann et al 2000). The clinical application and efficacy of these new strategies for treatment are still unclear; however, if found to be useful, they may act in combination or instead of antimicrobials to decrease recurrent infections and increase treatment efficacy.

SPECIFIC CLINICAL SITUATIONS

Asymptomatic bacteriuria

This is the presence of 10^5 organisms/ml in clear voided specimens in the absence of clinical symptoms. If left untreated, 60–80% of patients will spontaneously clear infection without long-term sequelae. However, there are several situations where treatment is advisable. In the young there is a high association with renal tract abnormality and infection which may result in renal scarring. Before urological surgery treatment of asymptomatic bacteriuria will reduce postoperative complications such as bacteriuria.

There has been much debate on the benefits and cost effectiveness of screening pregnant women for ASB. The prevalence of asymptomatic bacteriuria has been reported to range from 2% to 13% (Norden & Kass 1968). There is an association with premature birth and low birth weight (Andriole & Patterson 1991) as well as an increased risk of developing pyelonephritis. In a study of 5000 antenatal patients it was reported that in women with asymptomatic bacteriuria in pregnancy, 36% progressed to acute pyelonephritis if untreated versus 5% if treated (Little 1965). However, it has been suggested that in a population with a low prevalence of ASB, screening and treatment with antibiotics to prevent the potential sequelae of acute pyelonephritis are not worthwhile or cost effective, especially in view of the fact that the patient can be treated promptly and effectively if symptoms of upper tract infection occur. Also there is evidence to suggest that the standard reagent strip testing for urinary protein, nitrite and leucocyte esterase is not sensitive enough for detecting ASB in pregnancy and to justify the cost and time taken for screening using this method (Tincello & Richmond 1998).

If treatment is felt to be necessary the recommended antibiotics include amoxycillin or a cephalosporin, nitrofurantoin or nalidixic acid. Sulphonamides, tetracycline and trimethoprim are contraindicated due to effects on the developing fetus.

Recurrent infections

Up to 20% of women with acute cystitis develop recurrent urinary tract infection which is defined as three or more laboratory-confirmed infections per year. These occur due to either reinfection or a relapse of persistent infection. In cases of confirmed urine infection, prophylactic trimethoprim, nitrofurantoin or norfloxacin therapy reduces the risk of recurrent attacks by 95% when compared to placebo without an increase in drug resistance or side-effects (Nicolle & Ronald 1987).

There are several strategies for treatment. Postcoital prophylaxis with trimethoprim-sulphamethoxazole (40/200 mg) can be used if infection is related to intercourse. Acute self-treatment with a 3-day dose of standard therapy can also be used when symptoms occur. Alternatively continuous daily prophylaxis with nitrofurantoin 50–100 mg per day, trimethoprim-sulphamethoxazole (40/200mg), trimethoprim 100 mg per day, norfloxacin 50–100 mg per day or cephalexin 250 mg per day can be used. Following discontinuation of prophylaxis, recurrence rates are similar to preprophylaxis rates therefore prophylaxis does not alter the natural history of infections.

Acute pyelonephritis

Treatment should be commenced if necessary prior to the results of urine culture to avoid delay and worsening of infection. Potential complications of pyelonephritis include Gram-negative bacteraemia, endotoxic shock and disseminated intravascular coagulation. In general, acute pyelonephritis resolves without long-term renal damage in the majority of women. However, in the presence of obstruction, such as with stones, infection may result in papillary necrosis, renal or perinephric abscess or xanthogranulomatous pyelonephritis (Cattell 1998). Treatment consists of aggressive supportive treatment including rehydration and intravascular volume expansion.

Drugs of choice for parenteral therapy include cefotaxime, a quinolone or an aminoglycoside which should be instituted without delay. After results of culture are available, treatment may be changed to the appropriate antibiotic and should ideally be done after consultation with the microbiologists. The duration of treatment is usually 10–14 days (Bailey 1998, Cattell 1998).

Imaging of the renal tract is usually not necessary unless there has been no response to antibiotics after 48 hours or if there is a strong clinical suspicion of renal tract obstruction. The IVU will be normal in 75% of cases of uncomplicated acute pyelonephritis (Fraser et al 1995), as well as the renal ultrasound. CT imaging is usually normal unless infection is severe when changes include renal enlargement, focal swelling and parenchymal attenuation.

Catheter–associated infection

A UTI is reported to occur in approximately a third of patients catheterized in hospital (Hayley et al 1985). The risk of a UTI after an in-out catheter is 1–2% (Turck et al 1962), but higher in pregnancy, with a high bladder residual and in the immuno-compromised. In these cases single-dose antibiotic prophylaxis with nitrofurantoin, trimethoprim or trimethoprim-sulphamethoxazole would be advisable. As well as resulting in significant morbidity, such UTI are also associated with a threefold increased risk of mortality compared to non-bacteriuric patients (Platt et al 1982).

In contrast, a UTI is seen in up to 90% of patients with long-term indwelling catheters. A closed catheter system significantly reduces infection rates. If the catheter system is closed and the patient has no symptoms or signs of infection, then empirical treatment is not required. However, in 10% of cases there is a risk of bacteraemia and Gram-negative septicaemia and here aggressive antimicrobial treatment is required. Quinolones are particularly effective in these cases as they are active against pseudomonas. If possible, the catheter should be removed and a freshly voided urine sample sent for culture. To reduce the risk of UTI, indwelling catheters should be changed every 8–12 weeks and, if appropriate, intermittent self-catheterization employed instead. Prophylactic treatment is not usually advisable.

Urinary tract tuberculosis

This is usually caused by *Mycobacterium tuberculosis* or, more rarely, by *M. bovis* or *M. africanum*. Bloodborne spread occurs from the initial primary site, usually the lung but occasionally the gut. This form of tuberculosis tends to affect young adults and presents as a miliary tuberculosis or a nodular or cavitating tuberculosis affecting one kidney. Three early morning specimens should be sent for Lowenstein–Jensen culture for acid-fast bacilli as routine culture is sterile and usually reveals a pyuria and haematuria only. Renal function is usually normal unless there is widespread parenchymal damage. All patients should therefore have urea and creatinine levels assessed and renal imaging to reveal the extent of the disease. An IVU and cystoscopy should also be performed to assess the presence of urethral strictures, pyocalyx, pyonephrosis or a non-functioning kidney. Characteristic appearances on IVU and ultrasound include hydronephrosis and/or a small bladder. Bladder biopsies may be taken which culture more readily than urine which can take up to 8 weeks till considered truly negative. A chest radiograph should also be performed.

After diagnosis antituberculous therapy should be commenced. This consists of a four-drug treatment regime usually with isoniazid, rifampacin, ethambutol and pyrazinamide, modified to two drugs when the sensitivities of the tubercle bacilli are known. In total, if rifampacin is used, then treatment should continue for 9 months.

Contact tracing should be performed as tuberculosis is a notifiable communicable disease and contacts need prophylaxis.

Urolithiasis

In the presence of a stone a UTI must be treated and the urinary tract drained before removal of the stone. If a pyonephrosis or perirenal abscess is complicating the stone, immediate drainage using a percutaneous nephrostomy is required. A xanthogranulomatous pyelonephritis is a rare complication of a UTI in the presence of a stone. This usually presents with loin pain, intermittent fever, anaemia and malaise. A palpable unilateral renal mass is usually present and as well as a positive urine culture, liver function may be deranged. These cases are often resistant to antibiotics and a nephrectomy will be required.

Histologically the affected kidney will show a diffuse replacement of the renal parenchyma with lipid-filled macrophages, neutrophils, plasma cells and necrotic debris.

Schistosomiasis

Schistosoma haematobium is a freshwater parasite found in Africa and Asia. It penetrates the skin, migrating to and then reproducing in the liver. The eggs are then laid in the bladder and rectum and may erode through the bladder and result in chronic inflammation. Once passed into the urine, they leave the body and enter the water where the lifecyle enters the asexual phase.

The classic presentation is haematuria. The changes affecting the urinary tract include fibrosis and calcification of the bladder, ureteric strictures and an obstructive uropathy. In view of this an IVU should be performed to exclude obstruction. The diagnosis can be made on the findings of ova in the urine or on biopsy of the bladder or rectal mucosa.

CONCLUSIONS

Urinary tract infections are the most common cause of infection in women and a significant cause of distress and morbidity. The aetiology is multifactorial and treatment strategies are based on identifying any predisposing causes and eradicating pathogenic organisms adaquately to prevent recurrence of infection and long-term sequelae.

The management of women presenting with symptoms includes a detailed and stepwise diagnosis and investigation strategy with institution of appropriate antimicrobial treatment. Antimicrobial therapy should be tailored to the individual patient, accounting for local drug resistance patterns, antimicrobial sensitivities and whether the infection is complicated or uncomplicated. All antimicrobial regimes should be combined with advice on preventing recurrence of infection and if treatment fails, further investigations and treatment should be considered.

KEY POINTS

1. Urinary infections are a significant cause of morbidity in women aged 20–65 years.
2. Infections can present with only 10^2 or 10^3 organisms per ml of urine and even in the presence of sterile urine.
3. Up to 80% of recurrent infections are reinfection.
4. Between 10% and 30% of women with asymptomatic bacteriuria develop acute pyelonephritis during pregnancy.
5. Predisposing factors include diabetes mellitus, foreign body, instrumentation of the urinary tract and incomplete bladder emptying.
6. Prevention entails a high standard of perineal hygiene, avoidance of vaginal deodorants and bubble baths.
7. Management includes drinking at least 2 litres of fluid a day, regular and complete bladder emptying and voiding after intercourse.
8. Asymptomatic bacteriuria may not require treatment unless there is vesicoureteric reflux, renal scarring or failure to thrive in an infant.
9. Symptomatic lower urinary infection requires at least a 3-day course of antibiotics and follow-up within 2–3 weeks.
10. Urinary tract infection in a patient with a neuropathic bladder, indwelling catheter or ileal conduit should only be treated when it is symptomatic or there is proven bacteriuria.
11. Note that certain antibiotics may reduce the effectiveness of the oral contraceptive pill.

REFERENCES

Andriole VT, Patterson TF 1991 Epidemiology, natural history and management of urinary tract infections in pregnancy. Medical Clinics of North America 75:359–373
Arnold E 2000 Investigation. In: Stanton SL, Dwyer P (eds) Urinary tract infection in the female. Martin Dunitz, London, pp 36–59
Avorn J, Monane M, Gurwitz JH, Glynn RJ, Choodnovskiy I, Lipsitz LA 1994 Reduction of bacteriuria and pyuria after ingestion of cranberry juice. Journal of the American Medical Association 271:751–754
Bailey RR 1998 Vesicoureteric reflux and reflux nephropathy. In: Schrier RW, Gootschalk GW (eds) Diseases of the kidney, 4th edn. Little, Brown, Boston, pp 748–783
Boscia JA, Kaye D 1987 Asymptomatic bacteriuria in the elderly. Infectious Diseases Clinics of North America 1:892–903
Bryan CS, Reynolds KL 1984 Hospital acquired bacteraemic urinary tract infection: epidemiology and outcome. Journal of Urology 132:494
Cardozo L 1996 Postmenopausal cystitis. British Medical Journal 313:129
Cardozo L, Benness C, Abbott D 1998 Low dose oestrogen prophylaxis for recurrent tract infections in elderly women. British Journal of Obstetrics and Gynaecology 105:403–407
Cattell WR 1998 The patient with urinary tract infections. In: Davison AM, Cameron JS, Grunfeld J, Kerr DNS, Ritz E, Winearls CG (eds) Oxford textbook of clinical nephrology, 2nd edn. Oxford University Press, New York, pp 1252–1259
Ditchburn RK, Ditchburn JS 1990 A study of microscopical and chemical tests for the diagnosis of urinary tract infections in general practice. British Journal of General Practice 40:241–243
Fihn SD, Stamm WE 1983 Management of women with acute dysuria. In: Rund, Wolcot BW (eds) Emergency medicine annual. Appleton-Century-Crofts, Norwalk, p 225
Foxman B, Chi JW 1990 Health behavior and urinary tract infection in college-aged women. Journal of Clinical Epidemiology 43:329–337
Foxman B, Frerichs RR 1985a Epidemiology of urinary tract infection. I. Diaphragm use and sexual intercourse. American Journal of Public Health 75:1308–1313
Foxman B, Frerichs RR 1985b Epidemiology of urinary tract infections. II. Diet, clothing and urinary habits. American Journal of Public Health 75:1314–1317
Foxman B, Marsh J, Gillespie B et al 1997 Condom use and first-time urinary tract infection. Epidemiology 8:637–641
Fraser IR, Birch D, Fairley KF et al 1995 A prospective study of corticol scarring in acute febrile pyelonephritis in adults: clinical and bacteriological characteristics. Clinics in Nephrology 47:13–18
Grüneberg RN 1994 Changes in urinary pathogens and their antibiotic sensitivities, 1971–1992. Journal of Antimicrobial Chemotherapy 33 (suppl A):1–8
Hamilton-Miller JMT 1994 The urethral syndrome and its management. Journal of Antimicrobial Chemotherapy 33(suppl A):63–73
Hansson S, Martinell J, Stokland E, Jodal U 1997 The natural history of bacteriuria in childhood. Infectious Diseases Clinics of North America 11:499–512
Harding GKM, Ronald AR, Nicolle LE, Thomson MJ, Gray GJ 1982 Long term antimicrobial prophylaxis for recurrent urinary infection in females. Review of Infectious Diseases 4:438–443
Hayley RW, Culver DH, Waite JW, Morgan WM, Emori TG 1985 The national nosocomial infection rate. A new need for new vital statistics. American Journal of Epidemiology 121:159–167
Hooton TM, Scholes D, Hughes JP et al 1996 A prospective study of risk factors for symptomatic urinary tract infection in young women. New England Journal of Medicine 335:468–474
Johnson JR, Stamm WE 1987 Diagnosis and treatment of acute urinary tract infection. Infectious Diseases Clinics of North America 1:773–791
Johnson JR, Stamm WE 1989 Urinary tract infections in women: diagnosis and treatment. Annals of Internal Medicine 111:906
Kass EH 1956 Asymptomatic infections of the urinary tract. Transactions of the Association of American Physicians 69:56–64
Kunin CM 1987 Detection, prevention and management of urinary tract infections, 4th edn. Lea and Febiger, Philadelphia, pp 57–124
Langermann S, Mollby R, Burlein JE et al 2000 Vaccination against FimH adhesin protects cynomolgus monkeys from colonisation and infection by uropathogenic Escherichia coli. Journal of Infectious Diseases 181:774–778
Lewis-Jones HG, Lamb GHR, Hughes PL 1989 Can ultrasound replace the intravenous urogram in the preliminary investigation of urinary tract disease? British Journal of Radiology 62:977–980
Little PJ 1965 Prevention of pyelonephritis of pregnancy. Lancet i:567–569
Lomberg H, Cedergren B, Leffler H et al 1986 Influence of blood group on

the availability of receptors for attachment of uropathogenic Escherichia coli. Infection and Immunology 51:919–926

Maclean A 2000 Pregnancy In: Stanton SL, Dwyer PL (eds) Urinary tract infection in the female. Martin Dunitz, London, pp 145–160

Mansour M, Azmy AF, MacKenzie JR 1987 Renal scarring secondary to vesicoureteric reflux. Critical assessment and new grading. British Journal of Urology 70:32–34

Mooreville M, Fritz RW, Mulholland SG 1983 Enhancement of the bladder defence mechanism by an exogenous agent. Journal of Urology 130:607–609

Nicolle LE, Ronald AR 1987 Recurrent urinary infection in adult women: diagnosis and treatment. Infectious Diseases Clinics of North America 1:793–806

Nicolle LE, Harding GKM, Preiksaitis J, Ronald AR 1982 The association of urinary tract infection with sexual intercourse. Journal of Infectious Diseases 146:579–584

Norden CW, Kass EH 1968 Bacteriuria of pregnancy – a critical appraisal. Annual Reviews in Medicine 19:431–470

Norrby SR 1990 Short-term treatment of uncomplicated urinary tract infections in women. Review of Infectious Diseases 12:458–467

Parsons CL 1982 Prevention of urinary tract infection by the exogenous glycosaminoglycan sodium pentasanpolysulfate. Journal of Urology 127:942–947

Patel N, Daniels IR 2000 Botanical perspectives on health: of cystitis and cranberries. Journal of the Royal Society of Health 120:52–53

Patterson JE, Andriole VT 1997 Bacterial urinary tract infections in diabetes. Infectious Disease Clinics of North America 11:735–750

Raz R, Stamm WE 1993 A controlled trial of intravaginal estriol in postmenopuasal women with recurrent urinary tract infections. New England Journal of Medicine 329:753–756

Remis RS, Gurwith MJ, Gurwith D, Hargett-Bean NT, Layde PM 1987 Risk factors for urinary tract infection. American Journal of Epidemiology 126:685–694

Rubin UH, Shapiro ED, Andriole VT, Davis RJ, Stamm WE 1992 Evaluation of new anti-infective drugs for the treatment of urinary tract infection. Clinics in Infectious Diseases 15:S216–227

Rushton HG 1997 Urinary tract infections in children. Pediatric Clinics of North America 44:1133–1169

Sheinfeld J, Schaeffer AJ, Cordon-Cardo C, Rogatko A, Fair WR 1989 Association of Lewis blood-group phenotype with recurrent urinary tract infections in women. New England Journal of Medicine 320:773–777

Spencer J, Lindsell D, Mastorakou I 1990 Ultrasonography compared with intravenous urography in the investigation of urinary tract infection in adults. British Medical Journal 301:221–224

Stevens M 1989 Screening urine for bacteriuria. Medical Laboratory Science 46:194–206

Talner CB, Davidson AJ, Lebowitz RI, Dalla-Palma L, Goldman SM 1994 Acute pyelonephritis: can we agree on terminology? Radiology 192:297–305

Tincello DG, Richmond DH 1998 Evaluation of reagant strips in detecting asymptomatic bacteriuria in early pregnancy: prospective case series. British Medical Journal 316:435–437

Turck M, Giffe B, Petersdorf RG 1962 The urethral catheter and urinary tract infection. Journal of Urology 88:834–837

Winstanley TG, Limb DI, Eggington R et al 1997 A 10 year survey of antimicrobial susceptibility of urinary tract isolates in the UK: the microbe base project. Journal of Antimicrobial Chemotherapy 40:591–594

Zafiri D, Gron Y, Einstein BI et al 1987 Growth advantages and enhanced toxicity of Escherichia coli adherent to tissue culture cells due to restricted diffusion of products secreted by cells. Journal of Clinical Investigations 79:1210

Zhanel GG, Harding GKM, Guay DRP 1990 Asymptomatic bacteriuria: which patients should be treated? Archives of Internal Medicine 150:1389–1396

59

Lower intestinal tract disease

Alexander G. Heriot   Devinder Kumar

INTRODUCTION

There is a significant overlap and interaction between lower intestinal tract disease and gynaecological conditions. The close anatomical, physiological and functional relationship between the pelvic organs and the pelvic floor results in direct interaction and is reflected by overlapping symptoms and the fact that interventions can have an effect on a variety of systems.

PELVIC FLOOR ANATOMY

The rectum

The rectum commences at the point where the taeniae coli of the sigmoid colon spread and fuse to form a continuous longitudinal muscle coat. This is usually at the level of the 3rd sacral segment and the rectum follows the curve of the sacrum in the pelvis until it meets the pelvic floor where it turns posteriorly and downwards to meet the anal canal. The upper third of the rectum is almost completely covered by peritoneum other than its vascular supply posteriorly; the middle third is only covered anteriorly; and the lower third has no peritoneal covering. The peritoneum is reflected forward and up over the bladder in the male or the upper vagina in the female, forming the rectovesical or rectouterine pouch of Douglas.

Posteriorly the rectum is related to the sacrum, coccyx and puborectal muscles and in the upper rectum, the sacral plexus and autonomic nerve fibres, which pass down and lateral to the rectum. Other lateral relations include the uterine appendages above the peritoneal reflection and the ureters, iliac vessels and middle rectal artery. More inferiorly lies the pelvic floor. The posterior vaginal wall lies anterior to the inferior rectum, with the pouch of Douglas more superiorly. Loops of small bowel may pass down into the pouch of Douglas.

The rectal mucosa is folded longitudinally when the rectum is empty but as it distends two or three transverse folds, the valves of Houston, appear caused by the circular muscle of the rectum. The rectum is enveloped by its own fascial envelope and great care is taken during rectal mobilization to avoid malignant disease breaching this 'package'. The lower part of the rectum is attached to the sacrum by Waldeyer's fascia, which covers the presacral fascia and must be divided to mobilize the rectum. Anteriorly, the fascial envelope is continuous with the rectovesical fascia of Denovilliers. This thickened fascia extends from the peritoneal reflection to the urogenital diaphragm and forms part of the rectovaginal septum. Fascia may also be condensed lateral to the rectum, forming the lateral rectal ligaments.

Anal canal

The anal canal commences at the anorectal ring, where the rectum passes through the pelvic floor, and passes to the anal verge. It is around 4 cm long and passes back and down from the rectum from a point where the rectum is pulled forward by the sling-like puborectalis muscle. The anal canal sits like a tube within a funnel, the sides of the funnel formed by levator ani, with the stem of the funnel formed by the external sphincter. The latter is a continuous, circumferential band of striated muscle, up to 10 mm thick, encircling the anal canal. It attaches to the perineal body anteriorly, the coccyx posteriorly via the anococcygeal raphe and the ischiorectal fossae lie laterally. Superiorly the fibres of the external sphincter blend with puborectalis. The internal sphincter lies within the external sphincter and is formed by thickening of the circular smooth muscle fibres of the rectum. The anal canal is lined by columnar epithelium above the level of the dentate line and squamous epithelium below. At the dentate line there is an epithelial transition zone as the mucosa changes from columnar to squamous. This area is important for sensory function of the anal canal. The anal glands lie at the level of the dentate line in the intersphincteric plane. The anal lining is important to seal the anal canal to prevent leakage. Prolapse of the anal lining down from the high-pressure sphincter zone can lead to incontinence.

Pelvic floor

The pelvic floor is formed by levator ani and consists of a muscle funnel arising from the pelvic side walls through which the urethra, vagina and rectum pass down into the perineum. It supports the pelvic contents and prevents excessive descent of the perineum with tonic contraction as a postural reflex on standing. The levator ani is composed of four parts: puborectalis, pubococcygeus, ischiococcygeus and iliococcygeus. The puborectalis fibres compose the base of the funnel and form a sling, arising from and inserting into the symphysis pubis, extending around the vagina (or prostate) and the anorectum. This helps create the anorectal angle by pulling the rectum towards the symphysis, creating an angle of between 90° and 135° on straining. Some fibres fuse with the perineal body anterior to the anorectum, forming a fibromuscular mass providing additional support to the pelvic floor. The sides of the funnel are formed by the other components of levator ani. Pubococcygeus arises from the symphysis and the fascia over obturator internus and inserts into the coccyx. It is overlapped by iliococcygeus, arising from the arcus tendineus on the lateral pelvic wall and inserting into the coccyx and the anococcygeal raphe. Ischiococcygeus arises from the ischial spine and inserts into the coccyx and lower part of the sacrum.

Levator ani receives a direct motor supply from the perineal branch of the 3rd and 4th sacral nerves as they pass through the pelvic floor into the perineum. The peripheral part of levator ani is supplied by the pudendal nerve formed from the anterior divisions of S2, 3 and 4. The nerve passes out of the pelvis between piriformis and ischiococcygeus and has a short course in the buttock, lying on the posterior surface of the ischial spine. It passes back into the pelvis through the lesser sciatic foramen and runs in Alcock's canal in the lateral aspect of the ischiorectal fossa. It passes beneath levator ani and divides into the inferior rectal nerve, which passes down and supplies the external anal sphincter, the perineal nerve, which supplies the external sphincter and puborectalis, and the dorsal nerve of the penis/clitoris. The internal sphincter is supplied by excitatory sympathetic fibres running in the· hypogastric nerves and parasympathetic fibres in the sacral nerves.

PHYSIOLOGY OF DEFAECATION

Defaecation is a complicated mechanism that is first initiated as the rectum begins to fill following sigmoid colon contractions.

As the rectum distends, there is an urge to defaecate, initially transient, then constant as the rectum distends further, and then uncomfortable. The initial urge is mediated by stretch receptors in the rectal wall and stimulates a reflex relaxation of the internal sphincter (rectoanal inhibitory reflex). If it is not convenient to defaecate, the external sphincter contracts, allowing the internal sphincter time to recover, and then pelvic floor contractions push the rectal contents cranially. If it is convenient, defaecation is initiated. Intra-abdominal pressure is increased by diaphragmatic and abdominal wall contraction. Relaxation of puborectalis straightens the anorectal angle from around 90° to 120° and it is straightened further by pelvic floor descent initiated by pelvic floor relaxation. Prolonged inhibition of the internal and external sphincters allows emptying of the rectum.

INVESTIGATIONS

The application of physiological investigations to the management of anorectal problems has introduced the concept of physiology-directed treatment. Though inexact, it does allow the possibility of evidence-based treatment.

Manometry

The mechanisms of defaecation and continence are complicated and involve mechanical, neural and higher centre aspects. Production of a high-pressure zone by the anal sphincter is an important aspect of these mechanisms and measurement of this function provides valuable information. Pressures can be measured using either a balloon recording system or a perfusion system. The former consists of an air- or fluid-filled balloon connected to a pressure transducer. It is inserted into the rectum, with the patient usually in the left lateral position, and then withdrawn through the anal canal, with pressure recordings made at different positions both at rest and with the patient contracting the anal sphincter. Perfusion systems consist of a multichannel catheter that is perfused with water. Multiple side holes in the catheter allow pressures to be recorded at various sites along the catheter and the data can be recorded on paper charts or on a computer.

Static manometry allows measurement of resting anal pressure, maximum squeeze pressure, the length of the sphincter and the presence or absence of the anorectal reflex. The resting anal pressure is predominantly provided by the internal sphincter which is in a state of spontaneous contraction (Frenckner & von Euler 1975). Resting pressures tend to be lower in women than men and also in elderly patients. Reduction can also be noted in neurogenic faecal incontinence and with sacral nerve damage. The internal sphincter relaxes with rectal distension and this may occur spontaneously up to seven times per hour (Kumar et al 1989). This is thought to be a 'sampling' reflex, allowing discrimination between stool and flatus in the rectum (Duthie & Bennett 1963). This sphincter relaxation is accompanied by a spontaneous recovery in pressure. This sphincter relaxation and recovery in response to distension is termed the anorectal reflex. It can be demonstrated by rapidly introducing air into a rectal balloon whilst recording sphincter pressures and is mediated by an internal neural pathway in the wall of the rectum. It is absent in Hirschsprung's disease and may also be absent in cases of megarectum or following excision of the rectum, though the latter may recover.

The voluntary squeeze pressure is due to external sphincter contraction. It tends to be higher in men than women and reduces with age. It is reduced in patients with external sphincter damage and also in neurogenic incontinence. Measurements are usually performed at rest though ambulatory manometry is possible. This may give a more physiological series of measurements and may demonstrate abnormalities not detected on static manometry, such as reduced sphincter pressures in patients with incontinence though with normal pressures at rest.

Electrophysiology, electrosensitivity and electromyography

Electrophysiological tests of anal sphincter function provide important information regarding the cause of sphincter weakness and may influence whether surgery is appropriate. It can be divided into motor nerve conduction studies, electrosensitivity of the anal mucosa and electromyography of the sphincters.

The pudendal nerve is vulnerable to injury in its distal part where it is mobile. It is susceptible to damage from stretching during chronic straining or vaginal delivery, but may also be damaged by perineal descent resulting from pelvic nerve damage. Damage may be detected by extended pudendal nerve motor latency. With the patient in the left lateral position, the pudendal nerve is stimulated near the ischial spine using a St Mark's electrode attached to a gloved finger inserted into the rectum (Rogers et al 1988a). Motor nerve latency can be recorded on a standard EMG machine. Increased latency is considered to be a reflection of nerve damage and has been demonstrated following difficult vaginal delivery, with abnormal perineal descent and with chronic straining (Henry et al 1982). Increased latency following vaginal delivery has been shown to correlate with increased risk of developing faecal incontinence (Snooks et al 1985). Evidence of pudendal nerve damage has been shown to influence long-term results of postanal repair for faecal incontinence and is of value when surgery is considered (Tetzschner et al 1995). In other conditions, such as solitary rectal ulcer syndrome, the results are unlikely to influence management, as it is likely to be the same whether the latency is increased or not.

Anal mucosal electrosensitivity can be measured and may provide useful information, particularly in patients with faecal incontinence (Fig. 59.1). A lubricated electrode is placed in the anal canal and the supplying current increased up to 20 mA until a tingling sensation is reported. This is repeated in the upper, middle and lower anal canal. It is reproducible and may be abnormal in patients with neurogenic faecal incontinence, though this may reflect pudendal nerve damage (Roe et al 1986).

Electromyography has been applied to both the external anal sphincter and to the pelvic floor, particularly puborectalis and pubococcygeus. It can qualitatively assess the muscle function using surface electrodes or a concentric needle electrode (a bipolar electrode within a single cannula) or, by using a

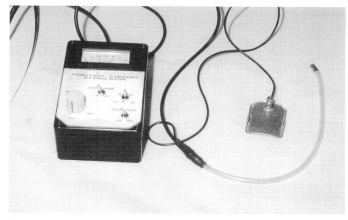

Fig. 59.1 Apparatus for anal mucosal electrosensitivity showing recording device, electrode and earth plate.

single fibre electrode, allows assessment of muscle denervation and reinervation. It is possible to map the distribution of functional muscle in a patient with a sphincter defect but this has not been shown to have an advantage over qualitative assessment. Increased EMG activity has been demonstrated in a number of conditions, all of which are associated with chronic straining at stool (Rutter 1974). It was presumed that obstructed defaecation would also be associated with excessive EMG activity and a failure of relaxation of puborectalis but this has not been shown.

Single-fibre electromyography allows recordings to be made from individual muscle fibres. The electrode is a modification of the concentric needle electrode and by reducing low-frequency response, recordings from single muscle fibres can be made. Fibre density can be measured by assessing the number of action potentials within the uptake of the electrode. Denervation and reinervation result in an increase in fibre density and so may be increased in neurogenic faecal incontinence (Lubowski et al 1988). Neuromuscular jitter indicated by variability in interval between two successive components of a multicomponent motor unit may also be indicative of nerve damage. Fibre density is also increased by age and by conditions that result in pudendal nerve damage such as solitary rectal ulcer syndrome. Single-fibre electromyography is not performed routinely but may in fact be more sensitive than pudendal nerve latency in detecting neurogenic pathology.

Rectal sensation

The rectum is sensitive to distension and it is possible to measure this. Insertion and distension of a rectal balloon produces a 'pelvis' sensation of distension. The volume at which this is first perceived by the patient is called the threshold volume. If distension continue the patient will then feel an urge to defaecate. Further distension will result in pain and the volume at which this is unbearable is the maximum tolerated volume. Patients with slow-transit constipation tend to have reduced sensation (Keighley & Shouler 1984). Sensation tends to be normal in patients with incontinence (Rogers et al 1988b).

Motility studies

Proctography

Evacuation proctography is a contrast radiological study of rectal emptying and can provide valuable information on both structural and functional aspects of defaecation. The rectum is filled with contrast such as barium paste and images are taken during normal defaecation consisting of a resting, evacuation and recovery phase (Mahieu et al 1984). The resting phase allows assessment of the resting anorectal configuration and the position of the pelvic floor. The resting anorectal angle can be measured and can be noted to widen by approximately 20° during evacuation, as the pelvic floor descends and the distal rectum empties. During the recovery phase the pelvic floor returns to its resting position, restoring the anorectal angle and closing the anal canal. Plain films can be taken at intervals or videoproctography can be performed. The degree of perineal and pelvic floor descent can be measured relative to the pubococcygeal line.

Structural abnormalities can be detected during any phase of evacuation. Rectocoeles may be detected by bulging of the anterior rectal wall and are considered pathological if greater than 2 cm (Shorvon et al 1989). They may retain barium and be associated with incomplete evacuation though barium retention has not been shown to be correlated with symptoms. Intussusception of the rectum, ranging from a few millimetres to full-thickness prolapse into the anal canal, can be noted though care must be taken to confirm true intussusception. Prolapse of the pelvic floor itself can be observed with the presence of a cystocoele or enterocoele though instillation of contrast into either organ may be necessary to confirm this (Altringer et al 1995). Normal pelvic floor descent can be measured and excess pelvic floor descent can be recorded though its significance is uncertain. Functional abnormalities of defaecation may also be detected such as failure of the anorectal angle to increase or excessive duration of defaecation. Anismus can be detected by rate of evacuation though there may be other supplementary signs such as failure of the pelvic floor to lower. Proctography may provide hard structural and functional information related to defaecation.

Isotope defaecography

Evacuation proctography can provide structural and qualitative functional information on defaecation but it is unable to provide quantitative information. Isotope defaecography can, however, provide quantitative measurements of the dynamics of defaecation. Radiolabelled simulated stool 100 ml is inserted into the rectum. The subject is then asked to sit on a commode and pass the simulated stool. Five-second frames are obtained during the entire act of defaecation. Using a gamma camera and recording the activity in the rectum before, during and after defaecation can measure the precise quantity remaining in the rectum following defaecation. Similarly, the total percentage evacuation and the rate of evacuation can be calculated from the gamma camera images (Fig. 59.2). Anatomical abnormalities such as a rectocoele can also be identified on the images obtained (Figs 59.3, 59.4). Any amount retained in a rectocoele can also be recorded (Fig. 59.5) and this can provide useful information in selection of patients for surgery.

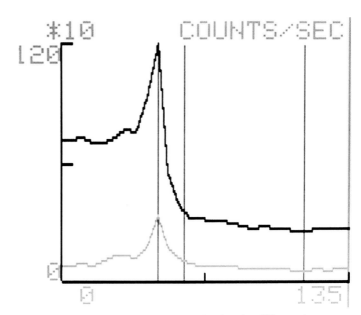

Fig. 59.2 Normal isotope defaecography showing filling and excretion with a minimal amount remaining in the rectum.

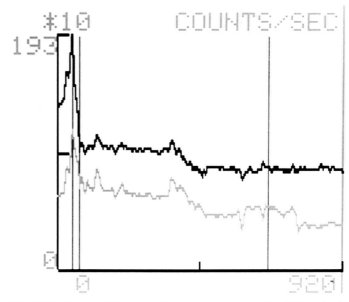

Fig. 59.3 Isotope defaecography showing a rectocoele with impaired emptying of both rectum and rectocoele.

Colonic motility

Disorders in colonic transit are common and constipation is usually the presenting symptom. If mechanical causes have been excluded, the cause may be abnormal colonic motility. Quantitative assessment of colonic motility can be obtained using either radio-opaque markers or radio-isotopes. Ingestion of radio-opaque markers and assessment of their passage by plain abdominal film is a useful screening tool for abnormal colonic transit (Fig. 59.6). Eighty per cent of markers are usually passed by 5 days following ingestion but if less is passed, transit can be considered abnormal though the site of abnormality,

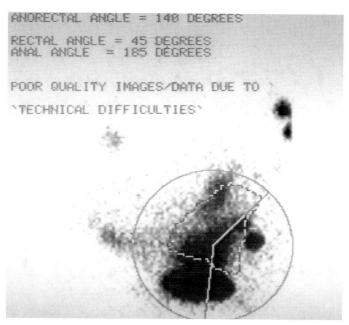

Fig. 59.4 Isotope defaecography illustrating the anatomical presence of the rectocoele.

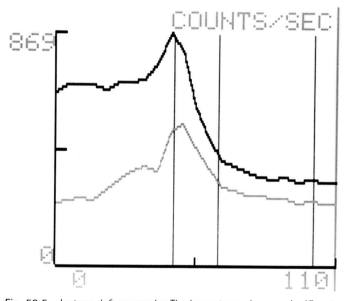

Fig. 59.5 Isotope defaecography. The lower trace shows a significant amount of material remaining in the rectocoele following defaecation.

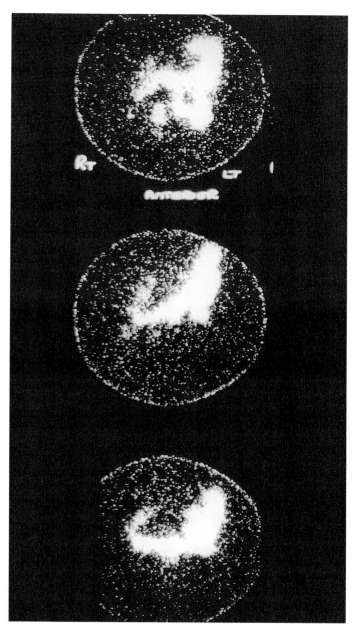

Fig. 59.6 Scintigraphic radiography transit study showing hold-up at the splenic flexure.

whether gastric, small bowel or colonic, cannot be determined (Hinton et al 1969). Segmental colonic transit can be measured by taking serial radiographs on successive days following ingestion of three different sets of markers over 3 days and recording which segment of colon is associated with delay (Metcalf et al 1987).

Radio-isotope studies involve ingestion of a radio-isotope such as In-III-DTPA, bound to cellulose, and recording of the proportion of isotope in each part of the colon over successive days. This can reduce radiation exposure and allows the colon to be divided into analytical segments and precise measurements of motility to be made (Notghi et al 1993). It can be very valuable in identifying slow-transit constipation as compared to simple symptomatic normal-transit constipation that is vital for appropriate management, particularly for selection for subtotal colectomy.

Anal ultrasonography

Anal ultrasonography has become a valuable tool for assessment of the anal canal and sphincters. A rotating 10 MHz ultrasound probe can be inserted into the anal canal and with longitudinal movement gives 360° cross-sectional images of the anal canal. The normal image in the anal canal is of four

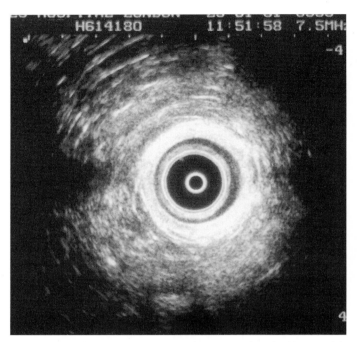

Fig. 59.7 Anal ultrasonography showing a normal anal sphincter with intact external and internal sphincter.

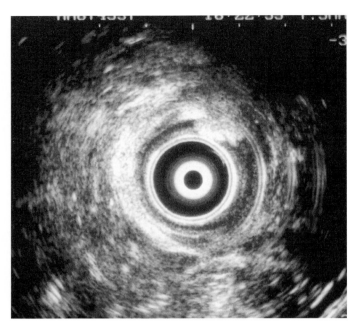

Fig. 59.8 Anal ultrasonography showing anterior tear of the external and internal anal sphincter.

concentric rings consisting of subepithelium, internal sphincter, longitudinal muscle and external sphincter (Fig. 59.7). The internal sphincter appears hypoechoic and is usually 2–3 mm thick (Burnett & Bartram 1991). The longitudinal muscle lies outside this and is moderately hyperechoic. The external sphincter has a more complex appearance. Superficially it is hypoechoic, more so in the male, though subcutaneously it is more reflective in both sexes. An apparent defect can be noted high in the anal canal in females though this is actually due to the muscle fibres being cut in cross-section as they run forward to form an anterior muscle bundle in the lower anal canal.

Increased thickness of the internal sphincter is pathological and may be associated with intussusception, solitary rectal ulcer (Halligan et al 1995) or anal pain though traumatic damage to the internal sphincter is the most common pathology. This can be identified by a defect in the ring (Fig. 59.8). It may be iatrogenic and well defined, such as following a lateral sphincterotomy (Sultan et al 1994), or may be iatrogenic and diffuse, such as following dilatation. The most common cause is obstetric trauma which often occurs in combination with external sphincter defects. Tears in the muscle appear poorly reflective as the muscle is replaced by fibrous tissue and anal ultrasonography is very effective in detecting tears. One-third of vaginal deliveries are associated with some degree of sphincter damage (Sultan et al 1993a) and forceps delivery increases the risk of this (Sultan et al 1993b). Repairs following third degree tears can often be shown to be incomplete on ultrasonography (Nielsen et al 1992).

Anal sepsis can be readily identified by anal ultrasonography. It may show a collection that may not be clinically identifiable or can demonstrate the pathway of a fistula. Its accuracy is similar to examination under anaesthetic.

CONDITIONS

Faecal incontinence

Faecal incontinence is a distressing problem and its prevalence is probably underreported and may be as high as 7% (Talley et al 1992). The degree of incontinence can range from incontinence to flatus, to liquid stool or to solid stool. Risk factors include increasing age and female gender. Maintenance of continence is a complex activity resulting from an interaction between the higher centres, spinal cord, peripheral nerves, sphincter complex and pelvic floor. Maintenance is usually subconscious, though there may be conscious influence. Deficiencies in any of the integral components can cause incontinence and management is directed at identifying and treating the specific abnormality.

Aetiology
Cerebral degeneration can contribute to incontinence and is one of the factors affecting incontinence in the elderly in combination with decreased rectal sensation. Continence during episodes of raised intra-abdominal pressure is mediated by a spinal reflex and so, though unaffected by an upper motor neurone lesion such as spinal cord damage, may be caused by a lower motor neurone lesion, for example affecting the pudendal nerve. Local or general pathology causing diarrhoea may result in incontinence. This may be local, such as inflammatory bowel disease or a rectal tumour producing excess mucus, or general, such as diabetes mellitus. Diabetes may cause a pudendal neuropathy, resulting in anal sphincter weakness and incontinence, and disorders of the anal sphincters and pelvic floor are common causes of incontinence, particularly in women.

Disruption of the anal sphincter mechanism is most commonly caused by obstetric injury and the risk of this is increased by forceps delivery, episiotomy or perineal laceration (Sorensen et al 1993, Sultan et al 1993a). Sultan et al (1993a) showed that 35% of vaginal deliveries result in sphincter disruption. External sphincter defects may be occult but still result in an increased risk of incontinence later. Internal sphincter damage is often associated with external sphincter damage, most commonly with anterior defects, though they may present in isolation (Law et al 1991). Obstetric trauma may result in perineal body disruption or even a rectovaginal fistula if extreme. Prolonged vaginal delivery can result in pudendal neuropathy directly, probably due to stretching of the nerve trunk and compression in the pudendal canal. This is reversible in 60% of women but can become established (Snooks et al 1986). It is also thought that sympathetic supply to the internal sphincter may also be stretched, resulting in an autonomic neuropathy (Speakman et al 1990). Neuropathy may result in incontinence directly through sphincter weakness though injury may be more subtle, causing reduced anal sensation, which may not become apparent until a woman becomes elderly. Damage may contribute to rectal prolapse which may itself cause incontinence due to stretching of the sphincters. Abnormal perineal descent, which itself can cause pudendal neuropathy, may also be a important factor.

Causative factors for incontinence may be iatrogenic. Radiotherapy may cause poor sphincter function and surgical trauma, particularly an overenthusiastic lateral sphincterotomy by an inexperienced surgeon, may cause significant sphincter damage.

Assessment

Clinical evaluation of the patient by history and examination is vital and will determine the necessity of further investigation. The degree of incontinence and the affect on life must be assessed and a continence scale is very useful in this respect (Miller et al 1988). The degree may be recorded with respect to incontinence to flatus, to liquid stool or to solid stool. Obstetric history is obviously vital. Local examination may demonstrate perineal soiling, scarring from a previous episiotomy or evidence of a fistula. Rectal examination will reveal overloading and allow assessment of the anal sphincter tone and defects in the sphincter that may be palpable. Perineal sensation should be recorded, along with degree of perineal descent and the effect of straining. Bimanual examination allows assessment of the rectovaginal septum. Proctoscopy and rigid sigmoidoscopy will reveal anorectal and rectal pathology such as proctitis and fibreoptic endoscopy may be required to examine the colon more proximally. Further investigation consists primarily of anorectal physiology and endoanal ultrasound. This may demonstrate and localize internal and external sphincter damage and the presence of any neuropathy.

Management

Non-operative management should be offered to patients with minor incontinence, no identifiable pathology or even initially for more severe incontinence with identifiable pathology. A spectrum of treatment is available and should be tailored for each patient. Patient education and dietary advice can be valuable and medication such as loperamide hydrochloride can contribute by increasing internal sphincter tone or by thickening loose stool. Biofeedback has been demonstrated to improve sphincter tone and can produce very satisfactory results with carefully selected patients when applied in conjunction with a therapeutic team (Ferrara et al 1995).

Patients with passive incontinence secondary to internal anal sphincter dysfunction or defect respond unfavourably to surgical repair. Recently, we have developed a non-surgical method of treating these patients using sphincter bulking with collagen. The results of sphincter bulking for faecal incontinence are similar to those for urinary incontinence and appear to be maintained at 5 years.

Surgery is appropriate in patients with severe incontinence and a correctable abnormality. The outcome varies, however, and is influenced both by the extent of damage and by the presence of pudendal neuropathy. The extent of operative intervention is dependent on the underlying defect and may include formation of a stoma if repair is impossible. Simple external anal sphincter defects such as following vaginal delivery can usually be repaired by an overlapping sphincter repair performed through a perineal incision. This may be performed as a primary repair at the time of the injury if it is recognized and the patient is stable. It is often, however, performed as a secondary repair as the injury was not recognized or the woman presents months or years later with incontinence. Following mobilization, the sphincter ends are overlapped and sutured with 2/0 polyglactin sutures. Damage to the anterior pelvic floor may be repaired at the same time with plication of levator ani as an anterior levatoroplasty. Results from direct repair range from 60% to 90% success (Londono-Schimmer et al 1994, Pezim et al 1987, Yoshioka & Keighley 1989) and are influenced by the degree of neuropathy present. Plication of defects in the internal sphincter in conjunction with external sphincter repair has failed to demonstrate any further benefit (Deen et al 1995).

Patients with a degree of neuropathy may undergo postanal repair of the pelvic floor. This was thought to reduce the anorectal angle, but though short-term success rates are up to 80% (Parks 1975), only a quarter of the patients show a sustained improvement (Setti Carraro et al 1994). This may be combined with an anterior levatoroplasty, producing a total pelvic floor repair, though longer term benefits remain limited (Deen et al 1993). The extreme end of the spectrum is insertion of an artificial sphincter or formation of a skeletal muscle neosphincter. This may be indicated if the sphincter is congenitally absent, damaged beyond repair or with severe neuropathy. Results with the artificial sphincter are promising but early and with limited numbers (Wong & Rothenberger 1994). Results of formation of a gracilis neosphincter do have larger numbers and have shown up to 75% long-term continence (Baeten et al 1995). Stoma formation remains a final option, can give good long-term results and should not be considered a failure of management.

Diarrhoea

Diarrhoea as a chronic symptom is not a common presentation but can be a manifestation of either organic pathology or of a functional abnormality such as irritable bowel syndrome (IBS). The pathophysiology of diarrhoea can be considered as resulting from osmotic, secretory or motor abnormalities, which may be due to a number of pathologies. These abnormalities may be present in the small bowel, colon or both. Gastrointestinal infection such as giardiasis or idiopathic bowel inflammation due to Crohn's disease or ulcerative colitis may increase fluid secretion and reduce absorption. Hypersecretion may be induced by dietary intolerance such as hypolactasia and malabsorption such as with chronic pancreatitis may have an osmotic effect from the bowel. Rapid transit, either drug induced such as from laxatives or iatrogenic from previous bowel resection or gastric surgery, may reduce the available time for fluid to be reabsorbed from the bowel, resulting in diarrhoea. Colorectal neoplasms may alter motility or secrete large quantities of mucus, both of which may result in diarrhoea.

Assessment of a patient with diarrhoea needs a careful balance of allowing identification of organic disease if present without overinvestigating the patient. A detailed history is vital, including stool consistency and frequency and the presence of pathological symptoms such as rectal bleeding, weight loss and fatty stools. Identification of symptoms consistent with irritable bowel syndrome, such as abdominal bloating and discomfort, small-calibre stools or incomplete evacuation, is valuable. Clinical examination may identify pathology, particularly when followed by selective investigations. This may include colonic biopsy to identify microscopic colitis and in complicated cases, measurement of stool fat and plasma hormones such as vasoactive intestinal polypeptide. The latter investigations are not routinely applied and once the majority of organic pathologies have been excluded, if the symptoms are consistent with a functional abnormality, the patient may be reassured and treated symptomatically. In cases of intractable diarrhoea, small and large bowel motility studies may be indicated.

Constipation

Constipation is a symptom and there can be a wide spectrum in the frequency of motions ranging from every few days to every few weeks. Colonic motility can be influenced by a number of factors. Colonic factors include function of the enteric muscle and intrinsic nerves as well as the luminal contents. The extrinsic nerve supply to the colon is important, as are circulating gastrointestinal and non-gastrointestinal hormones. Pelvic floor abnormalities can cause constipation resulting in abnormal evacuation.

There are multiple possible causes of constipation that influence motility through the factors above. Aetiology may be organic or functional. Organic causes may directly affect the structure of the colon, rectum or anus and include any pathology that may cause a stricture, distal mucosal inflammation, colonic neuromuscular abnormalities such as Hirschsprung's disease and anal lesions including fissures and infection. Multiple pathologies outside the colon may be involved: neurological abnormalities, of the central or peripheral nervous system; psychological pathology such as depression; systemic metabolic disorders such as hypothyroidism or uraemia; or drug induced. Constipation may often, however, be functional. Individuals may have reduced bowel frequency alone and can be considered to be at the 'slow' end of the normal spectrum. Irritable bowel syndrome may result in symptoms such as bloating along with

constipation, though colonic transit time is normal. 'Functional' anorectal pathology including solitary rectal ulcer or rectal prolapse may cause constipation and abnormal pelvic floor function alone may cause difficulty with evacuation despite normal transit time. These patients are usually female (Read et al 1986, Shouler & Keighley 1986) and may spend hours trying to evacuate and this may involve vaginal or perineal digitations. Pelvic surgery including hysterectomy or anorectal surgery may be associated or worsen the condition. Elderly or pregnant patients are commonly constipated. Young adults with a normal-sized colon may have severe idiopathic constipation. These patients are almost universally female and have a long history of constipation. Patients may have dilated rectum or colon (megarectum, megacolon) which itself forms a characteristic clinical group. Functional constipation, when pathological, tends to be the result of either disordered colonic motility or obstructed defaecation.

Assessment

A precise history, including frequency of motion and dietary intake, is vital. This should include age of onset which may give an indication whether the problem is congenital, functional or the first presentation of an organic pathology. Past medical and drug history is important. Examination may demonstrate general causes such as hypothyroidism and rectal examination will indicate the presence of faecal impaction and any anorectal pathology. Often, no investigations are indicated if the symptoms are mild in young patients. A plain abdominal film or water-soluble contrast enema will demonstrate megacolon or megarectum or a narrowed segment with proximal dilatation that may be consistent with Hirschsprung's disease and older patients may need colonoscopy or barium enema to exclude a stricture. The vast majority of patients do not require any further investigations. In severe cases, investigations are targeted to identify disorders of colonic transit and disorders of pelvic floor function, which may co-exist. Radio-opaque marker studies or radio-isotope studies can assess colonic transit. Proctography can demonstrate rectal emptying and may identify pathology such as a rectocoele or intussusception. Failure of pelvic floor relaxation may be indicated by anorectal physiology with sphincter contraction during straining or inability to expel a balloon. Absence of the anorectal reflex may indicate Hirschsprung's disease that may necessitate a full-thickness rectal biopsy to demonstrate absence of ganglia in the rectal wall.

Management

Patients can usually be managed conservatively with dietary modification and judicious use of laxatives. The application of the latter may vary and can range from occasional use of a simple osmotic laxative such as lactulose to repeated use of a stimulant such as sodium picosulphate though this is rare. As a principle, the minimum laxatives should be used as infrequently as possible. Enemas are also useful. Biofeedback can be valuable for patients with abnormal pelvic floor contraction and has demonstrated encouraging results (Bleijenberg & Kuijpers 1987, Koutsomanis et al 1995). Injection of botulinum toxin can be beneficial in cases of puborectalis spasm (Hallan et al 1988). Surgery is only indicated for a very select group of patients and careful, combined assessment by a gastroenterologist and a surgeon is vital. Severe abnormalities of colonic transit can be treated by subtotal colectomy and ileorectal anastomosis though this represents a very small group of patients (Kamm et al 1988, Pemberton et al 1991). Identifiable anatomical pelvic floor defects can be repaired which can improve pelvic floor function but the difficulty lies in identifying the cases where the anatomic defect is causing the obstructed defaecation rather than just being present alongside the functional abnormality.

Rectal prolapse

Rectal prolapse is 10 times more common in women than men and there is an increased incidence with increasing age (Loygue et al 1984) though the sex ratio is less extreme in younger patients. High parity and chronic straining are both associated with higher incidence. The pathophysiology of rectal prolapse is mixed. Pelvic floor weakness and the presence of a mobile rectum are both important. Previous hysterectomy is associated with rectal prolapse but is probably associated rather than causative. Pelvic floor weakness, a weakened sphincter mechanism and a mobile rectum are all likely to be influential.

The prolapse itself will directly result in symptoms and is usually associated with mucosanguinous discharge. Incontinence is present in over half of the more elderly patients. The prolapse is often visible on inspection though it may only be seen on straining. It may be necessary for the patient to strain on the toilet to demonstrate the prolapse. Assessment of the proximal bowel may be required to exclude other pathologies and videoproctography may reveal excessive pelvic floor descent. Resting and squeeze pressures are often reduced. The differential diagnosis includes mucosal prolapse though this is normally only anterior. Prolapsed haemorrhoids may also be mistaken but can be distinguished from rectal prolapse by absence of a sulcus between the lateral aspect of the prolapse and the anal verge.

The initial approach to management is conservative though in the majority of cases, surgery is necessary. Patients with chronic straining are encouraged towards strain-free regular evacuation with the application of advice and enemas. Surgery needs to be combined with medical management to avoid constipation in order to reduce the risk of recurrence. The aim of the surgery is to control the prolapse whilst avoiding constipation and obstructed defaecation and the decision over choice of operation is predominantly between a perineal and an abdominal approach. Anal encircling devices such as the Thiersch wire are now no longer applied as, though easy to perform, they had an unacceptable recurrence rate.

The most common perineal approach is the Delorme's procedure. The bowel is prolapsed and the mucosa is dissected free from 1 cm proximal to the dentate line, down to the apex of the prolapse and then up the lumen of the bowel for a distance equivalent to the length of the prolapse. The mucosa is then excised following application of stay sutures. The prolapsed muscle is then plicated with a series of longitudinal sutures, apposing the two edges of mucosa that are sutured together. The procedure is well tolerated with minimal systemic upset and is very applicable to elderly patients. Results are acceptable

with a recurrence rate between 5% and 13.5% (Abulafi et al 1990, Lechaux et al 1995). Resection of the prolapse is indicated in some cases such as for a gangrenous or incarcerated prolapse. Rectosigmoidectomy can be performed via a perineal approach and involves amputation of the prolapse, repair of levator ani anteriorly and then coloanal anastomosis of the two ends of bowel. Recurrence rates are low though this must be tempered by the advanced age of the majority of the patients (Altemeier et al 1971, Ramanujan & Venkatesh 1988).

An abdominal approach is based on the principle of rectal mobilization and fixation. The recurrence rate is usually lower than with a perineal approach though the systemic effects of the surgery itself are more significant and the risk of obstructed defaecation is higher. The rectum is mobilized to the pelvic floor and is then fixed through a variety of possible techniques. Posterior fixation is often considered to be the procedure of choice with the rectum fixed to the sacrum with sutures or by insertion of synthetic mesh. Surgery can be performed laparoscopically (Graf et al 1995). Resection of redundant sigmoid colon prior to reanastomosis and fixation is also used in the presence of excess colon (Luukkonen et al 1992). Recurrence rates following abdominal procedures are low and usually less than 10% (Keighley et al 1983, Loygue et al 1984). Incontinence is usually improved but one problem that does arise is that of constipation postoperatively. This may be a combination of pre-existing slow transit, the mechanical effects of surgery and possible denervation of the left side of the colon. Though there are randomized trials in progress between abdominal and perineal approaches, none are yet at a point of reporting. There are long-term results regarding abdominal procedures as the patients tend to be younger and it appears that this approach probably has a lower long-term recurrence rate than a perineal procedure. The perineal approach is most appropriate for elderly patients as it has acceptable results with limited morbidity. Large prolapses, in particular in young patients, are probably more appropriately managed by an abdominal approach.

Descending perineum syndrome

Descending perineum syndrome is a condition where individuals constantly strain at stool but are unable to completely evacuate their rectum. The perineum descends abnormally low, well below the plane of the ischial tuberosities, and this is thought to be due to sacral nerve injury. This is secondary to either childbirth or chronic straining and is aggravated by chronic straining. It can result in denervation of the external anal sphincter that may lead to incontinence. There is no role for surgery in this condition and biofeedback is the appropriate management.

Perineal pain syndrome

There are a number of ill-defined conditions that can result in chronic rectal pain. The principal syndromes are proctalgia fugax, coccygodynia and chronic idiopathic anal pain. All cause chronic episodes of pain. In the case of proctalgia fugax, this is episodic, of sudden onset and usually self-resolving after around 30 minutes. Coccygodynia causes a constant burning pain, with occasional exacerbations, which is concentrated in the rectum and sacrum. Chronic idiopathic anal pain is a vague term that is applied to perineal pain which is usually described as a feeling of obstruction of the rectum (Todd 1985). These conditions are more common in women and there is an increased incidence of emotional instability. Examination is normal but must be complete to confidently exclude any pathology. Adequate assessment of the colon is important and anorectal physiology may be beneficial to exclude other pathology. If other pathology can be confidently excluded, patients should be reassured. However, the conditions can be very difficult to manage and avenues such as biofeedback have shown potential (Grimaud et al 1991).

Solitary rectal ulcer syndrome

This is a functional disorder that results in a physical manifestation and it can occur at almost any age, with a peak in the 20s (Madigan 1969). It is three times more common in women and patients describe multiple fruitless attempts at defaecation daily, accompanied by straining and a feeling of incomplete defaecation. This is often associated with mucus discharge, bleeding and tenesmus. Sigmoidoscopy demonstrates mucus in the rectum with mucosal reddening or ulceration. This is usually on one of the rectal valves and anterior. Diagnosis can be confirmed on histology with the appearance of fibromuscular replacement of the mucosa and splaying of muscle fibres into the lamina propria (Madigan 1969). The pathology remains uncertain but it is considered to be associated with chronic straining. Over 50% of cases will also have evidence of internal rectal intussusception (Mackle et al 1990).

Management should be conservative if possible. This should aim to reduce straining and may involve the use of laxative and biofeedback but may often fail. Surgery should be reserved for the most severe cases and should be avoided in the background of symptoms indicative of irritable bowel syndrome or major psychological components. The available options are rectopexy, excision of the mucosa prolapse or, in the extreme cases, stoma formation. The symptomatic success rate for rectopexy, which is the most successful approach, is around 50% (Sitzler et al 1996).

Irritable bowel syndrome

Irritable bowel syndrome is a condition where the patient has a variety of symptoms but there is no identifiable organic pathology. It is a very common condition with over 40% of patients attending gastroenterology outpatients having features of the symptoms (Harvey et al 1983). The main symptoms are of abdominal pain that is relieved by defaecation, along with abdominal distension, frequent stools and passage of mucus. Patients may be anywhere along the spectrum from constipation to diarrhoea. Patients tend to have a number of symptoms which may include non-specific ones such as depression, anxiety and sleep disturbance. The history tends to be very characteristic and examination is normal. Investigations demonstrate no abnormality though it is appropriate to assess the whole colon to exclude any organic pathology. The pathophysiology of the syndrome is uncertain but is associated with a widespread motility disorder affecting the smooth muscle of the whole gastrointestinal tract (Kumar & Wingate 1985). The aetiology of this remains uncertain.

Having confirmed that there is no underlying organic pathology, management should be conservative. Discussion with the patient may be beneficial as there is a major psychological component to the syndrome. Dietary modification with increased fibre can be useful, as may the use of smooth muscle relaxants such as mebeverine or hyoscine. Management can be difficult and is usually undertaken by gastroenterologists or general practitioners.

Rectovaginal fistula

Rectovaginal fistula is a very distressing condition. The passage of stool and flatus via the vagina is diagnostic in itself and identification of the underlying pathology is important. Diverticular disease can cause this with the connection usually at the vault of the vagina. This is more common in patients who have previously undergone a hysterectomy. Surgery is required with excision of the diverticular segment and reanastomosis of the bowel. It is not necessary to close the hole in the vagina.

Obstetric trauma may result in a rectovaginal fistula in combination with sphincter damage. In the third world, this is likely to be due to prolonged obstructed labour with pressure necrosis of the rectovaginal septum. In the Western world, it is more common following failed repair of a 4th-degree tear. It may close spontaneously but repair may be required as a delayed procedure and should be with concomitant sphincter repair. Iatrogenic injury is a further cause of rectovaginal fistula and the most common iatrogenic cause is gynaecological surgery. It is more common in the presence of extensive disease such as endometriosis and may be noticed and repaired at the time of surgery. It may, however, present postoperatively such as following necrosis of a diathermy burn. This requires surgical repair, which is urgent if the patient develops peritonitis.

Pelvic floor clinic

There is an extensive overlap between gynaecological and anorectal conditions associated with pelvic floor disorders. The value of a joint assessment through a combined pelvic floor clinic is therefore substantial and in 1994 St George's Hospital opened the first regular pelvic floor clinic in the United Kingdom. It was staffed by a consultant coloproctologist (Devinder Kumar) and a consultant urogynaecologist (Stuart Stanton). The team comprised research fellows and a pelvic floor nurse specialist. The patient is referred to either clinician, investigations are performed and then the patient is seen jointly to discuss the results of investigations and decide on treatment which may be collaborative.

The full range of anorectal physiology investigations is available including anal sphincter endosonography, electrosensitivity and electromyography and motility studies, including isotope defaecography, and anal manometry. Urodynamic studies include cystometry or videocystourethrography, uroflowmetry, urethral pressure profilometry, pelvic floor ultrasound, ambulatory monitoring and dynamic pelvic floor fluoroscopy. Fifty-two per cent of patients had anorectal symptoms which comprised faecal incontinence, defaecation problems and constipation. The remaining patients had urological symptoms which were largely associated with urge incontinence, stress incontinence and voiding difficulties.

An audit of treatments showed that 32% of patients underwent conservative treatment, 26% had anorectal and urogynaecological operations, 25% had anorectal operations with conservative urogynaecological treatment and 17% had operative urogynaecology with conservative anorectal treatment.

The joint clinic has been beneficial by providing joint consultations for patients, a single hospital admission for complex joint surgery, the interchange of ideas on research, e.g. the clinic was the first centre to use bulking agents for the treatment of faecal incontinence, and the training of junior staff in both anorectal and urogynaecological disorders.

KEY POINTS

1. Anal manometry, electrophysiology, and rectal sensation can provide valuable functional information on the anorectal complex. Combined with structural information from endoanal ultrasound, this allows the possibility of evidence based management.
2. Evacuation proctography, isotope defaecography, and colonic motility studies allows structural and functional assessment of defecation which is vital for patient selection for surgery
3. Faecal incontinence is an underreported problem and there are multiple aetiologies. Obstetric injury is the commonest cause of anal sphincter disruption and though anal sphincter repair can be very successful, results are influenced by the extent of injury and the presence of pudendal neuropathy.
4. Assessment of constipation should include a detailed history and examination, combined with selective investigations. Management is predominantly conservative.
5. Joint assessment of patients with pelvic floor disorders in a combined pelvic floor clinic by a colorectal surgeon and a urogynaecologist is extremely valuable. Benefits include combined assessment, single hospital admission for complex joint surgery, and exchange of research ideas.

REFERENCES

Altemeier W, Cuthbertson W, Schowengerdt C, Hunt J 1971 Nineteen years experience with one stage perineal repair of rectal prolapse. Annals of Surgery 173:993–1001

Altringer W, Saclarides T, Dominguez J et al 1995 Four-contrast defecography: pelvic 'floor-oscopy'. Diseases of the Colon and Rectum 38:695–699

Abulafi A, Sherman I, Fiddian R, Rothwell-Jackson R 1990 Delorme's operation for rectal prolapse. Annals of the Royal College of Surgeons 72:382–385

Baeten C, Geerdes B, Adang E et al 1995 Anal dynamic graciloplasty in the treatment of intractable fecal incontinence. New England Journal of Medicine 32:1600–1605

Bleijenberg G, Kuijpers H 1987 Treatment of spastic pelvic floor syndrome with biofeedback. Diseases of the Colon and Rectum 30:108–111

Burnett S, Bartram C 1991 Endosonographic variations in the normal internal anal sphincter. International Journal of Colorectal Diseases 6:2–4

Deen K, Kumar D, Williams J et al 1995 Randomized trial of internal anal sphincter plication with pelvic floor repair for neuropathic fecal incontinence. Diseases of the Colon and Rectum 38:14–18

Deen K, Oya M, Ortiz J, Keighley M 1993 Randomized trial comparing three forms of pelvic floor repair for neuropathic faecal incontinence. British Journal of Surgery 80:794–798

Duthie H, Bennett R 1963 The relations of sensation in the anal canal to the functional anal sphincter: a possible factor in anal continence. Gut 4:179–182

Ferrara A, Lord S, Larach S et al 1995 Biofeedback with Home Trainer Program is effective for both incontinence and pelvic floor dysfunction. Diseases of the Colon and Rectum 38:17

Frenckner B, von Euler C 1975 Influence of pudendal nerve block on the function of the anal sphincters. Gut 16:482–489

Graf W, Stefansson T, Arvidsson D, Pahlman L 1995 Laparoscopic suture rectopexy. Diseases of the Colon and Rectum 38:211–212

Grimaud J-C, Bouvier M, Naudy B, Guien C, Salducci J 1991 Manometric and radiologic investigations and biofeedback treatment of chronic idiopathic anal pain. Diseases of the Colon and Rectum 34:690–695

Hallan R, Williams N, Melling J et al 1988 Treatment of anismus in intractable constipation with Botulinum A toxin. Lancet 2:714–716

Halligan S, Sultan A, Rottenberg G, Bartram C 1995 Endosonography of the anal sphincters in solitary rectal ulcer syndrome. International Journal of Colorectal Diseases 10:79–82

Harvey R, Salih S, Read A 1983 Organic and functional disorders in 2000 gastroenterology outpatients. Lancet ii:623–634

Henry M, Parks A, Swash M 1982 The pelvic floor musculature in the descending perineum syndrome. British Journal of Surgery 69:470–472

Hinton J, Lennard-Jones J, Young A 1969 A new method for studying gut transit times using radio-opaque markers. Gut 10:842–847

Kamm M, Hawley P, Lennard-Jones J 1988 Outcome of colectomy for severe idiopathic constipation. Gut 29:969–973

Keighley M, Fielding J, Alexander-Williams J 1983 Results of Marlex mesh abdominal rectopexy for rectal prolapse in 100 consecutive patients. British Journal of Surgery 67:54–56

Keighley M, Shouler P 1984 Outlet syndrome: is there a surgical option? Journal of the Royal Society of Medicine 77:559–563

Koutsomanis D, Lennard-Jones J, Roy A, Kamm M 1995 Controlled randomised trial of biofeedback versus muscle training alone for intractable constipation. Gut 37:95–99

Kumar D, Williams N, Waldron D, Wingate D 1989 Prolonged manometric recording of anorectal motor activity in ambulant human subjects: evidence of periodic activity. Gut 30:1007–1011

Kumar D, Wingate D 1985 The irritable bowel syndrome: a paroxysmal motor disorder. Lancet i:973–980

Law P, Kamm M, Bartram C 1991 Anal endosonography in the investigation of faecal incontinence. British Journal of Surgery 78:312–314

Lechaux J, Lechaux D, Perez M 1995 Results of Delorme's procedure for rectal prolapse. Advantages of a modified technique. Diseases of the Colon and Rectum 38:301–307

Londono-Schimmer E, Garcia-Duperly R, Nicholls R et al 1994 Overlapping anal sphincter repair for fecal incontinence due to sphincter trauma: five-year follow-up functional results. International Journal of Colorectal Diseases 9:110–113

Loygue J, Nordlinger B, Cunei O et al 1984 Rectopexy to the promontory for the treatment of rectal prolapse. Diseases of the Colon and Rectum 27:356–359

Lubowski D, Nicholls R, Burleigh D, Swash M 1988 Internal anal sphincter in neurogenic fecal incontinence. Gastroenterology 95:997–1002

Luukkonen P, Mikkonen U, Jarvinen H 1992 Abdominal rectopexy with sigmoidectomy vs. rectopexy alone for rectal prolapse: a prospective, randomised study. International Journal of Colorectal Diseases 7:219–222

Mackle E, Mills J, Parks T 1990 The investigation of anorectal dysfunction in the solitary rectal ulcer syndrome. International Journal of Colorectal Diseases 5:21–24

Madigan M, Morson B 1969 Solitary ulcer of the rectum. Gut 10:871–881

Mahieu P, Pringot J, Bodart P 1984 Defecography: 1. Description of a new procedure and results in normal patients. Gastrointestinal Radiology 9:247–251

Metcalf A, Phillips S, Zinsmeister A et al 1987 Simplified assessment of segmental colonic transit. Gastroenterology 92:40–47

Miller R, Bartolo D, Locke-Edmunds J, Mortensen N 1988 Prospective study of conservative and operative treatment for faecal incontinence. British Journal of Surgery 75:101–105

Nielsen M, Hauge C, Rasmussen O et al 1992 Anal endosonographic findings in the follow-up of primarily sutured sphincteric ruptures. British Journal of Surgery 79:104–106

Notghi A, Kumar D, Panagamuwa B 1993 Measurement of colonic transit time using radionucleotide imaging: analysis by condensed images. Nuclear Medicine Communications 14:204–211

Parks A 1975 Anorectal incontinence. Proceedings of the Royal Society of Medicine 68:681–690

Pemberton J, Rath D, Ilstrup D 1991 Evaluation and surgical treatment of severe chronic constipation. Annals of Surgery 214:403–413

Pezim M, Spencer R, Stanhope C et al 1987 Sphincter repair for fecal incontinence after obstetrical or iatrogenic injury. Diseases of the Colon and Rectum 30:521–525

Ramanujam P, Venkatesh K 1988 Perineal excision of rectal prolapse with posterior levator ani in elderly high-risk patients. Diseases of the Colon and Rectum 31:704–706

Read N, Timms J, Barfield L et al 1986 Impairment of defaecation in young women with severe constipation. Gastroenterology 90:53–60

Roe A, Bartolo D, Mortensen N 1986 New method for assessment of anal sensation in various anorectal disorders. British Journal of Surgery 73:310–312

Rogers J, Henry M, Misiewicz J 1988a Disposable pudendal nerve stimulator: evaluation of the standard instrument and new device. Gut 29:1131–1133

Rogers J, Henry M, Misiewicz J 1988b Combined sensory and motor deficit in primary neuropathic faecal incontinence. Gut 29:5–9

Rutter K 1974 Electromyographic changes in certain pelvic floor abnormalities. Proceedings of the Royal Society of Medicine 67:53–56

Setti Carraro P, Kamm M, Nicholls R 1994 Long term results of postanal repair in the treatment of faecal incontinence. British Journal of Surgery 81:140–144

Shorvon P, McHugh S, Diamant N et al 1989 Defecography in normal volunteers: results and implications. Gut 30:1737–1749

Shouler P, Keighley M 1986 Changes in colorectal function in severe idiopathic constipation. Gastroenterology 90:414–420

Sitzler P, Kamm M, Nicholls R 1996 Surgery for solitary ulcer syndrome. International Journal of Colorectal Diseases 11:136

Snooks S, Setchell M, Swash M, Henry M 1985 Injury to the innervation of the pelvic floor musculature in childbirth. Lancet 2:546–550

Snooks S, Swash M, Henry M, Setchell M 1986 Risk factors in childbirth causing damage to the pelvic floor inervation. International Journal of Colorectal Diseases 1:20–24

Sorensen M, Tetzchner T, Rassmusen O et al 1993 Sphincter rupture in childbirth. British Journal of Surgery 80:392–394

Speakman C, Hoyle C, Kamm M et al 1990 Adrenergic control of the internal anal sphincter is abnormal in patients with idiopathic faecal incontinence. British Journal of Surgery 77:1342–1344

Sultan A, Kamm M, Hudson C et al 1993a Anal sphincter disruption during vaginal delivery. New England Journal of Medicine 329:1956–1957

Sultan A, Kamm M, Bartram C, Hudson C 1993b Anal sphincter trauma during instrumental delivery. International Journal of Gynaecology and Obstetrics 43:263–270

Sultan A, Kamm M, Nicholls R, Bartram C 1994 Prospective study of the extent of internal anal sphincter division during lateral sphincterotomy. Diseases of the Colon and Rectum 37:1031–1033

Talley N, O'Keefe E, Zinsmeister A, Melton J 1992 Prevalence of gastrointestinal symptoms in the elderly: a population based study. Gastroenterology 102:895–901

Tetzschner T, Sorensen M, Rasmussen O et al 1995 Pudendal nerve damage increases the risk of faecal incontinence in women with anal sphincter rupture after childbrith. Acta Obstetrica et Gynecologica Scandinavica 74:434–440

Todd I 1985 Clinical evaluation of the pelvic floor. In: Henry M, Swash M (eds) Coloproctology and the pelvic floor. Butterworth, London, pp 187–188

Wong W, Rothenberger D 1994 Artificial anal sphincter. In: Fielding L, Goldberg S (eds) Surgery of the colon, rectum, and anus, 5th edn. Butterworth-Heinemann, Oxford, 773–777

Yoshioka K, Keighley M 1989 Sphincter repair for fecal incontinence. Diseases of the Colon and Rectum 32:39–42

Section 5
WOMEN'S REPRODUCTIVE HEALTH

60
Chronic pelvic pain

R. William Stones

INTRODUCTION

Chronic pelvic pain is recognized as a difficult or unsatisfactory area of clinical practice, by both patients and doctors. Women report problems in communicating the impact of their long-standing symptoms to their gynaecologist and clinicians trained in a surgical model of care may feel frustrated at their inability rapidly to identify a causal pathological process and institute curative therapy. This chapter aims to draw together current knowledge on the condition. While it would be impossible to attempt comprehensive elucidation of all the related subject areas, the aim is to present an overview which at least acknowledges the key elements of an integrative bio-psychosocial approach to understanding the pathophysiology and management of the condition.

BIOLOGY OF PAIN

Pain is defined by the International Association for the Study of Pain as 'an unpleasant sensory and emotional experience associated with actual or potential tissue damage, or described in terms of such damage' (IASP Task Force on Taxonomy 1994). The emphasis in this definition is that pain is an experience rather than a neurophysiological process and is therefore subjective. There is no such thing as 'objective' pain. This does not mean, however, that pain cannot be studied or that reproducible experimental models cannot be devised. Neuroscience has taken forward knowledge of the biological processes underlying pain. It is no longer appropriate to discuss the subject in terms of 'pain pathways', by analogy with a wiring diagram, or even to consider that the nervous system conveys *perceptions* such as touch or pain. Rather, the elements of the nervous system, comprising the 'different fibres, tracts, pathways and nuclei *process and convey information about bodily stimulus events*' (Berkley & Hubscher 1995). In this model, pain is a central nervous system construct derived from the totality of sensory input rather than from the activation of a particular pathway. Even the anatomy of neural pathways in the adult cannot be considered immutable: plasticity of the central nervous system has been clearly demonstrated in reproducible animal experimental models, such that a nerve injury leads to sprouting of afferent fibres within the dorsal horn of the spinal cord (Woolf et al 1992).

Special features of chronic and visceral pain

The processes underlying the transition from a single or repeated acute painful episode to a chronic pain state are of great potential clinical significance: patients often relate the onset of their chronic condition to an event such as an acute infection or surgical procedure. Moreover, visceral sensory mechanisms differ in certain respects from those found in cutaneous tissues. Key mechanisms potentially underlying the transition from acute to chronic visceral pain states are the activation of silent afferents in viscera (McMahon 1997) and central sensitization (Woolf 1983). There are certain similarities but also important differences in the context of visceral sensation between central sensitization and *wind-up*, where the response to repeated C-fibre stimulation is progressively augmented (Herrero et al 2000). It is possible that the development of central sensitization and/or wind-up can be modulated by analgesics or other agents, which has led to the therapeutic strategy of pre-emptive analgesia (Dickenson 1997) although clinical applications of this concept have been disappointing.

Vascular pain and pelvic congestion

By analogy with the pathogenesis of cerebral migraine, it has been suggested that pain associated with pelvic congestion might arise through vascular perturbation at the ovarian or uterine arteriolar level, resulting in the release of endothelial factors such as ATP which act by exciting sensory nerves in the outer muscle coat of venules and veins and which also cause vasodilatation through the release of nitric oxide (Stones 2000).

Sex differences in pain

There is a marked sex difference in the prevalence of a number of chronic painful conditions unrelated to the reproductive tract in the general population, such as irritable bowel syndrome, temporomandibular dysfunction and interstitial cystitis, which has prompted research on the potential underlying mechanisms using animal models such as bladder irritation (Bon et al 1997), uterine and vaginal distension (Bradshaw et al 1999).

Studies of human volunteers have investigated pain thresholds in women at different stages of the menstrual cycle using electrical stimulation, pressure dolorimetry on the skin, thermal stimulation and induced ischaemic pain. Patterns of variation in response seen in studies using these modalities were different and a meta-analytical review of pain perception

across the menstrual cycle (Riley et al 1999) estimated the effect size for menstrual cycle fluctuation of pain sensitivity between the most and least sensitive phase to be 0.40. The effect size for sex difference was around 0.55, indicating that hormone variability could account for a substantial proportion but not all of the observed differences.

Illustrating some of the possible underlying mechanisms, a study of the discrimination of thermal pain in male and female volunteers showed that women had a lower pain threshold and tolerance, as also noted in a number of other studies (Fillingim et al 1998). A further complexity to be considered when interpreting studies of human volunteers is that subjects may well have prior pain experience which could influence responses to experimental pain (Fillingim et al 1999). Finally, the potential influence on pain perception of exogenous hormone therapy needs to be considered. In 87 postmenopausal women consulting for chronic orofacial pain, hormone replacement therapy was associated with greater reported levels of pain with substantial effect sizes between 0.39 and 0.62 (Wise et al 2000). The possibility of increased pain as a result of HRT use has not been addressed prospectively but may be clinically important, especially in women with vulval pain where oestrogen deficiency changes are thought to co-exist.

Genetic variation in susceptibility to pain

Evidence for a genetic basis for the variation in response to painful stimulation is emerging in animal experimental studies (Mogil et al 1999a,b). There is clearly a long way to go before conclusions clinically relevant to pain in humans can be drawn, but there are already some important and relevant observations. For example a twin study showed that whereas 39% of the variance in reported menstrual flow was accounted for by genetic factors, the corresponding figure for dysmenorrhoea was 55% and for functional limitation from menstrual symptoms 77% (Treloar et al 1998).

EPIDEMIOLOGY OF PELVIC PAIN: POPULATIONS, CONSULTING AND REFERRAL PATTERNS

The first assessment of the prevalence and economic burden associated with chronic pelvic pain was based on extrapolation from hospital practice in the UK and estimated the prevalence in women at 24.4 per 1000. The annual direct treatment cost was estimated at £158 million, with indirect costs of £24 million (Davies et al 1992). The above prevalence now appears an underestimate since data from population-based studies have become available. A telephone survey was undertaken in the USA using a robust sampling methodology (Mathias et al 1996). Women aged 18–50 were interviewed about pelvic pain-related symptoms. 17 927 households were contacted, 5325 women agreed to participate and of these 925 reported pelvic pain of at least 6 months' duration, including pain within the past 3 months. Having excluded those pregnant or postmenopausal and those with only cycle-related pain, 773/5263 (14.7%) were identified as suffering from chronic pelvic pain. Direct costs of healthcare, estimated from Medicare tariffs and hence very conservative, were

$881.5 million, patients' out-of-pocket expenses were estimated at $1.9 billion and indirect costs due to time off work were estimated at $555.3 million.

In the UK, the population perspective was provided by a postal survey of 2016 women randomly selected from the Oxfordshire Health Authority register of 141400 women aged 18–49 (Zondervan et al 2001b). Chronic pelvic pain was defined as recurrent pain of at least 6 months' duration, unrelated to periods, intercourse or pregnancy. For the survey, a 'case' was defined as a women with chronic pelvic pain in the previous 3 months and on this basis the prevalence was 483/2016 (24.0%). Among those with pelvic pain, dysmenorrhoea was reported by 81% of those who had periods and dyspareunia was reported by 41% of those who were sexually active. Among women who did not have chronic pelvic pain as defined above, dysmenorrhoea was reported by 58% of those who had periods and dyspareunia was reported by 14% of those who were sexually active.

An estimate of the consulting pattern associated with pelvic pain was obtained using a national database study of UK general practices (Zondervan et al 1999b). Data relating to 284162 women aged 12–70 who had a general practice contact in 1991 were analysed to identify subsequent contacts over the following 5 years. The monthly prevalence rate was 21.5/1000 and the monthly incidence rate was 1.58/1000. These prevalence rates are comparable to those for migraine, back pain and asthma in primary care. Older women had higher monthly prevalence rates: for example, the rate was 18.2/1000 in the 15–20 year age group and 27.6/1000 in women over 60 years of age. This association is thought to be due to persistence of symptoms in older women, the median duration of symptoms being 13.7 months in 13–20 year olds and 20.2 months in women over the age of 60 (Zondervan et al 1999a). It is clear that future population-based studies need to include older women.

Among 483 women with chronic pelvic pain participating in the Oxfordshire population study discussed above, 195 (40.4%) had not sought a medical consultation, 127 (26.3%) reported a past consultation and 139 (28.8%) reported a recent consultation for pain (Zondervan et al 2001b). Of those women identified as cases of pelvic pain in the national general practice database, 28% were not given a specific diagnosis and 60% were not referred to hospital (Zondervan et al 1999a). The US population-based study discussed above also drew attention to the large numbers of women who have troublesome symptoms but do not seek medical attention: 75% of this sample had not seen a healthcare provider in the previous 3 months. It might be thought that not seeking care would be an indicator of milder symptoms and indeed, in the US study those who did seek medical attention had higher pain and lower general health scores than those who did not. However, among those not seeking help, scores for pain and functional impairment were still substantial. Lack of use of medical services might reflect sociocultural factors but could equally reflect previous unsatisfactory experiences of investigation and treatment as discussed later in this chapter.

Among women referred to a UK gynaecology outpatient clinic with chronic pelvic pain of at least 6 months' duration, the impact of the condition on quality of life was assessed

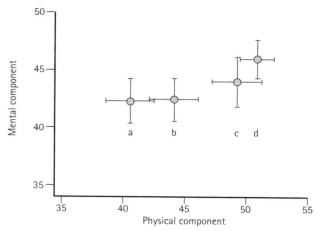

Fig. 60.1 Means +/– 95% confidence interval for the SF-36 mental component and physical component summary scales. Women with pelvic pain **a** seen in a general gynaecology clinic (Stones et al 2000) or in a postal survey (Zondervan et al 2001b) reporting **b** a recent consultation, **c** a previous consultation or **d** no medical consultation. Arbitrary units such that 50 represents the mean of a normal population.

using the SF-36 questionnaire (Stones et al 2000). Figure 60.1 shows a comparison of physical and mental component summary scores derived from the eight SF-36 subscales (Jenkinson et al 1996a) in this hospital population with the data from the Oxfordshire population study described above. These summary scores are adjusted such that 50 represents a normal population mean. It will be noted that, as might be expected, the hospital sample is consistent with the trend, evident in those who have previously or recently sought medical advice subscales compared to those who have not, to greater impairment of function on both physical and mental component.

PSYCHOLOGICAL FACTORS IN CHRONIC PELVIC PAIN

Many writers on pelvic pain have attempted to characterize an adverse psychological profile which might help the clinician to distinguish between 'organic' and 'psychogenic' pain, a distinction not in keeping with current neurophysiological understanding as discussed above. It is likely that some of the psychological disturbance that can be identified in women with chronic pelvic pain is the result of long-standing pain symptoms and unsatisfactory treatments, rather than the cause of pain (Slocumb et al 1989). Pain may contribute to or confirm a sense of helplessness or a tendency to engage in catastrophic thoughts and may itself be exacerbated by them (Horn & Munafo 1997). On the other hand, it is clear that concomitant mood disturbance or specific psychopathology may impair the patient's ability to cope with her symptoms and contribute to functional impairment and recognition is important but often neglected in the hurried setting of a gynaecology clinic (Yonkers 1995).

Depression

Women presenting with multiple pain symptoms are at especially high risk for current mood disturbance: the likelihood of an associated mood disorder was increased sixfold in individuals with two pain complaints and eightfold in those with three complaints (Dworkin et al 1990). In keeping with the irrelevance of the organic/psychogenic distinction for diagnosis, the absence of laparoscopically visible pathology was not associated with a higher probability of depression (Peveler et al 1995, Waller & Shaw 1995). In these studies no differences in mood-related symptoms were identified in women with chronic pelvic pain with and without endometriosis. Antidepressant therapy may be indicated in order to alleviate depression, but sertraline was not effective for pelvic pain in a recent small but well-conducted randomized trial (Engel et al 1998).

Abuse and somatization

Child sexual or physical abuse may be an antecedent for chronic pelvic pain but many individuals have suffered such abuse without this or other consequence in later life and the research literature is beset with the problem of appropriate comparison groups. A study from a tertiary referral multi-disciplinary clinic setting reported on the full assessment of psychological factors in three groups of 30 women with chronic pelvic pain, chronic pain of other types or women without pain identified from general practitioner records. Twelve (40%) of those with chronic pelvic pain reported sexual abuse compared to five (17%) in each of the two comparison groups. Experience of physical violence was similar in the three groups, but women with chronic pelvic pain had higher scores for somatization, meaning the experience and communication of distress and physical symptoms without clear underlying pathology. In women with pelvic pain, abuse histories were evenly distributed among those with and without identified pelvic pathology such as endometriosis, but somatization scores were higher among those with identified pathology (Collett et al 1998). It has been suggested that the potential link between sexual abuse and pelvic pain might be that abuse is an observable marker for childhood neglect in general (Fry et al 1997) and this might explain the association in some studies with physical rather than sexual abuse (Rapkin et al 1990).

Identification of patients with features suggesting somatization disorder is important as failure to do so will lead to further inappropriate investigation and treatment directed towards physical symptoms which are in fact manifestations of psychological distress. There are limited data as to the prevalence of frank somatization disorder in clinic populations; in a study comparing the medical assessment with a standardized questionnaire, doctors identified 19% of patients as being potential somatizers and around 5% met questionnaire criteria for overt somatization disorder (Peveler et al 1997).

Hostility

Hostility may be defined as an attitudinal bias that predisposes the individual to view others as 'untrustworthy, undeserving and immoral' (Barefoot 1992). It has been suggested that the cardiovascular risk associated with hostility is mediated through excessive sympathetic drive but another important factor may be that hostile individuals find difficulty in forming supportive relationships, one special type of which being the doctor–patient relationship. Where the patient is hostile the doctor, unless prepared, will find it difficult to establish an appropriate therapeutic relationship. The relevance to consultations for pelvic pain was investigated in a tertiary referral setting where the patient's rating of the medical consultation was shown to be related to a dimension of hostility expressing its inward or outward direction (Fry & Stones 1996). Again, the question of causality remains, as cynical hostility may either reflect adverse early life experiences or might be a consequence of the negative experience of pelvic pain over many years, together with frustrating and inconclusive medical encounters. A feature of special interest is the potential for hostile attitudes to engender further unsatisfactory medical consultations, thus perpetuating the patient's isolation and distress. It should be noted that there are uncertainties about the validity and reliability of some of the instruments used to assess hostility and this is an area where further research is needed.

SOCIOCULTURAL FACTORS IN CHRONIC PELVIC PAIN

It could be argued that in life-threatening medical conditions or conditions where a technical solution gives excellent results, the patient's experience of care and the quality of doctor–patient communication are not critical to the outcome. In contrast, in ill-defined, chronic conditions where a technical solution is unlikely to provide relief, sociocultural factors have a major influence on the patient's decision to seek care and the referral pathway subsequently followed. The population-based studies cited above provide an indication of the size of the iceberg of symptoms below the waterline of care seeking. Similarly, in general practice many women remain undiagnosed and unreferred. This is not necessarily inappropriate but the determinants of presentation and referral are unlikely to be disease factors alone. Once seen in a gynaecology clinic, the interaction between disease states and the consultation setting can be identified in statistical models: the presence of endometriosis was a factor predicting continuing pain 6 months after an initial hospital outpatient consultation but so also were the patient's initial report of pain interfering with exercise, her rating of the initial medical consultation as less satisfactory (Fig. 60.2) and the individual clinician undertaking the consultation (but not the doctor's grade or gender) (Selfe et al 1998a).

These statistical observations are consistent with women's descriptions of their experiences during the referral and treatment process. Sometimes news of the absence of specific pathology at laparoscopy is received not as reassurance but as a dismissal. The patient's loss of confidence is expressed in these words obtained during focus group interviews:

'Well – I suppose they must have done their job but they said to me that I probably had endometriosis and I felt all my symptoms related to that and that's what it was going to be – it seems strange that they don't actually find anything but obviously they're looking and they know what they can see ...'.

Often, problems are encountered not just with a particular individual clinician or aspect of care, but tend to accumulate

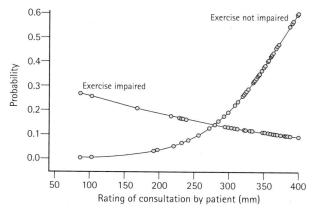

Fig. 60.2 Fitted probabilities of complete pain resolution with and without exercise impairment in relation to the patient's rating of the initial hospital consultation (Selfe et al 1998a). In women without exercise impairment a favourable rating of the initial consultation is associated with a higher probability of pain resolution, but the consultation has no effect in those with impairment.

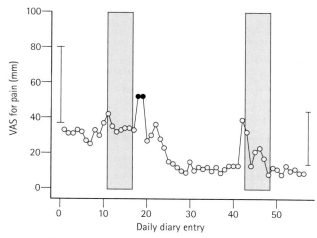

Fig. 60.3 Visual analogue pain scores (circles) from a daily pain diary completed over 8 weeks by a patient undergoing treatment as part of a clinical trial (Stones et al 2001). Vertical bars show the recalled 'usual' (lower end of bars) and 'most severe' (upper end of bars) pain scores from the previous 4 weeks. Hatched areas show days of menstruation and filled circles indicate days when intercourse occurred.

for some patients as they move through the system. This seems to be more of a problem for women of low socioeconomic status (Grace 1995). A solution to this mismatch between women's needs and the structures through which care is provided may be the multidisciplinary approach which at least works against the crude compartmentalized organic/psychological causation model, although it has been suggested that a more fundamental reconsideration of the medical paradigm is required (Grace 1998). Meanwhile, within the practical constraints of time, lack of continuity of care in the hospital setting and very limited access to multidisciplinary resources, gynaecologists can at least recognize the potential impact of their own attitudes and communication styles (Selfe et al 1998b).

CLINICAL ASSESSMENT

The conventional gynaecological history needs to be supplemented in consultations for chronic pelvic pain by additional information to aid understanding of the impact of symptoms and diagnosis.

Pain history

The history needs to include the onset and duration of symptoms, the location and radiation of pain, factors associated with exacerbation and relief and the relationship of pain to the menstrual cycle. Dysmenorrhoea may be a separate or related symptom. Dyspareunia may include pain during intercourse but for many women a particularly unpleasant symptom is postcoital pain and specific enquiry should be made about this.

A number of validated pain assessment measures are available for use in research and clinical practice, the most convenient of which are the 10 cm visual analogue scale, the Brief Pain Inventory (BPI) and the McGill Short Form pain questionnaire. The McGill questionnaire is included in the International Pelvic Pain Society's assessment form, available

for downloading at www.pelvicpain.org and the BPI may be downloaded at prg.mdanderson.org/bpi.htm. Patients' recall of pain symptoms over the previous month seems to be adequate and it is probably unnecessary to ask for a daily pain diary: 10 cm visual analogue scales for 'usual' and 'most severe' intensity of pain recalled over the past 4 weeks correlated very well with mean and maximal diary records (Fig. 60.3) (Stones et al 2001).

Impact on quality of life

At present a validated illness-specific instrument is not available for assessing quality of life and functional impairment in women with pelvic pain. Simple questions about the effect of the pain on work, leisure, sleep and sexual relationships are nevertheless useful. A generic quality of life measure such as the SF-36 may be used for monitoring outcomes. The SF-36 is somewhat problematic when used in episodic conditions such as menorrhagia (Jenkinson et al 1996b) but has face validity and reliability in chronic pelvic pain (Stones et al 2000). A manual describing the application of the UK version of the questionnaire and the calculation of the physical and mental component summary scales as used in Figure 60.1 may be obtained at hsru.dphpc.ox.ac.uk/newsf36.htm.

Sexual and physical abuse

The extent to which clinicians can or should attempt to elicit a history of sexual or physical abuse during a gynaecological consultation is a matter for judgement in relation to the setting, in particular the follow-up and support that are available to women following such disclosure. The history may be volunteered by the patient unprompted, especially so during a subsequent consultation when rapport has been established. Some women may even find it easier to raise the subject with an unfamiliar specialist than with a general practitioner with whom they have regular consultations for other matters. It may be useful to incorporate questions on abuse into a self-completion questionnaire, such as that provided by the International Pelvic Pain Society, or in a multidisciplinary clinic to address the topic during a consultation with the nurse or psychologist.

Systems review

The history should be thorough with regards to symptoms potentially indicative of irritable bowel syndrome: the poor outcome of patients with IBS referred to gynaecology clinics has been emphasized (Prior & Whorwell 1989). It is unlikely that dyspareunia can be attributed to IBS: bowel spasm perhaps accounts for the experience of those patients who describe an interval between the end of intercourse and the onset of acute pain (Whorwell 1995) associated with the urge to defaecate and abdominal distension. Pain associated with micturition or a full bladder should be enquired about, as there may be some overlap between chronic pelvic pain and the interstitial cystitis spectrum discussed in Chapter 56.

Physical examination

Observing the patient as she walks may give an indication of a musculoskeletal problem and examination of the back is relevant in those giving a history of pain radiating or originating there. The abdominal examination may reveal specific sites of tenderness. One-finger 'trigger point' tenderness will suggest a nerve entrapment, often involving the ilioinguinal or iliohypogastric nerves. These can develop spontaneously as well as following surgery. The diagnosis is confirmed after obtaining appropriate consent by infiltration of local anaesthetic into the tender area. 'Ovarian point' tenderness has been described as a feature of pelvic congestion syndrome (Beard et al 1988) but this sign is problematic in patients with irritable bowel syndrome who often have similar abdominal tenderness. A general neurological examination is appropriate to exclude a systemic neuropathy or demyelination and if abnormalities are present, a neurology opinion should be sought.

Vaginal examination should commence with a careful inspection of the vulva and introitus, paying particular attention to the presence of erythema which might suggest primary vulval vestibulitis (Gibbons 1998) (see Chapter 40). More frequently, no erythema is evident but a gentle touch with a cotton-tipped swab in the area just external to the hymeneal ring elicits intense sharp pain, even in patients who do not complain of dyspareunia. This allodynia in the absence of visible erythema probably represents referred sensation from painful areas higher in the pelvis but for some women represents the primary problem. Vulval varices may indicate incompetence of valves in the pelvic venous circulation; this subgroup of patients may benefit from radiological assessment and treatment (see below).

A gentle one-finger digital examination commences with palpation of the pelvic floor muscles. Focal tenderness may be present, indicating a primary musculoskeletal problem that should prompt referral to a pelvic floor physiotherapist for further assessment. As with 'vestibulitis', pelvic muscle tenderness may be a residual secondary response to pain from other parts of the pelvis, for example a previous episode of pelvic infection. Further digital examination may reveal nodularity in the pouch of Douglas or restricted uterine mobility suggestive of endometriosis. Adenomyosis may be suggested by a bulky tender uterus. Uterine retroversion should be noted although its relevance to dyspareunia is debatable. Adnexal rather than uterine tenderness may point to pelvic congestion syndrome. In the UK clinic setting, pelvic tenderness is unlikely to indicate chronic pelvic inflammatory disease although this diagnosis will be more likely among populations where early and appropriate antibiotic treatment for acute pelvic sepsis is less readily given.

INVESTIGATIONS

It is helpful to discount active pelvic infection, especially the presence of chlamydia, early in the assessment by taking endocervical swabs. Ultrasound examination may be useful in identifying uterine or adnexal pathology. The presence of dilated veins may indicate pelvic congestion (Stones et al 1990) but a recent study using power Doppler suggested that the primary value of sonography was to identify the characteristic multicystic ovarian morphology seen in this condition (Halligan et al 2000). Transuterine venography is of limited value in routine clinical practice but is technically simpler than selective catheterization of the ovarian vein. MRI provides the opportunity to identify adenomyosis but is not routinely indicated.

Laparoscopy is commonly undertaken as the primary investigation for chronic pelvic pain in many countries. The aim of laparoscopy is to aid diagnosis but also increasingly to provide 'one-stop' treatment for endometriosis and adhesions where these are identified. This approach is cost effective for endometriosis treatment, as the expense of a second procedure or hormonal treatment is obviated (Stones & Thomas 1995). However, given the potential for confusion arising from a 'negative' laparoscopy (Howard 1996) and the lack of a clear impact of recourse to laparoscopy on outcome at the referral population level (Peters et al 1991, Selfe et al 1998b), arguments in favour of deferring laparoscopy, at least until initial symptomatic treatment has failed, take on some force. The impetus for treatment using GnRH agonists without laparoscopic diagnosis has emanated from the US-managed care environment (Winkel 1999) and in the UK from retrospective assessment of outcomes (Lyall et al 1999). The outcome of prospective studies is awaited with interest. For clinical practice the timing of laparoscopy is a matter for discussion with the patient based on her needs for diagnosis and treatment and the overall context of treatment modalities available.

Pain mapping by laparoscopy under conscious sedation can be a useful procedure, particularly where the site of pain is unilateral, allowing comparison with a 'control' area, to assess the significance of adhesions, to identify unrecognized occult inguinal or femoral hernias and in the negative sense to identify individuals with a generalized hyperalgesic chronic pain state for whom further surgical intervention would be hazardous. The choice of instrumentation represents a trade-off between the lower quality field of view available from a 2 mm laparoscope and patient discomfort associated with a larger trocar and cannula. In practice, a 5 mm laparoscope does not cause significantly more pain than the smaller instruments. The role of this procedure remains to be clarified in the overall context of pain assessment and management but reports of experience are now available in the literature (Howard 1999).

DIAGNOSIS AND TREATMENT: SPECIFIC CONDITIONS

There is limited evidence from randomized clinical trials on which to base treatment decisions for women with chronic pelvic pain (Stones & Mountfield 2000). An approach to specific conditions is outlined below.

Pelvic congestion syndrome

This condition may be considered a clinical syndrome based on the characteristic symptom complex described by Beard and colleagues (1988). Pelvic congestion is typically a condition of the reproductive years and, in contrast to endometriosis, is equally prevalent among parous and nulliparous women. There may be an underlying endocrine dysfunction although peripheral hormone levels are not abnormal: the associated ovarian morphology is characterized by predominantly atretic follicles scattered throughout the stroma, while in contrast to polycystic ovary syndrome the volume of the ovary is normal. The thecal and rostenedione response to LH was increased as in PCO but granulosa cell estradiol production was reduced compared to normal tissue (Gilling-Smith et al 2000).

Symptoms include exacerbation of pain with prolonged standing, dyspareunia and postcoital aching and a fluctuating localization of pain. Patients may derive reassurance from being given the diagnosis as an explanation of their pain in terms of a functional condition similar to cerebral migraine. Therapy includes identification of stressors and the use of hormonal treatment in combination with stress and pain management, with the aim of encouraging the patient to make appropriate lifestyle changes so that on completion of a course of hormonal treatment her symptoms are less likely to recur. Medroxyprogesterone acetate 50 mg daily has been shown to be effective (Farquhar et al 1989) and GnRH agonists with oestrogen 'add-back' are increasingly used in this indication although so far randomized trial data are lacking. Hysterectomy and bilateral salpingo-oophorectomy followed by long-term oestrogen replacement therapy is an option for those who have extreme symptoms partially or temporarily relieved by hormonal therapy but this is naturally a treatment of last resort (Beard et al 1991).

Patients with peripheral venous disease and vulval varicosities are probably manifesting a different clinical entity from those described above. A surgical approach involving extraperitoneal dissection of the ovarian veins has been described (Hobbs 1976) and this group of patients may benefit from current interventional radiology techniques for vein occlusion (Fig. 60.4). However, the evidence for useful benefit in those without vulval or lower limb varices remains anecdotal.

Endometriosis

Endometriosis is discussed in detail in Chapter 34. From the perspective of clinical practice in chronic pelvic pain, endometriosis presents special problems at both ends of the spectrum of disease severity. Women with endometriosis have poor outcomes compared to those with other conditions in terms of pain relief (Selfe et al 1998a) and they require careful attention to the provision of effective pain relief. Many women have undergone laparoscopy with the expectation of endometriosis being confirmed and have difficulty coming to terms with the lack of a positive diagnosis when endometriosis is not found, as illustrated in the extract from a patient's comments presented above.

Treatments which suppress or ablate endometriosis are, in general, associated with relief of pain. In the case of hormonal therapies a major benefit is the suppression of menstruation, resulting in the prevention of dysmenorrhoea. Laparoscopic surgical ablation of deposits in stage I–III disease is associated with reduction in pain as demonstrated in the single available randomized trial (Sutton et al 1994) and laparoscopic surgery for late-stage endometriosis also improves pain symptoms, quality of life and sexual function (Garry et al 2000). There are insufficient data to make clear recommendations about the different available surgical approaches, for example laser vaporization versus excision and diathermy.

The place of laparoscopic uterine nerve ablation, as opposed to ablation of visible deposits, remains unclear. More positive results have been reported for presacral neurectomy (PSN) in primary dysmenorrhoea (Chen et al 1996, Nezhat et al 1998) which perhaps reflects the greater potential for interrupting sensory pathways to the uterus offered by this procedure. There is significant surgical risk associated with PSN and an incidence of complications, especially constipation, and the importance of high-level surgical skills has been emphasized (Perry & Perez 1993). In the light of the discussion of pain mechanisms earlier in this chapter, efforts to achieve pain relief by interruption of nerve pathways are probably naïve as they do not take into account the central nervous system contribution to the maintenance of chronic pain states following an initial inflammatory insult, of which endometriosis represents a good example.

Adhesions

Critical studies of the relationship between adhesions and pain suggest that they are often likely to be coincidental rather than causal (Rapkin 1986). Adhesiolysis is only effective for adhesions that are dense, vascularized or adherent to bowel (Peters et al 1992). As discussed above, pain mapping by laparoscopy under conscious sedation may be useful in identifying adhesions that are tender rather asymptomatic, with due regard to the complexities of visceral sensory pathways previously reviewed and the sensitivity and discrimination of sensations from the pelvic organs under normal conditions (Koninckx & Renaer 1997). Laparoscopic adhesiolysis needs to be undertaken with particular care so as to avoid bowel injury and with appropriate preoperative counselling and bowel preparation.

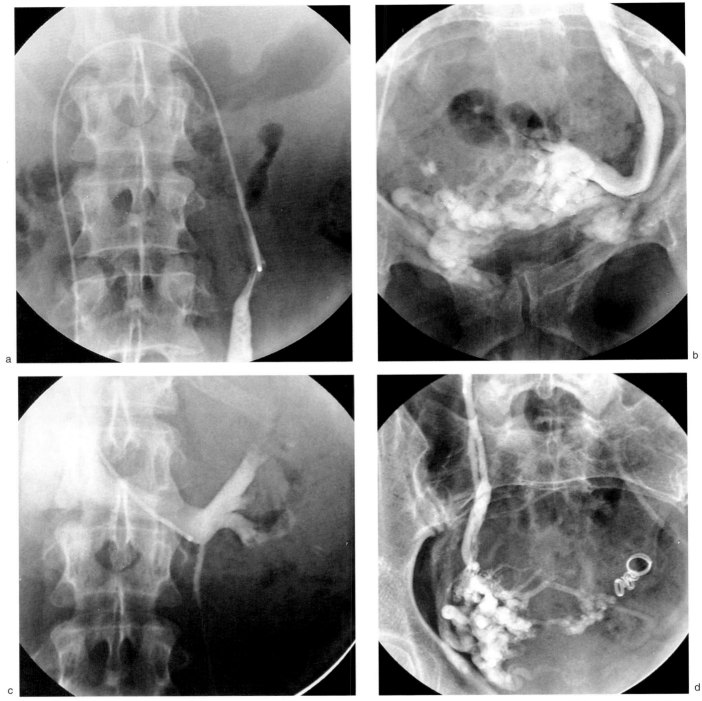

Fig. 60.4 Selective catheterization of the ovarian veins in a patient who presented with aching vulval varicosities which were successfully treated by embolization. **a** Transfemoral approach to the proximal left ovarian vein. **b** Distal left ovarian vein. Note dilatation and extensive communications to the uterine veins despite previous left oophorectomy. **c** Transjugular approach 2 months post embolization. Note occluded left ovarian vein. **d** Right ovarian vein showing residual collaterals. Note embolization coils visible on the patient's left. Images courtesy of Dr Nigel Hacking, Consultant Radiologist, Southampton General Hospital.

Chronic pelvic inflammatory disease

In UK clinical practice, chronic PID should be a laparoscopic diagnosis based on the finding of tubal damage and signs of active infection. Depending on the referral population, the true prevalence will vary but a diagnosis based on a clinical impression of pelvic tenderness and partial response to repeated courses of antibiotics is likely to be incorrect. This observation is also relevant for regions with a higher background

Fig. 60.5 Abdominal wall anatomy illustrating the course of the ilioinguinal and iliohypogastric nerves (after von Bahr 1979).

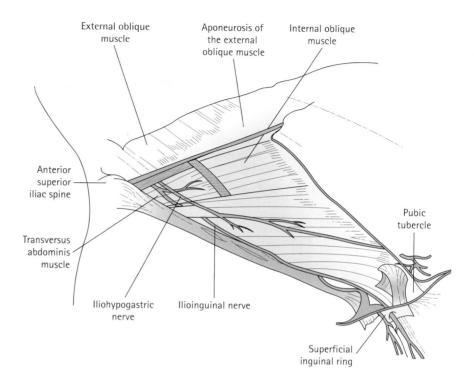

External oblique muscle

Aponeurosis of the external oblique muscle

Internal oblique muscle

Anterior superior iliac spine

Transversus abdominis muscle

Iliohypogastric nerve

Ilioinguinal nerve

Pubic tubercle

Superficial inguinal ring

prevalence of pelvic inflammatory disease such as sub-Saharan Africa (Kasule 1991). Apart from not resolving her problem, incorrect labelling of a patient as suffering from chronic PID may lead the patient to adopt an extremely negative self-image and inflict on her inappropriate anxiety about future fertility.

Where the diagnosis is confirmed, surgery in the form of salpingectomy or salpingo-oophorectomy may well be indicated rather than conservative management. Efforts to prevent continuing pain from ovarian adhesions have included ovariopexy and the use of barrier films but evidence in the literature of actual pain relief is scanty.

Nerve entrapment

The finding of abdominal wall tenderness which is consistently localized to a particular point should lead to consideration of a nerve entrapment. These predominantly involve the ilioinguinal and iliohypogastric nerves whose anatomy is illustrated in Figure 60.5, but genitofemoral nerve entrapment has also been described. A typical protocol for management includes establishing the diagnosis by infiltration of bupivacaine 0.25% and demonstrating complete relief of pain and tenderness. This can be followed by one or two injections 1 month apart of bupivacaine and a long-acting corticosteroid such as Depo Medrone 40 mg. Surgical exploration and excision of the nerve can be undertaken with around 70% success (Hahn 1989, Lee & Dellon 2000). The response to an initial infiltration of bupivacaine is often much more prolonged than would be expected from the duration of action of the local anaesthetic, perhaps because minor perineural adhesions are broken down by the volume of the infiltration or surrounding muscle spasm is relieved.

Neuropathic and postsurgical pelvic pain

Whereas abdominal nerve-related pain can often be clearly localized to a particular site, post-hysterectomy pain at the vaginal vault and vaginal pain following childbirth may be more difficult to evaluate. It is likely that the nerves involved are small unmyelinated fibres travelling in the nervi erigentes to the sacral segments and branches of the pudendal nerve. While nerve latency studies may be of value in assessing injury to the pudendal nerve, local anaesthetic nerve blockade is singularly unsuccessful. There may be the potential for surgery to decompress Alcock's canal where this is identified as the specific area of nerve compression, but case definition remains controversial.

In post-hysterectomy pain, pain mapping may be useful to delineate the extent of tenderness at the vaginal vault but this is usually with a view to aiding acceptance of a multidisciplinary pain management approach to treatment including drugs such as gabapentin and cognitive-behavioural psychology (see below) rather than with an expectation of identifying a focal lesion amenable to surgery. Patients with more extensive neuropathy should be referred for a neurology opinion.

A special instance of postsurgical pain where further surgery is indicated is ovarian remnant syndrome, where a fragment of active ovarian tissue generates pain through continued ovulatory activity. The diagnosis can be made by withdrawing oestrogen replacement therapy and demonstrating endogeneous hormone production and the lesion localized by the administration of clomiphene or human menopausal gonadotrophin prior to imaging. The surgery is technically challenging and is best approached by laparotomy rather than laparoscopy (Richlin & Rock 2001).

Hernias

Occult inguinal hernias have been recognized in women presenting with pain but without the normal swelling or cough impulse (Herrington 1975) but surgeons have naturally been reluctant to operate in the absence of more definite physical signs. Current surgical thinking on inguinal and femoral hernias and rarities such as spigelian and obturator hernias is discussed in a recent review (Daoud 1998). Inguinal and femoral hernias can readily be evaluated during pain mapping laparoscopy as the anatomy can be easily visualized and localized tenderness detected and laparoscopic repair can subsequently be undertaken.

Diagnostic overlap and 'no diagnosis'

Despite the best efforts of clinicians to identify specific causes of pelvic pain, it will be unclear how to classify many patients. In a consecutive series of 98 patients referred for investigation by their general practitioner, diagnoses were endometriosis (n = 12), adhesions (n = 10) and other gross pathology (n = 15). No positive diagnosis could be established in 29 patients. Three or more irritable bowel syndrome symptoms were present in 15 patients but in 13 there was overlap with other diagnoses. A symptom complex suggestive of pelvic congestion syndrome was present in 57 patients, but this overlapped with seven cases of endometriosis, six of adhesions, eight of gross pathology and nine of irritable bowel syndrome (Selfe et al 1998b). Similar findings of no positive diagnosis and diagnostic overlap were noted in women consulting in primary care (Zondervan et al 1999a) and self-reports of symptoms and received diagnoses in a population survey (Zondervan et al 2001a).

MANAGEMENT SETTINGS AND STRATEGIES

The general approach to treatment of chronic pelvic pain needs to reflect the patient population and to meet the different needs of individual women. Diagnostic and treatment plans need to be able to accommodate the spectrum of chronicity and severity of symptoms: it would probably be inappropriate to enrol every patient referred from general practice into a comprehensive multidisciplinary pain management programme but it would be equally inappropriate to subject a patient who has undergone multiple previous investigations and treatments for long-standing disabling pain to a brief clinical encounter with an inconclusive outcome. If data from a UK hospital outpatient population can be regarded as typical, approximately 25% of women referred by general practitioners still had significant pain 6 months after an initial consultation: perhaps this represents the scale of unmet need for a multidisciplinary service. Very few hospitals in the UK at present provide adequate services for women with chronic pelvic pain in the spirit of the Clinical Standards Advisory Group report on services for patients with pain (CSAG 2000).

An important step in formulating a management plan for any patient is to establish her treatment goals, especially whether she is primarily concerned with identifying a cause for her pain or is less concerned with causation but desires rapid symptomatic relief. In the former instance further investigation such as laparoscopy may help the patient towards her goal, whereas in the latter case initial symptomatic treatment may be more appropriate. Further clarification may be required as to the relative priority the patient gives to pain relief and restoration of normal function. The impact of a well-conducted and sympathetic consultation may itself be therapeutic based on some of the research discussed above and indeed, ultrasonography has been used effectively as a means of providing reassurance (Ghaly 1994).

For patients at the more severe end of the illness spectrum the elements of a pain management approach become more important and indeed, randomized trial evidence supports multidisciplinary care (Peters et al 1991). Multidisciplinary care may include contributions from other disciplines including anaesthesia, psychology, physiotherapy, nursing and liaison psychiatry. The analgesic regimen is optimized, bearing in mind that 6–10% of the Caucasian population are unable to metabolize codeine (Eckhardt et al 1998), and full use is made of adjunctive agents such as amitriptyline 10–50 mg at night or gabapentin in an incremental regimen from 400 to 3600 mg daily. The latter agent is indicated for neuropathic pain and does not interact with the oral contraceptive pill but has adverse effects of giddiness and drowsiness. Randomized trials have shown gabapentin to be of benefit for pain relief in diabetic neuropathy and trigeminal neuralgia (Backonja et al 1998, Rowbotham et al 1998).

Regular scheduled follow-up is an important element of a pain management programme, as distinct from pain-contingent consultations, and every effort must be made to provide continuity of care. Transcutaneous electrical nerve stimulation can be offered in appropriate circumstances and advice given on its correct use. The neurophysiological basis for TENS is that transmission of impulses via unmyelinated C fibres is inhibited at the level of the dorsal horn of the spinal cord by the activation of cutaneous myelinated afferents using electrical stimulation. Evidence from randomized trials suggests that while ineffective in labour pain and acute postsurgical pain, there may well be benefit in dysmenorrhoea. Formal trials of TENS in the context of chronic pelvic pain are lacking.

Where mood disturbance is identified, concomitant antidepressant therapy should be suggested and where there are indications of more complex psychopathology, in particular somatoform disorder, then a liaison psychiatry opinion is appropriate. The rate of attendance by gynaecological patients referred to psychiatric departments is extremely low and there are considerable advantages to service models which enable cross-referral on the same premises at short notice, but these often present practical problems. Psychological assessment itself has therapeutic value (Price & Blake 1999) and a psychologist or psychotherapist can provide guidance on pain and/or stress management and motivate patients to move from passivity to active participation in their treatment. Wherever possible, patients should be offered the opportunity of a structured programme of cognitive-behavioural therapy as evidence for the benefit of this approach is strong (CSAG 2000).

KEY POINTS

1. Pain is a central nervous system construct.
2. The organic/psychogenic categorization is obsolete.
3. The central nervous system exhibits plasticity.
4. Hormonal, sex and genetic factors influence pain perception.
5. Chronic visceral pain may involve activation of silent afferents and hyperalgesia.
6. Chronic pelvic pain is common among the general population and those consulting GPs.
7. Consultation rates are influenced by social class.
8. Mood disturbance, sequelae of abuse and hostility may be associated factors.
9. Women with multiple unexplained physical symptoms may have somatoform disorder.
10. Women with pelvic pain often find their experience of care unsatisfactory.
11. Pelvic congestion symptoms include dyspareunia and postcoital aching.
12. Pain mapping may be useful in the assessment of adhesions.
13. Chronic PID should only be diagnosed at laparoscopy and is uncommon in UK practice.
14. In many women the diagnosis is unclear or diagnoses overlap.
15. Multidisciplinary care is more effective than standard care.
16. The model of care needs to meet the individual needs of women.
17. Experience of care can influence clinical outcome.
18. Ultrasonography can be used to provide reassurance.

REFERENCES

Backonja M, Beydoun A, Edwards K et al 1998 Gabapentin for the symptomatic treatment of painful neuropathy in patients with diabetes mellitus – a randomized controlled trial. Journal of the American Medical Association 280:1831–1836

Barefoot J 1992 Developments in the measurement of hostility. In: Friedman H (ed) Hostility, coping and health. American Psychological Association, Washington DC, pp 13–31

Beard RW, Reginald PW, Wadsworth J 1988 Clinical features of women with chronic lower abdominal pain and pelvic congestion. British Journal of Obstetrics and Gynaecology 95:153–161

Beard RW, Kennedy RG, Gangar KF et al 1991 Bilateral oophorectomy and hysterectomy in the treatment of intractable pelvic pain associated with pelvic congestion. British Journal of Obstetrics and Gynaecology 98:988–992

Berkley K, Hubscher CH 1995 Are there separate central nervous system pathways for touch and pain? Nature Medicine 1:766–773

Bon K, Lanteri-Minet M, Menetrey D, Berkley KJ 1997 Sex, time-of-day and estrous variations in behavioral and bladder histological consequences of cyclophosphamide-induced cystitis in rats. Pain 73:423–429

Bradshaw HB, Temple JL, Wood E, Berkley KJ 1999 Estrous variations in behavioral responses to vaginal and uterine distention in the rat. Pain 82:187–197

Chen FP, Chang SD, Chu KK, Soong YK 1996 Comparison of laparoscopic presacral neurectomy and laparoscopic uterine nerve ablation for primary dysmenorrhea. Journal of Reproductive Medicine for the Obstetrician and Gynecologist 41:463–466

Clinical Standards Advisory Group 2000 Service for patients with pain. Department of Health, London

Collett BJ, Cordle CJ, Stewart CR, Jagger C 1998 A comparative study of women with chronic pelvic pain, chronic nonpelvic pain and those with no history of pain attending general practitioners. British Journal of Obstetrics and Gynaecology 105:87–92

Daoud I 1998 General surgical aspects. In: Steege JF, Metzger DA, Levy BS (eds) Chronic pelvic pain: an integrated approach. WB Saunders, Philadelphia 329–336

Davies L, Gangar KF, Drummond M, Saunders D, Beard RW 1992 The economic burden of intractable gynaecological pain. Journal of Obstetrics and Gynaecology 12(suppl 2):S54–S56

Dickenson AH 1997 Plasticity: implications for opioid and other pharmacological interventions in specific pain states. Behavioral and Brain Sciences 20:392–403

Dworkin SF, Von-Korff M, LeResche L 1990 Multiple pains and psychiatric disturbance. An epidemiologic investigation. Archives of General Psychiatry 47:239–244

Eckhardt K, Li SX, Ammon S, Schanzle G, Mikus G, Eichelbaum M 1998 Same incidence of adverse drug events after codeine administration irrespective of the genetically determined differences in morphine formation. Pain 76:27–33

Engel CC, Walker EA, Engel AL, Bullis J, Armstrong A 1998 A randomized, double-blind crossover trial of sertraline in women with chronic pelvic pain. Journal of Psychosomatic Research 44:203–207

Farquhar CM, Rogers V, Franks S, Pearce S, Wadsworth J, Beard RW 1989 A randomized controlled trial of medroxyprogesterone acetate and psychotherapy for the treatment of pelvic congestion. British Journal of Obstetrics and Gynaecology 96:1153–1162

Fillingim RB, Edwards RR, Powell T 1999 The relationship of sex and clinical pain to experimental pain responses. Pain 83:419–425

Fillingim RB, Maixner W, Kincaid S, Silva S 1998 Sex differences in temporal summation but not sensory-discriminative processing of thermal pain. Pain 75:121–127

Fry RPW, Stones RW 1996 Hostility and doctor–patient interaction in chronic pelvice pain. Psychotherapy and Psychosomatics 65:253–257

Fry RPW, Beard RW, Crisp AH, McGuigan S 1997 Sociopsychological factors in women with chronic pelvic pain with and without pelvic venous congestion. Journal of Psychosomatic Research 42:71–85

Garry R, Clayton R, Hawe J 2000 The effect of endometriosis and its radical laparoscopic excision on quality of life indicators. British Journal of Obstetrics and Gynaecology 107:44–54

Ghaly AFF 1994 The psychological and physical benefits of pelvic ultrasonography in patients with chronic pelvic pain and negative laparoscopy. A random allocation trial. Journal of Obstetrics and Gynaecology 14:269–271

Gibbons JM 1998 Vulvar vestibulitis. In: Steege JF, Metzger DA, Levy BS (eds) Chronic pelvic pain: an integrated approach. WB Saunders, Philadelphia pp 181–187

Gilling-Smith C, Mason H, Willis D, Franks S, Beard RW 2000 In-vitro ovarian steroidogenesis in women with pelvic congestion. Human Reproduction 15(12):2570–2576

Grace VM 1995 Problems of communication, diagnosis, and treatment experienced by women using the New Zealand health services for chronic pelvic pain: a quantative analysis. Health Care for Women International 16(6):521–535

Grace VM 1998 Mind/body dualism in medicine: the case of chronic pelvic pain without organic pathology – a critical review of the literature. International Journal of Health Services 28:127–151

Hahn L 1989 Clinical findings and results of operative treatment in ilioinguinal nerve entrapment syndrome. British Journal of Obstetrics and Gynaecology 96:1080–1083

Halligan S, Campbell D, Bartram CI et al 2000 Transvaginal ultrasound examination of women with and without pelvic venous congestion. Clinical Radiology 55(12):954–958

Herrero JF, Laird JMA, Lopez-Garcia JA 2000 Wind-up of spinal cord neurones and pain sensation: much ado about something? Progress in Neurobiology 61:169–203

Herrington JK 1975 Occult inguinal hernia in the female. Annals of Surgery 181(4):481–483

Hobbs JT 1976 The pelvic congestion syndrome. The Practitioner 216:529–540

Horn S, Munafo M 1997 Pain theory, research, and intervention. Open University Press, Buckingham

Howard FM 1996 The role of laparoscopy in the evaluation of chronic pelvic pain: pitfalls with a negative laparoscopy. Journal of the American Association of Gynecologic Laparoscopists 4(1):85–94

Howard FM 1999 Pelvic pain. In: Thomas EJ, Stones RW (eds) Gynaecology highlights 1998–99. Health Press, Oxford 53–63

IASP Task Force on Taxonomy 1994 Classification of chronic pain, 2nd edn. IASP Press, Seattle

Jenkinson C, Layte R, Wright L, Coulter A 1996a The UK SF-36: an analysis and interpretation manual. Health Services Research Unit, University of Oxford, Oxford

Jenkinson C, Peto V, Coulter A 1996b Making sense of ambiguity: evaluation of internal reliability and face validity of the SF-36 questionnaire in women presenting with menorrhagia. Quality in Health Care 5:9–12

Kasule J 1991 Laparoscopic evaluation of chronic pelvic pain in Zimbabwean women. East African Medical Journal 68:807–811

Koninckx PR, Renaer M 1997 Pain sensitivity of and pain radiation from the internal female genital organs. Human Reproduction 12:1785–1788

Lee CH, Dellon AL 2000 Surgical management of groin pain of neural origin. Journal of the American College of Surgeons 191:137–142

Lyall H, Campbell-Brown M, Walker JJ 1999 GnRH analogue in everyday gynecology: is it possible to rationalize its use? Acta Obstetricia et Gynecologica Scandinavica 78:340–345

Mathias SD, Kuppermann M, Liberman RF, Lipschutz RC, Steege JF 1996 Chronic pelvic pain: prevalemce, health-related quality of life, and economic correlates. Obstetrics and Gynecology 87:321–327

McMahon SB 1997 Are there fundamental differences in the peripheral mechanisms of visceral and somatic pain? Behavioral and Brain Sciences 20:381–391

Mogil JS, Wilson SG, Bon K et al 1999a Heritability of nociception I: responses of 11 inbred mouse strains on 12 measures of nociception. Pain 80:67–82

Mogil JS, Wilson SG, Bon K 1999b Heritability of nociception II. 'Types' of nociception revealed by genetic correlation analysis. Pain 80:83–93

Nezhat CH, Seidman DS, Nezhat FR, Nezhat CR 1998 Long-term outcome of laparoscopic presacral neurectomy for the treatment of central pelvic pain attributed to endometriosis. Obstetrics and Gynecology 91:701–704

Perry CP, Perez J 1993 The role for laparoscopic presacral neurectomy. Journal of Gynecologic Surgery 9:165–168

Peters AA, van Dorst E, Jellis B, van Zuuren E, Hermans J, Trimbos JB 1991 A randomized clinical trial to compare two different approaches in women with chronic pelvic pain. Obstetrics and Gynecology 77:740–744

Peters AAW, Trimbos-Kemper GCM, Admiraal C, Trimbos JB 1992 A randomized clinical trial on the benefit of adhesiolysis in patients with intraperitoneal adhesions and chronic pelvic pain. British Journal of Obstetrics and Gynaecology 99:59–62

Peveler R, Edwards J, Daddow J, Thomas EJ 1995 Psychosocial factors and chronic pelvic pain: a comparison of women with endometriosis and with unexplained pain. Journal of Psychosomatic Research 40:305–315

Peveler R, Kelkenny L, Kinmonth A-L 1997 Medically unexplained physical symptoms in primary care: a comparison of self-report screening questionnaires and clinical opinion. Journal of Psychosomatic Research 42:245–252

Price JR, Blake F 1999 Chronic pelvic pain: The assessment as therapy. Journal of Psychosomatic Research 46:7–14

Prior A, Whorwell PJ 1989 Gynaecological consultation in patients with the irritable bowel syndrome. Gut 30:996–998

Rapkin AJ 1986 Adhesions and pelvic pain: a retrospective study. Obstetrics and Gynecology 68:13–15

Rapkin AJ, Kames LD, Darke LL, Stampler FM, Naliboff BD 1990 History of physical and sexual abuse in women with chronic pelvic pain. Obstetrics and Gynecology 76:92–96

Richlin SS, Rock JA 2001 Ovarian remnant syndrome. Gynaecological Endoscopy 10(2):111–117

Riley JL, Robinson ME, Wise EA, Price DD 1999 A meta-analytic review of pain perception across the menstrual cycle. Pain 81:225–235

Rowbotham M, Harden N, Stacey B, Bernstein P, Magnus Miller L 1998 Gabapentin for the treatment of postherpetic neuralgia – a randomized controlled trial. Journal of the American Medical Association 280:1837–1842

Selfe SA, Matthews Z, Stones RW 1998a Factors influencing outcome in consultations for chronic pelvic pain. Journal of Women's Health 7:1041–1048

Selfe SA, van Vugt M, Stones RW 1998b Chronic gynaecological pain: an exploration of medical attitudes. Pain 77:215–225

Slocumb JC, Kellner R, Rosenfeld RC, Pathak D 1989 Anxiety and depression in patients with the abdominal pelvic pain syndrome. General Hospital Psychiatry 11:48–53

Stones RW 2000 Chronic pelvic pain in women: new perspectives on pathophysiology and management. Reproductive Medicine Review 8:229–240

Stones RW, Mountfield J 2000 Interventions for treating chronic pelvic pain in women. The Cochrane Library, issue 3

Stones RW, Thomas EJ 1995 Cost-effective medical treatment of endometriosis. In: Bonnar J (ed) Recent advances in obstetrics and gynaecology 19. Churchill Livingstone, Edinburgh pp 139–152

Stones RW, Rae T, Rogers V, Fry R, Beard RW 1990 Pelvic congestion in women: evaluation with transvaginal ultrasound and observation of venous pharmacology. British Journal of Radiology 63:710–711

Stones RW, Selfe SA, Fransman S, Horn SA 2000 Psychosocial and economic impact of chronic pelvic pain. Baillière's Clinical Obstetrics and Gynaecology 14:27–43

Stones RW, Bradbury L, Anderson D 2001 Randomized placebo controlled trial of lofexidine hydrochloride for chronic pelvic pain in women. Human Reproduction 16(8):1719–1721

Sutton JG, Ewen SP, Whitelaw N, Haines P 1994 Prospective, randomized, double-blind, controlled trial of laser laparoscopy in the treatment of pelvic pain asociated with minimal, mild and moderate endometriosis. Fertility and Sterility 62:696–700

Treloar SA, Martin NG, Heath AC 1998 Longitudinal genetic analysis of menstrual flow, pain, and limitation in a sample of Australian twins. Behavior Genetics 28:107–116

von Bahr V 1979 Local anaesthesia for inguinal herniorrhaphy. In: Eriksson E (ed) Illustrated handbook in local anaesthesia, 2nd edn. Lloyd-Luke, London pp 52–54

Waller KG, Shaw RW 1995 Endometriosis, pelvic pain, and psychological functioning. Fertility and Sterility 63:796–800

Whorwell P 1995 The gender influence. Women and IBS 2:2–3

Winkel CA 1999 Modeling of medical and surgical treatment costs of chronic pelvic pain: new paradigms for making clinical decisions. American Journal of Managed Care 5:S276–S290

Wise EA, Riley JL, Robinson ME 2000 Clinical pain perception and hormone replacement therapy in postmenopausal women experiencing orofacial pain. Clinical Journal of Pain 16:121–126

Woolf CJ 1983 Evidence for a central component of post-injury pain hypersensitivity. Nature 306:686–688

Woolf CJ, Shortland P, Coggeshall RE 1992 Peripheral nerve injury triggers central sprouting of myelinated afferents. Nature 355:75–78

Yonkers KACSJ 1995 Recognition of depression in obstetric/gynecology practices. American Journal of Obstetrics and Gynecology 173(2):632–638

Zondervan KT, Yudkin PL, Vessey MP, Dawes MG, Barlow DH, Kennedy SH 1999a Patterns of diagnosis and referral in women consulting for chronic pelvic pain in UK primary care. British Journal of Obstetrics and Gynaecology 106:1156–1161

Zondervan KT, Yudkin PL, Vessey MP, Dawes MG, Barlow DH, Kennedy SH 1999b Prevalence and incidence of chronic pelvic pain in primary care: evidence from a national general practice database. British Journal of Obstetrics and Gynaecology 106:1149–1155

Zondervan KT, Yudkin PL, Vessey MP et al 2001a Chronic pelvic pain in the community – symptoms, investigations, and diagnoses. American Journal of Obstetrics and Gynecology 184(6):1149–1155

Zondervan KT, Yudkin PL, Vessey MP et al 2001b The community prevalence of chronic pelvic pain in women and associated illness behaviour. British Journal of General Practice 51(468):541–547

61

Pelvic inflammatory disease

Jorma Paavonen   Pontus Molander

Pelvic inflammatory disease (PID) refers to infection of the uterus, fallopian tubes and adjacent pelvic structures not associated with surgery or pregnancy. PID comprises a spectrum of inflammatory disorders of the upper female genital tract, including any combination of endometritis, salpingitis, tubo-ovarian abscess and pelvic peritonitis. PID is associated with high morbidity. Long-term sequelae of PID, specifically tubal factor infertility (TFI) and ectopic pregnancy, are common and cause major problems to reproductive health in later life. Repeated episodes of PID are associated with a steep increase in the risk of permanent tubal damage.

It is apparent that PID poses a major threat to the reproductive health of young women and drains healthcare resources. It also represents an often neglected area of modern medical practice. However, it should be emphasized that PID and its sequelae are largely preventable.

EPIDEMIOLOGY

The exact incidence of PID is unknown because the disease cannot be diagnosed reliably from clinical symptoms and signs. PID is often asymptomatic or subclinical. Hospital discharge registries are poor surrogate markers for the true prevalence of PID. Factors associated with PID mirror those for sexually transmitted infections. Risk factors and risk markers for PID include young age, multiple sexual partners, intra-uterine device (IUD) insertion, vaginal douching, tobacco smoking, chlamydial and gonococcal cervicitis and vaginitis. Barrier contraceptive use protects against PID. Oral contraceptive (OC) use modifies the manifestations of PID towards less symptomatic disease and OC use may in fact protect against manifest PID.

The topic of intrauterine device (IUD) and upper genital tract infection has recently been systematically reviewed (Grimes 2000). Concern about upper genital tract infection related to intrauterine devices limits their wider use. Methodological flaws in early observational studies exaggerated the risk of PID associated with IUD use. This misunderstanding has inadvertently affected women's health around the world by limiting access to a highly effective contraceptive and thus indirectly adding to the burden of unintended pregnancy. Choice of an inappropriate comparison group, overdiagnosis of PID in IUD users and inability to control for the confounding effects of risk-taking sexual behaviour have exaggerated the apparent risk. Women with symptomless gonorrhoea or chlamydial infection having an IUD inserted have a higher risk of salpingitis than do uninfected women having an IUD inserted. However, the risk appears similar to that of infected women not having an IUD inserted. Furthermore, unbiased evidence indicates no important effect of IUD use on the risk for tubal infertility.

One important current trend is the shift from inpatient PID towards outpatient PID. Hospitalization of women with PID has rapidly decreased (Fig. 61.1). For instance, in Finland hospitalization for acute PID has decreased by 50% in 1990–99 although the rate of sexually transmitted chlamydial infections has not fallen (Fig. 61.2). However, this does not necessarily mean that the overall incidence of PID has decreased and may reflect only the change in clinical manifestations of PID. A

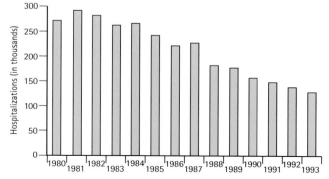

Fig. 61.1 Pelvic inflammatory disease (PID) hospitalizations of women aged 15–44 in the United States, 1980–93 (STD Surveillance, NIH, 1995).

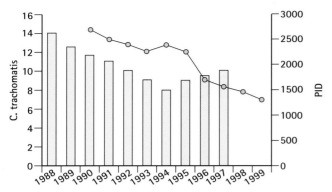

Fig. 61.2 *Chlamydia trachomatis* rates and inpatient PID rates in Finland.

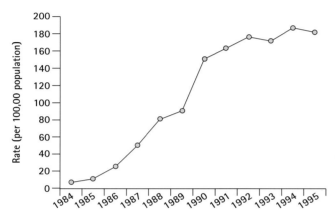

Fig. 61.3 *Chlamydia trachomatis* reported rates in the United States, 1984–95 (STD Surveillance, NIH, 1995).

Box 61.1 Recent prevalence rates of *C. trachomatis* among asymptomatic women and men in Finland

Women*
- Student health/family planning clinic   53/1090 (4.9%)
- Adolescent clinic   12/306 (3.9%)
- Antenatal clinic   10/401 (2.5%)

Men*
- Army recruits   25/963 (2.6%)

* First void urine: PCR or LCR

Table 61.1 Prevalence of *C. trachomatis* in PID. Modified from Simms & Stephenson (2000)

Setting	Rate (95% CI)	No. of studies
● STD clinic	40% (25–55)	1
● Gynaecological inpatients	32% (21–43)	9
● Gynaecological outpatients	31% (18–46)	3
● Emergency clinic	43% (26–61)	3
● Primary care clinic	25% (13–40)	1

chlamydial cervicitis develop PID if left untreated (Stamm et al 1984). However, this is probably an overestimation for *C. trachomatis* infection. For example, the models have used probabilities and assumptions for the consequences of untreated *C. trachomatis* infection which have been derived from a group of women who were culture positive for *C. trachomatis*. The assumption is that being culture positive is the same as being positive in a nucleic acid amplification (NAA) based test, which is unlikely in relation to bacterial load alone. None of the models have used primary data from a cohort of women who have been screened for *C. trachomatis* using a sensitive NAA-based diagnostic test and then followed over time.

Bacterial vaginosis (BV) is the most common cause of abnormal vaginal discharge. BV is characterized by a complex change in vaginal ecology. The concentration of hydrogen peroxide-producing lactobacilli is decreased together with a massive increase in the concentration of *Gardnerella vaginalis*, *Mobiluncus* species, other anaerobic Gram-negative rods and genital mycoplasms. On the other hand, aerobic vaginitis (AV) is characterized by an overgrowth of virulent aerobic bacteria, most notably *Escherichia coli*, group B streptococci and enterococci. Both vaginitis types lead to a massive increase in the concentration of microbial byproducts which are thought to destroy cervical host defence barriers, leading to ascent of micro-organisms and their byproducts to the upper genital tract (McCormack 1994). Non-chlamydial non-gonococcal micro-organisms detected in the upper genital tract of women with laparoscopically proven PID are mostly micro-organisms known to be associated with BV or AV (Paavonen et al 1987). Other less commonly associated micro-organisms include *Actinomyces* spp. which are typically linked to IUD usage. In less developed countries or populations with a high prevalence of tuberculosis, PID may be associated with *Mycobacterium tuberculosis*, due to dissemination of the micro-organism via

rapid change in the characteristics of hospitalized PID patients has also taken place in developed countries. These patients are now older, have more severe disease and longer duration of symptoms before seeking care. Furthermore, a new clinical PID entity, so-called 'silent' or 'subclinical' PID, has recently been described.

Another recent trend in developed countries is the shift in the microbial aetiology of PID. The relative role of *Chlamydia trachomatis* in the causation of PID has increased, whereas the role of *Neisseria gonorrhoeae* has decreased. In many developed countries, gonorrhoea is now a rare disease (van der Heyden et al 2000), whereas chlamydia rates are still high or on the rise (Fig. 61.3). Recent screening studies have shown strikingly high rates of *C. trachomatis* among asymptomatic populations (Box 61.1). Thus, *C. trachomatis* is now the predominant sexually transmitted organism causing PID (Table 61.1).

MICROBIOLOGY

The most important causative micro-organisms are *C. trachomatis*, *N. gonorrhoeae* and bacteria associated with vaginitis (McCormack 1994). The proportion of PID caused by *C. trachomatis* or *N. gonorrhoeae* reflects the background prevalence of these organisms in the target population. It has been estimated that 10–30% of women with gonococcal or

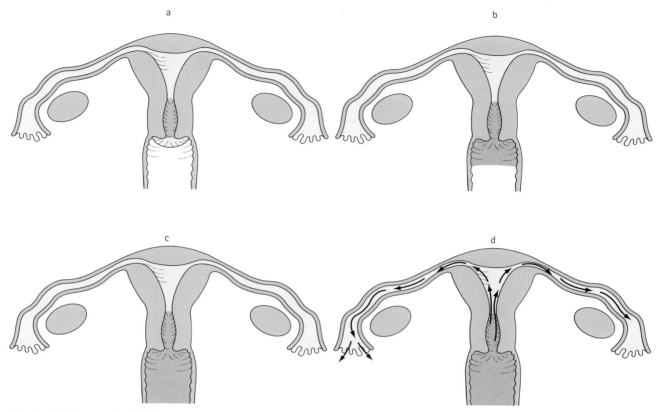

Fig. 61.4 Pathogenesis of PID. PID begins with chlamydial and/or gonococcal cervicitis **a**. This is followed by an alteration in the cervicovaginal microenvironment **b**, leading to bacterial vaginosis **c**. Finally, the original cervical pathogens, the flora causing vaginitis or both ascend into the upper genital tract **d**. The cross-hatched areas indicate the affected portions of the genital tract (modified from McCormack 1994).

the bloodstream rather than via ascending spread from the lower genital tract. In some areas of the world, granulomatous salpingitis may also be caused by organisms such as *Schistosoma* spp.

PATHOGENESIS

PID is an ascending infection in which pathogenic microorganisms ascend from the lower genital tract to the upper genital tract (Fig. 61.4). Endometritis is an early manifestation of PID and most but not all women with PID have plasma cell endometritis. Next, salpingitis develops, which can lead to pyosalpinx or tubo-ovarian abscess formation. Perihepatitis is associated with PID in 10–20% of cases.

Cervical mucus may be the most important natural barrier to the ascending spread of micro-organisms into the uterus. The mechanism for the extension of infecting micro-organisms into the upper female genital tract may vary according to the organism and continues to be a complex topic. In the setting of gonococcal PID, it is thought that infection probably extends via a direct intracavitary ascent from the endocervix into the endometrium and subsequently into the fallopian tubes. This causes oedema and induces an intense polymorphonuclear leucocyte response. In studies of gonococcal PID, the organism is more frequently recovered during and immediately after the menstrual period. Gonococci readily

attach to the microvilli of non-ciliated mucosal epithelial cells, which they enter, resulting in cell damage and sloughing of ciliated cells.

Animal models have been developed to study the pathogenesis of chlamydial PID (Patton & Lichtenwalner 1998). Experimental chlamydial infection induced in non-human primates has been defined as a complex process of immune-mediated responses leading to overt tubal damage. Chlamydial organisms attach to non-ciliated epithelial cells. Intracellular replication of *Chlamydia* results in the release of infectious elementary bodies by rupture of the infected cells. No good data are available on the pathogenesis of non-gonococcal, non-chlamydial PID.

Several studies have suggested that the risk for developing PID may increase at menses and that hormonal factors may play a role in the pathogenesis of PID by affecting the structural and functional barriers preventing infection of the upper female genital tract. It has been postulated that initial exposure to *C. trachomatis* or *N. gonorrhoeae* or both increases the risk for developing endometritis by the ascending spread of these micro-organisms and the concomitant or subsequent ascending infection with vaginal bacteria, including organisms associated with BV or AV.

Since age is an important risk factor for PID, specific age-related hormonal or other host immune response-related factors in the cervix or cervical mucus may also determine whether or not a cervicovaginal infection ascends to the upper genital tract causing manifest PID.

CLINICAL MANIFESTATIONS

The clinical spectrum of PID ranges from asymptomatic or subclinical endometritis to symptomatic salpingitis, pyosalpinx, tubo-ovarian abscess, pelvic peritonitis and sometimes perihepatitis. Bilateral lower abdominal pain is the most common presenting symptom. Perihepatitis causes right quadrant upper abdominal pain mimicking acute cholecystitis. Other common symptoms are abnormal vaginal discharge, metrorrhagia, postcoital bleeding, dysuria, fever and nausea. However, symptomatic PID only represents the tip of the iceberg. Increasing attention has recently been focused on so-called 'atypical' or 'silent' PID. For instance, only a fraction of women with TFI have history of frank PID, suggesting that silent PID may also lead to the development of permanent tubal damage. Women with chlamydial cervicitis and no symptoms or signs of PID can have plasma cell endometritis on endometrial biopsy consistent with subclinical PID. Furthermore, minimally symptomatic patients usually seek medical care late which increases the risk for tubal damage and long-term sequelae.

In developed countries, only a minority of patients with PID are HIV positive but in African countries, the HIV positivity rate may be as high as 30–40%. HIV-positive patients with PID are more likely to have pelvic abscesses, require prolonged hospitalization, respond more slowly to antimicrobial therapy and more often require change of antibiotics. Hospitalization and intravenous antimicrobial therapy are recommended for all HIV-positive patients with PID. However, much of the information on this topic has been derived from retrospective observations, case reports or limited cohort studies of PID in HIV-infected women.

DIAGNOSIS

The major criteria for the clinical diagnosis of PID are history of low abdominal pain, cervical motion tenderness, uterine tenderness, bilateral adnexal tenderness and negative pregnancy test (Box 61.2). The CDC criteria for the diagnosis of PID are listed in Box 61.3. The clinical diagnosis of PID has severe limitations since the clinical criteria have low diagnostic accuracy. Thus, false-positive and false-negative diagnoses are common. Multiple studies (Munday 2000) have shown that the sensitivity of the clinical diagnosis based on history and pelvic examination is low or very low when laparoscopy is used as the gold standard for diagnosis (Table 61.2). Therefore, clinicians should have a high index of suspicion of PID when

Box 61.2 Criteria for syndrome diagnosis of PID

- History of low abdominal pain
- Cervical motion tenderness
- Uterine tenderness
- Bilateral adnexal tenderness
- Negative pregnancy test

Box 61.3 Centers for Disease Control and Prevention criteria for the diagnosis of pelvic inflammatory disease

Minimum criteria
- Lower abdominal tenderness
- Adnexal tenderness
- Cervical motion tenderness

*Additional criteria**
- Oral temperature >38.3°C (101°F)
- Abnormal cervical or vaginal discharge
- Elevated erythrocyte sedimentation rate
- Elevated C-reactive protein
- Laboratory documentation of cervical infection with *Neisseria gonorrhoeae* or *Chlamydia trachomatis*

Definitive criteria†
- Histopathologic evidence of endometritis on endometrial biopsy
- Tubo-ovarian abscess on sonography or other radiologic tests
- Laparoscopic abnormalities consistent with PID

* More elaborate diagnostic evaluation is often needed because incorrect diagnosis and management might cause unnecessary morbidity. These additional criteria may be used to increase the specificity of the diagnosis of the minimum criteria listed previously.
† The definitive criteria for diagnosing PID are warranted in selected cases.

Table 61.2 Proportion of laparoscopically proven PID cases of those with clinically suspected PID. Modified from Munday (2000)

Author and reference	Year	Setting	Country	Proven/total (%)
Jacobson	1969	Gyn	Sweden	532/814 (65)
Chaparro	1978	Gyn	USA	103/223 (46)
Sweet	1979	Emergency room	USA	26/29 (90)
Murphy	1981	Gyn	Australia	8/22 (36)
Allen	1983	Gyn	S. Africa	63/103 (61)
Wasserheit	1986	STD/emergency room/gyn	USA	22/36 (61)
Brihmer	1987	Gyn	Sweden	187/359 (52)
Paavonen	1987	Gyn	Finland	36/45 (67)
Brunham	1988	Gyn	Canada	44/69 (64)
Heinonen	1989	Gyn	Finland	33/40 (83)
Sellors	1991	General practice	Canada	28/95 (30)
Rousseau	1991	Gyn	Canada	41/54 (76)
Livengood	1992	Emergency room/gyn	USA	23/33 (70)
Weström	1992	Gyn	Sweden	1186/1679 (71)
Morcos	1993	Gyn	USA	134/176 (76)
Stacey	1994	STD	UK	7/32 (22)
Soper	1994	Emergency room/gyn	USA	84/102 (82)
Bevan	1995	STD/emergency room/gyn	UK	104/147 (71)
Tukeva	1999	Gyn	Finland	27/30 (70)

evaluating women with pelvic pain. A treatment delay of just a few days seems to increase the risk for late sequelae (Hillis et al 1993).

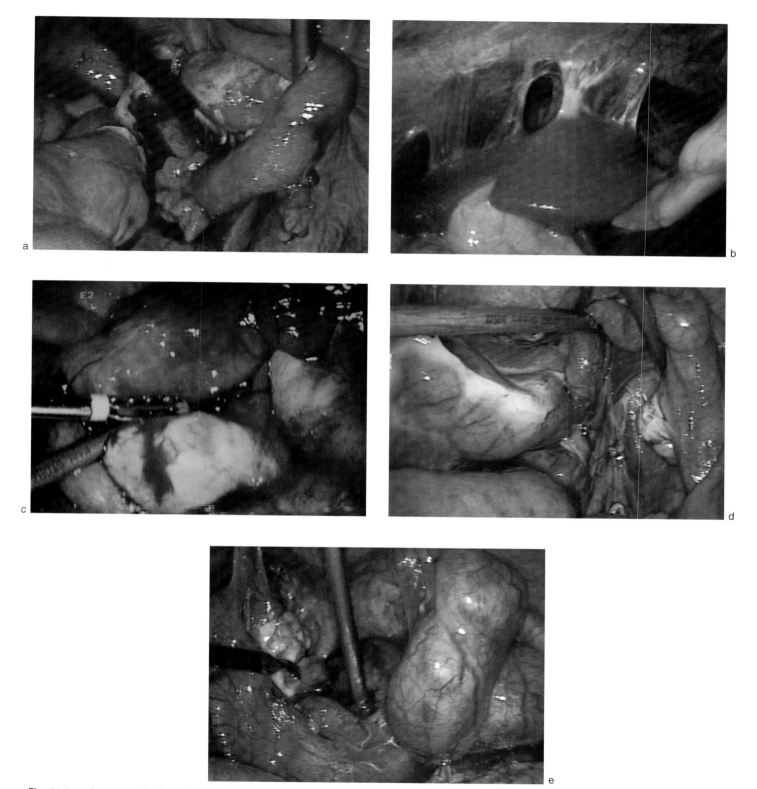

Fig. 61.5 **a** Laparoscopic view of acute salpingitis. Note swollen hyperaemic fallopian tube next to a normal right ovary. The right tube has just been detached from the pelvic peritoneum. **b** Laparoscopic view of perihepatitis. Note perihepatic adhesions formed after chlamydial infection. The patient developed acute symptoms with severe pain in the right upper quadrant. **c** Laparoscopic view of severe PID. Note pyosalpinx formation with a phimotic fimbrial end. Normal ovary is visualized underneath the infected fallopian tube. **d** Laparoscopic view of severe PID. Note a unilateral left-sided tubo-ovarian abscess. **e** Laparoscopic view of severe PID. Note large bilateral pyosalpinx formation.

Increasing concern about silent PID has changed the recommendations for PID diagnosis from laboratory-based and laparoscopy-based diagnosis towards so-called syndrome diagnosis (Box 61.2). Syndrome diagnosis may increase diagnostic sensitivity and lead to earlier therapy, although on the other hand it may also lead to unnecessary antimicrobial therapies due to low specificity (Dallabetta et al 1998). The syndrome diagnosis of PID is clearly broad and imprecise.

Laparoscopy, endometrial biopsy, transvaginal sonography (TVS), TVS with power Doppler and magnetic resonance imaging (MRI) can be used to obtain a more accurate diagnosis of PID. However, these facilities are not readily available in the vast majority of clinical settings where patients with suspected PID are seen or may not be justifiable in clinically mild disease. For instance, although laparoscopy was introduced in 1960s as the gold standard for PID diagnosis, direct visual diagnosis by laparoscopy is not always feasible, requires general anaesthesia and is costly.

Laparoscopy is still considered the 'gold standard' for confirming a diagnosis of PID because it not only allows direct inspection of the fallopian tubes and surrounding pelvic anatomy but also enables microbiologic sampling from the upper genital tract (e.g. fallopian tube, ovary and peritoneal fluid). Laparoscopy can be used to characterize and grade the severity of PID (Fig. 61.5). However, the routine use of laparoscopy to confirm a diagnosis of PID is limited by cost and availability, especially in the outpatient clinic settings where most PID is diagnosed. On the other hand, the accuracy or reproducibility of laparoscopy may not be 100% because of expectation bias or because laparoscopy may not detect subtle endosalpingitis. It should be emphasized that although laparoscopy is generally accepted as the gold standard for the diagnosis of PID, it has never been properly validated (Sellors et al 1991). Therefore the interobserver and intraobserver reproducibility of laparoscopic diagnosis is not known. Such observer reproducibility studies of laparoscopic diagnosis of PID are needed.

Endometrial biopsy obtained with an aspiration catheter is a simple outpatient procedure for histopathologic diagnosis of PID (plasma cell endometritis). Although the results are not readily available, endometrial biopsy can provide confirmatory histopathologic diagnosis of PID. In contrast to laparoscopy, endometrial biopsy can be performed on an outpatient basis and is considerably less invasive. Studies have found reasonable correlation between the results of endometrial biopsy and laparoscopic findings (Paavonen et al 1987).

Clinically PID must be differentiated from other abdominal and pelvic conditions, including life-threatening conditions, such as acute appendicitis (Fig. 61.6). Thus, laparoscopy should be performed if there is any doubt of the diagnosis. In addition, operative procedures can be performed during laparoscopy, such as liberation of adhesions, peritoneal lavation, drainage and lavage of abscesses, which shortens the hospital stay and may improve outcome (Molander et al 2000). Operative laparoscopy facilitates management of other conditions that cause differential diagnostic problems. For instance, endometriomas, ruptured ovarian cysts, adnexal torsions and appendicitis can all be managed laparoscopically (Figs 61.7, 61.8). Thus, laparoscopy also augments the management of

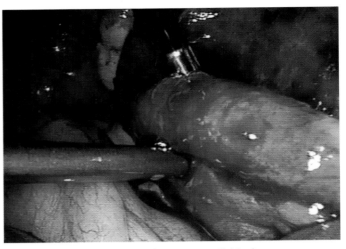

Fig. 61.6 Laparoscopic view of acute appendicitis. A gangrenous appendix situated deep in the pelvis can be seen next to normal right tube and ovary.

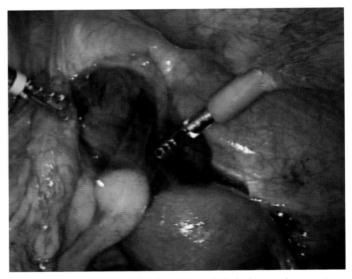

Fig. 61.7 A large haemorrhagic endometriotic lesion can be seen to the left of the uterus and the bladder. The omentum is attached to the lesion as a result of inflammation.

non-PID cases which are difficult to discriminate from acute PID by clinical examination alone. In conclusion, laparoscopy plays an important role in the management of conditions that cause acute pelvic pain in women of reproductive age. It facilitates the diagnosis and allows surgical intervention when indicated. Acute-phase laparoscopy may prevent long-term complications and help preserve fertility.

TVS and MRI are other techniques introduced to augment the clinical diagnosis of PID. TVS with power Doppler is a powerful tool in the diagnosis of PID but it requires special skills and is therefore highly observer dependent. MRI seems to be as accurate as TVS in the diagnosis of inpatient PID when laparoscopy is used as the gold standard (Tukeva et al 1999). However, MRI is seldom available in settings where PID cases are seen. Tubal enlargement can be easily seen on MR images

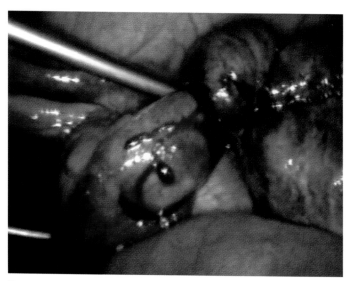

Fig. 61.8 Torsion of the right fallopian tube caused by an old sactosalpinx formation. The twisted tube was removed laparoscopically.

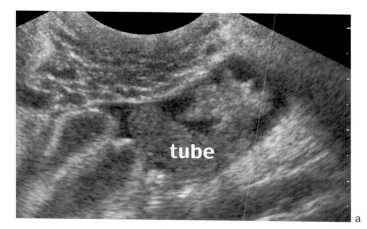

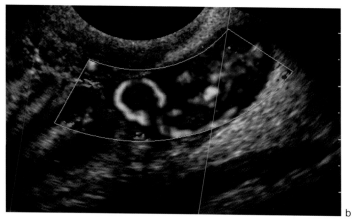

Fig. 61.9 Power Doppler TVS image of acute salpingitis. The thickened fallopian tube is entirely visualized because of surrounding cul-de-sac fluid. Note hyperaemia associated with acute inflammation.

and is characterized by tortuous folding of fluid-filled structures on T_2-weighted images. In one recent study the sensitivity of MRI in the diagnosis of PID was 95%, the specificity was 89% and the overall accuracy was 93% (Tukeva et al 1999). The MRI findings consistent with PID diagnosis included fluid-filled tube, pyosalpinx, tubo-ovarian abscess or polycystic-like ovaries in the presence of free pelvic fluid.

TVS is a non-invasive bedside procedure that is routinely performed in patients with pelvic pain. Earlier studies have shown that TVS performs well in the diagnosis of PID when the criteria include thickened fluid-filled tubes. TVS is superior to transabdominal sonography in the diagnosis of pelvic abnormalities. Recent innovation in the sonographic Doppler technique, i.e. power Doppler, improves the detection of blood flow, particularly low-velocity flow. The detection of inflammation-induced hyperaemia by power Doppler has so far been little studied even though early results are encouraging (Molander et al 2001). Power Doppler has already gained a variety of applications in obstetrics and gynaecology.

Specific TVS findings, including wall thickness >5 mm, cog-wheel sign, incomplete septa and the presence of cul-de-sac fluid, distinguish women with acute PID from women with no PID (Molander et al 2001). Power Doppler TVS reveals hyperaemia in women with acute PID, since it is rarely present in women without acute PID (Fig. 61.9). Pulsatility indices are significantly lower in the acute PID group than in control women without PID (Molander et al 2001). Thus, combined use of TVS and power Doppler augments the diagnosis of PID among women referred for low abdominal pain.

Power Doppler TVS can also distinguish between acute appendicitis and PID, avoiding the limitations of transabdominal ultrasound. In a preliminary study of six patients with laparoscopically proven acute appendicitis, power Doppler TVS showed either a typical submucosal ring with thick walls or a heterogeneous complex with surrounding hyperechogenic soft tissue. Hyperaemia was present in all cases and normal

adnexal structures could be visualized next to the inflamed appendix (Molander et al 2002).

Laboratory studies

The detection of *C. trachomatis* or *N. gonorrhoeae* in patients with lower abdominal pain, vaginal discharge and pelvic tenderness is highly suggestive of PID. The endocervical Gram-stained smear, if positive for typical Gram-negative, intracellular diplococci, may assist in the diagnosis of PID. In routine clinical practice, the laboratory diagnosis of *N. gonorrhoeae* is still based on culture although several non-culture tests, including DNA probes and enzyme immunoassays (EIA), have been developed for the detection of *N. gonorrhoeae* in clinical specimens.

Cell culture has long been the 'gold standard' for the confirmatory diagnosis of *C. trachomatis*. However, recently developed NAA techniques, such as PCR and LCR, have largely replaced cell culture and antigen tests in the diagnoses of *C. trachomatis* infection. NAA techniques, especially LCR and PCR on first void urine (FVU), are highly effective at detecting both symptomatic and asymptomatic chlamydial infection. Cell culture or antigen tests which are still used in many clinics miss a large proportion of cases. If screening for chlamydia is to be efficient such programmes should detect as many cases as possible. Therefore, NAA methods on FVU would be the best option. New techniques are constantly being introduced and evaluated. In general, NAA techniques are nearly ideal diagnostic tests with high accuracy (Wilson et al 2002).

Other laboratory tests, which are not specific for PID but are often abnormal or elevated in an acute infection or inflammation and which may help in the diagnosis and monitoring of PID, include the erythrocyte sedimentation rate (ESR), quantitative C-reactive protein (CRP) and the total white blood cell (WBC) count. Combining ESR and CRP increases the ability to discriminate severe PID from moderate to mild PID. Evaluation of laboratory markers in the diagnosis of PID based on multiple studies shows reasonable accuracy for ESR and CRP, but not for WBC (Munday 2000).

A simple algorithm developed for primary care bedside diagnosis could augment the management of women with clinical findings consistent with PID. Such an algorithm can be based on the assumption that the presence of lower genital tract infection is a prerequisite for the diagnosis of PID (Fig. 61.10). Thus, the presence or absence of cervical mucopus on speculum examination and presence or absence of abnormal findings on wet mount examination of vaginal discharge are the key steps of such a flow chart. Systematic use of these simple observations

during clinical bedside evaluation is likely to increase the accuracy of the clinical diagnosis of PID.

TREATMENT

Due to the complex microbiology of PID, broad-spectrum antimicrobial coverage is recommended. Problems that often complicate the management of PID include a difficult clinical diagnosis, inaccessibility of clinical sites for microbiologic tests, patient compliance in taking prescribed medications and delayed access to healthcare providers skilled and trained in the management of PID. It is fair to say that in real life PID patients are often managed badly by physicians with little interest in the condition.

The antimicrobial regimen should include agents known to be active against C. trachomatis, N. gonorrhoeae and the broad spectrum of aerobic and anaerobic bacteria commonly detected in the UGT of women with PID (Centers for Disease Control and Prevention 1997, Hemsel et al 2001). The choice of antimicrobial therapy should therefore be guided by knowledge of underlying or presumed aetiologic agents and data on the incidence and prevalence of antimicrobial resistance in PID pathogens, such as N. gonorrhoeae. For instance, in the USA in vitro resistance to penicillin and tetracycline occurs in 20–25% of isolates tested.

The CDC provides recommendations for the outpatient and inpatient therapy of PID. For example, recommended outpatient regimens include a single dose of ceftriaxone 250 mg intramuscularly plus oral doxycycline 100 mg twice daily for 10–14 days. Inpatient therapy regimens recommended by the CDC include cefoxitin (or a comparable cephalosporin) plus doxycycline or clindamycin plus gentamicin, in appropriate doses. Male sex partners should receive prophylactic treatment for gonococcal and chlamydial infection and should be counselled on the proper use of condoms to reduce further exposure to and transmission of STDs. PID patients and their sex partners should also receive information and counselling on the prevention of HIV infection as well as STDs and should be offered confidential HIV testing.

The decision to choose outpatient management rather than hospitalization for PID should ideally be based on specific clinical criteria. Regardless of the decision to treat PID on an outpatient or inpatient basis, all women with PID should be re-evaluated within 48–72 hours following the initiation of therapy and again following completion of therapy. All recommended antibiotic therapies are effective in achieving short-term clinical cure, but their success in preventing long-term sequelae is not known. The guidelines have not yet been critically evaluated in large, randomized, clinical trials. Another problem is that the guidelines have not been effectively implemented and are often not followed by clinicians.

Combination treatment with doxycycline plus metronidazole is usually effective for both inpatient and outpatient PID; it is well tolerated, easy to administer (orally or intravenously), rarely causes enterocolitis and is not very costly. One important disadvantage is that it does not provide adequate coverage against gonococci which may be a problem in populations with high background prevalence of N.

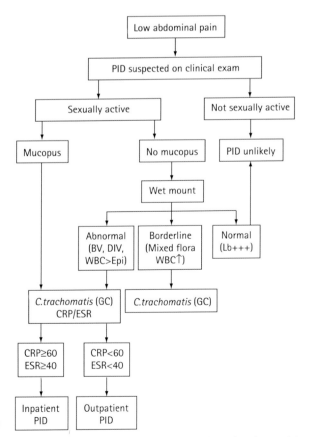

Fig. 61.10 Flow chart of the bedside evaluation of patients with suspected PID in primary care, based on speculum findings and wet mount examination.

gonorrhoeae. In this case, a single-dose therapy for gonorrhoea should be given (for instance, ciprofloxacin 500 mg). Recent data, although limited, show somewhat lower microbiological and clinical cure rates for doxycycline and metronidazole than other antibiotic combination regimens (Walker et al 1993). Limited bacteriological coverage to non-gonococcal non-chlamydial aerobic bacteria can explain lower success rates (Hasselquist & Hillier 1991).

Most patients with PID are managed as outpatients. Hospitalization of PID patients is recommended if the diagnosis is in doubt, pelvic abscess is diagnosed, severe symptoms preclude outpatient treatment or if there is no response to outpatient treatment. IUD should be removed once antimicrobial treatment is started and contraceptive counselling should be provided. Whether inpatient treatment improves the long-term outcome of PID is currently not known. Information on the effectiveness and cost-effectiveness of currently recommended treatment guidelines of PID in relation to long-term reproductive sequelae is needed. Most regimens of parenteral followed by oral antibiotic treatment are effective in resolving the acute symptoms and signs associated with PID. However, there is no good evidence on the optimal duration of treatment or comparing oral with parenteral treatment. Similarly, there is no evidence to support or refute empirical antibiotic treatment for suspected PID.

Surgical management of PID ranges from laparoscopy to laparotomy that is sometimes used to manage cases of ruptured tubo-ovarian abscess and severe peritonitis. Radical bilateral adnexectomy and hysterectomy is rarely indicated in the management of acute PID today.

Conservative laparoscopic modalities include procedures such as irrigation and drainage of the infected complex (de Wilde & Hesseling 1995, Molander et al 2001). However, controlled clinical trials are needed to evaluate the short-term and long-term response rates including preservation of fertility of acute-phase laparoscopic procedures.

OUTCOME

The worldwide increase in the incidence of PID during the past few decades has led to the secondary epidemics of TFI and ectopic pregnancy. PID and its sequelae account for a large proportion of the morbidity associated with sexually transmitted infections and the direct and indirect costs associated with PID are enormous. The proportion of TFI of all infertility ranges from approximately 37% in developed countries to up to 85% in developing countries (WHO 1995). After a single episode of PID, the risk for tubal factor infertility is approximately 7%. Each repeat episode of PID doubles or triples the risk (Weström 1980). TFI remains the leading indication for in vitro fertilization in developed countries and ectopic pregnancy is the main cause of maternal mortality in the first trimester of pregnancy in developing countries. Women with a history of PID have an approximately sixfold increased risk of tubal pregnancy compared to women with no history of PID and chronic pelvic pain occurs in a large proportion. They are also approximately 10 times more likely to be admitted for pelvic pain and hysterectomy rates are eight times higher than in other women. Thus, women with PID suffer substantial long-term gynaecological morbidity later in their lives (Buchan et al 1993).

PREVENTION STRATEGIES

Determination of risk factors for PID, especially those that are modifiable, is an essential step towards successful disease prevention (Simms & Stephenson 2000). Demographic and social indicators of risk such as race, socioeconomic status, age and marital status are markers of disease risk but are not modifiable. However, behavioural risk factors can be modified and should be targeted in campaigns for the prevention of PID.

Clinicians have an important role in the primary prevention of PID through lifestyle counselling and health education and by asking questions about risk-taking sexual behaviour, encouraging screening tests for those at risk, ensuring that male sex partners are evaluated and treated and by counselling about safe sex practices. However, primary prevention by health education has not proven to be very effective. More emphasis should be directed towards primary prevention. Effective school health education programmes should be implemented, especially among adolescents.

Secondary prevention by screening for *C. trachomatis* is likely to have the most critical role in the prevention of PID. Because *C. trachomatis* is the major cause of PID in developed countries, it is logical to focus PID prevention efforts on chlamydia (Scholes et al 1996). Chlamydial infections fill the general prerequisites for disease prevention by screening because they are highly prevalent, are associated with significant morbidity, can be diagnosed and are treatable. One recent randomized controlled trial showed that intervention with selective screening for chlamydial infections effectively reduced the incidence of PID by 64% during 1 year of follow-up (Scholes et al 1996). Use of FVU specimens (or vulvar or vaginal swabs) and NAA tests for diagnosis and a single dose of azithromycin for treatment should further enhance these efforts. However, it remains to be seen whether such intervention has a significant effect on the incidence of ectopic pregnancy and TFI.

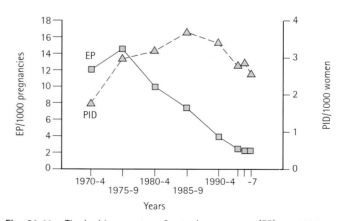

Fig. 61.11 The incidence rates of ectopic pregnancy (EP) per 1000 pregnancies and acute pelvic inflammatory disease (PID) per 1000 women in Örebro county, Sweden, from 1970 to 1997. Incidences were calculated per 5-year period from 1970–94 and then per year 1995–7 (Kamwendo et al 2000).

High *C. trachomatis* screening activity in Sweden resulted in a dramatic decrease of *C. trachomatis* rates, followed by a rapid decrease in the rates of hospitalizations for PID (Kamwendo et al 1998). Even more important, 5–10 years later this was followed by a significant fall in the rate of ectopic pregnancies, especially in young age groups (Egger et al 1998, Kamwendo et al 2000) (Fig. 61.11). These examples show that *C. trachomatis* screening is effective in a real-life situation. However, it is not yet known whether it produces a corresponding fall in the related incidence of TFI. Although *C. trachomatis* screening seems to be a straightforward approach, many research questions need to be addressed before nationwide screening programmes can be implemented.

Tertiary prevention includes treatment that prevents upper genital tract infection from leading to tubal dysfunction or obstruction. Early diagnosis and therapy can reduce the need for surgical intervention. The role of acute-phase laparoscopic intervention in combination with antimicrobial therapy should be evaluated in future clinical trials.

KEY POINTS

1. PID is a sexually transmitted infection with potentially harmful sequelae often managed suboptimally by physicians with little interest in the condition.
2. PID is the only preventable cause of infertility.
3. Screening for *C. trachomatis* is the most effective method of preventing PID.
4. The accuracy of syndrome diagnosis of PID should be improved by simple tests for the presence of lower genital tract infection.

REFERENCES

Buchan H, Vessey M, Goldacre M et al 1993 Morbidity following pelvic inflammatory disease. British Journal of Obstetrics and Gynaecology 100:558–562

Centers for Disease Control and Prevention 1997/1998 guidelines for treatment of sexually transmitted diseases. Morbidity and Mortality Weekly Report 47:1–111

Dallabetta GA, Gerbase AC, Holmes KK 1998 Problems, solutions, and challenges in syndromic management of sexually transmitted diseases. Sexually Transmitted Infections 74(suppl 1):S1–S11

de Wilde R, Hesseling M 1995 Tube-preserving diagnostic operative laparoscopy in pyosalpinx. Gynaecological Endoscopy 4:105–108

Egger M, Low N, Smith GD et al 1998 Screening for chlamydial infections and the risk of ectopic pregnancy in a county in Sweden: ecological analysis. British Medical Journal 316:1776–1780

Grimes DA 2000 Intrauterine device and upper-genital-tract infection. Lancet 356:1013–1019

Hasselquist MB, Hillier S 1991 Susceptibility of upper-genital tract isolates from women with pelvic inflammatory disease to ampicillin, cefpodoxime, metronidazole, and doxycycline. Sexually Transmitted Diseases 18:146–149

Hemsel DL, Ledger WJ, Martens M et al for the International Infectious Disease Society for Obstetrics and Gynaecology USA 2001 Concerns regarding the Centers for Disease Control's published guidelines for pelvic inflammatory disease. Clinical Infectious Diseases 32:103–107

Hillis SD, Joesoef R, Marchbanks PA 1993 Delayed care of pelvic inflammatory disease as a risk factor for impaired fertility. American Journal of Obstetrics and Gynecology 168:1503–1509

Kamwendo F, Forslin L, Bodin L, Danielsson D 1998 Programmes to reduce pelvic inflammatory disease – the Swedish experience. Lancet 351(suppl III):25–28

Kamwendo F, Forslin L, Bodin L et al 2000 Epidemiology of ectopic pregnancy during a 28 year period and the role of pelvic inflammatory disease. Sexually Transmitted Infections 76:28–32

McCormack WM 1994 Pelvic inflammatory disease. New England Journal of Medicine 330:115–119

Molander P, Cacciatore B, Sjöberg J, Paavonen J 2000 Laparoscopic management of acute pelvic inflammatory disease. Journal of the American Association of Gynecologic Laparoscopy 7:107–110

Molander P, Sjöberg J, Paavonen J, Cacciatore B 2001 Transvaginal power Doppler findings in laparoscopically proven acute PID Ultrasound in Obstetrics and Gynecology 17:233–238

Molander P, Paavonen J, Sjöberg J, Savelli L, Cacciatore B 2002 Transvaginal sonography in the diagnosis of acute appendicitis. Ultrasound in Obstetrics and Gynecology (in press)

Munday PE 2000 Pelvic inflammatory disease – an evidence-based approach to diagnosis. Journal of Infections 40:31–41

Paavonen J, Teisala K, Heinonen PK et al 1987 Microbiological and histopathological findings in acute pelvic inflammatory disease. British Journal of Obstetrics and Gynaecology 94:454–460

Patton DL, Lichtenwalner AB 1998 Animal models for the study of chlamydial infections. In: Chlamydial infections. Proceedings of the 9th International Symposium on Human Chlamydial Infection. Napa, California, USA, p 641

Scholes D, Stregachis A, Heidrich FE et al 1996 Prevention of pelvic inflammatory disease by screening for chlamydial infection. New England Journal of Medicine 334:1362–1366

Sellors J, Mahony J, Goldsmith C et al 1991 The accuracy of clinical findings and laparoscopy in pelvic inflammatory disease. American Journal of Obstetrics and Gynecology 164:113–120

Simms I, Stephenson JM 2000 Pelvic inflammatory disease epidemiology: what do we know and what do we need to know? Sexually Transmitted Infections 76:80–87

Stamm WE, Guinan ME, Johnson C 1984 Effect of treatment regimens for Neisseria gonorrhoeae on simultaneous infections with Chlamydia trachomatis. New England Journal of Medicine 310:545–549

Tukeva TA, Aronen HJ, Karjalainen PT et al 1999 MR imaging in pelvic inflammatory disease: comparison with laparoscopy and US. Radiology 210:209–216

van der Heyden JHA, Catchpole MA, Paget WJ, Stroobant A, the European Study Group 2000 Trends in gonorrhoea in nine western European countries, 1991–1996. Sexually Transmitted Infections 76:110–116

Walker CK, Kahn JG, Washington AE et al 1993 Pelvic inflammatory disease: metaanalysis of antimicrobial regimen efficacy. Journal of Infectious Diseases 168:969–978

Weström L 1980 Incidence, prevalence and trends of acute pelvic inflammatory disease and its consequences in industrial countries. American Journal of Obstetrics and Gynecology 138:880–892

Wilson J, Honey E, Templeton A et al 2002 The prevalence of Chlamydia trachomatis infection and screening practice in European women. Human Reproduction (submitted)

World Health Organization Task Force for the Prevention and Management of Infertility 1995 Tubal infertility: serologic relationship to past chlamydia and gonococcal infection. Sexually Transmitted Diseases 22:71–77

62

Sexually transmitted infections (STI)

Phillip Hay

INTRODUCTION

Sexually transmitted infections (STI) are one of the commonest reasons for seeing a doctor worldwide. A recent estimate from the UK is that 1.5% of young women have been treated in a genitourinary (G-U) medicine clinic for chlamydia in the last year. Despite this high incidence of detected infection, many STIs can be carried without symptoms for months or years. Most women experience an infection of the urogenital tract during their lifetime. The most common symptomatic infections are vulvovaginal candidiasis (thrush) and urinary tract infections, which are sexually associated rather than sexually transmitted. Viral infections such as human papilloma virus and herpes simplex virus may persist for life.

The stigma attached to STIs remains, despite the sexual revolution of the 1960s. The major morbidity of STIs include the sequelae of upper genital tract infection damaging the fallopian tubes, and cervical cancer as a result of HPV infection. The long-term sequelae of damage to the fallopian tubes include ectopic pregnancy and tubular factor infertility. Worldwide, human immunodeficiency virus (HIV) infection is predominantly sexually acquired and in some parts of the world as many as one-quarter to a one-third of pregnant women are now infected. Gynaecologists need to be aware of the way that HIV alters the manifestations of, and host susceptibility to, other infections. The current sexual health strategy recognizes that most people with STIs remain undiagnosed and seeks to increase the uptake of testing in general practice, family planning, gynaecology and other settings. Liaison can then occur with the established network of genitourinary medicine clinics for treatment, follow-up and partner notification. We now have the opportunity to screen non-invasively for infections such as chlamydia using DNA detection tests. This is being evaluated by pilot studies for the Department of Health and is likely to be adopted nationally.

EPIDEMIOLOGY

There was a dramatic increase in the reported incidence of STIs following the sexual revolution of the 1960s. This was followed by a fall, particularly in homosexual men in the late 1980s, following the safer sex campaigns that resulted from awareness of the acquired immune deficiency syndrome (AIDS) epidemic. In the last 5 years, however, there has been a rise in the incidence of STIs in the UK, particularly in the younger population. This is demonstrated by the incidence of gonorrhoea shown in Figure 62.1.

In the UK pilot studies of chlamydia screening the prevalence of chlamydia was 14% in women under 20 years of age. The sexual revolution of the 1960s was facilitated by the wider availability of reliable contraception and changing sexual mores. This trend was augmented by earlier sexual maturity in

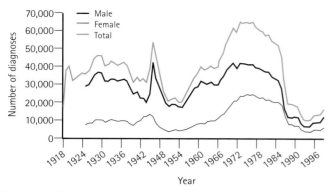

Fig. 62.1 Diagnoses of gonorrhoea seen in GUM clinics in England, Scotland and Wales from 1918 to 1996. The equivalent Scottish data are only available from 1922 onwards. As Northern Ireland data from the period 1918 to 1922 is incomplete they have been excluded from this figure.

Table 62.1 Markers for women at risk of STI

Age	15–34 years (maximal incidence 20–24)
Marital status	Single, separated or divorced
	Married before the age of 20
Occupation	Patient or consort with mobile job
Medical history	Previous STI
	Previous termination of pregnancy
	Multiple pregnancies before age 20
	Previous parasuicide or drug abuse
	Previous abnormal cervical cytology
Social history	Newly living away from home
	Disturbed family background
	Previously in care of local authority
	History of prostitution
	Late booking for antenatal care
	Self-applied tattoos

girls and earlier age of onset of sexual activity in both sexes. The change in sexual behaviour among young women is manifest as a falling ratio of male:female patients for most STIs, which now approaches 1. In the UK the importance of commercial sex workers (CSWs) as vectors of STI transmission has declined, although they remain of major importance in disease transmission in developing countries. Drug use often linked to commercial sex work, and the exchange of sex for drugs is particularly risky.

Other sociological changes that contribute to the increased incidence of STI include urbanization, increased mobility among the young, and the greater ease of international travel. Sexual tourism is increasingly common. This last factor has also promoted the importation of tropical STIs and antibiotic-resistant infections. It is a strange paradox that, despite the availability of effective treatment during the past 40 years, STIs have become more common in many countries.

The advent of AIDS has focused attention upon sexual behaviour and emphasised the importance of STI control. In most countries the commonest method of HIV transmission is by heterosexual intercourse. In sub-Saharan Africa and Southeast Asia there is widespread infection among young women, and consequent vertical transmission in pregnancy. Currently, the epidemic appears poised to spread through Russia and the old Eastern bloc. This is described in detail in the chapter on HIV (Chapter 63).

The major risk groups show considerable overlap with those of other medical conditions, e.g. women requesting termination of pregnancy or with increased obstetric hazards (Table 62.1).

Changed sexual behaviour as a consequence of the HIV threat dramatically reduced the incidence of all STIs among gay men, although a recent increase in the incidence of gonorrhoea in this group suggests that a new generation needs to be educated about safe sex. However, there has been far less of a change among heterosexuals. A high rate of sexual partner change, which is the single most important factor in determining risk for STI, remains common in many groups of young people. It is not necessarily related to social class, to educational attainment or to standards of personal hygiene. STIs not infrequently occur in apparently stable relationships, where neither partner admits infidelity. It is important to recognize that many STIs have long latent phases and that there are asymptomatic carriers in both sexes.

PRINCIPLES OF MANAGEMENT OF SEXUALLY TRANSMISSIBLE INFECTIONS

Many gynaecological infections are sexually transmissible. It takes practice to be comfortable taking a sexual history from a patient. If the clinician is embarrassed, this is quickly transmitted to the patient. It is also difficult to take a sexual history if there are friends or relatives present or in a ward or cubicle in which there is inadequate privacy and soundproofing. It is sometimes necessary therefore to postpone seeking a detailed history until the right atmosphere can be provided. A good history will contain details of the presenting symptoms, associated local or constitutional features. Parity, previous obstetric, medical and surgical history are noted; current drug therapy, including self-medication, and drug allergies are also recorded. In order to assess the risk of an individual having acquired a sexually transmitted disease, and to determine which samples to take to screen adequately we need to find out:

- When sexual intercourse last took place;
- Whether this was oral, vaginal or anal;
- What contraception was used;
- When the woman last had a different sexual partner, and any others in the previous 3 months;
- A travel history and knowledge about the origin of partners which may indicate a risk of a tropical infection seldom seen in the UK;
- Menstrual history (particularly to ascertain any risk of pregnancy).

Enquire about possible intravenous drug use by the patient and her partners. Do not assume that a woman is heterosexual until you have ascertained the sex of her partners.

Examination is best performed in the lithotomy position to allow adequate inspection of the external genitalia, perineum and perianal area, noting any ulcers, scars or warts. Palpate the inguinal lymph nodes, noting enlargement, asymmetry or tenderness. After passing a speculum note the quantity, colour and consistency of vaginal and cervical discharge. Contact bleeding of the cervix can be an indicator of cervicitis. Cervical motion tenderness, adnexal tenderness and masses may be indicative of pelvic inflammatory disease on bimanual examination.

If one sexually transmissible infection is present or suspected then there may be others. Ideally, therefore, a full screen should be performed for chlamydia, gonorrhoea, vaginal infections and serological tests for syphilis and hepatitis B, HIV and hepatitis C if indicated. Current practice is to only perform testing for HIV after a full pre-test discussion, although some units may move to providing written information for individuals without identified high-risk factors. If facilities are not available for such a screen, refer the patient to a genitourinary medicine (GUM) clinic.

If drug treatment is required simple regimens, preferably single dose are usually preferred to ensure adherence, particularly when treating asymptomatic infections. To break the chain of infection and prevent re-infection of the patient, it is essential that she avoids intercourse until she is sure that her partner(s) has been screened and received appropriate treatment. Follow-up evaluation and tests of cure are essential for individuals with gonorrhoea. There are psychological and social consequences for each affected individual which require additional management. Education and counselling should be performed in a non-judgemental manner.

CLINICAL PRESENTATIONS

Patients present with clinical syndromes rather than microbiological presentations. Thus chlamydia and gonorrhoea cause a similar spectrum of disease, although gonorrhoea may produce more florid discharge and have a shorter incubation period. The most common presentation of STIs is none, i.e., asymptomatic infection that may be picked up by screening, through partner notification or by chance when presenting with another condition.

In women the most common symptomatic presentations include abnormal vaginal discharge which might arise from vaginal infection or cervicitis. Cervicitis may also present as post-coital bleeding. Endometritis might produce inter-menstrual bleeding and pelvic pain. Salpingo-oophoritis presents as pelvic inflammatory disease (PID) with pelvic pain and deep dyspareunia. Fitz-Hugh Curtis syndrome presents as fever and right hypochondrial pain. Genital ulcers are most likely to be due to herpes simplex infection, but have a wide differential diagnosis. Immunosuppression due to HIV can alter the presentation of many STIs. If unrecognized, the late presentation of chlamydial or gonococcal PID is ectopic pregnancy, tubal factor infertility and chronic pelvic pain.

In many resource-poor settings STIs are managed by syndromic management. The wide differential diagnosis of vaginal discharge means that women are treated with combinations of antibiotics to cover bacterial vaginosis and trichomoniasis (metronidazole), as well as cervicitis from chlamydia (tetracycline or macrolides) and gonorrhoea (depending on local sensitivity patterns and availability). This results in the use of antibiotics that are not specifically indicated in many cases.

Table 62.2 The differential diagnosis of genital ulcers

Infective	Non-Infective
Herpes simplex virus	Aphthous ulcers
Primary syphilis	Trauma
Lymphogranuloma venereum	Skin disease e.g. lichen sclerosis
Chancroid	et atrophicus
Donovanosis	Behçet's Syndrome
HIV	Other Multisystem Disorder e.g.
	Sarcoidosis
	Dermatitis artefacta

GENITAL ULCERS

Herpes is the commonest cause of genital ulcers. In many tropical areas other STIs: chancroid; lymphogranuloma venereum; and Donovanosis present as ulceration. Underlying HIV infection may alter the presentation of any of these conditions. Non-infective causes of genital ulceration include traumatic ulcers, aphthous ulcers and Behçet's syndrome (Table 62.2).

Genital herpes

The human herpes viruses are characterized by life-long persistence of infection and the potential for reactivation, resulting in repeated disease episodes. The chronic nature of the infection means that many people know that it is 'incurable' and feel particular distress on being diagnosed with it. In the UK there has been a large increase in the reported cases of genital herpes since the early 1980s. This is partially a reflection of increased awareness and better diagnostic methods, but is principally a true increase in incidence matching those of other STIs.

Biology
Genital herpes is caused by the herpes simplex virus (HSV) types 1 and 2, which are large complex DNA viruses. Transmission occurs by contact with a person who is shedding virus, with or without symptomatic lesions. The incubation period is 2–14 days. Apparently longer incubation periods are usually due to 'non-primary first episodes'. It is becoming apparent from seroprevalence studies employing type-specific antibody tests that asymptomatic acquisition of HSV-2 infection may be the rule rather than the exception. In the UK, HSV-1 accounts for more than 50% of first episodes. This may reflect changes in sexual practices. HSV-1 may be transmitted in monogamous relationships from oro-labial lesions to the genitals of the partner, especially if they have pre-existing candida infection or vulval skin disease.

Clinical features
First episodes are often severe in women. They are less severe in those previously infected with oro-labial herpes. Symptoms are both local and constitutional. Pain, dysuria and discharge are commonly associated with flu-like symptoms.

The lesions begin as erythematous plaques, which vesiculate and then form extremely tender superficial ulcers that possess an erythematous halo and a yellow or grey base. These are

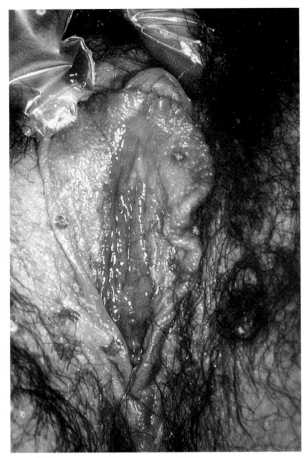

Fig. 62.2   Primary genital herpes: multiple painful ulcers are present on the labia minora.

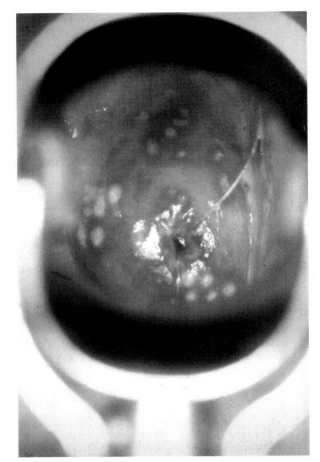

Fig. 62.3   Primary genital herpes: ulcers on the cervix.

often accompanied by bilateral inguinal lymphadenopathy. Lesions may be widespread in women and affect the introitus, labia majora, perineum, vagina and cervix (Figures 62.2 and 62.3). Without treatment, a primary episode lasts for 3–4 weeks.

Complications of first episodes are common. There may be secondary bacterial infection of lesions. Autoinoculation to distant sites occurs, especially to the fingers and eyes. Local neurological complications include a sacral radiculomyelopathy causing self-limiting hyperaesthesia in the buttocks, thighs or perineum, decrease in sensation over the sacral dermatomes and difficulty in bladder and bowel emptying. Acute urinary retention can occur as a result of this neuropathy, or simply due to severe pain (Figure 62.4). A self-limiting meningitis is sometimes seen. Severe, potentially fatal encephalitis is an extremely rare complication more typical in immunosuppressed individuals. Fulminating disseminated HSV infection is a very rare complication of primary infection in the third trimester of pregnancy.

Recurrent episodes occur in about 50% of patients. HSV-1 is less likely to cause recurrent disease than HSV-2. Recurrences are shorter, lasting 5–10 days, less severe, and are usually unilateral. Prodromal symptoms preceding the outbreak by 1–2 days consist of neuralgic-type pain in the buttocks, ankles or groin, or hyperaesthesia at the site of the lesion. Constitutional symptoms are less frequent. Psychological symptoms are often marked in those with frequent recurrences, and may be accompanied by emotional and relationship difficulties. Stress, dietary factors, menstruation, exposure to sunlight or sunbeds, and local trauma associated with intercourse may precipitate recurrences. Often no precipitating factor is identified. In the immunosuppressed patient recurrences can be frequent and prolonged. Herpetic ulceration persisting for more than 1 month is AIDS defining in someone with HIV infection. These individuals are also most at risk for developing aciclovir resistant herpes, which may require treatment with topical or intravenous foscarnet.

Diagnosis

The diagnosis should be confirmed by isolation of the virus in tissue culture or by detection of virus antigen in immuno-fluorescent or ELISA assays. Recently assays have been developed which detect type-specific antibodies to HSV-2 glycoprotein G; these have proved useful in epidemiological studies. Type-specific serological tests are now available, although their place in clinical management has not been defined. Screening tests for other STIs are essential, but may have to be delayed in first episodes because of severe discomfort preventing adequate examination. A negative culture does not exclude the diagnosis in someone with a typical ulcer. S/he should be asked to return for further testing if there are future recurrences.

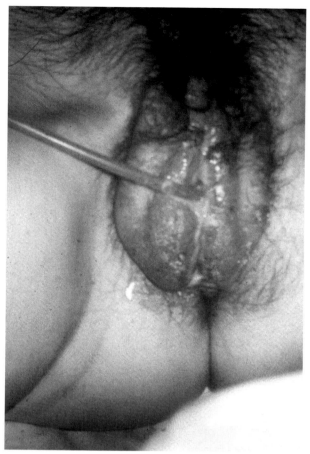

Fig. 62.4   Primary genital herpes: urinary retention and vulval oedema.

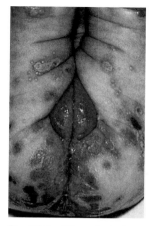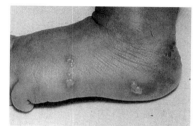

Fig. 62.5   Disseminated neonatal herpes: the lesions on the napkin area are haemorrhagic and ulcerated but vesicles are present on the foot.

Treatment

The general management should be as for other STIs. Patients need counselling as well as both symptomatic and specific therapy. Rest, and systematic and local analgesia are important in severe primary cases. Secondary bacterial infection may require antibiotics. Frequent saline bathing is not only soothing but also controls infection in most cases. Passing urine in the bath reduces pain and lessens the risk of retention.

Specific therapy is with aciclovir tablets 200 mg five times day for 5 days. Recurrences are usually self-limiting in 3–5 days. Antiviral agents do not usefully reduce their duration and should not be prescribed unless the patient is immunosuppressed, or the episode is unusually prolonged. In the few patients with frequent recurrences; more than 6–8 per year, suppressive treatment with aciclovir 400 mg twice daily can be effective in reducing the frequency of symptomatic recurrences, but does not eliminate completely the risk of transmission to partners during asymptomatic shedding. The need for such therapy should be re-evaluated after 6–12 months. New antiviral agents: famciclovir and valaciclovir; with improved bioavailability and half lives allow less frequent dosing, and appear as effective. The concept of using immune stimulants such as imiquimod is being studied. Several subunit vaccines have been developed and are currently being evaluated for the prophylaxis of HSV

infection. The possibility of a therapeutic vaccine is also being investigated.

Neonatal herpes

Neonatal herpes is a well-recognized complication of maternal genital herpes at the time of labour. The majority of cases of neonatal HSV infection arise from primary, often undetected, maternal infection (Fig. 62.5); the risk of transmission from a recurrent attack or from asymptomatic shedding is much lower (1–4%). Transmission is more likely if the neonate has suffered skin trauma from scalp electrodes or instrumental delivery. The best way to manage herpes in pregnancy is not clear.

One strategy is to carefully examine the vulva and cervix for herpes lesions in all women in labour. In cases of primary genital herpes a caesarean section should be performed. Where there is a history of genital herpes most obstetricians would recommend a caesarean section if the woman has a clinically apparent recurrence of prodromal symptoms at delivery, and the membranes have not been ruptured for more than 4 hours. Others feel that with recurrent lesions the risk of transmission is so low that vaginal delivery is safe. If this approach is taken, the neonate should be monitored closely and viral cultures taken; if HSV is isolated aciclovir should be started. Another approach being evaluated is the use of aciclovir in late pregnancy to suppress recurrences and asymptomatic shedding. Aciclovir appears to be safe and may be effective, although it is not yet licensed for this purpose.

The new type-specific antibody assays have shown the seroprevalence of HSV-2 to be around 30%; this adds weight to the evidence that the risk of transmission from non-primary maternal HSV infection is very low. The possibility of identifying high-risk women who are seronegative for HSV-2 but whose partners are seropositive, holds much promise for the future.

Syphilis

Syphilis is a chronic, systemic sexually transmissible infection caused by *Treponema pallidum*. In vitro, *T. pallidum* venereum causing venereal syphilis cannot be distinguished from *T. pertenue* which causes yaws, *T. pallidum* endemicum causing endemic syphilis, and *T. carateum* causing pinta. These three tropical treponematoses are not sexually transmitted, but pass between children and household contacts. A description of them is beyond the scope of this chapter. Clinicians in the UK must be aware that they occur in Sub-Saharan Africa, the Caribbean and most of the humid tropics (yaws), in desert regions (endemic syphilis), and isolated parts of Central and South America (pinta). Following such an infection the sero-logical tests for syphilis may remain positive for life, causing diagnostic confusion. The tropical treponematoses have become less common following mass treatment campaigns in the 1950s and 1960s, but they still occur, particularly in rural areas. If venereal syphilis cannot be excluded in someone with positive serological tests originating from one of these areas it is safest to administer treatment for syphilis. In developing countries syphilis remains a significant cause of morbidity and mortality among women and neonates. There have been local epidemics of syphilis in the Russia, the USA and the UK in the last 15 years related to homosexual men, and heterosexual spread particularly related to commercial sex work and crack cocaine use.

Clinical features

Syphilis is a chronic disorder, in which periods of florid clinical manifestations are interspersed by periods of latency. Early syphilis includes the primary, secondary and early latent stages in the first 2 years following infection, when sexual trans-mission can occur. Subsequently only vertical transmission occurs.

The first manifestation of venereal syphilis is a chancre at the site of inoculation, usually the external genitalia. Sometimes multiple lesions are seen. Chancres are usually painless, raised, well circumscribed ulcers (Fig. 62.6). The regional lymph nodes become enlarged, but not tender. Primary syphilis usually occurs 3 to 6 weeks after infection, but up to 3 months, and resolves spontaneously without treatment after a few weeks.

Presentation with secondary syphilis is more common in women when the primary lesion has been hidden in the vagina or on the cervix. Secondary syphilis can arise as the chancre disappears or up to 6 months later. This is manifest by a systemic eruption, most often a non-itchy maculopapular rash. It is symmetrical and involves the palms of the hands and soles of the feet. It may subsequently become nodular (Fig. 62.7). More florid lesions resembling warts, condylomata lata are seen in intertriginous areas, particularly perianally. Mucous patches and linear (snail track) ulcers are seen on the mucosal surfaces. There may be generalized lymphadenopathy. Other manifestations include fever, headache, bone pain, alopecia, arthritis, and meningitis. A sensorineural deafness can occur early in the infection, due to destruction of the hair cells in the inner ear.

Following resolution of secondary syphilis a period of latency occurs. There are no outward manifestations of infection, which is only detected on serological testing. There is a potential for lesions of secondary syphilis to relapse for up to 2 years, during which infection can be transmitted to a sexual partner. This is therefore called early latent syphilis.

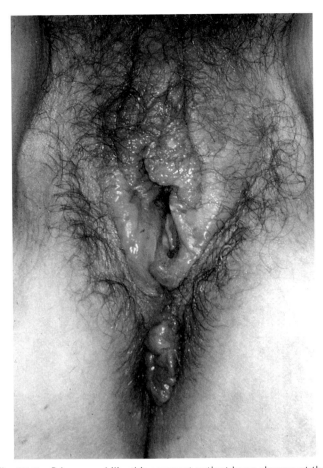

Fig. 62.6 Primary syphilis: this pregnant patient has a chancre at the fourchette with local oedema in the labia. She also has a trichomonal discharge.

Primary and secondary syphilis are not life threatening. The importance of the diagnosis rests on the risk of late tertiary syphilis. Neurosyphilis can be manifest within 5 years of infection in the form of meningovascular syphilis presenting with a stroke. This may subsequently progress to tabes dorsalis or general paresis of the insane. Approximately 10% of men and 5% of women develop neurosyphilis if not treated in the early stages. Approximately 20% will develop cardiovascular syphilis manifest as thoracic aortic aneurysm or aortic regurgitation, which can present many years later.

Congenital syphilis

Maternal syphilis often has an adverse effect on the pregnancy. T. pallidum can infect the fetus transplacentally at any time, typically leading to intrauterine death and mid-trimester abortion. The risk of congenital infection is greatest, as high as 70%, with primary and secondary syphilis but can occur even 5 to 10 years later. In surviving fetuses intrauterine growth retardation and prematurity are likely. Congenital infection may be readily apparent at birth. In less severely infected infants clinical manifestations can be delayed for weeks, months or years. The stigmata of late congenital syphilis include Hutchinson's triad of interstitial keratitis leading to corneal scarring, nerve deafness and notched permanent incisor

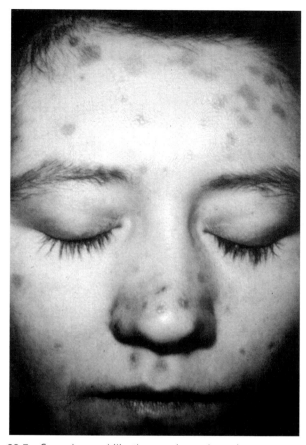

Fig. 62.7 Secondary syphilis: the maculopapular rash.

Table 62.3 Common patterns of syphilis serology

VDRL	TPHA	FTA	Likely diagnosis
+	–	–	False positive – repeat to exclude primary syphilis
+	+/–	+	Primary syphilis – dark-ground may be positive
+	+	+	Untreated or recently treated syphilis – probably beyond primary stage
–	+	+	Treated or partially treated syphilis – any stage Untreated latent or late syphilis
–	+	–	Treated syphilis
–	–	+	Very early primary syphilis

Treatment

T. pallidum replicates slowly, with an estimated doubling time of 20 hours. Sustained treponemicidal levels of antibiotic are needed for a minimum of 12 days in early syphilis. The treatment of choice is penicillin. A variety of regimens are used:

- Procaine penicillin 1.2 MU daily by intramuscular injection for 12 days;
- Benzathine penicillin 2.4 MU by intramuscular injection, repeated after 7 days;
- Doxycycline 100 mg two times/day for 14 days;
- Erythromycin 500 mg four times/day for 14 days.

In the UK daily administration of procaine penicillin 1.2 MU daily is prescribed commonly. If the infection has been present for more than 1 year treatment is extended to 21 days for penicillin regiments and 28 days for oral regimens. Only intravenous penicillin or high doses of procaine penicillin (2.4 MU daily) combined with probenecid (500 mg four times/day) produce adequate levels of penicillin in the CSF to treat neurosyphilis. In pregnancy the absorption of erythromycin is unreliable. Consider intravenous treatment for penicillin allergic pregnant women, or desensitization to penicillin.

Partner notification is essential. Review the sexual history. In some cases partners from a few years previously should be contacted when possible. Children may need to be tested, and siblings if congenital infection is possible. This may be arranged most easily with the help of a GUM clinic.

Ceftriaxone and azithromycin are being evaluated as potential treatments at present.

Congenitally infected babies are treated with procaine penicillin 500 mg/kg intravenous injection daily for 10 days. Babies born to mothers treated with penicillin at any stage of pregnancy do not need additional therapy.

teeth which may not present until childhood. These effects of late congenital syphilis are not necessarily prevented unless the mother is treated before 20 weeks of gestation in pregnancy.

Diagnosis

In primary and secondary syphilis the diagnosis is rapidly confirmed with dark-ground microscopy by demonstrating motile T. pallidum in serum from abraded lesions. Serological tests become positive in late primary disease, reach maximal titres in the secondary stage and decline slowly during the latent phase. Request an FTA specifically if primary syphilis is suspected, as it is the earliest test to become positive. Table 62.3 shows common patterns of syphilis serology. It is unusual for the highly sensitive, specific treponemal antibody tests such as the TPHA and fluorescent treponemal antibody (FTA-absorbed) to become completely negative, even after treatment. Biological false positive reagin tests are occasionally seen during pregnancy. This can be an indicator of anti-phospholipid syndrome or systemic lupus erythematosis. The specific treponemal tests will generally be negative, although false positive FTA-absorbed tests have been reported. The serological tests should always be repeated to exclude early syphilis.

Recently developed enzyme immunoassay (EIA) tests to detect anti-treponemal IgM and IgG appear to be both sensitive and specific. Because they can be automated, they are likely to be used increasingly for screening purposes.

Prevention

A further fall in the incidence of acquired syphilis will depend upon adoption of safer sexual practices. Congenital syphilis is totally preventable and antenatal testing remains cost-effective despite the low prevalence of syphilis in developed countries. If the incidence of syphilis is high repeat testing in the third trimester of pregnancy may identify a number of women who have seroconverted during pregnancy.

Table 62.4 Treatment for bacterial genital ulcers

Antibacterial Agent	Primary Syphilis	Lymphogranuloma venereum	Chancroid	Donovanosis
Azithromycin	Active, but not fully evaluated	Active, but not fully evaluated	1 Gram Stat	
Ceftriaxone	Active, but not fully evaluated		250 mg Stat IM	
Ciprofloxacin	Not active	Not reliable	500 mg twice/day for 3 days	750 mg twice/day for 21 days minimum
Cotrimoxazole	Not active		May be used, but resistance is common in some areas	960 mg twice/day for 21 days minimum
Doxycycline	100 mg twice/day for 14 days	100 mg twice/day for 21 days		100 mg twice/day for 21 days minimum
Erythromycin	500 mg four times/day for 14 days	500 mg four times/day for 21 days	500 mg four times/day for 7 days	500 mg four times/day for 21 days minimum
Penicillin	Procaine penicillin 1.2 MU/day for 12 days			

Tropical genital ulcer disease

Sexually transmitted infections causing genital ulcer disease present considerable diagnostic difficulty. In some cases more than one infecting agent may be present. Most of the aetiological agents cannot be cultured in standard microbiological media. Histological examination of tissue is sometimes the only means of confirming the diagnosis. In many resource-poor tropical countries a syndromic approach is taken to treatment of genital ulcers. Recommended treatments are shown in Table 62.4.

Lymphogranuloma venereum

Lymphogranuloma venereum (LGV) is caused by specific serovars (L1-L3) of Chlamydia trachomatis. It is found in the Far East, Sub-Saharan Africa and South America. In the early stages there is often a small superficial ulcer that can slowly increase in size, but often goes unnoticed. More obvious are the enlarged nodes, which become compressed by the inguinal ligament leading to the so-called groove sign. The nodes can become matted together and discharge pus, forming a bubo. In women a severe proctocolitis can progress to fistulae and strictures. The diagnosis can be confirmed serologically by a complement fixation test.

Chancroid

Chancroid is an infection caused by *Haemophilus ducreyii*. The geographical distribution is similar to that of LGV. It starts with small shallow ulcers which are usually multiple and painful. The edges are irregular and there is localized lymphadenopathy. The sores may persist for several months and the glands can suppurate through the skin. The organism can only be grown on specialized culture medium and ideally the medium should be inoculated directly from the patient. Even so it may be difficult to obtain a positive culture. There is a characteristic appearance on biopsy when Ducreyii's bacillus may be seen.

Granuloma inguinale (donovanosis)

Granuloma inguinale is an infection caused by *Klebsiella granulomatis* (previously called *Calymmatobacterium granulomatis*). It is

endemic in India, Papua New Guinea and Southern Africa. It is usually a slowly progressive infection starting with discrete papule on the skin or vulva which can enlarge to form 'beefy red' painful ulcers. These spread slowly around the genitalia and perineum. As they heal, fibrosis can develop which may lead to lymphoedema and elephantiasis. Diagnosis is best confirmed by biopsy or a crush preparation in which Donovan bodies are visible.

Gonorrhoea

Gonorrhoea and chlamydia infect the same tissues and cause a similar spectrum of disease. Up to 50% women with gonorrhoea have concomitant chlamydial infection. The causative agent of gonorrhoea, *Neisseria gonorrhoeae* was described by Albert Neisser in 1879. It reached a peak incidence in the UK during the mid 1970s, declined in the late 1980s/1990s but is again on the increase (Fig. 62.1). In some studies in Sub-Saharan Africa, 1–2% of men and women have been found to harbour apparently asymptomatic infection. Gonorrhoea remains a common cause of morbidity in women and neonates worldwide, and antibiotic resistance is increasingly encountered in developing and developed countries.

The organism is highly infectious and is transmissible prior to the onset of symptoms. Gonorrhoea has a short incubation period, usually 2–5 days. Asymptomatic infections are common in women, especially during pregnancy, and also occur in men. This results in late presentation with complications, and facilitates disease transmission.

Biology

Neisseria gonorrhoeae is a Gram-negative diplococcus bacterium. It colonizes columnar or cuboidal epithelium. In chronic infection there is a complex interaction with the host immune system. The expression of antigenic surface proteins changes over time in the face of an effective antibody response. Protective immunity does not appear to develop. Reliable serological tests for gonorrhoea have not been developed. Strains resistant to antibiotics emerge rapidly, where antibiotic use is not controlled adequately.

Chromosomal mutations conferring reduced sensitivity to penicillin emerge slowly in an incremental way. High level

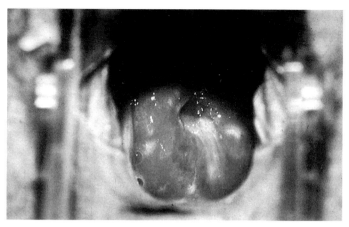

Fig. 62.8   Gonococcal cervicitis: the purulent endocervical discharge.

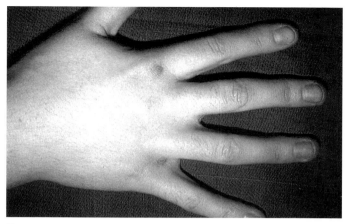

Fig. 62.9   Skin lesions caused by systemic gonococcal infection.

resistance to penicillin is mediated by a plasmid. The first one described encoded a penicillinase enzyme (PPNG strains). There is similarly a Tet-M plasmid conferring resistance to tetracyclines. Chromosomal mutations conferring resistance to quinolone antibiotics have emerged in the last decade.

Clinical features

At least half of all infected women have no symptoms and present as the result of contact-tracing procedures. When present, symptoms are similar to those of other lower genital tract infections, consisting of excessive vaginal discharge and dysuria.

Examination may reveal no abnormality but there may be signs of cervicitis, with a mucopurulent cervical discharge (Fig. 62.8). It is unusual to observe a urethral discharge in women. Rectal and pharyngeal infections are asymptomatic in the majority of cases and are more difficult to eradicate.

Complications

Complications may be local, ascending or distant. Acute local complications include skenitis, resulting in pain and swelling at the urinary meatus, and bartholinitis, causing painful unilateral vulval swelling which is fluctuant if an abscess has formed. The major ascending complication is pelvic inflammatory disease, which occurs in about 15% of infected women.

Distant complications consist of perihepatitis and septicaemia. Gonococcal perihepatitis results from spread of infection to the liver capsule, which may then form adhesions to the abdominal wall. Patients complain of pain in the right upper abdomen which is worse on coughing, deep breathing and on flexing the trunk. The pain may be referred to the right shoulder and may be accompanied by nausea and vomiting. Pyrexia, abdominal tenderness and signs of lower genital tract infection are usually present, and pelvic inflammatory disease may coexist.

Septicaemia is most often due to gonococci with particular growth requirements; these organisms are usually very sensitive to penicillin. Pregnancy appears to be a predisposing factor. This is usually a relatively benign illness, characterized by low-grade fever, asymmetrical arthralgia, tenosynovitis and arthritis

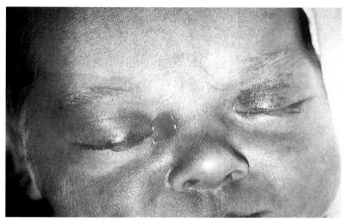

Fig. 62.10   Gonococcal ophthalmia neonatorum.

affecting wrists, elbows, knees and small joints of the hand. A peripheral skin rash may occur with crops of pink papules which become pustular with central necrosis (Fig. 62.9).

In pregnancy, gonorrhoea may be associated with early abortion, intrauterine growth retardation, prematurity and postpartum sepsis. Gonococcal opthalmia neonatorum usually begins 2–7 days after birth, with severe bilateral conjunctivitis (Fig. 62.10). This can lead to keratitis and blindness unless promptly treated. Gonococcal ophthalmia is a notifiable disease.

Although many men with gonorrhoea develop an overt urethritis with dysuria and a urethral discharge, the male consorts of women with complicated gonorrhoea are often asymptomatic carriers of N. gonorrhoeae.

Diagnosis

Typically the organism infects columnar epithelium. In GUM clinics the diagnosis is made presumptively by observing typical Gram-negative intracellular diplococci on Gram stained smears of urethral, cervical and rectal swabs. It is a fastidious organisms, requiring a CO_2 concentration of 7%, specific media such as blood agar and antibiotics to inhibit the growth of other organisms. Particularly if transport to the laboratory is delayed it may fail to grow on culture. Microscopy of clinical samples from women is only 50% sensitive at best. DNA-based detection tests are available for screening, but culture remains essential to allow antibiotic sensitivity testing.

Treatment

Gonorrhoea can usually be cured with a single dose of a suitable antibiotic. In the UK penicillin remains effective; it is usually given as amoxycillin and probenecid. Elsewhere in the world, due to either plasmid-borne β-lactamase production or chromosomally mediated factors, penicillin resistance is the rule, rendering the drug useless. This is often accompanied by resistance to aminoglycosides, tetracyclines, sulphonamides and other antibiotics. Suitable single-dose regimens are shown in Table 62.5. Recently the incidence of quinolone (ciprofloxacin) resistance in the UK has risen exponentially (Fig. 62.11). Cephalosporins are currently reliable in such cases.

In complicated infections continuous therapy is given. In gonococcal pelvic inflammatory disease it is important to remember that concurrent infection with Chlamydia, mycoplasmas, anaerobes and other facultative pathogens is common. Thus, initial antibiotic regimens usually include metronidazole, and will change from penicillin-based to tetracycline-based after the first 2–3 days.

Gonococcal ophthalmia is preventable and prophylaxis should continue in developing countries where infection rates remain high and antenatal maternal screening is not possible. Erythromycin (1%) or 1% tetracycline eye ointments can be used. Established neonatal disease is treated with a β-lactam stable antibiotic such as cefotaxime 100 mg/kg/day IV in three divided doses. It is probably unnecessary to use additional topical antibiotics, although regular saline irrigation to remove inflammatory exudate from the eyes is required.

It is essential that contact tracing is performed in all gonococcal infections, and both parents of infected babies should be examined as a matter of urgency.

Chlamydia

Chlamydia trachomatis is probably the commonest sexually transmitted bacterial pathogen in developed countries. This unusual Gram-negative bacterium behaves like a virus in that it replicates intracellularly. It is responsible for at least half of all cases of non-specific genital infection, which includes non-specific urethritis in the male and related conditions in the female.

Biology

C. trachomatis is a small bacterium, which is an obligate intracellular pathogen. Serovars A–C cause trachoma, infecting the conjunctiva. Serovars D–K cause genital infections. Specific LGV serovars (L1–L3) cause lymphogranuloma venereum. The infectious particle is the elementary body, which infects columnar epithelial cells in the genital tract. It gains entry to the cells by binding to specific surface receptors. Once inside the cell, inclusion bodies form. These contain the metabolically active reticulate bodies. These divide by binary fission. After a 48-hour life cycle, reticulate bodies condense into elementary bodies which are released from the cell surface. Heavily infected cells die, but it is the inflammatory response to infection that contributes most to damaging the epithelial surface. Humoral immunity may protect from reinfection, but antibodies are serovar specific and the protection is short lived. Cell-mediated immunity, with activation of cytotoxic T-cells and production of interferon-γ is more important for controlling established infection.

Clinical features

In women, early chlamydial infections are often silent and may remain so for months and possibly years. Most women are diagnosed as a result of routine screening, if complications occur, or if their partner presents with non-gonococcal urethritis (NGU). Symptomatic chlamydial infection may present with a wide variety of manifestations. Urethral involvement may lead to dysuria and frequency; Chlamydia is a cause of the urethral syndrome in young women. Sterile pyuria should alert the Clinician to the possibility of chlamydial infection. Cervical infection may be associated with an excessive discharge and postcoital or intermenstrual bleeding. Examination may show congested, oedematous cervical ectopy with small follicles, or there may be unexpected contact bleeding from the endocervical canal (Fig. 62.12). Mucopurulent cervicitis is regarded as the female equivalent of urethritis in men by some authorities. A purulent discharge from the cervix, often accompanied by contact bleeding after swabbing, arises due to infection from chlamydia, gonorrhoea or other organisms. Often, however, there are no abnormal signs.

Complications of local infection include skenitis and bartholinitis. Ascending infection may cause endometritis, which may manifest as painful and excessive menstrual loss.

Table 62.5 Single-dose regimens for gonorrhoea

Medication	Dosage
Spectinomycin	2–4 g IM
Amoxycillin with probenecid 1 g by mouth	3 g by mouth
Cefuroxime	1 g by mouth
Ciprofloxacin	250 mg by mouth
Doxycycline	300 mg by mouth
Minocycline	300 mg by mouth

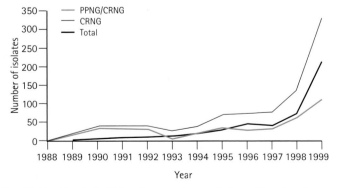

Fig. 62.11 Trends in *Neisseria gonorrhoeae* strains with reduced susceptibility to ciprofloxacin for England and Wales, 1988 to 1999. This shows the increase in resistant strains, particularly in the late 1990s.
PPNG/CRNG, penicillinase producing *N. gonorrhoeae* with decreased susceptibility to ciprofloxacin; CRNG, *N. gonorrhoeae* with decreased susceptibility to ciprofloxacin: MIC ≥0.05mg/l.

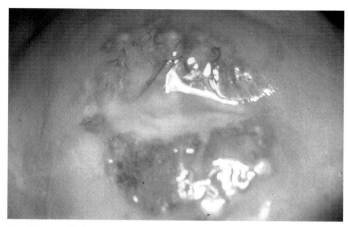

Fig. 62.12 Chlamydial cervicitis: a purulent discharge and inflamed follicles are seen.

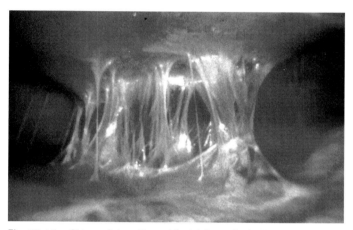

Fig. 62.13 Chlamydial perihepatitis: 'violin-string' adhesions are visible.

The most important complication of Chlamydia infection is PID, which may be acute, subacute or 'silent'. Chlamydia is now recognized to be associated with at least 50% of cases of acute PID in developed countries. It is also a more common cause of perihepatitis (Fitz-Hugh Curtis syndrome) than is the gonococcus (Fig. 62.13). Periappendicitis, in which inflammation begins in the serosal layer and adhesions form between the appendix and adjacent structures, is recognized as another chlamydial complication presenting as right iliac fossa pain in young sexually active women.

Late sequelae of PID are chronic pelvic pain and tubal damage, the latter potentially resulting in infertility or ectopic pregnancy. The risk of tubal damage increases with delayed treatment or multiple episodes of PID. Early treatment can result in complete functional resolution, but serological evidence of previous Chlamydia infection has been found in a high proportion of women with tubal infertility.

Disseminated infection with chlamydia may cause Reiter's syndrome or sexually acquired reactive arthritis (SARA). This probably occurs in fewer than 1% cases, and is associated with the HLA-B27 haplotype. There is usually an asymmetrical oligoarthritis, affecting large joints of the lower limb, or peripheral joints of the upper limb. In Reiter's syndrome the arthritis is accompanied by uveitis, and a rash that may be similar to psoriasis if florid.

In pregnancy, chlamydial infection may be asymptomatic or may present as vaginal discharge, bleeding or the urethral syndrome as in non-pregnant women. However, it has also been associated with chorioamnionitis, spontaneous abortion, intrauterine growth retardation, premature rupture of membranes, preterm birth, perinatal death, and puerperal sepsis. It has been suggested that acute infection during pregnancy, as evidenced by a specific IgM response, is more damaging than pre-existing infection.

The incidence of Chlamydia infection in women attending for termination of pregnancy (TOP) is 5–28%. Untreated, these women are at least three times more likely to develop post-TOP sepsis than untreated women. Tragically, some of these may later present with infertility. Current guidelines from the Royal College of Obstetrics and Gynaecology recommend administering anti-chlamydial treatment to young women before termination to protect against upper genital tract infection. This pragmatic approach, which does not involve screening for chlamydia, leaves women vulnerable to re-infection from an undiagnosed partner if the sexual relationship continues.

Chlamydia is also a common cause of neonatal disease. There is a 50–70% risk of transmission from an infected mother to the neonate during delivery. The associated conjunctival infection presents later than that due to the gonococcus – between 4 and 14 days, often after discharge from hospital (Fig. 62.14). An accompanying nasopharyngeal infection may later progress to afebrile pneumonitis and otitis media.

Diagnosis

Chlamydial infection is diagnosed by specific tests. Initially cell culture techniques were used. ELISA tests are used commonly, but their sensitivity is only approximately 60%. It is essential that samples are collected from the endocervix and areas of cervical ectropion so that columnar epithelial cells are harvested. A direct fluorescent antibody (DFA) test can be performed on cervical smears rolled onto a specific collecting slide and fixed in alcohol. Whilst relatively sensitive and specific it is operator dependent. ELISA tests cannot be used reliably on rectal or conjunctival swabs, when DFA is more appropriate.

Tests which detect DNA, such as the polymerase chain reaction (PCR), and the ligase chain reaction (LCR) are much more sensitive. They can be applied to urine samples or vaginal swabs with detection rates superior to ELISA tests on cervical swabs. This means that non-invasive screening for chlamydia is now possible. Most hospitals are now moving to using DNA detection tests.

Serological tests are not performed routinely in the diagnosis of chlamydial infections. Micro-immunofluorescence can be used to detect serum antibodies, which are not present in all infected individuals. The highest antibody titres are found in women with PID or disseminated infection. They are present in 60% women with tubal factor infertility.

Treatment

Because available tests for the detection of C. trachomatis infections are not 100% sensitive, if only those sexual partners who were Chlamydia positive were treated it is likely that a

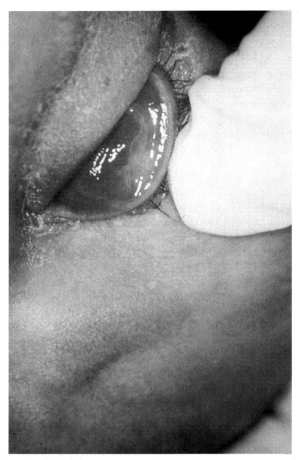

Fig. 62.14 Chlamydial ophthalmitis: the conjunctiva is swollen and inflamed.

significant number of infections would be missed, increasing the risks of reinfection and complications. Therefore in GUM clinics contact tracing is vigorously pursued and the index patient's sexual partner(s) will be treated whether or not Chlamydia is detected.

Uncomplicated Chlamydia infections are usually treated with systemic tetracyclines or macrolides. The failure rate of 2.5% can mostly be attributed to a failure to treat both partners concurrently, or poor adherence to treatment. Recently, three related cases of multi-drug resistant chlamydia were described in the USA. Antibiotic resistance can only be proved if transport medium for culture is available, and a reference laboratory continues to make culture available.

The following treatments are effective for uncomplicated chlamydial infection:

- Doxycycline 100 mg twice a day for 7 days.
- Erythromycin 500 mg twice a day for 14 days (used in pregnancy).
- Azithromycin 1 g as a single dose.
- Ofloxacin 400 mg daily for 7 days.

It is essential that sex partners are screened fully for sexually transmitted infections and prescribed treatment for chlamydia, before sexual intercourse is resumed.

Women who are pregnant or lactating should be given erythromycin stearate. This may be poorly tolerated. Clindamycin appears to be effective but is not yet licensed in the UK for use in pregnancy.

Chlamydial disease of the neonate requires prolonged systemic therapy with oral erythromycin ethyl succinate suspension 50 mg/kg/day in four divided doses before feeds for 3 weeks. Tetracycline eye ointment can be added in the treatment of conjunctivitis and may speed up healing. Both parents should be investigated.

Mycoplasma genitalium

This organism has emerged as a sexually transmitted pathogen that causes urethritis in men, and pelvic inflammatory disease in women. The incidence of symptomatic infection is lower than that of chlamydia. It grows very slowly in specialized medium so that studies rely on PCR to demonstrate infection. Its full disease spectrum, prevalence and transmission are still being elucidated, and routine diagnostic tests for it are not yet available. It usually responds to courses of tetracyclines or macrolides as prescribed for chlamydial infections. The difficulty of growing it in culture means that antibiotic sensitivity testing is difficult to perform.

Ureaplasma urealyticum

This bacteria from the Mycoplasma family causes NGU in men. It is commonly found in the vagina, but it has not been convincingly associated with vaginitis, cervicitis or pelvic inflammatory disease in women. It is usually sensitive to macrolide antibiotics, but there is no clear indication for its treatment in women.

OTHER VIRAL DISEASES

Genital warts

Genital warts (condylomata acuminata) are the commonest viral STI in the UK. They are caused by sexually transmitted human papilloma viruses (HPV). Subclinical infection is very common. Trigger factors for the appearance of warts are not known. Vertical transmission may also occur. Common wart viruses rarely cause warts in the genital area. The incubation period of genital warts varies from a few weeks to 9 months, perhaps longer in some cases.

Biology

HPV are these are small, non-enveloped icosahedral DNA viruses that have a particular tropism for epithelial cells. At least 100 different types have been recognised. Genital warts are almost always associated with infection caused by HPV types 6 or 11. Types 16 and 18 are the commonest oncogenic strains leading to cervical cancer. These infections are usually asymptomatic, or cause atypical flat warts. HPV have not been cultured successfully in vitro. Our understanding of their transmission and natural history therefore relies on DNA detection technologies.

Clinical features

Warts vary in appearance according to their site and causative viral type. In women they can occur anywhere in the ano-

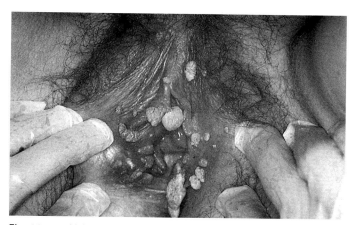

Fig. 62.15 Vulval warts.

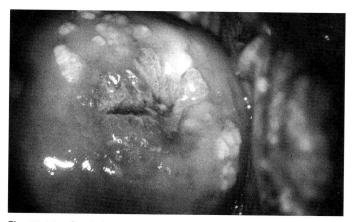

Fig. 62.16 Cervical warts.

genital region, but most commonly appear on the vulva at sites of maximal trauma during intercourse (Fig. 62.15). In warm moist areas they are filiform but tend to be flatter upon keratinized skin. Although some women complain of an associated itch, this is usually the result of concomitant infections.

Warts often proliferate in pregnant women, rarely posing obstetric problems, and regress spontaneously in the puerperium. Cervical warts are seen in less than 1 in 10 affected women, although a third will have evidence of warty change on cervical cytology or colposcopy (Fig. 62.16). Warts in men may be equally difficult to visualise, and show a wide variety of appearances and sites.

Patients presenting with warts should be screened for other STIs, which will be found in 25%. Colposcopic examination of the cervix and vagina is recommended if warts are present on the cervix.

Complications

It is generally accepted that genital HPV infection plays an important role in the development of malignant epithelial transformation of the cervix, vagina, vulva and anus, although other cofactors are necessary. Subclinical and latent infections with HPV types 16 or 18 appear to have the highest risk. Bowen's disease and Bowenoid papulosis may be mistaken for genital warts. In men, HPV-6 and 11 infections can rarely develop into a giant Buschke–Lowenstein tumour, which is a locally aggressive non-metastasising verrucous carcinoma prone to secondary bacterial infection.

Vertical transmission may uncommonly cause anogenital warts to appear within the first year of life. Very rarely, juvenile laryngeal papillomatosis may develop. The appearance of anogenital warts in older infants must raise the possibility of sexual abuse.

Treatment

Genital warts resolve when the HPV is suppressed by cell-mediated immunity. Destructive and chemical treatments can remove established lesions, but the virus remains in the surrounding tissue for months or years after resolution. Most non-surgical treatments produce complete resolution in about 40–60% of patients within 6 weeks. Immunosuppressed individuals, such as those with HIV infection, often have persistent and recurrent warts. Most Gum clinics offer cryotherapy or chemical methods as first line treatment.

Podophyllin   A plant extract applied to warts as a paint, is no longer recommended because of concerns about toxicity and variable potency between batches. It is potentially teratogenic and systemic absorption has resulted in serious maternal toxicity, affecting the liver, heart, kidneys and nervous system.

Podophyllotoxin   This is the main active ingredient of podophyllin. Liquid and cream preparations are now available for self-treatment. Courses are twice a day for 3 days, repeated after a 4-day break, up to 4 times.

Trichloroacetic acid   In 90–100% saturated solution this is a caustic agent which is useful to treat isolated, keratinized flat warts which respond poorly to podophyllin. Injudicious application can result in scarring.

Destructive methods   These include cryotherapy, curettage, diathermy and laser therapy.

Other chemical treatments   These include 5-fluorouracil, which has been used successfully to treat intra-urethral warts.

Immune modulation   Imiqimod cream applied three times per week stimulates cell mediated immunity leading to an inflammatory response and resolution of warts after 4–16 weeks of treatment. It appears to stimulate release of TH-1 cytokines, although the receptor is not yet identified. Interferons applied locally or systemically are expensive and produced modest results. They are not in routine use.

The partners of individuals with warts should always be examined, if necessary using a colposcope.

Molluscum contagiosum

This is caused by a large pox virus. In young adults it occurs on the genitalia as a sexually transmitted infection, although it can occur in children on the face, neck, upper limbs and trunk, spread by non-sexual close contact. Lesions on the genitals are found particularly on the pubis, thigh and labia majora. They are easily mistaken for genital warts, but close inspection of the small papular lesions shows a characteristic central umbilication. Expressed material shows a myriad of inclusion bodies.

Table 62.6 Characteristics of the known hepatitis viruses

Hepatitis virus	Transmission	Clinical features	Chronic infection
A	Faecal-oral Oroanal in homosexual men	Silent in 90% Fulminant hepatitis very rare	No
B	Parenteral Sexual Vertical Horizontal in endemic areas	Silent in 90% Children more often asymptomatic Fulminant hepatitis in 1%	10% in adults 90% in perinatal infection Can lead to: Chronic active hepatitis Cirrhosis Hepatocellular carcinoma
C	Parenteral Sexual transmission uncommon	Silent in 95% Fulminant hepatitis very rare	60% Chronic hepatitis Cirrhosis Hepatocellular carcinoma
D	Parenteral Sexual Only in those infected with HBV	Coinfection or superinfection with hepatitis B Fulminant hepatitis 20%	60% Effects as for HBV
E	Faecal-oral Oroanal possible	? limited to Africa/Asia Fulminant hepatitis common in pregnant women (10%)	No

Treatment consists of disrupting the papule, expressing the core and applying phenol with a sharpened orangestick to the residual lesion. Cryotherapy is equally successful. The fluid from the vesicles is infectious, and patients should be warned not to pick at them. In immunosuppressed individuals widespread large confluent lesions may develop. These are currently almost untreatable, as resolution requires an immune response. Nucleotide analogue drugs, such as cidofovir, show in vitro activity against the virus, offering the prospect of specific antiviral treatment.

Viral hepatitis

Several viruses can cause hepatitis, including cytomegalovirus (CMV) and Epstein-Barr virus. The major viral causes are the hepatitis viruses A, B, C, D and E. The major characteristics of these viruses are given in Table 62.6. The parenterally transmitted viruses B, C and D may also be sexually transmitted.

Hepatitis A This is an RNA virus, which is spread through the faecal-oral route. Approximately 50% of the UK population have antibodies from childhood infection but the prevalence is falling. The majority of individuals in developing countries acquire infection during childhood. It is usually a benign illness, but occasionally fulminating hepatitis has been described in pregnant women. It has not been associated with congenital abnormalities.

Hepatitis B Hepatitis B is a more severe infection that may be followed by chronic carriage and disease ending in cirrhosis and hepatocellular carcinoma. It is transmitted sexually, through blood products or vertically to the fetus from an infected mother. The majority of acute infections are not clinically recognized as only 20% of individuals develop jaundice. The earlier in life the infection occurs the more likely the person is to become a carrier. Approximately 80% of infants infected perinatally become carriers. Infection is particularly common in China and South-East Asia but prevalent in most tropical countries.

During acute infection hepatitis B surface antigen and e antigen are detectable in serum. Hepatitis B core antibody appears after approximately 6 weeks and remains detectable thereafter as a marker of exposure. As immunity develops anti-e antibody develops and the e antigen becomes undetectable. With clearance of the virus, the surface antigen disappears and surface antibody becomes detectable. When the e antigen is present the individual is highly infectious. Thus to screen for chronic infection anti-core antibody is sought. If this is positive the other markers are tested to define the stage of infection.

Some people do not clear the acute infection and go on to develop chronic hepatitis. Treatment with a combination of interferon, adefovir and lamivudine is being introduced at present. Vertical transmission can be prevented by vaccination of neonates born to mothers with hepatitis B. Additional Hepatitis B immune globulin is given at birth if the mother is e antigen positive. Many countries with a higher prevalence of hepatitis B infection than the UK, and several European countries have a policy of universal vaccination of all infants.

Hepatitis C (HCV) This is another RNA virus which causes chronic hepatitis. Acute infection often passes asymptomatically but more than 50% of infected individuals have active hepatitis which may progress to cirrhosis and possibly hepatocellular carcinoma. The prevalence varies widely across the world with the highest incidence in Egypt, possibly associated with the use of contaminated needles for mass treatment for schistosomiasis. In the UK infection is highly prevalent in those with a history of intravenous drug use. It may be transmitted sexually but transmission is not very efficient with only 1–2% of long-term partners becoming infected. Vertical transmission is uncommon and appears to correlate with hepatitis C RNA viraemia. The risk of transmission is, however, increased in those co-infected with HIV. Treatment with interferon and ribavirin can clear the infection in some infected individuals.

Hepatitis D This is a defective virus that can only replicate in the presence of hepatitis B. Those who have this super infection are more likely to develop severe hepatitis.

Table 62.7   Serological diagnosis of viral hepatitis

Hepatitis virus	Markers of acute infection	Markers of past infection	Markers of chronic infection
A	IgM anti-HAV	IgG anti-HAV	
B	HBV DNA	IgG anti-HBc	HBV DNA
	HBsAg	anti-HBe	HBsAg
	HBeAg	anti-HBs	HBeAg (indicates high infectivity)
	IgM anti-HBc	(infectivity)	anti-HBe (indicates low infectivity)
C	anti-HVC	PCR HCV RNA	anti-HCV
			PCR HCV RNA
D	IgM anti-HDV	IgG anti-HDV	
E	IgM anti-HEV	IgG anti-HEV	

Table 62.8   The differential diagnosis of the common causes of vaginal discharge

Symptoms and signs	Candidiasis	Bacterial vaginosis	Trichomoniasis	Cervicitis
Itching or soreness	++	–	+++	–
Smell	May be 'yeasty'	Offensive, fishy	May be offensive	–
Colour	White	White or yellow	Yellow or green	Clear or coloured
Consistency	Curdy	Thin, homogeneous	Thin, homogeneous	Mucoid
pH	< 4.5	4.5–7.0	4.5–7.0	< 4.5
Confirmed by	Microscopy and culture	Microscopy	Microscopy and culture	Microscopy, tests for chlamydia and gonorrhoea

Hepatitis E   Hepatitis E virus is transmitted by the faeco-oral route, causing usually an acute and self-limiting infection. It causes a high mortality rate in pregnant women, of the order of 17–30%, and occurs in epidemic form in India, Central and South-East Asia, the Middle East and North Africa.

Diagnosis

Table 62.7 shows the major tests available for the diagnosis of hepatitis infections, and their significance. Epstein–Barr virus and cytomegalovirus infections can be diagnosed by tests for specific serum immunoglobulin M antibodies.

Prevention

Those at risk of hepatitis A and B through lifestyle include: homosexual men and intravenous drug users, while those at risk through occupation include healthcare workers (hepatitis B). Sewage workers (hepatitis A) should be screened for prior infection and vaccinated.

VAGINAL INFECTIONS

Physiological discharge

Normal vaginal discharge is white, becoming yellowish on contact with air, due to oxidation. It consists of desquamated epithelial cells from the vagina and cervix, mucus originating mainly from the cervical glands, bacteria and fluid which is formed as a transudate from the vaginal wall. More than 95% of the bacteria present are lactobacilli. The acidic pH, below 4.5, is maintained through the production of lactic acid by the vaginal epithelium metabolizing glycogen and by the lactobacilli. Physiological discharge increases due to increased mucus production from the cervix in mid-cycle. It also increases in pregnancy, and sometimes when women start a combined oral contraceptive pill. The differential diagnosis is of the common causes of vaginal discharge are summarized in Table 62.8.

Bacterial vaginosis (BV)

Bacterial vaginosis, previously known as anaerobic vaginosis and Gardnerella vaginitis, is the commonest cause of abnormal vaginal discharge in women of childbearing age. Its prevalence is about 12–15% in most UK populations. It is an imbalance in the vaginal flora, in which the normally dominant lactobacilli are replaced by an overgrowth of anaerobic commensal organisms. The bacteria involved include *Gardnerella vaginalis*, *Prevotella* (Bacteroides) species, *Peptostreptococcus* species, *Mycoplasma hominis* and *Mobiluncus species*. They produce volatile amines, such as trimethylamine, putrescine and cadaverine that give rise to the characteristic fishy smell of the condition. Probably the rise in pH that is found in BV is crucial to allowing these organisms to overcome inhibitors such as hydrogen peroxide that are produced by many Lactobacillus species.

Although BV is more common in sexually active women, it is also found in virgins and lesbians. There is no good evidence that it is an STI. It is more common in users of the IUCD and other non-barrier methods of contraception. It is also commoner in black women than white. In some studies in rural Sub-Saharan Africa the prevalence has been as high as 50%. Symptoms often develop following menstruation or sexual intercourse, and it is possible that hormonal changes and semen, among other factors, may trigger its onset.

Clinical features

The cardinal symptom of BV is a smell, usually described as fishy. This is associated with a thin grey or white homogeneous adherent vaginal discharge, which is sometimes frothy (Fig. 62.17). It is seldom associated with mucosal

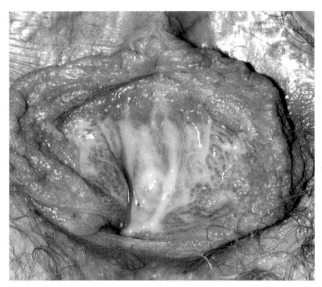

Fig. 62.17   Bacterial vaginosis.

inflammation or with irritation. About 50% of women with bacterial vaginosis are asymptomatic. Relapse after treatment is common, and frustrating for both the woman and her physician.

Complications

BV may cause psychological distress and disruption to sexual activity in some women, particularly if recurrences are frequent. BV is associated with serious sequelae in women undergoing surgery and in pregnancy. Metronidazole or clindamycin cream can reduce the incidence of endometritis/PID after termination of pregnancy in women with BV. In pregnancy, BV is strongly associated with second trimester miscarriage, preterm premature rupture of membranes, preterm birth and post-Caesarean section endometritis. These arise as a result of chorioamnionitis leading to amniotic fluid infection and ultimately fetal infection. Studies of the treatment in pregnant women are being undertaken, but have produced conflicting results.

Diagnosis

The clinical diagnosis of BV can usually be confirmed by simple tests on the vaginal discharge, using four composite (Amsel) criteria. The thin homogeneous discharge is recognizable in most women with BV. The pH is greater than 4.5. A drop of 10% potassium hydroxide added to a drop of secretion on a glass slide releases the fishy odour of volatile amines. Microscopy of a wet film shows masses of small bacteria coating epithelial cells ('clue cells').

On a Gram stain preparation the replacement of lactobacilli by large numbers of small Gram-positive and Gram-negative bacteria is readily recognized. Culture can be misleading as G. vaginalis can be found in up to 50% of women without BV. Commercially available tests detect specific enzymes, such as proline aminopeptidase or sialidase, or utilize PCR to quantify *Gardnerella* DNA and generally have a sensitivity of about 80%.

Management

A 5-day course of metronidazole 400 mg twice daily is used most commonly in the UK. A single 2 g dose is nearly as effective.

Topical treatment with either metronidazole or clindamycin cream is also effective. Clindamycin 300 mg twice daily for 5 days has been used in some studies in pregnancy, but is not licensed for this indication. Whatever treatment is used, BV recurs in 30% women following the next menstrual period. Although concerns remain about potential mutagenicity with metronidazole its use in pregnancy is no longer contra-indicated.

In randomized controlled trials treating male partners with metronidazole, tinidazole or clindamycin did not significantly reduce the rate of recurrnece of BV. BV is, however, associated with chlamydial infection in some studies, and has been associated with NGU in male partners in one study. Male partners of women with recurrent or persistent BV should therefore have a screen for STIs.

Trichomoniasis

This is caused by Trichomonas vaginalis, a flagellated protozoan. It is usually sexually transmitted but may be carried asymptomatically for months or years, Vertical transmission occurs, but usually resolves in the first month as the effects of maternal oestrogens on the infant's vagina wane. Non-sexual transmission is theoretically possible, as the organism can survive in moist secretions, mineral baths and toilets for several hours, but it is likely to be an exceptional means of acquisition. Trichomoniasis is frequently associated with other STIs.

Unlike the other causes of vaginitis, the incidence of trichomoniasis has fallen since the mid 1980s. T. vaginalis is more common in young sexually active girls, in women in their 40s and in users of nonhormonal, non-barrier methods of contraception. Before the introduction of metronidazole it could be a chronic persistent and very troublesome condition.

Clinical features

Trichomonas causes an offensive mucopurulent vaginal discharge with accompanying symptoms of dysuria and vulval soreness. On examination there is often a severe vulvovaginitis, with perivulval intertrigo and petechial haemorrhage on the vaginal wall and ectocervix (Fig. 62.18). It is usually associated with an elevated pH and often with bacterial vaginosis.

Diagnosis

Trichomonas can be identified on wet mount microscopy of vaginal fluid, through its movement and characteristic form. It can also be seen in cervical smears, but does not stain well on Gram stain. Culture requires a specialized medium such as Feinberg-Whittington. Microscopy is only 50–60% sensitive compared to culture. Clinical diagnosis is unreliable in milder cases as the discharge can be mistaken for bacterial vaginosis.

Treatment

Metronidazole is the drug of choice using regimens similar to those in bacterial vaginosis. Other nitroimidazole drugs, such as tinidazole, are also successful in single- or multiple-dose courses. True metronidazole resistance in T. vaginalis is extremely rare. Failures are more often related to utilisation and degradation of the drug by other vaginal bacteria, or by failure to absorb the drug after oral administration. Combination broad-

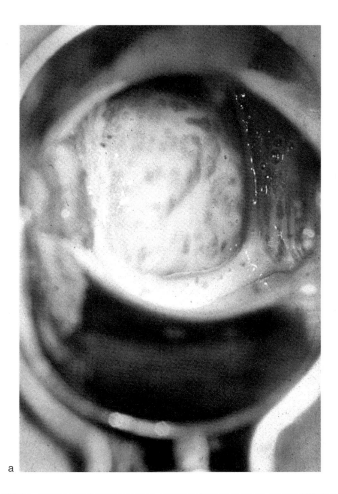

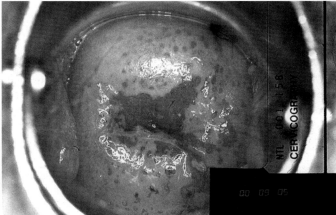

Fig. 62.18 Trichomoniasis: **a** grey, watery discharge and **b** 'strawberry cervix' with petechial haemorrhage.

spectrum antibiotic metronidazole regimens will usually eradicate the organism. Occasionally it proves necessary to give intravenous metronidazole on 5 consecutive days. Imidazole pessaries used for candidal infections, such as clotrimazole, have some activity in suppressing Trichomonas.

Male partners usually have asymptomatic urethral infection with T. vaginalis but some develop urethritis or balanitis. The organism may be detected in at least one-third of all sexual partners. All male partners should receive treatment with metronidazole before intercourse resumes.

Candidiasis

Vulvovaginal candidiasis occurs worldwide. Over three-quarters of women have at least one episode of vaginal candidiasis, often during pregnancy or following a course of antibiotics. A few women get frequent recurrences. The organism is carried in the gut, under the nails, in the vagina and on the skin. The yeast Candida albicans is implicated in more than 80% cases. *Candida glabrata, C. krusei* and *C. tropicalis* account for most of the rest. Sexual acquisition is rarely important, although the physical trauma of intercourse may be sufficient to trigger an attack in a predisposed individual. About 20% of women attending GUM clinics harbour vaginal yeasts. In most of these it represents asymptomatic carriage.

Predisposing causes

C. albicans is an opportunistic pathogen which requires an underlying deficit in host local or systemic immunity in order to invade the vagina and cause disease. Local immunity is compromised by the disturbance of commensal bacterial flora induced by broad-spectrum antibiotics; by other genital infections causing inflammation or ulceration of epithelial surfaces; by local trauma induced by intercourse or skin sensitisers; and by genital dermatoses.

Vulvovaginal candidiasis is a well-recognized complication of the reduced cellular immunity in late pregnancy, and in all pathological states associated with immunosuppression (Box 62.1) It is also more common in endocrine disorders such as diabetes mellitus and thyroid, parathyroid and adrenal disease. Although iron deficiency and other anaemias predispose to chronic mucocutaneous candidiaisis, their association with vulvovaginal candidiasis is unproven.

Clinical features

The cardinal symptom is an intense vulval itch, worse with warmth and at night. This may be associated with external dysuria and dyspareunia. Excessive vaginal discharge is not a consistent feature. When present it is classically thick 'cottage cheese' in type, but in some women can be thin and muco-purulent.

The physical signs vary widely – some women with disabling symptoms have little to see other than mild vulval erythema and a few introital fissures. In the most acute cases there is a

Box 62.1 Factors predisposing to vaginal candidiasis

Immunosuppression
- HIV
- Immunosuppressive therapy, e.g., steroids

Diabetes mellitus

Vaginal douching, bubble bath, shower gel, tight clothing, tights

Increased oestrogen
- Pregnancy
- High dose combined oral contraceptive pill

Underlying dermatosis, e.g. eczema

Broad spectrum antibiotic therapy

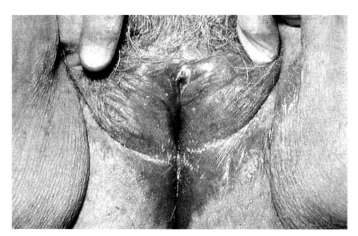

Fig. 62.19 Candida vulvitis.

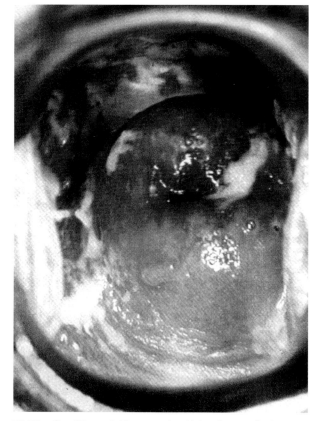

Fig. 62.20 Candida vaginitis: note the thick adherent discharge.

pronounced vulvovaginitis, with peripheral vulval satellite lesions, vulval oedema and vaginitis with adherent mycotic plaques on the vaginal wall and ectocervix (Figs 62.19 and 62.20).

Diagnosis

Clinical features should not be relied upon. The diagnosis should be confirmed and other pathogens excluded by thorough microbiological investigation. Microscopy of the vaginal discharge shows fungal elements in either 10% potassium hydroxide or

Gram stain. A high vaginal swab cultured for Candida will give a positive result in carriers, as well as from women with symptomatic vulvovaginal candidiasis.

Treatment

Underlying causes should be corrected if possible. Drugs of the polyene group, such as nystatin, or of the imidazole group, such as clotrimazole, miconazole and econazole, are commonly employed as creams and pessaries in topical treatments lasting 1–14 days. Yeast resistance to these drugs is virtually unknown and topical sensitivity is rarely encountered. Acute isolated episodes are usually successfully treated in this way. The systemic antifungal drugs fluconazole and itraconazole are effective in a single or double oral treatment respectively and appear to be free from serious toxicity. Many patients find these drugs more acceptable than topical treatments, although they are considerably more expensive.

Chronic recurrent candidiasis is often a therapeutic problem. All currently available antifungal agents are fungistatic than fungicidal, so elimination of the causative agent is unlikely to occur. In women in whom the underlying cause cannot be identified, or eliminated regular treatment for a period of 3 to 6 months can be successful. Regimens include an initial 7-day course of fluconazole 50 mg daily, followed by prophylactic treatment with 150 mg single doses at fortnightly or monthly intervals for 3–6 months. Clotrimazole 500 mg pessaries can be used as an alternative.

ECTOPARASITIC INFESTATIONS

Both pediculosis pubis and scabies are common infestations in sexually active adults. Their presence should stimulate investigation for accompanying STI.

Pediculosis pubis

The pubic louse, Phthirus pubis, has greatly enlarged middle and hind legs with claws adapted to match the diameter of pubic and axillary hair. The louse has also been recovered from the beard area, eyelashes and eyebrows. Adult lice are sedentary, move slowly and survive up to 24 hours when removed from their host. The adult female lays up to four eggs daily, cemented to hairs, and these hatch within 5–10 days. Sexual transmission is usual, although infestations acquired from shared beds and clothing are recorded.

Clinical features

Allergic sensitization to louse bites results in itching, which develops within a week in some individuals whereas others remain asymptomatic for weeks or months. Characteristic blue spots occur at bite sites. Adult lice situated at the base of hairs are often mistaken for freckles or crusts. Nits on hair shafts are more obvious.

Treatment

Topical preparations should kill both adults and their eggs. After application, the drug should remain in contact with eggs for at least 1 hour. There are several proprietary preparations which, as lotions, creams or shampoos, usually have as their active constituents either g-benzene hexachloride or malathion. Vaseline applied to the eyelashes and eyebrows will smother lice by obstructing their breathing apparatus.

Scabies

Scabies is caused by the itch mite Sarcoptes scabiei. Adult females measure 400 mm in length, move rapidly, and burrow into the horny layer of the skin where they lay up to three eggs daily. These develop, via larval stages, into adult mites within 10 days.

Epidemiology

Scabies affects all age groups. Non-sexual transmission occurs in families and particularly affects children. Sexual transmission should be suspected in young adults, especially when genital lesions occur.

Clinical features

Although individuals may remain asymptomatic for months, the usual development of intense itching, which is worse at night, occurs 1–8 weeks after infestation. A rash develops symmetrically on the trunk and limbs. Lesions on the head and neck occur rarely. Thread-like linear burrows, crossing skin creases, most commonly affect the fingers, wrists, axillae and nipples. Characteristic excoriated papules occur on the genitals.

Complications include secondary bacterial infection of excoriated lesions. In the mentally retarded, steroid-treated or immunologically compromised individual, massive infestations resulting in a generalized psoriasiform dermatosis may occur, sometimes called Norwegian scabies. The diagnosis is readily confirmed by identification of the mite on microscopy of material removed from burrows.

Treatment

It is important to treat the patient and all close family and sexual contacts. Topical applications are applied with a paintbrush to all skin areas from the neck down and left for 24 hours. Prior bathing should be avoided as it may increase the risk of systemic toxicity.

g-Benzene hexachloride does not sting and can be used on eczematized skin, but should be avoided in children and pregnant women because of possible neurotoxicity. Malathion, in aqueous or alcoholic solution, has an unpleasant smell and stings on application to broken skin. Monosulfiram, 25% solution in methylated spirit, is diluted in 2–3 parts of water and applied on 3 successive nights. Alcohol should be avoided during treatment because of the risk of 'antabuse-like' reactions.

Secondary bacterial infection will require appropriate antibiotics. Post-treatment pruritus will usually respond to topical hydrocortisone and reassurance.

KEY POINTS

1. STIs are not necessarily related to social class, to educational attainment or to standards of personal hygiene.

KEY POINTS (CONTINUED)

2. A patient with one STI is likely to have another; screening for other infections is essential.
3. STIs are common in women undergoing termination of pregnancy, and are associated with an increased risk of sepsis.
4. The incidence of bacterial STIs in developed countries is no longer declining, whereas viral STIs are increasing.
5. Antenatal screening for syphilis remains cost effective.
6. The commonest sexually transmitted bacterial pathogen in developed countries is Chlamydia trachomatis.
7. Chlamydial infections are often silent and may remain so for months, and possibly years. Long-standing infection is a frequent cause of tubal damage and infertility.
8. Genital warts are the commonest viral STI; subclinical HPV infection is even more common.
9. The majority of cases of neonatal HSV infection arise from maternal first-episode genital herpes. Classic lesions may be absent.
10. All pregnant women should be examined at delivery for evidence of herpes lesions. If present, delivery should be by caesarean section.
11. The commonest vaginal infections are associated with bacterial vaginosis, Candida albicans ('thrush') and Trichomonas vaginalis.
12. STIs increase transmission of HIV; STI control is an essential element of an AIDS control programme.
13. DNA-based tests such as polymerase chain reaction (PCR) or ligase chain reaction (LCR) offer the possibility of non-invasive sample collection to screen for infections such as chlamydia and gonorrhoea.
14. A national screening programme will reduce the incidence of chlamydia, pelvic inflammatory disease, and subsequent ectopic pregnancy and infertility.
15. Screening for and treating genital infections such as bacterial vaginosis in pregnancy may significantly reduce the incidence of miscarriage, preterm birth and subsequent neurological impairment.
16. The development of antiviral drugs continues. New agents are being developed which are likely to be effective against human papilloma viruses, herpes viruses and HIV. Novel immune stimulators that can be applied topically are also being evaluated.
17. Vaccines are being developed for the same chronic infections. If successful this approach should reduce the incidence of carcinoma of the cervix related to HPV infection.

FURTHER READING

Adler MW 1995 ABC of sexually transmitted diseases, 2nd edn. British Medical Journal, London
Arya OP, Osoba AO, Bennett FJ 1988 Tropical venereology, 2nd edn. Churchill Livingstone, Edinburgh
Center for Disease Control 1989 Sexually transmitted diseases treatment guidelines. Morbidity and Mortality Weekly Report 38 (suppl)
Holmes KK, Mardh PA, Sparling PF, Weisner PJ 1989 Sexually transmitted diseases, 2nd edn. McGraw Hill, New York

Kinghorn GR, Spencer RC (eds) 1993 Sexually transmitted diseases. Medicine International 21:73–148

Morse SA, Moreland AA, Thompson SE 1989 Atlas of Sexually Transmitted Diseases. Gower, Aldershot

Robertson DHH, McMillan A, Young H 1989 Clinical practice in sexually transmitted disease. Churchill Livingstone, Edinburgh

Sweet RL (ed) 1993 Bacterial vaginosis. American Journal of Obstetrics and Gynecology (suppl) 169:441–482

Thin RH 1988 Management of genital herpes simplex infections. American Journal of Medicine 85:3–6

White TS, Coda FA, Ingram DL, Pearson A 1983 Sexually transmitted diseases in sexually abused children. Paediatrics 72:16–20

Wisdom A 1989 A colour atlas of sexually transmitted diseases. Wolfe, London

Zurhausen H 1987 Papillomaviruses in human cancer. Cancer 15:1692–1696

63
HIV

Antonia Moore   Margaret Johnson

Twenty per cent of HIV-infected individuals in Europe and the USA are women. Whilst HIV itself has no major specific gynaecological manifestations it does impinge heavily on gynaecological practice. Some problems, such as recurrent, severe vaginal candidiasis, florid HPV infection and an increased prevalence of cervical intraepithelial neoplasia, are the result of increasing immune suppression. However, many of the current gynaecological issues encountered in the HIV-positive woman, such as contraception, pregnancy and infertility management, are the result of dramatic improvements in available therapy and consequent improvement in overall prognosis.

BACKGROUND

HIV is a retrovirus, a double-stranded RNA virus that uses the enzyme reverse transcriptase to form DNA and integrate itself into the host cell which then becomes a 'factory' for producing more virus (Fig. 63.1). T-cell helper lymphocytes bearing the CD4 receptor, pivotal in the cell-mediated immune response, are targeted by the virus and destroyed.

The natural history of HIV is characterized by gradual clinical deterioration. Decreasing CD4 lymphocyte count and increasing levels of virus in the blood plasma are used in monitoring the course of the disease in conjunction with clinical events. Most evidence regarding natural history of HIV infection is based on studies of men and it is not clear whether this is directly applicable to women. Seroconversion, the development of antibodies to HIV detectable in the serum, usually occurs within 3 months of infection and false-negative results, although

rare, usually occur during this period. Re-testing should be offered if the original negative test was taken during this interval. Up to 50% of patients may experience an acute infectious mononucleosis-like syndrome, the primary HIV infection (PHI), at the time of seroconversion with rash, fever, myalgia, arthralgia, headache, diarrhoea and sore throat.

AIDS diagnoses represent a range of disorders including infection and neoplasia (Centers for Disease Control 1992). The risk of severe immune deficiency and AIDS increases with duration of infection. The median time to development of AIDS in untreated HIV-positive patients is approximately 7–10 years. Prior to the development of AIDS, patients may either be asymptomatic or experience persistent generalized lymphadenopathy (enlarged lymph nodes in at least two extrainguinal sites, lasting for at least 3 months and not attributable to any other cause) or symptoms due to immune deterioration that has many manifestations.

Early in the epidemic, before the widespread use of antiretroviral therapy and prophylaxis against opportunistic infections, median survival after an AIDS-defining illness was 11 months. Some studies suggested a worse prognosis for women with HIV and with AIDS though this finding is likely to have been the result of inequalities in access to care rather than biological gender differences. The course of infection varies between individuals and there are 'long-term non-progressors' who are infected for long periods of time but manifest no evidence of immune compromise, in terms of either peripheral CD4 count or clinically detectable disease.

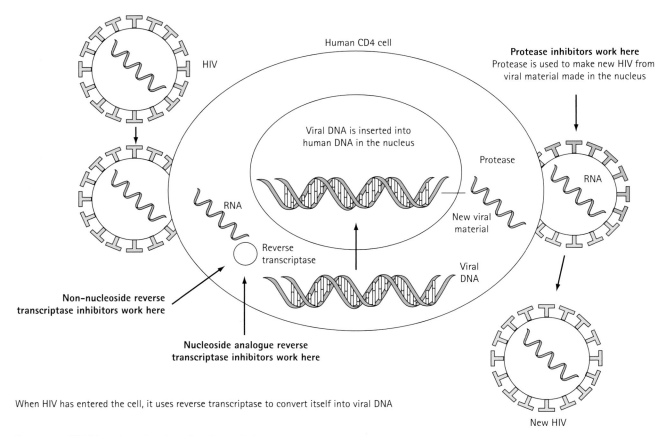

When HIV has entered the cell, it uses reverse transcriptase to convert itself into viral DNA

Fig. 63.1   HIV lifecycle and action of antiretroviral agents.

TREATMENT

Over the last 5 years, widespread use of combination anti-retroviral therapy in Europe and USA has reduced substantially the rate of progression to AIDS and improved survival. The death rate in 1995 was 29.4/100 person-years but had reduced to 8.8/100 person-years by mid 1997 (Palella et al 1998). Three main categories of antiretroviral agents are in general usage: nucleoside reverse transcriptase inhibitors (NRTIs), protease inhibitors (PIs) and non-nucleoside reverse transcriptase inhibitors (NNRTIs) all of which interrupt the virus' lifecycle (Fig. 63.1). The aim of highly active antiretroviral therapy (HAART), a combination of three or more drugs usually including a PI or an NNRTI, is to slow progression of the disease by reducing viral load and so increasing CD4 count. The British HIV Association has published guidelines on when to start HAART (BHIVA 2001a,b). On treatment, viral load should reach 'undetectable' levels, usually less than 50 copies/ml. The CD4 count should rise, levels of below $200 \times 10^6/l$ representing a significant risk of development of an opportunistic infection. Compliance with HAART regimes needs to be in excess of 95% (Paterson et al 1999) for treatment to be effective and to reduce the chances of the emergence of resistant virus.

TRANSMISSION

HIV has been isolated in blood, seminal fluid, vaginal secretions, cerebrospinal fluid, saliva, lacrimal secretions and breast milk.

The concentration in different body fluids varies. The virus may be transmitted by sexual intercourse, intravenous drug use, transfusion or occupational exposure and vertically, from mother to child. The predominant route of infection worldwide is heterosexual sex and, with the great majority of the affected population being in their reproductive years, vertical transmission is an increasing problem. Proper use of condoms is known to reduce greatly the risk of transmission (de Vincenzi et al 1994). Male-to-female transmission is more efficient than female to male, the mucous membrane of the vagina being more permeable and the surface area being greater, though a partner receptive to anal intercourse is at greatest risk. It is difficult to quantify the risk of sexual transmission 'per act', as a constellation of factors are involved, although higher levels of viral load and intercurrent sexually transmitted infection (Wasserheit 1992), particularly ulcerative conditions, in either partner make transmission more likely. Use of barrier methods should also be encouraged in concordant HIV-positive couples to reduce the risk of transmission of resistant virus.

Although transmission of HIV between women who have sex with women (Monzon & Capellon 1987) is rare, cases have occurred. Use of dental dams (latex barriers) should be encouraged to reduce oral contact with vaginal secretions and shared sex toys should be cleaned appropriately. Salivary hypotonicity is thought to inactivate HIV-infected lymphocytes and hence salivary transmission is rare. Oral sex, though less risky than vaginal or anal sex, may result in transmission and this may in part be the result of the isotonic nature of seminal fluid overcoming the inactivation of infected cells by hypotonic saliva.

Since 1983 all those at increased risk of HIV in the UK have been asked not to donate blood. Transfusion and administration of blood products prior to the initiation of blood screening and heat treatment of blood products in 1985 lead to HIV infection in some recipients of transfusion, haemophiliacs and their sexual partners, the association between administration of infected factor VIII and HIV first being recognized in 1982.

Vertical transmission rates vary from country to country but in the UK are between 15% and 20% in the non-breast feeding, untreated, HIV-positive woman. Although not completely preventable, the risk of mother-to-child transmission (MTCT) can be reduced dramatically and is addressed later in this chapter.

HIV TESTING

HIV testing should be performed only with the woman's consent after pre-test counselling by a trained healthcare worker. Medical care and support for those diagnosed HIV positive should be arranged immediately after diagnosis. As with all medical care, patient confidentiality should be respected. Enzyme-linked immunosorbent assay (ELISA) is the method most commonly used to screen for HIV antibody and is highly sensitive.

Although a cure for HIV remains elusive, the advent of effective treatment has resulted in a significantly more optimistic outlook for infected patients. There are clear advantages to knowledge of HIV status, not only in terms of accessing medical monitoring and treatment but also regarding protection of sexual partners and reduction of risk of MTCT. Antenatal testing, previously offered only to women deemed at high risk of infection, should now be offered universally as part of the package of routine investigations offered to women in early pregnancy (see below).

THE HIV EPIDEMIC

Worldwide, the epidemic continues to grow and there are now thought to be in excess of 33.4 million people living with HIV/AIDS, 22.5 million of those living in sub-Saharan Africa and 5.6 million in south and south-east Asia. Over 20% of those aged 15–49 in South Africa and over 35% of adults in Burundi are HIV positive. The epidemic in Europe and the USA is on a much smaller scale but the resources available to these patients are enormous by comparison (UNAIDS 2000).

UK data show that women infected with HIV are generally of child-bearing age and that the majority are infected as the result of heterosexual sex abroad. In 2000, the median age for heterosexually acquired HIV infection was 31 years for women and 35 years for men. This has gradually increased from a median age of 28 years in 1991 among women. More than 50% of the women whose ethnicity is known are of black African origin, the majority of these women at present (>80%) living in London, whilst the majority of the 28% who are white live outside the capital (PHLS). Physicians should be aware, however, that government plans to disperse refugees around the country may affect this distribution and all should be aware of the possibility of HIV in women presenting for investigation and treatment.

GYNAECOLOGICAL SYMPTOMATOLOGY

Women with HIV experience the same range of gynaecological symptoms as their HIV-negative counterparts. As with any woman, it is important that she is treated with compassion and understanding and that investigation and treatment of gynaecological problems are thorough and tailored to the woman's individual situation. Problems that might in the past not have been of real significance to women coping with a terminal disease are now increasingly relevant with women realistically expecting a longer lifespan. By and large, HIV status should not alter treatments available to women, although there are a few caveats to this which are discussed below. As with all medical care, good communication with accurate information is essential.

Menstrual cycle

Intuitively it might be expected that women with HIV, as with any chronic disease, might experience menstrual irregularity or periods of amenorrhoea, perhaps associated with weight loss or deteriorating health and it is certainly true that associated medical problems such as thrombocytopenia may result in menorrhagia while liver or renal insufficiency may cause amenorrhoea.

Whilst anecdotally women with HIV are often said to suffer menstrual disturbance, evidence to support an effect of HIV itself on menstrual pattern is sparse and often conflicting, the consensus being that there is no direct HIV effect though increasingly disturbed cycles may occur in women with severe immune compromise (CD4 count <200) (Harlow et al 2000).

The clinical impression of a high prevalence of an abnormal bleeding pattern may be biased in two ways.

- Women with HIV routinely see their doctors at frequent (usually 3 monthly) intervals and so have more opportunity to consult their physicians regarding any perceived problem.
- The majority of infected women are of black African origin and are therefore more likely to have fibroids.

HIV shedding into cervical fluid is lowest in the follicular phase and peaks during menstruation (Reicheldorfer et al 1999) with obvious implications for sexual transmission.

Little information is available on endocrine function in females with HIV. In men, no striking differences have been found when the men are well but hypogonadotrophic hypogonadism has been reported as a common feature in those who have AIDS. It has been suggested that this may relate to chronic ill health and weight loss rather than to HIV infection itself.

In general, menstrual abnormality should be investigated and treated as in the HIV-negative population although caution should be exercised when intercurrent disease or treatment affects liver function and may alter metabolism of drug therapy or hormones. In the severely immune-compromised patient, abnormal uterine bleeding may be the result of an HIV-related condition, opportunistic infection or neoplasm and investigation should be tailored appropriately.

Genital infection

Vaginitis

Recurrent vaginal candidiasis is the most common initial clinical manifestation of HIV infection (Carpenter et al 1991) and is a problem even at relatively well-maintained CD4 counts. Iman et al (1990) suggested a hierarchy of risk of candidal infection, with recurrent vaginal candidiasis becoming more common with early systemic immunosuppression, oral candidiasis becoming common at moderate immunosuppression and oesophageal candidiasis (an AIDS-defining diagnosis) typically occurring with severe immunosuppression. Not only are HIV-infected women more prone to recurrence but yeasts other than *Candida albicans* (e.g. *Torulopsis glabrata*) are isolated more frequently and there is a shorter time before recurrence (Spinollo et al 1994). Response to treatment is usually good, but relapses frequently require retreatment or maintenance therapy.

Pelvic sepsis

Studies of HIV-infected women show no significant difference in the prevalence rates of gonorrhoea and chlamydia among HIV-positive and HIV-negative women (Minkoff et al 1999). Patients should be treated using standard therapy and referred to genitourinary medicine clinics for initiation of contact tracing and follow-up. Pelvic sepsis is probably more common in patients with HIV but presentation can be varied with less severe symptoms and lesser rises in lymphocyte count sometimes occurring at lower levels of immune competence (Korn et al 1993). In general terms, early treatment with standard antibiotics is appropriate and effective.

Syphilis

Syphilis should be treated similarly to HIV-negative patients though some suggest either CSF examinations before treatment or treatment that will cross the blood–brain barrier as HIV-positive patients may experience neurological manifestations earlier in the course of the disease.

HSV and genital ulceration

Frequency, duration and severity of HSV attacks may be increased in HIV-positive women, particularly in those with immune compromise. Attacks may be avoided or treated with oral aciclovir though resistance can occur and culture and sensitivity testing is sometimes useful. In resistant cases of genital ulceration directed biopsy may be necessary to exclude neoplasia. Where infective and neoplastic causes have been excluded, thalidomide may be a useful adjunct in the treatment of resistant genital ulceration (Paterson et al 1995).

Genital warts

Human papilloma virus (HPV), usually types 6–11, are common in HIV-infected women and may be more extensive and florid than is typical in HIV-negative patients. Treatment is along standard lines and in those with severe immune compromise, resolution may be seen with increasing CD4 count resulting from systemic antiretroviral therapy.

Cervical intraepithelial neoplasia

Cervical intraepithelial neoplasia (CIN) is common in women with HIV (Adachi et al 1993, Massad et al 1999) and the prevalence increases with advancing immunosuppression (Johnson et al 1992, Schafer et al 1991). HIV-positive women are more likely to be infected with HPV (Palefsky et al 1999) and more of this infection is the result of 'high-risk' HPV than in the HIV-negative population. Notably HPV has been found in women who have sex exclusively with women and therefore even this population must undergo cervical screening.

Data from the pre-HAART era suggested that CIN disease was more often of higher grade and more often aggressive compared with seronegative women and that dysplasia was more likely to persist and progress than in seronegative women (Andieh et al 1999). Treatment with HAART may influence cervical dysplasia although results are not consistent across studies, with some suggesting that women treated with HAART experience early regression of lesions (Heard et al 1998) and others showing no convincing evidence of an effect (Moore et al 2002).

There have been concerns about the usefulness of cervical cytology in HIV-infected women and the optimal method and frequency of screening of this population remain unresolved. Larger studies have validated the use of cervical cytological screening combined with a low threshold for colposcopy and directed biopsy. RCOG guidelines advocate annual smears for women with HIV with no history of abnormality. Screening intensity should continue unaltered even in women with excellent CD4 and viral load responses to HAART. High-grade cervical lesions should be treated appropriately whilst women with low-grade abnormalities who are likely to adhere to follow-up may safely be monitored on a 6-monthly basis. The clinical usefulness and cost-effectiveness of HPV typing incorporated in routine clinical practice in women with HIV remain uncertain.

Cancer of the cervix

This diagnosis is a gender-specific AIDS diagnosis added to the AIDS definition in 1993. In the UK we have not seen a great rise in the number of cases of cervical carcinoma in HIV-positive women and this may represent either effective screening or long latency of the disease, with more effective antiretroviral therapy likely to play a role. One study has shown that 2.5% of HIV-positive women aged 15–49 in is European countries have presented with this malignancy as a first AIDS-defining event (Serraino et al 2002).

Other genital neoplasia

Vulval and anal intraepithelial neoplasia have also been reported more commonly in HIV-infected women (Williams et al 1994) though the possible role of screening has not been evaluated.

PREGNANCY

Fertility does not seem to be affected by HIV infection. Women (and men) with HIV are just as keen to pursue pregnancy as the HIV-negative population. Even before the advent of HAART, termination rates were no higher amongst those who were HIV positive. Pregnancy does not appear to have any major effect on the rate of progression of HIV disease and HIV infection itself (unless very advanced) does not affect pregnancy outcome. The main concern is the risk to the baby of becoming HIV infected. Of infected babies, about one-third present early with symptoms and progress rapidly, one-third experience a relapsing–remitting course with the remainder having a more chronic infection and living well into their teenage years.

In order to prevent vertical transmission, the diagnosis of HIV must first be made. The UK's record on antenatal diagnosis has been extremely poor and the majority of mothers of children vertically infected with HIV discovered their own diagnosis only when the child developed AIDS (PHLS 1999). The Department of Health subsequently issued guidelines that all pregnant women should be offered an HIV test with the aim that uptake of the test be 90% by the end of 2002 and the number of vertically HIV-infected babies reduced by 80% (DOH 1999). Great progress has already been made towards this goal with more than double the number of new cases of HIV diagnosed in women cited as having been the result of antenatal testing in 2000 compared to 1999 (DOH 2001).

Factors known to be associated with increased risk of MTCT are increasing viral load, decreasing CD4 count, increasing duration of rupture of membranes, vaginal route of delivery, younger gestational age at delivery, the presence of other sexually transmitted infections, invasive medical procedures such as amniocentesis, fetal blood sampling and assisted delivery, and breastfeeding.

Care of a pregnant, HIV-positive woman has two main aims: first, to ensure the good health of the mother and second, to attempt to reduce the risk of transmission to the baby to a minimum.

Antiretroviral therapy

If the mother is not yet on HAART but requires antiretroviral therapy, then this should be given in accordance with BHIVA guidelines for non-pregnant women. Some women choose to defer treatment until after the period of organogenesis after discussion with their HIV physician. Women already taking HAART will often choose to continue their therapy although uncertainty regarding the long-term effects of intrauterine exposure to antiretrovirals at any gestation may be a cause for anxiety.

In developed countries most studies have shown a transmission rate of 15–25% in the absence of treatment but the use of antiretroviral therapy in pregnancy has significantly reduced transmission rates. Use of AZT (a nucleoside) monotherapy was a breakthrough in reducing vertical transmission (Connor et al 1994). AZT commenced prior to the third trimester, given to the mother intravenously during delivery and to the neonate orally reduced transmission by 67% in a placebo-controlled trial. AZT monotherapy does not reduce viral load to undetectable levels and so does not prevent vertical transmission solely by an effect on viral load. Its precise mechanism of action remains uncertain. For this reason, although AZT monotherapy is still a regime recommended by the BHIVA, there is a trend towards use of short-term antiretroviral therapy 'START' regimes (combination therapy taken from around

28 weeks' gestation for the duration of the pregnancy only) even in mothers who do not require antiretroviral therapy for themselves (i.e. have a CD4 count of >350). Unlike AZT monotherapy, START regimes aim to reduce viral load to undetectable levels to reduce levels of transmission as far as possible.

The potential for simplified regimes has been assessed and neviripine (an NNRTI) monotherapy given in two doses, one to the mother during labour and the other to the neonate at 48–72 hours, has been shown in Africa to be more effective than a single dose of AZT (Guay et al 1999). However, evidence of subsequent neviripine resistance (which will compromise effective treatment regimes available to the mother) continues to emerge and use of neviripine monotherapy is generally not advised.

Obstetricians should be aware of possible side-effects occurring in women receiving antiretroviral therapy. Protease inhibitors may lead to glucose intolerance and an increasing likelihood of gestational diabetes whilst two of the nucleoside agents (DD1 and D4t) have been associated with the development of lactic acidosis (three fatal cases), which may mimic the HELLP syndrome. These agents should probably be avoided if possible. Those women with greater immune compromise may be taking antibiotic prophylaxis against opportunistic infection. Septrin, the agent most commonly used, is a folate antagonist and prescription of folate supplements should prevent developmental abnormalities.

All women should be registered prospectively on the Antiretroviral Pregnancy Registry (managed by GlaxoSmithKline), set up to monitor long- and short-term side-effects. Women and their children should also be registered with the RCOG and the British Paediatric Surveillance Unit (BSPU). Current French data suggest possible mitochondrial dysfunction in children of mothers who took antiretroviral therapy in pregnancy (10 confirmed cases in 2209 children exposed to antiretrovirals and no cases in 1874 children not exposed to therapy in utero) (Delfraissy et al 2001) but the UK register has not demonstrated any adverse effects of therapy to date. Efavirenz (an NNRTI also known as DMP) has been shown to cause a range of defects of varying severity in cynomolgus monkeys and its use should be avoided if at all possible. In counselling women in this area, it is important to weigh up the uncertainty regarding toxicity against the undisputed benefits of preventing vertical transmission.

Delivery route

In the majority of cases transmission occurs at the time of delivery but a small percentage will occur in utero. There is now conclusive evidence to recommend pre-labour lower segment caesarean section. Meta-analysis of 15 prospective cohort studies showed a 50% reduction in transmission (International Perinatal HIV Group 1999) and a 70% reduction was found in the European controlled trial (European Mode of Delivery Collaboration 1999). There is uncertainty whether there is a persistent benefit in caesarean section when the mother has undetectable viral load (<50 copies/ml).

Breastfeeding further increases the risk of transmission of HIV by between 7% and 22% (Dunn et al 1992). In the developed world the majority of postpartum transmission is the result of breastfeeding and its avoidance significantly reduces rates of infection (Kreiss 1997). If a woman decides to breastfeed despite this evidence she should be advised to breastfeed exclusively as transmission rates are highest when mixed feeding is employed. There may well be considerable cultural difficulties around not breastfeeding and women need support and advice as to how to deal with this.

Transmission rates

Transmission rates of between 1% and 2% can be achieved by a combination of antenatal treatment with antiretrovirals, AZT infusion at a pre-labour caesarean section, avoidance of breastfeeding and infant antiretroviral therapy. Treatment and follow-up of the infant should be undertaken by a specialist paediatric team.

PREGNANCY CONTROL

Contraception

All patients should be advised to use barrier contraception to protect against transmission of HIV, transmission of resistant HIV, other infections and pregnancy. Many women decide to use a 'belt and braces' approach, using an additional method to reduce the risk of unplanned pregnancy further although there is some evidence that condom use declines in HIV-positive women who use combined oral contraception (COC). Women taking antiretroviral therapy which may induce or suppress liver enzymes to varying degrees should be made aware of the possible risk of subtherapeutic levels of their combined contraceptive pill and advice to also use condoms should be reinforced. Those using depot injections and taking HAART should have injections every 10 weeks. HAART regimes containing protease inhibitors have been associated with elevations in blood triglycerides and cholesterol which should be closely monitored in those taking COC.

Previous advice was for women with HIV to avoid use of the IUD because of potential risks of infection and possible increase in risk of transmission to male partners resulting from increased duration and heaviness of menses. This has not been substantiated (European Study Group on Heterosexual Transmission of HIV 1992) and in carefully selected candidates this may well be a method of choice (Sinei et al 1998). We are increasingly using the progestogen intrauterine system (IUS) for women with HIV with the benefits of excellent contraception and a reduction in blood flow.

Sterilization should be undertaken under the same guidelines as apply to other women. However, care needs to be taken around the time of diagnosis of HIV when women have not had sufficient opportunity to adjust to the diagnosis and may subsequently regret the procedure.

Spermicides, such as nonoxynol-9, appear to inactivate HIV in vitro but may not be so effective in vivo. Unfortunately there is evidence that nonoxynol-9 may cause mucosal inflammation that might lead to an increased risk of HIV transmission. The contraceptive implant Implanon has not been evaluated in these women although it is likely to have a role. All women should be made aware of emergency contraception (Levonelle and emergency IUD insertion) and where this can be accessed.

Termination of pregnancy

Women requesting termination of pregnancy should be referred to an appropriate clinic where both medical and surgical options may be offered as appropriate. As for HIV-negative women who have had unprotected sexual intercourse, sexually transmitted infection screening may also be appropriate at this time.

PLANNING PREGNANCY

Any woman planning pregnancy should be advised to stop smoking and reduce alcohol consumption and folate supplements should be prescribed. It is sensible to assess the woman's overall state of health and in the HIV-positive woman this will include checking recent levels of viral load and CD4 count. HAART regimes containing a known teratogen such as efavirenz should be altered if possible.

Both partners may be HIV infected or only one. Where only the woman is infected, the entirely safe method of artificial insemination using the partner's semen can be employed. Advice should be given regarding timing of ovulation and the optimum time of insemination, some women preferring to buy commercially available ovulation predictor kits.

An HIV-negative woman may have an HIV-positive male partner. HIV does not appear to directly infect sperm. Therefore, if sperm can be isolated from the white blood cells and seminal plasma in a 'sperm-washing' procedure it should be possible to inseminate a woman safely. Semprini et al (1992), Gilling-Smith (2000) and Marina et al (1998) have experience of more than 3000 cycles of sperm washing and intrauterine insemination or in vitro fertilization (resulting in 300 live births) with no reported seroconversions. The sperm-washing procedure is expensive and not currently freely available and some couples may decide to pursue 'unsafe' insemination with unprocessed semen or to practise 'unsafe' sex. Mandelbrot et al (1997), however, have published results of a study of 92 HIV-negative women whose partners were HIV positive and who had 104 pregnancies. All couples had unprotected intercourse during the fertile period as determined with commercial ovulation predictor kits. There were only four seroconversions, all in couples who did not use condoms consistently during the rest of the cycle.

Even when both partners are infected with HIV, condom-free intercourse cannot be recommended because of the possibility of transmission of resistant virus. Couples may choose to perform the possibly less risky home insemination.

INFERTILITY

This has been a contentious but important area. Women and their partners should not automatically be denied access to treatment because of HIV infection. As with HIV-negative women with potentially life-shortening conditions such as complicated diabetes, post transplant or a history of cancer, HIV-infected women must be equipped with information and allowed to make their own reproductive decisions (Gilling-Smith et al 2001).

Continuing childlessness can be extremely distressing and factors such as current state of health and long-term prognosis, support networks and motivation to pursue often stressful investigations and treatments should be discussed and counselling given. Advice regarding HIV, treatment and prevention of vertical transmission should be accurate, up to date and given in conjunction with expert HIV physicians.

Infertility may present in a number of different situations with one or both partners being infected with HIV. Where IVF is necessary, the possible emotional and financial costs should be discussed and this treatment should be carried out only where there are provisions to perform treatment safely and without risk of infection to others.

PREPARATION FOR GYNAECOLOGICAL SURGERY

Most HIV-infected women will tolerate surgery well, even if their CD4 count is low. Chest and wound infections are more common, but with prophylactic antibiotics and physiotherapy will not usually present serious problems. Where surgery is indicated HIV status itself should not affect the decision to operate.

NOSOCOMIAL TRANSMISSION

Occupational transmission to healthcare workers

Most occupational transmission has occurred following needle-stick or other sharps injury and there have been a very few documented seroconversions after contamination of broken skin or mucous membranes. The risk of acquiring HIV from a single accidental parenteral exposure to infected blood has been estimated at around 0.3%. Those performing surgical procedures should employ universal precautions, bearing in mind the prevalence of undiagnosed HIV, hepatitis B and C infection. The last two conditions are much more readily transmitted than HIV. A woman with HIV should not be subjected to any unnecessary and discriminatory infection control procedures which could isolate her or draw attention to her before other patients or relatives.

Postexposure prophylaxis (PEP)

Immediately after a percutaneous or mucous membrane exposure to potentially HIV-infected blood, thorough washing with warm running water and soap and clinical evaluation of the injury should be performed. Any bleeding should be encouraged. Consultation with local HIV experts should be as rapid as possible in order that appropriate prophylactic antiretroviral therapy can be commenced, preferably within an hour, to reduce the risk of seroconversion (DOH 2000).

HIV-infected healthcare workers

The Department of Health, Medical Defence Union and UKCC are clear that HIV-positive health workers should not take part in invasive 'exposure-prone' procedures and the individual should inform their occupational health department of their status. In addition, the General Medical Council recommends that staff who think they have been at risk should be tested confidentially.

CONCLUSION

The national strategy for sexual health and HIV (DOH 2001) aims to reduce transmission of HIV, increase diagnosis of prevalent cases, improve the health and social care of people with HIV and reduce the stigma attached to the diagnosis. Rates of HIV infection continue to increase and the number of women affected is rising. Use of HAART has dramatically improved the prognosis for patients with HIV. Obstetricians and gynaecologists should be aware of the possibility of HIV infection in their patients and should facilitate HIV testing in order that women are able to experience the benefits of therapy.

KEY POINTS

1. Increasing numbers of incident infections and improvement in treatments available have lead to an increase in prevalence of HIV infection in women.
2. Whilst HIV remains an incurable condition, currently available therapy has improved the prognosis dramatically.
3. Women with HIV experience the same range of gynaecological problems as their HIV-negative counterparts and their HIV status itself should not influence the treatment they receive.
4. CIN is more common in this population and women with HIV should be screened annually.
5. Mother-to-child transmission rates are 15–20% in untreated women but this can be reduced to under 2% with appropriate intervention.
6. HIV infection should not influence the availability of fertility investigation and treatment.
7. Obstetricians and gynaecologists should be aware of the possibility of HIV in their patients and should facilitate testing to monitor infection rates and to alert infected women to their need for treatment.

REFERENCES

Adachi A, Fleming I, Burk RD, Ho CYF, Klein RS 1993 Women with human immunodeficiency virus infection and abnormal Papanicolaou smears: a prospective study of colposcopy and clinical outcome. Obstetrics and Gynecology 81:372–377

Andieh L, Munoz A, Vlahov D et al 1999 Cervical neoplasia and the persistence of HPV infection in HIV+ women. The 6th Conference on Retroviruses and Opportunistic Infections, January 31–February 4, Chicago, Illinois. Abstract 463

British HIV Association 2001a Guidelines for the treatment of HIV-infected individuals with antiretroviral therapy. (http://www.aidsmap.com/about/bhiva/guidelines.pdf)

British HIV Association 2001b Guidelines for the management of HIV-infected pregnant women and the prevention of mother to child transmission. British HIV Association. (http://www.aidsmap.com/about/bhiva/BHVA%202001%20Final.pdf)

Carpenter CCJ, Mayer KH, Stein MD, Leibman BD, Fisher A, Fiore TC 1991 Human immunodeficiency virus infection in North American women: experience with 200 cases and a review of the literature. Medicine 70:307–325

Centers for Disease Control 1992 Revised classification system for HIV infection and expanded surveillance case definition for AIDS among adolescents and adults. Morbidity and Mortality Weekly Report 41(RR-17):1–19

Connor EM, Sperling RS, Gelber R et al 1994 Reduction of maternal–infant transmission of human immunodeficiency virus type 1 with zidovudine treatment. New England Journal of Medicine 331:1173–1180

Delfraissy JF, Blanche S, Tardieu M et al 2001 Mitochondrial and mitochondrial-like symptoms in children born to HIV-infected mothers. Exhaustive evaluation in a large prospective cohort. The 8th Conference on Retroviruses and Opportunistic Infections, February 4–8, Chicago, Illinois. Abstract 625B

Department of Health 1999 Targets aimed at reducing the numbers of children born with HIV. DOH, London

Department of Health 2000 HIV post-exposure prophylaxis: guidance from the UK chief medical officer's Expert Advisory Group on AIDS. DOH, London

Department of Health 2001 The national strategy for sexual health and HIV. DOH, London

de Vincenzi I, for the European Study Group on Heterosexual Transmission of HIV 1994 A longitudinal study of human immunodeficiency virus transmission by heterosexual partners. New England Journal of Medicine 331:341–346

Dunn DT, Newell M-L, Ades AE, Peckham C 1992 Estimates of the risk of HIV-1 transmission through breast feeding. Lancet 320:585–588

European Mode of Delivery Collaboration 1999 Elective caesarean section versus vaginal delivery in prevention of vertical HIV-1 transmission: a randomised clinical trial. Lancet 353:1035–1039

European Study Group on Heterosexual Transmission of HIV 1992 Comparison of female to male and male to female transmission of HIV in 563 stable couples. British Medical Journal 304:809–813

Gilling-Smith C 2000 Assisted reproduction in HIV discordant couples. AIDS Reader 10:581–587

Gilling-Smith C, Smith JR, Semprini AE 2001 HIV and infertility: time to treat. There's no justification for denying treatment to parents who are HIV positive. British Medical Journal 322:566–567

Guay LA, Musoke P, Fleming T et al 1999 Intrapartum and neonatal single-dose nevirpine compared with zidovudine for prevention of mother-to-child transmission of HIV-1 in Kampala, Uganda: HIVNET 012 randomised trial. Lancet 354:795–802

Harlow SD, Schuman P, Cohen M et al 2000 Effect of HIV infection on menstrual cycle length. Journal of the Acquired Immune Deficiency Syndrome 24:68–75

Heard I, Schmitz V, Costagliola D, Orth G, Kazatchkine MD 1998 Early regression of cervical lesions in HIV-seropositive women receiving highly active antiretroviral therapy. AIDS 12:1459–1464

Iman N, Carpenter CCJ, Mayer K et al 1990 Hierarchical pattern of mucosal Candida infections in HIV-seropositive women. American Journal of Medicine 89:142–146

International Perinatal HIV Group 1999 Mode of delivery and vertical transmission of HIV-1: a meta-analysis from 15 prospective cohort studies. New England Journal of Medicine 340:977–987

Johnson JC, Burnett AF, Willet GD et al 1992 High frequency of latent and clinical human papillomavirus cervical infections in immunocompromised human immunodeficiency virus infected women. Obstetrics and Gynecology 79:321

Korn AP, Landers DV, Green JR, Sweet RL 1993 Pelvic inflammatory disease in human immunodeficiency virus-infected women. Obstetrics and Gynecology 82:765–768

Kreiss J 1997 Breast feeding and vertical transmission of HIV-1. Acta Paediatrica 421(suppl):113–117

Mandelbrot L, Heard I, Henrion-Geant E, Henrion R 1997 Natural conception in HIV-negative women with HIV-infected partners (letter). Lancet 349:850–851

Marina S, Marina F, Alcolea R et al 1998 Human immunodeficiency virus type I-serodiscordant couples can bear healthy children after undergoing intrauterine insemination. Fertility and Sterility 70:35–39

Massad LS, Riester KA, Anastos KM et al 1999 Prevalence and predictors of squamous cell abnormalities in Papanicoloaou smears from women infected with HIV-1. Journal of the Acquired Immune Deficiency Syndrome and Human Retrovirology 21:33–41

Minkoff HL, Eisenberger-Matityahu D, Feldman J, Burk R, Clarke L 1999 Prevalence and incidence of gynecologic disorders among women infected with human immunodeficiency virus. American Journal of Obstetrics and Gynecology 180:824–836

Monzon OT, Capellan JMB 1987 Female to female transmission of HIV. Lancet 2:40–41

Moore AL, Sabin CA, Madge S et al 2002 Highly active antiretroviral therapy and cervical intraepithelial neoplasia. AIDS 16:927–929

Palefsky JM, Minkoff H, Kalish LA et al 1999 Cervicovaginal human papillomavirus infection in human immunodeficiency virus-1 positive and high risk HIV-negative women. Journal of the National Cancer Institute 91:226–236

Palella FJ Jr, Delaney KM, Moorman AC et al 1998 Declining morbidity and mortality among patients with advanced human immunodeficiency virus infection. HIV Outpatient Study Investigators. New England Journal of Medicine 338:853–860

Paterson DC, Georghiou PR, Allworth AM, Kemp RJ 1995 Thalidomide as treatment of refactory aphthous ulceration related to human immunodeficiency virus. Clinical Infectious Diseases 20:250–254

Paterson DC, Swindells S, Mohr J et al 1999 How much adherence is enough? A prospective study of adherence to protease inhibitor therapy using MEMSCaps. The 6th Conference on Retroviruses and Opportunistic Infections, January 31–February 4, Chicago, Illinois. Abstract 92

PHLS 1999 http://www.phls.co.uk/facts/HIV/hiv.htm

Reicheldorfer P, Coombs R, Wright KD et al 2000 Effect of menstrual cycle on HIV-1 levels in the peripheral blood and genital tract. WHS 001 Study Team. AIDS 14:2101–2107

Richardson BA, Morrison CS, Sekadde-Kigondu C et al 1999 Effect of intrauterine device use on cervical shedding of HIV-1 DNA. AIDS 13:2091–2097

Rudin C, Laubereau B, Lauper U 1998 Attitudes towards childbearing and adherence to safer sex rules in a cohort of HIV infected women. The 12th World AIDS Conference, June 29–July 3, Geneva, Switzerland. Abstract 14111

Schafer A, Friedmann W, Meikle M, Schwartlander B, Koch MA 1991 The increased frequency of cervical dysplasia-neoplasia in women infected with the human immunodeficiency virus is related to the degree of immunosuppression. American Journal of Obstetrics and Gynecology 164:593–599

Semprini AE, Levi-Setti P, Bozzo M et al 1992 Insemination of HIV-negative women with processed semen of HIV-positive partners. Lancet 340:1317–1319

Sinei SK, Morrison CS, Sekadde-Kigondu C, Allen M, Kokonya D 1998 Complications of use of intrauterine devices among HIV-1-infected women. Lancet 351:1238–1241

Spinollo A, Michelone G, Cavanna C, Colonna L, Cadyzzi E, Bucika S 1994 Clinical and microbiological characterisation of symptomatic vulvovaginal candidiasis in HIV-seropositive women. Genitourinary Medicine 70:268–272

Serraino D, Dal Maso L, La Vecchia C et al 2002 Invasive cervical cancer as an AIDS-defining illness in Europe. AIDS 16:781–786

UNAIDS 2000 Report on the global HIV/AIDS epidemic. Joint United Nations Programme on HIV AIDS. (http://www.unaids.org/epidemic_update/report/Epi_report.pdf)

Wasserheit JN 1992 Epidemiological synergy. Interrelationships between human immunodeficiency virus infection and other sexually transmitted diseases. Sexually Transmitted Diseases 19:61–77

Williams AD, Darragh TM, Vraniazn K et al 1994 Anal and cervical human papillomavirus infection and risk of anal and cervical epithelial abnormalities in human immunodeficiency virus-infected women. Obstetrics and Gyecology 83:205–211

64

Forensic gynaecology

Camille de San Lazaro   Helen M. Cameron

INTRODUCTION

Sexual offences constitute 5–6% of reported violent crime in England and Wales with 75% of cases of sexual assault being rape or indecent assault on females (Home Office 2000). In a global context, it is known that conclusions drawn from crime statistics are virtually useless for estimating the incidence of sexual assault because women are universally reluctant to report rape to the authorities.

Sexual exploitation of children is now well recognized as part of the spectrum of maltreatment of children. It is important that the examining doctor should be experienced in general clinical forensic examination and should be familiar with the range of normal genital and anal findings in the age range of victims being examined.

The first part of this chapter explores the issues of child sexual abuse relevant to the gynaecologist while the second part covers adult forensic gynaecology and the medicolegal aspects relating to sexual offences.

CHILD SEXUAL ABUSE

Child sexual abuse has been most clearly defined by Shecter & Roberge (1976) as the 'involvement of dependent, developmentally immature children and adolescents in sexual activities which they do not fully comprehend and to which they are unable to give informed consent or that violate the social taboos of family roles'.

The most recent comprehensive United Kingdom study conducted by the NSPCC (2000) presented findings of a survey of 2869 18–24 year olds. Seven per cent had suffered serious physical abuse, 6% physical neglect, 4% had been sexually abused by a parent or relative, 1% had experienced penetrative sex by people known but unrelated to them.

One in three of the respondents had never told anyone of the abuse. Contrary to common belief, the most likely relative to abuse within the family is a brother or stepbrother.

In England in the year 2000, 30 300 children were on child protection registers; of these 5600 were registered for sexual abuse.

Presentation

Acute presentations are rare. They may be fortuitous, i.e. there is discovery of bleeding or bruising or the child makes a comment which raises suspicion. In these circumstances or in situations where a child makes a clear allegation of recent assault, skilled urgent examination by a practitioner(s) with paediatric and forensic skills is indicated. More commonly, suspicions are raised by a child's behaviour, a history of contact with a known offender or genitourinary symptoms reflecting longer exposure to sexual abuse.

Box 64.1 Symptoms suggesting abuse

Emotional:	Clinging anxiety, nightmares, loss of bowel or urinary control
Physical:	Rectal and vaginal bleeding, genitourinary complaints
Psychiatric:	Self-injury, poisoning, depression, eating disorders
Behavioural:	Promiscuous behaviour, truancy, delinquency

Older children and adolescents may present to genitourinary clinics, drop-in advisory centres or to gynaecologists for suspected pregnancy. Health professionals may fear that engaging with a child protection system may jeopardize their ability to provide sexual health advice in these circumstances.

The welfare of the young person is of paramount importance, as they may be powerless to protect their own interests. The need to preserve confidentiality must be balanced with the need to offer protection.

Medical practitioners are also increasingly being asked to assist the police in investigating crimes involving procurement, pornography and paedophilic material on the Internet. Visual images of sexual acts against children require analysis in respect of the pubertal status of the children and anatomical evidence of penetration.

Child sexual abuse rarely takes place in a vacuum. Much sexual abuse occurs within a background of other disadvantage, including emotional abuse, neglect, physical abuse, geographical instability, family violence or substance abuse and these factors have obvious implications for interpretation of symptoms of distress.

Consent

A common area of contention, particularly in cases involving adolescents, is the issue of consent. It should be recognized that consent should always be based on choice and should involve an active decision to participate. This is only possible if the adolescent knows that saying 'no' will not demean them or endanger them.

Elements of consent can be summarized as:

- understanding the request
- knowing the standard (i.e. societal definition/regard) of that behaviour; being aware of the possible consequences
- knowing that any decision will be respected.

It is important that young adolescents are helped to explore their feelings fully to determine what elements of consent and competence are present within their sexual engagement. Physical examination findings or a history suggesting force or instrumentation should never be seen as acceptable.

Difficulties do arise when both victim and alleged assailant are young. It is helpful to understand that normal childhood exploratory behaviour does not involve aggressive penetrative acts or serious coercion on the part of one child. The age and sex of the children involved also help to guide the practitioner to a sensible evaluation of likely power differentials and possible victimization. In general, if any child is affected emotionally and physically by the sexual behaviour of another, the matter should be referred for investigation, as there is at least one victim. It should also be clear that the aggressor may well be displaying learned behaviour because of victimization and there is likely to be adult involvement somewhere in the chain.

Multidisciplinary working

Child protection systems in the UK are guided by the Children Act 1989 and Department of Health guidelines. A multidisciplinary framework involving health services, social services, police and education underpins all investigations in child abuse. The health component includes primary care, school health and paediatrics. However, all health professionals who deal with children have an overriding duty to the child whose needs should always be paramount.

All health professionals need to be familiar with child protection guidelines, their legal responsibilities and the referral process (BMA 1994, DOH 1999, GMC 2000a,b,c).

Assessment of the sexually abused child

It is widely accepted that every child in whom sexual abuse is suspected should be offered a full paediatric assessment. This may include anogenital examination and this latter decision should be taken following a face-to-face discussion with the child and family and a preliminary engagement within which the history, symptoms and the child's consent are evaluated.

The practitioner should always remember that the child's initial account to a parent or child protection worker is unlikely to be comprehensive. Children who have been told they will be punished or not believed if they tell are likely to test adult reaction with minimal information. If the response is adverse, the child may well retreat into silence and denial. Even in the best of circumstances, the child's embarrassment, limited vocabulary or fear of the perpetrator are powerful disincentives to full disclosure.

The medical assessment should take account of these issues. It is possible to acknowledge them by an open approach, e.g. 'We know that children find it very hard to talk about these things. You don't have to say anything to me now – just tell someone when you are ready or remember. But we know that a full body check helps a lot of children feel better.'

The timing of the assessment is most influenced by the time since the last incident of molestation. Clearly if this was several months previously there is no urgency but, in general, family distress and the child's anxiety about the examination itself make expediency desirable.

If the child has not made a formal statement to the police by the time of the examination, care should be taken to collect such history as is known, outside the child's presence. Alternatively, a free narrative account from the child without leading questions may be taken, if the child is comfortable with this. There are no firm rules about the order of investigation; the medical examination may well inform the police interviewing process and vice versa. With careful liaison, the best outcome for the child should be sought in planning the order of events. The examiner must ensure sufficient consultation time. It is unreasonable to fit in a 'quick genital check' within a busy pre-existing schedule. Likewise, it is not

Box 64.2   Medical assessment aims and objectives

Healing	An accepting, non-judgemental approach, a focus on the whole child when taking the history, offering the child choices, providing information, toys and books.
Assessing health	Examining all systems, assessing growth and development, immunization status, education progress and peer relationships.
Gathering evidence	Skilled anogenital examination, recording findings, sampling for trace evidence and sexually transmitted disease.
Planning for aftercare	Evaluating family strengths and support systems, referral for psychosocial counselling, psychiatric referral when needed.
Arranging review	Re-evaluate physical signs as needed, re-testing for STD, ensuring aftercare in place.

helpful to offer a time of day when a child may be tired or hungry or an appropriate relative cannot be present.

The child's needs must be paramount when deciding on the nature and timing of medical input.

Clinical approach

Medical assessments should take place in an environment which is child friendly, well lit and fully equipped with all material that may be required. It is highly desirable that a designated area is furnished for such assessments and that this should be separate from other areas of busy emergency activity.

A non-clinical environment will reduce fear and intimidation. Early attention should be given to presenting toys, books and music and the approach should be unhurried and welcoming. The child should be allowed to familiarize herself with the equipment and the examination process should be explained. Involving the child in choosing the colour of stethoscope, which body part will be examined first and assisting in switching equipment on and off will give her a sense of control. The practitioner should engage in non-threatening conversation about hobbies, friends, likes and dislikes. This is specially helpful during genital examination (San Lazaro 1995).

A full top-down examination should be aimed for, undressing and dressing as one proceeds. Adolescents are best left to undress in privacy behind screens and offered a gown and sheet.

Genital examination

Procedure

The child is best examined on a firm couch with the head resting on a carer's lap. The supine, frog leg or lithotomy position is usually adequate. Following inspection of the labia majora, lateral separation will reveal the hymen and orifice if there are no labial adhesions. Gentle posterior traction directed towards the bed or anterior traction (grasping the labia majora and pulling gently anteriorly) will stretch the hymenal free edge and expose the orifice with clarity.

The knee–chest posture is favoured by some examiners. It is usually used if there are minor hymenal irregularities, especially shallow notches; these may flatten out with gravity in the knee–chest position though most will do so with patience and firm anterior traction techniques.

Digital or speculum examination is not indicated in young children. While digital examination of the sexually active adolescent is sometimes desirable, the anxious, recently assaulted adolescent often responds with considerable vaginismus and such examinations may not provide evidence or otherwise of vaginal capacity. Caution should be exercised in giving the view that 'penile penetration is unlikely or impossible'.

A colposcope does provide an excellent fibre-optic light source and a useful facility for still or videotape images but it is clearly intrusive, creates a clinical atmosphere and may increase anxiety. There should be secure storage of such images and children, especially adolescents, should be made aware that they could be copied and used in a court. Informed consent should be obtained. While it is virtually impossible to conduct an accurate examination of a child without her co-operation and consent, some practitioners include a formal written consent within the examination record.

Acute examination

An urgent forensic evaluation is required in any child or adolescent where the history suggests contact abuse less than 96 hours previously.

The persistence of trace materials is dependent on:

- time since the event
- any washing or bathing
- whether a condom was used
- whether the subject is mobile.

Drainage of vaginal contents would be relatively slow in a child who is immobile for any reason.

Trace material such as blood, semen, fibres or saliva may be available from clothing, bites, genital, rectal and mouth swabs.

The history is critical; for example, skin swabs may identify adhesive, if taken from the wrists or ankles of a victim who alleges being strapped down.

The forensic process is very similar to the adult format (see later). However, the younger the child, the more likely it is that trace material may be found in extragenital sites like the abdomen and thighs. A Woods light may assist in defining areas of abnormal fluorescence. It should be used with caution.

The examination should consist of the following elements:

- Assessing demeanour, signs of toxicity, visible injury.
- Assessing items of clothing for tears and staining.
- A general inspection for signs of trauma or trace material.
- An anogenital examination.
- Collection of specimens as below.

Signs of acute sexual assault include:

- aggressive bites and suction bites
- bruising, abrasions and lacerations
- tears to the hymen and fourchette, oedema and bleeding
- anal lacerations, oedema, swelling and bruising
- haemorrhages or contusions in the mouth/palate.

In young children presenting with significant trauma, forensic swab collection is likely to be frightening and poorly tolerated. Examination under anaesthesia should be considered in these circumstances, which are rare.

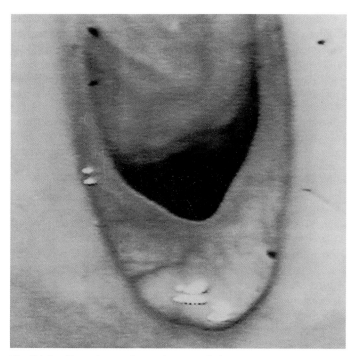

Fig. 64.1   Normal, prepubescent crescentic hymen.

Hymenal examinations in sexual abuse

The newborn hymen is oestrogenized and thickened, often with leucorrhoeic secretions. This appearance may persist in the first 2 years of life. In infancy and toddlerhood the hymen in appearance is often full and frilly, with the orifice obscured.

An atrophic, sharp-edged annular or crescentic hymen (Fig. 64.1) tends to be the pattern seen in mid childhood, though there may be minor variations. Symmetrical deficiencies of the anterior hymen are common.

The most common congenital variant seen in practice is a septate hymen.

In the non-abused prepubescent child the free edge is usually smooth and well defined. Shallow notches or small remnant tags (bumps) may be seen in normal children (Berensen et al 2000).

The pubescent hymen is more difficult to evaluate. With increasing oestrogenization, the tissue becomes fleshy and redundant, leucorrhoeic secretions are present and the orifice less easy to define with simple inspection. The free edge of the hymenal orifice is less sensitive to contact than in prepubescence and manipulation with a cotton-tipped swab is usually well tolerated.

The size of the hymenal orifice has been subject to numerous studies, but is now recognized to be so variable as to be an unreliable single marker for sexual abuse. It is generally agreed that a transverse orifice size greater than 1 cm is not commonly seen in non-abused prepubertal children (RCP 1997).

Gardner (1992) found a small proportion of non-abused children to have diameters greater than 1 cm and in practice, large-sized orifices are not uncommonly seen in obese children.

Abnormal genital findings

Physical signs of sexual abuse are much rarer than one might be led to expect from children's accounts. Even when these

Box 64.3   Signs suggesting abuse

Blood staining
Acute bruising
Bites
Hymenal loss/attenuation
Healed tears/scars
Sexually transmitted disease
Lacerations or scarring beyond the skin of the anus

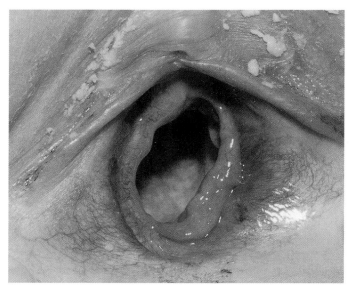

Fig. 64.2   Attenuated hymen in a 4 year old ('Daddy hurt my rudies'). Note transection at 7 o'clock (right of posterior midline).

accounts include penetration, symptoms of pain and dysuria, there may be little to see. Adams et al (1994) studied 236 children where there had been perpetrator convictions (86% of perpetrators confessed to abuse) and found definite genital abnormality in only 14%. Abnormal anal findings were found in only 1% of cases. Two factors which influenced the likelihood of abnormal findings were a history of bleeding and the time since the last incident of abuse (Box 64.3).

Healing of hymenal injuries is rapid and comparable to healing patterns of any mucosal injury, for example in the mouth. Superficial abrasions may resolve in hours. Penetrative trauma (Fig. 64.2) may result in tears which may heal, resulting in residual deep notches or angulated clefts, which most often affect the posterior hymen. Narrowing of the hymenal ring at a point in the posterior hymen or complete loss in areas of the hymen are of significance. Frequent blunt penetrative acts may result in 'wearing away' of the hymen of the immature child, leaving an overall depleted narrow strip of hymen. If the hymen is narrower than 1 mm, this is likely to reflect abusive trauma. An attenuated hymen is likely to contribute to a 'gaping' hymenal orifice, i.e. a view may be obtained of the vagina without labial traction and separation.

Substantial healed lacerations through the hymen may involve the posterior vaginal wall and fourchette. Composite scarring through these structures may be seen in elective examinations. Scarring of the fourchette must be distinguished from an avascular linear pale area which is a midline variant and of no significance (linear vestibularis).

A lax anus with poor gripping ability should raise concern if there is a history of risk. Similarly, well-defined scarring beyond the anal verge may be an indicator of blunt penetration. Such scarring may be seen years after abuse.

Other changes such as labial adhesions, urethral dilatation, altered vascularity, anal venous congestion and dilatation may be seen in abused children. They are, however, non-specific and may not be used as sole diagnostic markers for sexual abuse.

Historical abuse

When months or years have elapsed since the last event of abuse, the likelihood of abnormal relevant findings diminishes. The hymen may smoothen out and unless there has been complete loss in one area, it may be difficult to identify specific markers for trauma. Oestrogenization will mask smaller deficits. Minor anal scars will disappear. However, the practitioner should bear in mind that some signs do persist despite these confounding factors; the examination process may also give the victim a sense of being believed and contribute to a sense of body integrity whatever the outcome. It is also perhaps appropriate to note at this point that tampon use does not produce classic signs of hymenal penetrative trauma in adolescents (Emans et al 1994).

Anogenital symptomatology and differential diagnosis

One of the commonest problems in general practice relates to vulval symptoms. In infants in nappies, ammoniacal dermatitis, poor hygiene and secondary candidiasis are the most frequent causes of a vulval rash.

In middle childhood, vulval symptoms of intermittent discomfort, redness and discharge appear to be non-specific and most likely related to oestrogen-dependent vulvitis in this group. Though they are commonly managed with antifungal creams, there is little research to support a chronic infective cause and bacterial isolates are more likely to be secondary or contaminants (Steele & San Lazaro 1994). Contact sensitivity to detergents and other noxious agents, eczema or psoriasis may be factors in vulvitis in this age group.

A bloodstained discharge must raise the suspicion of a foreign body; the object may be a fragment of toilet paper or cotton wool or a small toy. These scenarios are largely benign, but findings of hymenal trauma or repetitive aggressive self-placement of foreign objects should raise suspicion of exposure to sexual abuse.

Lichen sclerosus et atrophicus is a rare disorder affecting the vulva. Characteristic atrophic changes with pallor and haemorrhaging may be seen and may raise the suspicion of an acute assault. The hymen is not involved in this condition, which may be linked to autoimmune disease in the family. It is important to recognize that lichen sclerosus et atrophicus may co-exist with sexual abuse and that the well-recognized Koebner phenomenon is as relevant in children. A large study of prepubescent children (Warrington & San Lazaro 1996) found a history of accidental or sexual trauma to have preceded the development of lichen sclerosus in 17 of 42 cases.

Anal symptoms of soreness, itchiness, constipation and bleeding are similarly not uncommonly benign. Superficial fissuring associated with perianal inflammation may be secondary to threadworms, eczema, poor hygiene and lichen sclerosus. Secondary stool withholding may result in large hard stooling, causing further fissures and setting in chain a cycle of chronic constipation. Most of these presentations are too ubiquitous to be useful markers for sexual abuse but the possibility should always be borne in mind.

In adolescents who are not sexually active, chronic vulval symptoms are comparatively rare. Symptoms may relate to eczema, psoriasis, poor hygiene or lichen sclerosus.

In all ages acute vulvitis secondary to group A *Streptococcus pyogenes*, *Haemophilus influenzae* or *Staphylococcus aureus* may occur as a single event. Repeated infection requires investigation for latent diabetes, immune deficiency or carrier status in a family member.

Sexually transmitted disease

Symptoms of STD in children include discharge, itching, genital pain and dysuria. As in adults, infection may be asymptomatic. STD screening is indicated in all children with a history of contact abuse and those where findings indicate penetration regardless of the history. Persistent symptoms also mandate screening.

The presence of sexually transmitted disease is potent evidence for sexual contact and the rules of evidence for chain of custody should be used to transport elective samples to the laboratory.

Transmission of infection may occur:

- from mother to child, e.g. HIV, HPV, *C. trachomatis*, *N. gonorrhoeae* or herpes simplex virus
- from fomites and auto inoculation, e.g. HPV and possibly HSV and rarely *Trichomonas vaginalis*
- Via sexual contact.

Testing should take into account the incubation period of the range of common organisms and interval testing after an acute assault gives a more reliable outcome. A careful maternal history should be taken in each case.

N. gonorrhoeae in children other than neonates should be assumed as a strong indicator of sexual contact. Unless the child is severely symptomatic it is wise to confirm the isolate with a second culture under optimum forensic conditions. Children may be non-symptomatic (de Jong 1986).

Chlamydia trachomatis
Perinatal transfer is documented to result in prolonged colonization in the first year of life (Bell et al 1986).

The finding of this organism in any age group beyond infancy, however, should raise the strongest suspicion of sexual abuse. Asymptomatic infection may occur.

Trichomonas vaginalis
This organism may cause offensive vaginal discharge in adolescents. It is not recognized to infect the pre-oestrogenized child, though newborns may acquire it from infected maternal secretions. It is a strong marker for sexual contact.

Herpes simplex virus

The legal significance of HSV is less certain. Both type 1 and 2 may present in young children and may be associated with significant systemic illness. Autoinoculation and benign transfer cannot be excluded. Recurrent genital herpes is not expected in young children. The presence of genital HSV in adolescents has the same implications as for adults and sexual contact is likely.

Human papilloma virus

This extremely ubiquitous infection in adults has been widely studied in children. Transfer may be perinatal and the variable incubation period to manifestation of skin lesions makes assessment fraught with uncertainty.

Perianal condylomata is the commonest manifestation in young children. Preliminary (unpublished) research in Newcastle upon Tyne suggests that exclusive vulval or vaginal lesions are more suspicious of abusive contact. The presence of anogenital warts mandates a search for other STDs; 65% of children in one study showed other sexually transmissible organisms (Herman-Giddens et al 1988).

Most children are asymptomatic. Some may present with itching or bleeding.

Other sexually transmitted disease

Screening for syphilis, HIV or hepatitis B is not automatically indicated in most sexual abuse scenarios. A history suggesting multiple perpetrators, the involvement of drugs or procurement for prostitution contributes to an assessment of risk for such infections. The timing of such tests should be judicious and should follow appropriate counselling of the child and the carers.

Methods

Diagnostic methods should use the most specific test available for each organism. In the prepubescent child, fine ENT swabs will enable vaginal sampling without hymenal contact if the child is well relaxed (Steele & San Lazaro 1994). An alternative is to collect a vaginal rinse. C. trachomatis can be reliably tested for using urine PCR (polymerase chain reaction)? though it is wise to confirm positive tests with formal cultures. Prior to puberty vaginal epithelium is essentially columnar. After puberty, columnar sites are at the endocervix and urethra, vaginal epithelium becoming stratified squamous. The ideal for adolescents is urethral and cervical sampling using a small speculum. High vaginal swabs may suffice but are not as reliable.

Child sexual abuse sequelae

Finklehor (1986) describes the trauma genesis of sexual abuse within four dynamics.

Traumatic sexualization. Refers to a process in which a child's sexuality is shaped in an inappropriate and dysfunctional fashion. It occurs through the misconceptions and confusions about sexual behaviour and morality transmitted to the child by the offender. Children emerge from their experience with an inappropriate repertoire of sexual behaviours and unusual emotional associations to sexual activities.

Betrayal When children discover that someone on whom they are dependent has caused them harm. Some children

who have become inured to and who have actually felt loved because of the abuse are deeply damaged when they realize what is really happening.

Powerlessness The child's body space is repeatedly invaded and there may be threat. The child feels trapped within a secret system that they may not alter.

Stigmatization This dynamic refers to shame and guilt, increased by the secret nature of their experience.

These four dynamics contribute to long-term effects of:

- sexual precociousness, reckless sexual behaviour and sexual dysfunction
- difficulties in trust, isolation and a dislike of intimacy
- depression, phobias and re-victimization
- self-harm, substance abuse, delinquent behaviour.

Studies into the long-term consequences of sexual abuse are complicated by the marked variability in prevalence statistics, variations in definitions and the confounding factors of other adverse life experiences.

Ferguson et al (1997) reported on a long-term study over 18 years of a birth cohort of 520 young women. They were able to assign subjects to different groups depending on the extent of abuse. Results showed clear association between sexual abuse and later risk-taking sexual behaviours and re-victimization. The worst outcomes were in the group reporting penetrative abuse.

There is much evidence to suggest that adults who experienced sexual abuse as children are more likely to suffer psychopathology. Mullen and co-workers (1993) found higher symptoms of depression, anxiety and eating disorders. They also found that negative family factors increased the risks of these outcomes.

Banyard (1997), who studied 430 low-income single-parent mothers, found lowered parenting self-esteem and more use of violence in those who had experienced sexual abuse.

Sexual dysfunction is another parameter which has been studied by several researchers. Women who experienced sexual trauma as children are significantly more likely to experience diminution in sexual desire and other difficulties (Sarwer & Durlak 1996).

It is certainly true that not all child sexual abuse victims develop adverse outcomes. Extensive research suggests that many factors mediate or mitigate the effects. Good parental and peer support appear to be protective. In any individual case, the direction of therapy and other services is far more dependent on a thorough and holistic evaluation of all the social dynamics in the child's sphere than on details of the abusive experience.

ADULT FORENSIC GYNAECOLOGY

There seems to be an escalating epidemic of rape globally and it is known that the majority of sexual assaults are not reported to the police and domestic or spousal rape is even less commonly reported. This reluctance is thought to be due in part to the low frequency of convictions. In the USA the 1996 Federal Welfare Reform Law promoted an aggressive enforcement of statutory rape laws at the local and state level. There have been concerns expressed that with increased enforcement, victims of rape, especially teenagers, would be discouraged from seeking help (Miller et al 1998, 1999).

Most rape allegations do not proceed to court; in 1982–5 in Oslo only 20% of the reported cases went to court (Bang 1993). The conviction rate as a percentage of complaints is approximately 10% (Craven 1996). Thus, in effect, there is a pyramid of consequences of sexual assault.

Reasons for failure to report sexual assault

- Fear of becoming involved in complicated police investigations and subsequent court proceedings
- Anxiety, guilt, shame
- Fear of reprisal
- USA state mandatory reporting of sexual assault acting as a deterrent

It is important that all the professionals involved with victims of sexual assault recognize that the assault may be followed by rape-related posttraumatic stress disorder (RR-PTSD).

One of the principal aims of those involved in medical examination of sexual assault victims should be to minimize the mental and physical trauma to the woman whilst endeavouring to collect useful forensic evidence in as dignified and understanding a manner as possible.

The clinician must take an accurate enough account of the event to ensure that an appropriate examination is undertaken and that the collection of forensic evidence is complete. It is, however, the police officer's role to obtain a detailed investigative history so the examining doctor must avoid playing detective. The use of a record of examination with checklists and body diagrams to illustrate the findings provides invaluable assistance to the examining doctor who is not infrequently called to a complainant in the middle of the night.

Consent to forensic examination

Consenting to a medical and forensic examination may be perceived as allowing the victim a sense of control over the examination (Hampton 1995). The General Medical Council (GMC) emphasizes the principles of confidentiality, indicating that 'Patients have a right to expect that information about them will be held in confidence by their doctors' (GMC 2000a,b,c). However, the GMC does accept that doctors may have contractual obligations to third parties such as in their work as police surgeons and in such circumstances disclosure may be expected. In such circumstances the GMC recommends that the doctor is 'satisfied that the patient has been told at the earliest opportunity about the purpose of the examination and/or disclosure, the extent of the information to be disclosed and the fact that relevant information cannot be concealed or withheld'. Thus standard consent forms require major modification to accommodate details about disclosure of evidence to the relevant authorities.

Details of consent to forensic medical examination include:

- medical examination – non-genital/genital
- recording of the details of the examination
- retention of relevant items of clothing for forensic examination

- collection of forensic evidence
- disclosure of details of medical record and/or laboratory tests to police/ Crown Court/Crown Prosecution Service for use in evidence.

The woman should also be made aware that the examination could be discontinued at any stage if she so wishes. The stage of the examination reached and the time at which she decides against further examination should be recorded. It is often the case that the woman is already in the acute phase of the RR-PTSD, exhibiting shock, disbelief, anger and possibly memory blocking. The examiner may question whether such a woman is able to give 'informed' consent to all aspects of the forensic medical examination. It may be appropriate, in this case, to complete the consent for examination and sample collection and defer the consent to disclosure of the medical details until a later date.

The complainant may agree to a 'qualified consent', i.e. to the release of information to the prosecution without allowing scrutiny by the defence. If she does not consent to release of the medical details then the examiner may be ordered to disclose information by a judge, in which case 'disclose only information relevant to the request for disclosure: accordingly you should not disclose the whole record' (GMC 2000a,b,c). In the absence of a court order, a request for the disclosure by a third party, e.g. solicitor, is not sufficient justification for disclosure without the patient's consent.

If the woman is a non-police referral or does not wish to involve the police initially she should be informed that she could pursue a formal complaint subsequently. The medical record should be completed in the same detailed way as if there were consent to disclosure, in case the woman decides at a later date to report the incident to the police, at which stage additional consent should be sought.

Examination of the female rape victim

Who should undertake the examination?
In ideal circumstances the victim of sexual assault should be allowed to choose the gender of the examining doctor. The gender of the examining physician is not always felt to be a factor affecting the victim's response to the medical examination (Hockbaum 1987).

Training in sexual assault examination
Few doctors have received any formal training in the principles of clinical forensic medicine and now that more gynaecologists are entering clinical forensic roles, the necessity of formal education becomes increasingly important. Training in the collection and maintenance of the integrity of forensic evidence is essential as mishandling of evidence leaves the prosecution powerless.

To ensure optimal care for the victims of sexual assault, a co-ordinated multidisciplinary approach should be made to tackle the theoretical and practical training issues. Local programmes should be developed at all levels from undergraduates and specialist registrars through to continuing medical education (CME) of those actively involved in rape examination. These programmes should be validated. One area of training that is especially valuable is court witness skills. Professional networking is particularly important in the field of rape examination.

The Rape Examination, Advice, Counselling and Help (REACH) Project

In 1983 Northumbria Police initiated a scheme whereby a number of women doctors from a variety of professional backgrounds (gynaecology, general practice, etc.) volunteered to undertake the examination of victims of sexual assault. In England and Wales several other schemes also provide a similar service to these women. Many police forces have specially designed and equipped centres, often on hospital sites, to provide a comprehensive support for the victims.

The REACH Project was opened in 1991 to provide a service to women in the Northumbria region who have been sexually assaulted. The Rhona Cross Centre in Newcastle upon Tyne and the Ellis Fraser Centre in Sunderland each offers a unique range of services. The services that REACH provides include:

- experienced women doctors able to conduct the medical examination in the purpose-built suite
- confidential access to experienced counsellors regardless of whether the woman reports the assault to the police or not
- for those women who wish to involve the police, specially trained women police officers to conduct the interview and statement taking
- referral may be through the police, GP, hospital doctor or by self-referral
- dedicated 24-hour helpline.

Role of the police officer

The police officer has an important role in the rape victim's experiences and decision to further pursue legal prosecution. At the time of the examination the trained woman police officer offers advice and information about the criminal justice process as well as taking the formal statement. In addition to the main role of the police officer of taking the detailed statement, the officer accompanies the complainant to the examination centre, ensuring that she takes a change of clothes with her.

Prior to the doctor taking a history of the assault the officer provides a summary of the allegation for the doctor. During the examination the officer not only chaperones the examining doctor but also assists in a discreet manner with the collection of the significant items of clothing and also ensures that each forensic sample is correctly labelled and sealed. The police officer assists with completion of the documentation, recording the time the examination commences and finishes and the time the blood alcohol sample is taken. The forensic samples are then sent to a central submissions unit for later dispatch of the appropriate samples to the scientific AIDS laboratory. The police officer is responsible for arranging the transport of the forensic specimens and will assist with the follow-up arrangements for the victim.

The severely injured patient

The medical needs of the victim must take priority over the need to achieve forensic samples and urgent medical advice should be sought where necessary, in an appropriately equipped setting, e.g. accident and emergency department. The reason for delay in undertaking the forensic examination should be carefully documented in the medical record. Where possible a police photographer (of the same gender) should be involved. A supply of examination kits may be available in the examination centre and in addition to using these kits at outreach facilities, they can be used to facilitate the examination of inpatient victims.

The incidence of major non-genital injuries may be as high as 5% of rape victims (Marchbanks 1990) and the majority of female victims (approximately 80%) will have some form of physical injury, although most will be of a minor nature (Bowyer & Dalton 1997).

The examining doctor

The examining doctor must be objective and non-judgemental and must avoid giving even the smallest cues of suspicion or disbelief which may heighten the victim's anxiety and emotional trauma (Dupré et al 1993) and cause a spiralling decline as her guilt and shame increase and her story is shaken.

A record of the initial examination and forensic specimens should be kept and this record should contain contemporary notes. Since the Northumbria Police Record of Medical Examinations was first used in 1983 there have been many alterations to the style and content to accommodate changes in certain elements of the examination and forensic techniques. Other centres have also devised protocols. In the late 1980s the US Department of Justice sponsored a programme to establish protocols for forensic and medical examinations of victims of sexual assault and subsequently states such as New Hampshire and Michigan have developed their own protocols based on this national model (Hockbaum 1987, Young et al 1992).

Medical details

Certain medical facts should be recorded, such as the last menstrual period (LMP), date and time of last coitus, previous pregnancies and outcome, present contraception, serious medical or psychiatric problems and current medication.

Account of the event

An account of the incident allows the doctor to adapt the standard forensic examination according to the circumstances of the assault, limited to the information necessary to treat any possible injuries and collect appropriate specimens for evidence. The complainant may be unable to recall the details of the assault, possibly due to the influence of alcohol/drugs at the time of the assault or subsequently. The use of drugs in 'date' or acquaintance rape is increasingly common with drugs such as flunitrazepam (Rohypnol) being used to 'spike' drinks. Drugs impair the recollection of events surrounding the sexual assault, making identification and prosecution of the assailant even more difficult. The victim may be naturally reticent, as in the elderly victim, or already suffering 'memory block' associated with the RR-PTSD. Hence it is safer practice to complete the full forensic sampling at this, usually the only opportunity afforded to the doctor to collect evidence. Specific questions can be asked to clarify the details of the assault.

Medical examination

The examination must be undertaken in a good light using an ancillary light for the genital examination. A sexual examination kit with all necessary equipment should be to hand. The medical record should contain a reference to any area that is omitted. A magnifying lens should be available for closer examination of any surface markings.

All injuries should be described and drawn with relevant measurements on the body chart. For complex injuries it is very important to consider photography.

Delay in reporting sexual assault

Delay in reporting of a sexual assault may affect the historical detail given by the victim, especially if she has begun to block the memory of the event. The examination findings may also be affected with alteration to the emotional state and healing of minor injuries. The forensic evidence may be severely limited.

Persistence of spermatozoa after sexual assault

The persistence of forensic evidence (e.g. spermatozoa in the vagina) is very variable.

- Vaginal intercourse – up to 10 days (Wilson 1982) or 7–10 days in the cervix
- On rectal swabs – up to 65 hours (Willott & Allard 1982)
- On anal swabs – up to 46 hours (Willott & Allard 1982)
- After oral intercourse – 12–14 hours (Willott & Crosse 1986)

There is considerable variation between individuals with respect to the probability of detecting spermatozoa at different times after intercourse and this should be taken into consideration when deciding on the appropriateness of samples and evaluating the results (Davies & Wilson 1974). It is important to note that motile sperm are only seen in those postmenopausal women who are examined within 6 hours of the rape (Ramin et al 1992).

Description of wounds

The doctor examining a complainant of sexual assault may experience difficulty with the nomenclature when describing wounds and may be daunted by the medicolegal significance of the lesions. Even more difficulty may be encountered when asked to give an opinion as to how they may have been caused.

The following recommended classification was formulated by Crane (1996).

Bruises

A bruise is caused by the application of blunt force to the skin that damages small blood vessels beneath the skin surface. The blood then spreads through the tissue spaces. Bruises resolve over a variable period of time. On the whole, blue and black bruises are indicative of recent trauma but estimating the age of a bruise is a risky undertaking and should be avoided at all costs especially if one is asked to do so in court.

Petechiae Pinhead-sized haemorrhages *within* the skin. Causes:

- mechanical trauma, with underlying clothing leaving imprint of the material's texture as petechiae
- sucking as in 'love-bites'

- congestion/mechanical asphyxiation on face, upper neck, conjunctiva as in childbirth and strangulation.

Purpura Larger haemorrhages *within* the skin, often seen in the elderly.

Haematoma Blood that collect as a mass beneath the skin.

Factors to remember about bruising

- Bruising may be delayed in its appearance
- May not reflect the size of object impacting with skin
- May not represent the point of impact due to tracking along tissue planes
- May not represent the severity of the blow due to age or frailty of tissues
- Can vary according to the site, e.g. underlying bone
- Can assist in interpretation of causation, e.g. finger-tip bruising on inner aspect of upper arms

Abrasions

Abrasions, also known as scratches or grazes, are injuries involving only the outer layers of skin – partial-thickness tears. The skin injury of an abrasion is at the site of the impact with injuring force. Abrasions are usually linear in nature but may be curved due to fingernails or a human bite.

Lacerations

Lacerations, also known as cuts or tears, occur when the injuring blunt force causes full-thickness splitting of the skin in a ragged way. They are often associated with bruising and there may be flaps of skin due to a shearing force being applied.

Incisions

Incisions are caused by sharp cutting weapons and are seen less commonly in the genital injuries of rape and sexual assault although the genitalia and breasts may be the target of the assailant wielding a knife or similar sharp weapon. The tissues are cleanly divided and the cut is long and less deep than a stab wound.

Stab wounds

A stab wound is a penetrating deep injury and with respect to transvaginal impalement, there is considerable risk of damage to extravaginal sites. Identification of possible extensive injury may be difficult and would require multidisciplinary involvement.

Absence of genital injury

Data about the genital injuries sustained by victims of sexual assault are derived only from women who choose to report the incident and so the results of studies reporting the presence or absence of injury must be interpreted with care due to this self-reporting bias.

The absence of genital injuries should not negate an allegation of sexual assault/rape but the presence of genital injury is thought to carry more weight in obtaining a successful conviction. In a retrospective view of case records of women from Northumbria Police area, only 22 out of 83 women had genital injuries (27%) but 68 out of 83 had some form of

Table 64.1   Assessment of injury

Type of injury	Site of injury	Likely mechanism	Alternative causes
Non-genital			
Reddening	Face, arms, back, etc.	Frictional Blunt force – slap	Dermatographia, irritant substances Response to fear, embarrassment
Bruising			
Petechiae	Neck, breasts	Sucking of love-bites (non-consensual)	Consensual love-bites
	Face, upper neck, conjunctiva	Strangulation	Straining as in childbirth
	Legs, arms, buttocks, trunk	Mechanical trauma often leaving petechial clothes pattern	Accidental, e.g. straps, blood disorders
	Roof of the mouth	Blunt force of penis	Sucking hard sweets
Bruises			
Fingertip bruises <2 cm in dia, usually >2 marks	Upper arms, legs, breasts	Blunt force of finger grip Associated with resistance	Non-sexual assault
	Neck	Manual strangulation	None
Medium sized (2–4 cm)	Inner thighs, inner aspect of knees	Assailant's knees/thumbs as blunt force to separate legs	Accidental – unlikely
	Mouth and lips	Blunt force of hand applied over face to keep victim quiet	None
Streaky, linear purple bruising	Neck, wrists, ankles	Application of a ligature	Accidental – watch strap, jewellery
>4 cm diameter, roughly oval	Face and trunk	Blunt force of a punch	Accidental fall onto protruding object, unlikely if multiple and same age
Any size or shape	Back, buttocks, arms, legs, elbows, knees	Being pushed onto hard surface or blunt, protruding object during struggle	Accidental; however, unlikely if multiple and of same age
Ovoid or elliptical pattern of small bruises	Neck, breasts, abdomen, arms, thighs	Full mouth bite	May be voluntary; alternative implement may be possible (shoe heel, etc.)
Pairs of similar bruises	Neck, shoulders, cheeks, breasts	Pinch marks	Accidental pinching unlikely
Abrasions			
Linear parallel abrasions	Back, arms, shoulders, trunk	Fingernails dragged over skin with force or movement away from grip by victim	Possible during consensual sexual activity; self-inflicted (note direction of scratches), attempt by victim to tear away hands or ligature at strangulation
Multiple scratches running in different planes	Back, buttocks, back of legs	Being pulled through bushes	Accidental unlikely
Pattern of small curved abrasions	Neck	Manual strangulation – fingernail marks	None
Ovoid or elliptical pattern of small abrasions	Neck, breasts, abdomen	Full mouth bite	May be voluntary; fall against door knob may be possible
Streaky abrasions (+associated bruising)	Neck, wrists, ankles	Application of a ligature	Accidental – watch strap, jewellery
Genital			
Reddening	Posterior fourchette, labia minora	Friction – penile or digital Penetration of unlubricated genitalia	Mild vulvovaginitis, consensual sexual activity, non-specific finding
Bruising	Vulva, clitoris, hymen, fourchette, perineum, mons pubis	Violent attempts at digital penetration or forceful insertion of object	Bleeding disorder, associated with other atypical bruises Very unlikely in consensual sexual activity, due to pain
Abrasions	Posterior fourchette, labia minora, introitus, hymen	Violent attempts at penile penetration, violent insertion of objects or fingers	Childbirth Extremely unlikely in consensual sexual activity, due to pain except possibly in postmenopausal atrophy

Table 64.1 *(Continued)*

Type of injury	Site of injury	Likely mechanism	Alternative causes
	Anal	Violent attempts at penile penetration, violent insertion of object or fingers	Childbirth, painful passage of very large, hard stool, consensual activity unlikely
	Rectal mucosa	Violent insertion of object or fingers	Consensual activity unlikely
Lacerations	Posterior fourchette, hymen, perineum	Violent attempts at penile penetration, violent insertion of objects or fingers	Childbirth
	Vagina	Violent insertion of foreign body	Penile impact post menopausally, postoperatively and post radiation
	Anal (fissure)	Stretching due to forceful insertion of object or fingers	Childbirth, penile impact postmenopausally or post operatively
	Rectal with extension, perforation and sphincteric injury	Violent insertion of foreign body Fist fornication	None
Incisions	Vagina, with impalement causing extravaginal injury	Sharp cutting weapon	None

physical injury (Bowyer & Dalton 1997). It was concluded that the 'absence of genital injury should not be used as pivotal evidence by the police or Crown Prosecution Service'. Similar incidence of genital injury was reported in a study of 440 cases of reported sexual assault where 16% of all the victims had visible genital injury (Cartwright et al 1986). By the same token, absence of genital injury in no way implies consent by the victim nor the absence of vaginal penetration by the assailant (Cartwright et al 1986).

Reasons for absence of genital injury may include:

- verbal threats to victim, intimidation and threats that failure to comply with assailant's demands will result in physical injury/death to herself or another person, e.g. child. Coercion may play a significant role in marital rape
- force used is insufficient to produce an injury (especially in sexually active parous women)
- Bruises may not become apparent for 48 hours
- delay in reporting assault, allowing healing of lesions
- use of lubricant at time of rape.

A common tactic of the barrister defending a suspect in a rape trial is not to deny that sexual intercourse between their client and the complainant took place but rather to claim that she consented to the encounter (Cartwright et al 1986). Continuing with this approach, the defending barrister may point out to the examining gynaecologist and jury that there are no injuries to the victim's genitalia and he may ask the doctor how a victim of an alleged rape could escape injury unless, of course, she actually consented to intercourse. Cartwright found that 75 victims in a review of 440 cases of reported rape showed objective evidence of non-compliance (injuries to non-genital sites) and vaginal penetration (sperm in the vagina) and only 28% of these women had sustained genital injury. Thus the absence of genital injury does not imply consent by the victim.

Forensic sampling

The evidence collected during the examination is used to help prove three points:

- the occurrence of sexual contact
- the lack of consent on the part of the victim
- the identity of the assailant.

Postexamination follow-up

There are many factors that may negatively influence a rape victim's use of the follow-up services, such as avoidance behaviour, denial and disorganization. Follow-up may genuinely not be required or her low socioeconomic status may be a barrier to traditional follow-up.

At best, a follow-up rate of 31% was achieved in a sexual assault follow-up evaluation clinic, despite efforts to encourage female victims to use the clinic (Holmes et al 1998). Our ability to reduce the occurrence of the long-term effects of sexual assault is limited by the low rates of reporting and lack of focused follow-up for those who do report their assault. However, the doctor can significantly enhance the uptake of counselling in the aftermath of an assault.

- Consider antibiotic prophylaxis against gonorrhoea and chlamydia if victim unlikely to attend for follow-up
- Genitourinary medicine (GUM) clinic referral:
  - HIV testing and hepatitis screening
  - examination at 1–3 days.

Follow-up at 7–14 days:

- counsellor referral 7–14 days
- re-examination occasionally indicated if:
  - genital injuries not visible
  - examination shortly after incident
- Tenderness on examination
- Emergency contraception
- Hormonal up to 72 hours after the incident (levonorgestrel)
- IUCD if > 72 hours have already elapsed
- Statement preparation and submission to officer in charge
- GP letter
- Photography – consent should be sought and documented on the victim consent form
- Take-home literature

Photographs of injuries, especially complex skin trauma, should be an adjunct to the description to the findings. It has been claimed that a carefully observed, well-documented description of any injury or group of injuries is worth many photographs (Bunting 1996). Others claim that a photograph can be worth a thousand words if the assailant is claiming consent and the attorney has pictures of the victim with a black eye or worse (Ledray 1993).

Rape-related pregnancy

In the USA unintended pregnancy has been identified as a national epidemic and substantial resources have been dedicated to addressing this problem. To date, rape-related pregnancy has not been identified as a contributing factor in the unintended pregnancy rate. The risk of rape-related pregnancy has been estimated at approximately 5% of rape victims of reproductive age in the USA (Holmes et al 1996) where there are an estimated 32101 pregnancies a year resulting from rape. In Mexico the pregnancy rate was estimated as 10% (Martinez et al 1999). Of the 34 known cases of rape-related pregnancy in Holmes's study, the majority occurred among adolescents and resulted from assault by a known, often related perpetrator.

In the USA, DNA typing has significantly altered the conviction rate but sometimes it is unclear from a victim's history if a pregnancy has been achieved by the assailant or by a consensual partner. Resolution of pregnancy parentage in such circumstances may allow a couple to make an informed decision regarding continuation of the pregnancy. Blood can be taken from the woman and her consensual partner and cultured amniotic or chorion villus cells can be submitted for fetal genetic analysis (Hammond et al 1995).

Paternity testing can thus positively exclude an alleged father or provide a high likelihood of paternity.

Should a victim proceed with termination of a presumed rape-related pregnancy, abortion material can be submitted for genotyping which can be undertaken immediately or the tissues stored for subsequent analysis.

Chorion villus sampling (CVS) provides an uncontaminated source of fetal tissue for genotyping, compared with surgical abortion material which consists of ruptured tissue of fetal and maternal origin. Undertaking a CVS in such fraught circumstances may increase the victim's trauma but one could consider CVS under general anaesthetic immediately prior to the surgical termination of pregnancy. Medical termination of pregnancy might offer an alternative, less contaminated source of fetal material.

Sexually transmitted diseases following sexual assault

The frequency of sexually transmitted diseases (STD) in victims of sexual assault is difficult to estimate due to the low reporting and follow-up of victims. In Mexico the frequency of STD was 20% amongst 213 patients (Martinez et al 1999). With respect to HIV infection, no true seroconversion for HIV was found in 108 victims who agreed to HIV testing at follow-up (Holmes et al 1998).

Patterns of injury in postmenopausal women

One of the factors influencing the type of injury sustained is the victim's age. Postmenopausal women represent only a small percentage of the number reporting sexual assault – 2.2% in Dallas County between 1986 and 1991 (Ramin et al 1992) – while 3.3 per cent of female victims of sexual assault referrals to the REACH Project are aged 50 years or over.

There is no significant difference in the relative proportion of women experiencing non-genital injuries; trauma in general occurred as frequently in the older woman (67%) as in the younger group. Genital trauma is more common – 43% in the postmenopausal group compared with 18% in younger women. Almost one in five older women had genital lacerations. Other authors have also reported an increased frequency of genital injuries in the older victim of sexual assault (Cartwright & Moore 1989).

The increased genital trauma rate is presumably due to postmenopausal atrophy causing increased genital tissue susceptibility.

The differences between stranger and acquaintance rape

Victims of acquaintance rape are known to be less likely to report the attack to the police. A degree of social interaction is more likely to have occurred immediately prior to an acquaintance assault than where a stranger is involved. Verbal aggression is more likely in acquaintance assault together with the use of threatening behaviour such as warning of the consequences to herself or her family of reporting the attack. It has been found that 95% of acquaintance rapists interact with their victims after the rape, with 43% trying conciliatory, non-threatening behaviour such as falling asleep beside the victim or even helping her to get dressed!

In stranger rape the encounter is more likely to have occurred outdoors or in a vehicle (a feature of the predatory behaviour of the rapist) and the assailant is more likely to display or use a weapon. Stranger rapists are less likely to interact with their victim after the sexual part of the assault than acquaintance rapists, with 63% of stranger rapists abandoning their victims immediately (Bownes et al 1991). Physical resistance is more strongly related to injury when the rapist is a stranger than when the rapist is known to the victim (Ruback & Ivie 1988).

The influence of age of the victim and the injuries sustained

Adolescent victims

A pre-existing relationship between a victim and the assailant may explain other elements that distinguish an adolescent victim from her adult counterpart, with 19% of adolescents reporting a previous sexual assault (Muram et al 1995). Weapons and physical force are used less frequently where adolescent victims are involved but alcohol and drug use is prevalent in adolescent victims (47% of cases). There are conflicting opinions about the frequency of physical, non-genital injuries in adolescents versus older victims of sexual assault. The frequency of extra-genital trauma may be increased in younger victims who are more likely to sustain injuries to the head and neck together with more scratches and lacerations.

Adult victims

With respect to adult victims, the perpetrator is more likely to be a stranger than in cases of adolescent assault; also adult victims are more likely to be abducted than adolescent victims. Weapons, especially firearms, are more often used in adult victims to carry out the victim's capture. Older victims tend to live alone, are often robbed and are more likely to raped by a stranger (Tyra 1993).

Advanced techniques of examination

Ultraviolet light

Several studies have shown that ultraviolet light induced fluorescence (UVI) may be used as a part of forensic medical examinations (Lynnerup & Hjalgrim 1995, Stoilovic 1991, West et al 1992). Disturbance within the skin of the various components, including haemoglobin, melanin, fibroproteins, collagen and fatty tissues, results in changes in fluorescence so that traumatized skin illuminated with UV light in a dark room fluoresces (Barsley et al 1990, David et al 1994). Body fluids such as semen and saliva also fluoresce. UVI can be used to detect stains at crime scenes and on items of clothing or bedding but further studies are required to evaluate whether or not it is a valuable tool in finding faint signs of skin trauma or locating stains, thus enabling retrieval of material for forensic analysis.

Colposcopic examination of the genitalia

The role of the colposcope has yet to be established in the United Kingdom but descriptive studies from the United States have revealed that 87% of women examined within 48 hours of sexual assault had positive findings (Slaughter & Brown 1992). It was felt that the technique is so simple, quick and efficacious that it should be included in rape examination protocols. A later study compared colposcopic examination undertaken within 24 hours of penile penetration during sexual assault with consensual sexual intercourse. This revealed that 89% of the 142 women who experienced non-consensual sex had genital injuries whereas only 11% of 75 women who had voluntary sexual intercourse had genital colposcopic findings (Slaughter et al 1997).

The Foley catheter technique in adolescent girls

A 12- or 14-gauge Foley bladder catheter with a 5–10 ml balloon can be used to evaluate the margins of the hymen in adolescents (Starling & Jenny 1997). The moistened tip of the catheter is introduced into the vaginal canal and the balloon inflated. The examiner then applies gentle traction until the balloon reaches the hymenal margins and so the redundant folds attenuate, providing a clear view of the hymenal folds. Starling does not recommend the technique on prepubertal girls and suggests that the speculum examination precede the catheter test.

Toluidine blue dye testing

Prior to insertion of a speculum or examining finger, a 1% aqueous solution of toluidine blue can be applied to the posterior fourchette and perineum using cotton tip applicators (Lauber & Souma 1982). After drying for a few seconds the excess dye is removed either by spraying with 1% acetic acid or by gently wiping with a cotton ball moistened with lubricating gel. In this way toluidine blue can help to detect lacerations in the genital area.

Lauber reported an increase in the detection rate of posterior fourchette lacerations from 16% to 40% in adult rape victims. However, a positive toluidine blue test is supportive but not conclusive evidence of sexual assault. As the toluidine blue is applied prior to the speculum examination and thus the collection of forensic evidence, there were concerns that it may have adverse effects on the recovery of material for DNA analysis. However, the quantity and quality of the extractable DNA obtained after application of toluidine blue were comparable with those from uncontaminated swabs (Hochmeister et al 1997).

COURT PROCEEDINGS

Medical witness statement

The minimum requirement for a doctor's statement is in the form of a 'witness to the fact' document providing a basic interpretation of the findings only. It is a wise practice to complete a statement as soon as possible after the examination and include an interpretation and opinion at the end of the statement either using lay terms where possible or including a glossary of the medical terminology.

Aims of the statement
- Documentation of findings – normal/abnormal
- Causation of injuries
- Mechanisms leading to injury
- Degree of force required to produce the injury
- Other possible causes for findings
- Exclude unlikely causes
- Consistency of findings
- Opinion – using a sliding scale to describe the degree of certainty

The victim in court

The victim may be called to give evidence as a witness at a Crown Court if the attacker pleads not guilty. In addition to the support of the police officers and counsellors involved, they can also seek the support of the Crown Court Witness Service. Arrangements can be made for the complainant to visit the court before the trial and information on police and court procedure, liaison with other organizations on behalf of the victim and assistance in application for compensation from the Criminal Injuries Compensation Board (CICB) can all be provided.

Doctor in court

The examining doctor will be expected to read through the notes carefully before attending court and may be called to a pre-trial discussion with solicitors, Crown Prosecution Service (CPS) and counsel for the prosecution. The defence usually ask for an independent medical expert report and they will have access to copy statements from the complainant, the examining doctor and the defendant and even transcripts of interviews; they may also request the contemporaneous medical notes. It is important that the examining doctor has access to the defence medical expert's reports before the trial and be able to discuss this opinion with counsel.

Examination-in-chief

The examining doctor may be called to court as a professional witness. Addressing the jury, the doctor will be asked by the counsel for the prosecution (barrister) to describe what was found at the time of the examination. The doctor is usually asked to give an opinion as to the possible causation for the findings.

Cross-examination

Counsel for the defence then conducts the cross-examination of the professional witness.

Youth Justice and Criminal Evidence Act 1999

The Youth Justice and Criminal Evidence Act 1999 will significantly alter the court proceedings for rape and sexual assault cases. However, there may prove to be difficulties in implementation of certain sections of the Act, especially with respect to the restrictions placed on questioning the complainant.

Chapter I deals with the eligibility for and the granting of 'special measures' direction in the case of vulnerable witnesses. Children under 17 at the time of the hearing are automatically eligible and victims of sexual offences will be eligible for special measures such as screens, live TV links and video recording of evidence.

Chapter II creates protection for certain witnesses, such as a complainant in a sexual offence case, by prohibiting an unrepresented defendant from cross-examining the witness in person.

Chapter III covers the protection of such complainants in circumstances in which the evidence can be led or questions asked about the complainant's previous sexual behaviour.

CONCLUSION

There is growing international concern about the low conviction rate for rape. The criminal justice systems in the USA and UK have introduced initiatives in an attempt to improve the response to rape cases. It is important to recognize that there is need for improvement in the clinical/forensic management of sexual assault cases including:

- improved levels of support for complainants at all stages
- improved levels of communication between the forensic physician, GP, counsellors, police, CPS and the complainant
- continuing improvements in evidence gathering
- the establishment of training programmes and continuing multidisciplinary education for all concerned in the care of rape victims.

In addition, it is very important that there is rapid implementation of the new laws which aim to protect the vulnerable

witnesses in rape trials and that research programmes are established to gain a better understanding of why complainants withdraw their allegation or, indeed, why there is a high rate of charge reduction.

KEY POINTS

1. There may be many reasons for failure to report sexual assault.
2. Consent to forensic medical examination differs from the standard consent forms and must accommodate details about disclosure of evidence.
3. The estimation of the age of a bruise should be avoided.
4. The absence of genital injury does not imply consent by the victim.
5. Following the examination the victim should be offered appropriate medical advice, counselling and follow-up.
6. When interpreting the findings, the professional witness should comment upon whether the appearances are normal or abnormal and describe their degree of certainty about the likely cause of any injuries.

REFERENCES

Adams J, Harper K, Knudson S, Revilla J 1994 Examination findings in legally confirmed child sexual abuse – it's normal to be normal. Paediatrics 4(3):310–317

Bang L 1993 Rape victims – assaults, injuries and treatment at a medical rape trauma service at Oslo Emergency Hospital. Scandinavian Journal of Primary Health Care 11:15–20

Banyard VL 1997 The impact of childhood sexual abuse and family functioning on four dimensions of women's later parenting. Child Abuse and Neglect 21(11):1095–1107

Barsley RE, West MH, Frair J 1990 Forensic photography, ultraviolet imaging of wounds on skin. American Journal of Medicine and Pathology 11(4):300–308

Bell TA, Stamm WE, Kuo CC et al 1986 Chronic chlamydia trachomatis infections in infants. In: Onel D, Ridgeway G, Schacter J et al (eds) Chlamydial infections. Cambridge University Press, Cambridge

Berensen A, Clarke M, Werimann C et al A case control study of anatomic changes resulting from sexual abuse. American Journal of Obstetrics and Gynecology 182(4):820–834

Bownes IT, O'Gorman EC, Sayers A 1991 Rape – a comparison of stranger and acquaintance assaults. Medical Science and Law 31(2):102–109

Bowyer L, Dalton ME 1997 Female victims of rape and genital findings. British Journal of Obstetrics and Gynaecology 104:617–620

Bunting R 1996 Clinical examination in the police context. In: McLay WDS (ed) Clinical forensic medicine. Greenwich Medical Media, London, pp 59–73

Cartwright PS, Moore RA 1989 The elderly victim of rape. South African Medical Journal 82:988–989

Cartwright PS, Moore RA, Anderson JR, Brown DH 1986 Genital injury and implied consent to alleged rape. Journal of Reproductive Medicine 31(11):1043–1044

Crane J 1996 Injury. In: McLay WDS (ed) Clinical forensic medicine. Greenwich Medical Media, London, pp 143–162

Craven SA 1996 Assessment of alleged rape victims – an unrewarding exercise. South African Medical Journal 86(3):237–238

David TJ, Sobel DDS, Sobel MN 1994 Recapturing a five month old bite mark by means of reflective ultraviolet photography. Journal for Science 39(6):1560–1567

Davies A, Wilson E 1974 The persistence of seminal constituents in the human vagina. Forensic Science 3:45–55

De Jong AR 1986 Sexually transmitted disease in sexually abused children. Sexually Transmitted Disease 13:123–126

Department of Health, British Medical Association and Conference of Medical Colleges 1994 Child Protection: Medical Responsibilities. Guidance for Doctors Working with Child Protection Agencies. Addendum to 'Working Together – Under the Children Act 1989', HMSO

Dupré AR, Hampton HL, Morrison H, Meeks GR 1993 Sexual assault. Obstetrical and Gynaecological Survey 48(9):640–648

Evans SJ, Woods ER, Alfred EN, Gracia E 1994 Hymenal findings in adolescent women: impact of tampon use and consensual sexual activity. Journal of Paediatrics 125(1):153–160

Ferguson D, Horwood LJ, Lynskey MT 1997 Childhood sexual abuse, adolescent sexual behaviours and sexual revictimisation. Child Abuse and Neglect 21(8):789–803

Finklehor DA et al 1986 A sourcebook on child sexual abuse. Sage Publications, London

Gardner J 1992 Descriptive study of genital variation in healthy non-abused premenarchal girls. Journal of Paediatrics 120(2):251–256

General Medical Council 2000a Section 1 – Patients' right to confidentiality. In: Confidentiality: protecting and providing information. General Medical Council, London, p 4

General Medical Council 2000b Section 5 – Putting the principles into practice. In: Confidentiality: protecting and providing information. General Medical Council, London, pp 14–15

General Medical Council 2000c Section 38 – Children and other patients who may lack competence to give consent. In: Confidentiality: protecting and providing information. General Medical Council, London, p 17

Hammond HA, Redman JB, Caskey CT 1995 In-utero paternity testing following alleged sexual assault. A comparison of DNA-based methods. Journal of the American Medical Association 273(22):1774–1777

Hampton HL 1995 Care of the woman who has been raped. New England Journal of Medicine 332(4):234–237

Herman-Giddens ME, Gutman LT, Berson N and the Duke Child Protection Team 1988 Association of co-existing vaginal infections in female children with genital warts. Sexually Transmitted Diseases 15:63–67

Hochmeister MN, Whelan M, Borer UV et al 1997 Effects of toluidine blue and destaining reagents used in sexual assault examinations on the ability to obtain DNA profiles from postcoital vaginal swabs. Journal of Forensic Science 42(2):316–319

Hockbaum SR 1987 The evaluation and treatment of the sexually assaulted patient. Emergency Medicine Clinics of North America 5(3):601–622

Holmes MM, Resnick HS, Kilpatrick DG, Best CL 1996 Rape-related pregnancy: estimates and descriptive characteristics from a national sample of women. American Journal of Obstetrics and Gynecology 175(2):320–325

Holmes MM, Resnick HS, Frampton D 1998 Follow-up of sexual assault victims. American Journal of Obstetrics and Gynecology 179:336–342

Home Office, Department of Health, Department of Education and Science and Welsh Office 1991 Working together under the Children Act 1989. A Guide to Arrangements for Inter-Agency Co-operation for the Protection of Children from Abuse.

Home Office 2000 Statistical bulletin, notifiable offences. Research and Statistics Department. Home Office, Croydon, pp 20–22

Lauber AA, Souma ML 1982 Use of toluidine blue for documentation of traumatic intercourse. Obstetrics and Gynecology 60:622–648

Ledray L 1993 Sexual assault nurse clinician: an emerging area of nursing experience. AWHONN's Clinical Issues 4(2):180–190

Lynnerup N, Hjalgrim H 1995 Routine use of ultraviolet light in medico-legal examinations to evaluate stains and skin trauma. Medical Science Law 35(2):165–168

Marchbanks PA, Lui KJ, Mercy JA 1990 Risk of injury from resisting rape. American Journal of Epidemiology 132:540–549

Martinez AH, Villanueva LA, Torres C, Garcia LE 1999 Sexual aggression in adolescents. Epidemiologic study. Ginecologia y Obstetricia de Mexico 67:449–453

Miller HL, Miller CE, Kenny L, Clark JW 1998 Issues in statutory rape law enforcement: the views of district attorneys in Kansas. Family Planning Perspectives 30(4):177–181

Miller C, Miller HL, Kenny L, Tasheff J 1999 Issues in balancing teenage clients' confidentiality and reporting among Kansas Title X clinic staff. Public Health Nursing 16(5):329–362

Mullen PE, Martin JL, Anderson JC, Romans SE, Herbison GP 1993 Childhood sexual abuse and mental health in adult life. British Journal of Psychiatry 163:721–732

Muram D, Hostetler BR, Jones CE, Speck PM 1995 Adolescent victims of sexual assault. Journal of Adolescent Health 17(6):372–375

National Society for the Prevention of Cruelty to Children 2000 Survey finds hidden victims of child abuse. NSPCC, London

Ramin SM, Satin AJ, Stone IC, Wendel GD 1992 Sexual assault in postmenopausal women. Obstetrics and Gynecology 80:860–864

Royal College of Physicians of London 1997 Physical signs of sexual abuse in children, 2nd edn. RCP, London

Ruback RB, Ivie DL 1988 Prior relationship, resistance and injury in rapes: an analysis of crisis center records. Violence and Victims 3(2):99–111

San Lazaro C 1995 Making paediatric assessments in sexual abuse a therapeutic experience. Archives of Disease in Childhood 73:174–176

Sarmer DB, Durlak JA 1996 Childhood sexual abuse as a predictor of adult female sexual dysfunction: a study of couples seeking sex therapy. Child Abuse and Neglect 20(10):963–972

Schecter MD, Roberge L 1976 Sexual exploitation. In: Helfer RE, Kempe CH (Eds) Child abuse and neglect: the family and the community. Ballinger, Cambridge, MA

Slaughter L, Brown CRV 1992 Colposcopy to establish physical findings in rape victims. American Journal of Obstetrics and Gynecology 166:83–86

Slaughter L, Brown CRV, Crowley S, Peck P 1997 Patterns of genital injury in female sexual assault victims. American Journal of Obstetrics and Gynecology 176:609–616

Starling SP, Jenny C 1997 Forensic examination of adolescent female genitalia: the Foley catheter technique. Archives of Pediatric and Adolescent Medicine 151:102–103

Steele AM, San Lazaro C 1994 Transhymenal cultures for sexually transmissible organisms. Archives of Disease in Childhood 71(5):423–427

Stoilovic M 1991 Detection of semen and blood staining using polight as a light source. Science International 51:289–296

Tyra PA 1993 Older women: victims of rape. Journal of Gerontology Nursing 19(5):7–12

Warrington S, San Lazaro C 1996 Lichen sclerosus et atrophicus and sexual abuse. Archives of Disease in Childhood 75:512–516

West MH, Barsley RE, Hall JE, Hayne S, Cimrancic M 1992 The detection and documentation of trace wound patterns by use of an alternative light source. Journal of Forensic Science 37(6):1480–1488

Willott GM, Allard JE 1982 Spermatozoa – their persistence after sexual intercourse. Forensic Science International 19:135–154

Willott GM, Crosse MM 1986 The detection of spermatozoa in the mouth. Journal of the Forensic Science Society 26:125–128

Wilson EM 1982 A comparison of the persistence of seminal constituents in the human vagina and cervix. Police Surgeon 22:44–45

Young W, Bracken A, Goddard M, Matteson S 1992 The New Hampshire Sexual Assault Medical Examination Protocol Project Committee. Sexual assault: review of a national model protocol for forensic and medical evaluation. Obstetrics and Gynecology 80:879–883

65

Violence against women

Mary Hepburn

BACKGROUND

Violence against women is prevalent worldwide and is most commonly inflicted by men. Such violence takes many forms in different settings, sometimes legally sanctioned by the state and/or morally sanctioned by the society within which it occurs. However, while women can be at risk in many settings the most common form of violence against women is domestic violence or abuse inflicted by the woman's partner or ex-partner and the violence usually takes place in the home.

While the term 'domestic violence' could imply violence or abuse from either partner in a heterosexual or homosexual relationship, a United Nations report in 1995 recognized that the most common manifestation is violence against women by male partners (United Nations 1975). In the 1992 British Crime Survey (Mayhew et al 1993) domestic violence constituted the single largest category of assaults, with 80% directed against women. In the United States it is estimated that 95% of battered partners are women (Jones 1997). The United Nations report highlighted the range of types of physical abuse suffered worldwide by women at the hands of their partners, including battering, marital rape, dowry violence, domestic murder, forced pregnancy, abortion and sterilization and forced prostitution. During pregnancy violence may also cause miscarriage or fetal injury and/or death. Women also experience non-physical abuse in the form of psychological, emotional and economic abuse.

Domestic violence or abuse is difficult to define but a definition such as 'the psychological, emotional and economic as well as physical and sexual abuse of women by male partners or ex partners' (SNAP 1997) indicates the range of ways and circumstances in which women can be abused by their partners. Thus while society's perception is that the greatest risk of violence comes from strangers outside the home, statistics confirm that for women this is not the case. Nevertheless, in addition to beating of a wife by her husband, violence against women includes other types of abuse such as abortion of female fetuses, female genital mutilation, forced prostitution by non-partners, rape (including rape and sexual violence as a war strategy) and murder. Women are also at risk of violence or abuse from any relationship or interaction with men in which sex is a factor; thus while forced prostitution by a partner is itself a form of partner violence women working as prostitutes, whether for a partner, another man or independently, are also at risk of violence from their clients.

Violence against women is important to those providing reproductive healthcare. Women experiencing or at risk of violence are particularly vulnerable during pregnancy. Domestic violence often starts or escalates during pregnancy and since the circumstances that drive a woman to commercial sex do not change because she has become pregnant, prostitution continues throughout pregnancy. Violence during pregnancy has obvious implications for the health of both mother and baby and consequently relevance for those providing maternity care (although recognition of this has been slow to develop). The relevance of violence to non-pregnant women is often viewed only in terms of rape. However, violence can cause or affect other gynaecological conditions as well as having implications for other types of reproductive healthcare. It is therefore important to recognize that the entire spectrum of violence against women is of relevance to all aspects of reproductive healthcare.

PREVALENCE

The true prevalence of violence against women is difficult to determine. This is largely because of underidentification but also because prevalence will depend on the definition of violence adopted. Studies in many countries have produced a range of estimates of prevalence for various categories of domestic violence and/or abuse. While the figures vary according to the type of abuse recorded, all are likely to be underestimates. In the USA estimates ranged between 2 000 000 (United Nations 1995) and 4 000 000 battered women with 2 000 women murdered each year (30% of female homicides) in association with battering (Jones 1997). In a Canadian survey of 12 300 women, 29% reported having experienced violence from a current or previous marital partner since the age of 16 (Johnson & Sacco 1995). In the UK the Home Affairs Select Committee Report on Domestic Violence (1993) concluded that domestic violence is 'common'. While the 1992 British Crime Survey (Mayhew et al 1993) found that 11% of women reported physical violence in their relationships, a 1993 crime survey in Islington, London (Mooney 1994) found that one in four women reported a lifetime experience of domestic violence. In a study of 930 women in San Francisco 12% reported rape by their husbands (Russell 1982) while in a UK study of 1000 women, one in four reported having experienced marital rape. The prevalence of violence to prostitutes from both clients and pimps (whether or not the latter is the regular sexual partner) is also difficult to assess. Nevertheless, its occurrence is well recognized by those who work with prostitutes although not necessarily by the criminal justice system whose response has often been inappropriate (Kennedy 1993).

THE ABUSER, THE ABUSED AND PATTERNS OF ABUSE

Many of the forms of violence described above occur in the UK. It is widely believed that such violence is largely confined to the lower social classes but this is a misconception. Domestic abuse occurs across the social spectrum and is inflicted by men who are not necessarily mentally ill but who have a range of personality defects (Mezey 1997). Various factors may co-exist with violence either as cause or effect. While abuse occurs throughout society, socioeconomic deprivation, unemployment and lack of education are cited as precipitating and perpetuating factors (Kennedy & Dutton 1989). Whatever the precise relationship, women from backgrounds of socioeconomic deprivation may have fewer resources and fewer options for dealing with the abuse.

Problem drug and alcohol use are often thought to be linked to abuse and are often offered as an excuse or justification. While men with substance misuse problems may be more likely to abuse their partners, this may not be because they are intoxicated and they may do so while sober. The 1996 British Crime Survey showed that intoxication of the perpetrator with alcohol or drugs was less common in the case of domestic violence than in stranger and acquaintance violence (Mirrlees-Black et al 1996). Additionally abusive men may cite substance misuse by the partner as the cause or justification for their abusive behaviour. While there is no evidence to support this, it is true that women suffering abuse may develop drug and/or alcohol problems as a consequence of the abuse (Plichta 1992, Stark & Flitcraft 1991).

Women working as prostitutes experience poverty and many have drug or alcohol problems. Many such women will have a history of abuse including sexual abuse by a family member, partner or other person. Their partner may also have problem substance use financed by the prostitution. The more chaotic the woman's lifestyle, the greater her financial need, the less she is paid, the more clients she has to service to raise the necessary money, the more dangerous the circumstances in which she must work and the greater her exposure to the risk of violence. However, while associations with various factors do exist and some groups of women are consequently at increased risk of violence it is important to remember that these factors are not necessarily obvious and, moreover, there is no typical abuser and no typical abused woman.

REPRODUCTIVE HEALTH CONSEQUENCES

Women who experience violence are more likely to suffer a number of consequences relevant to reproductive health services. Violence often begins or escalates during pregnancy (Bohn 1990, Hillard 1995). During pregnancy the injury sites include breasts and abdomen with consequent risk of injury to the fetus, including miscarriage, premature delivery and fetal death (Mezey & Bewley 1997). Women who have experienced violence are more likely to have suffered miscarriage (Stark & Flitcraft 1996). Pregnancy, genital tract infections and genital tract injury are possible consequences of sexual violence while other persistent gynaecological problems, especially abdominal pain, may be the presentation of abuse. Such women may find it difficult to undergo pelvic examination.

Obviously in all of these situations the converse does not apply and not all women with such problems or difficulties have been abused. Equally many women who have been abused demonstrate no obvious problems or stigmata which might indicate a history of abuse.

PRESENTATION

Women may present because of violence in a number of ways. They may specifically report physical violence, including rape (see Chapter 64), or may present for treatment of physical injuries sustained (with or without admission of the circumstances), in which case the setting is most commonly the accident and emergency department or the general practitioner's surgery. Injuries sustained include bruises, cuts, fractured bones and internal injuries (Dobash & Dobash 1980). In pregnancy injuries include maternal rupture of the uterus, spleen or liver, placental abruption, premature spontaneous rupture of the membranes, miscarriage and fetal death (James-Hanman & Lang 1994). Abused women may present later with psychological problems such as anxiety, depression (including suicide attempts) and drug or alcohol problems (Hillard 1985, Stark et al 1979). They may present to reproductive health services, including obstetric and gynaecology departments, in various ways. Immediate problems prompting attendance include obstetric complications and injuries, including genital tract injuries. Women may present with clinical problems secondary to the violence such as possible genital tract infection, the need for emergency contraception or subsequently with a pregnancy. Many women only present later with chronic gynaecological problems such as chronic pelvic pain.

Violence, domestic or otherwise, may therefore be highly relevant to women's attendance at obstetric and/or gynaecology services. However, irrespective of the immediacy or directness of the association and no matter how obvious the markers, the possibility will not necessarily be recognized. Moreover, women who present in these ways rather than with a specific complaint of violence and/or rape, whether or not the perpetrator is the partner, are unlikely to admit the abusive circumstances unless asked directly. Violence and/or abuse may therefore not be identified unless healthcare workers ask; since in such situations the occurrence of abuse is often not suspected, routine direct enquiry will be necessary for effective identification and management of this problem.

IDENTIFICATION

Violence against women is often not identified within healthcare services because women may not volunteer the information but also are often not asked about it. In one study of 290 pregnant women in which a total of 23% reported battering past or present, none had been questioned about violence by any of the healthcare providers (Helton et al 1987). Many women do not want to involve authorities such as police or law courts and the authorities may not consider the problem within their remit – and indeed, may not even consider it a problem at all. In the UK until 1829, a man had a right to 'chastise' his wife provided he used a stick 'no thicker than his thumb'. The possible existence of rape within marriage was only recognized in Scotland in 1989 and in England and Wales in 1991. Since commercial sex is widely viewed as voluntary, with the women morally responsible, violence against prostitutes is often considered an unavoidable risk of this activity that does not justify legal pursuit. Even when the violence extends to murder this is seen as different from murder of a 'respectable' woman (Kennedy 1993).

Women who experience violence from a partner often feel ashamed. They also often feel they are at least partly to blame and must in some way have deserved the abuse. They are also afraid that if they disclose the abuse to a third party their partner will find out and they will suffer even more violence. Similarly, women working as prostitutes are also often ashamed of their involvement in prostitution and do not want to admit it. While not necessarily believing they deserve violence, they may feel their activities invite it and they therefore bear some responsibility. Whatever their feelings, however, most prostitutes believe a report of violence would not be sympathetically received by the relevant services, would not lead to an effective response and would therefore be pointless. Similarly, many women suffering partner violence do not expect a sympathetic or helpful response from services. Nevertheless, evidence shows that despite their reluctance to raise the subject and report the violence, and despite the inadequacy of responses, women who suffer violence or abuse want to be asked about it and to be given an opportunity to disclose it. In one American primary care survey 75% of women favoured routine enquiry about physical abuse and 97% of female and male respondents said they would answer truthfully if asked directly but only 7% said they had ever been asked (Friedman et al 1992).

There are various reasons why healthcare workers do not ask about violence (Sugg & Inui 1992). They may be unaware of the possibility of abuse or think it is rare; they may not perceive violence, domestic or otherwise, as their responsibility; or they may be unwilling to ask either because they feel they lack the necessary skills, because they fear they may cause offence or because they are afraid of broaching a problem they

would not have the time or the knowledge to deal with. In many areas there are also insufficient or inadequately resourced support services to which women could be offered referral. The advice given is often limited to a recommendation to leave the batterer and frustration is expressed when women do not follow this advice. Consequently many healthcare workers feel unhappy about asking about abuse and would do so only if there were obvious evidence of abuse. Any injury might be expected to raise suspicion but in particular injuries at various sites, of different ages and for which no good explanation is offered should indicate possible abuse. However, even in the presence of obvious markers of abuse healthcare workers do not always make the connection and, whether consciously or unconsciously, do not recognize the possibility of abuse or enquire about it. Moreover, many abused women will not demonstrate any of the recognized markers while those who do will not all have been abused.

Risk markers are therefore insufficiently sensitive or specific and should not be used as a basis for selective enquiry. As well as being ineffective, selective enquiry – if obviously selective – can also be offensive whether or not the woman has suffered abuse. Any awkwardness on the part of the health worker will be conveyed to the woman. The way the question is posed is therefore important. A statement such as 'I know this probably doesn't apply to you but we have to ask everyone' gives a clear indication of the 'correct' response and does not encourage disclosure. Identification of violence is important in reproductive healthcare and given the nature of services provided, it is entirely appropriate to take an adequate sexual and social history, including direct enquiry about violence and abuse in all cases.

MANAGEMENT OF ABUSE

While all women should be asked about abuse the circumstances must be conducive to disclosure. Privacy is essential and all women should have at least part of any reproductive health consultation conducted on a one-to-one basis with the doctor, nurse or midwife. The presence of a partner who is reluctant to leave will not only prevent enquiry but may be an indicator of abuse. There should be recognition that not all abused women will admit this on routine enquiry; a negative response will not preclude violence and if there are strong suspicions some support can often be provided in the absence of an explicit admission. Disclosure may then occur during a later consultation.

All women presenting in pregnancy should be asked about the circumstances of the pregnancy, whether the pregnancy is planned, intended and/or wanted, their relationship with their partner (or man who accompanies them) and whether he is the baby's father. In this context it is simple to ask the woman about the quality of the relationship and specifically whether her partner has ever been violent to her. She should also be asked whether anyone else has ever been violent to her and whether she has ever been forced to have sex with someone against her wishes. Women presenting with a gynaecological problem should similarly have a full sexual history taken. All women, pregnant or non-pregnant, presenting for any type of reproductive healthcare should have a social history taken. This should include questions about lifestyle, including use of tobacco, alcohol and illicit drugs, all of which can directly affect reproductive health. Women who disclose illicit drug use should be asked how this is financed, including specific enquiry about involvement in commercial sex.

There are several important aspects to management (Heath 1992). It is important that a woman who discloses a history of violence is reassured that she is believed and that she is not responsible for nor deserving of the violence. In the reproductive health setting management of the relevant injuries or medical problems with which she presents will be a priority (management of women presenting with a present history of rape or sexual abuse is described in Chapter 64) but the healthcare worker's responsibility does not end there. Details of the violence together with the woman's circumstances should be elicited and an assessment made of immediate risk to the woman and/or her children or others in her immediate circle. The information she provides should be accurately documented together with details of examination findings including injuries if present and any treatment given. Such information may be required for future legal action. She should be reassured that any information she provides will be treated with confidentiality but there should also be discussion about the meaning of and limits to confidentiality. Should the healthcare worker envisage having to disclose the information, for example to ensure child protection, this should be discussed with the woman at the outset.

There should be discussion with women experiencing domestic violence or abuse about the possibility of leaving the abuser. Information including contact telephone numbers should be provided about services both residential and non-residential for women experiencing violence as well as availability of any other alternative accommodation. However, it is important to recognize that it is often not feasible for women to remove themselves from the situation. For example, they may be financially, emotionally or otherwise dependent on the abuser or for various reasons it might not be possible for them to take their children with them. Moreover, when the woman appears to be at significant and imminent risk of further violence, leaving the situation may increase that risk and women are especially likely to suffer significant injury or even be killed when they leave a violent domestic environment (Browne 1987, Geberth 1992). It is therefore essential that women are reassured that there is recognition of and sympathy for limitations to their options and are not given the impression that they are expected to leave or will be considered stupid or weak if they fail to do so.

Regardless of their circumstances or chosen action, women should be provided with information about services and also the offer of direct referral. Where specific problems (whether cause or effect) are identified, such as for example mental health or substance misuse problems, appropriate referral for specialist management will be helpful even if it does not resolve the problem of violence. Moreover, problem drug and/or alcohol use can have direct effects on reproductive health which in their own right merit treatment of the problem. This is therefore discussed later.

MANAGEMENT OF PROSTITUTION

Women experiencing violence in non-domestic settings should receive similar support. Women seen at reproductive health services who admit involvement in commercial sex will invariably have attended for some other reason and the presenting problem will obviously need to be dealt with. Nevertheless, an admission of prostitution should prompt a full relevant history including details of type of services offered and clients buying them. Sexual behaviour and consequent risks together with relevant signs and symptoms should be explored. In the obstetric context women engaging in commercial sex will often claim that paternity is not in doubt and the pregnancy is definitely to their partner. However, clients often pay more for unprotected intercourse and a carefully taken sexual history may indicate such confidence is misplaced. Nevertheless, such self-deception by a woman and/or her partner, whether conscious or unconscious, is often an essential coping strategy so it is not necessarily helpful to comment on it unless specifically asked to do so when it should be discussed with the woman on her own. Even if not explicitly admitted, however, uncertainty or concern about paternity may increase the risk of violence to the woman from her partner. It is of course entirely reasonable and appropriate to discuss with non-pregnant women involved in prostitution strategies for risk reduction regarding both sexually transmitted infections and unplanned and unwanted pregnancies. In this context it would also be appropriate to discuss possible paternity problems if the woman is not pregnant but keen to conceive to her partner. Preconceptual counselling about risks to a pregnancy from sexually transmitted infections (including bloodborne viruses such as HIV) would also be desirable in this situation.

Women engaged in commercial sex will escape the consequent violence by ceasing prostitution. For those women whose prostitution is directed and controlled by their sexual partner, this may be achieved by leaving the partner as in other domestic abuse situations but for similar reasons this may be difficult or impossible. In addition, some such women and many working independently will still have to continue working because of their own financial needs. There is a social hierarchy of prostitution. At the upper end of the market, in saunas and other indoor settings, there is less risk, often less financial pressure but greater financial rewards while at the more risky lower end financial need is often greater or more acute but income relatively lower. Amongst the most vulnerable women working on the streets factors such as problem drug and/or alcohol use that necessitate prostitution are also much more common. Nevertheless all women engaged in prostitution, regardless of the circumstances, are at risk of violence. An approach similar to that described for domestic abuse should be adopted. An adequate history and examination are essential as is accurate documentation of relevant information. Immediate healthcare needs should be assessed and appropriate management instigated, in this situation the presence of any genital tract trauma or infection, whether the woman is pregnant and consequently whether she requires maternity care, a termination of pregnancy, effective contraception or preconceptual care.

While some women working as prostitutes might be able to leave the violent situation by leaving a violent partner or pimp for whom they were earning money, most would only be able to stop prostituting if their own financial needs were resolved. For many this in turn would require effective management of their drug or alcohol problem.

MANAGEMENT OF PROBLEM SUBSTANCE USE

Problem drug and/or alcohol use is often associated with poor nutrition which in turn may cause amenorrhoea. Heroin use can also cause amenorrhoea with or without anovulation. Methadone substitution therapy improves social stability and general health including nutrition and commencement of therapy is often followed by return of fertility which can precede return of menstruation.

Many drug-using women incorrectly assume their amenorrhoea indicates infertility but they must be warned this is not so and provided with effective contraception if they do not want to become pregnant. Conversely, however, drug-using women who experience difficulty in conceiving should be advised that stabilization of their drug use and consequently of their lifestyle with methadone substitution therapy where appropriate will increase their chances of conception. Such measures would also improve the baby's health as well as the mother's parenting abilities. This advice also holds true for their partners since in association with use of sedative drugs including benzodiazepines and opiates/opioids (including methadone), reduced sperm motility is often observed. Although the precise functional significance of this is uncertain, in the absence of successful conception it seems reasonable to give both partners general advice about reduction in levels of drug use and for those on substitute medication to recommend stabilization at the lowest level compatible with stability.

Management of the drug problem per se is obviously not the clinical responsibility of reproductive healthcare professionals. However, if such a problem is identified, whether incidentally or in association with prostitution, violence or reproductive health problems, women should be given appropriate information about possible effects on pregnancy fertility and effective contraception if indicated. This should be provided together with information about and the offer of referral to specialist services.

SEXUAL VIOLENCE IN WAR

The use of sexual violence as a strategy in war has been observed and reported by healthcare workers, humanitarian organizations and others working in such settings (Shanks et al 2001). Women who have experienced such violence may move to other countries as refugees or asylum seekers and may then present to healthcare workers who do not have direct experience of such problems. Refugees presenting for reproductive healthcare may have experienced violence; their trauma may be exacerbated by being in a culturally unfamiliar environment, possibly without the support of family or friends, often with language and communication difficulties and encountering workers who are unaware of or have no understanding of their previous circumstances and experiences. Some such women may be in the country illegally or awaiting the outcome of an asylum application. They may consequently be unable or afraid to access services or to admit or discuss their problems when they do so. Similarly, other black or ethnic minority women may be reluctant to seek help because of previous experience of racism from public services or institutions (Mama 1989) and expectation of repetition and/or fear of deportation. They may

also have problems in accessing services or obtaining financial support, making it even more difficult for them to leave an abusive partner.

HEALTH SERVICE PROVISION

There is now a wide range of literature on various aspects of domestic abuse. There is increasing recognition of the need to acknowledge the impact of abuse on health, the need to deal with the problem effectively and the need for adequate training to do so. There is also recognition that this requires a multidisciplinary approach. These issues have been strategically addressed on a national level (DoH 2000, Scottish Executive 2000). The British Medical Association (1998) has considered the problem of domestic violence in relation to health and healthcare in general while in common with many other professional bodies, the Royal College of Obstetricians and Gynaecologists has dealt with the issue from a specialty viewpoint and examined domestic violence in the context of reproductive health (Bewley et al 1997).

SUMMARY

Violence against women is common and is relevant to all aspects of reproductive healthcare. Women are often reluctant to admit that they have experienced abuse but most want to be asked about it and to have an opportunity to discuss it. While there are some indicators that indicate the possibility of abuse they are insufficiently sensitive or specific to form the basis for selective enquiry. All women presenting for any type of reproductive healthcare but especially pregnant women should have a full sexual and social history taken which includes routine direct enquiry about violence or abuse from their partner or other individual.

Women who volunteer a history of abuse should have their experience validated. In addition to treatment of the immediate health consequences, they should have their current situation and level of risk assessed and be given information about available services, including the offer of direct referral. Limitations of options, including difficulties in removing themselves from the abusive situation, should be recognized. Careful documentation is essential for future use, including possible legal action. Effective management of this problem requires not only adequate availability of suitable services but adequate training of healthcare professionals. Both require adequate resources.

KEY POINTS

1. Most violence against women is inflicted by men, most commonly partners or ex-partners, and usually occurs in the home.
2. Domestic abuse occurs throughout the social spectrum but women from disadvantaged backgrounds may have fewer resources to deal with it.
3. Abuse experienced by women may be physical, psychological, emotional or economic.

KEY POINTS (*CONTINUED*)

4. Women are at risk of violence in any situation involving sex, including commercial sex which carries a risk of violence both from partners (and/or men controlling their prostitution) and from clients.
5. Domestic abuse often begins or escalates during pregnancy.
6. Domestic abuse has gynaecological and obstetric consequences and should therefore be addressed by those providing reproductive healthcare.
7. Mental health and behavioural problems including depression and substance misuse are more commonly effects rather than causes of domestic abuse.
8. Markers of abuse are insufficiently specific or sensitive to be used as indicators for enquiry and all pregnant women should be routinely asked about domestic abuse.
9. Healthcare workers require training in social history taking, identification and management of domestic abuse.
10. The possibility that healthcare workers may themselves be experiencing domestic abuse must be borne in mind.

REFERENCES

Bewley S, Friend J, Mezey G 1997 Violence against women. RCOG Press, London

Bohn DK 1990 Domestic violence and pregnancy. Implications for practice. Journal of Nurse-Midwifery 35:86–98

British Medical Association 1998 Domestic violence: a health care issue? British Medical Association, London

Browne A 1987 When battered women kill. Collier Macmillan, London

Department of Health 2000 Domestic violence: a resource manual for health care professionals. DoH, London

Dobash RE, Dobash RP 1980 Violence against wives. Open Books, London

Friedman LS, Samet JH, Roberts MS, Hudlin M, Hans P 1992 Inquiry about victimization experiences. A survey of patient preferences and physician practices. Archives of Internal Medicine 152:1186–1190

Geberth VJ 1992 Stalkers. Law and Order October: 138–143

Heath I 1992 Domestic violence: the general practitioner's role. In: Royal College of General Practitioners Members Reference Book. Sabrecrown, London

Helton AS, McFarlane J, Anderson ET 1987 Battered and pregnant: a prevalence study. American Journal of Public Health 77:1337–1339

Hillard PJA 1985 Physical abuse in pregnancy. Obstetrics and Gynecology 66:185–190

Home Affairs Select Committee 1993 Domestic violence (2 vols). HMSO, London

James-Hanman D, Long L 1994 Crime prevention: an issue for midwives? British Journal of Midwifery 2:29–32

Johnson H, Sacco V 1995 Researching violence against women: Statistics Canada's national survey. Canadian Journal of Criminology July 281–304

Jones RF 1997 Domestic violence – a physician's perspective. In: Bewley S, Friend J, Mezey G (eds) Violence against women. RCOG, London

Kennedy H 1993 Eve was framed. Vintage, London

Kennedy LW, Dutton DG 1989 The incidence of wife assault in Alberta. Canadian Journal of Behavioural Sciences 21:40–54

Mama A 1989 The hidden struggle: statutory and voluntary responses to violence against black women in the home. Runnymede Trust, London

Mayhew P, Maung NF, Mirrlees-Black C 1993 The 1992 British Crime Survey. HMSO, London

Mezey GC 1997 Perpetrators of domestic violence. In: Bewley S, Friend J, Mezey G (eds) Violence against women. RCOG, London

Mezey GC, Bewley S 1997 Domestic violence and pregnancy. British Medical Journal 314:1295

Mirrlees-Black C, Mayhew P, Percy A 1996 The 1996 British Crime Survey: England and Wales. The Stationery Office, London

Mooney J 1994 The hidden figure: domestic violence in North London. Islington Council, London

Plichta S 1992 The effects of woman abuse on health care utilisation and health status: a literature review. Women's Health Issues 2:154–163

Russell D 1982 Rape in marriage. Indiana University Press, Bloomington

Scottish Executive 2000 Scottish partnership on domestic abuse: national strategy to address domestic abuse in Scotland. Scottish Executive, Edinburgh

Scottish Needs Assessment Programme (SNAP) 1997 SNAP report on domestic violence. Scottish Forum for Public Health Medicine, 69 Oakfield Avenue, Glasgow G12 8QQ

Shanks L, Ford N, Schull M et al 2001 Responding to rape. Lancet 357:304

Stark E, Flitcraft A 1996 Women at risk. Sage, London

Stark E, Flitcraft A, Frazier W 1979 Medicine and patriarchal violence. The social construction of a private event. International Journal of Health Services 9:41–93

Stark E, Flitcraft AH 1991 Spouse abuse. In: Rosenberg M, Mercy J (eds) Violence in America: a public health approach. Oxford University Press, New York

Sugg NK, Inui T 1992 Primary care physicians' response to domestic violence: opening Pandora's box. Journal of the American Medical Association 267:3194–3195

United Nations 1995 Violence against women: a world-wide report. United Nations, New York

66

Lesbian health issues

Tamsin Wilton   Susan Bewley

INTRODUCTION

Lesbians are like other women; there is nothing distinctive about lesbian physiology. Sexual activity between women does not result in any unique health problems and lesbians experience broadly the same range of obstetric and gynaecological problems as non-lesbian women (Skinner 1996). It is, nevertheless, increasingly recognized that medicine fails to meet the needs of lesbian patients (Gruskin 1999, Solarz 1999, Stern 1993, Wilton 1997, 2000).

Research into this professional deficiency highlights two causes for concern: simple ignorance or misinformation and prejudicial or discriminatory attitudes (Das 1996, Stevens 1993). Since it is a professional responsibility to help *all* patients, professional bodies such as the Royal Colleges of Nursing and Midwifery in the UK and the Institute of Medicine in the USA have called for lesbian issues to be incorporated into the training of all health professionals (RCM 2000, RCN 1994, 1998, Solarz 1999). In order to help their lesbian patients, gynaecologists need accurate information and to address any thoughtless or discriminatory attitudes which result in poor clinical practice.

SOCIAL CHANGE

Attitudes towards sexuality underwent a dramatic change during the twentieth century, at least in the industrialized West. Lesbians have benefited from this and no longer endure the extremes of social exclusion and criminalization that were the norm until recently (Cruikshank 1992, Healey & Mason 1994). However, the impact of change is not consistent. Whole-hearted acceptance exists alongside organized campaigns against equality and bigoted individuals continue to commit acts of extreme violence – such as the nail-bombing of a gay bar in London (Fanshaw 1999) – against those whom they believe to be lesbian or gay (Cant & Hemmings 1988, Comstock 1991, Schulman 1994, Wilton 2000).

Clinicians, accustomed to thinking in terms of 'prevalence', often seek to know what percentage of their patients are likely to be lesbian. This is an unhelpful approach for two reasons. First, research into sexuality is dogged by complex methodological issues and there are simply no reliable data. Estimates range widely, from less than 1% to nearer 20%, depending on sample and method (Solarz 1999). Second, the notion of prevalence assumes that sexual orientation is fixed and measurable and this is simply not the case (see below).

It is a mistake to categorize lesbians under the generic label 'homosexual', as most authorities agree that gender is as significant a difference in this group as it is for heterosexuals. For example, lesbians tend to be poorer than gay men, as the labour market is still segregated along gender lines (Gluckman & Reed 1997). The distinctiveness of the lesbian experience has only recently been acknowledged and material on 'homosexuality' has tended to take the male as the norm (Wilton 1995). This chapter focuses exclusively on the lesbian experience and particularly those aspects which relate to gynaecology.

ATTITUDES IN HEALTHCARE

The contradictory pace of change is reflected in healthcare. Depending on factors such as user demand or the kind of service provided, different healthcare professionals have been quicker or slower to recognize that lesbians constitute a distinct group with specific needs. In primary care and nursing, for example, the generic nature of the work has required an effective response to the requirements of lesbian patients (Deevey 1990, Harrison 1996, Platzer 1993, Rankow 1997, Stevens 1994, White & Levinson 1993). There is now a demand that all practitioners be 'culturally competent' in their professional interactions with lesbians, a demand which has exposed serious weaknesses in medical education (Das 1996, Solarz 1999).

The culturally competent practitioner must acquire basic understanding in three areas:

- lesbian identity and how it relates to sexual practice
- the social position of lesbians and its likely impact on the individual patient
- the historical role of the medical profession in pathologizing homosexuality, a factor which continues to influence doctor–patient relationships.

A study conducted at eight London medical schools which investigated medical students' attitudes towards lesbians found examples of extreme prejudice. Thirty-seven per cent of respondents did not think it was important to acknowledge a lesbian patient's partner and almost 40% thought that lesbians want to be men. When asked how they would feel if a patient revealed herself to be lesbian, comments included: 'I'd ask if I could watch', 'Wouldn't affect me at all – particularly if the woman was ugly as many lesbians are', and one respondent thought that medical education about lesbians should be 'in the context of euthanasia' (summarized from Das 1996:6–8)

Evidence from the UK, the USA, Canada, South Africa, Australia and New Zealand suggests that healthcare is, for many lesbians, a game of chance (de Pinho 1994, Michigan Organization for Human Rights 1991, Rankine 1999, Rose & Platzer 1993, Trippet & Bain 1993a,b). Whilst there are informed and sympathetic practitioners, lesbians are equally likely to face problems, ranging from simple ignorance on the part of their carers to outright hostility and even negligent treatment (Stevens & Hall 1988, 1990).

There are important consequences for gynaecology. Lesbians may delay seeking medical advice or opt for complementary therapies in preference to conventional treatment (Rankine 1999, Sheffield Health 1996, Trippet & Bain 1993a). Studies have shown that this may be particularly true for gynaecological symptoms. For example, Trippet & Bain (1993b: 59) found that 'the most prevalent problems lesbian women encountered for which they did not seek [conventional] health care were menstrual, sexually transmitted diseases, reproductive, bladder or kidney and breast problems'. Although gynaecology is here implicated as a problematic area of healthcare for lesbians, it seems that relatively minor improvements may therefore produce disproportionately beneficial outcomes.

WHAT IS HOMOSEXUALITY?

The term 'homosexuality', only coined in 1869, implies that sexual orientation is a fixed and intrinsic characteristic and this notion persists to the present day (Weeks 1985, Wilton 2000). In particular, as we shall see, it justifies biomedical research. Such research posits a biological 'cause' for the putative distinction between 'heterosexuals' and 'homosexuals', with the residual category 'bisexual' to mop up anyone left over (Herdt & Boxer 1995, Rosario 1997).

The evidence does not support this approach. Sociologists, historians and anthropologists point to huge diversity between cultures and throughout history in the social organization of sexuality (Bremmer 1989, Caplan 1987, Duberman et al 1989, Fradenburg & Freccero 1996, Herdt 1984). In classical Greece, for example, adult, free, male citizens were at liberty to enjoy sex with women, boys, slaves or foreigners. Sex was primarily concerned with sociopolitical status, gender preference was a matter of taste and the Greeks did not recognize a distinction between 'homosexual' and 'heterosexual' (Halperin 1989).

Nor, as theologians point out, did Biblical Hebrew tribes (Doe 2000, Helminiak 1994). Old Testament proscriptions against sexual activity between men (sex between women is not mentioned) are based on the reason that sex is primarily for procreation and 'wastage of semen' is condemned. There is no concept of a distinct type of individual, whether 'heterosexual' or 'homosexual'.

However, researchers have found close correlation among healthcare professionals between religiosity and prejudice against lesbians (Stevens 1993). It is important to recognize that there is lively disagreement within all the major religions concerning the correct interpretation of sacred texts on this matter and that such interpretations may change dramatically from generation to generation (Doe 2000). For example, there is certainly evidence that early Christian societies celebrated same-sex unions (Boswell 1995, Helminiak 1994, Pharr 1988).

The influence of religion also varies between different cultural contexts. During their conquest of Africa, India and the Americas, for example, Christian missionaries forcibly suppressed indigenous customs of same-sex marriage, such as the 'female husbands' of African tradition or the 'two-spirit' people of many native American tribes (Gay 1985, Nanda 1993, Whitehead 1993). The strong association between 'development' and the religious teachings of the colonizing nations has lead to a situation where, for example, Christian communities in some African countries are now far more illiberal than those in Britain or mainland Europe (Doe 2000). It seems that same-sex attraction is found everywhere and most societies seem to have had little trouble accepting and managing it. The extent to which such behaviours may come to be associated with a division between different categories or types of individual varies. Yet, despite the lack of evidence for such a division, it continues to underpin the medical model of sexuality.

THE MEDICAL MODEL

Many biomedical researchers have attempted to identify a symptomatology, locate a cause and (sometimes by implication) find a cure. In the 21st century, the focus is on brain structure or chromosomal abnormality (Hamer & Copeland 1994, LeVay 1993, 1996). As aetiological explanations have shifted, so 'cures' involving aversion therapy, excision of brain tissue or electroconvulsive shock have given way to debate on the ethics of aborting 'gay fetuses' (Wilton 2000).

Biomedicine cannot account for the fact that most men who meet other men for casual sex in public toilets are heterosexual, many of them happily married (Humphreys 1970). Researchers now believe that the majority of gay men have occasional sex with women (Davies et al 1990, Fitzpatrick et al 1990). As we shall see, most lesbians have had sex with men at some time in their lives, suggesting that sexuality is fluid.

It is important that doctors recognize the inaccuracy of myths concerning the 'mannish' or 'unnatural' lesbian. Biomedical theories of sexual orientation all depend on the claim that sexual object-choice is a marker of gender identity. Thus, in order to desire other women, a lesbian must harbour some bodily or psychological element of masculinity. There is no evidence whatsoever to support this notion. Yet wrong assumptions about a lesbian's attitude to her body and its reproductive functions, particularly her uterus and ovaries, or her sex life after prolapse surgery, may result in insensitive or unkind care.

HETEROSEXUAL EXPERIENCE

Even within the 'first world', there is great diversity among lesbians (Blackwood & Wieringa 1999, Gay 1985). Of particular importance to gynaecology is the fact that lesbians differ greatly in the extent to which they relate sexually to men, a fact which may surprise those unaccustomed to questioning the biomedical model.

Some lesbians only ever experience attraction to women and have no sexual contact with men. To these women the notion of having sex with a man may be as repugnant as it is to some heterosexual men. However, the majority of lesbians have had at least some sexual experience with male partners (Cassingham & O'Neil 1993, Whisman 1996). This may have been during early adulthood, at a time when they perhaps did not recognize their attraction to women or felt unable to act on it for social, religious or cultural reasons. Others may have tried to deny their feelings and endured unhappy heterosexual relationships or even marriage. Such women may feel strongly that they are 'born' lesbians.

The growing emancipation of women during the second half of the 20th century resulted in a qualitatively distinct approach to a lesbian identity. Many women who had lived conventionally happy heterosexual lives chose to explore the very different intimacy of a lesbian lifestyle and while some returned to partnerships with men, others did not (Clausen 1997, Menasche 1999). Different again are 'political lesbians', primarily characterized by withdrawal from sexual contact with men, who may or may not engage in sex with other women. While 'political lesbianism' was an historical moment that seems to have passed, it remains not uncommon for women to experience lesbianism as a positive choice, rather than an innate drive (Cassingham & O'Neil 1993, Whisman 1996).

Following the upheaval wrought by HIV in lesbian and gay subcultures came a different notion again, that of 'queer'. As a deliberately reclaimed term of abuse (and still offensive when used as such), 'queer' signals a move away from the desire to be assimilated into mainstream society. Those who call themselves 'queer' argue that the division into heterosexual and homosexual is anachronistic and that it constrains everyone, not simply lesbians and gay men. They see sexual pluralism and gender fluidity as radicalizing. Younger female members of such 'queer' subcultures may, therefore, be sexually active with both women and men (Smyth 1992), as may their partners. Such behaviour norms may increase the likelihood of exposure to STDs, including HIV infection, although urban gay communities do tend to be well informed about safer sex (O'Sullivan & Parmar 1992).

Finally, lesbians share the economic disadvantage of their heterosexual peers. At every level of the sex industry some of the women struggling to support themselves, their children and/or a drug habit are lesbians (Frank 1998, Pyett & Warr 1996) and some have penetrative sex with male clients.

IMPLICATIONS FOR GYNAECOLOGICAL HEALTH

This diversity of sexual behaviour among lesbians may have different outcomes for their gynaecological health. Awareness of and sensitivity to this range of experiences is likely to be of benefit to *all* gynaecology patients and there are three key areas where this is so.

Clinical examination

All women dislike vaginal and speculum examinations, but lesbians may find the experience particularly distressing. Indeed, experience of insensitive or painful vaginal examination is one reason why some lesbians may avoid seeking help for gynaecological symptoms (Wilton 1997). Even lesbians who have given birth may never have had penetrative vaginal intercourse. Sensitive vaginal examination, giving the patient as much control as possible, should therefore be routine and is recommended by the Royal College of Obstetrics and Gynaecology (RCOG 1997).

Cervical screening

Since their history may include past or current sexual activity with men, lesbians need cervical screening as much as other women. This is borne out by research in lesbian specialist GUM clinics in London, which found rates of cervical abnormality comparable to what might be expected in similar samples of non-lesbian women (Farquhar et al 2001). This is important, since lay knowledge in many lesbian communities holds that lesbians do *not* require smears. Moreover, many primary care physicians also believe this to be the case and are known to advise their patients accordingly (Farquhar 1999, Mugglestone 1999, Wilton 1999a).

Sexually transmissible diseases

Sex between women is a largely ineffectual transmission route for HIV (Richardson 2000). The rarity of HIV transmission between women does not mean that lesbians are not at risk. Unprotected heterosexual intercourse or unsafe use of street drugs pose the same degree of risk regardless of women's sexual identity. Yet widespread misinformation about lesbianism has led to a general perception that lesbians are a 'low-risk' group (O'Sullivan & Parmar 1992, Richardson 1994, 2000).

Similarly, although sex between women carries a relatively low risk of transmitting STDs such as gonorrhoea, syphilis and chlamydia, other infections, such as bacterial vaginosis, do appear to be transmitted in this way (Farquhar et al 2001). Moreover, since past or current heterosexual contact cannot be ruled out, symptoms which may be indicative of pelvic inflammatory disease, or of its sequelae, should be taken as seriously in the lesbian patient as in any other woman.

WHAT DOES 'SEX' MEAN?

It is often necessary for a patient to discuss sexual activity with her gynaecologist. The gynaecologist may need to know when the patient last had intercourse or to advise her on resuming sex after surgery or on the likely effects of treatment on sexual sensation or function. It is clearly important that both parties share a common understanding of what 'having sex' means. If a gynaecologist regards every patient as heterosexual by default, the assumption will be that 'sex' means penile penetration of the vagina. In this scenario, the lesbian patient who does not feel safe enough to disclose her sexual preference is not likely to receive much useful information. Nor is her gynaecologist (Hemmings 1987).

Communication problems may remain even if the patient is confident enough to 'come out'. Her gynaecologist may be ill-informed about lesbian sexual practices, perhaps assuming, for example, that lesbians have no penetrative sex. Notions of what is 'acceptable' sexual behaviour tend to shift quite rapidly and this is as true of lesbians as of anyone else. Like heterosexuals, many lesbians enjoy different forms of penetrative sex – with fingers, hands, tongues or sex toys – but many others do not. Advice always needs, therefore, to be based on frank and relaxed discussion with individual patients, not on stereotypical beliefs which may be inaccurate.

Attitudes to sex toys are also as varied among lesbians as among heterosexuals. Following genital or pelvic surgery it is important to reduce the risk of infection, so patients may need clear advice on their use. Those used for penetration should not be shared unless a new condom is used for each woman and nothing used for anal stimulation should *ever* be inserted into the vagina. It is safer to buy purpose-made sex toys rather than to improvise and devices made of leather should be avoided, as leather is difficult to clean (Califia 1988).

Such topics are seldom addressed in medical schools and some individuals (doctors and nurses as well as patients!) may find explicit discussion challenging. Embarrassment may cause laughter or other inappropriate responses. It may therefore be preferable to prepare a simple printed sheet with guidance on a wide range of sexual activities, to be available to all patients who need this information. Detailed advice on the 'health and safety' aspects of sex play may be found in lesbian health handbooks or sex manuals (e.g. Califia 1988, Wilton 1997), and such handouts should include contact details of local lesbian helplines.

Sexuality is a sensitive issue. However, if advice about sexual behaviour is to be useful, doctors must develop an approach which combines respect for sexual diversity with calm explicitness. Following hysterectomy and most vaginal surgery, for example, clitoral stimulation may safely be resumed before vaginal penetration. Such information is useful regardless of sexual orientation. Gynaecological ill-health may be damaging to women's self-esteem and emotional well-being and resuming sexual activity can be an important element in recovery.

TOWARDS GOOD PRACTICE

Understanding the social position of lesbians is important on many levels. First, a degree of awareness and empathy must underpin the good doctor–patient relationship. Second, information about a lesbian patient's sexuality should remain confidential and some understanding of the possible consequences of breaking confidentiality is useful in ensuring this. Third, recovery from illness and/or surgery is a complex process, influenced by social and psychological factors such as the emotional state of the patient, her resilience or the degree of support she is able to access.

Stigma and vulnerability

It is important to take account of the likely impact of social stigma. As a group, for example, lesbians have been found to be at disproportionately high risk of suicide, attempted suicide and other markers of emotional distress (Gibson 1989, Hammelman 1993, Millard 1995). Such findings give an insight into the emotional pressures which may make the lesbian patient unusually vulnerable when exposed to the stresses of illness, a hospital stay or surgery (Gruskin 1999).

This likely vulnerability means that sensitivity around close relationships, friendship communities and next-of-kin issues is of particular importance. Many lesbians refer to their close friendship circle as their family (Weston 1998) and many have strained or dysfunctional relationships with blood relatives (Griffin & Mulholland 1997), making the support of a partner and/or close friends still more important. Yet research into the healthcare experiences of lesbians continues to uncover instances of disrespectful and unprofessional behaviour towards partners. Typically this takes the form of refusing to acknowledge the relationship or denying partners visiting rights or information about the patient's condition. One lesbian living in a large city in the south of England reported that, when she was hospitalized following an accident, 'My partner was not allowed to be with me, because she was not my family or my husband' (Wilton 1999a), an experience frequently reported in the literature.

Seeing it from her perspective

The stresses of everyday lesbian life are unfamiliar to most non-lesbians (Griffin & Mulholland 1997, Harvard Law Review 1990, Kaufman & Lincoln 1991, Mason & Palmer 1996, Rosembloom 1996). It should be borne in mind that many women have lost their jobs, their homes, access to or custody of their children and contact with their family of origin simply because they are lesbians. Moreover, all lesbians, however privileged in terms of income, class or education, are vulnerable to abuse or actual physical assault (Mason & Palmer 1996).

The hostile hospital

Even where such prejudice (often referred to as 'homophobia') is not experienced, lesbians live in a world which by and large seems unaware of their needs. Such lack of awareness may cause the hospital environment to be experienced as hostile, uncaring or unsafe. For example, many who design or carry out routine administrative procedures, such as the completion of booking-in forms, presume that patients are heterosexual unless proven otherwise. From the point of view of a lesbian patient, anyone who make these thoughtless assumptions is not 'safe', since they may prove to be judgemental or condemnatory. Such fears make concealment more likely, thus perpetuating the general ignorance about lesbians.

It should also be borne in mind that the distribution of lesbians working in healthcare is likely to be concentrated in traditionally female-dominated areas, such as nursing and midwifery. However, it is as risky for them to be 'out' as it is for lesbian patients. It is likely that both their colleagues and the patients they work with will remain in ignorance. Sadly it may be very difficult for lesbians, at every level of the profession, openly to support lesbian patients or to challenge the attitudes of their colleagues.

Finally, if lesbians have reason to believe that gynaecology services are ill-equipped to offer them high standards of care, they may look elsewhere, with potentially harmful consequences. Women with sinister gynaecological symptoms may delay seeking help, whilst those who choose informal donor insemination may be at greater risk of infections, including HIV (Palmer et al 1990, Saffron 1994, Wilton 1997). Some degree of preparedness to meet the needs of lesbians is therefore basic to good gynaecological care.

LESBIAN MOTHERS

As we have seen, the anachronistic model of homosexuality as a form of *disordered gender* remains influential in medicine (Hemmings 1987, Wilton 1997). In particular, it still influences attitudes to lesbian mothers. If 'lesbian' means 'masculine' and if the mothering instinct is quintessentially feminine, lesbian motherhood becomes a contradiction in terms (Richardson 1993). Such attitudes, together with ill-informed concerns that lesbians make bad parents, present difficulties for lesbians who wish to become pregnant and for those who are already mothers (Wilton 1999b). In Britain, for example, lesbians have been prevented from accessing clinical services in assisted reproduction (Rosenbloom 1996), a situation now open to challenge under European human rights legislation.

There is no connection between gender, sexual preference and desire for children. Like heterosexual women, lesbians can become mothers in different circumstances. Some are single parents, by choice or force of circumstances, while others are in stable, long-term co-parenting relationships. Many have children from a previous marriage, whilst others become pregnant via donated semen or unprotected heterosexual intercourse. Whatever the circumstances of conception, researchers have found no evidence that the children of lesbians are harmed in any way by their mothers' sexuality (Flaks et al 1995, Golombok & Tasker 1996, Golombok et al 1983, Green et al 1986).

In Britain the Human Fertilization and Embryology Act 1990 made it a statutory responsibility for clinics to consider the welfare of any potential child, including the need for a father. The statute has been used primarily to exclude women without male partners, including lesbians. However, the suggestion that absence of a male parent is per se harmful to the development or well-being of children is not supported in the literature (Gruskin 1999, Saffron 1994, Solarz 1999). Other complex issues, such as the right of donor insemination children to know the identity of their sperm donor, apply to all recipients of assisted reproductive services.

Some continue to question the fitness of lesbians to parent. They should be reassured that several decades of research on lesbian mothers and their children have concluded that the parenting skills of lesbians are in no way inferior to those of heterosexuals and that their children are as well adjusted in every way as those from more mainstream backgrounds. Indeed, the findings of one recent British study suggest that being brought up by lesbians may be of positive *benefit* to children (Dunne 1997).

BENEFITS OF A LESBIAN LIFESTYLE

Focusing on lesbianism as a deviation from the norm tends both to obscure the health hazards of heterosexuality and to overshadow the potential health benefits of lesbian lifestyles. It is perhaps unsurprising that researchers have, to date, paid little attention to the beneficial aspects of lesbian life. However, research into the damaging consequences of heterosexual activity for women's health suggests that there may be health benefits to women whose sexual preference is for female partners. They avoid the risks associated with heterosexual intercourse, such as unwanted pregnancy, ectopic pregnancy, abortion, sexually transmitted infections, pelvic inflammatory disease and cervical intraepithelial neoplasia (Doyal 1995, Graham 1993, Smyke 1993). Further research into the positive aspects of lesbian health may yield unexpected benefits in terms of promoting the sexual and gynaecological health of all women.

CONCLUSION

Lesbians seeking healthcare commonly meet with ignorance, prejudice and hostility. Even where attitudes are more tolerant, the lesbian patient often finds herself having to educate and inform those responsible for her care. This unacceptable situation obliges many lesbians to protect themselves by not 'coming out' in healthcare interactions. Contrary to popular myth, it is only possible to know that a woman is a lesbian *if she wants you to know*. If the attitude of health professionals leads women to conceal their sexual orientation, it is likely that gynaecologists are usually unaware when they treat lesbian patients.

The gynaecologist who strives for the best possible outcome for every patient needs, therefore, to develop sensitive strategies both for encouraging lesbian patients to feel confident in disclosing their sexuality and for discussing openly any other relevant issues. After all, doctors who are unable to deal effectively with such matters are likely to have difficulty with other sensitive issues. Gynaecologists should also inform themselves about relevant matters, such as the support services available to lesbians in their locality. Because the existence of lesbians is routinely ignored, something as simple as displaying contact details of local lesbian community services in clinic waiting areas can make a disproportionately effective statement about inclusion and respect.

The healthcare profession is taking steps to rectify its previous failures in relation to the lesbian patient. In Britain, for example, the Royal Colleges of Nursing and of Midwifery have taken the lead in establishing guidelines for good practice and teaching materials are now available to support the education of nurses, social workers and others (e.g. Wilton 2000). It appears that those involved in the 'caring' rather than the 'curing' side of the profession have found themselves having to take the initiative and respond effectively to the concerns of patients and policy makers.

There is increasing support available to those seeking to update their knowledge of these issues. Experienced educators are available to facilitate training sessions or address groups of concerned professionals and there is a growing literature (see Further Reading section below).

As the speciality with direct responsibility for the healthcare of women, gynaecology is in a key position in relation to improving the health of lesbians and gynaecologists are well placed to demand effective support from nursing, midwifery and ancillary staff. The fact that lesbians are particularly unwilling to seek medical help for gynaecological symptoms suggests that the profession has failed this vulnerable group. On the other hand, attempts to remedy past failures may offer great and lasting benefit.

KEY POINTS

1. Lesbians are as diverse as non-lesbian women and there is great overlap between the two.
2. Lesbians face social stigma, prejudice and legal discrimination, so will often hide their sexuality.
3. Lesbians may avoid or delay seeking medical help, particularly with gynaecological symptoms.
4. Doctors who consider lesbianism a disorder should rethink this non-evidence-based belief.
5. Simple changes in attitudes and practice may substantially improve doctor–patient relationships.
6. Common health concerns include menstrual problems, bladder, breast and reproductive disorders.

REFERENCES

Blackwood E, Wieringa S (eds) 1999 Female desires: same-sex relations and transgender practices across cultures. Columbia University Press, New York

Boswell J 1995 The marriage of likeness: same-sex unions in pre-modern Europe. Harper Collins, London

Bremmer J (ed) 1989 From Sappho to de Sade: moments in the history of sexuality. Routledge, London

Califia P 1988 Sapphistry: the book of lesbian sexuality. Naiad, Tallahassee

Cant B, Hemmings S (eds) 1988 Radical records: thirty years of lesbian and gay history. Routledge, London

Caplan, P (ed) 1987 The cultural construction of sexuality. Routledge, London

Cassingham, B, O'Neil, S 1993 And then I met this woman: previously married women's journeys into lesbian relationships. Mother Courage Press, Racine

Clausen J 1997 Beyond gay or straight: understanding sexual orientation. Chelsea House, Philadelphia

Comstock G 1991 Violence against lesbians and gay men. Columbia University Press, New York

Cruikshank M 1992 The gay and lesbian liberation movement. Routledge, London

Das R 1996 The power of medical knowledge. Paper presented at Teaching to Promote Women's Health International Conference at Women's College Hospital, University of Toronto

Davies P, Hunt A, Macount M et al 1990 Longitudinal study of the sexual behaviour of homosexual males under the impact of AIDS: a final report to the Department of Health. Project SIGMA Working Papers. Department of Health, London

de Pinho H 1994 Placing lesbian health issues on the policy agenda. Paper presented to the Reproductive Health Priorities' Conference, Faculty of Medicine, University of Natal, Durban

Deevey S 1990 Older lesbian women: an invisible minority. Journal of Gerontological Nursing 16(5):35–37

Doe M 2000 Seeking the truth in love: the church and homosexuality. Darton, Longman and Todd, London

Doyal L 1995 What makes women sick: gender and the political economy of health. Macmillan, London

Duberman MB, Vicinus M, Chauncey G (eds) 1989 Hidden from history: reclaiming the gay and lesbian past. Penguin, Harmondsworth

Dunne G 1997 Lesbian lifestyles: women's work and the politics of sexuality. Macmillan, London

Fanshaw S 1999 April bombings: from bullies to bombs. Stonewall Newsletter 8(1):2–3

Farquhar C 1999 Lesbian sexual health: deconstructing research and practice. Unpublished PhD thesis. South Bank University, London

Farquhar C, Bailey J, Whittaker D 2001 Are lesbians sexually healthy? Report on the lesbian sexual health and behaviour questionnaire. Social Science Research Papers no 11. South Bank University, London

Fitzpatrick R, McLean J, Boulton M et al 1990 Variation in sexual behaviour in gay men. In: Aggleton P, Davis P, Hart G (eds) AIDS: individual, cultural and policy dimensions. Taylor and Francis, London

Flaks DK, Ficher I, Masterpasqua F et al 1995 Lesbians choosing motherhood: a comparative study of lesbian and heterosexual parents and their children. Developmental Psychology 31(1):105–114

Fradenburg L, Freccero C (eds) 1996 Premodern sexualities. Routledge, London

Frank K 1998 The production of identity and the negotiation of intimacy in a "gentleman's club". Sexualities 1(2):175–202

Gay J 1985 Mummies and babies and friends and lovers in Lesotho. Journal of Homosexuality 2(3–4):97–116

Gibson P 1989 Gay and lesbian youth suicide. In: Feinlieb M (ed) Prevention and intervention in youth suicide: report of the Secretary's Task Force on Youth Suicide, vol. III. US Department of Health and Human Services, Washington DC, pp 109–142

Gluckman A, Reed B (eds) 1997 Homo economics: capitalism, community and lesbian and gay life. Routledge, London

Golombok S, Spencer A, Rotter M 1983 Children in lesbian and single-parent households: psychosexual and psychiatric appraisal. Journal of Child Psychology and Psychiatry 24:551–572

Golombok S, Tasker F 1996 Do parents influence the sexual orientation of their children? Findings from a longitudinal study of lesbian families. Developmental Psychology 32(1):3–11

Graham H 1993 Hardship and health in women's lives. Harvester Wheatsheaf, London

Green R, Mandel J, Hotvedt M et al 1986 Lesbian mothers and their children: a comparison with solo parents, heterosexual mothers, and their children. Archives of Sexual Behaviour 15:167–184

Griffin K, Mulholland L (eds) 1997 Lesbian motherhood in Europe. Cassell, London

Gruskin EP 1999 Treating lesbians and bisexual women: challenges and strategies for health professionals. Sage, Thousand Oaks

Halperin D 1989 Sex before sexuality: pederasty, politics and power in classical Athens. In: Duberman MB, Vicinus M, Chauncey G (eds) Hidden from history: reclaiming the gay and lesbian past. Penguin, Harmondsworth

Hamer D, Copeland P 1994 The science of desire: the search for the gay gene and the biology of behaviour. Simon and Schuster, New York

Hammelman TL 1993 Gay and lesbian youth: contributing factors to serious attempts or considerations of suicide. Journal of Gay and Lesbian Psychotherapy 2(1):77–89

Harrison AE 1996 Primary care of lesbian and gay patients: educating ourselves and our students. Family Medicine 28(1):10–23

Harvard Law Review 1990 Sexual orientation and the law. Harvard University Press, Cambridge, Mass

Healey E, Mason A (ed) 1994 Stonewall 25: the making of the lesbian and gay community in Britain. Virago, London

Helminiak D 1994 What the Bible really says about homosexuality. Alamo Square Press, San Francisco

Hemmings S 1987 Overdose of doctors. In: O'Sullivan S (ed) Women's health: a Spare Rib reader. Pandora, London

Herdt G 1984 Ritualized homosexuality in Melanesia. University of California Press, Berkeley

Herdt G, Boxer A 1995 Bisexuality: towards a comparative theory of identities and culture. In: Parker R, Gagnon J (eds) Conceiving sexuality: approaches to sex research in a postmodern world. Routledge, London

Humphreys L 1970 Tearoom trade. Duckworth, London

Kaufmann T, Lincoln P (eds) 1991 High risk lives: lesbian and gay politics after the clause. Prism Press, Bridport

LeVay S 1993 The sexual brain. MIT Press, London

LeVay S 1996 Queer science: the use and abuse of research into homosexuality. MIT Press, London

Mason A, Palmer T 1996 Queer bashing: a national survey of hate crimes against lesbians and gay men. Stonewall Press, London

Menasche A 1999 Leaving the life: lesbians, ex-lesbians and the heterosexual imperative. Onlywomen Press, London

Michigan Organization for Human Rights (MOHR) 1991 The Michigan Lesbian Health Survey (executive summary). MOHR, Michigan

Millard J 1995 Suicide and suicide attempts in the lesbian and gay community. Australian and New Zealand Journal of Mental Health Nursing 4:181–189

Mugglestone J 1999 Are you sure you don't need contraception? Report of the Bolton and Wigan Lesbian Health Needs Assessment. Specialist Health Promotion Service, Bolton

Nanda S 1993 Hijras as neither man nor woman. In: Abelove H, Barale M, Halperin D (eds) The lesbian and gay studies reader. Routledge, London

O'Sullivan S, Parmar P 1992 Lesbians talk (safer) sex. Scarlet Press, London

Palmer DJL, Cuthbert J, Mukoyogo J et al 1990 Micro-organisms present in donor semen. British Journal of Sexual Medicine April:114–121

Pharr S 1988 Homophobia: a weapon of sexism. Chardon Press, Little Rock

Platzer H 1993 Nursing care of gay and lesbian patients. Nursing Standard January 13:34–37

Pyett P, Warr D 1996 When "gut instinct" is not enough: women at risk in sex work. Report to the Community. Centre for the Study of STDs, La Trobe University, Melbourne

Rankine J 1999 New lesbian survey shows poorer health. Women's Health Update 3(2):2

Rankow EJ 1997 Primary medical care of the gay or lesbian patient. North Carolina Medical Journal 58(2):92–96

Richardson D 1993 Women, Motherhood and Childrearing. Macmillan, London

Richardson D 1994 Inclusions and exclusions: lesbians, HIV and AIDS. In: Doyal L, Naidoo J, Wilton T (eds) AIDS: setting a feminist agenda. Taylor and Francis, London

Richardson D 2000 The social construction of immunity: HIV risk preception and prevention among lesbians and bisexual women. Culture, Health and Sexuality 2(1):33–49

Rosario V (ed) 1997 Science and homosexualities. Routledge, London

Rose P, Platzer H 1993 Confronting prejudice. Nursing Times August 4:52–54

Rosenbloom R (ed) 1996 Unspoken rules: sexual orientation and women's human rights. Cassell, London

Royal College of Midwifery 2000 Maternity care for lesbian mothers. Position paper no. 22. RCM, London

Royal College of Nursing 1994 The nursing care of lesbians and gay men: an RCN statement. RCN, London

Royal College of Nursing 1998 Guide for nurses on "next-of-kin" for lesbian and gay patients and children with lesbian or gay parents. Issues in Nursing and Health no. 47. RCN, London

Royal College of Obstetrics and Gynaecology 1997 Intimate examinations: report of a working party. RCOG Press, London

Saffron L 1994 Challenging conceptions: planning a family by self-insemination. Cassell, London

Schulman S 1994 My American history: lesbian and gay life during the Reagan/Bush years. Cassell, London

Sheffield Health 1996 Lesbian health needs assessment: report of a participatory research study. Healthy Sheffield Team, Sheffield

Skinner CJ 1996 A case-controlled study of the sexual health needs of lesbians. Genitourinary medicine 72(4):277–280

Smyke P 1993 Women and health. Zed Books, London

Smyth C 1992 Lesbians talk queer notions. Cassell, London

Solarz A 1999 Lesbian health: current assessment and directions for the future. Institute of Medicine/National Academy Press, Washington DC

Stern PN (ed) 1993 Lesbian health: what are the issues? Taylor and Francis, London

Stevens PE 1993 Lesbian health care research: a review of the literature from 1970 to 1990. In: Stern PN (ed) Lesbian health: what are the issues? Taylor and Francis, London

Stevens PE 1994 Lesbians health-related experiences of care and non-care. Western Journal of Nursing Research 16(6):639–659

Stevens PE, Hall JM 1988 Stigma, health beliefs and experiences with health care of lesbian women. Image: Journal of Nursing Scholarship 20(2):69–73

Stevens PE, Hall JM 1990 Abusive health care interactions experienced by lesbians: a case of institutional violence in the treatment of women. Response: to the Victimization of Women and Children 13(3):23–27

Terry J 1995 Anxious slippages between "us" and "them": a brief history of the scientific search for homosexual bodies. In: Terry J, Urla J (eds) Deviant bodies: critical perspectives on difference in science and popular culture. Indiana University Press, Bloomington

Trippet S, Bain J 1993a Reasons American lesbians fail to seek traditional health care. In: Stern PN (ed) Lesbian health: what are the issues? Taylor and Francis, London

Trippet S, Bain J 1993b Physical health problems and concerns of lesbians. Women and Health 20(2):59–60

Weeks J 1985 Sexuality and its discontents: meanings, myths and modern sexualities. Routledge and Kegan Paul, London

Weeks J 1986 Sexuality. Routledge, London

Weston K 1998 Families we choose. In: Nardi P, Schneider B (eds) Social perspectives in lesbian and gay studies: a reader. Routledge, London

Whisman V 1996 Queer by choice: lesbians, gay men and the politics of identity. Routledge, London

White J, Levinson W 1993 Primary care of lesbian patients. Journal of General Internal Medicine 8(1):41–47

Whitehead H 1993 The bow and the burden strap: a new look at institutionalized homosexuality in Native North America. In: Abelove H, Barale M, Halperin D (eds) The lesbian and gay studies reader. Routledge, London

Wilton T 1995 Lesbian studies: setting and agenda. Routledge, London

Wilton T 1997 Good for you: a handbook on lesbian health and wellbeing. Cassell, London

Wilton T. 1999a Second best value: lesbian, gay and bisexual life in Bristol. Summary report published by Bristol City Council and Bristol Lesbian, Gay and Bisexual Forum

Wilton T 1999b Towards an understanding of the cultural roots of homophobia in order to provide a better midwifery services to lesbian clients. Midwifery 15(3):154–164

Wilton T 2000 Sexualities in health and social care: a textbook. Open University Press, Buckingham

FURTHER READING

Gruskin EP 1999 Treating lesbians and bisexual women. Sage, London

Solarz A 1999 Lesbian health: current assessment and directions for the future. Institute of Medicine/National Academy Press, Washington

Stein E 1999 The measure of desire: The science, theory and ethics of sexual orientation. Oxford University Press, Oxford

Stern NP (ed) 1993 Lesbian health: what are the issues? Taylor and Francis, London

Wilton T 1997 Good for you: a handbook on lesbian health and wellbeing. Cassell, London

Wilton T 2000 Sexualities in health and social care: a textbook. Open University Press, Buckingham

67

Gynaecology in old age

Tara Cooper   D. Gwyn Seymour

DEMOGRAPHIC AND OTHER TRENDS

In the last two decades, gynaecologists have seen an increasing number of older women in their outpatient clinics and hospital wards (Seymour 1999a). For example, Hitzmann & Heidenreich (1994) reported that, over a 10-year period, gynaecological surgery in patients aged 80 years and over increased fourfold, from 1.1% to 4.6%.

Some of this increased activity can be accounted for by demographic change, as the relative and absolute numbers of older people have been increasing in developed societies in recent decades. Initial changes were seen in the age group 65–74 and 75–84 but the main changes are currently being experienced in the over-85s (Grundy 1998). Such demographic changes need to be considered when future health provision in gynaecology is being planned, but emotive terms such as 'demographic time bombs' have been overused (Frankel et al 2000). The percentage of the population aged 80 and over is projected to increase from 4% to 5.7% in the UK (3% to 4% in the USA) between the years 1994 and 2020 but this hardly amounts to an 'explosion' and these changes are much less than those anticipated in developing countries (Butler et al 1998).

Such demographic changes have a disproportionate effect on the practice of gynaecologists, however, because many gynaecological problems, both benign (Olsen et al 1997, Parazzini et al 2000, Samuelsson et al 1999, Scotti et al 2001, Swift 2000) and malignant (Schwartz & Rutherford 2001, Lawton 1999) become commoner with age. Older women already account for a significant proportion of gynaecological and genitourinary consultations in primary care and the rate of consultation is increasing (McCormick et al 1995). In the case of gynaecological cancer, Lawton (1999) has estimated that patients aged 65 and over account for half the deaths from carcinoma of the cervix, over 60% of deaths from carcinoma of ovary and almost 80% of deaths from carcinoma of the endometrium.

In addition, as Seymour (1998) has pointed out, factors over and above those related to demographic change are tending to increase the number of specialist surgical procedures being performed in old age. Improvements in surgical and anaesthetic techniques (including minimally invasive procedures) and advances in the therapy of advanced gynaecological malignancy (Podratz 1999, Schwartz & Rutherford 2001) have extended the range of interventions available to the specialist and there appears to be a greater willingness among older patients and referring doctors to consider surgical therapy (Seymour & Garthwaite 1999). If ageism is avoided in screening programmes (Sutton 1997) and if gynaecologists take a more proactive approach to the problems of older women, a major expansion in 'gynogeriatrics' (Stenchever 1997) is to be anticipated.

PATHOPHYSIOLOGY OF AGEING AND EFFECT ON VULVAL AND PELVIC ORGANS

The physiological ageing process in the female accelerates after the menopause, particularly in the genital tract. The ovary has a finite number of primordial follicles which are exhausted by an average age of 51. This results in falling oestrogen production and the ovary becomes less responsive to gonadotrophins which results in a gradual increase in the circulating levels of follicle-stimulating hormone (FSH) and later luteinizing hormone (LH) and a subsequent decrease in estradiol concentrations. FSH levels can fluctuate markedly several years before menses cease, but eventually follicular development fails completely, oestradiol production is no longer sufficient to stimulate the endometrium, amenorrhoea ensues and FSH and LH levels are persistently elevated.

The vagina and distal urethra are oestrogen-dependent tissues and the physiological changes which occur after the menopause are particularly linked to atrophic changes in this region. These changes may affect 10–20% of patients within

3 years and increases to 40–50% within 8 years of the menopause (Whitehead & Godfree 1992). Lack of oestrogen results in a thinning of the vaginal epithelium with loss of vascularity and elasticity. The vagina becomes shorter and narrower and there is an overall vaginal dryness which makes the region more susceptible to trauma and infection. Similar effects on the distal urethra may lead to urinary frequency, urgency and dysuria. Oestrogen and progesterone receptors are present throughout the pelvic floor (Haardem et al 1991) and oestrogen deprivation has marked effects on the urethral and anal sphincter. Urge and stress incontinence and faecal incontinence all increase in incidence with increasing age (Olsen et al 1997).

Does oestrogen deficiency predispose older women to urinary tract infection and more importantly from a practical point of view, does oestrogen treatment help prevent recurrent urinary tract infections?

A systematic review by Cardozo et al (2001) has given us a partial answer to these questions. Cardozo and colleagues refer to published evidence that the prevalence of urinary tract infections increases with increasing age so that among post-menopausal women as many as 15% of those seeking advice from their primary care doctor in the UK are suffering from urinary tract infections. However, this does not by itself prove that oestrogen deficiency is a causal factor. As early un-controlled trials had reported a beneficial effect of oestrogen on the management of recurring urinary tract infections but case control studies had come to the opposite conclusion, Cardozo et al evaluated only randomized controlled trials in their review. Five trials were considered, although there was the usual problem of different methodology and definitions of outcome, which made meta-analysis difficult. Two of the trials used oral oestrogen while three used the vaginal route but the oral doses used were not of the level used in high-dose systemic oestrogen replacement therapy. Looking at all the studies, Cardozo et al concluded that there was an overall beneficial effect of oestrogen supplementation in the prevention of recurrent urinary tract infections in postmenopausal women, with the most convincing results being obtained with the vaginal route of administration. They stressed, however, that the findings should be considered cautiously because only 384 subjects were considered in the five trials and because there were significant methodological differences. The recommendation was that a randomized placebo-controlled trial with sufficient power should be carried out in this area, although it was mentioned that such a trial might be difficult to perform because systemic oestrogen replacement therapy has now become standard postmeno-pausally in much of the developed world.

The cervix becomes more flush with the vaginal vault and stenosis of the external os is common. There is a marked reduction in uterine size so that the uterine body to cervix ratio alters from 4:1 to 2:1. The myometrium undergoes interstitial fibrosis and the endometrium regresses to a single layer of cuboidal cells with a few inactive glands. The postmenopausal ovary is small and sclerotic with absence of follicular activity. There is continuing steroidogenesis with estrone being the major postmenopausal oestrogen. Production of testosterone remains relatively unchanged and surgical oophorectomy will, therefore, result in decrease of serum testosterone levels of up to 50% (Judd et al 1994). Postmenopausal changes in the vulva include shrinkage of the skin, flattening of the labia majora and sparse greying hair.

Ageing encourages pelvic floor weakness. Research suggests that the collagenous connective tissue deterioration that is of relevance in postmenopausal osteoporosis also occurs in urogenital tissue (Jackson et al 1996). The pelvic floor musculature is also weaker after vaginal delivery and there is evidence of partial denervation occurring with childbirth which will lead to an increase in urogenital prolapse. The incidence of prolapse is difficult to define as many suffering women do not seek medical advice, but it does provide a sizeable workload for gynaecologists. A retrospective cohort study estimated that women have an 11.1% lifetime risk of undergoing a single operation for pelvic organ prolapse or urinary incontinence (Olsen et al 1997).

SEXUALITY AND AGEING

The importance of sexuality for older women is gaining recognition. Both physicians and patients are often embarrassed to bring the subject up and it is often a low priority in relation to other health problems. Longitudinal studies suggest that sexual activity remains relatively constant within a stable relationship over the years (George & Weiler 1981) and only declines with a negative life event, particularly for the male partner.

Sexuality is extremely complex and influenced by many different factors including age, self-image, physical appearance, culture, education and social attitudes. Sexual function can be a predictor of general health and affect quality of life. Age-related changes in sexual behaviour may also be the result of illness, medication, surgical procedures and pathophysiological changes.

As previously described, thinning and shortening of the vagina occur with loss of elasticity and reduced lubrication. These changes can lead to dyspareunia and avoidance of penetrative sexual activity even in the presence of desire. Urinary urgency and frequency will be aggravated by sexual activity and stress incontinence can be provoked, leading to embarrassment. Studies have also suggested a decrease in the capacity for orgasm after the menopause (McCoy & Davidson 1985) and sense of touch in the genital area may be reduced or experienced as unpleasant or painful, which can further inhibit or prevent orgasm.

Oestrogen replacement vaginally and/or systemically can improve sexual function but testosterone is also important, especially in women who have undergone surgical oophorectomy. Tibolone, an oral form of HRT, displays androgenic activity and has been shown to improve sexual symptoms including libido (Rymer et al 1994).

Dyspareunia and reduced orgasmic potential for the female partner may be influenced by modification in the physiology of the male erection (Pentimone & del Corso 1994), leading to difficulty with penetrative sex. In men over 75, 55% are impotent, commonly due to penile arterial insufficiency and/or a collateral effect of drugs such as antihypertensives and illnesses including diabetes. Physical ailments can also influence female sexual activity such as osteoarthritis, chronic lung disease and cardiovascular disease.

Body image is very important in Western cultures and ageing can influence this. Increasing grey hair, wrinkles, drooping breasts and middle-age spread do not accord with the accepted image of beauty. The addition of health aids such as glasses, hearing aids and dentures further detracts from the perception of attractiveness. Medical problems leading to procedures such as mastectomy or colostomy can also severely affect self-image although there are major improvements in breast reconstruction surgery and changes in attitude now make it more acceptable for older women to request this type of procedure.

Psychological issues are also relevant to sexuality in the elderly. Positive aspects include loss of fear of pregnancy, greater privacy from children who have left home and more free time if careers have ended. Conversely, this can result in women becoming nervous about spending extra time with their partner and being pressurized into sex, especially if they are suffering dyspareunia.

As women have a longer life expectancy than men there will always be more women living alone or in institutions. Little is known about masturbatory or same-sex activity amongst this group and it is often easier for carers to ignore the issue rather than ask embarrassing questions.

Physicians need to be more proactive in acknowledging that sexuality has an important part to play in older patients' lives and make it possible for patients to freely discuss it.

PATHOPHYSIOLOGICAL CHANGES AND RELATIONSHIP TO SURGICAL AND ANAESTHETIC RISK

The local anatomical and physiological age changes that occur in the genitourinary tract have been considered above. In this section we discuss the general systemic effects of age changes in physiology (Lakatta 1995, Lindeman 1995, Masoro 1995, Sparrow & Weiss 1995) and pathology (Seymour et al 1992) on postoperative outcome.

Studies of groups of older surgical patients tend to show a rising rate of post-operative morbidity and mortality with age (Seymour 1998, 1999b). However, as Seymour (1998) has pointed out, there is a complex relationship between age, surgery and postoperative outcome even in the absence of demographic changes.

- Many surgically treatable diseases become commoner with age.
- Age may affect surgical presentation.
- Ageist attitudes or misconceptions about the risks of surgery may lead to a low rate of elective referrals, but may result in an increased rate of non-elective referrals later on. This is worrying, as non-elective procedures tend to have higher rates of morbidity and mortality.
- Older patients may have one or more co-existing medical conditions, although this cannot be assumed in individual patients.
- Even in the absence of co-existing medical disease, there is evidence of a reduction in homeostatic reserve of most organ systems with age (Yates & Benton 1995) although this tends to influence outcome in conditions of extreme

stress (such as multiple trauma or severe sepsis), rather than in the more controlled situation found in most types of gynaecological surgery.

Attempts to disentangle these various factors have led to the overall conclusion that it is age-associated illness rather than the ageing process itself that is the main reason for the increase in postoperative morbidity and mortality often observed in groups of older people. The corollary of this is that every older patient in whom surgery is being considered needs to undergo an individual assessment. In those individuals in whom medical problems are absent, age by itself has only a minor effect on postoperative outcome (Dunlop et al 1993, Seymour 1998).

Anaesthesia

Anaesthetic methods for managing older people are becoming more and more sophisticated and are discussed in detail elsewhere (Crosby et al 1992, McLeskey 1997). Anaesthetic safety is steadily improving, although questions still remain in regard to postanaesthetic cognitive function in a small proportion of older people (Moller et al 1998).

In regard to anaesthetic drugs, Dodds (1995) has described anaesthesia in old age as 'applied clinical pharmacology with enough pathophysiology to confuse the picture'. He points out that:

- sensitivity to drugs tends to increase with age. For example, many older people are particularly sensitive to opiate analgesia and because of reduced neuronal density and reduced metabolic rate, older people also tend to be more sensitive to a given amount of any anaesthetic drug. On the other hand, neuromuscular blocking agents may have unpredictable effects in old age
- co-morbidity is important. Cardiorespiratory changes with age tend to have complex effects on the uptake of volatile gases although this is less pronounced when more insoluble gases are used. The presence of pre-existing ischaemic heart disease may complicate anaesthesia by exaggerating the effects of cardiac depressant anaesthetics. Metabolism and/or clearance of drugs by liver and kidney is also commonly affected by age but there is considerable interindividual variability
- adverse effects of drugs may also be commoner with age. For example, some anaesthetics are potentially nephrotoxic in older people and non-steroidal anti-inflammatory agents may present additional risks in old age.

Postoperative cardiorespiratory problems

While respiratory problems tend to be the leading cause of morbidity after surgery, cardiac problems together with thromboembolic problems tend to be the leading causes of mortality (Seymour et al 1992). The detailed prophylaxis of thromboembolic problems is not discussed here, but the topic is of particular interest to older women as both age and malignancy are significant risk factors for thromboembolism.

In regard to cardiac problems, for many years a major research effort has been made to identify patients with ischaemic heart disease before they undergo non-cardiac surgical procedures, so that appropriate methods of risk evaluation and therapy modification can be applied. Guidelines proposed by the American College of Cardiologists and the American Heart Association (1996) have suggested an algorithmic approach to patients in whom heart disease is suspected. Broadly, these guidelines aim to divide patients into:

- those with no or minimal cardiac risk in whom surgery can proceed straight away
- those at intermediate risk in whom non-invasive investigations are required
- those in high-risk groups in whom the main need is close monitoring and perhaps consideration of a non-surgical approach.

Postoperative respiratory complications often have their origins in atelectasis which becomes increasingly likely with age due to increased functional residual capacity. Other risk factors include preoperative lung disease, smoking and surgical incisions in the upper abdomen (Seymour 1998, 1999b). In this respect gynaecological patients are a relatively low-risk group except where major intra-abdominal procedures are being carried out. Postoperative hypoxaemia may occur within hours of surgery due to respiratory complications but a later-onset form of hypoxaemia has increasingly been recognized with the greater use of pulse oximetry. In some older patients this appears to be caused by a form of obstructive sleep apnoea which occurs with the return of rapid eye movement (REM) sleep. REM sleep tends to be suppressed in the first 2–3 days after surgery due to various factors including opiates and the stress of the operation. Prevention of this late form of hypoxaemia might require administration of oxygen for several days postoperatively. Prevention of early postoperative atelectasis is best achieved by inspiratory rather than expiratory manoeuvres and in high-risk patients these should be initiated prior to surgery (Seymour 1998, 1999b).

Postoperative cognitive function

While there appear to be no studies specifically confined to the older gynaecological patient, a number of recent studies of elective general surgical patients have explored the possibility that uncomplicated surgery and/or anaesthesia may still be associated with a permanent loss of cognitive function in a small proportion of older people. Many of the earlier studies could be criticized because they had no controls and/or because preoperative psychological testing was limited or absent. However, the first International Study of Postoperative Cognitive Dysfunction (ISPOCD) was specifically designed to meet these objections and still came to the worrying conclusion that 25.8% patients had postoperative cognitive dysfunction (POCD) 7 days after surgery and that 9.9% of all patients still had evidence of POCD on the repeat neuropsychological tests carried out at 3 months (corresponding values for controls were 3.4% and 2.8%) (Moller et al 1998). Contrary to expectations, no relationship was found between hypoxaemia and/or hypotension and the development of early or late POCD. Indeed, despite analyses of the effects of more than 25 other clinical parameters, only age showed a statistically significant

correlation with late POCD. Because the ISPOCD1 study did not provide the expected answers in regard to the prevention or treatment of POCD, ISPOCD2 is now under way looking at a variety of other factors that might be related to cognitive impairment and this is yet to report.

However, there is a more optimistic report that is available at the moment, because a subset of the ISPOCD1 patients has now been followed for 1–2 years (Abildstrom et al 2000). While about one patient in 10 still had cognitive impairment, this prevalence was now similar to the rate of cognitive impairment in non-operated controls, suggesting that some of the cognitive deficits noted 3 months after surgery were reversible. While numbers are small and confidence intervals correspondingly wide, Abildstrom et al suggest that POCD is a reversible condition in the majority of older patients undergoing non-cardiac surgery and their best current estimate for the long-term persistence of POCD is 1%.

Nutritional Problems

Malnutrition has a wide range of adverse clinical effects (Green 1999), but the benefits of preoperative and early postoperative therapy have mainly been demonstrated in severely malnourished patients with underlying gastrointestinal disease or hip fractures (Green 1999, Seymour 1998, 1999b). Detailed information on gynaecological patients is lacking, but extrapolation from general surgical patients would indicate that nutritional supplementation might be indicated in gynaecological patients who are underweight, particularly if there has been rapid weight loss immediately prior to surgery. As was stressed in a recent national audit of surgery in the over-90s, older people are also very susceptible to volume depletion on the one hand and fluid overload on the other (NCEPOD 1999). Minimally invasive surgical techniques have extended the possibilities of gynaecological therapy in patients of all ages, but may present unusual physiological challenges in older people (Peters & Katkhouda 2001).

Effect of age on surgical outcome

Do age-related changes in perineal tissues lead to a higher failure rate when reconstructive surgery is carried out to treat incontinence in older women? While age is not a reason for denying an individual reconstructive surgery, it is likely that failure rates are slightly higher in older women due to the anatomical features mentioned above. It is difficult to prove or quantify this association, however, as there are many methodological difficulties when carrying out randomized controlled trials of surgery and urinary incontinence (Black & Downs 1996, Black et al 1997) and the surgeon has many procedures to choose from (Black & Downs 1996, Black et al 1997, Jarvis 1994). In their review, Black & Downs (1996) mention age along with pathology, severity of stress incontinence, co-morbidity, previous surgery for stress incontinence, co-existence of other types of incontinence, parity and hormonal status as possible confounding factors when deciding whether a particular surgical procedure was successful or not. They point out, however, that few of these confounding factors were analysed by the majority of the 76 studies they reviewed, and they make no general statement on the effect of age.

Another factor that has a bearing on the success or otherwise of surgical treatment for incontinence is pre-existing detrusor instability (Khullar et al 1998). Detrusor instability tends to become more common with increasing age and might thus lead to a higher failure rate of incontinence procedures, particularly if bladder function was not assessed preoperatively.

SUMMARY

Women of all ages have a right to expect optimal gynaecological care and preventive and curative strategies should not be predetermined by arbitrary age limits. While fears about 'demographic time bombs' may have been exaggerated, there is a need for gynaecologists to prepare for likely changes in the range of age-related pathologies they encounter and in the legitimate expectations of their patients. These expectations are likely to include a more positive attitude to sexual activity. Many of the conditions discussed in this chapter can be managed by appropriate hormone replacement therapy. Where surgical treatment is required, an individual assessment of benefits and risks needs to be carried out: age by itself is not a contra-indication to surgical treatment.

KEY POINTS

1. Demographic change is only one of many factors that are tending to increase the number of older women consulting with gynaecologists.
2. Oestrogen deprivation has a wide range of adverse anatomical and physiological effects, but most of these are remediable.
3. There is no upper age limit for the expression of sexuality.
4. It is age-related disease rather than the ageing process itself that has the main adverse effect on postoperative outcome. Each older surgical patient requires and deserves an individual assessment of risks and benefits. Age by itself is not a contraindication to surgery or anaesthesia.

REFERENCES

Abildstrom H, Rasmussen LS, Rentowl P et al and the ISPOCD group 2000 Cognitive dysfunction 1–2 years after non-cardiac surgery in the elderly. Acta Anaesthesiologica Scandinavica 44:1246–1251

American College of Cardiology/American Heart Association 1996 Guidelines for perioperative cardiovascular evaluation for noncardiac surgery. A report of the American College of Cardiology/American Heart Association Task Force on Practice Guidelines. Circulation 93:1278–1317. For updates, see http://www.americanheart.org

Black NA, Downs SH 1996 The effectiveness for stress incontinence in women: a systematic review. British Journal of Urology 78:497–510

Black N, Griffiths J, Pope C, Bowling A, Abel P 1997 Impact of surgery for stress incontinence on morbidity: cohort study. British Medical Journal 315:1493–1498

Butler RN, Oberlink M, Schechter M 1998 The elderly in society: an international perspective. In: Tallis RC, Fillit HM, Brocklehurst J (eds) Brocklehurst's textbook of geriatric medicine and gerontology, 5th edn. Churchill Livingstone, London, pp 1445–1459

Cardozo L, Lose G, McClish D, Versi E, de Koning Gans H 2001 A systematic review of estrogens for current urinary tract infections: third report of the Hormones and Urogenital Therapy (HUT) Committee. International Urogynecology Journal 12:15–20

Crosby DL, Rees GAD, Seymour DG 1992 The ageing surgical patient. Anaesthetic, operative and medical management. John Wiley, Chichester

Dodds C 1995 Anaesthetic drugs in the elderly. Pharmacology and Therapeutics 66:369–386

Dunlop WE, Rosenblood L, Lawrason 1993 Effects of age and severity of illness on outcome and length of stay in geriatric surgical patients. American Journal of Surgery 165:577–580

Frankel S, Ebrahim S, Davey Smith G 2000 The limits to demand for health care. British Medical Journal 321:40–45

George L, Weiler SJ 1981 Sexuality in middle and late life. Archives of General of Psychiatry 38:919–923

Green CJ 1999 Existence, causes and consequences of disease-related malnutrition in the hospital and the community, and clinical and financial benefits of nutritional intervention. Clinical Nutrition 18 (suppl2):3–28

Grundy E 1998 The epidemiology of aging. In: Tallis RC, Fillit HM, Brocklehurst J (eds) Brocklehurst's textbook of geriatric medicine and gerontology, 5th edn. Churchill Livingstone, London, pp 1–17

Haardem K, Ling L, Ferno M, Graffner H 1991 Estrogen receptors in the external anal sphincter. Obstetrics and Gynecology 164:609–610

Hitzmann H, Heidenreich W 1994 Zunehmendes Lebensalter bei operativen Eingriffen. Zentralblatt fur Gynakologie 116:687–690

Jackson S, Avery N, Shepherd A, Abrams P, Bailey A 1996 The effect of oestradiol on vaginal collagen in postmenopausal women with stress urinary incontinence. Neurourology and Urodynamics 15:327–328

Jarvis GJ 1994 Surgery for genuine stress incontinence. British Journal of Obstetrics and Gynaecology 101:371–374

Judd HL, Judd GE, Lucas WE, Yen SSE 1994 Endocrine function of the post menopausal ovary: concentrations of androgens and oestrogens in ovarian and peripheral blood. Journal of Clinical Endocrinology and Metabolism 39:102–4

Khullar V, Cardozo L, Eoos K, Bidmead J, Kelleher C 1998 Effects of confounding variables and outcomes of incontinence surgery must be considered. British Medical Journal 317:143

Lakatta EG 1995 Cardiovascular system. In: Masoro EJ (ed) Handbook of physiology. Section 11, Ageing. Oxford University Press, New York, pp 413–474

Lawton F 1999 Gynaecological cancer surgery in elderly women. In: Year book of obstetrics and gynaecology, vol 7. RCOG Press, London, pp 122–128

Lindeman RD 1995 Renal and urinary tract function. In: Masoro EJ (ed) Handbook of physiology. Section 11, Ageing. Oxford University Press, New York, pp 485–503

Masoro EJ (ed) 1995 Handbook of physiology. Section 11, Ageing. Oxford University Press, New York, pp 413–474

McCormick A, Fleming D, Charlton J 1995 Morbidity statistics from general practice. Fourth national study 1991–1992. HMSO, London

McCoy NL, Davidson JM 1985 A longitudinal study of the effects of menopause on sexuality. Maturitas 7:203–210

McLeskey CH 1997 Geriatric anesthesiology. Williams and Wilkins, Baltimore

Moller JT, Cluitmans P, Rasmussen LS et al 1998 Long-term postoperative cognitive dysfunction in the elderly: ISPOCD1 study. Lancet 351:857–861

National Confidential Enquiry into Perioperative Deaths 1999 Extremes of age. NCEPOD, London

Olsen AL, Smith VJ, Bergstom JO, Colling JC, Clarke AL 1997 Epidemiology of surgically managed pelvic organ prolapse and urinary incontinence. Obstetrics and Gynecology 89:4501–4506

Parazzini F, Colli E, Origgi G et al 2000 Risk factors for urinary incontinence in women. European Urology 37:637–643

Pentimone F, del Corso L 1994 Male impotence in old age. Minerva Medica 85:261–264

Peters JH, Katkhouda N 2001 Physiology of laparoscopic surgery. In: Rosenthal RA, Zenilman ME, Katlic MR (eds) Principles and practice of geriatric surgery. Springer, New York, pp 1021–1035

Podratz KC 1999 Gynecologic oncology – on the eve of the new millennium. Gynecologic Oncology 74:157–162

Rymer JM, Chapman M, Fogelman I, Wilson P 1994 A study of the effect of tibolone on the vagina in postmenopausal women. Maturitas 18:127–133

Samuelsson EC, Victor FTA, Tibblin G, Svardsudd KF 1999 Signs of genital prolapse in a Swedish population of women 20–59 years of age and possible related factors. American Journal of Obstetrics and Gynecology 180:299–305

Schwartz PE, Rutherford TL 2001 Gynecologic malignancies in the elderly. In: Rosenthal RA, Zenilman ME, Katlic MR (eds) Principles and practice of geriatric surgery. Springer, New York, pp 834–844

Scotti RJ, Hutchinson-Colas J, Budnick LE, Lazarou G, Greston WM 2001 Benign gynecologic disorders in the elderly. In: Rosenthal RA, Zenilman ME, Katlic MR (eds) Principles and practice of geriatric surgery. Springer, New York, pp 817–833

Seymour DG 1998 Surgery and anaesthesia in old age. In: Tallis RC, Fillit HM, Brocklehurst J (eds) Brocklehurst's textbook of geriatric medicine and geronotology, 5th edn Churchill Livingstone, London, pp 235–254

Seymour DG 1999a Trends in surgery in the older patient with gynaecological problems. In: Year book of obstetrics and gynaecology, vol 7. RCOG Press, London, pp 115–221

Seymour DG 1999b The aging surgical patient – an update. Reviews in Clinical Gerontology 9:221–233

Seymour DG, Garthwaite PH 1999 Age, deprivation category and rates of inguinal hernia surgery in men. Is there evidence of inequity of access to health care? Age and Ageing 28:485–490

Seymour DG, Rees GAD, Crosby DL 1992 Introduction – demography, prophylaxis, surgical diagnosis, pathophysiology, and approach to anaesthesia. In: Crosby D, Rees G Seymour DG (eds) The ageing surgical patient: anaesthetic, operative and medical management. John Wiley, London, pp 1–90

Sparrow D, Weiss ST 1995 Respiratory system. In: Masoro EJ (ed) Handbook of physiology. Section 11, Ageing. Oxford University Press, New York, pp 475–483

Stenchever MA 1997 Gynogeriatrics: a challenge for the 21st century. Obstetrics and Gynecology 90:632–633

Sutton GC 1997 Will you still need me, will you still screen me, when I'm past 64? British Medical Journal 315:1032–1033

Swift SE 2000 The distribution of pelvic organs support in a population of female subjects seen for routine gynecologic health care. American Journal of Obstetrics and Gynecology 183:277–285

Whitehead M, Godfree V 1992 Hormone replacement therapy: your questions answered. Churchill Livingstone, Edinburgh.

Yates FE, Benton LA 1995 Loss of integration and resiliency with age: a dissipative destruction. In: Masoro EJ (ed) Handbook of physiology, Section 11, Ageing. Oxford University Press, New York, pp 591–610

68

Evidence–based medicine and effective care in gynaecology

Siladitya Bhattacharya   Allan Templeton

INTRODUCTION

Evidence-based medicine (EBM) has been defined as *'the judicious and conscientious use of current best evidence from medical care research for making medical decisions'* (Sackett et al 1996). In practice, this means finding the best available evidence, rating the quality of the published information and judging the applicability of the results of research in clinical practice. EBM views clinicians as scientists rather than inspired artists and relies on systematically reviewed evidence rather than intuitive interpretation of existing knowledge as the basis for clinical decisions. At the same time, it encourages a flexible clinical environment where preferences of patients and doctors are valued. The ideal clinical decision is a product of complex personal characteristics as well as objective research evidence (Eraker & Politser 1988). Effective implementation of EBM can only be possible if a proposed intervention has the approval of health professionals and patients.

Evidence-based care is not a new concept. What is new is its rapidly expanding role in clinical practice, including gynaecology, and its gradual acceptance by the medical fraternity. The Royal College of Obstetrics and Gynaecology (RCOG) has long acknowledged the need to update clinical practice on the basis of research findings. Since 1973, the RCOG has regularly convened study groups to address important growth areas within the specialty. These groups met, evaluated the results of recent research and conducted in-depth discussions on a variety of topics. These discussions shaped the development of clinical recommendations which were initially based on consensus but gradually gave way to genuine evidence-based guidelines. It was perceived that these would ensure the future of this discipline as a science, address inequalities of clinical care and ensure a uniform standard of excellence.

The aim of this chapter is to introduce the reader to the concept of EBM as applied to clinical gynaecology. Topics that will be covered in this context include:

- identification of evidence
- appraisal of evidence
- methods of implementing research evidence (the role of guidelines and audit)
- barriers to EBM

IDENTIFICATION OF EVIDENCE

In order to practise EBM, doctors should make use of research literature in their day-to-day clinical decision making. In actual fact, time constraints and the sheer diversity and volume of published literature make this impractical. One way of making the literature accessible to clinicians is through secondary research including systematic reviews and meta-analyses. A systematic review provides unbiased and complete exploration of evidence on a subject. It is an overview of scientific studies using explicit, systematic and therefore reproducible methods to locate, select, appraise and synthesize relevant and reliable evidence. Systematic reviews can be either quantitative or qualitative or contain elements of both. One of the main advantages of a systematic review is its ability to combine results from studies that may be too small to produce reliable results into a meta-analysis. A meta-analysis is a statistical analysis of

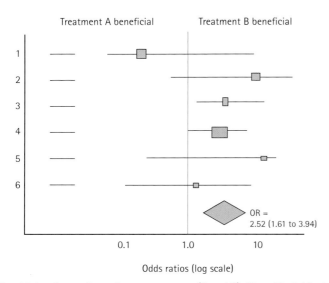

Fig. 68.1 Comparison of two treatments (A and B). Plot of individual effect estimates and pooled results expressed as odds ratio with 95% confidence intervals.

Table 68.1 Levels of evidence (US Agency for Health Care Policy and Research and SIGN)

Categories	Types of studies
Ia	Evidence obtained from meta-analysis of randomized trials
Ib	Evidence obtained from at least one randomized trial
IIa	Evidence obtained from at least one well-designed controlled study without randomization
IIb	Evidence obtained from at least one other type of quasi-experimental study
III	Evidence obtained from well-designed non-experimental descriptive studies, correlation studies and case studies
IV	Expert opinions

Table 68.2 Grading of recommendations

Grade	Recommendation
A	Requires at least one randomized controlled trial as part of the body of literature of overall good quality and consistency addressing the specific recommendation.
B	Requires availability of well-conducted clinical studies but no randomized clinical trials on the topic of recommendation.
C	Requires evidence from expert committee reports or opinions and/or clinical experience of respected authorities. Indicates absence of directly applicable studies of good quality.

the results of two or more scientific studies for the purpose of synthesizing their findings (Greenhalgh 1997, NHS CRD 1996). Thus for any intervention, a systematic review allows unbiased appraisal of outcomes across different populations and settings. A meta-analysis can then be used to make a precise estimate of the effects of a particular treatment. Its purpose is to obtain an overall ('pooled') estimate of an effect of a risk factor or intervention on the outcome of interest on the basis of data from a number of studies.

For each outcome investigated by a meta-analysis it is customary to construct a chart listing results from individual trials which have measured that particular outcome (see Fig 68.1). The odds ratio of the outcome for the experimental group compared with the control group is shown as a box with 95% confidence intervals around it. The size of the box is relative to the number of women included in each study so that it can be seen which studies should have the greater weight in the pooled analysis. The pooled summary estimate of the odds ratio is shown at the bottom of the chart as a diamond. The centre of the diamond represents the pooled odds ratio and the ends of the diamond the 95% confidence interval for the estimate.

Interpretation of findings from a systematic review are as important as for any piece of primary research. The implications for practice and for future research are important consider- ations. Systematic reviews of trials are well established and the Cochrane Collaboration represents the gold standard in the methodology of systematic reviews evaluating interventions. Systematic reviews of observational studies are also being undertaken although they present more difficulties with search strategies and techniques of meta-analysis. Clinicians and other health professionals now have access to a large volume of systematically reviewed research evidence including the Cochrane Library (The Cochrane Library. Update Software, Oxford, 2000) and DARE (Database of Reviews of Clinical Effectiveness) among others. These require regular updates and are therefore most suited to an electronic format.

APPRAISAL OF EVIDENCE

Much of the evidence in the literature is very uneven in quality and requires careful appraisal if it is to find clinical application. In selecting primary studies it is important to assess the suitability of the methodology used in the context of specific clinical questions. Randomized trials provide the best evidence for treatment but valid evidence for diagnosis, prognosis and causation may be derived from publications based on other study designs. Many common aspects of routine clinical practice have never been subjected to formal evaluation. Others are difficult to appraise due to a variety of practical and logistic reasons. These facts have to be considered while processing evidence to produce guidelines for good clinical practice.

The US Agency for Health Care Policy and Research has categorized the strength of evidence into four levels (Table 68.1). In a system adopted by the Scottish Intercollegiate Guidelines Network (SIGN) guidelines in Scotland (1995) and the recent Royal College of Obstetrics and Gynaecology (RCOG) guidelines (RCOG 1998), recommendations are graded from A to C depending on the quality of evidence on which they are based (Table 68.2). While clearly helpful in terms of classifying the strength of the evidence for each clinical intervention, this system has certain limitations. For example, since randomized controlled trials (RCTs) are not the best way to assess diagnostic tests, no recommendation regarding them can be graded as grade A, however strong the weight of evidence behind it.

Grade C includes both interventions which represent good practice but cannot be evaluated in the context of a controlled study but also those where the weight of the evidence is insubstantial. In both cases, the final decision is based on the approval of an 'expert panel'.

Despite the constraints of the grading system, this represents a relatively simple method of evaluating evidence of the majority of practising clinicians. An added feature of the RCOG guidelines is the inclusion of 'good practice points' within guidelines which, based on the clinical experience of the guideline development group, identify those interventions which are considered to represent best practice. New grading systems are being devised which address these issues, particularly in relation to diagnostic tests.

EFFECTIVE CARE: THE ROLE OF CLINICAL AUDIT AND GUIDELINES

Clinical effectiveness has been defined as: 'the use of specific clinical interventions which, when deployed in the field for a particular patient or population, do what they are intended to do – i.e. maintain and improve health and secure the greatest possible health gain from the available resources' (NHS CRD 1996). Effective care involves using treatments that combine efficacy, appropriateness and efficiency. In other words, the most desirable treatments are those which work in a real-life setting (and not just in the context of clinical trials) and are at least as effective as others of comparable cost. Systematic reviews can identify interventions that are effective but availability of research information is not enough to ensure that it is accessed and then applied in practice by clinicians (NHS CRD 1999). It is necessary to devise strategies for promoting the adoption of this evidence base by health professionals who can then incorporate it within their clinical practice. The NHS Executive's Clinical Effectiveness Initiative (1996) includes the following themes: inform, change and monitor. Essential elements of such an approach include guideline development, implementation strategies and clinical audit. These processes which are crucial for the practice of EBM have been brought together first within the Clinical Effectiveness Initiative and then more recently within the broader remit of clinical governance (Penney & Templeton 2001).

Guidelines

Clinical guidelines have been defined as 'systematically developed statements which assist clinicians and patients in making decisions about appropriate treatment for specific conditions' (Mann 1996). The aim of any guideline is to ensure that all women being considered for any gynaecological intervention should have access to a service of uniformly high quality across all relevant healthcare sectors. They are intended for gynaecologists as well as other professional groups caring for women with relevant conditions.

To be effective and relevant, guidelines must fulfil three essential criteria.

- They must be *multidisciplinary*, i.e. they must be developed by a multiprofessional working group including clinicians,

nurses and other health professionals and representatives of consumer groups.
- They must be *evidence based*: guideline development must include a systematic search for and synthesis of all available research evidence.
- They must be *evidence linked*: individual recommendations within a guideline must be explicitly linked to the strength and quality of the evidence on which they are based using a recognized grading scheme.

It is generally anticipated that national guidelines will in turn be used as a basis for the development of local protocols and guidelines in conjunction with local commissioners and providers of healthcare as well as service users. These should take into account specific needs of local service provision and the preferences of the local population. Examples of structured reviews relevant to gynaecology now abound in the literature. Recommendations from recent guidelines on infertility, menorrhagia, sterilization and induced abortion produced by the RCOG are shown in Table 68.3. The list is incomplete due to constraints of space and the reader is referred to the original documents for more information. Some examples are considered below.

Grade A recommendation

- Drug treatments for endometriosis in women with this condition and infertility do not improve conception rates and should not be prescribed for this purpose

This recommendation is based on robust evidence from a meta-analysis of randomized trials and as such there is less uncertainty about its implementation.

Grade B recommendation

- A midluteal plasma progesterone level should be checked in a regularly menstruating female as a test of ovulation

Despite the absence of randomized trials, these recommendations are supported by data from observational studies, nonrandomized experimental studies or case control studies.

Grade C recommendation

- The investigation of infertility should involve both partners from the outset

It would be unusual to find any studies addressing this issue and as such the recommendation is based on expert opinion. It is unlikely ever to be tested in a clinical trial but indicates good clinical practice.

Implementation strategies

Unfortunately methods of getting evidence into practice have lagged behind methodologies for clinical research (Freemantle et al 2000, NHS CRD 1999). A systematic review of trials of interventions aimed at helping health professionals deliver services more effectively (Oxman 1997) concluded that while all the interventions showed some effect, even relatively complex policies such as outreach visits and the use of opinion leaders have at best a limited effect. For an evidence-based system of medicine to work, it is important to identify

Table 68.3   Examples of RCOG recommendations

		Grade
Infertility		
1	The investigation of infertility should involve both partners from the outset	C
2	The female partner should be asked to take folic acid supplements	A
3	The female partner's rubella status should be checked	B
4	A general examination of both partners should be performed	C
5	A pelvic examination of the female partner should be performed	C
6	A genital examination of the male partner should be performed	C
7	A midluteal plasma progesterone level should be checked in a regularly menstruating female as a test of ovulation	B
8	Temperature charts are of limited use and couples should be discouraged from keeping them	B
9	Women with oligomenorrhoea or amenorrhoea should be referred to a gynaecologist regardless of the duration of their infertility	C
10	Diagnostic laparoscopy and dye transit rather than hysterosalpingography should be the primary investigation of the female genital tract	B
11	The initial investigation of the male partner should include two semen analyses at least 1 month apart	B
12	The postcoital test should not be used in the routine investigation of the infertile couple	B
13	Counselling by trained counsellors should be available to all couples	C
14	Drug treatments are ineffective in the treatment of idiopathic male infertility	A
15	Drug treatments for endometriosis in women with this condition and infertility do not improve conception rates and should not be prescribed for this purpose	A
16	Ovarian stimulation with intrauterine insemination is an effective treatment for couples with unexplained infertility	A
17	IVF is an effective treatment whatever the cause of infertility provided there is a reasonable likelihood that embryos can be created in vitro and then placed in the uterus with the expectation that implantation will occur	B
Male and female sterilization		
1	Both vasectomy and tubal sterilization should be discussed with all patients requesting sterilization	C
2	Vasectomy carries a lower failure rate in terms of postprocedure pregnancies and less risk related to the procedure	B
3	A history should be taken and an examination performed on all patients requesting vasectomy or tubal occlusion	C
4	Women should be informed that tubal occlusion is associated with a failure rate and that pregnancies can occur several years after the procedure. The rate should be quoted as approximately 1 in 200 lifetime risk	B

Table 68.3   (*Continued*)

		Grade
5	Mechanical occlusion of the tubes by either clips or rings should be the method of choice for tubal occlusion at laparoscopy	B
6	Local tubal anaesthesia should be used to provide additional postoperative pain relief even when a general anaesthetic is administered	A
7	Tubal occlusion should be performed after an appropriate interval following pregnancy whenever possible. Should tubal occlusion be requested in association with pregnancy, either post partum or post abortum, every effort should be made to make the woman aware of the increased regret rate and possible increased failure rate	B
Induced abortion		
1	The earlier in pregnancy an abortion is performed, the lower the risk of complications. Services should therefore offer arrangements which minimize delay	B
2	Verbal advice must be supported by accurate, impartial printed information which the woman considering abortion can understand and may take away and read before the procedure	B
3	There are no proven associations between induced abortion and subsequent infertility or preterm delivery	B
4	Abortion care should encompass a strategy for minimizing the risk of postabortion infective morbidity	A
5	Conventional suction termination should be avoided at gestations of <7 weeks	B
6	For early medical termination a dose of 200 mg mifepristone in combination with a prostaglandin is adequate	A
7	Misoprostol given vaginally is a cost-effective alternative for all abortion procedures where gemeprost is conventionally used	A
8	For women beyond 12 weeks gestation, medical abortion with mifepristone followed by prostaglandin has been shown to be safe and effective	B
9	Midtrimester abortion by dilatation and evacuation (D&E) preceded by cervical preparation is safe and effective when undertaken by specialist practitioners with access to the necessary instruments and who have a sufficiently large caseload to maintain their skills	A
Menorrhagia		
1	Full blood count should be obtained in all women complaining of menorrhagia	B
2	An endometrial biopsy is not essential in the initial assessment of menorrhagia	C
3	Tranexamic and mefenamic acid are effective treatments for reducing heavy menstrual blood loss	A
4	Antifibrinolytic drugs and non-steroidal anti-inflammatory drugs are both effective in reducing heavy menstrual blood loss in women with intrauterine contraceptive devices	A
5	Combined oral contraceptives can be used to reduce menstrual blood loss	A

Table 68.3 (Continued)

		Grade
6	A progesterone-releasing intrauterine device is an effective treatment for menorrhagia	A
7	Low-dose luteal administration of norethisterone is not an effective treatment for menorrhagia	A
8	Second-line drugs such as danazol, gestrinone and gonadotrophin-releasing hormone analogues are effective in reducing heavy menstrual blood loss but side-effects limit their long-term use	A
9	Endometrial ablative procedures are effective in treating menorrhagia	A
10	Hysterectomy is an established effective treatment for menorrhagia	A

mechanisms which can allow individual and organizational change. Multifaceted interventions targeting different barriers to change are more effective than single interventions.

Audit

Any systematic approach to changing professional practice should have at its heart plans to monitor and evaluate, maintain and reinforce any change. This cannot be accomplished without the help of clinical audit. Audit is defined as 'a clinically led initiative which seeks to improve the quality and outcome of patient care. It involves structured peer review whereby clinicians examine their practices and results against agreed standards and modify their practice where indicated' (NHS Executive 1996, (Burnett & Winyard 1998). Clinical audit performs a dual function. While it is a key component of the overall Clinical Effectiveness Initiative as a monitoring tool, it can also inform participants about standards of care, promote reflective practice and change where needed.

THE ROLE OF THE PATIENT

The practice of EBM involves more than the application of the results of research to patients. Individuals seen in a real-life clinical setting differ from the 'average' patient studied in a clinical trial (Glasziou & Irwig 1995, Lilford et al 1998). There are a number of patient-specific factors that affect the probability that the treatments will have the same effects as those measured in a trial. Differences in individual values or utilities affect the nature and severity of any potential side-effects that a person is prepared to trade off against the advantages of a treatment. To determine optimal care, clinicians should attempt to determine the risk:benefit ratio for a particular treatment targeted at a particular person. This should be done by using that person's baseline risk in conjunction with clinical prediction guidelines that can quantitate the expected potential benefit. In addition, it is necessary to incorporate the patient's own values into the decision-making process. The elements of satisfactory joint decision making include not just the disclosure of information about risks and benefits of therapeutic alternatives, but also exploration of the patient's values about both the therapy and potential outcomes (McAllister et al 2000).

Despite being accessed and appraised systematically, most research findings are currently applied intuitively. If EBM is to be seen through to its logical conclusion involving a synthesis of empirical evidence and human values then the current conflict between the explicit collection of data and its implicit use must be addressed. This area is being investigated and possible options are being evaluated. One of them is decision analysis which provides an intellectual framework for the development of an explict decision-making algorithm (Dowie 1996). When there are several treatment options which may have different effects on a patient's life, there is a strong case for offering patients a number of choices. It is possible that their active involvement in the decision-making process may actually increase the effectiveness of the treatment (Coulter et al 1999).

BARRIERS TO EVIDENCE-BASED CARE

Nature of evidence

One of the major limitations of EBM is the absence of evidence in certain key clinical areas. However, most good systematic reviews will highlight gaps in the literature that need to be addressed by suitably designed studies. Where studies do exist, the findings can be misleading due to design flaws leading to bias or poor generalizability. The results of a meta-analysis are inevitably influenced by the quality of the primary studies included in it. Poor studies exaggerate the overall estimate of treatment effect and may lead to incorrect inferences (Khan et al 1996). On the other hand, stringent inclusion criteria can lead to rejection of most of the published data in poorly researched areas. Failure to research the 'grey literature', i.e. unpublished abstracts, conference proceedings, PhD theses, or limiting the search to papers published in a specific language can also contribute to bias in study selection.

Inconsistencies in classification

Despite the use of explicit review protocols and grading systems, there are differences in the way evidence is processed by different review bodies. Even when the data are certain, recommendations for or against interventions will involve subjective value judgements by a guideline development group that may not necessarily be the right choice for individual patients (Woolf et al 1999). Recommendations based on evidence can also be influenced by opinions, clinical experience and composition of the guideline development group. This is reflected in differential grading of the available evidence and in the interpretations of the evidence base and can lead to confusion in interpretation by clinicians.

Consensus and expert opinion

Although necessary in dealing with areas that are unlikely to be researched adequately, the value of consensus of opinion and expert opinion can be and often is challenged. The beliefs to which experts subscribe can be based on misconceptions and personal recollections that may represent population norms (Kane 1995). This can be avoided by inclusion of other health professionals and consumers of healthcare within the guideline development group.

Traditional reliance on empirical therapy

In many clinical areas, there has been a long tradition of empirical therapy which is hard to break. Clinicians have traditionally tended to base their knowledge and practices on standards of practice generated by other clinicians – standards that are often at odds with the scientific evidence. In a 1998 study 76% of clinicians surveyed were aware of the concept of evidence-based practice but only 27% were familiar with methods of critical literature review and faced with a problem, most would consult a colleague rather than the evidence (Olatunbsun et al 1998).

Technological innovation

Occasionally, new developments in health technology are incorporated into clinical practice before being fully evaluated in terms of effectiveness and safety. Within gynaecology there are a number of examples in assisted reproduction and minimal access surgery where enthusiasm to adopt new techniques (often prompted by popular demand) has overtaken the need to assess the weight of evidence relating to them.

Costs and side-effects

Most trials continue to concentrate on clinical outcomes and this is where the evidence is strongest. Few primary studies and fewer systematic reviews have focused on cost-effectiveness as an outcome. This can lead to a situation where an effective treatment may not be affordable. Similarly, side-effects may limit the use of an otherwise successful treatment.

Patient preference

Individual preferences on the part of patients can compromise evidence-based practice due to rejection of effective treatments. On the other hand, it is clear that adoption of evidence-based care can be facilitated by empowering patients with appropriate information to allow them to drive clinical decision making along evidence-based lines.

CONCLUSION

The purpose of clinical research is to generate new knowledge on how to treat individual patients and how best to deliver healthcare services. The purpose of EBM and its component activities such as audit and clinical guidelines is to maximize the extent to which clinical practice is based on research evidence. Within gynaecology, recent years have seen considerable progress in strategies aimed at seeking and appraising evidence. The next hurdle involves dissemination of this evidence and its incorporation into routine clinical care. A comprehensive approach towards getting research evidence into practice is promoted by NHS clinical effectiveness and clinical governance initiatives. What is being challenged is the way doctors make clinical decisions and the way patients respond to them.

KEY POINTS

1. Evidence-based medicine involves the use of the best available evidence from medical care research to make clinical decisions.
2. Recommendations regarding clinical practice are best graded according to the quality of evidence on which they are based.
3. Guidelines are systematically developed statements which assist clinical decision making.
4. Effective care involves using treatments that combine efficacy, appropriateness and efficiency.
5. Strategies need to be developed to overcome existing barriers to the wider implementation of evidence-based medicine in gynaecology.

REFERENCES

Burnett AC, Winyard G 1998 Clinical audit at the heart of clinical effectiveness. Journal of Quality in Clinical Practice 18:3–19
Coulter A, Entwhistle V, Gilbert D 1999 Sharing decisions with patients: is the information good enough? British Medical Journal 318(7179):318–322
Dowie J 1996 The research–practice gap and the role of decision analysis in closing it. Health Care Analysis 4:5–18
Eraker SA, Politser P 1988 How decisions are reached: physician and patient. In: Dowie J, Elstein A (eds) Professional judgement: a reader in clinical decision making. Cambridge University Press, New York, pp 379–394
Freemantle N, Harvey EL, Wolf F, Grimshaw JM, Grilli R, Bero LA 2000 Printed educational materials: effects on professional practice and health care outcomes. Cochrane Database of Systematic Reviews. Issue 4
Glasziou PP, Irwig LM 1995 An evidence based approach to individualising treatment. British Medical Journal 311:1356–1359
Greenhalgh T 1997 Papers that summarise others (systematic reviews and meta-analysis). In: Greenhalgh T (ed) How to read a paper: The basics of evidence based medicine. British Medical Journal Books, London
Kane RL 1995 Creating practice guidelines: the dangers of over reliance on expert judgement. Journal of Law and Medical Ethics 23:62–64
Khan KS, Daya S, Jadad A 1996 The importance of quality of primary studies in producing unbiased systematic reviews. Archives of Internal Medicine 156(6):661–666
Lilford RJ, Pauker SG, Braunholtz DA, Chard J 1998 Getting research findings into practice: decision analysis and the implementation of research findings. British Medical Journal 317(7155):405–409
Mann T 1996 Clinical guidelines: using clinical guidelines to improve patient care within the NHS. NHS Executive, London
McAllister FA, Strauss SE, Guyatt GH, Haynes RB 2000 Users' guide to the medical literature. XX. Integrating research evidence with the care of the individual patient. Evidence Based Medicine Working Group. Journal of American Medical Association 283(21):2829–2836
National Health Service Centre for Reviews and Dissemination 1996 Undertaking systematic reviews of research on effectiveness. NHS CRD, University of York
National Health Service Centre for Reviews and Dissemination 1999 Getting evidence into practice. Effective Health Care 5:1
NHS Executive 1996 Promoting clinical effectiveness: a framework for action in and through the NHS. NHS Executive, London

Olatunbsun CA, Eduard L, Pierson RA 1998 British physicians, attitudes to evidence based obstetric practice. British Medical Journal 316:365–366

Oxman AD 1997 No magic bullets: a systematic review of 102 trials of interventions to help health care professionals deliver services effectively or efficiently. North East Thames Regional Health Authority, London

Penney GC, Templeton A 2001 The clinical impact of audit and guidelines. Advances in Obstetrics and Gynaecology 19:8–13

Sackett DL, Rosenberg WMC, Gray JAM, Haynes RB, Richardson WS 1996 Evidence based medicine: what it is and what it isn't. British Medical Journal 312:56–57

Woolf S, Grol R, Hutchinson A, Eccles M, Grimshaw J 1999 Potential benefits, limitations and harms of clinical guidelines. British Medical Journal 318:527–530

69

Medico-legal issues and clinical risk: how clinical governance improves care

Nick J. Naftalin   Christine McManus
Susanna Nicholls   Aidan Halligan

INTRODUCTION

There has been growing concern and effort to achieve a measurable improvement in the quality of health services in Britain over the last decade. A number of high-profile tragedies, often involving the repetition of the same mistakes by different people, have reconfirmed the desirability of a large-scale review of the quality of healthcare in the NHS.

With its White Paper in 1997 (DoH 1997) the government affirmed its commitment to improving quality and made individuals accountable for the delivery of high-quality, safe healthcare. The importance of clinical governance as a means to improve quality and build capacity for improvement into NHS organizations was further developed by Scally & Donaldson (1998) shortly after.

Since 1998 the means by which clinical governance will help make the delivery of continuous quality improvement inherent within all healthcare systems has become better understood. The support structures which underpin clinical governance and the new duty of quality – the National Institute for Clinical Excellence (NICE), the Commission for Health Improvement (CHI), the National Service Frameworks (NSFs), the National Clinical Assessment Authority, the Modernisation Agency – and mechanisms to ensure patient advocacy and empowerment are recognized as central elements in the delivery of quality.

In the autumn of 2000 the Chief Medical Officer published the results of work by an expert group which reviewed learning from adverse events in the NHS (DoH 2000a). The publication of this report sets the context for a review of risk, safety and the associated medico-legal issues.

PROFESSIONAL SKILLS AND CLINICAL NEGLIGENCE

Advances in knowledge and technology have in recent decades immeasurably increased the power of health care to do good, to prevent or treat illnesses against which there was previously no defence. Yet they have also immeasurably increased the complexity of health care systems ... and with such complexity comes an inevitable risk that at times things will go wrong. ... The great majority of NHS care is of a very high clinical standard ... serious failures are uncommon (but) ... in health care when things go wrong the stakes are higher than in almost any other sphere of human activity (DoH 2000a).

Clinical governance and a commitment to improving quality invite healthcare professionals to proactively protect patients, and confidence in the health service, by developing an awareness of their own competencies and limitations and the risks involved in delivering healthcare.

Clinical negligence

Negligence involves a 'lack of care' in some aspect of treatment provision. Where there is a 'lack of care' in some respect and that lack of care causes an adverse result, then there has been negligence. An unwanted outcome which was unpredictable, or was a known risk carefully guarded against, is not negligence.

Professionals accused of negligence (and their teams) can endure long-term stress as they become the 'second victim' (Wu 2000) of the event. Professionals and organizations need the skills and resources to adequately support teams when errors occur because those involved can find themselves isolated, castigated and unsupported. When staff 'find dysfunctional ways to protect themselves' the cycle of damage is perpetuated.

It helps that 'whistle blowing' is covered by the Public Interest Disclosure Act 1999. This Act gives significant statutory protection to employees who disclose information reasonably and responsibly in the public interest and who are victimized as a result.

A no-blame culture may be defined as one in which individual blame is levelled only for behaviour where:

- incidents have not been reported
- problems are recurrent for the individual despite support and counsel
- breaches of the law have occurred.

Dealing with actual and alleged clinical negligence costs the NHS several hundred million pounds each year in damages and legal costs. Some 60% of these litigation costs are generated within obstetrics. The most expensive component of these costs is the claims made on behalf of brain-damaged babies. Compensation in obstetric claims is substantial: sums of up to £3 million per case are not uncommon (with legal costs per case of up to £200 000).

Developing a memory

It is acknowledged not only that there are too many mistakes made in healthcare at present, but that the same mistakes are being made by different people. The NHS has a poor track

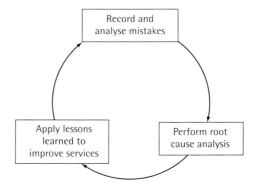

Fig. 69.1 The active learning cycle.

record when it comes to learning from experience. We need to learn how to complete an active learning cycle (Fig. 69.1).

To make proactive learning a reality requires a change in culture so that 'blame is no longer passed around until the music stops and someone has to face it' (Crossley 2000). We have to work towards a culture where there are no 'second victims', where there is effective communication, integrity and honesty and a comprehensive understanding of a whole-systems approach.

When avoidable accidents happen it is only right that compensation is awarded. The following section describes the main stages in the claim/litigation process (as they stand at the moment) and the possible interactions of the patient (claimant), clinicians and hospital (defendant) and the lawyers involved.

What constitutes negligence?

All healthcare professionals owe their patient a *duty of care;* that is to say, they must provide care to a reasonable standard. To prove negligence the claimant (based on her expert evidence) must demonstrate that there has been a breach of that duty of care. She must also then show that the breach of duty has caused her injury (known as 'causation'). Breach of duty and causation are collectively referred to by lawyers as 'liability.'

Breach of duty

In considering breach of duty one must ask whether the service provided fell below the reasonable standard. The 'reasonable standard' applied is formulated on the Bolam (1957) and Bolitho (1997) tests.

- *Bolam* – a surgeon must perform surgery to a reasonable standard, i.e. that which a recognized body of professional opinion (which does not have to be the majority) would agree was acceptable. He does not have to operate to the level of the leading specialist unless he purports to be such a specialist.
- *Bolitho* – the court also has to be satisfied that the expert(s) in a case, relying on a 'body of professional opinion' (i.e. a recognized school of thought in the particular clinical area), can show that such opinion has a logical basis. Where appropriate, the expert must have considered the comparative risks and benefits of a particular course of action and have reached a defensible (i.e. a logical) conclusion.

Causation

Once it has been shown that there has been a breach of duty it is then necessary to demonstrate that the breach caused the injury under consideration. Sometimes the case is not clear; pre-existing conditions and previously unknown circumstances (for example, abnormal anatomy) need to be taken into consideration. It is for the experts (see below) to confirm that any breach of duty which is discovered led to the injury in question.

Furthermore, the injury must have been 'foreseeable'. The test applied is one of 'the balance of probabilities,' i.e. was it more likely than not? Was there more than a 50% chance that this or a similar injury would occur as a consequence of the identified breach of duty?

If there are several causes it is sufficient that the negligent act or omission made a material or substantial contribution to the injury. However, a defendant will only be liable to compensate the patient/claimant to the extent that they caused the injury/disease (Holtby 2000).

Causation is difficult to establish in some cases where, for example, there has been a failure to prevent cervical cancer due to the misinterpretation of cervical smears. The experts have to analyse not only the contribution of the 'under-' or 'misreporting' to the eventual development of cancer, but also the type of cancer, the timeframes involved, the effect on health and survival had it been picked up earlier/treated appropriately and the effects of treatment ultimately necessary.

An injury can include, in certain circumstances, psychological trauma or psychiatric ill health. There must usually have been a physical injury linked to the psychiatric illness.

THE LITIGATION PROCESS

Ten key stages in a claim are identified in Box 69.1. These are typical or 'stagepost' events in the litigation process between the start of the patient journey at referral to hospital through the formal complaints procedure to a trial.

Not all claims follow the same pattern or include all the stages listed below. Some may start at stage 4, for example, if the patient goes straight to a solicitor. If there is a limitation problem (see below for an explanation of the time limits for bringing a claim) then proceedings (i.e. a claim form – stage 8) may be the first point of entry into the process.

The courts are managing cases far more proactively under the new Civil Procedure Rules (CPR) (April 1999). One of the aims of the CPR is to make litigation a course of last resort.

WHAT CREATES A CLAIM FROM AN EPISODE OF TREATMENT?

Despite the increasing trend towards litigation, most patients and their families still retain the highest regard for the healthcare professionals who treat them and are sympathetic to the pressures which doctors and nurses face. However, this goodwill is lost when they find, for example, that they have postoperative complications for which they were not prepared before surgery and for which there is no satisfactory explanation. Patients lose confidence when the doctor avoids their questions

Box 69.1 Clinical negligence: chronological events in negligence claim

1	Adverse event	Unexpected complication/event
2	Complaint	Made by the patient within 6 months of the incident or within 6 months of realizing that something went wrong, and in any event, within 12 months of the incident itself
3	Solicitor	Instructed by patient to initiate legal action
4	Disclosure	Of medical records to the patient and/or her advisers
5	Expert opinion	Requested by claimant's lawyer as to grounds for claim of negligence. If there are no grounds the claim should progress no further
6	Letter of claim	From patient to the defendant setting out the injury suffered, the allegations of negligence and the details of any proposed losses/expenses. The letter should be sent to the defendant in accordance with the pre-action clinical negligence protocol (see stage 6, p. 979) – there are then 3 months for the defendant to investigate and decide whether the claim is justified or defensible
7	Claim form/ particulars of claim	Proceedings commenced by the claimant
8	Defence	The defendant's formal response to the claim
9	Experts' meeting	The experts appointed by both claimant and defendant meet to discuss the issues in dispute and to resolve as much as is possible
10	Trial	If there remain issues in dispute

or appears to avoid the discussion. Frustration, fear and resentment build up if it seems that nobody listens.

Failure to recognize and address promptly a patient's concerns may transform a patient with anxieties into a patient contemplating litigation. By understanding and improving systems and by thinking through meaningful and effective communication, complaints and litigation can be reduced, with a consequent increase in satisfaction for patients and for staff.

INFORMED CONSENT: WARNING THE PATIENT OF RISKS

The General Medical Council (GMC) has issued detailed guidance to help professionals and patients achieve informed consent (GMC 1998). The guidance highlights the importance of an equal, trusting relationship between doctor and patient, one which is founded on ensuring and enabling patient autonomy. There are clear guidelines about how and what information should be shared and by whom. The importance of developing excellence in communication skills is emphasized and there is guidance about consent in relation to, for example, the mentally incapacitated, children and emergency treatment.

The following principles are important.

- There must be a shared understanding – this may involve consideration of appropriate language and any language barriers; the condition of the patient (for example, if the patient is in great pain or sedated, it may be appropriate to conduct the consent process in the presence of family/next of kin/witnesses) and ethnic and cultural differences. It is important that sufficient time is made available to ensure shared understanding because 'obtaining consent cannot be an isolated event: it involves a continuing dialogue' (GMC 1998).
- Consent should be obtained by a competent clinician capable of carrying out the procedure.
- The consent should be current in relation to the intervention. If consent is obtained some time in advance of the planned intervention then it is wise to check (and to document) that there have been no changes in the interim and that the patient recalls what was previously discussed.
- A contemporaneous record should be made in the patient's notes. In other words, it is not sufficient to 'just get the consent form signed'. An entry should be made in the medical notes of the conversation held, the risks which were explained and any particular features of the consent, for example the involvement of interpreters or presence of next of kin.

EVENTS IN CLINICAL NEGLIGENCE CLAIM

Stage 1: adverse event

Case Study

A surgical patient initiated a claim as a result of complications arising from a swab retained at an operation 1 year previously.

The history

Infection resulted in leg amputation being required some weeks postoperatively in another hospital. A retained swab was found in the amputated limb. When the claim was received and the notes were reviewed the surgeon's contemporaneous operation note described an uncomplicated procedure. Liability was therefore admitted by the surgeons involved and negotiation of a settlement was advised.

Investigation

Further investigation revealed that an incident report had been filed by the theatre sister following the first operation. This report was internal to the theatre department and was not mentioned in the patient's notes. It described a swab count which had indicated a missing swab and detailed how the wound had been reopened and explored immediately – with no swab found. An image intensifier had been brought into theatre and the operation site had been screened. A further wound exploration was carried out and when nothing was found the wound was closed for a second time.

New interpretation

Although the missing swab was never found appropriate action had been taken to give reasonable assurance that the swab was not in the wound.

Systems at fault

No written record of the events occurring in theatre after discovery that a swab was missing appeared in the patient's notes. This resulted in the delayed diagnosis and suboptimal management of the subsequent infection. The patient had not been informed of the events in theatre.

Learning issues arising from the case study

- Shared systems of incident reporting, collected centrally, are vital.
- When adverse events occur, help must be sought from seniors and from other staff in appropriate disciplines.
- All documentation must accurately reflect events as they occur and not become a 'routine' statement.
- Documentation is an important form of communication which is essential as reference and to inform and guide correct management.
- The subsequent management (rescue) of an adverse incident may influence the outcome as much as the incident itself.
- Verbal communication with the patient when adverse events occur is a protection against subsequent clinical and legal consequences.

Stage 2: complaints procedure

Most frequently it is poor communication which leads to complaints and subsequent litigation. A brief outline of the legal stages of the complaints procedure follows.

Complaints procedure (stage 1) is referred to as 'local resolution'. Under the Patient's Charter a patient has a right to a full written explanation of events from the trust's chief executive. This should usually be provided within 4 weeks' of receipt of the written complaint.

Complaints procedure (stage 2) is called 'independent review'. If the patient is not satisfied with the chief executive's response at stage 1, the matter can be referred to a special panel. Whether or not the matter should go to this panel for independent review is decided by the 'convenor' who assesses the case after stage 1 if the matter remains unresolved at that point. The two other options available to the convenor are to dismiss the claim or to refer it back for further local resolution. The health authority/trust must appoint one (or more) of its non-executives to act as convenor/s.

It is open to the patient to pursue the complaint to the Health Service Commissioner (the Ombudsman) if after independent review she is still dissatisfied or if independent review is denied. The complaints procedure is automatically halted if legal action is commenced.

Stage 3: instructing a solicitor

Clinical negligence claims are expensive to investigate. It is often not until several expert reports have been obtained on her behalf that a patient will know whether or not there has been negligence.

Very few patients can afford to fund a claim themselves. The Legal Services Commission (the successor to the Legal Aid Board) only funds cases run by firms of solicitors to whom they have granted a franchise in recognition of their experience in this field.

The NHS Litigation Authority (NHSLA) funds the defence of the larger claims against health authorities and trusts, i.e. where the claim involves NHS treatment. The various unions and medical defence societies fund the defence of claims against clinicians where the claim is made in relation to private patient treatments or 'Good Samaritan' treatment.

Stage 4: disclosure of medical records

For the claimant and her advisers to properly analyse the treatment given they need to have access to her medical records. The clinical negligence pre-action protocol (see stage 6 below) indicates that the records should be sent to the claimant within 40 days of the request.

The claimant is entitled to see her medical records. The exceptions to this general principle are:

- if it would be harmful to the patient (it is for this reason that clinician(s) must review the records and confirm that they can be disclosed) or
- if a document was created at a time when a claim was contemplated, as these may include reference to the claim. Such comments may be 'privileged', i.e. they might fall within the client/lawyer confidentiality relationship.

Similarly, when a defendant is dealing with a claim they too must have access to the claimant's medical records in order to fully investigate the allegations. Where there are other records not held by the defendant, for example GP notes, the claimant must consent to these being released to the defendant and his advisers.

On 2 October 2000 the Human Rights Act 1998 (the Act) came into force in England and Wales. It raises a number of questions. For example, does disclosure of a patient's medical records for review by the defendant's advisers constitute an infringement of the patient's right to privacy under Article 8? What happens when a patient refuses to disclose her records? A defendant is unlikely to be able to properly assess a case without considering the medical records.

Prior to the introduction of the Act courts had been prepared to 'stay' (i.e. suspend) a claim where the patient declined to give consent for disclosure of records. The impact of the Human Rights Act on this will become clearer as time passes and the law is tested.

Stage 5: the role of the medical expert

An 'expert' will be a practising clinician, usually one working in the same field as the clinician whose treatment is under scrutiny. He will usually be a recognized leader in that area – an experienced practitioner, an academic or an individual involved in research who has published or who has peer reviewed scientific/academic contributions on the topic.

The expert is asked to give an opinion about whether or not there has been a breach of the duty of care. Experts must remain impartial: their duty is to the court and not to the party who has instructed them. As causation can be very complex in clinical negligence cases, each party will usually instruct their own expert in any given field. However, where appropriate, the courts are actively encouraging parties to instruct one expert on a joint basis, who will send the report to both parties at the same time.

The expert must decide whether or not in his view there has been negligence. There may be some years between the incident and judgement on it and science, knowledge and thinking may have moved on. The expert's view, and any subsequent legal decisions, are always made in light of the information which was commonly available in the public and medical arena at the time of the event and what was standard practice at that time.

If the report of the expert appointed by the claimant does not support her claim she will usually choose not to disclose it. In that event her claim should go no further.

Stage 6: letter of claim

The pre-action clinical negligence protocol was introduced by the CPR to support the aim of making litigation a course of last resort. As the name suggests, its aim is to regulate the parties' conduct at the pre-action stage. It entails the following.

1. The claimant sends the defendant a letter of claim setting out the basis of the claim.
2. An acknowledgement must be made within 14 days of receipt.
3. A substantive response to the claim must be given within 3 months.

If the defendant persists in defending an indefensible claim, forcing the claimant to issue proceedings, the court may eventually order the defendant to pay penalty interest to the claimant.

If the matter cannot be resolved by the above means, proceedings are issued.

Stage 7: claim form/particulars of claim

Issuing proceedings

Proceedings are started in the civil courts by way of a 'claim form' which sets out the basis of the claim. This will be sent to the defendant. The allegations of negligence are specified in the 'particulars of claim' (which may be sent to the defendant at the same time as the claim form or which may follow separately, but which must be served within 4 months of the claim form being issued by the court). A claim for clinical negligence is a claim for 'personal injury'. The claimant must serve a medical report confirming details of the injury suffered.

Time limits: the 'limitation period'

Proceedings must be initiated within 3 years of the alleged negligent incident or within 3 years of the claimant realizing that an incident has occurred which occasioned injury. This is known as the 'limitation period'. However, the timing of legal proceedings in relation to events which set them in train can be difficult. It is not always immediately obvious that someone has suffered an injury: if sterilization clips have not occluded the lumen of a fallopian tube, for example, the failing may not be discovered until a pregnancy occurs which may be years after surgery.

In the case of a child the 3-year period begins when they reach 18 years. If they do not have the mental capacity to manage their affairs this 3-year period effectively never commences. So it is not uncommon to see claims notified for the first time many years after the original incident occurred which can make it difficult to trace all the healthcare professionals involved and to obtain complete sets of records.

Stage 8: the defence

On receiving the claim form and particulars of claim, the defendant NHS hospital, on behalf of the clinician(s) against whom the allegations are made, must prepare and serve a defence stating why the claim is defensible. If the claim is brought by a private patient against a clinician he must prepare a defence (but his defence union will want to arrange this). It is not sufficient simply to deny negligence: under the CPR the court can strike out frivolous claims and bare denials alike.

The clinician(s) against whom negligence is alleged should be closely consulted and statements taken from all concerned (if this has not already been done). Healthcare professionals should have full access to the medical records for this purpose.

The claim process can take anything from 12 months to several years to complete depending on the nature of the case.

Once the court receives the defence it fixes a timetable, in consultation with both parties, for the various stages in the proceedings to be completed. A hearing may be required for this.

Claims are allocated by the court to one of three process pathways ('tracks'):

- the small claims track, for claims up to £5000 (where the 'personal injury' element, as opposed to the losses caused by the injury, does not exceed £1000)
- the fast track, for claims between £5000 and £15 000 (where the 'personal injury' element exceeds £1000)
- the multi-track for cases which exceed £15 000 or are particularly complex in nature.

Clinical negligence claims are generally allocated to the multi-track process.

Stage 9: experts' meetings

It used to be the case that neither side saw the other's expert evidence until the trial. Today parties are encouraged to be more open.

Each side must obtain permission from the court to call experts to give evidence in specific areas of clinical practice. Expert reports must be disclosed to the other party; evidence that has not been disclosed in accordance with the timetable laid down by the court will generally be excluded by the judge at trial.

Usually experts in 'like' specialties are ordered by the court to meet to discuss the claim in an attempt to narrow the issues in dispute and so shorten the length of any trial. After such a meeting the experts are required to produce a joint statement confirming those issues on which they agree and those which remain in dispute.

Stage 10: trial

A trial is a traumatic experience for all concerned. The claimant will have to remember and relate events the telling of which may well be uncomfortable. She will have to face cross-examination by the barrister for the defendant. Healthcare professionals who were involved in some way in the original event will similarly have to give evidence and undergo cross-examination. All parties involved will be required to recall and recount, under some conditions of stress, an event which may be some distance past. It may be difficult to remember with clarity.

The hearing on liability

Assuming it has not been possible to resolve the dispute between the parties by negotiation, mediation or experts' meetings, the claim will proceed to a trial which will be before a judge: there is no jury.

The judge will then make a finding based on the evidence heard. If he finds for the claimant she will be entitled to compensation for the injury.

Damages/compensation

The purpose of compensation is to place the injured person in the same position they would have been in had the injury not occurred, to the extent that this is possible by financial means.

Damages are divided into the following categories.

- *General damages* – for 'pain, suffering and loss of amenity' resulting from physical injury itself. The actual amount is based on awards made in previous cases involving similar injuries (see the Judicial Studies Board Guidelines). At present the maximum award in this category is £200 000 and in the past this sort of figure has been awarded for the worst cases of brain damage.
- *Special damages* – in respect of expenses and losses which result from the injury and which have been incurred up to the date of settlement/trial.
- *Future loss* – damages are awarded under this heading for expenses/losses which will be ongoing in the future.

Structured settlements and lump sums

If a 'lump sum' is agreed investment decisions become important. The money needs to produce sufficient flow of income to cover all costs expenses detailed above, for the required period.

As an alternative to a lump sum figure, a 'structured settlement' may be agreed. A structured settlement is usually only appropriate where the compensation is substantial i.e. over £1 million. It entails annual payments to meet ongoing expenses. These are paid for the remainder of the claimant's life or for an agreed number of years. A structured settlement provides certainty for both sides and the annual payments are currently tax free.

SHOULD A CLINICIAN ADMIT TO A PATIENT THAT SOMETHING HAS GONE WRONG?

In some situations the matter is clear. If a patient has the wrong kidney removed or the wrong leg amputated the mistake is obvious. The clinicians and the hospital complaints/claims manager should be able to take swift action to investigate such an incident and should be prepared to provide an apology and an early explanation to the patient and her family and negotiate compensation (with the prior approval of the NHSLA or relevant professional body) where appropriate.

The full details of the systems breakdown which allowed such a catastrophic event to occur are often not immediately clear. Although an apology can be given, a full explanation is not possible until the matter has been investigated properly and the appropriate experts have considered all the relevant information. However, like the institutions which employ them, doctors owe their patients a professional duty of candour. This entails the patient being told whatever is known about what has happened to them and what is likely to happen in the future.

In 1997 the NHSLA issued a circular (97/C10) to the chief executives and finance directors of all NHS bodies outlining its views on giving explanations and apologies. In respect of explanations it states:

Arguably, greater care needs to be taken in the dissemination of explanations so as to avoid future litigation risk, but, for the avoidance of any doubt, NHSLA will not take a point against any NHS body or any clinician seeking NHS indemnity, on the basis of a factual explanation offered in good faith before litigation is in train. We consider the provision of such information to constitute good clinical practice ... provided that facts, as opposed to opinions, form the basis of the explanation nothing is likely to be revealed which would not subsequently be disclosable in the event of litigation.

In respect of apologies it states:

... it is both natural and desirable for those involved in treatment which produces an adverse result, for whatever reason, to sympathize with the patient or the patient's relatives and to express sorrow or regret at that outcome. Such expressions of regret would not normally constitute an admission of liability, either in part or in full, and it is not our policy to prohibit them, nor to dispute any payment, under any scheme, solely on the grounds of such expression of regret.

CLINICAL GOVERNANCE: IMPROVING QUALITY, AVOIDING MISTAKES

Clinical governance has been defined as 'a framework through which NHS organizations are accountable for continually improving the quality of their services and safeguarding high

standards of care by creating an environment in which excellence in clinical care will flourish' (Scally & Donaldson 1998). Its 'fit' in the government's framework for quality development is illustrated diagrammatically in Figure 69.2.

Clinical governance is a 'way of working' and a 'behaviour' which espouses teamwork, leadership and communication alongside clinical effectiveness and risk management as skills integral to the effective delivery of patient-centred, quality healthcare.

Previous approaches to quality have been fragmented. Obstetricians and gynaecologists have been in the forefront of quality improvement since 1957 when the Confidential Enquiry into Maternal Deaths was first introduced and they have continued to implement national quality development initiatives with more recently, for example, the Confidential Enquiry into Stillbirths and Deaths in Infancy (1989).

Even so, at a clinical team and directorate level, it is clear that action loops have not always been closed; the expected return from clinical audit has been disappointing overall. Initiatives such as patient-focused care, total quality management and process redesign (re-engineering) demonstrated a capacity for significant quality gain but failed to gain wide acceptance, perhaps because they were felt to be management rather than clinically led. The evidence-based medicine school which started in North America (Evidence Based Medicine Working Group 1992) continues to offer impetus and support to quality development but lacks the means of integration into the everyday delivery of healthcare.

Implicit in the implementation of clinical governance is a duty of care. Clinical governance is an integral component of the NHS Plan (DoH 2000b) and is supported by a robust framework to facilitate the delivery of quality and to review on an ongoing basis its effectiveness in practice (Box 69.2).

NATIONAL SUPPORT MECHANISMS FOR CLINICAL GOVERNANCE

The National Institute for Clinical Excellence (NICE) commissions experts to review best evidence and produces definitive guidelines which represent agreed best practice. At the time of writing these have not impacted significantly in obstetrics and gynaecology but inevitably as time passes and national guidance is translated for local use, they will begin to have a positive impact.

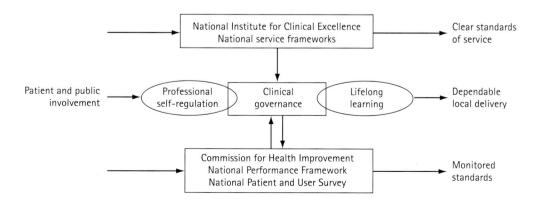

Fig. 69.2 Setting, delivering and monitoring standards. From *A first class service: quality in the new NHS*. Department of Health, 1998.

Box 69.2   Key elements of the NHS quality strategy

Standards
National Institute for Clinical Excellence
National Service Frameworks
National Performance Framework
Royal College clinical standards

Local duty of quality
Clinical governance
Clinical controls assurance

Assuring quality of individual practice
Annual appraisal
Revalidation
National Clinical Assessment Authority
GMC performance procedures

Scrutiny
Commission for Health Improvement
Royal College Accreditation for Training visits

Learning mechanisms
Adverse incident reporting
Learning networks
Continuing professional development

Patient empowerment
National Patient and User Survey
Complaints procedure
Patient forums

Underpinning strategies
Information and information technology
Research and development
Education and training

The Commission for Health Improvement (CHI) has begun the process of reviewing every health service organization in the country and will repeat this process every 3–4 years or more often should the initial review prove unsatisfactory. The Commission also evaluates the quality of care delivered by organizations and how the organizations are supporting continuous improvement. It will also address the difficult task of assessing the culture of organizations to ascertain whether the environment will enable the delivery of excellent care and lifelong learning.

The CHI will work with trusts and regional health authorities to create action plans which enable organizations to address issues arising out of the review process. It will also work with organizations such as the Modernisation Agency's Service Improvement Team, the Clinical Negligence Scheme for Trusts (CNST), Royal Colleges and the GMC to ensure that national standards which are promulgated by authoritative sources are being implemented. The CHI will have a role in evaluating the implementation of NICE guidelines and National Service Frameworks.

The Department of Health has also created a Clinical Governance Support Team (NCGST), a component of the Modernisation Agency. This team works with organizations at board and clinical team levels to first catalyse the cultural shift required to enable quality improvement initiatives and then to provide leaders with the skills and competencies which underpin change management so that they can steer practical devel-

opment of clinical governance 'on the ground'. The NHS comprises a wealth of vastly talented individuals, all of whom can make an invaluable contribution to improving service. Many ideas and inspirations have previously been allowed to 'wither on the vine' because NHS culture has not had the capacity or structure to support staff as they capture, develop, project manage, implement and monitor improvement change. The NCGST and the Modernisation Agency provide a mechanism and support to help organizations and clinical teams first change culture and then develop a vision and plan for its delivery.

LOCAL IMPLEMENTATION OF CLINICAL GOVERNANCE

Under the 1999 Health Act Trust chief executives are accountable for delivering the statutory duty of quality as represented by clinical governance, but clinical governance is the responsibility everyone who works in a healthcare environment. All trusts are obliged to create an agreed organizational strategy which is widely shared, understood and followed. The details of the strategy might vary from trust to trust but the principles will not. Patient and carer opinion, obtained through whatever mechanisms are appropriate – for example, patient forums, workshops, focus groups, analysis of complaints – must underpin the strategy.

A quality development strategy ensures that all aspects of care provided – corporate and team – are evaluated on an ongoing basis. Performance information must be regularly provided for those who need it (managers and clinical teams), in an accessible format which gives feedback on improvement initiatives and facilitates swift interpretation to inform future development.

Such strategic development information will provide the basis for the annual appraisals and job plan reviews which are now part of national policy. Objectives arising from annual appraisals will be aligned to quality improvement objectives of service and should be simply expressed and easily measured. For doctors, such objectives and their achievement will form part of their personal development plan and will become an integral part of the revalidation process of the GMC. It will be incumbent upon trusts to provide, at organizational level, the means by which agreed objectives can be achieved. This will be done through programmes of continuing professional development.

Learning 'systems lessons'

A number of important lessons about systems awareness were learned during the process (see case study).

- An ambiguous thromboprophylaxis guideline led to misinterpretation as to dose of heparin; this caused a number of cases of postoperative bleeding.
- Confusion between 'seniority' and 'competence' led to doctors in training being left with operations outside the scope of their ability.
- Lack of supervision in the outpatient clinic resulted in patients being listed without potential difficulties (recognizable to the more experienced practitioner) being highlighted.

- Overconfidence and an unwillingness to disturb senior staff out of hours led to delays in the recognition and early management of postoperative complications.

Using information to inform improvement action: a case study

The Gynaecology Directorate of a teaching trust

Case Study

A casual enquiry

For the second time in a month the afternoon theatre list started late. Enquiry revealed that a patient from the morning list had had to return to theatre and this had pushed back the afternoon's list. Theatre sister remarked that this was not uncommon – it had occurred perhaps four or five times in the previous month.

Further enquiry

The Clinical Director was notified. Ward staff concurred; they were aware that several patients had had to return to theatre. No such occurrences had been reported to the department's Risk Manager via the adverse incident system. An internal review was established and a consultant and the Risk Manager investigated.

The facts

Preliminary data showed 14 patients had been returned to theatre over the previous 4 months. An additional three patients had suffered significant operative complications.

The analysis

A departmental meeting was held and the problems and their origins were discussed. Whilst some of the complications were simple misfortune, there were some clear signs of system failures which the department addressed. A number of improvements in practice were agreed and implemented.

Closing the improvement action loop:

- The thromboprophylaxis policy was amended.
- The selection process for theatre cases was improved.
- Systems of delegation to doctors in training were improved.
- Improved communication mechanisms and data collection and analysis systems around postoperative complications were agreed.

Demonstration of improvement

A re-audit after implementation revealed that unscheduled returns to theatre had fallen by over 90% in the subsequent 6-month period.

An example: using information to guide practice

Table 69.1 summarizes a review of results at 6 months following endometrial ablation/resection (1995–97) broken down by operating surgeon (A–G).

The clear message from these data is that the performance of such procedures should be concentrated in the hands of one or two individuals and 'occasional operating' should be discouraged. Clear guidelines issued by the Royal College cover such areas as colposcopy and gynaecological oncology for the same reason (RCOG 1999a,b).

All too often audit is self-directed at areas where performance is already known to be excellent, rather than being directed towards fields of practice where both subspecialty interest and outcome measures are lacking. Obtaining a comprehensive information base at the individual/team level covering activity, compliance with guidelines, outcome measures and patient satisfaction will be fundamental to the deliverance of a clinical governance strategy and ultimately to revalidation.

Clinical governance encompasses and enhances previous quality initiatives and the systems set up to deliver them – clinical audit, clinical effectiveness and clinical risk management. Clinical governance must become part of the daily routine of healthcare. It should appear in one form or another on the agenda of every meeting in the hospital and its quality principles should inform every patient consultation, every intervention and every strategic decision. In the wake of recent service failures, and with obstetrics and gynaecology prominent in the league table of litigation expenses, it is a good time for obstetricians and gynaecologists to review how clinical governance can best serve their profession.

In 2000, the Chief Medical Officer chaired an expert group which has reviewed risk management in the NHS. The subsequent report (DoH 2000a) states that in a service which is working well.

- serious failures of standards of care are uncommon
- serious failures of a similar kind do not recur
- incidents where services have failed in one part of the country are not repeated elsewhere
- systems are in place which reduce to a minimum the likelihood of serious failure in standards of care
- attention is paid to monitoring and reducing levels of less serious incidents.

The NHS falls short of many of these challenges. The report reveals that:

- one-fifth of healthcare organizations do not have reporting systems covering the whole organization
- less than half provide specific training on risk management or incident reporting

Table 69.1

	A	B	C	D	E	F	G
Total number of patients	9 (8%)	17 (14%)	14 (12%)	22 (18%)	49 (42%)	3 (3%)	4 (3%)
Amenorrhoea	1 (11%)	1 (6%)	0 (0%)	0 (0%)	22 (45%)	0 (0%)	2 (50%)
Light period	3 (33%)	4 (24%)	0 (0%)	5 (23%)	15 (31%)	1 (33%)	1 (25%)
Repeat treatment	2 (22%)	4 (24%)	8 (57%)	11 (50%)	1 (2%)	1 (33%)	1 (25%)

- less than one-third provide guidance to staff on what to report
- one-third do not require clinicians to report unexpected operations, complications or unexpected events.

Addressing these issues will depend on both national and local policy and is of particular importance in obstetrics and gynaecology. Past NHS experience suggests that top-down initiatives alone cannot deliver and sustain quality improvement and all too often crisis or adverse publicity is the lever for change in practice. Clinical governance will seek to influence culture and attitudes and modify 'the way we do things around here' so that there is local flexibility to design and deliver best service within a clear and supportive framework. For development of a successful risk management strategy, and the consequent development of 'learning organizations', there must be an awareness and an understanding of systems.

A commitment to analysing and reviewing current systems is important. Clinical governance is an opportunity for professionals who can currently deliver quality care, despite existing systems, to challenge professional and agency barriers which have before been considered inviolable. Clinical governance offers a chance to forge new partnerships, to review pathways and methods of care and to redesign systems to make them effective and efficient for patients and for staff.

A 'NO-BLAME' CULTURE. NOT 'WHO WENT WRONG?' BUT 'WHAT WENT WRONG?'

All organizations have safety mechanisms which have grown up to protect against error and accident. Healthcare staff depend on these defences to shield them and their patients from service failures. Some defences are 'hard' (mechanical) – safety switches, for example, or computer software that does not allow entry of mismatched data. Some defences are termed 'soft' (to do with people and processes) – double checking drugs, countersigning instructions. Hard and soft defences together should ideally create an impregnable barrier and eliminate error. In reality some defences will be flawed and may fail.

When defences fail sequentially a 'gap' or 'channel' is created via which a hazard meets a victim (Fig. 69.3).

Understanding systems means realizing that in the past defence systems have failed staff and patients. Poor reporting mechanisms, lack of centralized information, a failure of 'active learning' (building in the lessons) has resulted in missing 'the learning experience'.

We can learn a great deal from non-healthcare organizations about risk management; industries such as mining, railways, sport and particularly airlines can demonstrate examples of learning from experience from which the NHS can benefit. The airline industry runs a Confidential Human Factors Incident Reporting Programme (CHIRPS) and its Mandatory Occurrence Reporting System (MORS) apportions blame only when incidents are not reported. British Airways has published figures showing how the numbers of critical incidents fell as reporting (and reviewing and learning) increased (Fig. 69.4).

Ten recommendations emerge from an *organisation with a memory* (DoH 2000).

- Introduce a mandatory reporting scheme for adverse healthcare events and specified near misses.
- Introduce a scheme for confidential reporting by staff of adverse events and near misses.
- Encourage a reporting and questioning culture in the NHS.
- Introduce a single overall system for analysing and disseminating lessons from adverse healthcare events and near misses.
- Make better use of existing sources of information on adverse events.
- Improve the quality of relevance of NHS adverse event investigations and inquiries.
- Undertake a programme of basic research into adverse healthcare events in the NHS.
- Make full use of the new NHS information systems to help staff access learning from adverse healthcare events and near misses.
- Act to ensure that important lessons are implemented quickly and consistently.
- Identify and address specific categories of serious recurring adverse healthcare events.

This last recommendation includes a challenge to 'by 2005 reduce by 25% the number of instances of negligent harm in the field of obstetrics and gynaecology which result in litigation'.

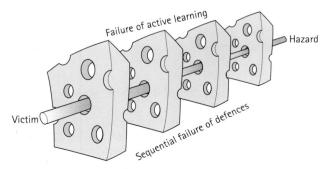

Fig. 69.3 How accidents happen.

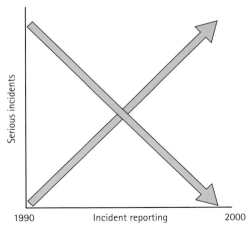

Fig. 69.4 The relationship between incident reporting and the number of serious incidents.

Work has already begun to design systems and guidelines to support staff as they implement these recommendations. Clinical governance initiatives will have facilitated the open, no-blame, shared learning environment which will make such structures meaningful and productive.

TRAINING AND DEVELOPMENT

It is well established that it is doctors in the early days of their postgraduate training who make the most mistakes (Lesar et al 1990, Wilson et al 1998, Wu 2000). In recognition that traditional didactic teaching may not adequately equip the new generation of doctors for the environment in which they will work, the GMC (1993) introduced problem-based learning into the undergraduate curriculum. This is now beginning to produce doctors who can see the whole picture, who are not afraid to say they don't know, who value the contributions of others and are used to working in teams and sharing experience to come to the wisest decision.

Postgraduate training, historically obtained by a combination of time and experiential learning, has been replaced by structured training (DoH 1993) with in-built processes of formative and summative appraisal which ensure that knowledge and skills are adequately and regularly assessed so that identified deficiencies can be addressed.

Work in the aviation industry revealed that most accidents were related to breakdowns in crew co-ordination, communication and decision making. Once these 'human factors' were recognized to be at least as important as the better known mechanical ones, the industry addressed training and selection of pilots. The ability to co-ordinate activities, learn from error and recognize shared contribution to problem solving were all seen to be important.

Box 69.3 CNST standard 10

- The arrangements are clear concerning which professional is responsible for the woman's care at all times.
- There are referenced, evidence-based, multidisciplinary policies for the management of all key conditions/situations on the labour ward. These are subject to review at intervals of not more than 3 years.
- There is an agreed mechanism for direct referral to a consultant or a midwife.
- There is a personal handover of care when medical shifts change.
- There is a labour ward forum, or equivalent, to ensure that there is a clear documented system for management and communication throughout the key stages of maternity care.
- All clinicians should attend 6-monthly multidisciplinary in-service education/training sessions on the management of labour and CTG interpretation.
- There is a lead consultant obstetrician and clinical midwife manager for labour ward matters.
- The labour ward has sufficient medical leadership and experience to provide a reasonable standard of care at all times.
- Emergency caesarean section can be undertaken rapidly and in a short enough period to eliminate unacceptable delay.
- There is a personal handover to obstetric locums, either by the post-holder or senior member of the team, and vice versa.

The industry began to train whole crews together, rather than individuals alone, as experience, research and analysis demonstrated that safety and quality performance were functions of how well the crew functioned as a whole.

The Clinical Negligence Scheme for Trusts (CNST) issues standards, which are organizational and generic; some are specific to maternity services (see Box 69.3). All hospital trusts in England subscribe and achievement of the standards at levels 1, 2 and 3 are rewarded by a commensurate discount on annual premium. The standards reflect excellence in risk management practice and should be familiar to all clinical staff.

LEADERSHIP

The key to successful roll-out of the clinical governance strategy — including improvement in risk management — is the development of leaders within our profession who have the skills and competencies to facilitate teamwork.

Resistance to change is potentially so strong that without consistent, unswerving commitment from leaders, programmes for change are unlikely to be successful

The skills required to manage a clinical department or a clinical team and to deliver on complex agendas such as the CNST standards are numerous. They include abilities in project leadership, change management, motivation and communication. A good leader needs appraisal skills — the ability to give and receive feedback, manage information, listen and counsel.

Training leaders in an important task for the NHS and the establishment of the NHS Leadership Centre is a recognition that this is an important development area. The profession needs time for reflection, and time to devote to learning from experience. In the past these have been areas which have not been afforded a high priority.

COMMUNICATION

Effective two-way communication is a key factor in obstetrics and gynaecology, as in other areas of healthcare. Deficiencies in communication are the most common underlying factor in complaints and litigation and by implication must be one of the most important factors in substandard care. Poor communication (mixed messages, failing to check understanding, not checking for possible communication barriers) during consultation or while obtaining consent has already been discussed. However, all communication between professionals, verbal or written, is a high-risk area.

Times of transition – the introduction of locums, periods when staff in training rotate – are times of particular risk. Guidelines and systems for effective communication, plus appropriate training and induction of staff, are vital. Organization of adequate handover on the delivery suite, for example, and instructions to report evolving clinical situations to senior staff should be relatively simple to facilitate with organizational guidelines. All too often baseline information to specify and illustrate the problems, and the appropriate guidelines, are lacking or are not consistently implemented.

Improving technology will help improve communication. Typed entries into case records, e.g. operation notes, help clarity and the introduction of an electronic patient record (EPR) will ultimately improve the quality, speed and accuracy of communication. It may, however, be many years before the widespread introduction of the EPR so self-help in the interim is essential.

ATTITUDE

Skills and knowledge are continually updated by most clinicians and are specifically addressed in continuing professional development programmes. Attitude, expressed particularly through verbal and non-verbal communication, may be less commonly updated throughout professional life. Recognition of changing patient and carer expectations and development of appropriate responses by accessing appropriate training programmes will aid the implementation of clinical governance and thereby reduce clinical risk.

ROLE OF THE ROYAL COLLEGES IN STANDARD SETTING

The Royal College of Obstetrics and Gynaecology's Clinical Standards Group has introduced 15 key standards relating to quality of care. Any department wishing to be accredited for teaching will have to comply with these (Box 69.4).

Thus the NHS and obstetricians and gynaecologists, with a concerted and substantive approach to improving quality through clinical governance, are beginning to reduce risk and improve safety for patients and staff. The revolution has begun!

Box 69.4 RCOG clinical standards (2001)

Labour ward: minimum standards
All labour wards should have a lead consultant obstetrician and clinical midwife manager.

Antenatal ultrasound scanning
The performance of the 20-week anomaly scan should be a minimum standard (defined in the RCOG report). If a unit cannot deliver to this minimum standard the woman should be referred to an appropriate unit.

Colposcopy
The colposcopy service should have a designated lead clinician and lead nurse.

Ovarian cancer
All patients suspected of having ovarian cancer should be operated on by a designated gynaecological surgeon or referred to a gynaecological oncologist.

Vulval cancer
Women with vulval cancer should receive their care in cancer centres staffed by the relevant multidisciplinary teams.

Induced abortion
Because the earlier in pregnancy an abortion is performed, the lower the morbidity, services should offer arrangements (e.g. telephone referral and direct access) which minimize delay.

Infertility
The secondary and tertiary management of infertility should take place in dedicated, specialist infertility clinics staffed by an appropriately trained multiprofessional team with facilities for investigating and managing problems in both partners.

Box 69.4 *(Continued)*

Menorrhagia
The initial investigation of menorrhagia should be according to a locally available protocol derived from the RCOG guideline.

Sterilization
Verbal and written information must be provided advising those requesting sterilization of the consequences, risks, failure rate and sequelae associated with the procedure.

Intimate examinations
A chaperone should be offered to all patients undergoing intimate examination in gynaecology and obstetrics irrespective of the gender of the gynaecologist. If the patient prefers to be examined without a chaperone this request should be honoured and recorded in the notes.

Outpatient times
Antenatal clinics: each unit should allow 15 minutes for each new and return visit. Thus during a 3-hour clinic session an experienced doctor, with no other commitments, might expect to see a maximum of 12 patients.
Gynaecology clinics: each unit should allow 20 minutes for new and 10 minutes for return visits. There should be approximately the same proportion of new and returning patients. Thus during a 3-hour clinic session an experienced doctor, with no other commitments, might expect to see 6 new and 6 returning patients.

Cervical and vaginal cancer
Women with cervical cancer should receive their care in cancer centres and be managed by the relevant multidisciplinary team.

Endometrial cancer
Women diagnosed with endometrial cancer should be carefully assessed preoperatively, including imaging to assess myometrial invasion and histopathology to assess tumour type and degree of differentiation.
Women with higher risk tumours should receive their care in cancer centres and be managed by the relevant multidisciplinary team.

Early pregnancy loss
All units should provide an early pregnancy assessment service with direct access for general practitioners and patients. Ideally, the service should be sited in a dedicated area with appropriate staffing. It should be available on a daily basis, at least during the normal working week.

Urogynaecology
All units providing urogynaecology should have local protocols in place for the initial management of patients in primary care.

KEY POINTS

1. What is Negligence?
2. Whistle blowing
3. No blame culture
4. Duty of Care – Causation – Liability
5. Bolam/Bolitho
6. The Litigation Process
7. The 'Pre-action protocol' – trying to avoid litigation
8. System approach to adverse event analysis

KEY POINTS (*CONTINUED*)

9. NICE/CHI/Clinical Governance Support Team
10. Organization with a Memory
11. Training and Development
12. Clinical Negligence Scheme for Trusts

REFERENCES

Bolam v Friern Hospital Management Committee 1957 Weekly Law Reports 1:582

Bolitho (deceased) v City and Hackney Health Authority 1997 Times Law Reports 13 November

Crossley T 2000 Doctors and nurses should monitor each other's performance. British Medical Journal 320:1070–1071

Department of Health 1993 Hospital doctors training for the future. Report of the Working Group in Specialist Medical Training. Stationery Office, London

Department of Health 1997 The new NHS. Stationary Office, London

Department of Health 2000a An organisation with a memory: report of an expert group on learning from adverse events in the NHS. Stationery Office, London

Department of Health 2000b The NHS plan. Stationery Office, London

Evidence-Based Medicine Working Group 1992 Evidence-based medicine: a new approach to teaching the practice of medicine. Journal of the American Medical Association 268:2420–2425

General Medical Council 1993 Tomorrow's doctors: recommendations on undergraduate medical education. General Medical Council, London

General Medical Council 1998 Seeking patients' consent: the ethical considerations. General Medical Council, London

Holtby v Brigham & Cowan (Hull) Ltd 2000 All England Law Reports 3

Lesar T, Briceland L, Delcoure K, Parmalee C, Masta-Gornic V, Pohl H 1990 Medication prescribing errors in a teaching hospital. Journal of the American Medical Association 263:2329–2334

Royal College of Obstetrics and Gynaecology 1999a Clinical recommendations for the management of vulval cancer. Royal College of Obstetrics and Gynaecology, London

Royal College of Obstetrics and Gynaecology 1999b Recommendations for service provision and standards in colposcopy, Royal College of Obstetrics and Gynaecology, London

Royal College of Obstetrics and Gynaecology 2001 Clinical standards. Royal College of Obstetrics and Gynaecology, London

Scally G, Donaldson LJ 1998 Clinical governance and the drive for quality improvement in the new NHS in England. British Medical Journal 317:61–65

Wilson D, McArtney R, Newcombe R et al 1998 Medication errors in paediatric practice: insights from a continuous quality improvement approach. European Journal of Pediatrics 157:769–774

Wu AW 2000 Medical error: the second victim. British Medical Journal 320: 726–727

Index

APC gene, 530, 531
Apocrine gland adenocarcinoma, vulva, 574, 616
Apologies, to patients, 979
Appendices epiploicae, 28
Appendicitis, acute, 896, 897
Appendix, mucinous cystadenoma, 667
Arcuate arteries, 459–460
Arcuate nucleus, *204*, 205
Arcus tendineus fasciae pelvis, 744, *817*
Argon laser, 75
Arias-Stella phenomenon, 375
Aromatase, 170, **171**, 298
    defects, 175
    gene (*CYP19*) mutations, 175
    inhibitors, in breast cancer, 717
    in ovarian steroidogenesis, 172
Arrhythmias, 121, 147
Arteriovenous malformations, uterine, 109
Arthritis, sexually acquired reactive (SARA), 911
Artificial anal sphincter, 873
Artificial urinary sphincter, 780, *781*
Ascites
    cytology, 683, 684
    drainage, 142, 255
    management of recurrent, 689
    ovarian tumours, 670, 682, 683
Asherman's syndrome (intrauterine adhesions)
    amenorrhoea/oligomenorrhoea, 232
    complicating hysteroscopy, 51
    diagnostic hysteroscopy, 38, 44, *45*
    hysteroscopic treatment, 49
Aspirin, low-dose, 125, 127, 354
Assisted reproduction treatments (ART)
    ectopic pregnancy risk, 374
    in endometriosis, 323, 324, 498–499
    ethics, 335–336
    future prospects, 336–337
    laboratory techniques, 321–322
    for lesbians, 955
    in male infertility, 310–312
    micromanipulation techniques, 310–312
        number of treatment cycles, 317, *318*
        see also Intracytoplasmic sperm injection
    number of attempts, 327
    oocyte collection, *see* Oocyte, recovery
    in ovarian failure, 240, 248–249
    ovarian stimulation, *see* Superovulation, for assisted conception
    perinatal outcome, 333–334
    potential health risks, 328–334
    preimplantation genetic diagnosis, 334–335
    selection of patients, 318–319
    sperm and oocyte donation, 327–328
    success rates/factors affecting, 322–328
    uterine fibroids and, 482
    see also In vitro fertilization
Association of Marital and Relationship Therapy, 457

Asthenozoospermia, 286, 305
Asthma, 121, 446
Asylum seekers, 949
Atelectasis, postoperative, 142, 145–146, 962
Athletic amenorrhoea, 233–234
Atrial natriuretic peptide, 403
Atropine, 794
Attitude, clinicians', 984
Audit, clinical, 969, 981
Autocrine action, 153, *154*
Autoimmune disease
    ovarian failure, 223, 236, 418
    recurrent miscarriage, 353–354
    vasectomy and, 444
Autoimmunity, in endometriosis, 498
Autonomic nerves, pelvic, 33–34, 745
    surgical damage, 591
Autonomic neuropathy, diabetic, 752
Axillary lymph nodes, 700
    dissection, 716
    radiotherapy, 716
    sentinel node biopsy, 716
Azithromycin, **908**, 912
Azoospermia, 285, 304–305
    aetiologies, 285
    hormonal induction, 442
    obstructive, 285, 303, 310, 311
    treatment, 311
AZT (zidovudine), 925
Azygos arteries (of vagina), 32

Baclofen, 810
Bacterial infections, vulva, 607–608
Bacterial vaginosis (BV), 610
    miscarriage and, 346, 352
    PID and, 892, 893
    vaginal discharge, 915–916
Bacterial virulence factors, 858
Bacteriuria, 857
    asymptomatic (ASB), 857, 862
Baden & Walker classification of prolapse, 813, *814*
Bad news
    breaking, 730–732
    definition, 730
Bag specimen retrieval systems, laparoscopic, 62
Balanitis xerotica obliterans, 604
Baldness, *see* Alopecia
Balloon tamponade
    laparoscopy-associated haemorrhage, 140
    post-hysteroscopy haemorrhage, 50
Barium enema, 93, 846
Barium meal and follow-through, 846
Bartholinitis, 607
    chlamydial, 910
    gonococcal, 909
Bartholin's (greater vestibular) glands, 26
    carcinoma, 624
Basal arteries, 32
Basal arterioles, 460
Basal body temperature (BBT), 287–288, 440

Basal cell carcinoma, vulva, 624
Basal ganglia, control of micturition, 746
Bathing, postoperative, 143
BAX protein, 539
Bayesian modelling, 181
BCG vaccine, intravesical therapy, 831
Bcl-2, 480, 539
Bedrest, in threatened miscarriage, 349
Behavioural changes, in PMS, 402
Behavioural therapy
    overactive bladder, 796
    psychosexual problems, 453, 456, 729
    in stress incontinence, 773–774
Benefits Enquiry Line, 737
γ-Benzene hexachloride, 919
Benzodiazepine receptors, peripheral, 169
Bereavement, 736–737
    sources of support, 737
β-adrenergic blocking drugs (β-blockers), 125, 409
β-adrenoreceptors, bladder, 745
β-human chorionic gonadotrophin (β-hCG), 656
    assays, 105, 656
    in early pregnancy, 106, 107
    in ectopic pregnancy, 164, 376, 377
        methotrexate therapy and, 381, 382
        serial measurements, 376
    ovarian tumours, 671, 691, 692
    vaccines, 441
    see also Human chorionic gonadotrophin; Pregnancy, tests
Bethanechol, 810
Betrayal, in child sexual abuse, 934
Bilharzia, *see* Schistosomiasis
Billings method of family planning, 439–440
Bimanual examination
    in cervical cancer, 589
    at colposcopy, 566
    ovarian tumours, 670
Binding assays, hormone, 160–161
Bioassays, 160
Biochemical tests, preoperative, 125–126
Biofeedback
    in anorectal disorders, 873, 874
    in overactive bladder, 796
    in stress incontinence, 773–774
Biological agents
    in breast cancer, 717
    in cancer therapy, 556
    in ovarian cancer, 690
Biopsy
    breast, 701–702, 703, 715
    cervix, 589
    cone, *see* Cone biopsy
    embryo, 334
    endometrial, *see* Endometrial sampling/biopsy
    fistula, 847
    lymph node, *see* Lymph nodes, biopsy
    testicular, 285, 308
    vulva, 573, 602

Hyperandrogenism, 387
  cutaneous signs, 390–391
  ovarian, 174–175
  in polycystic ovary syndrome, 264, 265
  recurrent miscarriage and, 353
  treatment, 396–398
  see also Hirsutism; Virilization
Hyperhomocysteinaemia, 354
Hyperinsulinaemia
  cutaneous signs, 391
  ovarian steroid synthesis and, 175
  in polycystic ovary syndrome, 251, 259, 265, 392
  pubertal development and, 219
Hyperlipidaemia, 265–266, 422
Hyperprolactinaemia, 234–235, 248
  causes, 235, 248
  diagnosis, 238, *239*
  drugs causing, **235**
  idiopathic, 235
  male infertility, 308
  in placental-site trophoblastic tumour, 657
  recurrent miscarriage and, 353
  treatment, 239–240, 248, 249–250
  see also Prolactinoma
Hypertension
  in congenital adrenal hyperplasia, 193
  HRT in, 422
  oral contraception and, 435, 436
  in polycystic ovary syndrome, 265
  preoperative assessment, 120
Hyperthyroidism
  amenorrhoea/oligomenorrhoea, 237
  in gestational trophoblastic disease, 656
  HRT, 423
  in struma ovarii, 666
Hypertrichosis, 388
Hypervolaemia, hysteroscopy-associated, 50
Hypnotherapy, in overactive bladder, 796
Hypogastric nerves, 745
Hypogonadism
  hypergonadotrophic, 233, 238–239, 248–249
    see also Ovarian failure
  hypogonadotrophic, 232–233
    delayed puberty, 223
    diagnosis/management, 238, 249
    idiopathic, 233
    male infertility, 285, 304
    management in males, 309
    ovulation induction, 252
  normogonadotrophic, 249
Hyponatraemia, hysteroscopy-associated, 50
Hypo-osmotic swelling test, 286
Hypopituitarism, 233
Hypospadias, 195, 312, 331
Hypothalamic–pituitary–adrenal axis, 173
Hypothalamic–pituitary axis
  anatomy, 203–204
  control during menstrual cycle, 212–213
  function, 204–207
  modulation by ovarian steroids, 209–210

neurotransmitters/second messengers modulating, 207–209
Hypothalamic–pituitary–ovarian (H–P–O) axis, 203–213, *232*
  disorders, 229, 232–237
  feedback control mechanisms, *212*
Hypothalamic–pituitary–testicular axis, 297–298
Hypothalamus
  anatomy, 203, *204*
  hormones, **205**
  neural connections, 204
  regulation of pituitary secretion, 204–207
  space-occupying lesions, 233, 249
  see also Gonadotrophin-releasing hormone
Hypothermia, postoperative, 145
Hypothyroidism
  amenorrhoea/oligomenorrhoea, 235, 237, 238
  HRT, 423
  menorrhagia, 465
  precocious puberty, 220
Hypoxaemia, postoperative, 962
Hysterectomy
  abdominal, 66, 131–132
    in endometrial cancer, 640
    in endometrial stromal sarcoma, 645
    in endometriosis, 509
    for menstrual disorders, 471
    ovarian tumours, 690
  avoiding bladder injury, 136–137
  in bladder outlet obstruction, 811
  in cervical adenocarcinoma in situ, 570
  cervical carcinoma after, 595
  chronic pelvic pain after, 887
  in CIN, 569
  in endometrial hyperplasia, 578
  fistulae complicating, 838–840, 842, 855
  haemorrhage after, 145
  HRT after, 419
  laparoscopic, 66
  laparoscopic-assisted vaginal (LAVH), 66
    for menstrual disorders, 471
    for uterine fibroids, 485
  for menstrual problems, 471, 473
  in ovarian borderline tumours, 684–685
  in ovarian cancer, 685–686, 687
  in pelvic congestion syndrome, 885
  in placental-site trophoblastic tumour, 662
  for PMS, 410
  premature ovarian failure, 418
  prolapse after, 819
  prophylactic, in familial cancer, 533
  radical (Wertheim)
    in cervical cancer, 590–592
    complications, 591–592
    in endometrial carcinoma, 641–642
    nerve-sparing, 591
    postoperative care, 591–592
    preoperative care, 590
    procedure, 590–591
    results, 592
    in vaginal cancer, 626

routes, 65–66, 131–132
  subtotal, carcinoma of cervical stump, 595
  for uterine fibroids, 484–485
  vaginal, 65–66, 131–132
    in endometrial cancer, 640
    for menstrual disorders, 471
    in uterine prolapse, 821–822
    VAIN after, 571, 572
  vs endometrial ablation, 49, 473
Hysterosalpingo contrast sonography (HyCoSy), 363
  see also Sonohysterography
Hysterosalpingography (HSG), 82, 83–84
  in adenomyosis, 86
  in fistula investigation, *844*, 846
  in infertility, 288, *289*
  in recurrent miscarriage, 351
  in tubal disease, 363–364
  in uterine malformations, 200
  vs hysteroscopy, 41
Hysteroscopes, 39–40
  disinfection/sterilization, 43
  flexible, 40
  operative, 39, *40*, 47–48
  rigid, 39
  sheaths, 40
Hysteroscopy, 37–52
  complications, 49–51
  contact, 40
  contraindications, 38–39
  diagnostic, 41–43
    anaesthesia, 42
    in endometrial cancer, 639
    endometrial preparation, 41–42
    indications, 37–38
    in menstrual disorders, 469
    normal appearances, 44
    pathology seen, 44, *45*, *46*
    positioning, 42
    postoperative care, 43
    procedure, 42–43
    uterine fibroids, 483
  distension media, 40–41
    hazards, 50
  future developments, 52
  in infertility, 289
  instrumentation, 39–40, 46–48
    inadequate, 39
  operative, 46–49
    consent issues, 51–52
    endometrial ablation, 472
    endometrial preparation, 49
    instruments, 46–48
    myomectomy, 48, 49, 486–487
    sterilization, 49
  outpatient, 43–44, 46
  pre-procedure imaging, 41
  skills, 44, **46**
  training and learning curve, 44–46
  uterine anatomy, 41, *42*
Hysterosonography, hystero-ultrasonography, *see* Sonohysterography

Weight (cont'd)
    in polycystic ovary syndrome, 263,
        266–267
Wein classification, lower urinary tract
        dysfunction, 770
Wexner scoring system, 748, **750**
'Whistle-blowing', 974
William's vulvovaginoplasty, 198, 224
Witnesses, medical, in rape/sexual abuse, 941
Wolffian duct, 2, 5, 6, 189–190
    development in male, 190
    regression in female, 190
    remnants, 6, 190
    see also Mesonephric duct
Wolffian system, in XY agonadal individuals,
        7, 8
Women's Health Initiative (WHI), 420
Women's International Study of Long
        Duration Oestrogen after the
        Menopause (WISDOM), 420
Wound
    care, 143
    classification, rape victims, 937,
        938–939
    dehiscence, 147
      radical vulvectomy, 621
    drains, 133

infections, 133, 143, 146
    radical vulvectomy, 621
WT-1 gene, 190
Wuchereria bancrofti, 609

X chromosome, *9*
    aneuploidy, 9
    fragile X premutation, 236
    inactivation, 9
    mosaicism, 9, **11**
    structural abnormalities, 9–10, **11**
    translocations, 11, *12*, 223
X monosomy (45 X karyotype), 9, **11**
    miscarriage, 344
    see also Turner's syndrome
X-rays, 79
    contrast studies, 79
    lateral chain, 762
    megavoltage, 545
    in ovarian tumours, 670
    in urethral sphincter incompetence, 773
    in urinary tract infections, 860
    in urogynaecological disorders, 761
    in voiding difficulties, 808
XX males, 194
46XX sex reversal, 194
X-X translocations, 11, *12*

XXX karyotype, 9, 223
XXXX karyotype, 9
XXY karyotype, *see* Klinefelter's syndrome
XY females (male pseudohermaphroditism),
        7–8, 193–195, 225
XYY syndrome, 7–8

Yaws, 906
Y chromosome, 190
    deletions/microdeletions, 302, 312
    translocations, 194
Yolk sac, 107, 377
    tumour, *see* Endodermal sinus tumour
Young people, consent, 118
Young's syndrome, 303
Youth Justice and Criminal Evidence Act,
        1999, 942

Zidovudine (AZT), 925
Zona binding/penetration tests, 287
Zona-free hamster egg penetration test, 287
Zona pellucida, 274, 276, 277
    vaccine, 441
Zona reaction, 277
Zona–sperm binding, 277
ZP1/ZP2/ZP3 proteins, 277
Z score, 427